Imaging in Rheumatology

A Clinical Approach

Imaging in Rheumatology

A Clinical Approach

FIRST EDITION

Adam Greenspan, MD, FACR
Professor of Radiology and Orthopedic Surgery
University of California, Davis School of Medicine
Former Director, Section of Musculoskeletal Imaging
Department of Radiology
University of California, Davis Medical Center
Sacramento, California

M. Eric Gershwin, MD, MACP, MACR
The Jack and Donald Chia Distinguished Professor of Medicine
University of California, Davis School of Medicine
Chief, Division of Rheumatology/Allergy and Clinical Immunology
Department of Internal Medicine
University of California, Davis Medical Center
Sacramento, California

Foreword by
Andrew J. Grainger, BM, BS, FRCP, FRCR
Consultant MSK Radiologist and Honorary Clinical Associate Professor
Leeds Teaching Hospitals and Leeds University
Leeds, United Kingdom

Wolters Kluwer

Philadelphia • Baltimore • New York • London
Buenos Aires • Hong Kong • Sydney • Tokyo

Acquisitions Editor: Sharon Zinner
Development Editor: Brendan Huffman
Editorial Coordinator: Alexis Pozonsky
Marketing Manager: Dan Dressler
Production Project Manager: Linda Van Pelt
Design Coordinator: Joan Wendt
Manufacturing Coordinator: Beth Welsh
Prepress Vendor: SPi Global

9 8 7 6 5 4 3 2 1

Printed in China

Library of Congress Cataloging-in-Publication Data
Names: Greenspan, Adam, author. | Gershwin, M. Eric, 1946- author.
Title: Imaging in rheumatology : a clinical approach / Adam Greenspan, M. Eric Gershwin ; foreword by Andrew J. Grainger.
Description: First edition. | Philadelphia : Wolters Kluwer, [2018] | Includes bibliographical references.
Identifiers: LCCN 2017025981 | ISBN 9781496367631
Subjects: | MESH: Rheumatic Diseases—diagnostic imaging
Classification: LCC RC927 | NLM WE 544 | DDC 616.7/23075—dc23 LC record available at https://lccn.loc.gov/2017025981

LWW.com.

CCS1017

Dedication

To my grandson Avi, who was born during work on this book.

A.G.

To my mother "Gary" on her 100th birthday. She set the stage for my entire life.

M.E.G.

Foreword

I am both honored and delighted to be writing the Foreword for this book. The honor stems from being associated with two authors who I hold in greatest esteem and who are superbly well equipped to write this book. They have a wealth of experience and knowledge of the subject matter and an enviable reputation as teachers of the highest order. My delight comes from the knowledge that this book is timely, much needed, and will be widely appreciated as a valuable resource to a readership from a wide variety of backgrounds.

In the time I have been studying and practicing medicine, I have seen dramatic changes in our understanding and management of rheumatic diseases. Nevertheless, as a radiologist, I find it gratifying that imaging continues to play a fundamental role in the diagnosis and management of these conditions. The continued relevance of imaging to this field is in no small part explained by the enormous strides that we have seen in the imaging techniques available for the assessment of joint-based disease. Furthermore, the application of imaging in rheumatologic research has played a significant role in advancing our understanding of joint diseases, and a review of contemporary publications in the rheumatologic and radiologic literature shows that this continues to be the case. It therefore makes sense that Drs. Greenspan and Gershwin have chosen to focus this text on imaging. While recognizing the important place advanced imaging techniques now have in the evaluation of rheumatologic disease, stressing their role where relevant, the authors have put a firm emphasis on conventional radiographic findings, which remain at the heart of the diagnostic workup. This results in a book which fulfills its purpose of being a clinically relevant text, highlighting how imaging is used in practice.

The great strength of this book comes from the breadth of knowledge brought by the authors combining their wealth of experience as radiologist and rheumatologist. The first section of the book discusses the clinical, pathologic, and imaging assessment of arthritides and arthropathies, and the very first chapter provides a wonderful overview of the clinical and laboratory evaluation of these diseases. This is particularly valuable for those readers who like myself have come to the book as radiologists, with rusty clinical skills and a hazy recollection of laboratory tests, allowing us to appreciate how imaging fits into the diagnostic process. On the other hand, the overview of imaging techniques provided by Chapter 2 will prove particularly helpful to those readers with a nonradiologic background, although many radiologists will like me benefit from the review of radiographic projections and advanced imaging techniques provided. A chapter highlighting the way in which clinical, laboratory, and imaging findings come together in making a diagnosis and a chapter discussing the treatment of arthritides and arthropathies complete this section.

Section 2 takes the reader through the most common arthritides and arthropathies, each chapter providing a clinically relevant and practical overview of the disease, its clinical and pathologic features, and its treatment. At the heart of these chapters is a comprehensive and extensively illustrated description of the imaging features of the condition. To fully understand the imaging features of a disease, it is vital to relate the imaging findings to the pathologic processes at work—we are ultimately simply viewing snapshots of these processes. By laying down the groundwork for the imaging findings through the discussion of pathologic processes, Drs. Greenspan and Gershwin emphasize this link admirably, with the relationship between "what is happening" and "what we see" clearly evident to the reader through description and illustration.

While it is important to understand the features of rheumatologic diseases, it is equally important to recognize a disease process masquerading as arthritis, and this is the objective of the final section of this book. Again, the authors are to be commended on the extensive illustration of this section and the drawing of parallels between the pathologic processes and the imaging findings.

As someone involved in teaching radiology, I know rheumatologic imaging is an area which trainee and experienced radiologists often find confusing and challenging. This book provides a clear and comprehensive review of the subject and will be an excellent resource for them. However, to suggest this is simply a radiology textbook is misleading in the extreme. In their preface, the authors state that the book is intended to be easy to read and something that will translate to everyday use. There is no doubt Drs. Greenspan and Gershwin have fulfilled their intention, and as a result, this book will prove invaluable not only to radiologists but also to rheumatologists and all physicians in this field of medicine as they undertake their day-to-day practice. Fundamentally, the authors have achieved the aim stated in their preface and produced a book that will help patients.

Andrew J. Grainger, BM, BS, FRCP, FRCR
Consultant MSK Radiologist and
Honorary Clinical Associate Professor
Leeds Teaching Hospitals and Leeds University
Leeds, United Kingdom

Preface

One hundred years ago, there were less than 10 known causes of arthritis. Indeed, rheumatoid arthritis could not be readily distinguished from osteoarthritis. Systemic lupus erythematosus was confused with rheumatoid arthritis. The concept of autoimmunity had not yet been defined, and, for the most part, arthritis was considered a disease of old people. We now distinguish arthralgia, which essentially means discomfort in the joints, from arthritis, which implies inflammation in the joints. In fact, as estimated by the Arthritis Foundation, currently in the United States alone, there are more than 50 million sufferers with arthritis. There are more than 300,000 children who have some form of arthropathy, which translates to 1 in 250 children. Overall, approximately 1 in 5 adults has been diagnosed as having arthritis by their physicians. There are 21 million people diagnosed with osteoarthritis and 2.1 million with rheumatoid arthritis. Moreover, arthritis and related conditions are the leading cause of disability and account for more than $156 billion annually in lost wages and medical expenses. Clearly, osteoarthritis is the most common form, but we should not forget that there are more than 100 different types of arthritides and arthropathies, with enormous sociologic and economic implications. The economic impact, the comorbidities, the reduction in physical activity, and the impacts on family life are immeasurable. Arthritis spares no one and affects all races and all gender groups. Fortunately, there have been enormous advances in our understanding of rheumatic diseases, and among these advances is an incredible increase in our knowledge and utility of radiologic imaging.

In this text, our focus is on imaging and, in particular, the clinical and pathologic correlations with the findings found on the radiographs, scintigraphic studies, CT scans, MRIs, and the array of newer diagnostic modalities. To this end, the text integrates the use of different imaging modalities in diagnosing various arthritides and arthropathies, stressing the application of conventional radiography as the most effective means of demonstrating an articular abnormality and making a specific diagnosis. The diagnosis of many rheumatologic disorders can be made solely on the basis of a particular discernible radiographic pattern using the most effective approach—recognizing characteristic radiographic morphology of the articular lesion and its distribution in the skeleton. These radiographic findings coupled with thorough clinical examination and laboratory results can lead to the correct diagnosis without using more advanced imaging techniques. Obviously, we are not completely disregarding the utility of MRI, which can detect the inflammatory process much earlier than any other imaging modality, thus allowing early treatment, so crucial to management of the rheumatologic diseases. Equally important are the newest techniques to evaluate the articular cartilage, such as delayed gadolinium-enhanced MRI of cartilage (d-GEMRIC), T1 in the rotating frame (T1-rho) imaging, and sodium (^{23}Na) MR imaging. The same can be said about dual-energy CT, the technique that in not so obvious cases is able to pinpoint the location of monosodium urate mineralization, thus confirming the presence of gouty arthritis. This text integrates the use of a variety of imaging techniques in diagnosing most common arthritic disorders with discussion of the most effective clinical tests, clinical appearance of these conditions, epidemiology, genetics, pathology, differential diagnosis, and treatment.

The text is organized in three parts. Part I is dealing with general evaluation of arthritic disorders from the clinical, pathologic, imaging, and therapeutic aspects, and part II is devoted to detailed description of the most common arthritides and arthropathies, whereas in part III, several articular and periarticular lesions that clinically may mimic arthritic process are discussed. Some of the figures used to illustrate these parts have been reprinted from the 6th edition of *Orthopedic Imaging* (Greenspan A, Beltran J. *Orthopedic Imaging: A Practical Approach.* Philadelphia, PA: Wolters Kluwer; 2015).

This book is meant to help patients. It is intended for physicians in a variety of subspecialties to have something at their fingertips, which is extremely easy to read and can be translated to everyday patients' use. In particular, this book has been written for the radiologists and rheumatologists, although it may also be beneficial to the orthopedic surgeons and other physicians interested in application of imaging techniques to the rheumatologic diseases. We have done our best to avoid any mistakes, but we are aware that in any volume of this depth, there will be errors, and, as such, we remind our readers that all clinical decisions should be made entirely based on a physician's acumen with appropriate specialist consultation. It is our hope that the data expressed herein will be a guide to help physicians in that direction.

Adam Greenspan, MD, FACR
M. Eric Gershwin, MD, MACP, MACR

Acknowledgments

We would like to express our sincere thanks and appreciation to many friends from Wolters Kluwer Health who helped us in preparation of this text. In particular, we are grateful to Ryan Shaw, the former Acquisition Editor, who was instrumental in launching this project, and to Sharon R. Zinner, the current Senior Acquisitions Editor, Medicine and Advance Practice Publishing, who closely supervised the production and completion of this work, and who guided us throughout the writing process. A special thankful note goes to Brendan Huffman, Developmental Editor, and Alexis (Lexi) Pozonsky, Editorial Coordinator, for pertinent editorial advice, attentive review of the manuscript, and eloquent suggestions during writing and revision of the text. We would like to acknowledge Joan Wendt for the beautiful design of the cover and interior of this book. We also would like to thank Julie Ostoich-Prather, Senior Photographer at the Department of Radiology, University of California, Davis Medical Center in Sacramento, California, for creating some of the digital images; Professor Carlo Francesco Selmi, MD, PhD, Director of Rheumatology and Clinical Immunology Unit, Humanitas Research Hospital, BIOMETRA Department at the University of Milan, Italy, for allowing us to use some of the clinical photographs from his private collection; and Samantha Greenspan and Michael Greenspan for their constant help with many technical problems. We are grateful to Andrew J. Grainger, BM, BS, FRCP, FRCR, Honorary Clinical Associate Professor and Consultant of Musculoskeletal Radiology at Leeds Teaching Hospitals and Leeds University, Leeds, United Kingdom, for writing such a meaningful and relevant Foreword for this book. We would also like to thank Linda Van Pelt, Wolters Kluwer Production Manager, and Remya Divakaran, Project Manager from SPi Global, for supervision and help during the final composition of this book. The prudent and dutiful effort of the many individuals acknowledged here helped us to successfully complete this project in a timely fashion.

Finally, we are indebted to all authors who have given permission to reproduce selective illustrations from their publications and private collections. Thank you for contributing to the advancement of scientific knowledge.

Ron Adler, MD, New York
Dr. Francisco Aparisi, Valencia, Spain
Robert Baran, Cannes, France
Cyrus Bateni, MD, Sacramento, California
Javier Beltran, MD, Washington, DC
Luis Beltran, MD, New York
Jenny Bencardino, MD, New York
Dariusz Borys, MD, Chicago, Illinois
Peter G. Bullough, MD, New York
Dr. Luis Cerezal, Santander, Spain
Abhijit Chaudhari, MD, PhD, Sacramento, California
Dr. Zbigniew Czyrny, Warsaw, Poland
Eva M. Escobedo, MD, Sacramento, California
Cameron Foster, MD, Sacramento, California
Lawrence Friedman, MD, Hamilton, Canada
Robert Goldfarb, MD, New York
Professor Andrew Grainger, Leeds, United Kingdom
John C. Hunter, MD, Sacramento, California
Professor Herwig Imhof, Vienna, Austria
Professor Gernot Jundt, Basel, Switzerland
Michael J. Klein, MD, New York
Dr. Jose Marcos-Robles, Madrid, Spain
Alex Norman, MD, New York
Kristian Reich, Hamburg, Germany
Professor Carlo F. Selmi, Milano, Italy
David K. Shelton Jr., MD, Sacramento, California
Lynne S. Steinbach, MD, San Francisco, California
Professor Iwona Sudol-Szopinska, Warsaw, Poland
Robert M. Szabo, MD, Sacramento, California
Jashmid Tehranzadeh, MD, Orange, California

Contents

PART I

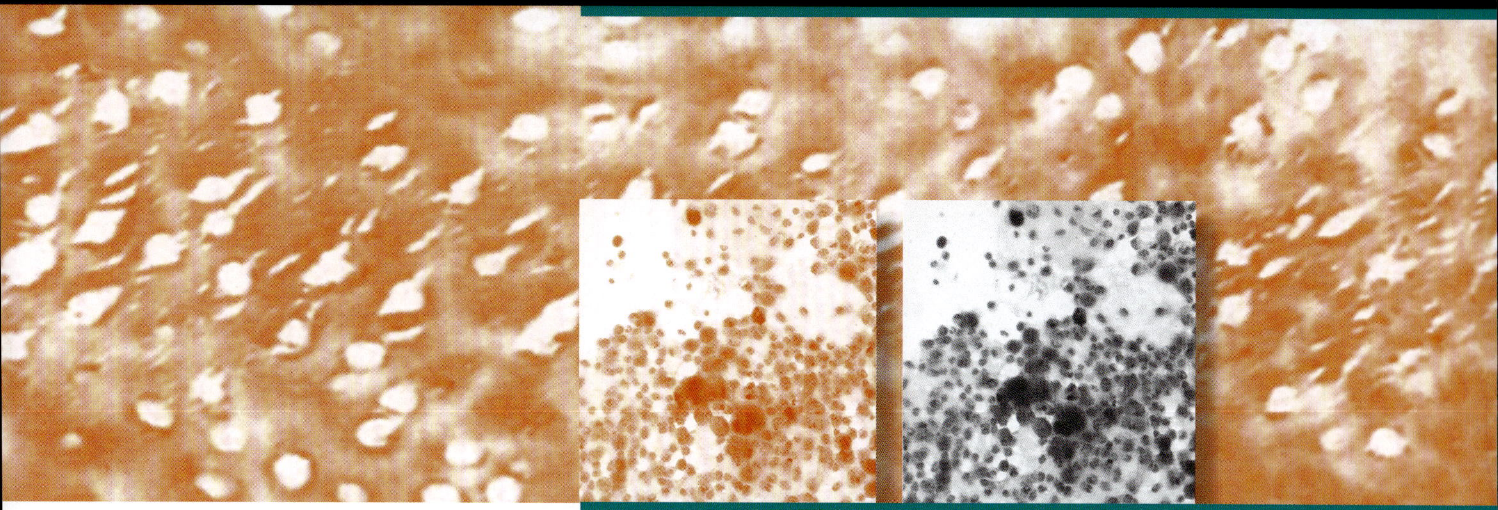

Clinical, Pathologic, and Imaging Evaluation of the Arthritides and Arthropathies

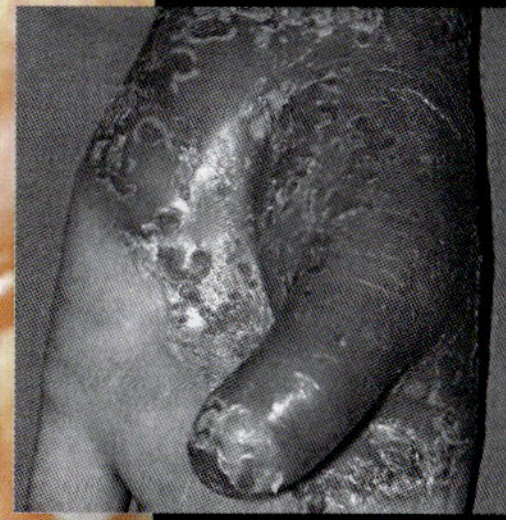

CHAPTER 1

Diagnostic Clinical Parameters

In its general meaning, the term *arthritis* indicates inflammation in the joint. It is not a specific diagnosis, and there are multiple etiologic agents and diseases that can produce inflammatory responses in joints. These include infections, but also a variety of autoimmune and metabolic disorders. Arthritis is distinguished from *arthralgias*, which implies aches and pains in the joint. Arthralgias are much more common and do not necessarily mean that the patient suffers from arthritis. Indeed, the most critical component of an examination in clinical practice is the determination of whether inflammation is present in the joint—that is, is it an inflammatory or noninflammatory process? The presence of inflammatory process is much more serious and in some cases, such as infection, creates rheumatology emergency. It should be clarified that the cardinal features of inflammation include the presence of pain (*dolor*), swelling (*tumor*), erythema (*rubor*), and warmth (*calor*), which are typically detected on physical examination, at least with respect to the peripheral joints. In addition, the elevation of white blood cell (WBC) count in the synovial fluid (>2,000 per mcL), elevated erythrocyte sedimentation rate (ESR), and a high C-reactive protein (CRP) level are also the reliable factors.

In addition to *arthritis* and *arthralgia*, there is also a term known as *arthropathy*, a generic term applied to more than 100 different genetic, autoimmune, metabolic, and other acquired diseases that produce pathologic processes of the joint or joints (Fig. 1.1). Distinguishing these different processes is key to proper imaging and treatment and plays a major role in the critical element of patient's care.

There are now a large number of standardized objective parameters that are useful to determine whether inflammation is present. The most important is a quality physical examination looking for the four key components of inflammation described in the text above. In addition, there are blood tests available that include the measurements of blood sedimentation rate (ESR) and C-reactive protein (CRP). ESR is a valuable but nonspecific test that measures the rate at which red blood cells sediment in standardized Westergren tube in a period of one hour. The CRP is a protein produced by the liver, induced and generated by cytokine interleukin-6 (IL-6) in response to infection or other cause of inflammation. An elevation of ESR or CRP is a clear indicator of the presence of an inflammatory systemic process and strongly implicates the need for further evaluation of the patient that must incorporate a thorough physical examination as well as synovial fluid analysis, including quantification of cells, the presence or absence of crystals, a Gram stain, and culture for microorganisms. These tests, in conjunction with careful clinical evaluation, provide the cornerstone for the diagnosis and management of patient with joint abnormalities. In this part of the book, we will focus our attention on the clinical aspect of a variety of joint diseases and also on imaging modalities by providing a framework for a logical and systematic approach to both the proper use of imaging techniques as well as their interpretation. In addition, we will place this analysis in the perspective of other diagnostic tests useful for the clinician. Our goal is to provide a structured approach to diagnosis by focusing on some of the common problems seen in several rheumatologic diseases. In doing so, we hope that the clinician will be able to interpret the imaging findings and the pathophysiology involved in the perspective of the patient's clinical history and physical examination. The cornerstone of rheumatology remains with the bedside examination; generally, the radiologists are at some distant radiologic office preventing the clinician from establishing the relationship between the physical examination and radiologic findings. Nevertheless, the use of imaging techniques is critical to the clinician, because standard radiographs and newly developed techniques, including among others CT, MRI, and PET, have added significantly to the clinician's armamentarium for evaluating the presence, type, and extent of involvement in various joint abnormalities.

(Continued on page 5)

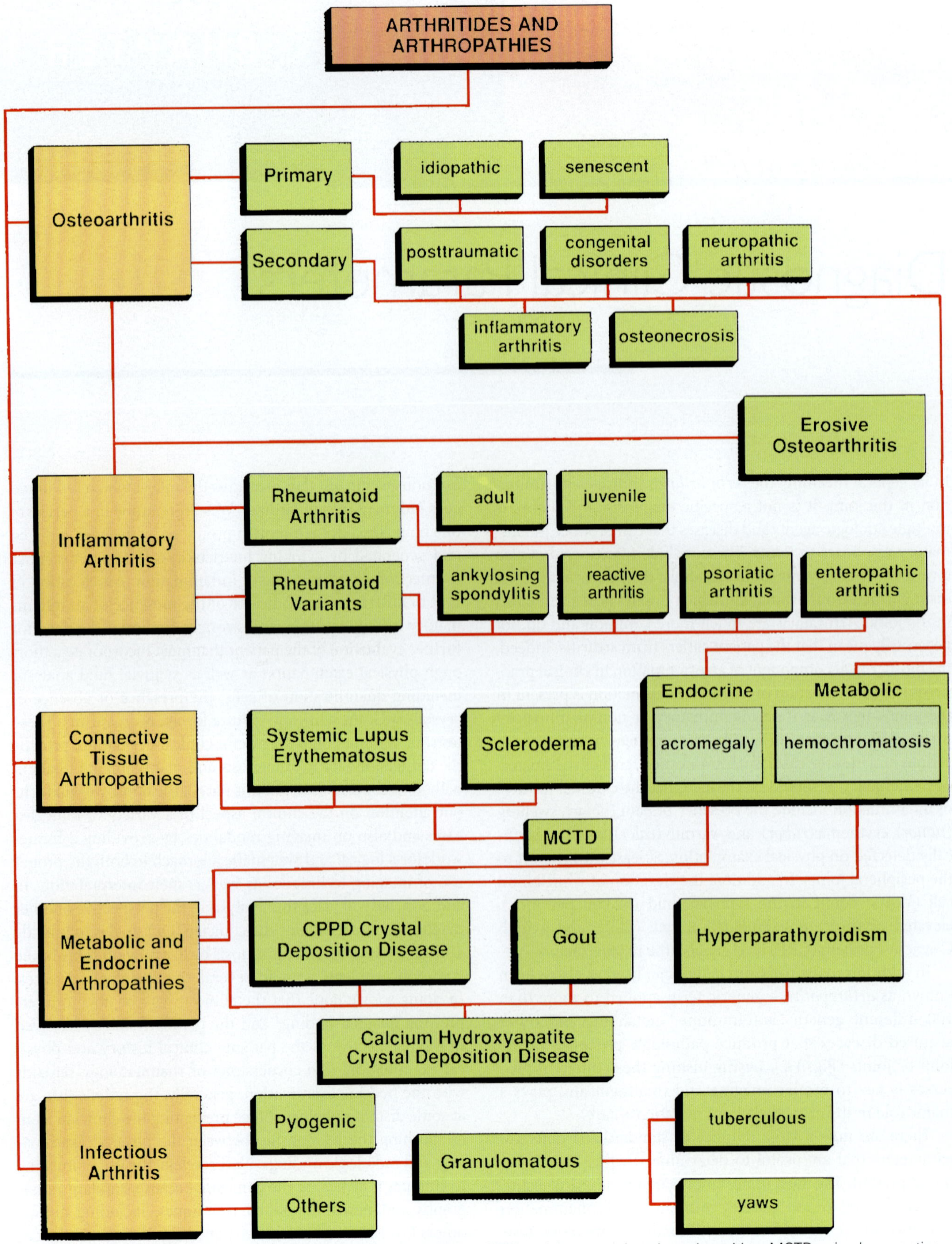

Figure 1.1 ■ **Classification of the arthritides and arthropathies.** CPPD, calcium pyrophosphate deposition; MCTD, mixed connective tissue disease.

CLINICAL HISTORY AND PHYSICAL EXAMINATION

Clinical history and physical examination are keys to diagnosis and prognosis in rheumatology. The importance of gaining a clear account and understanding of a clinical problem has long been recognized. Good clinical observation remains central to the management of several rheumatologic disorders. The manner of onset and evolution of symptoms over time is very helpful in establishing the correct diagnosis. A thoughtful and detailed clinical history plays a critical role in determining the nature of the patient's complaints and provides the focus to the clinical examination. The history should be structured in such a way as to be able to answer the specific questions regarding the symptoms, in particular if they are symmetric or asymmetric in location, and whether they are referred to the one particular region or are generalized. It is important to determine if the symptoms are acute, subacute, or chronic in nature and if they suggest a systemic process. The patient should be questioned regarding muscle weakness, joint pains and stiffness, limitation in joint motion, fever, fatigue, weight loss, anorexia, skin changes, paresthesias and other neurologic symptoms, photosensitivity, mouth and eyes dryness, and similar symptoms among others. It is of utmost importance to find out if there is a family history of similar or related problems.

The fundamentals of physical examination remain the cornerstone of rheumatology, and the examination technique is universally recognized as a sensitive detector of crucial abnormalities. The GALS (gait, arms, legs, spine) locomotor system was devised to rapidly screen the patient for musculoskeletal disorders. The physical examination should be focused among others on the following features: type of gait, joint swelling, deformities and contractures, joint movements (active and passive), skin changes including redness and rashes, and wasting of muscles. Each joint should be individually and systematically examined. Particular attention should be directed to the appearance of the hand, because distinctive patterns of hand involvement and several characteristic abnormalities can point to the specific diagnosis. Swelling of the joints and deformity of the digits resulting from loss of alignment may be consequence of destructive arthritis such as rheumatoid (Fig. 1.2). Swan-neck and boutonnière deformities have characteristic clinical appearance suggesting inflammatory arthritis (Fig. 1.3); the presence of Heberden or Bouchard nodes (see Fig. 5.58)

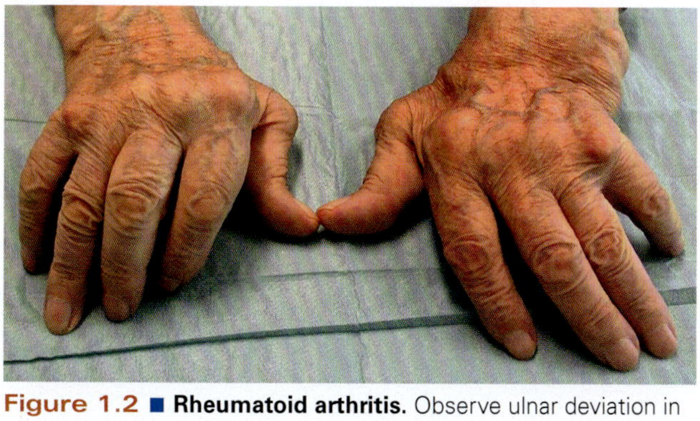

Figure 1.2 ■ Rheumatoid arthritis. Observe ulnar deviation in the swollen metacarpophalangeal joints of both hands and hyperextension of the thumbs ("hitchhiker's thumbs").

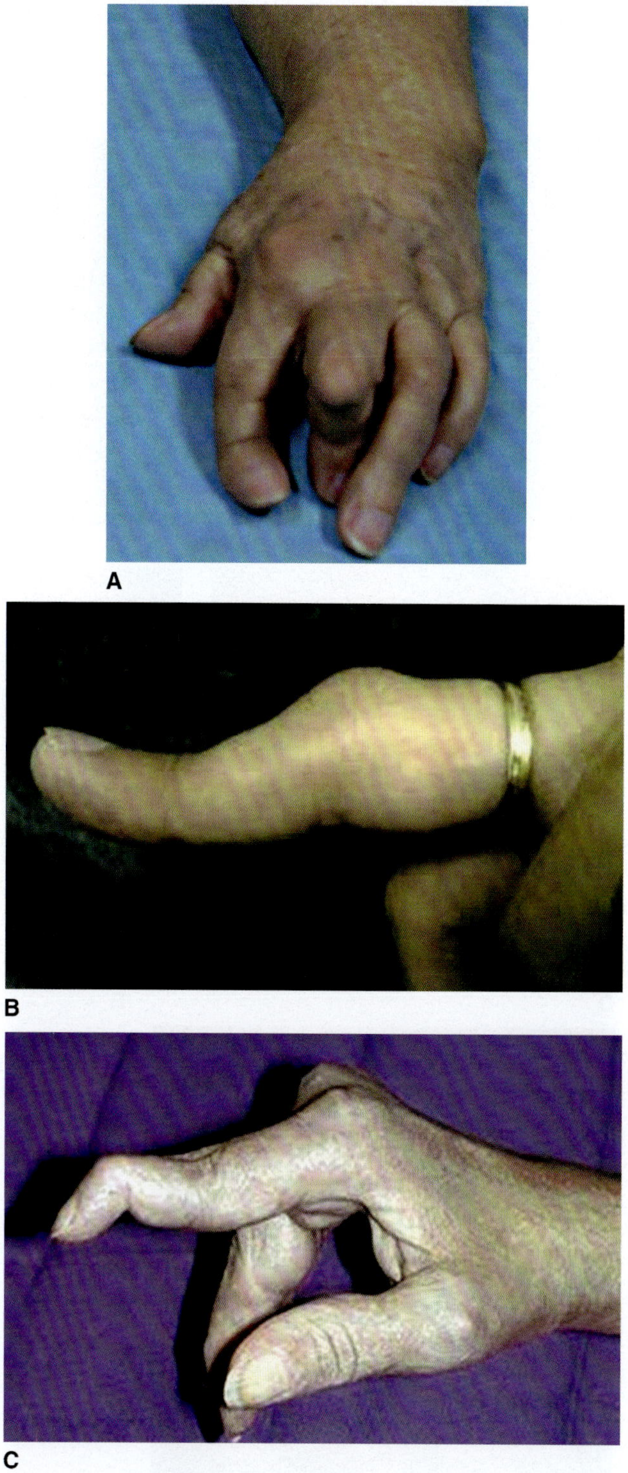

Figure 1.3 ■ Rheumatoid arthritis. A: Flexion in the proximal interphalangeal joints and extension in the distal interphalangeal joints of the index and middle fingers resulted in boutonnière deformity. **B:** In another patient, note characteristic boutonnière deformity of the index finger. **C:** Extension in the proximal and flexion in the distal interphalangeal joint is known as a swan-neck deformity.

may point to the diagnosis of interphalangeal osteoarthritis; swelling of the proximal and distal interphalangeal joints (Fig. 1.4A) and nail changes such as onycholysis (separation of the nail plate from the nail bed) (Fig. 1.4B), pitting of the nails (Fig. 1.4C), leukonychia (white nails, milk spots) (Fig.1.4D), splinting hemorrhages (Fig. 1.4E), subungual hyperkeratosis (Fig. 1.4F), and swelling of the entire finger (dactylitis or "sausage digit") (Fig. 1.4G) are commonly seen in psoriasis; flexible, easy-reducible joint contractures combined with redness and telangiectasia of the nail fold capillaries may be indicative of systemic lupus erythematosus; tapering of the ends of digits and sclerodactyly is characteristic of scleroderma. In the foot, the redness and swelling of the big toe may indicate the presence of gout (Fig. 1.5).

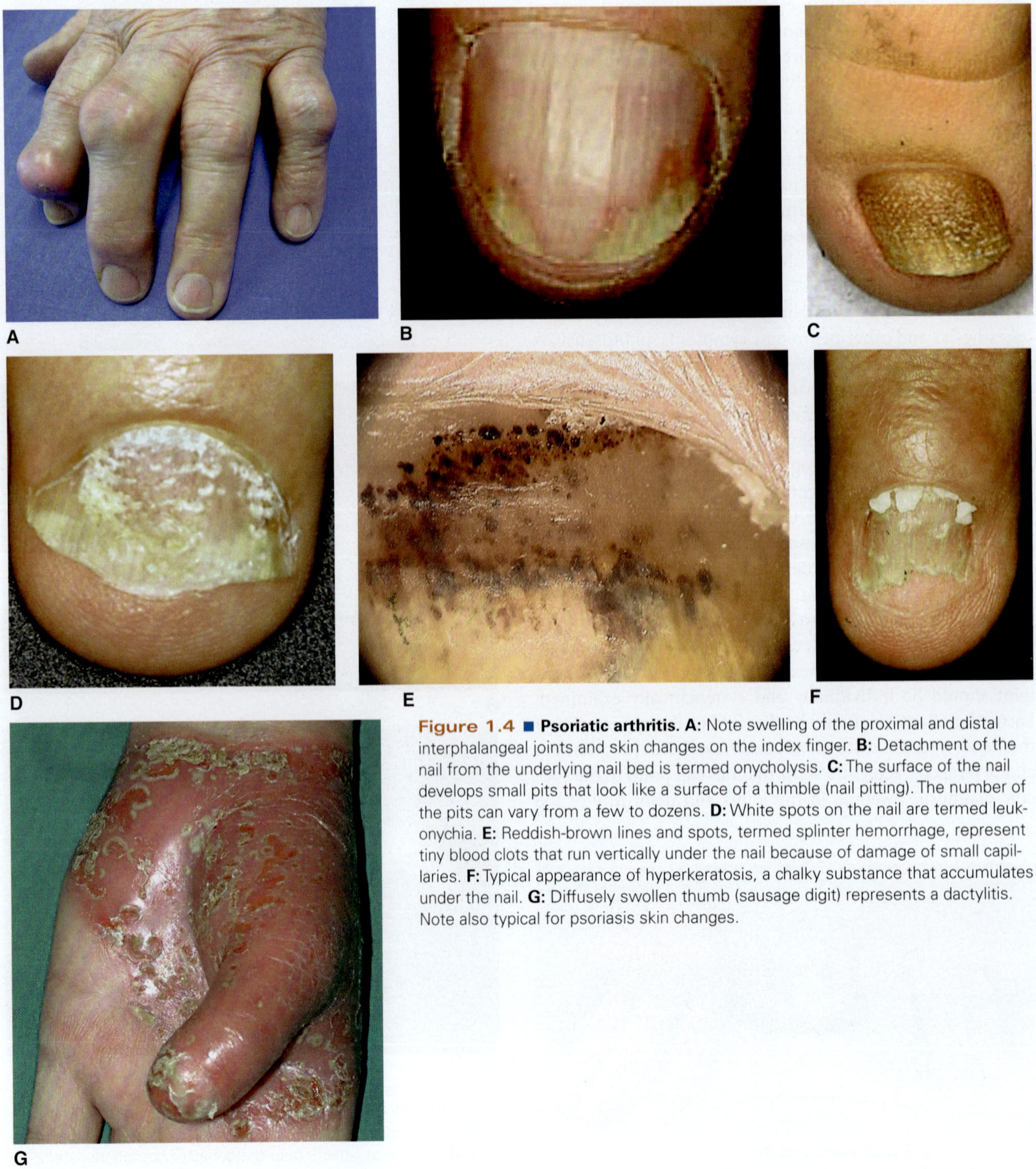

Figure 1.4 ■ **Psoriatic arthritis. A:** Note swelling of the proximal and distal interphalangeal joints and skin changes on the index finger. **B:** Detachment of the nail from the underlying nail bed is termed onycholysis. **C:** The surface of the nail develops small pits that look like a surface of a thimble (nail pitting). The number of the pits can vary from a few to dozens. **D:** White spots on the nail are termed leukonychia. **E:** Reddish-brown lines and spots, termed splinter hemorrhage, represent tiny blood clots that run vertically under the nail because of damage of small capillaries. **F:** Typical appearance of hyperkeratosis, a chalky substance that accumulates under the nail. **G:** Diffusely swollen thumb (sausage digit) represents a dactylitis. Note also typical for psoriasis skin changes.

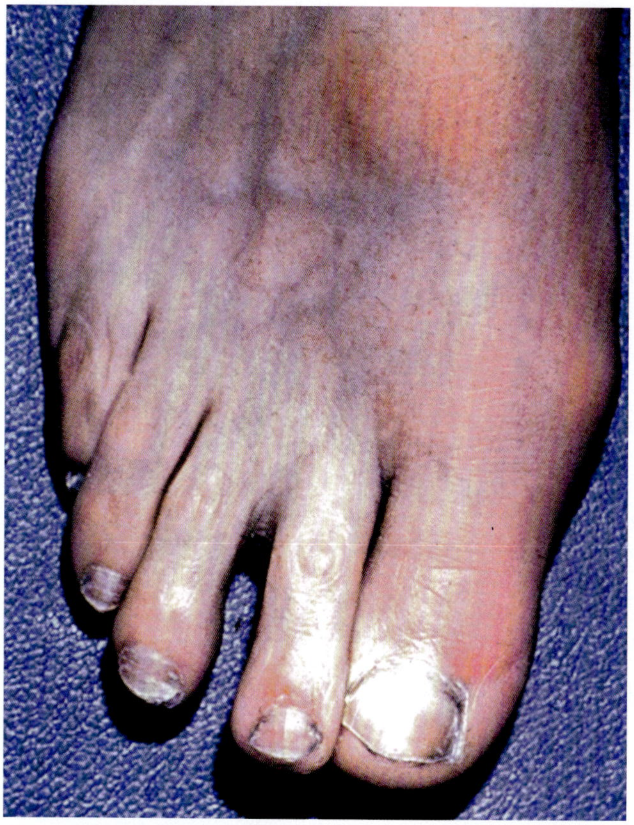

Figure 1.5 ■ **Gouty arthritis.** Observe the big toe swelling and dorsal mass at the site of the first metatarsophalangeal joint representing a tophus. (Reprinted from Klein MJ, Bonar SF, Freemont T, et al., eds. *Atlas of Nontumor Pathology. Non-neoplastic Diseases of Bones and Joints.* Washington, DC: American Registry of Pathology and Armed Forces Institute of Pathology; 2011, Fig. 8-206, with permission of the author and the Publishers.)

SYNOVIAL FLUID

Evaluation of synovial (joint) fluid, in terms of its physical, chemical, and microscopic characteristics, is of prime importance in the differential diagnosis of variety of arthritides. There are four elements to synovial fluid analysis: visual inspection, nucleated cell count, wet preparation, and cytocentrifuge preparation. On visual inspection, synovial fluid is examined for color, clarity, and viscosity. The color of the synovial fluid varies with its content (Fig. 1.6). Knowledge of the formation and composition of normal fluid is a requisite for an evaluation of abnormal findings. Synovial fluid is a dialysate of plasma to which hyaluronate–protein has been added as a result of synthesis by the synovial lining cells. Its lubricating behavior is dependent upon the reaction between the hyaluronans and protein within the fluid, one of the most important being the hyaluronan-binding protein lubricin. Normal synovial fluid is present in small quantities within the diarthrodial joints; it is transparent and almost colorless. It is highly viscous, its viscosity being dependent upon the content of hyaluronic acid, a long-coiled carbohydrate polymer. Normal synovial fluid does not clot, as fibrinogen and other clotting factors are absent; the walls of blood vessels and the normal barrier function of

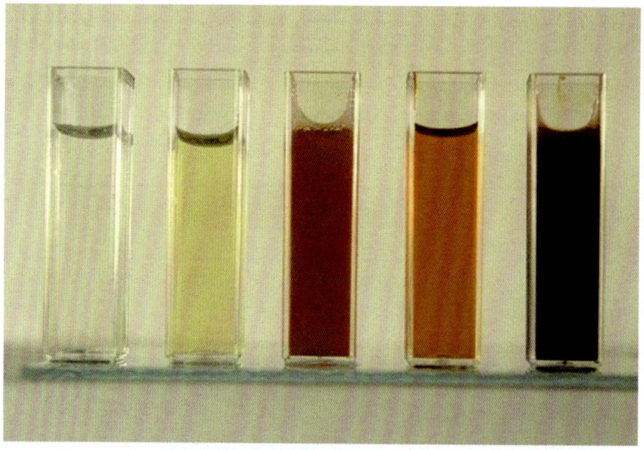

Figure 1.6 ■ **Synovial fluid.** Depending upon the content, the synovial fluids exhibit different colors. From left to right: normal, noninflammatory arthropathy, hemarthrosis, xanthochromic, and ochronotic. (Reprinted from Klein MJ, Bonar SF, Freemont T, et al., eds. *Atlas of Nontumor Pathology. Non-neoplastic Diseases of Bones and Joints.* Washington, DC: American Registry of Pathology and Armed Forces Institute of Pathology; 2011, Fig. 8-27, with permission of the author and the Publishers.)

the synovial membrane prevent these and other large molecules from entering the joint cavity. The total protein concentration is ~1.8 g%, with a relative increase in albumin as compared with globulin. The high molecular weight proteins, such as beta-2-macroglobulin and alpha-2-macroglobulin are usually absent or present in very small amounts. Small molecules such as glucose, uric acid, and bilirubin are found in a concentration in synovial fluid similar to that in plasma. Finally, synovial fluid normally is relatively acellular, with 200 to 300 primarily mononuclear cells per mcL (1 mm^3). Most of the cells are synoviocytes, fibrochondrocytes, and lymphocytes. As a guide to differential diagnosis, pathologic fluids can be divided into four general groups: class I—noninflammatory; class II—inflammatory; class III—purulent; and class IV—hemorrhagic (Table 1.1). Noninflammatory fluids, such as accompanied osteoarthritis, osteonecrosis, amyloidosis, or sarcoidosis, have fewer cells (<200 per mcL) and low protein content. Inflammatory fluids present in such conditions as rheumatoid arthritis (Fig. 1.7), seronegative spondyloarthropathies, systemic lupus erythematosus, crystal-induced arthropathies (Figs. 1.8 to 1.12), hemochromatosis (Fig. 1.13), dermatomyositis, or mixed connective tissue disease are more cellular with more polymorphs and abnormal cell morphology, protein count is high, and crystals and occasionally bacteria are present. Purulent fluids have white cell count often above 100,000 per mcL and are typically seen in septic arthritis caused by *Staphylococcus aureus*, streptococci, and gram-negative organisms. Hemorrhagic fluid is commonly posttraumatic, but also present in some neoplastic and tumor-like (such as pigmented villonodular synovitis) conditions.

The diagnostic and therapeutic indications for arthrocentesis are depicted in Table 1.2. The contraindications for arthrocentesis are shown in Table 1.3. In general, the diagnostic indications include evaluation of any joint with detectable increases in joint fluid where the exact diagnosis of such

(Continued on page 11)

Table 1.1 CATEGORIES OF JOINT FLUID AND DISEASE ASSOCIATIONS

Characteristic	Normal	Noninflammatory Group I	Inflammatory Group II	Purulent Group III	Hemorrhagic
Volume (mL) (knee)	<3.5	Often >3.5	Often >3.5	Often >3.5	Often >3.5
Color	Colorless	Xanthochromic	Xanthochromic to white	Depends on organism	Xanthochromic to frankly bloody
Clarity	Clear	Clear	Translucent to opaque	Opaque	Opaque (clear if centrifuged)
Viscosity	High	High	Low	Varies; may be high	High
Leukocytes (per mm^3)	<200	200–2,000	2000 – 100,000 (average 20,000)	20,000 – 200,000 (average 100,000)	Variable (usually)
Polymorphs (%)	<25%	<25%	About 75%	>75%	Variable (usually <75%)
Glucose (mg%; fasting)	Nearly equal to blood	Nearly equal to blood	Often lower than blood	Often >25 mg% lower than blood	Nearly equal to blood
Culture	Negative	Negative	Negative	Positive/Negative	Negative
Spontaneous clot	No	Occasionally	Often	Often	Often
Mucin clot	Firm	Firm	Friable	Friable	Friable

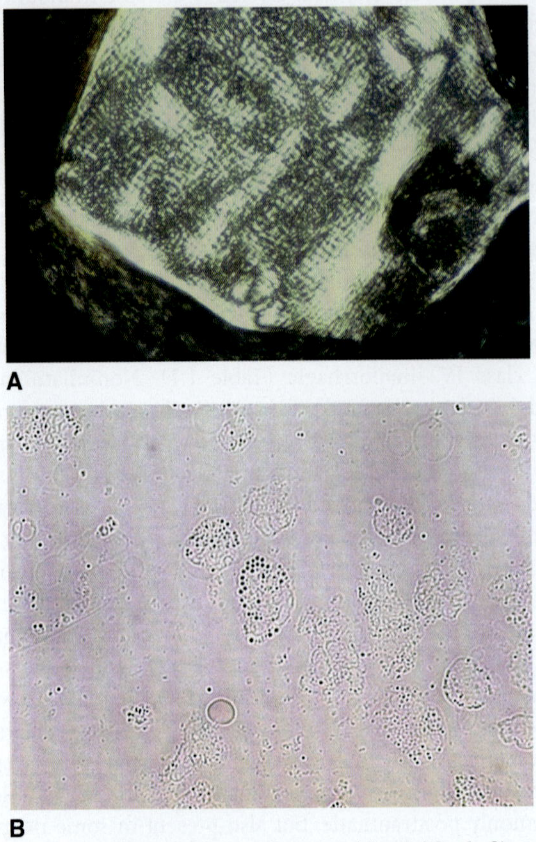

Figure 1.7 ■ Synovial fluid—rheumatoid arthritis. A: Clotted fibrin viewed between polarizers in a wet preparation of synovial fluid obtained from a patient with active rheumatoid arthritis. **B:** Ragocytes viewed in diffused light in a wet preparation of synovial fluid from the same patient. Observe characteristic large granules within the ragocytes, representing cytoplasmatic inclusions of ingested aggregated IgG immunoglobulin and fibrin. (Reprinted from Klein MJ, Bonar SF, Freemont T, et al., eds. *Atlas of Nontumor Pathology. Non-neoplastic Diseases of Bones and Joints.* Washington, DC: American Registry of Pathology and Armed Forces Institute of Pathology; 2011, Fig. 8-190, with permission of the author and the Publishers.)

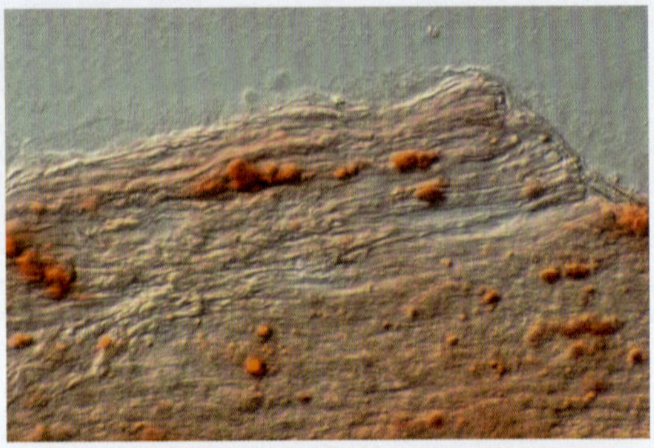

Figure 1.8 ■ Synovial fluid—hydroxyapatite crystals. The normally almost invisible crystalloids of hydroxyapatite within a fibrin clot form birefringent red complexes with the alizarin when stained with alizarin red. (Reprinted from Klein MJ, Bonar SF, Freemont T, et al., eds. *Atlas of Nontumor Pathology. Non-neoplastic Diseases of Bones and Joints.* Washington, DC: American Registry of Pathology and Armed Forces Institute of Pathology; 2011, Fig. 8-34, with permission of the author and the Publishers.)

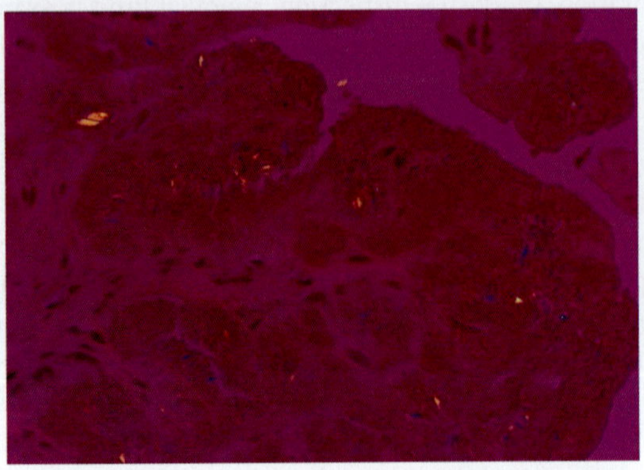

Figure 1.9 ■ Synovial fluid—pyrophosphate crystals. Pyrophosphate crystals (*blue* and *red*) are identified by polarizing microscopy with interference (compensating) plate in the path of light (H&E, polarized light). (Reprinted from Klein MJ, Bonar SF, Freemont T, et al., eds. *Atlas of Nontumor Pathology. Non-neoplastic Diseases of Bones and Joints.* Washington, DC: American Registry of Pathology and Armed Forces Institute of Pathology; 2011, Fig. 8-16, with permission of the author and the Publishers.)

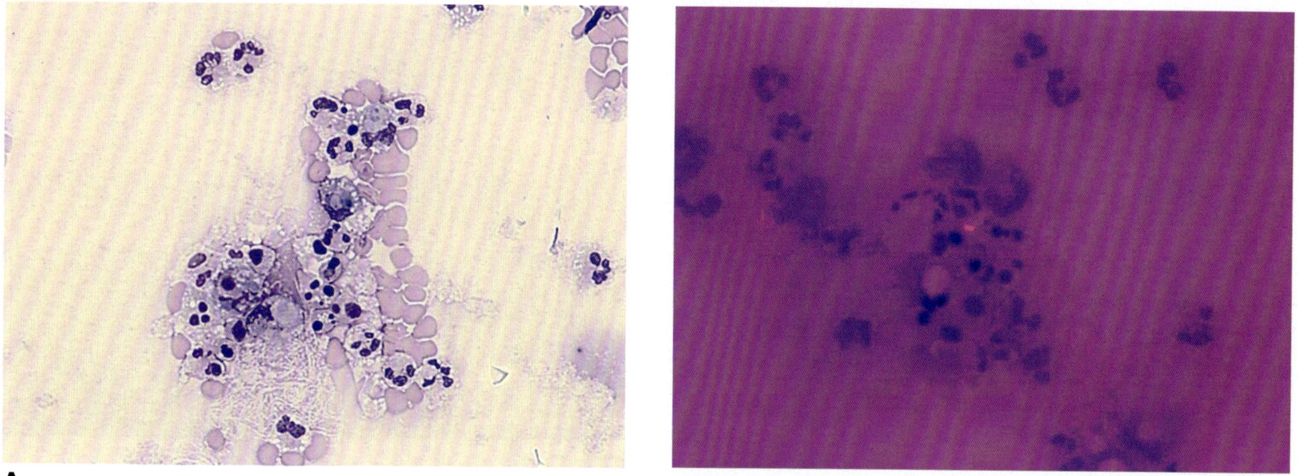

A B

Figure 1.10 ■ **Synovial fluid—pyrophosphate crystals. A:** Pyrophosphate crystals within the synovial fluid cytocentrifuge stained with Jenner-Giemsa. The unstained spaces contain the crystals. **B:** Same specimen viewed now in polarized light with a quarter-wave plate shows the crystals more clearly. (Reprinted from Klein MJ, Bonar SF, Freemont T, et al., eds. *Atlas of Nontumor Pathology. Non-neoplastic Diseases of Bones and Joints.* Washington, DC: American Registry of Pathology and Armed Forces Institute of Pathology; 2011, Fig. 8-222, with permission of the author and the Publishers.)

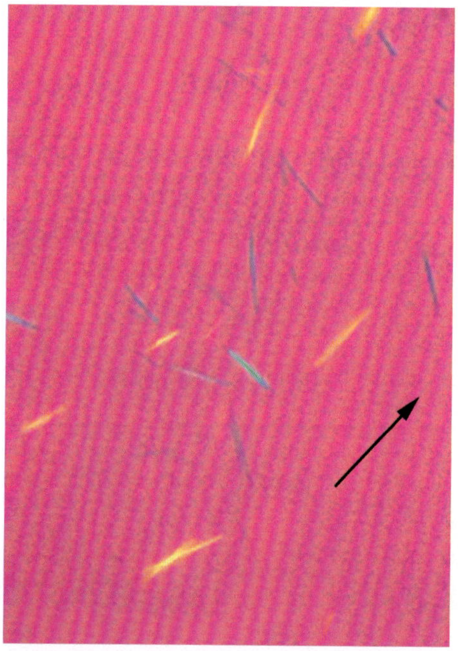

A

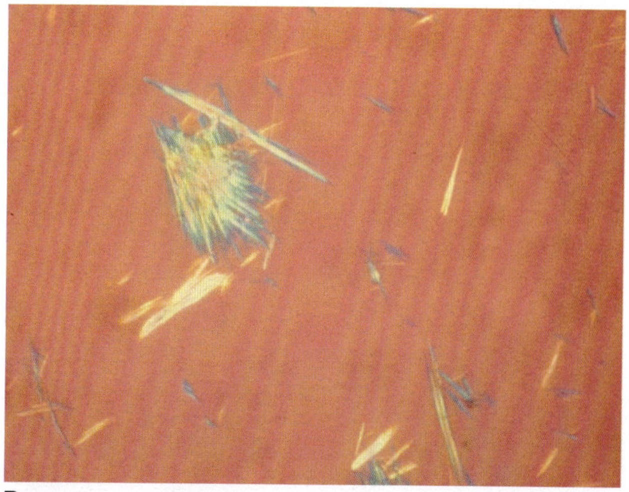

B

Figure 1.11 ■ **Synovial fluid—urate crystals. A:** The needle-shaped monosodium urate monohydrate crystals in synovial fluid aspirated from a patient with acute gouty arthritis are viewed here in polarized light with a quarter-wave compensating plate. The slow wave vector (the direction of the extraordinary axis of the compensating plate) is indicated by the *arrow*. **B:** In the synovial fluid obtained from another patient with acute gouty arthritis and viewed in polarizing light with an interposed quarter-wave plate, the urate crystals are clearly visible. **C:** Urate crystals within a neutrophil (Jenner-Giemsa stain). (**A** and **C** reprinted from Klein MJ, Bonar SF, Freemont T, et al., eds. *Atlas of Nontumor Pathology. Non-neoplastic Diseases of Bones and Joints.* Washington, DC: American Registry of Pathology and Armed Forces Institute of Pathology; 2011, Figs. 8-31 and 8-213, with permission of the author and the Publishers.)

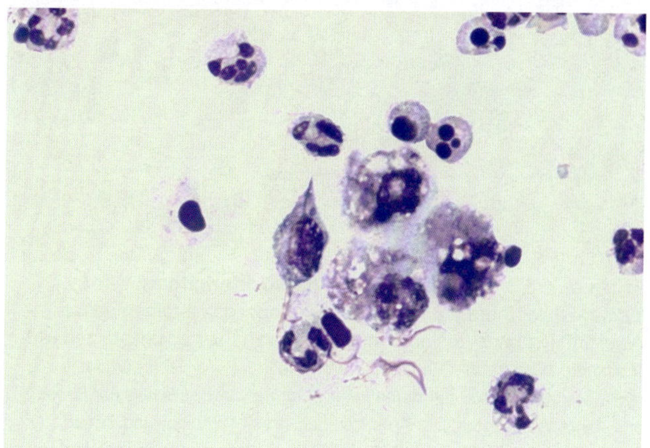

C

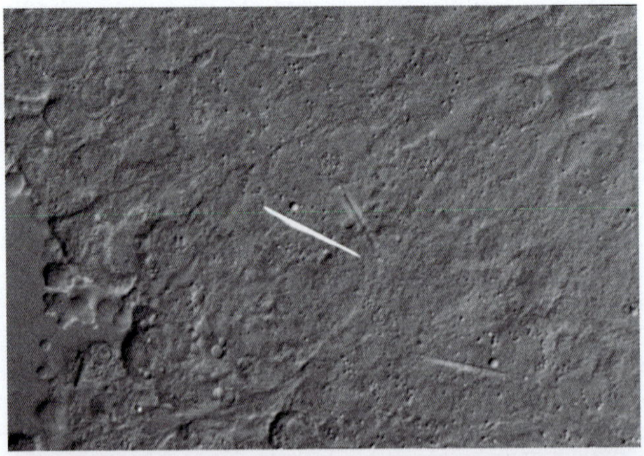

A

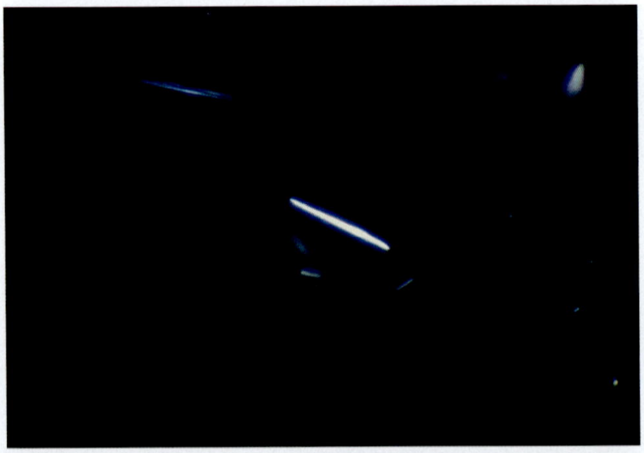

B

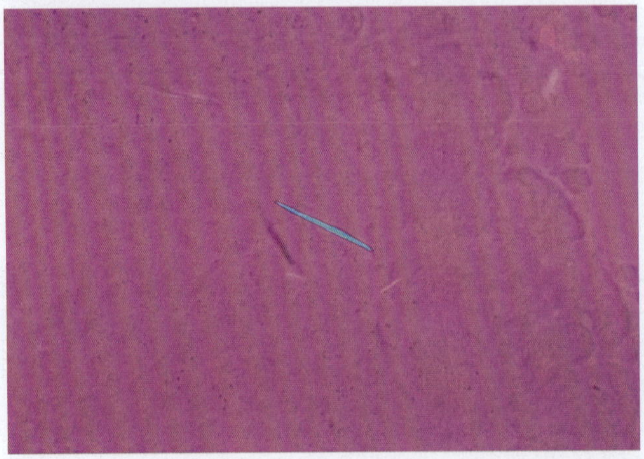

C

Figure 1.12 ■ Synovial fluid—urate crystals. Urate crystals in a fibrin clot viewed **(A)** in Nomarski phase, **(B)** in polarized light, and **(C)** with a quarter-wave plate. The *arrow* shows the orientation of the extraordinary wave. (Reprinted from Klein MJ, Bonar SF, Freemont T, et al., eds. *Atlas of Nontumor Pathology. Non-neoplastic Diseases of Bones and Joints.* Washington, DC: American Registry of Pathology and Armed Forces Institute of Pathology; 2011, Fig. 8-212, with permission of the author and the Publishers.)

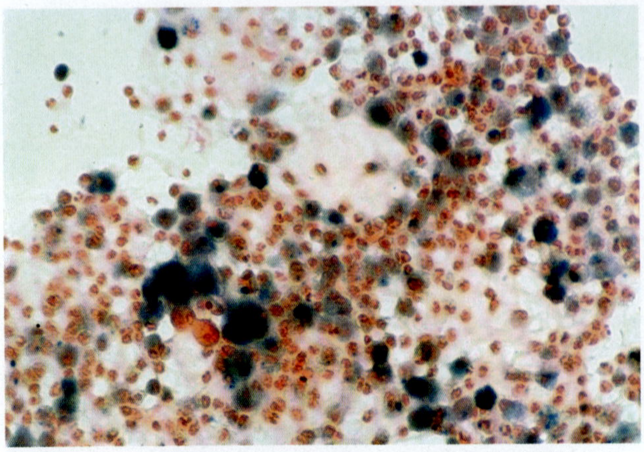

Figure 1.13 ■ Synovial fluid—hemochromatosis. Within synovial fluid, there are numerous macrophages (*stained dark blue*) and lymphocytes and neutrophils with their nuclei stained red (*Prussian blue stain*). (Reprinted from Klein MJ, Bonar SF, Freemont T, et al., eds. *Atlas of Nontumor Pathology. Non-neoplastic Diseases of Bones and Joints.* Washington, DC: American Registry of Pathology and Armed Forces Institute of Pathology; 2011, Fig. 8-62, with permission of the author and the Publishers.)

Table 1.2 INDICATIONS FOR ARTHROCENTESIS

Diagnostic	Therapeutic
1. Whenever the specific diagnosis of arthritis is in doubt	1. Provide rapid relief of pain in swollen joint
2. Confirmatory evidence for a clinical diagnosis	2. Removal of toxic bacterial and white blood cell substances in septic arthritis
3. Definition of pain as articular versus extraarticular	3. Provide maximum control of sterile inflammatory conditions with local corticosteroid injection when systemic anti-inflammatory drugs are contraindicated or ineffective
4. Provide additional diagnostic documentation for clinical studies	4. Aid in physical therapy (i.e., contractures) or in orthopedic problems (i.e., fracture extending into joint).

Table 1.3 CONTRAINDICATIONS FOR ARTHROCENTESIS

1. Local periarticular (skin or soft tissue) sepsis
2. Bacteremia
3. Severe articular instability
4. Arthritis in joints where entry into synovial space is not feasible (i.e., spinal joint or severely deformed joint)
5. Clotting abnormalities

Table 1.4 JOINT FLUID EXAMINATIONS

Gross Inspection—Aspirated Fluid

COLOR
- Normal: clear to slightly straw-colored
- Range: bloody, xanthochromic, yellow, milky, gray or green

CLARITY
- Normal: can read newsprint through filled test tube
- Range: cloudy to opaque with high white blood cell count

VISCOSITY
- Drop test: express drops slowly from needled syringe
  - Normal: strings several inches
  - Range: increasingly inflammatory fluid results in progressive loss of string
- String test: place drop between thumb and finger and slowly pull apart
  - Normal: string >3 cm
  - Range: increasing inflammation correspondingly shortens string
- Mucin clot: add fluid drop by drop to tube of dilute acetic acid, then agitate gently
  - Normal: firm clot at bottom
  - Range: increasing inflammation (or contamination with serum) results in friability of dot

Light Microscopic Examination—Heparin or EDTA Anti-coagulated

LEUKOCYTE COUNT (HEMOCYTOMETER WITH SALINE DILUENT—0.3 JV LYSES RED BLOOD CELLS).
- Differential cell count (Wright stain)
- Morphology
  - LE cells
  - Ragocyte (inflammatory cells)
  - Intracellular inclusions
- Red blood cell count (hemocytometer with 0.9 N saline).
- Particulate matter
  - Cartilage fibrils
  - Crystals
  - Cholesterol
  - Red blood cell and other cellular fragments
- Gram stain (bacteria)
- India ink prep (fungus)
- Special staining
  - Amyloid–Congo red
  - Fluorescent TB stain
- Crystal identification (polarized filters added)
  - Sodium urate (red filter differentiates from calcium pyrophosphate)
  - Calcium pyrophosphate
  - Corticosteroid
  - Starch
- Cultures
  - Bacterial
    - Aerobic
    - Anaerobic
    - Special media (e.g., chocolate agar in 10% CO_2 for GC)
  - Fungal
  - TB–guinea pig inoculation
  - Viral–yolk sac inoculation
- Chemistry
  - No anticoagulant added
    - Hyaluronic acid
    - Lipid
    - Enzymes–lactate dehydrogenase
  - Potassium oxalate anticoagulant
    - Glucose
    - Total protein
- Serology
  - Immune complexes
    - Rheumatoid factor
    - Antinuclear antibody
    - Immunoelectrophoresis and other immune complex assays
  - Complement
    - Total hemolytic complement—CH_{50}
    - Component assay
  - Quantitative immunoglobulins

effusion is in doubt. In most diagnostic and all therapeutic procedures, an attempt should be made to withdraw all fluid accumulated in the joint space. Nonetheless, although about 5 mL is sufficient for most of the necessary studies, as little as one drop may be diagnostic of gout or pyrophosphate dehydrate crystal deposition disease if the appropriate crystals are present (see Figs. 1.9 to 1.12). Furthermore, most studies can be minimized to scale down the amount of drowned fluid in pediatric patients. If there is doubt regarding the origin of fluid from a tap (i.e., blood vs. bloody tap or subcutaneous fluid vs. synovial fluid), this may be resolved with the mucin test or metachromatic staining for the presence of hyaluronate (Table 1.4).

ADDITIONAL LABORATORY TESTS

Erythrocyte Sedimentation Rate (ESR)

ESR is determined by allowing anticoagulated blood to sediment for one hour in a Westergren glass tube. Although it is nonspecific, it is a sensitive indication of inflammatory process. It is, however, age and gender dependent and can be increased in any conditions in which serum fibrinogen is elevated, such as pregnancy, diabetes mellitus, or end-stage renal disease.

C-reactive Protein (CRP)

CRP is a substance produced by the liver in response to inflammation. Serum level of CRP increases following interleukin-6 (IL-6) secretion by macrophages and T cells, and although an indicator of inflammatory process, similar to ESR, it is not a specific factor for diagnosis of rheumatologic disorders, because it may be abnormal in other conditions such as infections, malignancies, heart diseases, burns, and diabetes. CRP is age and gender dependent, and obesity and cigarette smoking may elevate its values.

Anti–cyclic Citrullinated Peptides Antibodies (Anti-CCP Abs)

Anti-CCP Ab are the autoantibodies produced by the patient's immune system and directed against three unique proteins: α-enolase, fibrinogen, and vimentin. They are found in patients with seropositive rheumatoid arthritis (RA) and are actually directed at a modification of these three proteins. Under normal circumstances, the amino acid arginine is present in α-enolase, fibrinogen, and vimentin; however, during inflammation, an alpha-amino acid called citrullin (originally isolated from watermelon) replaces the arginine. The switch of arginine to citrullin occurs in everyone's body and is accelerated by smoking, but in rheumatoid arthritis, this change is enough to elicit a loss of immune tolerance and thus the production of autoantibodies. These antibodies are useful for the diagnosis of RA and are even detectable many years before clinical onset of disease. They are more specific than rheumatoid factor (RF), and unlike RF, the immune response to these proteins is integrally related to the pathogenesis of RA. Anti-CCP Ab are measured by the enzyme-linked immunosorbent assay (ELISA) using synthetic citrullinated peptides. These antibodies are frequently detectable in early rheumatoid arthritis (RA), although they are not useful in the monitoring disease activity.

Rheumatoid Factor (RF)

RF is an antibody against the Fc portion of immunoglobulin G (IgG) produced by the immune system. It is detectable in the blood of ~80% of adults with rheumatoid arthritis. The presence of RF in serum, however, can also indicate the occurrence of autoimmune activity unrelated to RA, such as present in many other autoimmune diseases, chronic infections, sarcoidosis, and some malignancies and associated with tissue or organ rejection. The most common methods of detecting RF are latex fixation, using latex beads coated with human IgG, and nephelometry, using human IgG as the target antigen. For nearly 50 years, RF was felt to be a highly specific immunoassay for the detection of RA. It is, however, not nearly as specific as antibodies to Anti-CCP. Nevertheless, patients with high RF titer are more likely to have more severe disease and to suffer from extra-articular features of RA including Felty syndrome, rheumatoid disease of the lung, and lymphoma.

Antinuclear Antibodies (ANAs)

ANAs (also known as antinuclear factor or ANF) are a heterogeneous group of antibodies directed against components normally present in all nucleated cells. They bind to contents of the cell nucleus and are directed against histones, single- and double-stranded DNA, ribonucleoprotein (RNP) complexes, and other nuclear components. The common tests used to detect and to quantify ANAs are indirect immunofluorescence and ELISA. ANAs are found in many disorders, such as systemic lupus erythematosus (SLE), RA, Sjögren syndrome, scleroderma, dermatomyositis, polymyositis, multiple sclerosis, and other conditions. They are useful in the differential diagnosis of SLE, and changes in the titer of antibodies to DNA are useful in following disease activity.

Antineutrophil Cytoplasmic Antibodies (ANCA)

ANCA are autoantibodies (mainly of the IgG type) that react with the cytoplasmic granules of neutrophils and can be detected by immunofluorescence. The most common subsets of ANCA are those that target the proteins myeloperoxidase (MPO) and proteinase 3 (PR3). ANCA has a high positive predictive value for granulomatosis with polyangiitis (Wegener granulomatosis) and eosinophilic granulomatosis with polyangiitis (Churg-Strauss syndrome). Other autoimmune diseases, infections, and certain medications may cause occasionally positive ANCA tests.

Cryoglobulins

These are abnormal antibody proteins consisting of immunoglobulins that precipitate reversibly at reduced temperatures. In a variety of diseases, cryoglobulins bind with complement proteins and other peptides to form immune complexes. They come in three main types according to Brouet classification: type I (monoclonal immunoglobulins, commonly of the IgM isotype, directed against the Fc region of IgG), most common type II (a mixture of polyclonal IgG and monoclonal IgM), and type III (a combination of polyclonal IgG and polyclonal IgM molecules). Types II and III have RF activity and bind to polyclonal immunoglobulins. Cryoglobulins are not specific for any particular disorder; however, type I is linked to lymphoproliferative diseases and some malignancies, type II may be associated with chronic hepatitis C infection, and type III is associated with vasculitis, hepatitis C, subacute bacterial endocarditis, and autoimmune disorders such as SLE and RA.

SYNOVIAL BIOPSY

Although histologic confirmation is not commonly required for diagnosis or therapeutic purposes of the common forms of inflammatory arthritis, nevertheless, synovial biopsy has been found to be a valuable adjunct to conventional investigation of some of the arthritides. In clinical setting, this procedure is helpful in certain cases where routine clinical and imaging evaluation is equivocal or has failed to provide a definitive diagnosis. In infection arthritis, sometimes cultures of synovial tissue may be positive even when blood and synovial fluid cultures have been negative. Moreover, microscopic examination of synovial tissue can assist in diagnosis

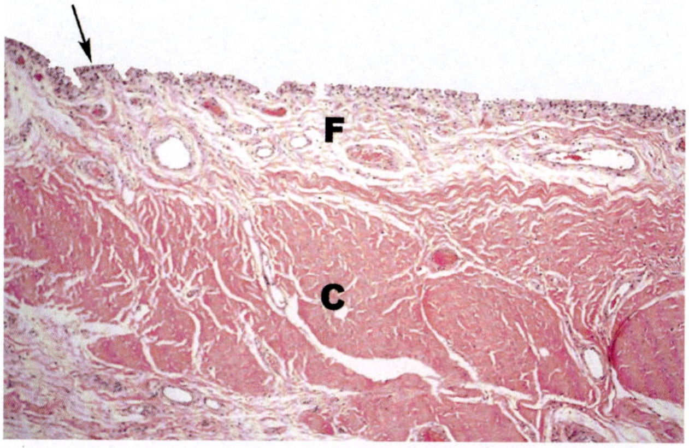

Figure 1.14 ■ **Normal synovium.** Normal synovium consists of a layer of synoviocytes (*arrow*) on the top of loose fibrovascular tissue (*F*) lining the inside of the fibrous joint capsule (*C*). (Reprinted from Klein MJ, Bonar SF, Freemont T, et al., eds. *Atlas of Nontumor Pathology. Non-neoplastic Diseases of Bones and Joints.* Washington, DC: American Registry of Pathology and Armed Forces Institute of Pathology; 2011, Fig. 1-45, with permission of the author and the Publishers.)

of atypical or rare synovial disorders. Synovial biopsy can be performed by the orthopedic surgeon through arthroscopy or by the interventional radiologist using ultrasound-guided needle technique. The microscopic diagnostic features usually evaluated include hypertrophy and hyperplasia of the synovial cells, proliferation of synoviocytes, proliferation of villi, presence of fibrin and its location (whether superficial or deep), type of inflammatory cells and their distribution, capillary proliferation, pannus formation, and presence of hemorrhage and hemosiderin pigment (Figs. 1.14 to 1.17).

PATHOLOGY

The synovial (diarthrodial) joint consists of two bone ends cupped by the articular cartilage, dense fibrous capsule lined by the synovium, and synovial fluid (Fig. 1.18A). The articular cartilage consists of a hyaline cartilage of various thickness (about 2 mm to 4 mm depending of the particular anatomic site), resting on and integrated with the subchondral plate, a layer of bone resembling the cortex (Fig. 1.18B). In young people, hyaline cartilage is translucent and bluish white, whereas in older individuals, it is opaque and slightly yellowish. On microscopic examination, it is composed of a dense extracellular matrix containing sparsely distributed chondrocytes, type II collagen, and hydrophilic sulfated proteoglycans including aggrecan (which contains highly negatively charged glycosaminoglycan chains), decorin, biglycan, and fibromodulin. The distribution of proteoglycans in the cartilage matrix varies from joint to joint, but generally the surface layers of the cartilage contain much less proteoglycan than do the deeper layers. In histologic sections stained with hematoxylin and eosin, the junction between calcified cartilage and noncalcified cartilage is marked by a basophilic line known as the tidemark (Fig. 1.19). Synovium, also referred to as synovial membrane, lines the inner surface of the joint capsule and all other intra-articular structures, with the exception of the articular cartilage. It consists of fibrous tissue and fat covered by an incomplete layer of two types of intimal cells: type A synoviocytes (deriving from macrophages) and type B synoviocytes (deriving from

(*Continued on page 15*)

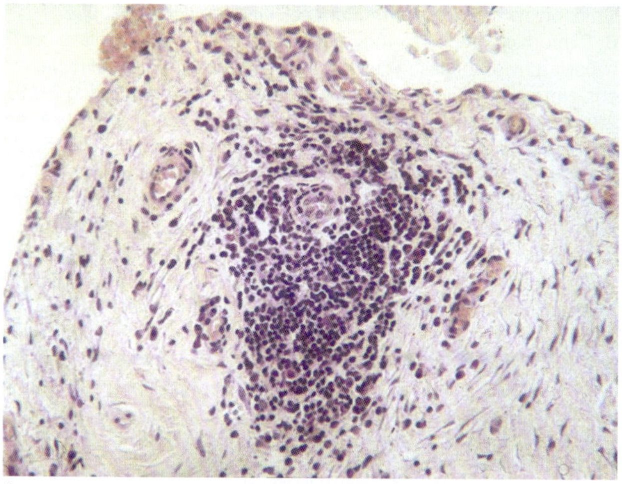

A

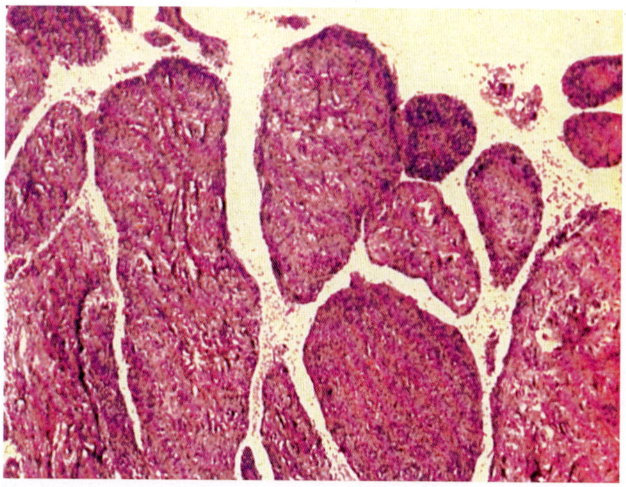

B

Figure 1.15 ■ **Noninflammatory arthropathy. A:** Synovial biopsy shows a perivascular aggregate of lymphocytes and occasional plasma cells (H&E, ×100). (Reprinted from Klein MJ, Bonar SF, Freemont T, et al., eds. *Atlas of Nontumor Pathology. Non-neoplastic Diseases of Bones and Joints.* Washington, DC: American Registry of Pathology and Armed Forces Institute of Pathology; 2011, Fig. 8-13, with permission of the author and the Publishers.) **B:** In another patient, microscopic examination of the synovial membrane shows the villous pattern of the synovium and hyperplasia of the synovial lining cells (H&E, ×4). (From Bullough PG. *Atlas of Orthopedic Pathology with Clinical and Radiologic Correlation.* 2nd ed. New York: Gower Medical Publishing; 1992:10.8, Fig. 10.23.)

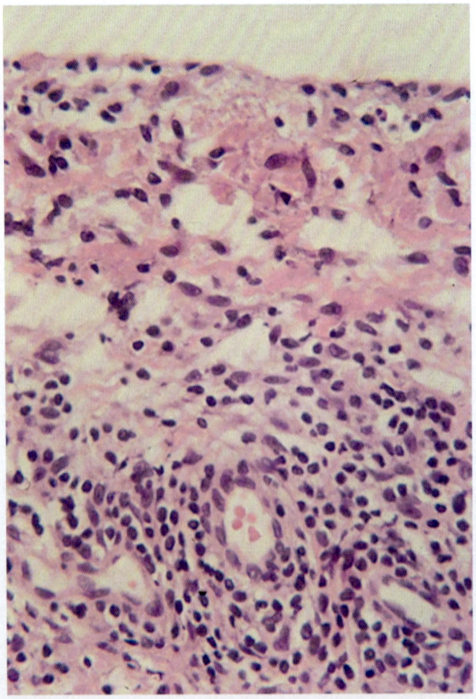

A

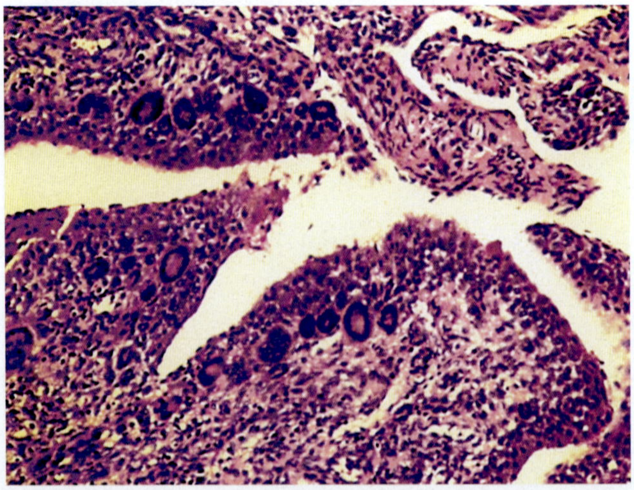

B

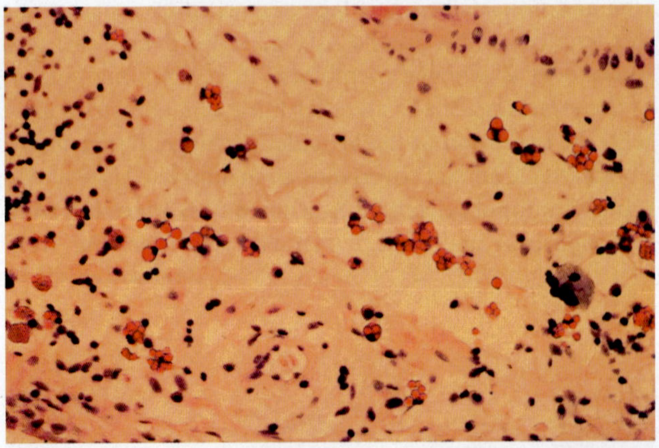

C

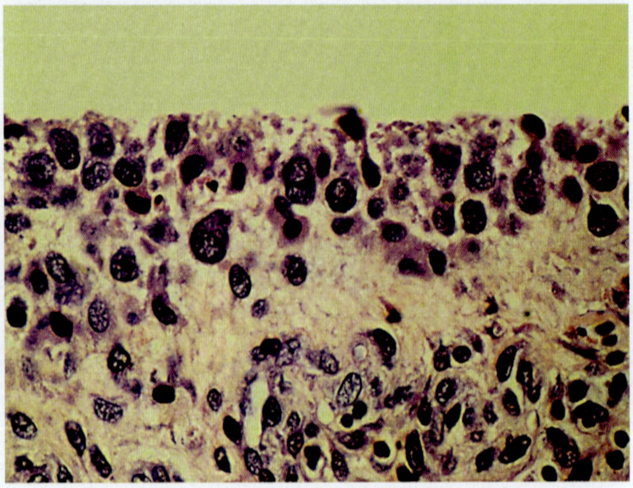

D

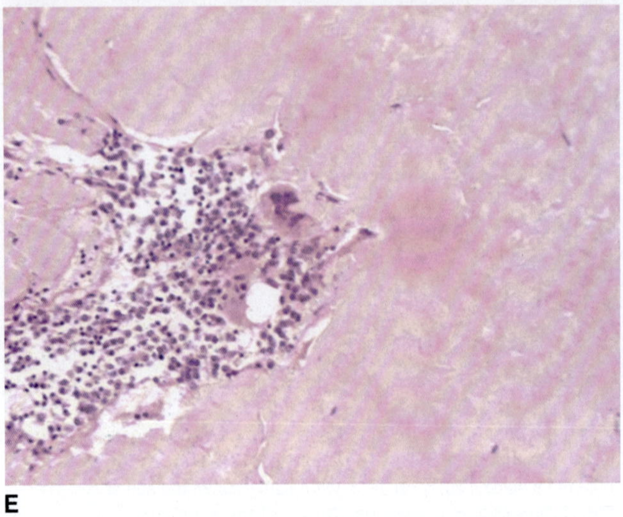

E

Figure 1.16 ■ **Inflammatory arthritis. A:** Synovial biopsy shows inflamed synovium with surface fibrin and a uniform diffuse lymphoplasmacytic inflammatory cell infiltrate (H&E, ×200). **B:** Photomicrograph of synovial membrane shows hyperplasia and hypertrophy of the lining cells. Numerous giant cells are also present. Note also inflammatory infiltrate in the subintimal tissue (H&E, ×10). **C:** In another field of view, inflammatory infiltrate reveals eosinophilic cytoplasmic inclusions (Russell bodies) within the plasma cells (H&E, ×10). **D:** Photomicrograph shows the hyperplasia of the synovial lining cells (H&E, ×40). **E:** Synovial amyloid in a patient with rheumatoid arthritis. Note a giant cell reaction (H&E). (**A** and **E** reprinted from Klein MJ, Bonar SF, Freemont T, et al., eds. *Atlas of Nontumor Pathology. Non-neoplastic Diseases of Bones and Joints. Washington*, DC: American Registry of Pathology and Armed Forces Institute of Pathology; 2011, Figs. 8-12 and 8-193, with permission of the author and the Publishers. **B, C,** and **D** reprinted from Bullough PG. *Atlas of Orthopedic Pathology with Clinical and Radiologic Correlation.* 2nd ed. New York: Gower Medical Publishing; 1992, Figs. 11.10, 11.12, and 11.9.)

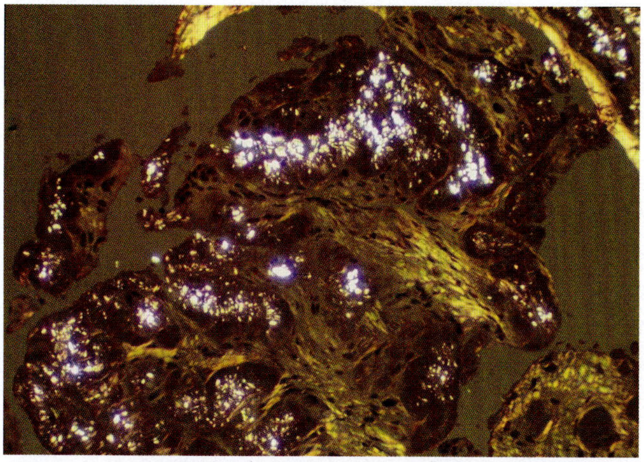

Figure 1.17 ■ CPPD crystal deposition disease. Synovial biopsy shows synovial aggregates of calcium pyrophosphate dehydrate crystals (H&E, polarized light). (Reprinted from Klein MJ, Bonar SF, Freemont T, et al., eds. *Atlas of Nontumor Pathology. Non-neoplastic Diseases of Bones and Joints.* Washington, DC: American Registry of Pathology and Armed Forces Institute of Pathology; 2011, Fig. 8-22, with permission of the author and the Publishers.)

fibroblasts) (see Fig. 1.14). The synovium has three principal functions: secretion of synovial fluid hyaluronate by B cells, phagocytosis of waste material derived from the various components of the joints by A cells, and regulation of the movements of solutes, electrolytes, and proteins from the capillaries into the synovial fluid.

In any of the arthritic conditions, there is anatomic and physiologic alteration of the joint's normal structure and function. In general, this includes loss of capacity of the articulating surfaces to move over one another and loss of joint stability. Regardless of the cause, joint injury is characterized by certain basic cellular and tissue responses. Usually, there is macroscopic and microscopic evidence of both degeneration and repair. The morphologic abnormalities of the articular cartilage and synovial membrane are depending upon the specific arthritic process. *Osteoarthritis* is characterized by damage and loss of articular cartilage, subchondral bone sclerosis, degenerative cysts, and osteophytosis (Fig. 1.20). The initial changes in articular cartilage are localized; however, the gradual damage and destruction of the cartilage eventually results in complete loss of articular cartilage exposing the underlying bone (Fig. 1.21). Microscopic findings include hypertrophy and hyperplasia of synoviocytes and synovial hypervascularity. The early changes within the cartilage include loss of proteoglycan (Fig. 1.22), followed by flaking and cracking of the cartilaginous surface with formation of the fissures (Fig. 1.23). In areas of residual cartilage, there is often irregularity, duplication, and reduplication of the tidemark (Fig. 1.24).

(Continued on page 18)

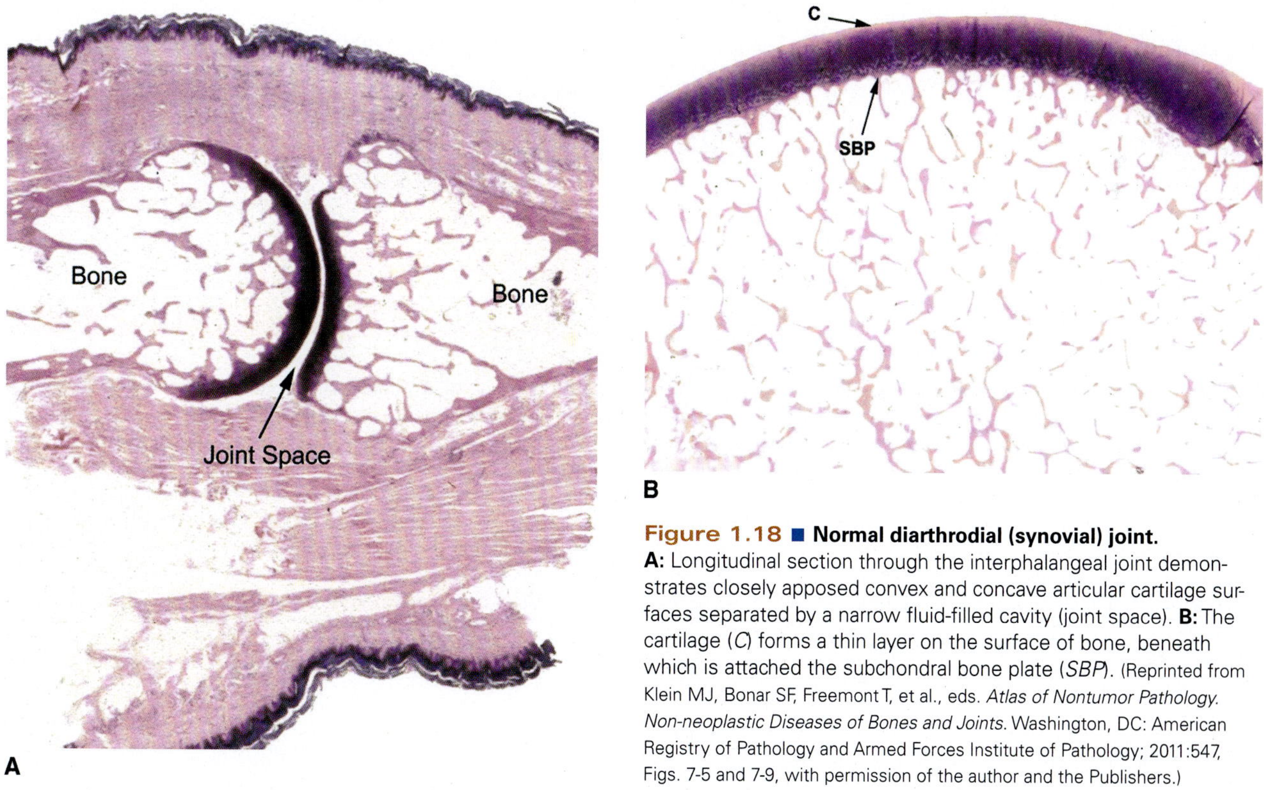

Figure 1.18 ■ Normal diarthrodial (synovial) joint. **A:** Longitudinal section through the interphalangeal joint demonstrates closely apposed convex and concave articular cartilage surfaces separated by a narrow fluid-filled cavity (joint space). **B:** The cartilage (*C*) forms a thin layer on the surface of bone, beneath which is attached the subchondral bone plate (*SBP*). (Reprinted from Klein MJ, Bonar SF, Freemont T, et al., eds. *Atlas of Nontumor Pathology. Non-neoplastic Diseases of Bones and Joints.* Washington, DC: American Registry of Pathology and Armed Forces Institute of Pathology; 2011:547, Figs. 7-5 and 7-9, with permission of the author and the Publishers.)

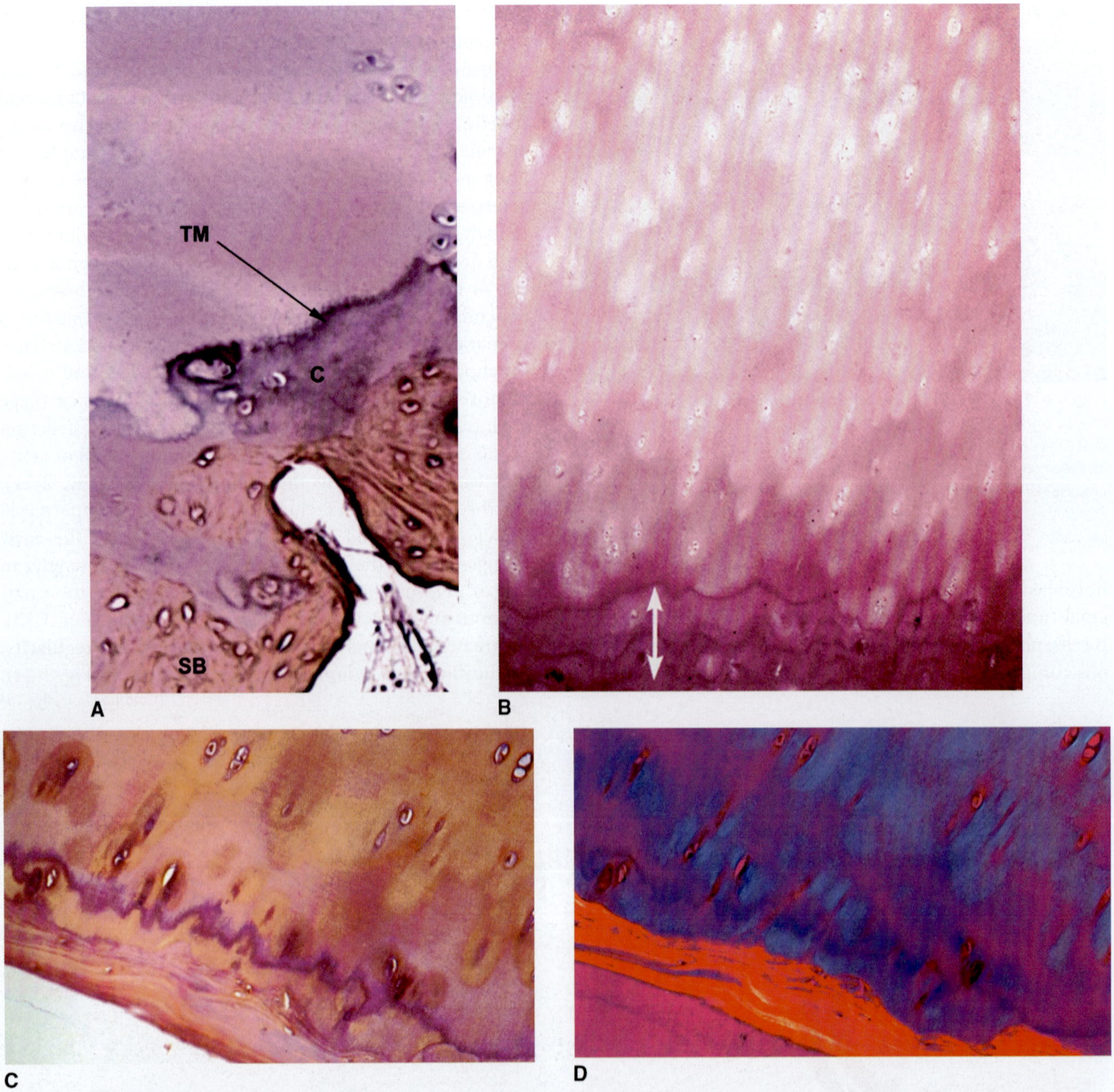

Figure 1.19 ■ **Normal articular cartilage. A:** On this photomicrograph, the cartilage (*C*) immediately adjacent to the subchondral bone (*SB*) exhibits calcified matrix demarcated from the rest of the cartilage by a wavy interface known as the tidemark (*TM*). **B:** Mature articular cartilage at its base contains a calcified zone (*double-headed arrow*) into which anchored are the collagen arcades of the cartilage. Because this area resembles high and low tidemarks on a beach, it is referred to as the "tidemark." **C:** Photomicrograph of the bone–cartilage interface demonstrates the tidemark, which is identified by a dark-red wavy line (H&E, ×10). **D:** When the same histologic field is viewed in a polarized light using a first-order red compensator filter, the bone–cartilage interface is visualized more clearly (H&E, ×10, polarized light). (**A** and **B** reprinted from Klein MJ, Bonar SF, Freemont T, et al., eds. *Atlas of Nontumor Pathology. Non-neoplastic Diseases of Bones and Joints.* Washington, DC: American Registry of Pathology and Armed Forces Institute of Pathology; 2011, Figs. 7-16 and 1-37, with permission of the author and the Publishers. **C** and **D** from Bullough PG. *Atlas of Orthopedic Pathology with Clinical and Radiologic Correlation.* 2nd ed. New York: Gower Medical Publishing; 1992:1.23, Fig. 1.54A,B.)

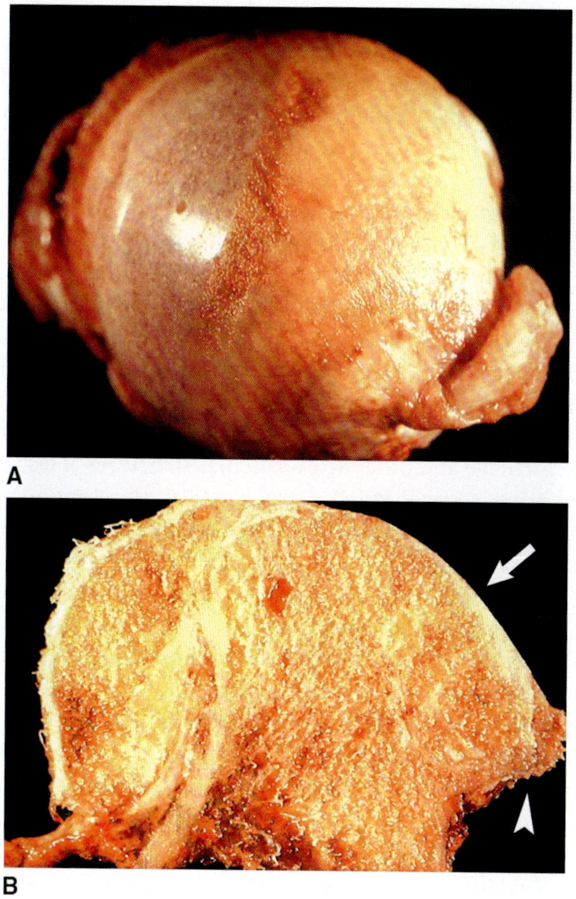

Figure 1.20 ■ **Pathology of osteoarthritis. A:** Photograph of the gross specimen of the femoral head shows absence of the articular cartilage on the superior and lateral aspects and "polish" appearance of the exposed subchondral bone (eburnation). The remaining cartilage exhibits yellowish color and roughened surface. **B:** Coronal section of resected femoral head shows marked thinning of the articular cartilage medially (*arrow*) and a large osteophyte (*arrowhead*). (Modified from Bullough PG. *Atlas of Orthopedic Pathology with Clinical and Radiologic Correlation.* 2nd ed. New York: Gower Medical Publishing; 1992, Figs. 10.8 and 9.11.)

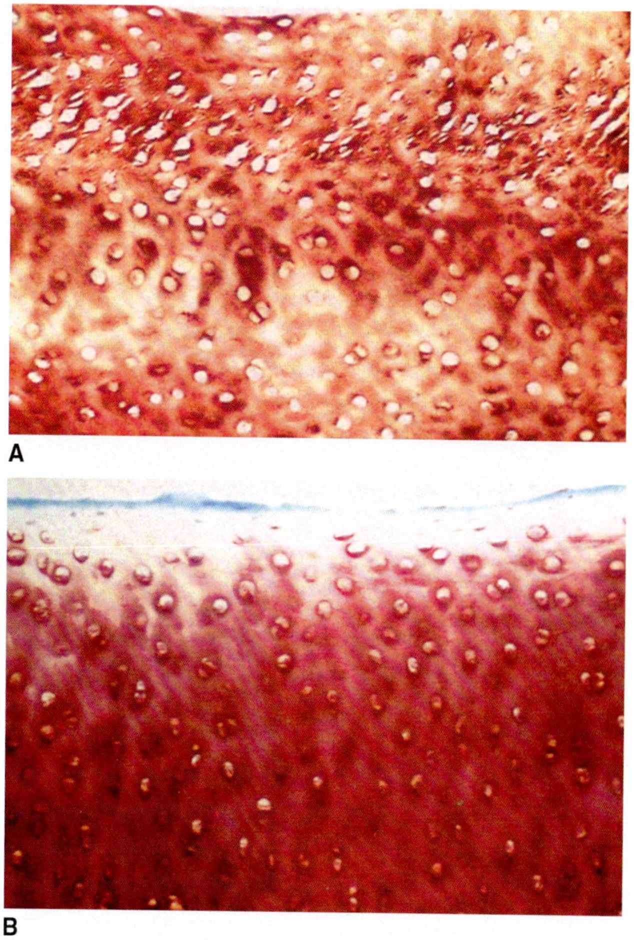

Figure 1.22 ■ **Pathology of chondromalacia. A:** The photomicrograph of normal articular cartilage shows intense staining of proteoglycan. **B:** In articular cartilage undergoing chondromalacia, there is loss of proteoglycan in the matrix seen by the decreased intensity of staining (safranin O, ×10). (From Bullough PG. *Atlas of Orthopedic Pathology with Clinical and Radiologic Correlation.* 2nd ed. New York: Gower Medical Publishing; 1992:9.9, Fig. 9.19A,B.)

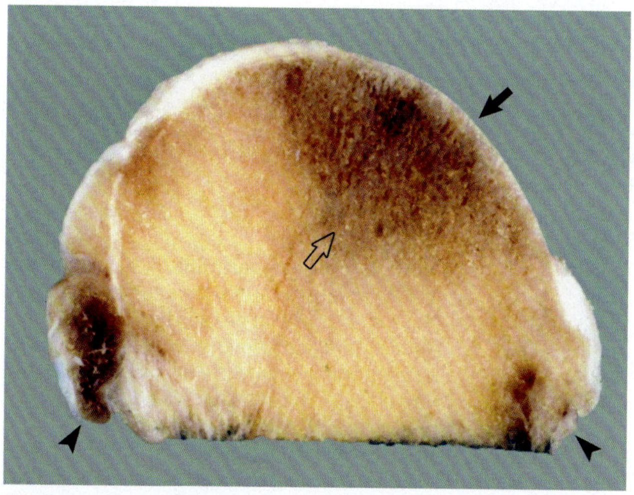

Figure 1.21 ■ **Pathology of osteoarthritis.** Coronal section through the femoral head shows marked thinning of articular cartilage (*arrow*), an area of eburnation (*open arrow*), and osteophytes (*arrowheads*). (Modified from Klein MJ, Bonar SF, Freemont T, et al., eds. *Atlas of Nontumor Pathology. Non-neoplastic Diseases of Bones and Joints.* Washington, DC: American Registry of Pathology and Armed Forces Institute of Pathology; 2011:604, Fig. 8-51, with permission of the author and the Publishers.)

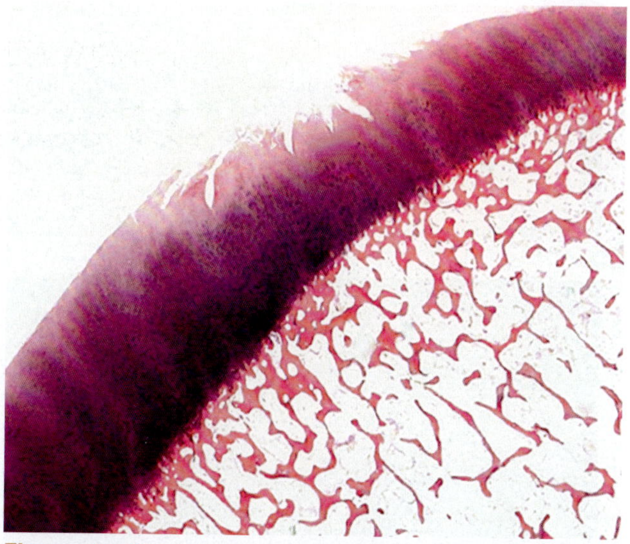

Figure 1.23 ■ **Pathology of osteoarthritis.** Early changes of osteoarthritis consist of focal clefts on the surface of articular cartilage (H&E). (Reprinted from Klein MJ, Bonar SF, Freemont T, et al., eds. *Atlas of Nontumor Pathology. Non-neoplastic Diseases of Bones and Joints.* Washington, DC: American Registry of Pathology and Armed Forces Institute of Pathology; 2011:627, Fig. 8-88, with permission of the author and the Publishers.)

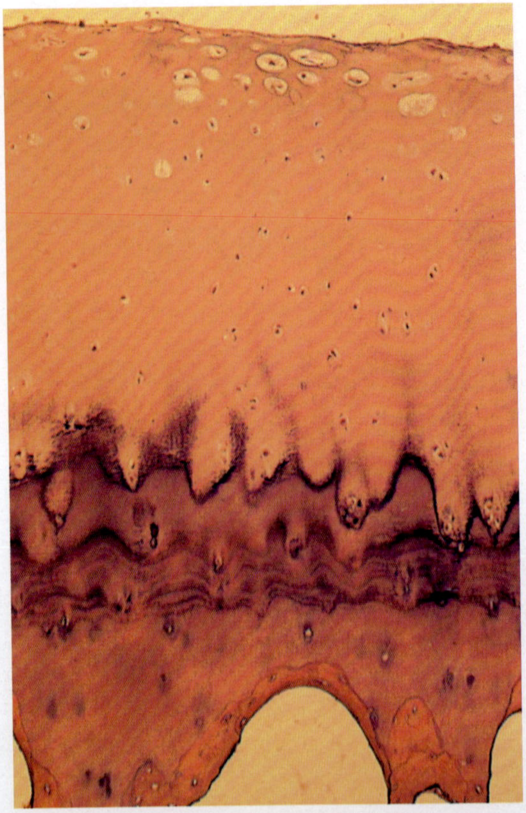

Figure 1.24 ■ Pathology of osteoarthritis. Photomicrograph of a portion of the articular cartilage shows irregularity and duplication of the tidemark (H&E, ×4). (From Bullough PG. *Atlas of Orthopedic Pathology with Clinical and Radiologic Correlation*. 2nd ed. New York: Gower Medical Publishing; 1992, Fig. 10.18.)

In subchondral bone, the marrow elements are replaced by granular, eosinophilic material lacking cellular elements. There is reduction in number of osteocytic lacunae, which in addition may become empty or may contain cellular debris. In more advanced stages, there is complete loss of the articular cartilage (Fig. 1.25A, B), increased endochondral ossification, increased vascular penetration of the calcified cartilage, and deposition if immature, woven bone at the bone–cartilage interface (Fig. 1.25C). *Inflammatory arthritis*, such as rheumatoid arthritis, has a particular predilection for synovium (Fig. 1.26). The synovial membrane becomes thickened, swollen, and red. The inflammatory pannus erodes first the parts of bone not covered by the articular cartilage (so called bare areas) and later destroys the cartilage and other intra-articular structures (Figs. 1.27 and 1.28). *Crystal-induced arthropathies* represent a spectrum of inflammatory articular abnormalities secondary to cellular reaction directed against deposited crystals (such as monosodium urate, calcium hydroxyapatite phosphate, or calcium pyrophosphate dihydrate) in the joints and periarticular tissues. For instance, the monosodium urate crystals accumulate in the synovial fluid and soft tissue tophi, whereas pyrophosphate crystals are found most commonly in fibrocartilaginous tissues, such as knee joint menisci (Fig. 1.29). In *septic arthritis*, the synovial fluid is opaque or frankly purulent. The nucleated cell count is very high (20,000 to 100,000 cells/mm^3), and there is progressive infiltrate in synovium, associated with vascular congestion, and increase in the number of type A and B synoviocytes.

(Continued on page 21)

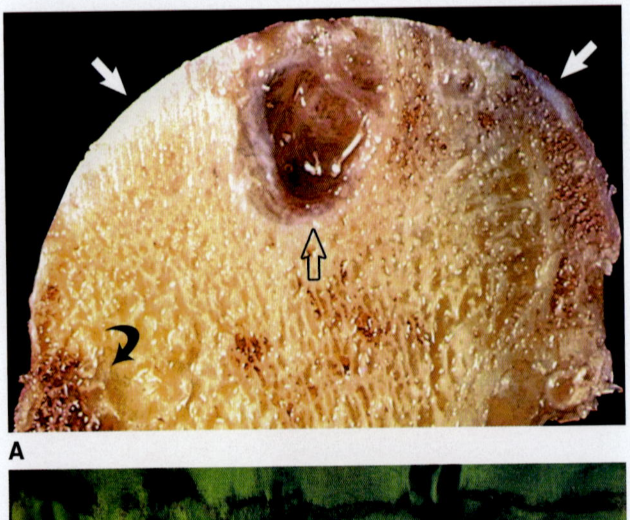

A

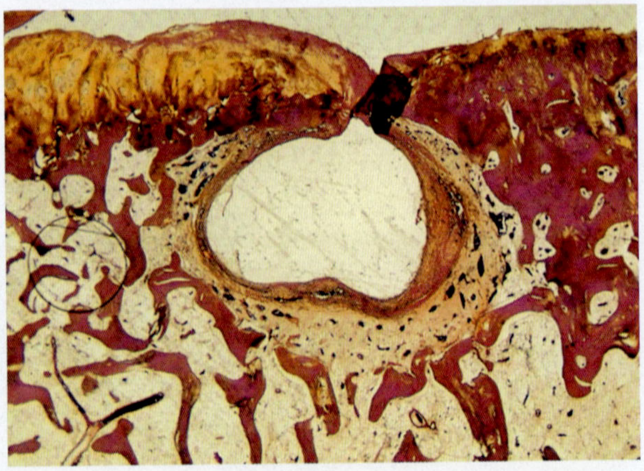

B

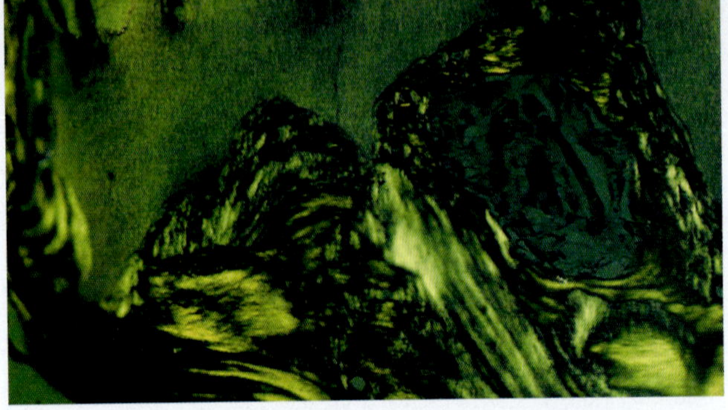

C

Figure 1.25 ■ Pathology of osteoarthritis. A: Coronal section of the femoral head resected from the patient with advanced osteoarthritis of the hip joint demonstrates lack of articular cartilage (*arrows*), large subchondral cyst (*open arrow*), and medial osteophyte (*curved arrow*). **B:** Photomicrograph shows absence of the articular cartilage and a subchondral cyst, which connects with a joint space through a short neck (phloxine & tartrazine, original magnification, ×2.5). **C:** Photomicrograph taken with polarized light shows woven bone formation in the subchondral region, indicative of accelerated remodeling (×25, polarized light). (Modified from Bullough PG. *Atlas of Orthopedic Pathology with Clinical and Radiologic Correlation*. 2nd ed. New York: Gower Medical Publishing; 1992, Figs. 9.32, 10.9, and 10.20.)

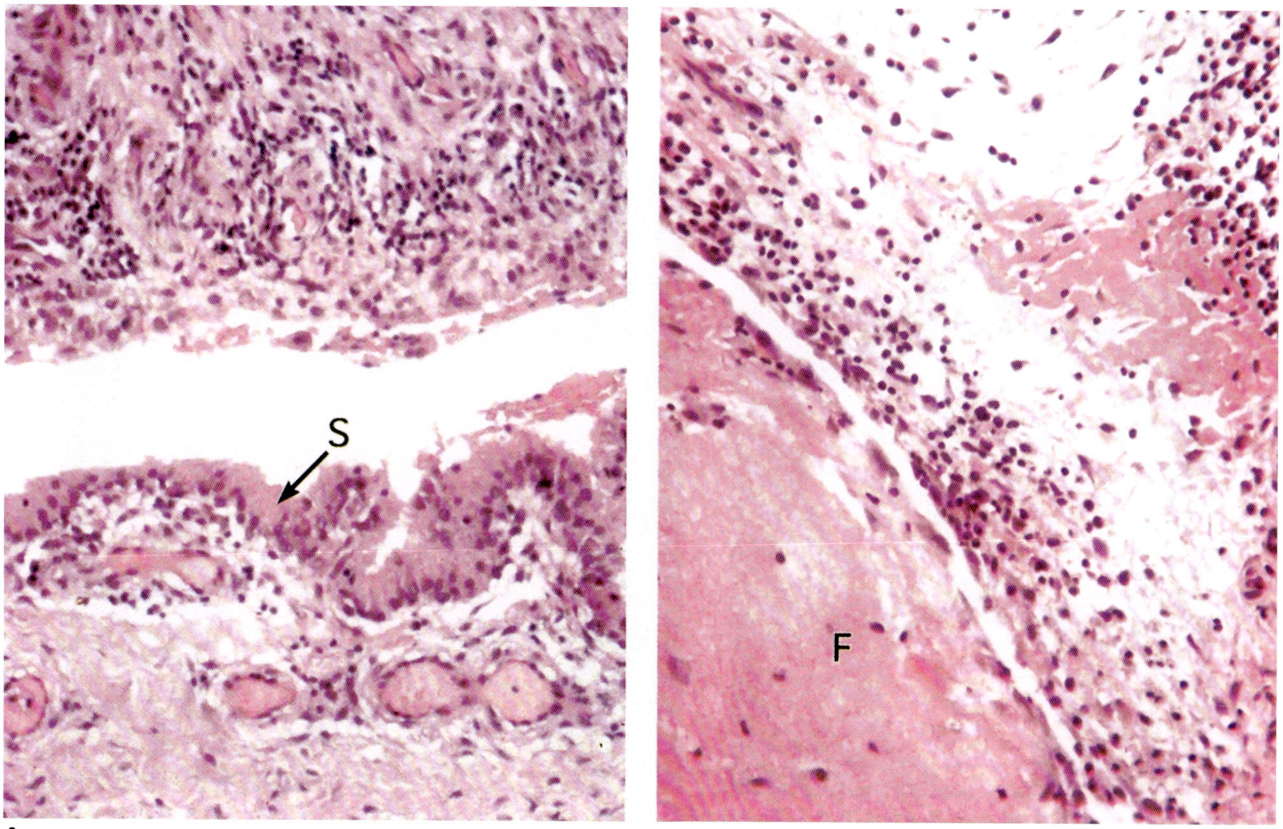

A B

Figure 1.26 ■ **Pathology of rheumatoid arthritis. A:** Synovium shows hypertrophy and hyperplasia of the synoviocytes (*S*). **B:** In another histologic section, observe that synoviocyte layer and adjacent subintima are replaced by granulation tissue. Fibrin (*F*) lies on the surface (H&E). (Reprinted from Klein MJ, Bonar SF, Freemont T, et al., eds. *Atlas of Nontumor Pathology. Non-neoplastic Diseases of Bones and Joints.* Washington, DC: American Registry of Pathology and Armed Forces Institute of Pathology; 2011:695, Fig. 8-176, with permission of the author and the Publishers.)

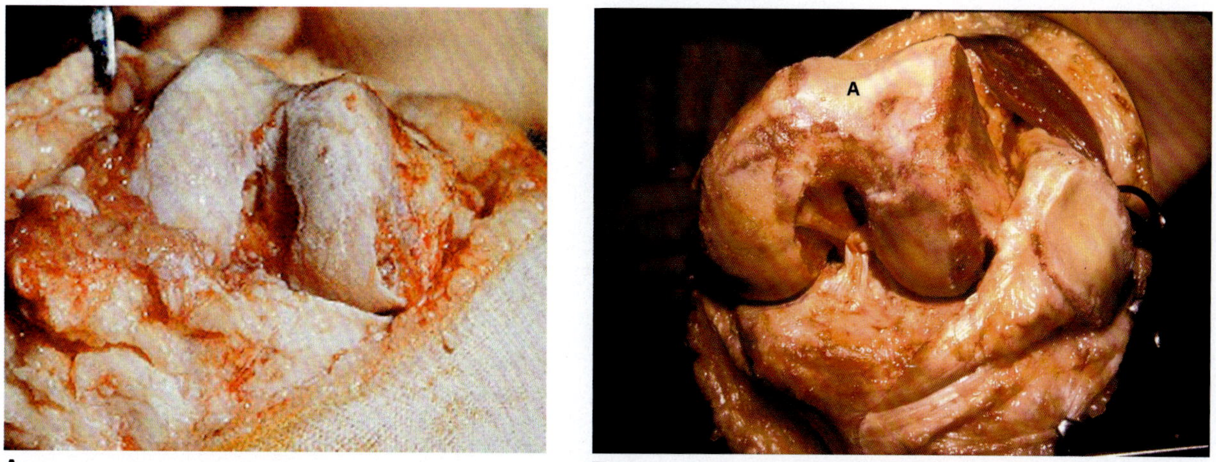

A B

Figure 1.27 ■ **Pathology of rheumatoid arthritis. A:** Photograph of the distal end of the femur shows inflammatory pannus and peripheral erosions of the articular cartilage of the femoral condyles. **B:** In another patient, observe erosion of the articular cartilage (*A*) by pannus invading the articular surface from periphery. (Reprinted from Klein MJ, Bonar SF, Freemont T, et al., eds. *Atlas of Nontumor Pathology. Non-neoplastic Diseases of Bones and Joints.* Washington, DC: American Registry of Pathology and Armed Forces Institute of Pathology; 2011, Figs. 8-52 and 8-171.)

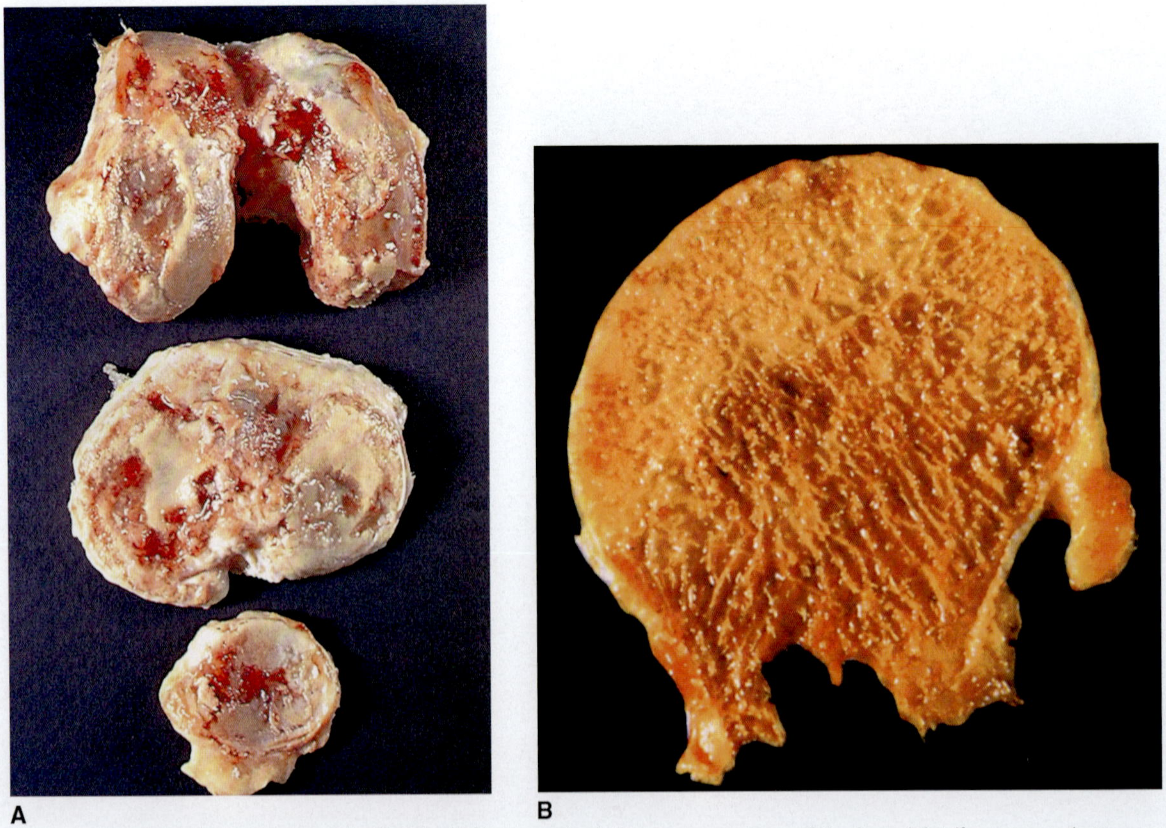

Figure 1.28 ■ **Pathology of rheumatoid arthritis. A:** Photograph of the gross specimen of the knee joint (from *top to bottom*: articular surfaces of the femoral condyles, tibial plateau, and fibular head) shows destruction of the articular cartilage. Note that articular cartilage is destroyed mostly at the periphery of the joint, with central areas somewhat spared. **B:** Coronal section of the femoral head shows destruction of the articular cartilage, but there is no evidence of subchondral sclerosis or osteophyte formation. (From Bullough PG. *Atlas of Orthopedic Pathology with Clinical and Radiologic Correlation*. 2nd ed. New York: Gower Medical Publishing; 1992, Figs. 11.5 and 11.6.)

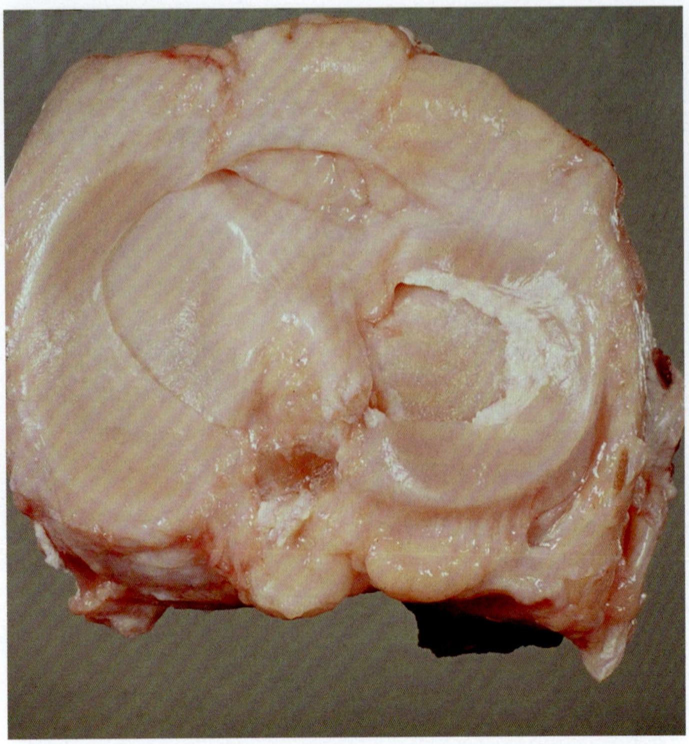

Figure 1.29 ■ **Pathology of calcium pyrophosphate crystal deposition disease.** Gross specimen of the knee shows deposit of the calcium pyrophosphate dihydrate within the lateral semilunar cartilage (meniscus). (Reprinted from Klein MJ, Bonar SF, Freemont T, et al., eds. *Atlas of Nontumor Pathology. Non-neoplastic Diseases of Bones and Joints.* Washington, DC: American Registry of Pathology and Armed Forces Institute of Pathology; 2011.)

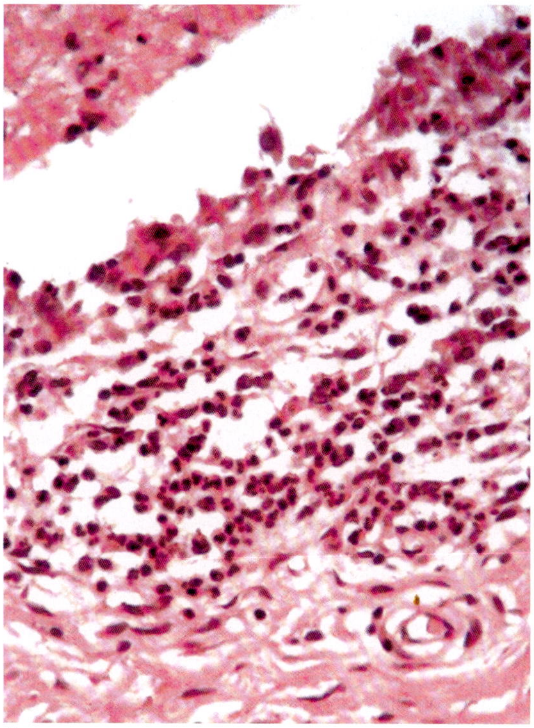

A

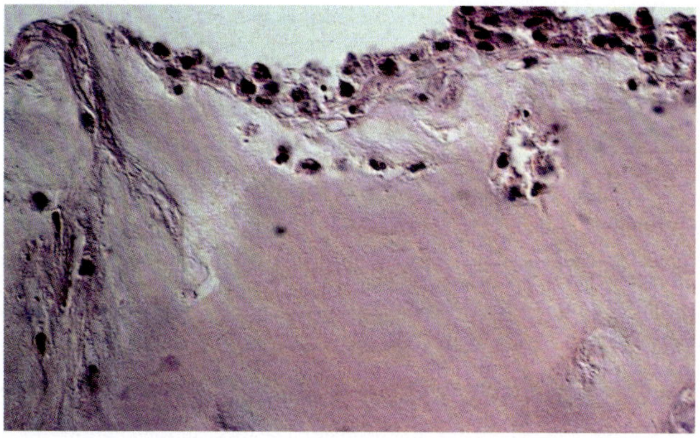

B

Figure 1.30 ■ Pathology of infectious arthritis. **A:** Synovium from the patient with septic arthritis exhibits ulceration of the synovial surface and proliferation of the neutrophils (H&E). (Reprinted from Klein MJ, Bonar SF, Freemont T, et al., eds. *Atlas of Nontumor Pathology. Non-neoplastic Diseases of Bones and Joints.* Washington, DC: American Registry of Pathology and Armed Forces Institute of Pathology; 2011:588, Fig. 8-15.) **B:** In another patient, photomicrograph of a portion of articular cartilage obtained from the septic joint shows polymorphonuclear leukocytes on the cartilage surface and underlying erosion of the cartilage (H&E, ×25). (From Bullough PG. *Atlas of Orthopedic Pathology with Clinical and Radiologic Correlation.* 2nd ed. New York: Gower Medical Publishing; 1992:4.11, Fig. 4.20.)

The synovium is inflamed, and there is inflammatory cell infiltrate in the subintima associated with presence of neutrophils within subintima and synoviocyte layer, often with aggregates amounting to microabscesses (Fig. 1.30). In addition, the inflamed granulation tissue is covered by fibrin and necrotic debris. The cartilage shows features of necrosis associated with loss of chondrocytes and irregularity of the surface due to damage from neutrophil-derived enzymes. There is extensive neutrophilic infiltrate with cells containing coarse ragocyte granules.

SUGGESTED READINGS

Aletaha D, Neogi T, Silman AJ, et al. 2010 Rheumatoid arthritis classification criteria: an American College of Rheumatology/European League Against Rheumatism collaborative initiative. *Arthritis Rheum.* 2010;62:2569–2581.

Altman R, Alarcon G, Appelrowth D, et al. The American College of Rheumatology criteria for the classification and reporting of osteoarthritis of the hip. *Arthritis Rheum.* 1991;34:505–514.

Archer CW, Morrison H, Pitsillides AA. Cellular aspects of the development of diarthrodial joints and articular cartilage. *J Anat.* 1994;184: 447–456.

Bayliss MT, Dudhia J. Articular cartilage: structure, function and physiology. In: Fitzgerald RH, Kaufer H, Malkani AL, eds. *Orthopaedics.* St. Louis, MO: Mosby; 2002:160–167.

Brannan SR, Jerrard DA. Synovial fluid analysis. *J Emerg Med.* 2006;30:331–339.

Bresnihan B. Are synovial biopsies of diagnostic value? *Arthritis Res Ther.* 2003;5:271–278.

Bridgen M. The erythrocyte sedimentation rate. Still a helpful test when used judiciously. *Postgrad Med.* 1998;103:257–262.

Brouet JC, Clauvel JP, Danon F, et al. Biological and clinical significance of cryoglobulins: a report of 86 cases. *Am J Med.* 1974;57:775–788.

Bruhlmann P, Michel BA. History and clinical examination in rheumatology—key to diagnosis and prognosis. *Ther Umsch.* 2006;63:485–490.

Bullough PG. *Atlas of Orthopedic Pathology with Clinical and Radiologic Correlation.* 2nd ed. New York: Gower Medical Publishing; 1992.

Castrejon I, McCollum L, Tanriover MD, Pincus T. Importance of patient history and physical examination in rheumatoid arthritis compared to other chronic diseases: results of a physician survey. *Arthritis Care Res.* 2012;64:1250–1255.

Chen LX, Clayburne G, Schumacher HR. Update on identification of pathogenic crystals in joint fluid. *Curr Rheumatol Rep.* 2004;6:217–220.

Cohen AS. Synovial membrane histopathology in the differential diagnosis of rheumatoid arthritis, gout, pseudogout, systemic lupus erythematosus, infectious arthritis and degenerative joint disease. *Medicine.* 1978;57:239–251.

de Crombrugghe B, Lefebvre V, Behringer RR, et al. Transcriptional mechanism of chondrocyte differentiation. *Matrix Biol.* 2000;19:389–394.

Doherty M, Dacre J, Dieppe P, Snaith M. The GALS locomotor screen. *Ann Rheumatol Dis.* 1992;51:1165–1169.

Engvall E, Perlmann P. Enzyme-linked immunosorbent assay (ELISA): quantitative assay of immunoglobulin G. *Immunochemistry.* 1971;8:871–874.

Eustace S, DiMasi M, Adams J, et al. *In vitro* and *in vivo* spin echo diffusion imaging characteristics of synovial fluid: potential non-invasive differentiation of inflammatory and degenerative arthritis. *Skeletal Radiol.* 2000;29:320–323.

Feng PH. Approach to rheumatic diseases. *Ann Acad Med Singapore.* 1989;18:5–7.

Fernandes JC, Martel-Pelletier J, Pelletier JP. The role of cytokines in osteoarthritis pathophysiology. *Biorheology.* 2002;39:237–246.

Ferri C, Zignego AL, Pileri SA. Cryoglobulins. *J Clin Pathol.* 2002;55:4–13.

Fremont AJ. The pathophysiology of cartilage and synovium. *Br J Rheumatol.* 1996;35(Suppl 3):10–13.

Gerlag D, Tak PP. Synovial biopsy. *Best Pract Res Clin Rheunatol.* 2005;19:387–400.

Goldenberg DL, Cohen AS. Synovial membrane histopathology in the differential diagnosis of rheumatoid arthritis, gout, pseudogout, systemic lupus erythematosus, infectious arthritis and degenerative joint disease. *Medicine (Baltimore).* 1978;57:239–252.

Goldenberg DL, Eustace S, DiMasi M, Adams J, et al. *In vitro* and *in vivo* spin echo diffusion imaging characteristics of synovial fluid: potential non-invasive differentiation of inflammatory and degenerative arthritis. *Skeletal Radiol.* 2000;29:320–323.

Gonzalez S, Martina-Barra J, Lopez-Larrea C. Immunogenetics. HLA-B27 and spondyloarthropathies. *Curr Opin Rheumatol.* 1999;11:257–264.

Greenspan A, Beltran J. *Orthopedic Imaging—A Practical Approach.* 6th ed. Philadelphia, PA: Wolters Kluwer; 2015:527–535.

Greenspan A, Gershwin ME. *Radiology of the Arthritides—A Clinical Approach.* Philadelphia, PA: JB Lippincott—Gower Medical Publishing; 1990:1.1–1.8.

Imboden JB. Approach to the patient with arthritis. In: Imboden JB, Hellmann DB, Stone JH, eds. *Current Diagnosis & Treatment: Rheumatology.* 3rd ed. New York: McGraw Hill; 2013:1–6.

Ingegnoli F, Castelli R, Gualtierotti R. Rheumatoid factors: clinical application. *Dis Markers.* 2013;35:727–734.

Iwanaga T, Shikichi M, Kitamura H, et al. Morphology and functional roles of synoviocytes in the joint. *Arch Histol Cytol.* 2000;63:17–31.

Kaplan PA, Helms CA, Dussault R, et al. *Musculoskeletal MRI.* Philadelphia, PA: WB Saunders Company; 2001:1–21.

Khan MA. An overview of clinical spectrum and heterogeneity of spondyloarthropathies. *Rheum Dis Clin N Am.* 1992;18:1–10.

Klein MJ. Radiographic correlation in orthopedic pathology. *Adv Anat Pathol.* 2005;12:155–179.

Klein MJ, Bonar SF, Freemont T, et al. *Atlas of Nontumor Pathology. Non-neoplastic Diseases of Bones and Joints.* Washington, DC: American Registry of Pathology and Armed Forces Institute of Pathology; 2011: 1–53, 545–575, 577–767.

Klein-Nulend J, Nijweide PJ, Burger EH. Osteocyte and bone structure. *Curr Osteoporos Rep.* 2003;1:5–10.

Korkusuz P, Dagdeviren A, Eksioglu F, Ors U. Immunohistological analysis of normal and osteoarthritic human synovial tissue. *Bull Hosp Jt Dis.* 2005;63:63–69.

Lajeunesse D, Reboul P. Subchondral bone in osteoarthritis: a biologic link with articular cartilage leading to abnormal remodeling. *Curr Opin Rheumatol.* 2003;15:628–633.

Leopold SS, Redd BB, Warme WJ, et al. Corticosteroid compared with hyaluronic acid injections for the treatment of osteoarthritis of the knee. A prospective, randomized trial. *J Bone Joint Surg Am.* 2003;85-A:1197–1203.

Leslie D, Lipsky P, Notkins AL. Autoantibodies as predictors of disease. *J Clin Invest.* 2001;108:1417–1422.

Lumbreras B, Pascual E, Frasquet J, et al. Analysis of the crystals in synovial fluid: training of the analysts results in high consistency. *Ann Rheum Dis.* 2005;64:612–615.

Lyon R, Sonali N. Effective use of autoantibody tests in the diagnosis of systemic lupus erythematosus. *Ann NY Acad Sci.* 2005;1050:217–228.

Mauri C, Ehrenstein MR. Cells of the synovium in rheumatoid arthritis. B cells. *Arthritis Res Ther.* 2007;9:205.

Mills JA. Physical examination of the musculoskeletal system. In: Imboden JB, Hellmann DB, Stone JH, eds. *Current Diagnosis & Treatment: Rheumatology.* 3rd ed. New York: Mc Graw Hill; 2013:1–6.

Morley JJ, Kushner I. Serum C-reactive protein levels in disease. *Ann NY Acad Sci.* 1982;389:406–418.

Nakamura MC, Imboden JB. Laboratory diagnosis. In: Imboden JB, Hellmann DB, Stone JH, eds. *Current Diagnosis & Treatment: Rheumatology.* 3rd ed. New York: Mc Graw Hill; 2013:15–25.

Nalbant S, Martinez JA, Kitumnuaypong T, et al. Synovial fluid features and their relations to osteoarthritis severity: new findings from sequential studies. *Osteoarthritis Cartilage.* 2003;11:50–54.

Niewold TB, Harrison MJ, Paget SA. Anti-CCP antibody testing as a diagnostic and prognostic tool in rheumatoid arthritis. *QJM (Oxford).* 2007;100:193–201.

Nikac V, Blazar P, Earp B, Weissman BN. Radiographic and surgical considerations in arthritis surgery of the hand. *Skeletal Radiol.* 2017;46:591–604.

Pasqual E, Jovani V. Synovial fluid analysis. *Best Pract Res Clin Rheumatol.* 2005;19:371–386.

Petri M. Review of classification criteria for systemic lupus erythematosus. *Rheum Dis Clin North Am.* 2005;31:245–254.

Punzi L, Oliviero F, Plebani M. New biochemical insight into the pathogenesis of osteoarthritis and the role of laboratory investigations in clinical assessment. *Crit Rev Clin Lab Sci.* 2005;42:279–309.

Puszczewicz M, Iwaszkiewicz C. Role of anti-citrullinated protein antibodies in diagnosis and prognosis of rheumatoid arthritis. *Arch Med Sci.* 2011;7:189–194.

Robinson DB, El-Gabalawy HS. Evaluation of the patient. A. History and physical examination. In: Klippel JH, Stone JH, Crofford LJ, White PH, eds. *Primer of the Rheumatic Diseases.* 13th ed. New York: Springer; 2008:6–41.

Roodman GD. Advances in bone biology: the osteoclast. *Endocr Rev.* 1996;17:308–332.

Schumacher HR. Synovial fluid analysis and synovial biopsy. In: Kelly WN, Harris ED, Ruddy S, Sledge CB, eds. *Textbook of Rheumatology.* 4th ed. Philadelphia, PA: WB Saunders; 1993:562–578.

Shmerling RH. Synovial fluid analysis. A critical appraisal. *Rheum Dis Clin North Am.* 1994;20:503–512.

Sigurdson LA. The structure and function of articular synovial membranes. *J Bone Joint Surg.* 1930;12:603–639.

Singhal O, Kaur V, Kalhan S, et al. Arthroscopic synovial biopsy in definitive diagnosis of joint diseases: an evaluation of efficacy and precision. *Int J Appl Basic Med Res.* 2012;2:102–106.

Sox HC Jr, Liang MH. The erythrocyte sedimentation rate: guidelines for rational use. *Ann Intern Med.* 1986;104:515–523.

Stewart SR, Gershwin ME. Diagnostic tests and procedures in rheumatic diseases. *Clin Med.* 1981;3:565–609.

Sun S-F, Chou Y-J, Hsu C-W, Chen W-L. Hyaluronic acid as a treatment for ankle osteoarthritis. *Cur Rev Musculoskeletal Med.* 2009;2:78–82.

Swan A, Amer H, Dieppe P. The value of synovial fluid assays in the diagnosis of joint disease: a literature survey. *Ann Rheum Dis.* 2002;61: 493–498.

Tan E, Feltkamp TE, Smolen JS, et al. Range of antinuclear antibodies in "healthy" individuals. *Arthritis Rheum.* 1997;40:1612–1618.

Taylor P, Gartemann J, Hsieh J, Creeden J. A systematic review of serum biomarkers anti-cyclic citrullinated peptide and rheumatoid factor as tests for rheumatoid arthritis. *Autoimmune Dis.* 2011;259:414–420.

Vervoordeldonk MJ, Tak PP. Cytokines in rheumatoid arthritis. *Curr Rheumatol Rep.* 2002;4:208–217.

Vigorita VJ. *Orthopaedic pathology.* Philadelphia, PA: Lippincott Williams & Wilkins; 1999.

Vordenbaumen S, Joosten LAB, Friemann J, et al. Utility of synovial biopsy. *Arthritis Res Ther.* 2009;11:256–265.

Vossenaar ER, Smeets TJ, Kraan MC, et al. The presence of citrullinated proteins is not specific for rheumatoid arthritis. *Arthritis Rheum.* 2004;50:3485–3494.

Wener MH, Daum PR, McQuillan GM. The influence of age, sex and race on the upper limit of serum C-reactive protein concentration. *J Rheumatol.* 2000;27:2351–2359.

White RH, Gershwin ME. Utility of common diagnostic tests, including arthrocentesis, in rheumatic diseases. *Med Rounds.* 1987;1:81–85.

Woolf AD, Akesson K. Primer: history and examination in the assessment of musculoskeletal problems. *Nat Clin Pract Rheumatol.* 2008;4:26–33.

Zendman AJW, Venroij V, Pruijn GJM. Use and significance of anti-CCP autoantibodies in rheumatoid arthritis. *Rheumatology.* 2006;45:20–25.

Zimmermann B III, Mikolich DJ, Ho G Jr. Septic bursitis. *Semin Arthritis Rheum.* 1995;24:391–410.

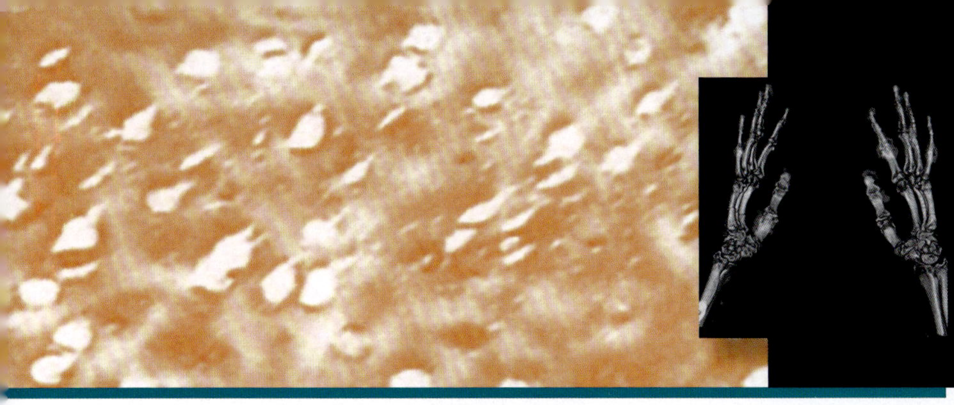

CHAPTER 2

Radiologic Imaging Modalities

RADIOGRAPHY AND DIGITAL RADIOGRAPHY (DR)

Among the variety of available imaging techniques, the most important modality for the evaluation of arthritis is conventional radiography. It is clearly the procedure of choice for the initial examination because of its effectiveness in evaluating the bone and joint changes associated with arthritic disorders, including diminution of the radiographic joint space, osteopenia, sclerosis, subchondral cysts, erosions, osteophytosis, periosteal reaction, and soft tissue calcifications. Characteristic radiographic features, when pathognomonic, may suggest a diagnosis or at least a differential diagnosis. The radiographs may provide objective evidence for the presence and extent of abnormalities, and serial studies may be utilized for recording progress or its lack during the course of a therapy and thus may influence the choice of treatment. In addition, correlation of the radiographic findings with clinical impressions may be useful in determining prognosis. Standard radiographic techniques with minor technical adjustments provide indirect and direct information regarding almost all the tissues within and surrounding the joint. Detailed features of osseous structures along with less well-defined visualization of soft tissues can be demonstrated. Although articular cartilage is not visible, its thickness can be gauged by determining the width of radiographic joint space, with thinning of the cartilage reflected by diminution of visible joint space.

Standard radiographs of the involved joint should be obtained in at least two projections at 90 degrees to each other. Special projections may at times be required to demonstrate destructive changes in the joint to better advantage. In *the shoulder*, the special posterior oblique view, known as the *Grashey projection*, permits the glenoid to be seen in profile. This variant of the anteroposterior (AP) projection in shoulder imaging is obtained by placing the patient in a 40-degree posterior oblique position and directing the center beam toward the glenohumeral joint. This projection shows the glenoid in true profile and clearly visualizes the glenohumeral joint space, which is obscure in the standard AP projection (Fig. 2.1). The Grashey view has been found to be particularly effective in demonstrating subtle shoulder joint erosions in inflammatory arthritides. A superoinferior view, known as the *axillary projection*, is helpful to determine the exact relationship of the humeral head and the glenoid (Fig. 2.2A,B) and is effective in demonstrating the degenerative and inflammatory abnormalities of the glenohumeral joint (Fig. 2.2C). This view, however, may at times be difficult to obtain, particularly if the patient is unable to abduct the arm, in which case a variant of the axillary projection known as the *West Point view* may be similarly effective (Fig. 2.3). Another useful variant of the axillary projection is the *Lawrence view*. The importance of this projection lies in the fact that it does not require full abduction of the arm because it can be compensated for by angulation of the radiographic tube (Fig. 2.4). Abnormalities of the *acromioclavicular joint* are best seen on the special view of this structure obtained with 15 degrees cephalad tilt of the radiographic tube (Fig. 2.5A,B). The key to this other variant of the AP view of the shoulder is a special low-kilovoltage technique in which the radiographic factors are reduced to ~ 33% to 50% of those used in the standard technique for the AP view. The excellent visualization of the acromial end of the clavicle, the acromion, and the acromioclavicular joint afforded by this projection can be helpful in demonstrating early resorptive changes of the distal end of the clavicle seen in rheumatoid arthritis (Fig. 2.5C) and hyperparathyroid arthropathy. In *the elbow*, the radial head–capitellum view, by eliminating overlap of the radial head and coronoid

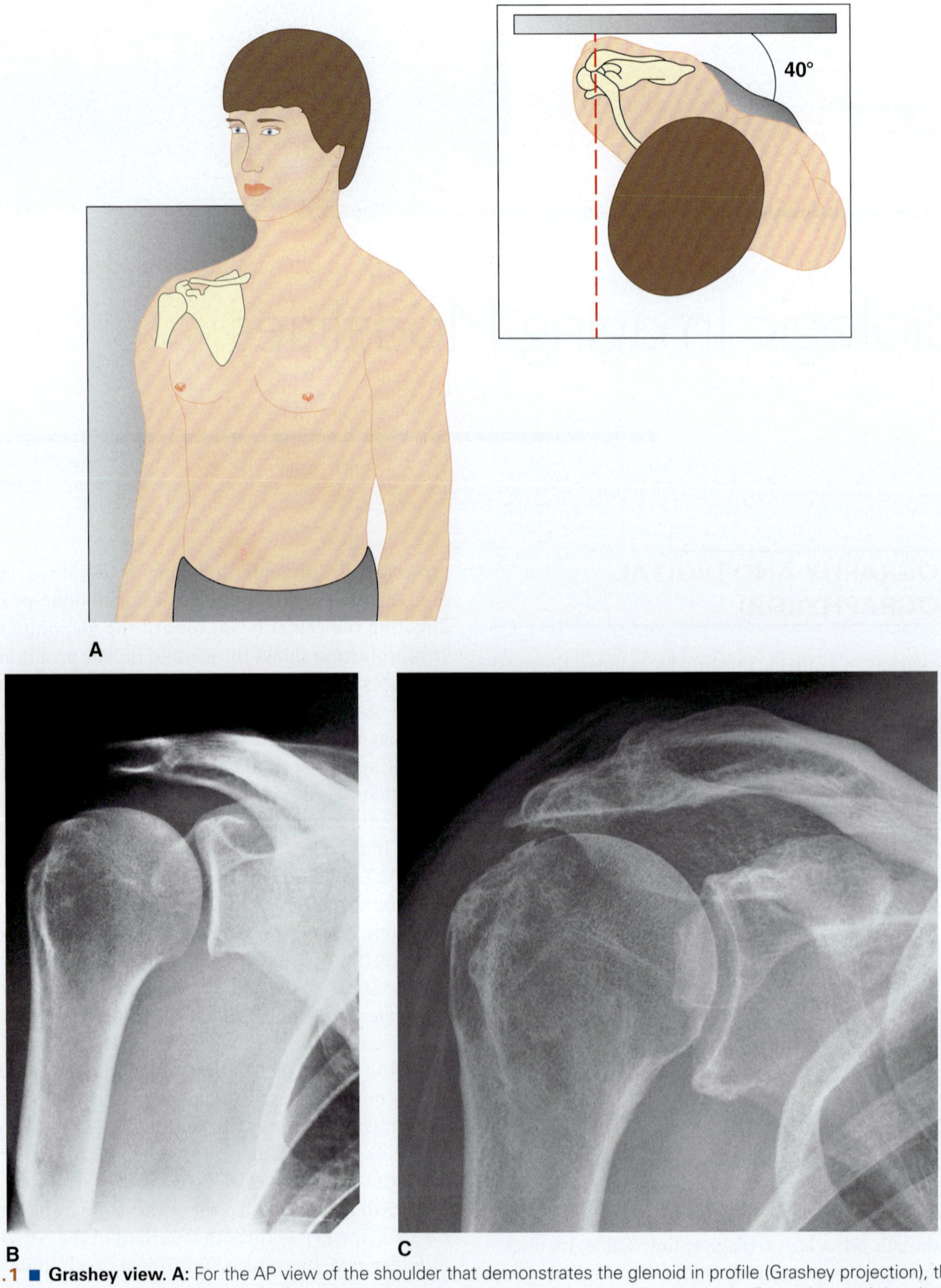

Figure 2.1 ■ **Grashey view. A:** For the AP view of the shoulder that demonstrates the glenoid in profile (Grashey projection), the patient may be either erect (as shown here) or supine. He or she is rotated ~ 40 degrees and the central beam is directed toward the glenohumeral joint. **B:** The radiograph in this projection (posterior oblique view) shows clearly the glenohumeral joint space. **C:** Narrowing of the joint space and subchondral sclerosis associated with formation of osteophytes are present in acromioclavicular and glenohumeral joints, reflecting osteoarthritis. Significant narrowing of the subacromial space is due to a chronic rotator cuff tear.

process and by more clearly demonstrating the humeroradial and humeroulnar joints, shows the inflammatory changes in the elbow joint to better advantage (Fig. 2.6). This projection has proved to be particularly useful in evaluating the capitellum, radial head, and coronoid process. The semisupinated oblique view of *the hand and wrist* (the so-called *ball-catcher view*), introduced by Nørgaard in 1965, effectively demonstrates the radial aspects of the

(*Continued on page 27*)

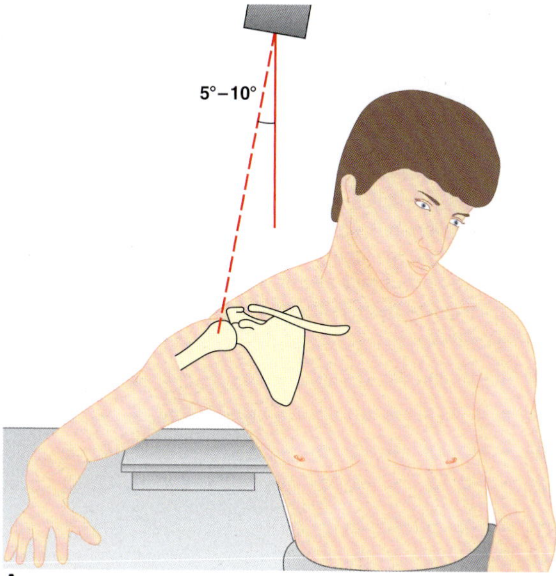

A

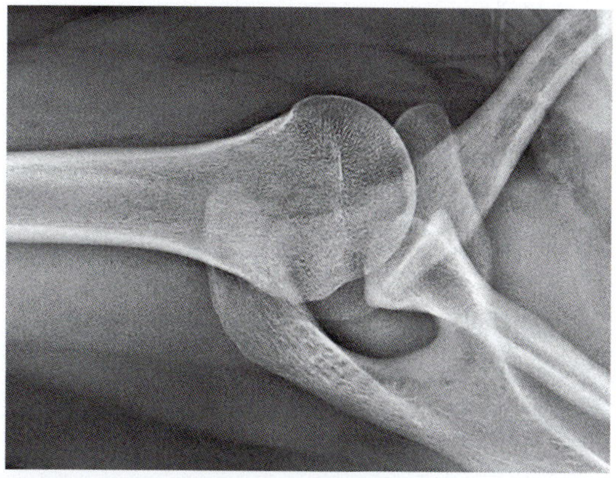

B

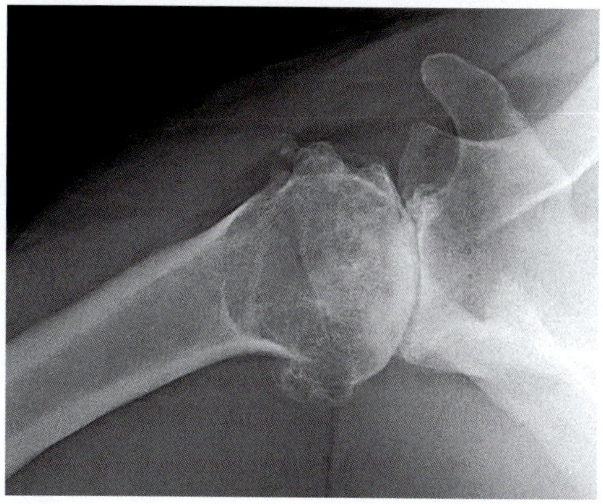

C

Figure 2.2 ■ **Axillary view. A:** For the axillary view of the shoulder, the patient is seated at the side of the radiographic table, with the arm abducted so that axilla is positioned over the film cassette. The radiographic tube is angled ~ 5 to 10 degrees toward the elbow, and the central beam is directed through the shoulder joint. **B:** The radiograph in this projection demonstrates the exact relationship of the humeral head and glenoid, and the glenohumeral joint space is clearly demonstrated. **C:** Advanced osteoarthritis is affecting the glenohumeral joint.

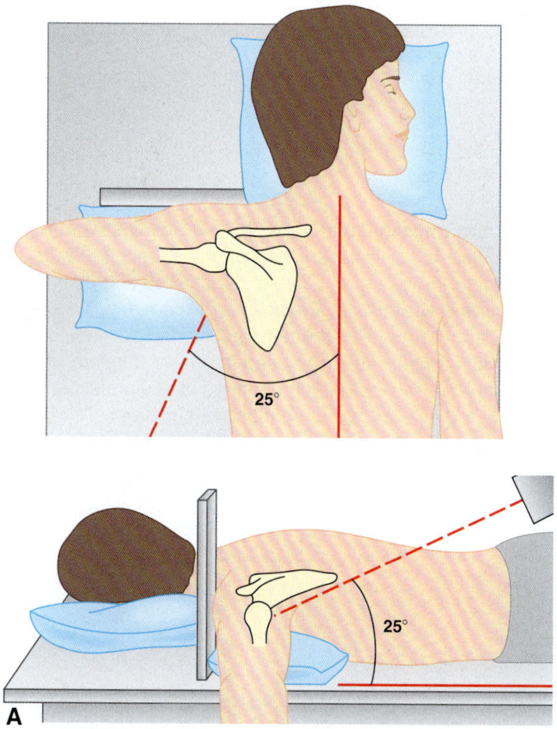

A

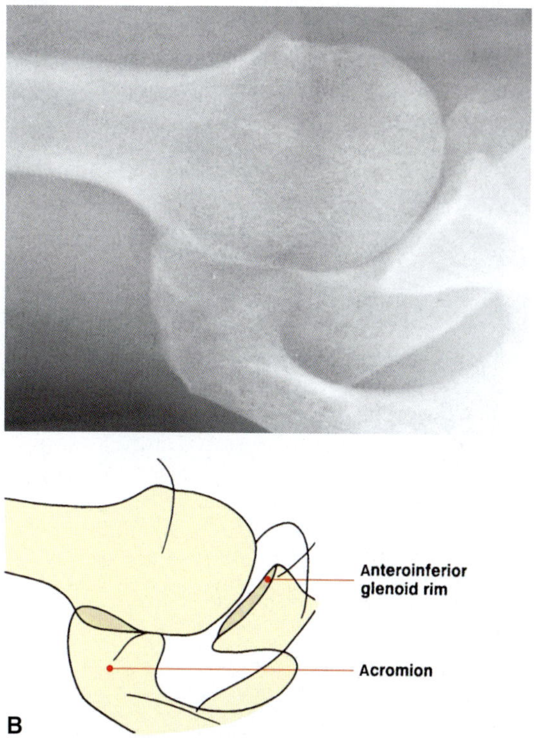

B

Figure 2.3 ■ **West Point view. A:** For the West Point view of the shoulder, the patient lies prone on the radiographic table, with a pillow placed under the examined shoulder to raise it ~ 8 cm. The film cassette is positioned against the superior aspect of the shoulder. The radiographic tube is angled toward the axilla at 25 degrees to the patient's midline and 25 degrees to the table's surface. **B:** On the radiograph in this projection, the relationship of humeral head and the glenoid can be sufficiently evaluated as on the axillary view, but the anteroinferior glenoid rim, which is seen tangentially, is better visualized.

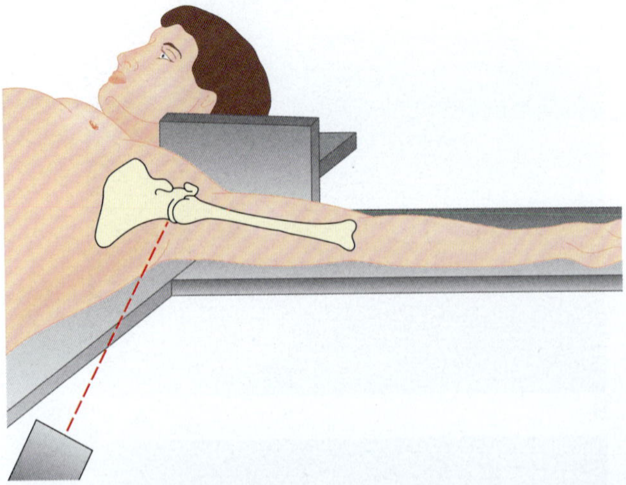

Figure 2.4 ■ Lawrence view. For the Lawrence variant of the axillary projection of the shoulder, the patient lies supine on the radiographic table with the examined arm abducted up to 90 degrees. The film cassette is positioned against the superior aspect of the shoulder with the medial end against the neck, which places the midportion of the cassette at the level of the surgical neck of the humerus. The radiographic tube is at the level of the ipsilateral hip and is angled medially toward axilla. The amount of angulation depends on the degree of abduction of the arm: less abduction requires increased medial angulation. The central beam is directed horizontally slightly superior to the midportion of the axilla. This view demonstrates the same structures as the standard axillary view.

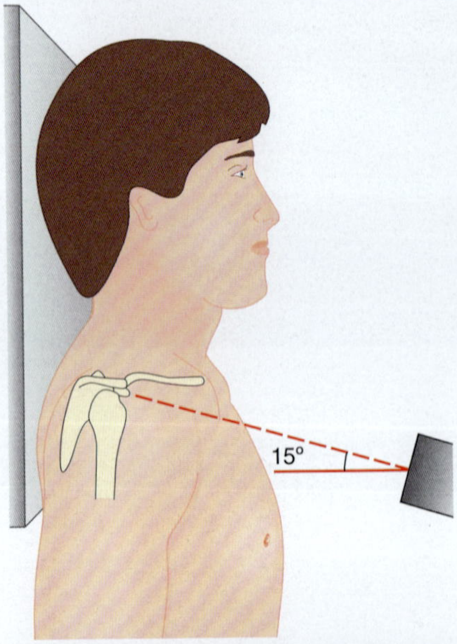

A

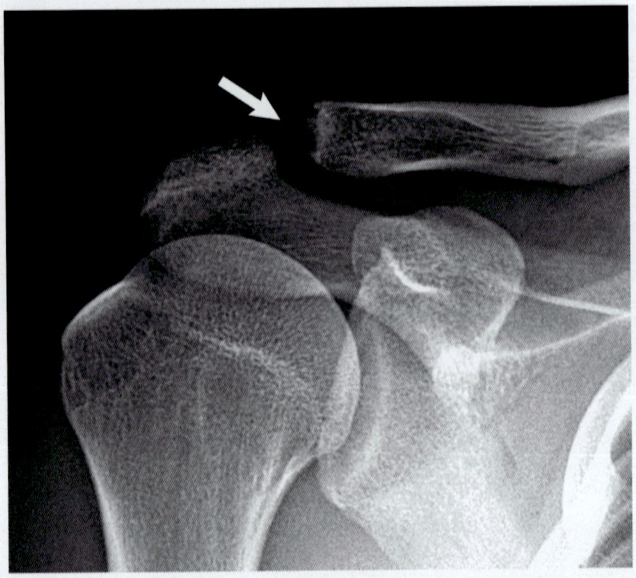

C

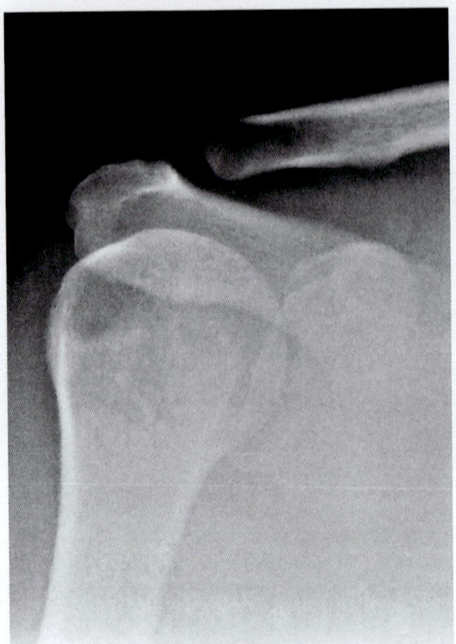

B

Figure 2.5 ■ Acromioclavicular view. A: To properly evaluate the acromioclavicular (AC) articulation, the patient is erect, with the arm in neutral position. The central beam is directed 15 degrees cephalad toward the clavicle. As overexposure of the film will make it difficult to evaluate the AC joint, the radiographic factors should be reduced to ~ 33% to 50% of those used to obtain standard AP view of the shoulder. **B:** The radiograph obtained in this projection shows clearly the AC joint. **C:** In a patient with clinically documented rheumatoid arthritis, there is early osteolysis of the acromial end of the clavicle (*arrow*).

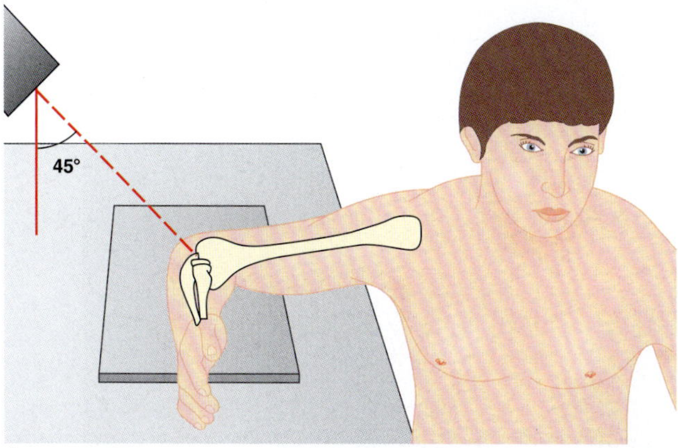

A

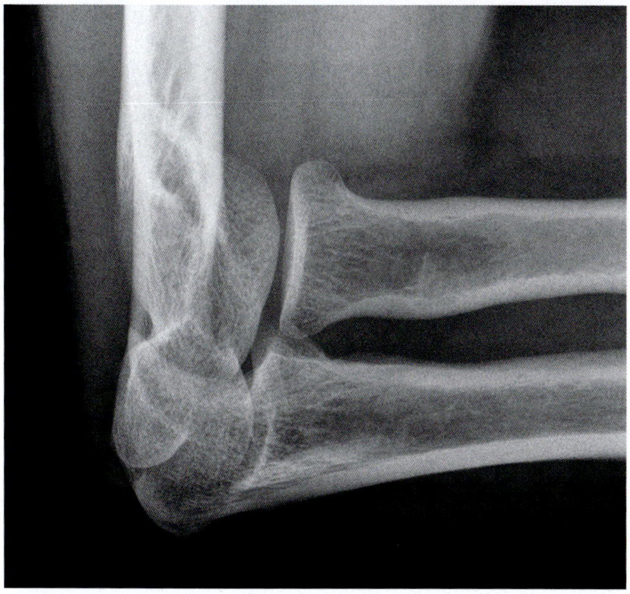

B

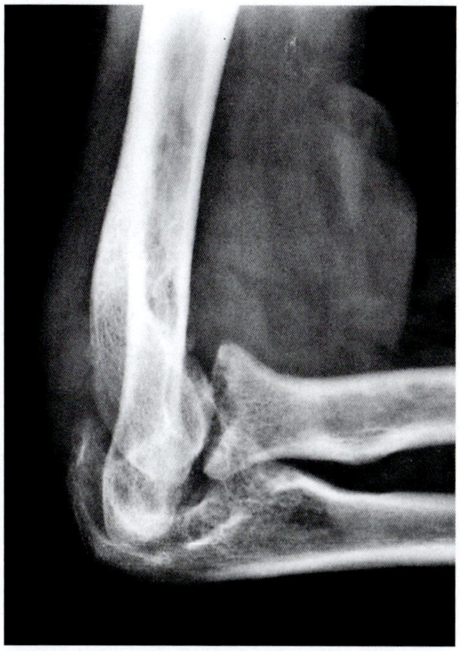

C

Figure 2.6 ■ **Radial head–capitellum view. A:** For the radial head–capitellum projection of the elbow, the patient is seated at the side of the radiographic table, with the forearm resting on its ulnar side, the elbow joint flexed 90 degrees, and the thumb pointing upward. The central beam is directed toward the radial head at a 45-degree angle to the forearm. **B:** The radiograph obtained in this projection shows the radial head projected ventrad, free of overlap by the coronoid process, which is also well demonstrated. This view is also effective in evaluating the capitellum and the humeroradial and humeroulnar articulations. **C:** In a patient with advanced rheumatoid arthritis, this projection effectively demonstrates the erosions of the humeroradial and humeroulnar joints.

metacarpal heads and of the base of the proximal phalanges in the hand and the triquetrum–pisiform joint in the wrist (Fig. 2.7). Because the earliest erosive changes of some inflammatory arthritides begin in these areas, the *Nørgaard view* may provide important information at the early stages of arthritides. It may also demonstrate subtle subluxations in metacarpophalangeal joints frequently seen in systemic lupus erythematosus (SLE). In *the hip*, demonstration of the anatomic structures of the proximal femur including the greater and lesser trochanters is facilitated by the *frog-leg lateral projection* (Fig. 2.8). Demonstration of the *sacroiliac joints* requires either a posteroanterior projection, which is obtained to greater advantage with 25 to 30 degrees caudal angulation of the radiographic tube, or an AP view with 30 to 35 degrees cephalad angulation, known as the *Ferguson view* (Fig. 2.9). In *the knee*, a weight-bearing view may be of value, particularly for a dynamic evaluation of any decrement in the joint space under the weight of the body (Fig. 2.10). On the *Merchant projection* (Fig. 2.11), the patellofemoral disorders are better evaluated than on the standard *sunrise view* (Fig. 2.12). This projection is especially effective in demonstrating the articular facets of the patella and femur and can be helpful in detecting subtle subluxations of the patella. In *the ankle*, the *Harris-Beath view* is effective in demonstrating the posterior and medial facets of the subtalar joint (Fig. 2.13), whereas *Broden's view*, in addition to clear visualization of the posterior facet of the subtalar joint, provides a good image of the sustentaculum tali, talofibular joint, and talofibular syndesmosis (Fig. 2.14). In *the cervical spine*, an *open-mouth view* provides effective visualization of the structures of the first two cervical vertebrae. The body of C2 is clearly imaged, as well as the atlantoaxial joints, the odontoid process, and the articular pillars of C1 (Fig. 2.15). If the open-mouth view is difficult to obtain, or the odontoid process is not clearly visualized, the *Fuchs*

(Continued on page 33)

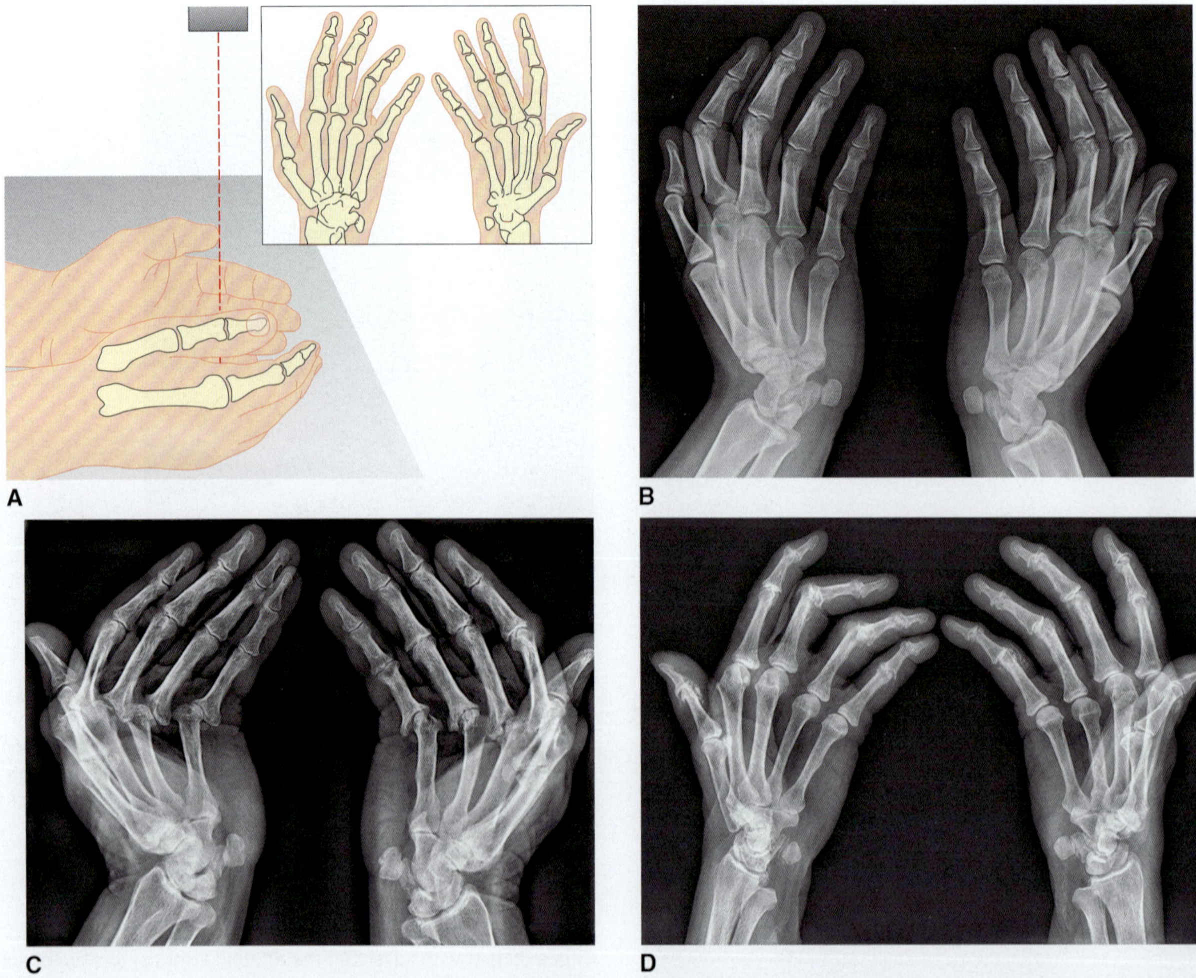

Figure 2.7 ■ **Nørgaard view. A:** For the ball-catcher view of the hands and wrists, the patient's arms are fully extended and resting on their ulnar sides, and the fingers are extended. The hands are in slight pronation, as when catching a ball. The central beam is directed toward the metacarpal heads. **B:** On the radiograph in this projection, the radial aspects of the base of the proximal phalanges, triquetrum, and pisiform bones, as well as triquetropisiform joints are well demonstrated. **C:** In a patient with rheumatoid arthritis, observe the periarticular osteoporosis, erosions of the metacarpophalangeal and proximal interphalangeal joints, and erosions of the triquetral bones. **D:** In another patient, this projection shows coexistence of gull wing–type erosive changes affecting the proximal and distal interphalangeal joints, typical for erosive osteoarthritis, with narrowing of the metacarpophalangeal joints together with chondrocalcinosis (particularly well demonstrated in the right triquetropisiform joint), characteristic for calcium pyrophosphate dihydrate (CPPD) crystal deposition disease.

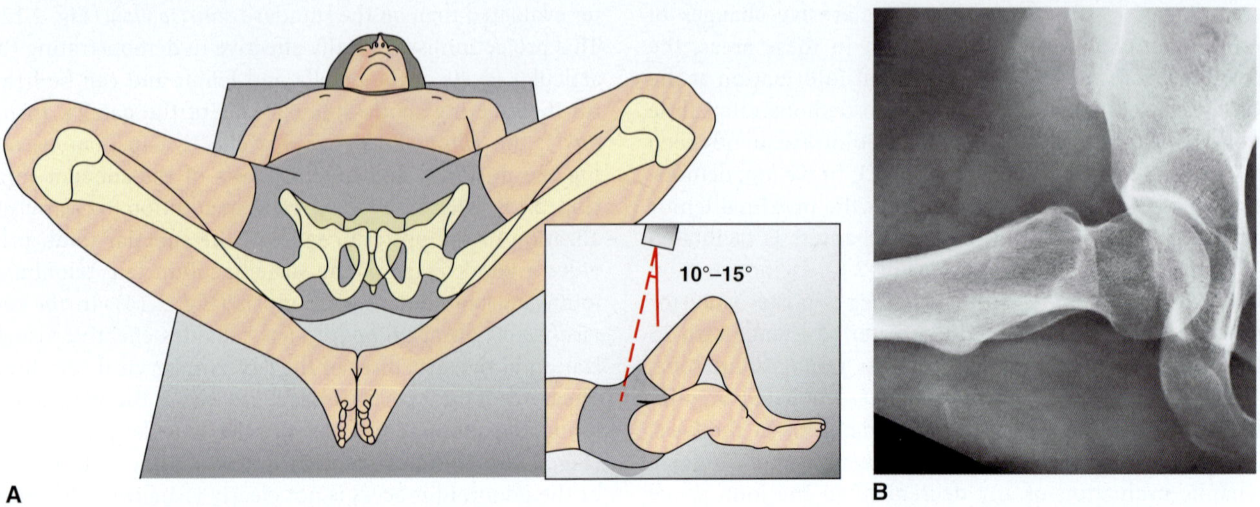

Figure 2.8 ■ **Frog-leg lateral view. A:** For the frog-leg lateral projection of the proximal femur and hip, the patient is supine with knee flexed, the soles of the feet together, and the thigh maximally abducted. For simultaneous imaging of both hips, the central beam is directed vertically or with 10 to 15 degrees cephalad angulation to a point slightly above the pubic symphysis (*inset*). For selective examination of one hip, the central beam is directed toward the affected hip joint. **B:** The radiograph obtained in this projection demonstrates the lateral aspect of the femoral head and both trochanters.

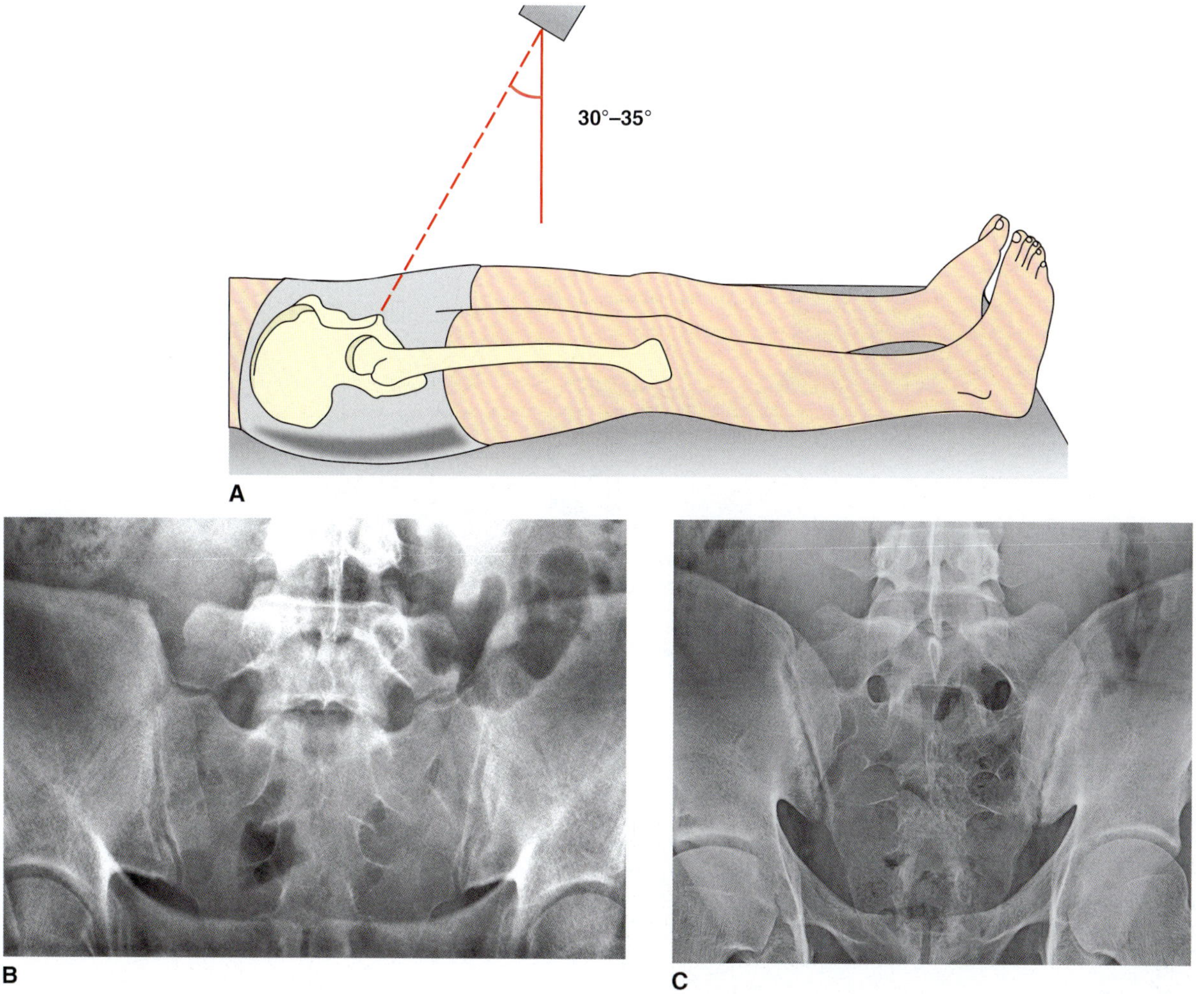

Figure 2.9 ■ **Ferguson view. A:** For the angled AP (Fergusson) view of the sacroiliac joints, the patient is in the same position as for the standard AP projection of the hips. The radiographic tube, however, is angled ~ 30 to 35 degrees cephalad and the central beam is directed toward the midportion of the pelvis. **B:** The radiograph in this projection provides a tangential view of the sacroiliac joints and the sacral bone. **C:** This view clearly shows bilateral sacroiliitis in a patient with Crohn disease.

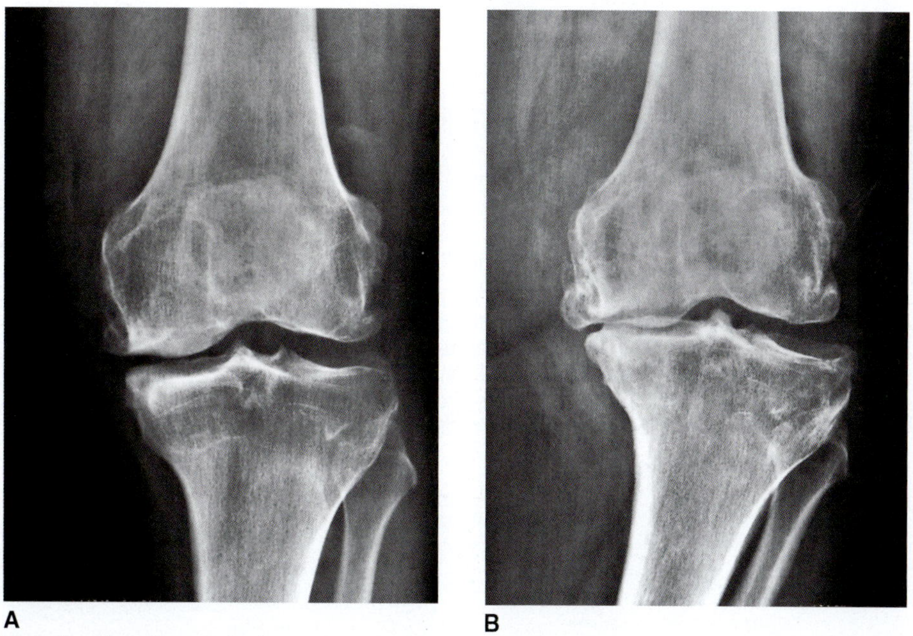

Figure 2.10 ■ **Weight-bearing view of the knee. A:** AP non–weight bearing radiograph of the left knee of the patient with osteoarthritis shows narrowing of the medial femorotibial joint compartment, subchondral sclerosis, and marginal osteophytes. **B:** With weight bearing, there is collapse of the medial compartment under the weight of the body that resulted in varus deformity of the knee.

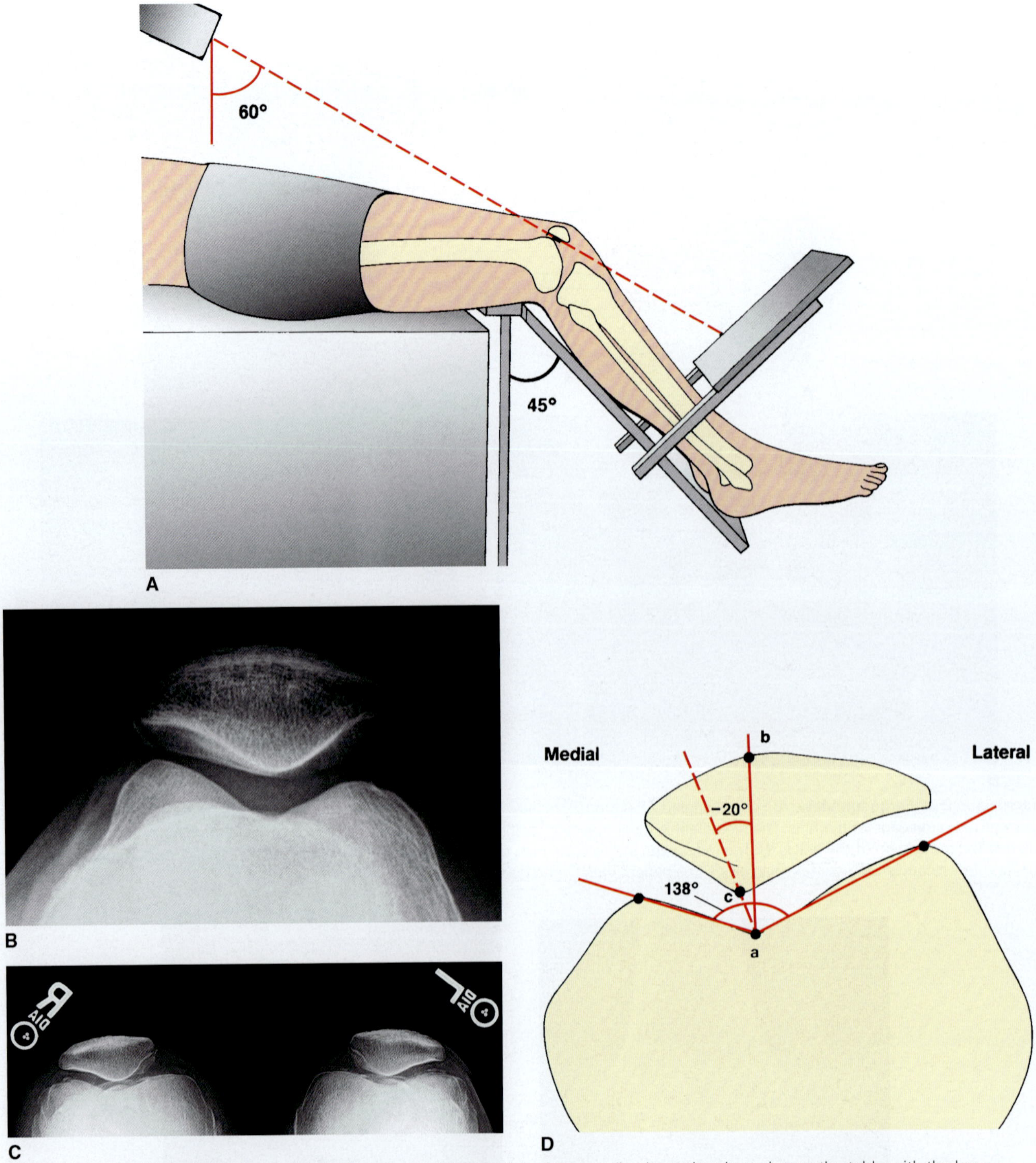

Figure 2.11 ■ **Merchant view. A:** For the Merchant axial projection of the patella, the patient is supine on the table with the knee flexed ~ 45 degrees at the table's edge. A device keeping the knee at this angle also holds the film cassette. The central beam is directed caudally through the patella at a 60-degree angle from the vertical. **B:** On the radiograph obtained in this projection, the articular facets of the patella are well demonstrated. **C:** Merchant view of both patellae shows chondrocalcinosis in a patient with CPPD crystal deposition disease. **D:** Sulcus and congruence angles can also be evaluated on this projection.

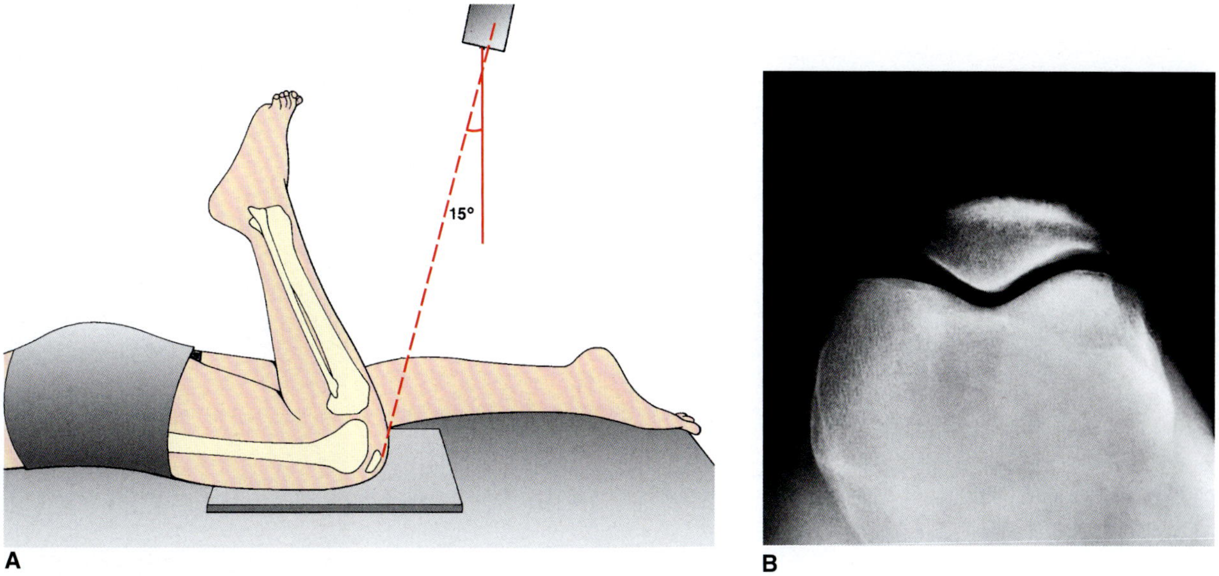

Figure 2.12 ■ **Sunrise view. A:** For an axial (sunrise, skyline) view of the patella, the patient is prone, with the knee flexed 115 degrees. The central beam is directed toward the patella with ~ 15-degree cephalad angulation. **B:** The radiograph in this projection demonstrates a tangential (axial) view of the patella. Note, however, the deep position of this structure within the intercondylar fossa, although the femoropatellar joint compartment is still well demonstrated.

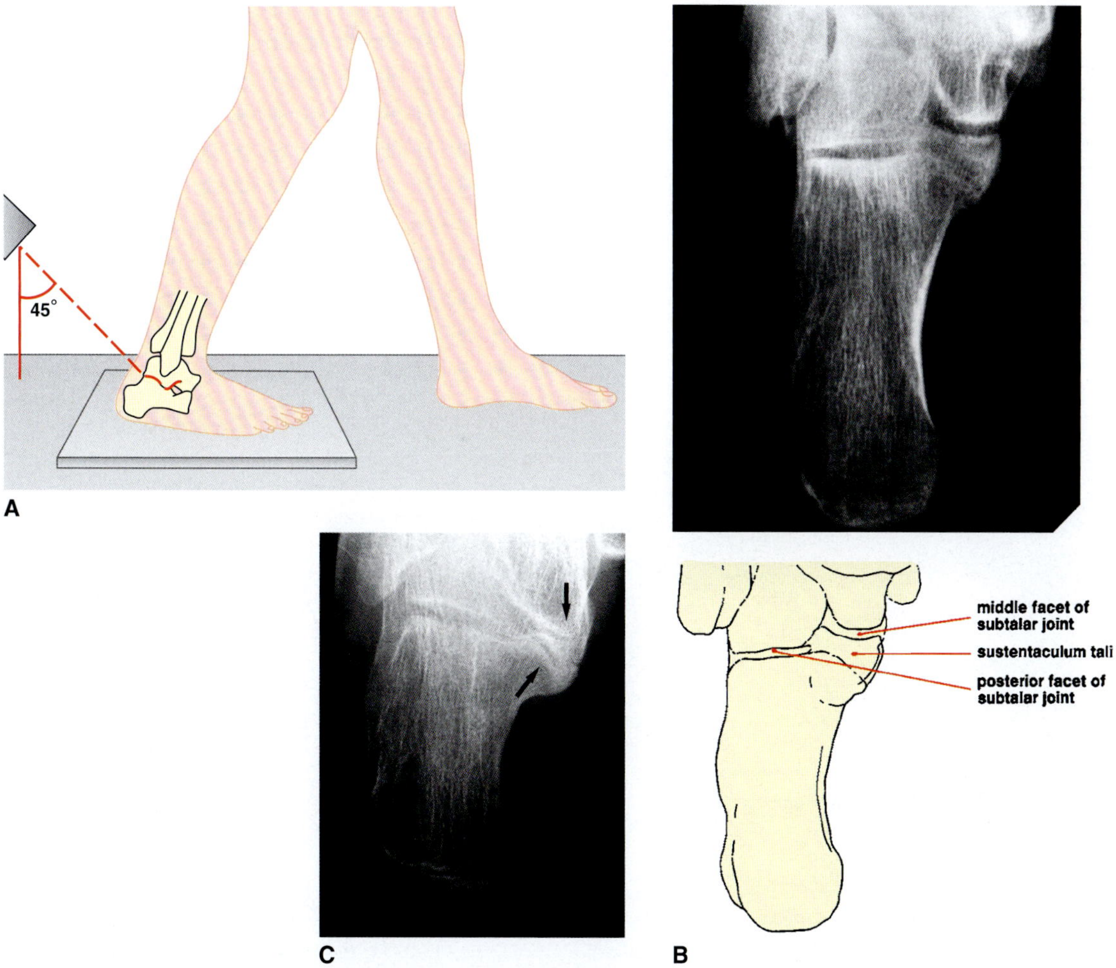

Figure 2.13 ■ **Harris-Beath view. A:** For the posterior tangential (Harris-Beath) view of the foot, the patient is erect, with sole of the foot flat on the film cassette. The central beam is usually angled 45 degrees toward the midline of the heel, but 35 or 55 degrees of angulation may also be used. **B:** On the radiograph in this projection, the middle facet of the subtalar joint is seen horizontally oriented, and the sustentaculum tali projects medially. The posterior facet projects laterally and is parallel to the middle facet. The body of the calcaneus is also well demonstrated. **C:** Tarsal (talocalcaneal) coalition at the middle facet of the subtalar joint is well demonstrated (*arrows*).

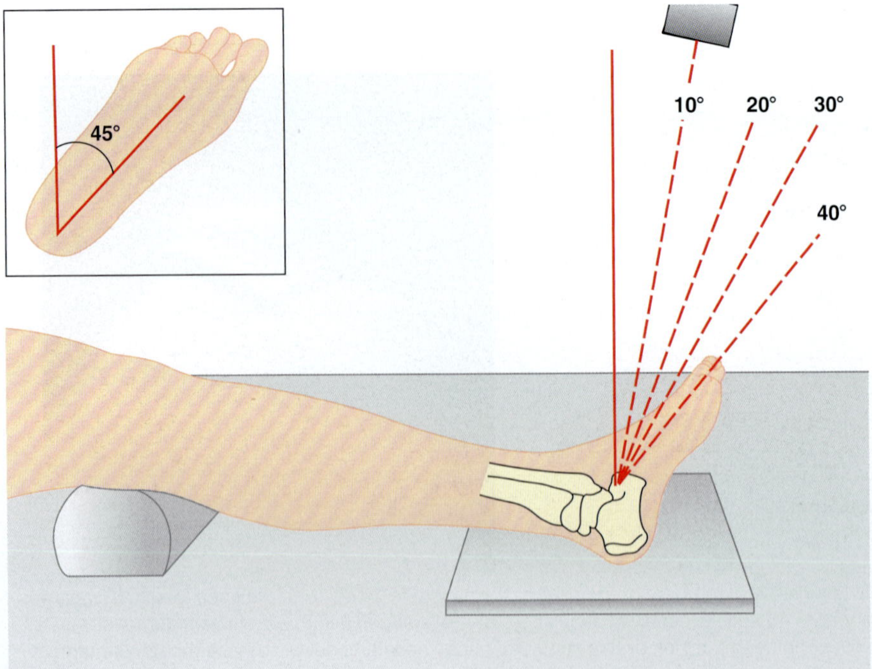

A

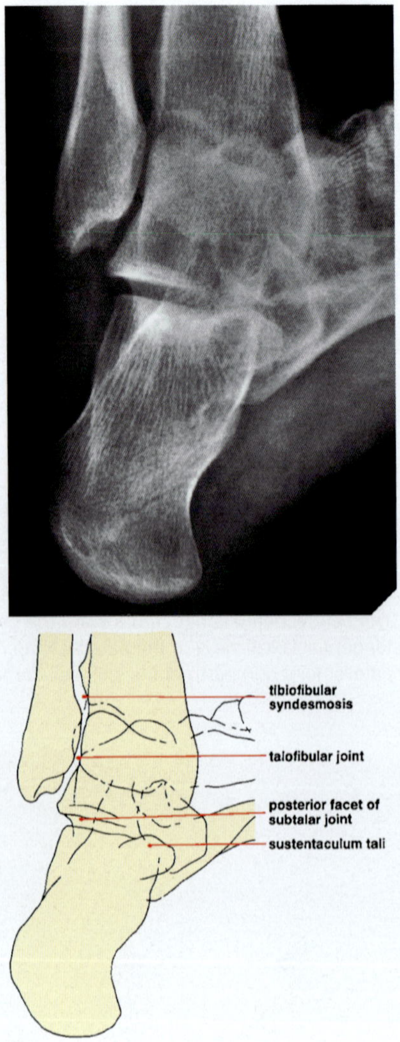

B

Figure 2.14 ■ Broden's view. A: For Broden's view of the foot, the patient is supine, with the knee slightly flexed and supported by a small sandbag. The foot rests on the film cassette, dorsiflexed to 90 degrees, and, together with the leg, is rotated medially ~ 45 degrees (*inset*). The central beam is directed toward the lateral malleolus. Radiographs may be obtained at 10, 20, 30, and 40 degrees of cephalad angulation of the tube. **B:** The radiograph obtained at 30-degree cephalad angulation demonstrates the posterior facet of the subtalar joint. Note also the good demonstration of the sustentaculum tali and the excellent visualization of the talofibular joint and the tibiofibular syndesmosis.

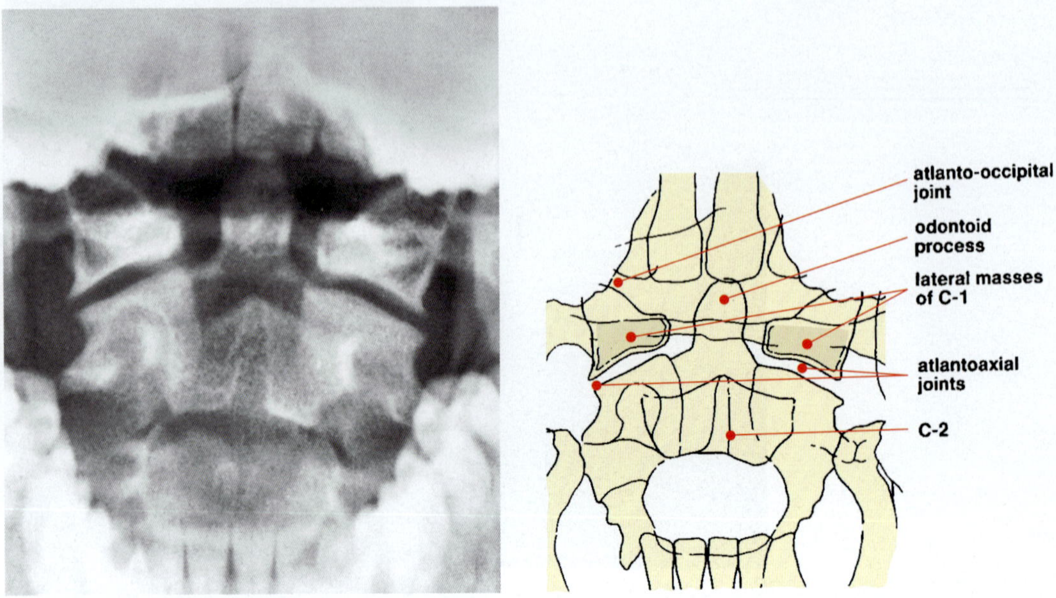

Figure 2.15 ■ Open-mouth view. For the open-mouth view, the patient is either erect or supine; the head is straight and in the neutral position. With the patient's mouth open as widely as possible, the central beam is directed perpendicular to the midpoint of the open mouth. During the exposure, the patient should softly phonate "ah" to affix the tongue to the floor of the mouth so its shadow is not projected over C1 and C2. On the radiograph obtained in this projection, the odontoid process, the body of C2, and the lateral masses of the atlas are well demonstrated; the atlantoaxial joints are seen to best advantage.

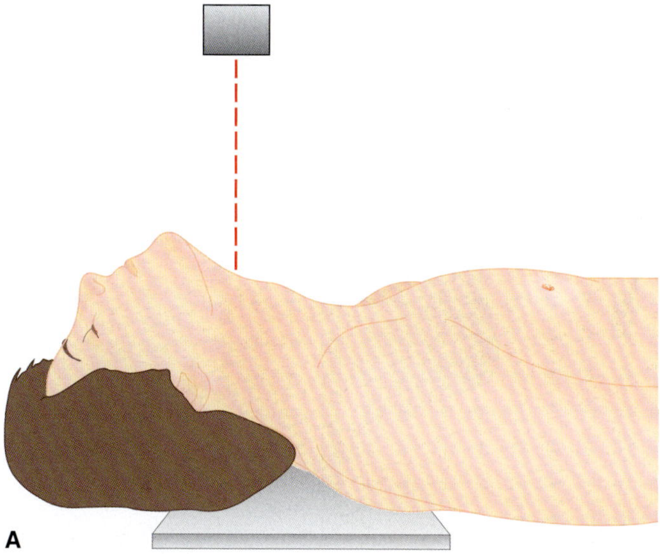

A

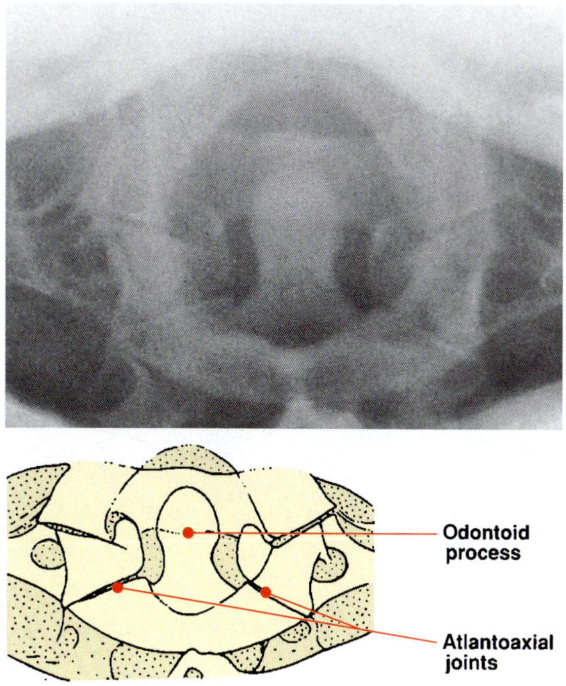

B

Figure 2.16 ■ **Fuchs view. A:** For the Fuchs view of the odontoid process, the patient is supine on the table, with the neck hyperextended. The central beam is directed vertically to the neck just below the tip of the chin. **B:** On the radiograph obtained in this projection, the odontoid, especially its upper half, is clearly visualized.

view may be helpful (Fig. 2.16). *Flexion–extension views* in the lateral projections are needed to evaluate stability of C1–C2 articulation and predental space and are particularly effective in demonstrating the abnormalities of these structures in the patients with rheumatoid arthritis affecting the cervical spine (Fig. 2.17). *Oblique view* is critical for evaluation of cervical neural foramina (Fig. 2.18). Because the visualization of C7 and T1 vertebrae is often obscured on the standard projections owing to overlap of the clavicle and soft tissues of the shoulder girdle, the swimmer's view provides the solution to this problem (Fig. 2.19). In *the thoracic spine*, to clearly demonstrate the vertebral bodies and disk spaces on the lateral projection, the special technique known as *autotomography* is used, which requires shallow breathing by the patient to blur the structures involved in respiratory motion and gives a clear view of the thoracic vertebral column (Fig. 2.20).

Digital (computed) radiography (DR or CR) is the name given to the process of digital image acquisition using an x-ray detector comprising a photostimulable phosphor imaging plate and image reader–writer that processes the latent image information for subsequent brightness scaling

(Continued on page 35)

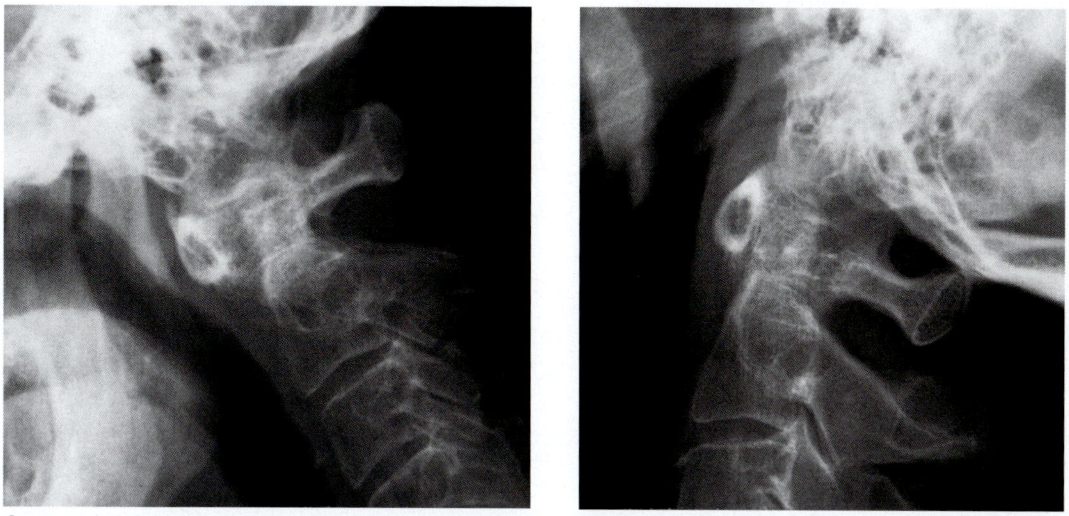

A B

Figure 2.17 ■ **Flexion–extension view of the cervical spine.** Flexion **(A)** and extension **(B)** lateral radiographs of the cervical spine demonstrate subluxation of C2 (widening of the atlanto-odontoid distance with flexion) in a 66-year-old woman with rheumatoid arthritis.

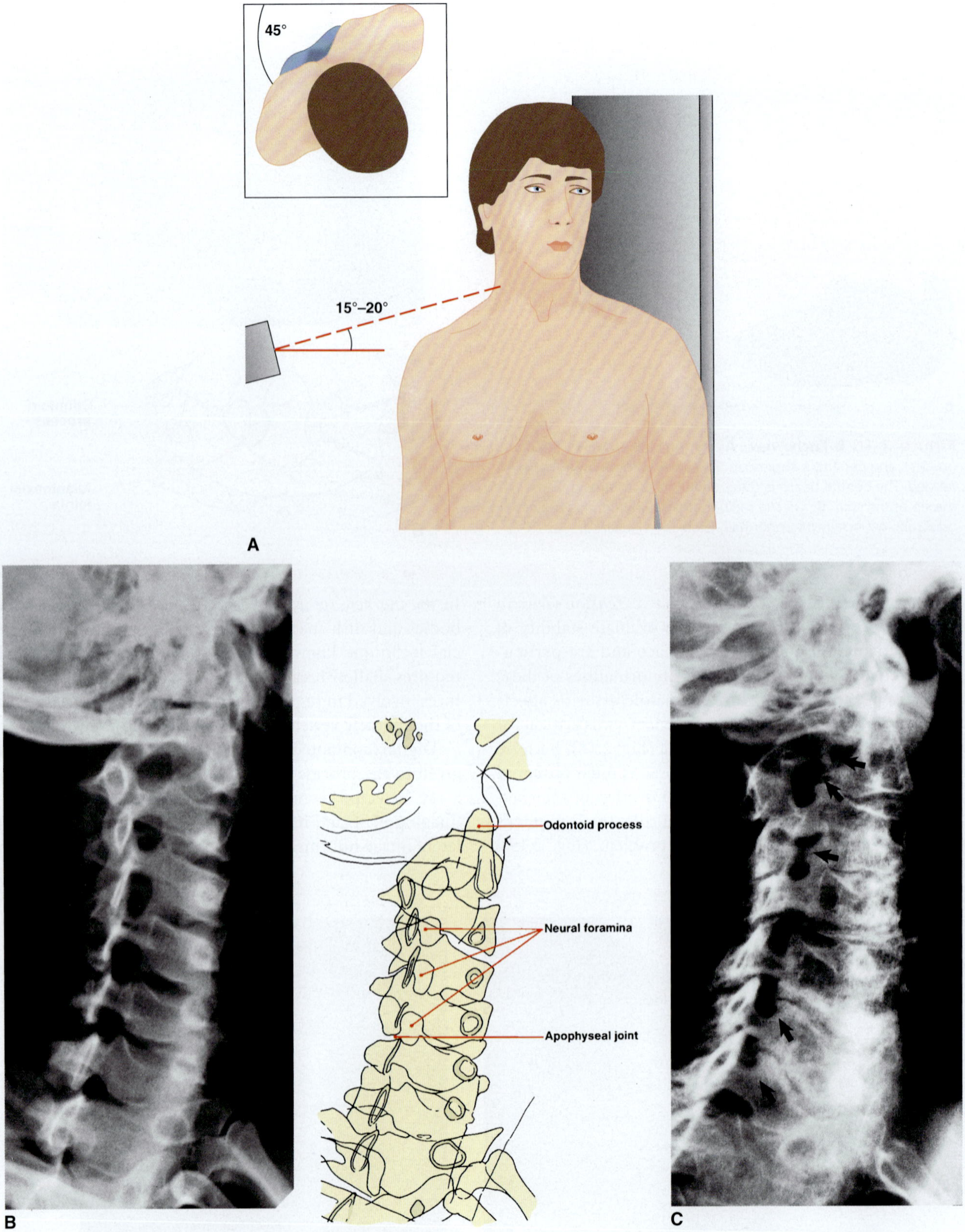

Figure 2.18 ■ **Oblique view of the cervical spine. A, B:** An oblique view of the cervical spine may be obtained in the anteroposterior (as shown here) or posteroanterior projection. The patient may be erect or recumbent, but the erect position (seated or standing) is more comfortable. The patient is rotated 45 degrees to one side—to the left, as shown here, to demonstrate the right-sided neural foramina and to the right to demonstrate the left-sided neural foramina. The central beam is directed to the C4 vertebra with 15- to 20-degree cephalad angulation. **B:** The radiograph obtained in this projection is effective primarily for demonstrating the intervertebral neural foramina. **C:** Oblique radiograph of the cervical spine in a 72-year-old woman who reported neck pain radiating to both shoulders reveals multiple posterior osteophytes encroaching on numerous neural foramina (*arrows*).

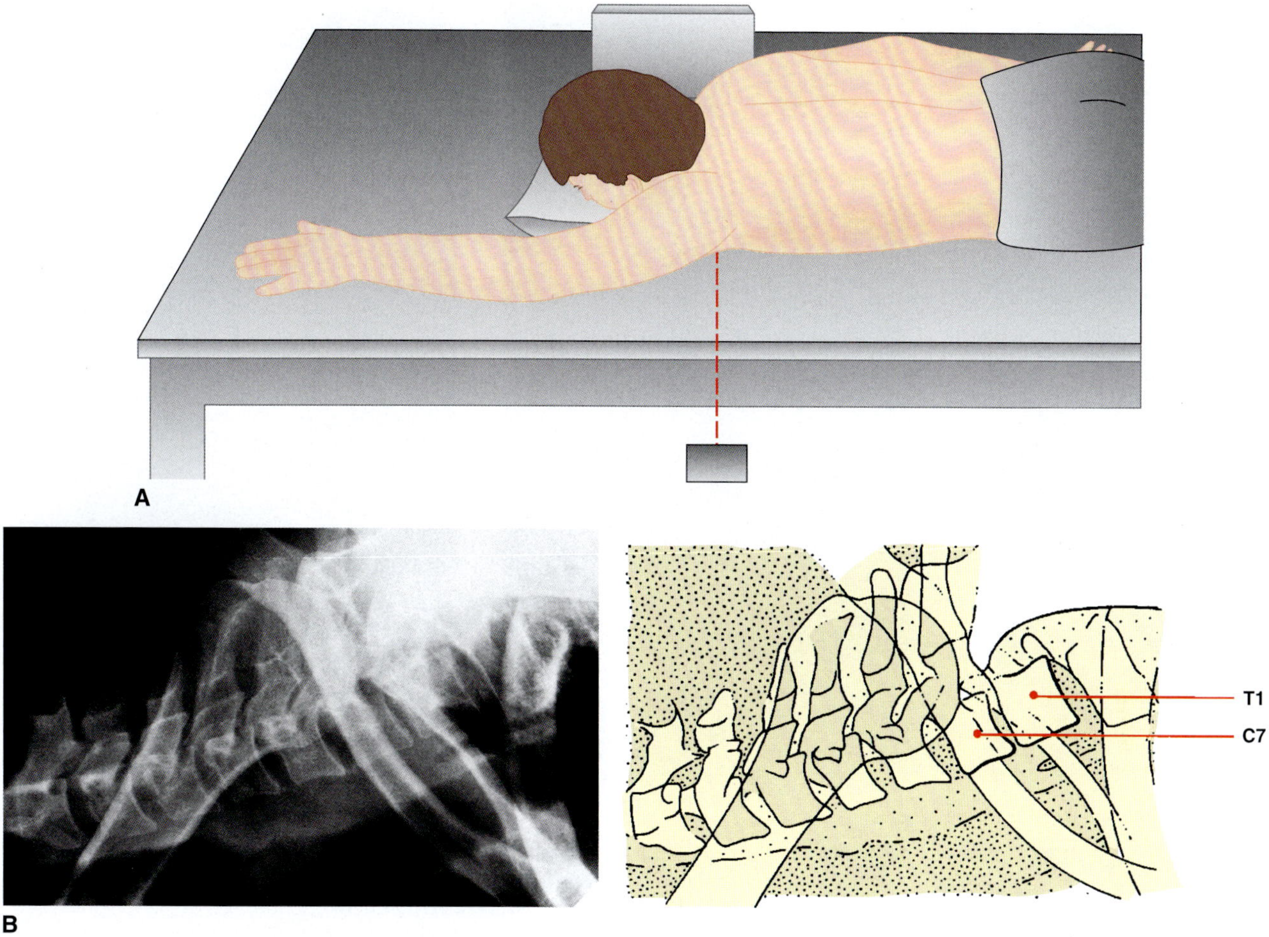

Figure 2.19 ■ **Swimmer's view. A:** For the swimmer's projection of the cervical spine, the patient is placed prone on the table with the left arm abducted 180 degrees and the right arm by the side, as if swimming the crawl. The central beam is directed horizontally toward the left axilla. The radiographic cassette is placed against the right side of the neck. **B:** The radiograph obtained in this projection provides adequate visualization of CT, T1, and occasionally T2 vertebrae, which would otherwise be obscured by the shoulders.

and laser printing on film (Fig. 2.21). The system works on the principle of photostimulated luminescence. When the screen absorbs x-rays, the x-ray energy is converted to light energy by the process of fluorescence, with the intensity of light being proportional to the energy absorbed by the phosphor. The stimulated light is used to create a digital image (a computed radiograph). A major advantage of DR/CR over conventional film-screen radiography is that once acquired, the digital image data are readily manipulated to produce alternative renderings. Moreover, advantages of digitalization include contrast and brightness optimization by the manipulation of window width and level settings as well as a variety of image processing capabilities, quantization of image information, and facilitation of examination storage and retrieval. Digital imaging has vastly replaced conventional radiography, and images are mostly viewed in a PACS (picture archive and communication system) workstation, allowing one to change contrast and orientation, choose magnification, and obtain measurements of linear distances and angles, among many other customizations.

TOMOGRAPHY AND COMPUTED TOMOGRAPHY

Among the ancillary imaging techniques, conventional tomography was used in the past, its major purpose being to demonstrate to better advantage the degree of joint destruction. Currently it has been replaced by computed tomography (CT).

CT is a radiologic modality containing an x-ray source, detectors, and a computer data processing system. The essential components of CT system include a circular scanning gantry, which houses the x-ray tube and image sensors; a table for the patient; an x-ray generator; and a computerized data processing unit. The patient lies on the table and is placed inside the gantry. The x-ray tube is rotated 360 degrees around the patient while the computer collects the data and formulates an axial image, or "slice." Each cross-sectional slice represents a thickness between 0.1 cm and 1.5 cm of body tissue. The newest CT scanners use a rotating fan of x-ray beams, a fixed ring of detectors, and predetector

(Continued on page 37)

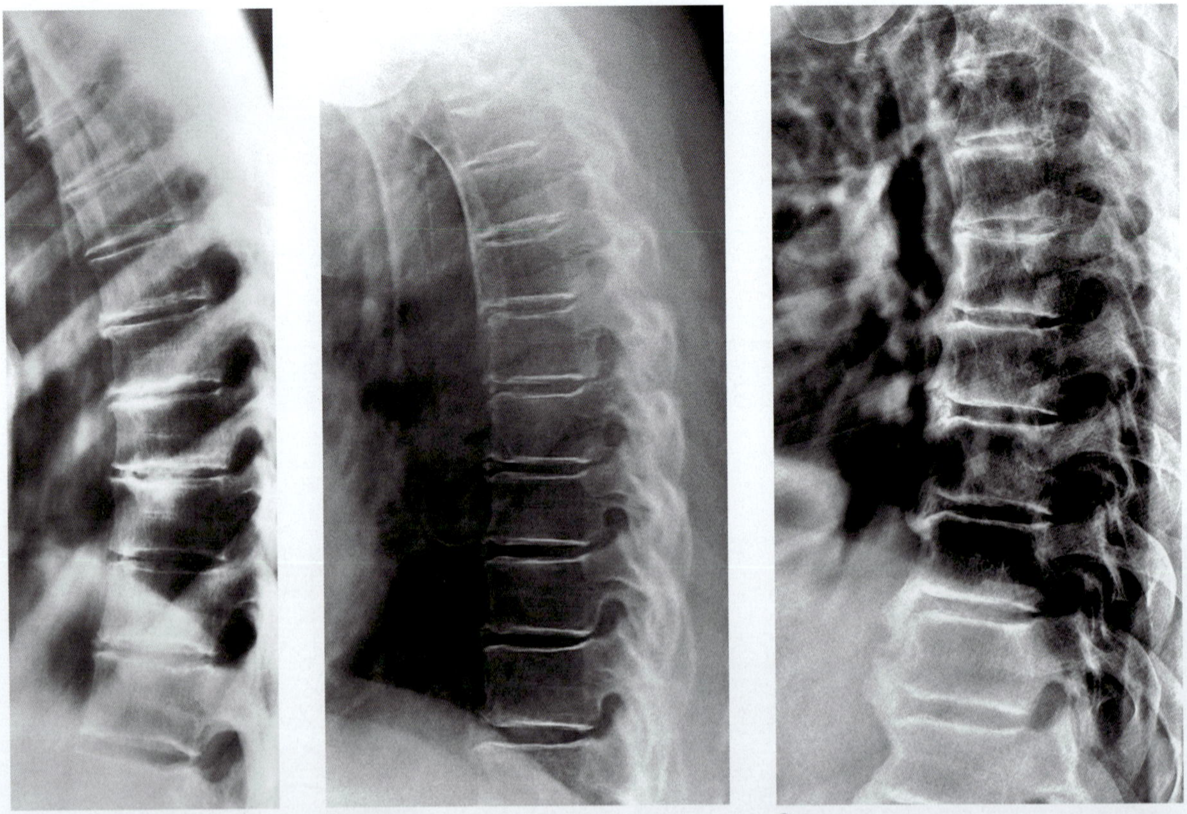

A B C

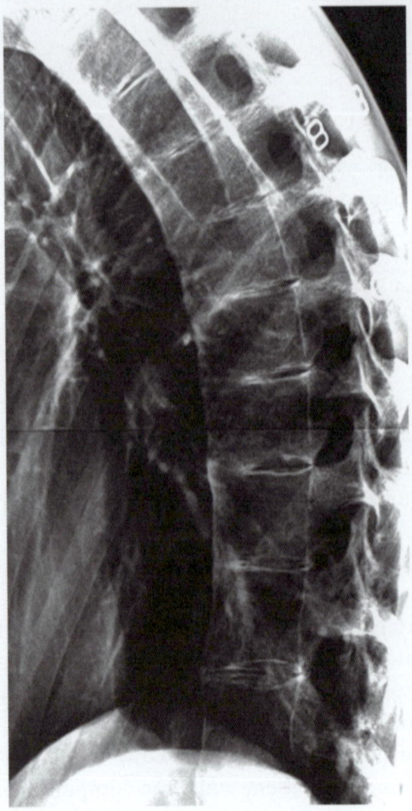

D

Figure 2.20 ■ **Lateral view of the thoracic spine, autotomography.** For the lateral view of the thoracic spine, the patient is erect with the arms elevated. The central beam is directed horizontally to the level of the T6 vertebra with about 10 degrees of cephalad angulation. To eliminate the structures that could obscure the bone elements of the thoracic spine, the patient is instructed to breathe shallowly during the exposure. **A:** The radiograph in this projection demonstrates a lateral image of the vertebral bodies and intervertebral disk spaces. **B:** In a patient with degenerative disk disease note narrowing of several intervertebral disk spaces, formation of anterior osteophytes, and focal calcifications of anterior longitudinal ligament. **C:** In a patient with diffuse idiopathic skeletal hyperostosis (DISH syndrome) observe characteristic anterior flowing hyperostosis and relative good preservation of the disk spaces. **D:** In a patient with ankylosing spondylitis, there is squaring of the vertebral bodies and formation of delicate anterior and posterior syndesmophytes, giving the appearance of "bamboo" spine.

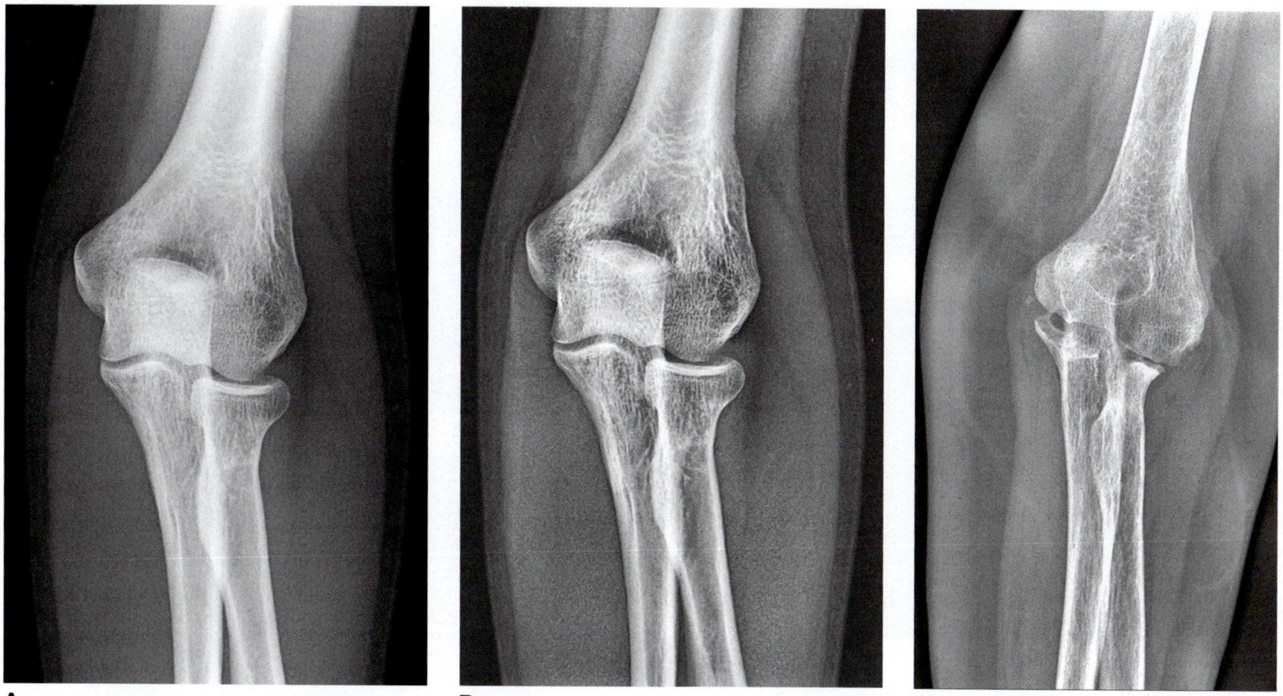

Figure 2.21 ■ **Digital radiography.** Digital radiograph of the elbow **(A)** without and **(B)** with edge enhancement. The bone and soft tissue details are better appreciated than on the standard radiographs. **C:** Digital radiograph of the elbow of a patient with advanced rheumatoid arthritis shows osteopenic bones and articular erosions.

collimator. A highly collimated x-ray beam is transmitted through the area being imaged. The tissues absorb the x-ray beam to various degrees depending on the atomic number and density of the specific tissue. The remaining, unabsorbed (unattenuated) beam passes through the tissues and is detected and processed by the computer. The CT computer software converts the x-ray beam attenuations of the tissue into a CT number (Hounsfield units) by comparing them with the attenuation of water. The attenuation of water is designed as 0 (zero) H; that of air is designated as −400 to −1,000 H, fat as −60 to −100 H, body fluid as +20 to +30 H, muscle as +40 to +80 H, trabecular bone as +100 toa300 H, and normal cortical bone as +1,000 H. Routinely, axial sections are obtained; however, computer-reformatted images taken in multiple planes or reconstructed with three-dimensional (3D) techniques may be generated if desired.

The introduction of spiral (helical) scanning was a further improvement of CT. This technique, referred to as *volume-acquisition CT*, has made possible a data-gathering system using continuous rotation of the x-ray source and the detectors. It allows the rapid acquisition of volumes of CT data and renders the ability to reformat the images at any predetermined intervals ranging from 0.5 mm to 10.0 mm. Unlike standard CT, in which up to a maximum of 12 scans could be obtained per minute, helical CT acquires all data in 24 or 32 seconds, generating up to 92 sections. This technology has markedly reduced scan times and has eliminated interscan delay and hence interscan motion. It also has decreased the motion artifacts, improved the definition of scanned structures, and markedly facilitated the ability to obtain 3D reconstructions generated from multiple overlapping transaxial images acquired in a single breath-hold. Spiral CT allows data to be acquired during the phase of maximum contrast enhancement, thus optimizing the detection of abnormality. The data volume may be viewed either as conventional transaxial images (Figs. 2.22 and 2.23) or as multiplane reformation (Fig. 2.24) and 3D reconstruction (Fig. 2.25).

Most recently, with the advent of multichannel multidetector-row CT (MDCT), images can be generated with subsecond gantry rotation times yielding high-resolution volume data sets, and at the same time minimizing the radiation dose to the patient. Even more advanced is high-resolution flat-panel volumetric CT (fpVCT), which uses digital flat-panel detectors and provides volumetric coverage as well as ultra-high spatial resolution in two-dimensional (2D) and 3D projections. Furthermore, it reduces metal and beam-hardening artifacts. In addition to the aforementioned features, fpVCT also allows dynamic imaging of time-varying processes.

Occasionally, iodinated contrast agents may be used intravenously to enhance the CT images. A contrast agent directly alters image contrast by increasing the x-ray attenuation, thus displaying increased brightness in the CT images.

CT is effective in evaluating degenerative and inflammatory changes of various joints (see Figs. 2.22B, C, 2.24, and 2.25), and in the spine to document spinal stenosis (see Fig. 2.23). In the assessment of spinal stenosis secondary to degenerative changes, CT examination may also be performed after myelography (Fig. 2.26), although myelography alone is often sufficient (see later and Fig. 2.38).

(Continued on page 41)

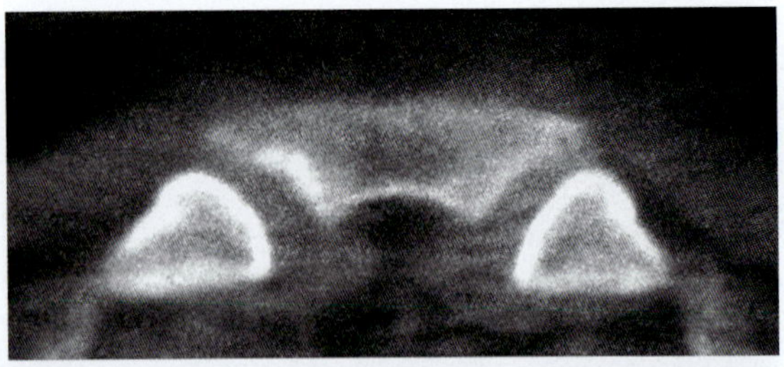

A

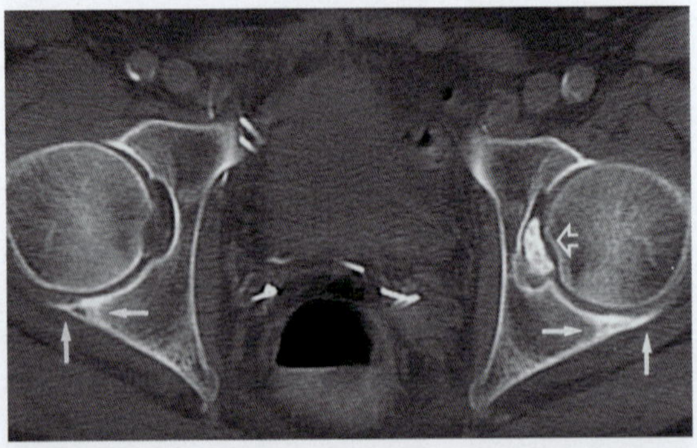

B

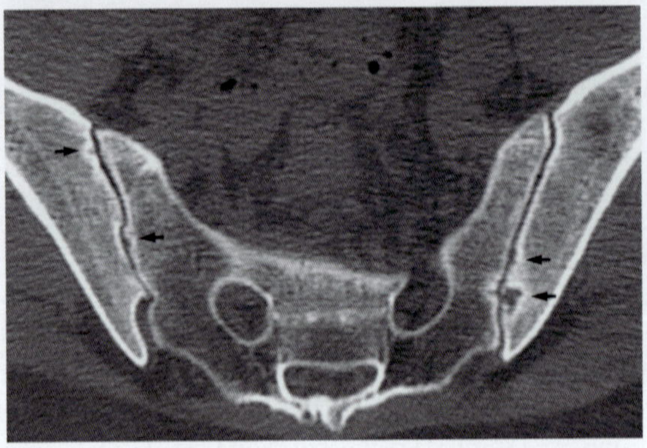

C

Figure 2.22 ■ Computed tomography, axial sections. **A:** In this direct transaxial image, the normal sternoclavicular joints are well depicted. **B:** Axial CT image of the hip joints of a 55-year-old man with osteoarthritis shows narrowing of the joint spaces, subchondral sclerosis, and osteophyte formation (*arrows*). In addition, there is an osteochondral body present within the medial joint compartment of the left hip (*open arrow*). **C:** Axial CT section through the sacroiliac joints of a 49-year-old man with psoriatic arthritis shows diffuse narrowing of the joints and articular erosions (*arrows*).

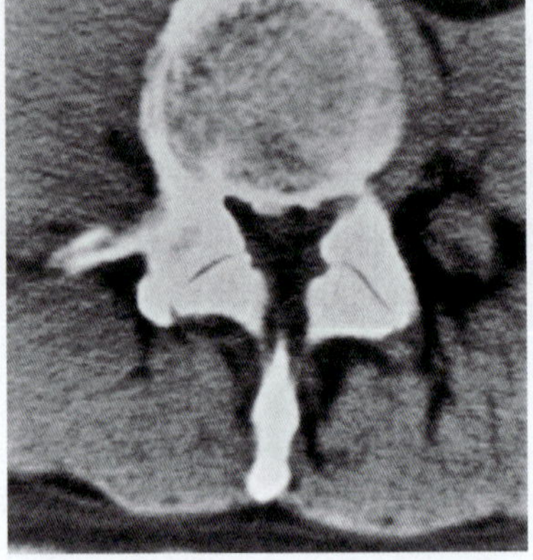

Figure 2.23 ■ Computed tomography of spinal stenosis. Axial CT section of the lumbar spine of a 66-year-old man with degenerative spine disease shows osteoarthritis of the facet joints and marked narrowing of the spinal canal.

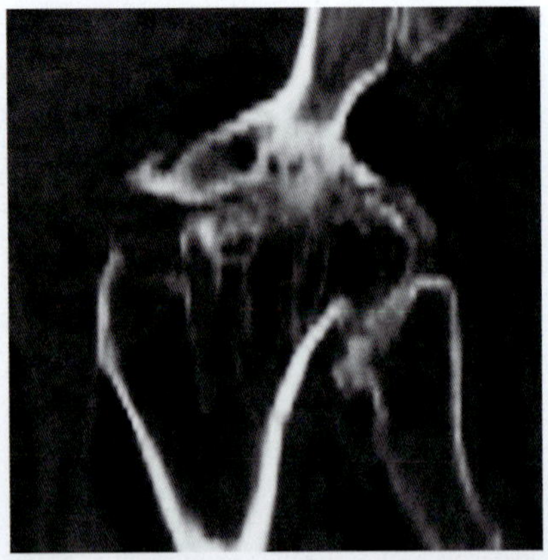

A

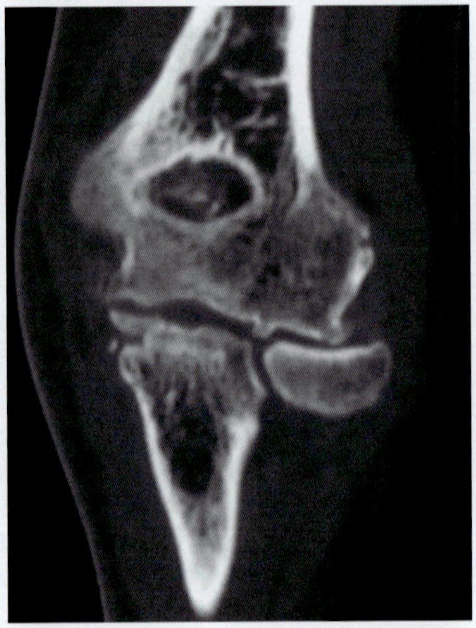

B

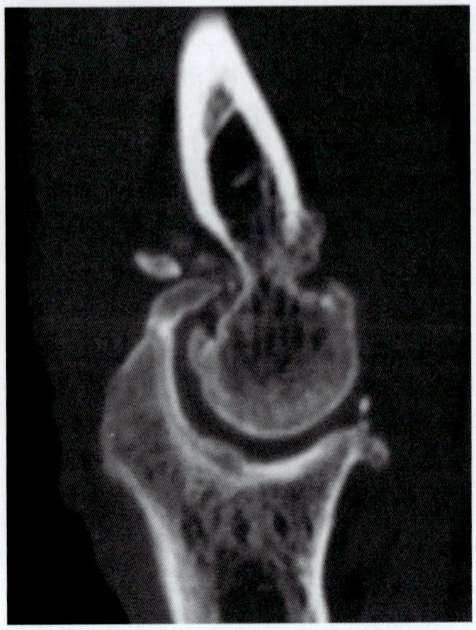

C

Figure 2.24 ■ Computed tomography, multiplane reformations. **A:** Reformatted in the coronal plane CT image of the right hip of a 64-year-old man with osteoarthritis shows narrowing of the joint space, subchondral sclerosis, and acetabular protrusio. Coronal **(B)** and sagittal reformatted **(C)** CT images of the elbow of another patient show joint space narrowing, osteophyte formation, and intra-articular osteochondral bodies typical for osteoarthritis.

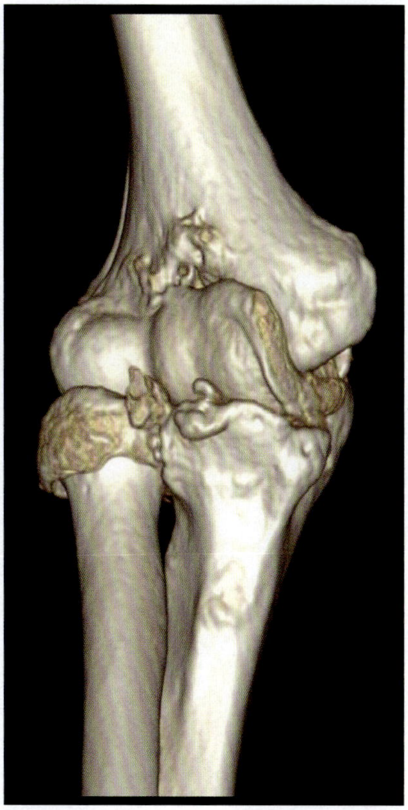

A

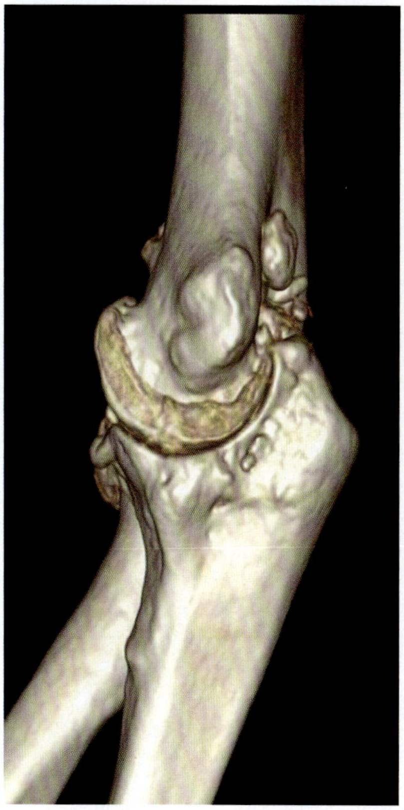

B

Figure 2.25 ■ **Computed tomography, 3D reconstruction. A, B:** 3D CT images of an elbow joint in shaded surface display demonstrate advanced osteoarthritis.

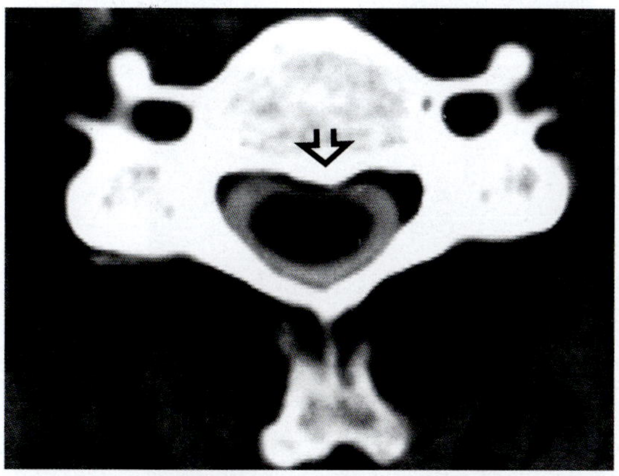

A

Figure 2.26 ■ **CT myelogram. A:** Axial CT section of the cervical spine obtained after myelography shows impingement of the posterior osteophyte on the thecal sac (*open arrow*). **B:** In another patient, sagittal reformatted CT image of the lumbar spine shows advanced degenerative disk disease at L2–L3 associated with vacuum phenomenon. Numerous osteophytes are seen arising from the vertebral bodies. Posterior osteophytes arising from the vertebral bodies L1 and L2 are impinging on the ventral aspect of the thecal sac filled with water-soluble contrast.

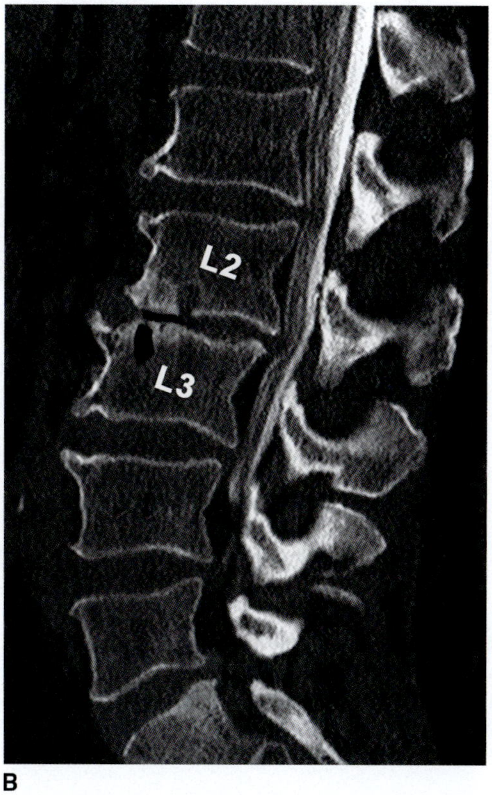

B

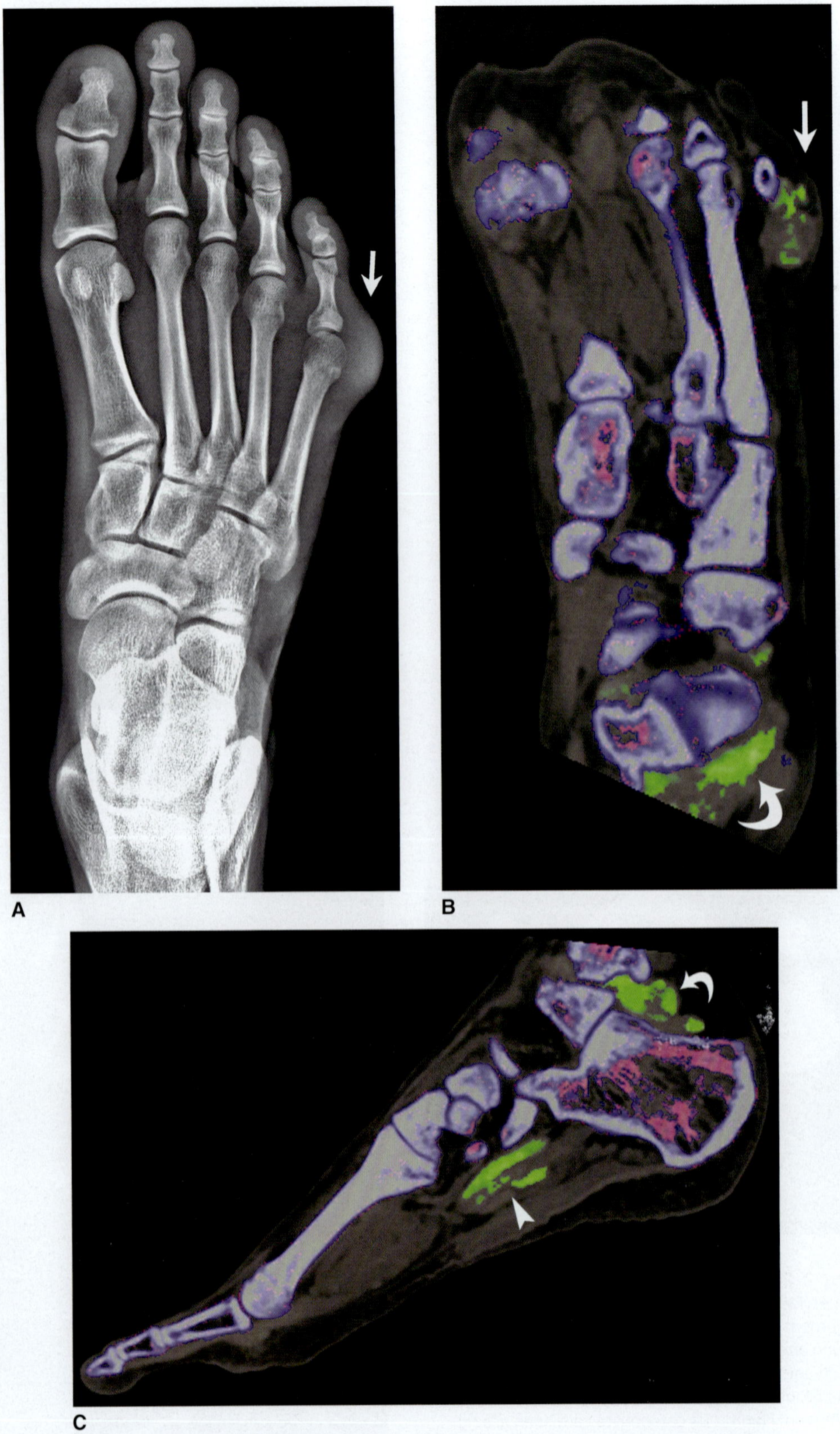

Figure 2.27 ■ **Dual-energy CT of tophaceous gout.** A 45-year-old man presented with a painful mass of the small toe of the left foot for past 4 months. **A:** AP radiograph shows a soft tissue mass at the lateral aspect of the fifth metatarsophalangeal joint (*arrow*); however, the osseous structures are intact and there is no evidence of erosions. Dual-energy coronal **(B)** and sagittal **(C)** reformatted color-coded CT images, in addition to the mass at the small toe (*arrow*), reveal unsuspected masses (*green areas*) in the plantar (*arrowhead*) and posterior aspects (*curved arrow*) of the hindfoot, consistent with uric acid crystal deposition within the gouty tophi in clinically occult sites.

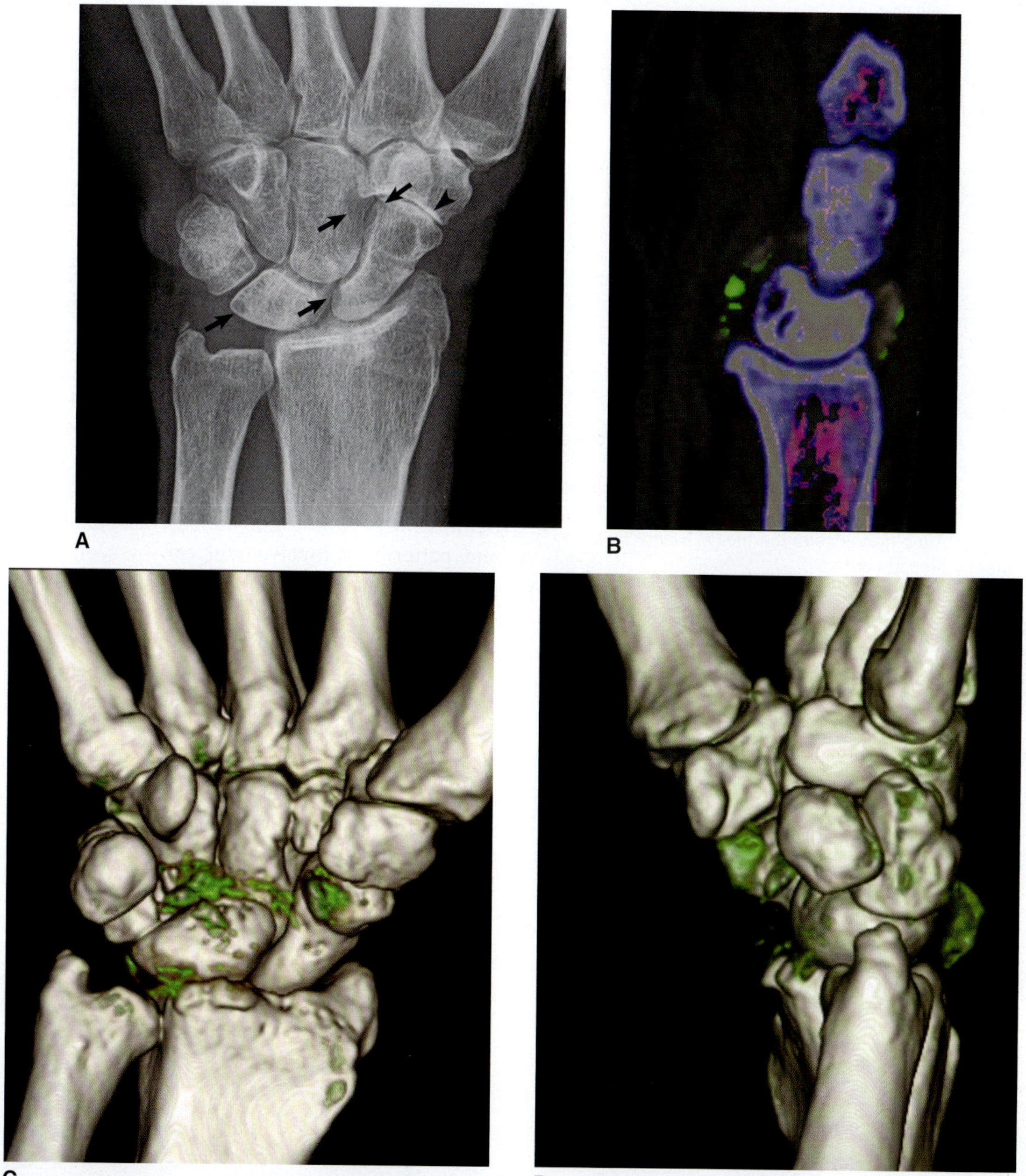

Figure 2.28 ■ **Dual-energy CT of tophaceous gout. A:** Anteroposterior radiograph of the right wrist of a 72-year-old man shows erosions of the capitate, scaphoid, and lunate (*arrows*) of unknown etiology. Osteoarthritis is noted of the scaphoid–trapezium–trapezoid joint (*arrowhead*). **B:** Sagital DECT color-coded image shows the presence of urate crystals (*green*). **C, D:** 3D reformatted CT images show the exact anatomic relationship between the monosodium urate–containing gouty tophi (*green*) and osseous structures.

Recently dual-energy CT (DECT) gained a wide acceptance as a modality used for detection or exclusion of tophaceous gout. The DECT system is equipped with two x-ray tubes with different peak kilovoltages (80 kVp and 140 kVp), thus allowing simultaneous acquisition of two sets of images of the desired anatomic region. The material-specific differences in attenuation of various elements enable classification of the chemical composition of scanned tissue, allowing accurate and specific characterization and separation of monosodium urate from calcium-containing mineralization. DECT data yield color-coded cross-sectional images, clearly depicting the foci of accumulation of urate crystals (Fig. 2.27). The 3D reconstructed images may also be generated (Fig. 2.28). In addition, in patients with known tophaceous gout, this technique may be used for serial volumetric quantification of subclinical tophus to evaluate response to treatment.

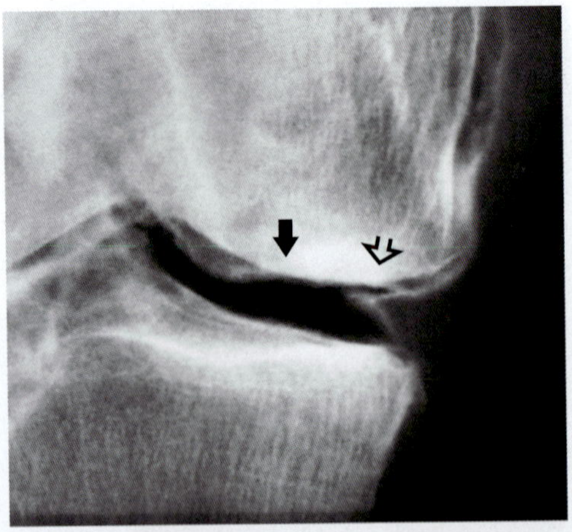

Figure 2.29 ■ Arthrography of osteoarthritis. Double-contrast arthrogram of the knee in a 62-year-old man with a history of progressive pain localized to the medial femorotibial joint compartment demonstrates destruction of the articular cartilage (*arrow*) and a degenerative tear of the free edge of the medial meniscus (*open arrow*), consistent with osteoarthritis.

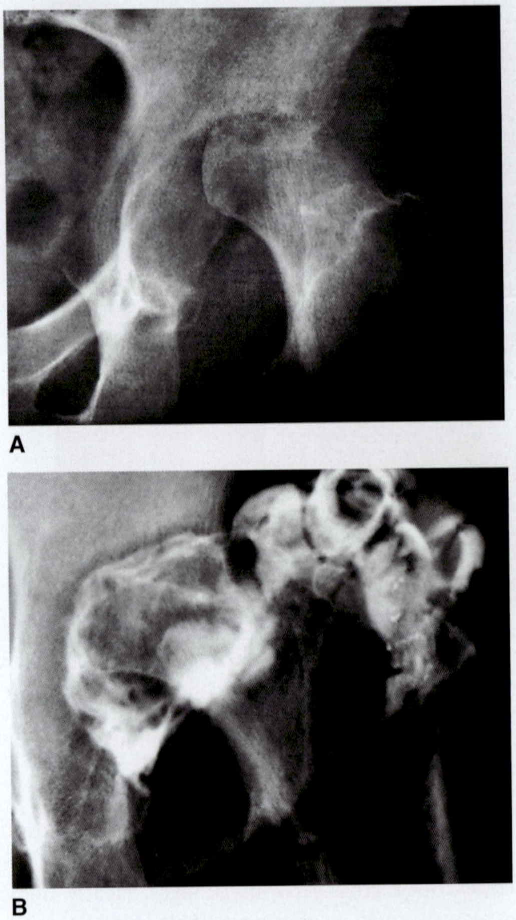

Figure 2.30 ■ Arthrography of infectious arthritis. A: Anteroposterior radiograph of the left hip of a 64-year-old woman who had had an upper respiratory infection 6 months before shows complete destruction of articular cartilage on both sides of the joint and erosion of the femoral head diagnostic of septic arthritis. **B:** Contrast arthrogram was performed primarily to obtain joint fluid for bacteriologic examination, which yielded *S. aureus*. The contras agent outlines the destroyed joint, showing a synovial irregularity consistent with chronic infectious synovitis.

ARTHROGRAPHY

Arthrography has some limited application in the evaluation of degenerative (Fig. 2.29), inflammatory, and infectious conditions of the joint (Fig. 2.30) and currently has been replaced by MR arthrography (see later).

ANGIOGRAPHY, CT ANGIOGRAPHY, AND MR ANGIOGRAPHY (MRA)

The use of contrast material injected directly into selective branches of both the arterial (arteriography) and venous (venography) circulation has aided greatly in assessing the involvement of the vascular system in systemic rheumatologic diseases and has provided a precise method for defining local pathology. Characteristic anatomic locations and patterns of involvement can be seen in such disorders as Takayasu arteritis, temporal arteritis, polyarteritis nodosa, and other forms of systemic vasculitis. Because generalized arteritis commonly involves the bowel, resulting in ischemia, necrosis, and hemorrhage, selective arteriography may be used diagnostically to differentiate diffuse from localized processes. Currently, instead of arteriography, CT angiography (Figs. 2.31, 2.32, and 2.33) and magnetic resonance arteriography (Figs. 2.34, 2.35, and 2.36) are more commonly performed. In particular, the latter imaging technique, with recent innovations in hardware and software and the advent of 3.0-Tesla magnets

(Continued on page 45)

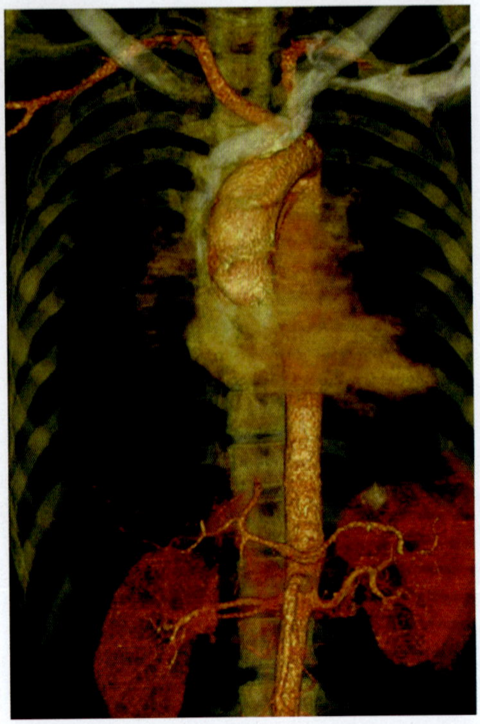

Figure 2.31 ■ CT angiography. Normal 3D CT angiogram of the chest.

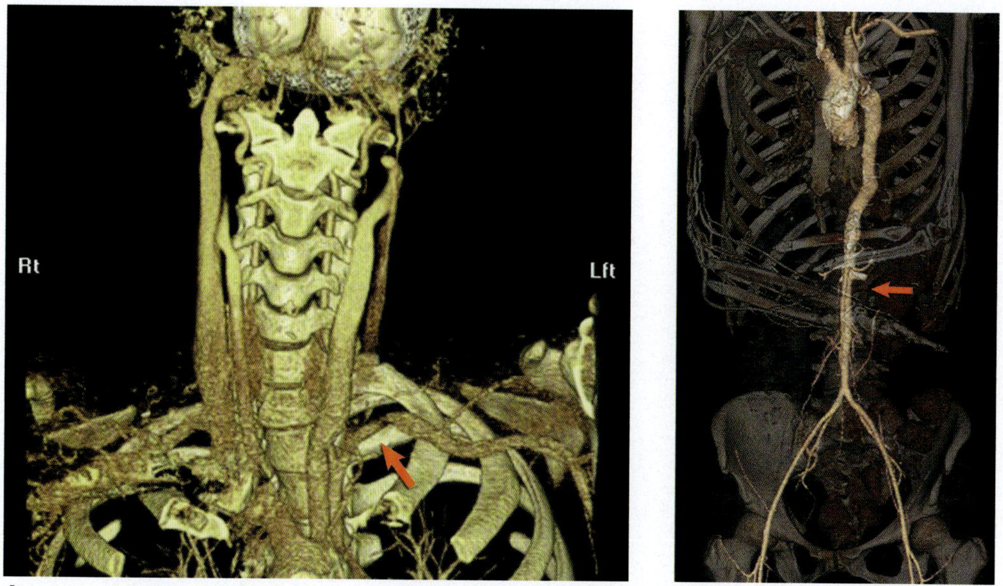

A B

Figure 2.32 ■ **CT angiography of Takayasu arteritis. A:** 3D reconstructed volume-rendering image of the neck of a 37-year-old woman obtained after intravenous administration of 125 mL of Omnipaque 350 shows narrowing of the left subclavian artery distal to the origin of the carotid artery (*arrow*). **B:** 3D CT reconstructed volume-rendering image of the thoracic and abdominal aorta shows diffuse narrowing of the abdominal aorta *(arrow),* calcified plaque at the diaphragmatic hiatus, stenosis at the origin of the celiac axis, and occlusion of the right main renal artery.

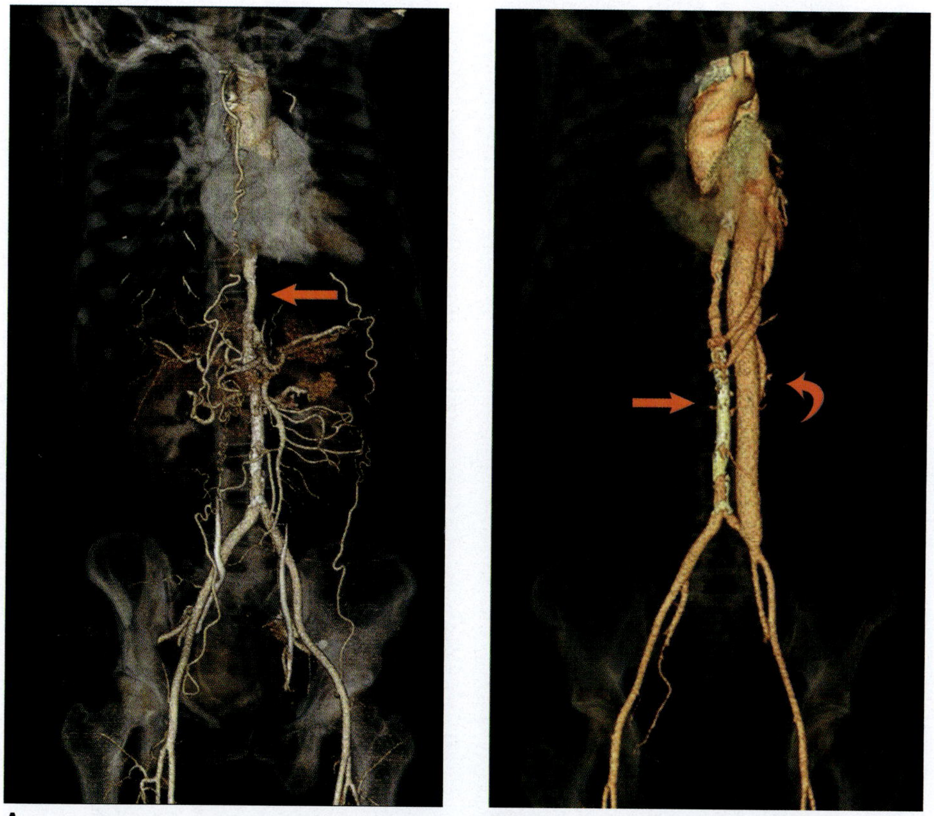

A B

Figure 2.33 ■ **CT angiography of Takayasu arteritis.** A 56-year-old woman, who was diagnosed with Takayasu arteritis three years before, presented with high blood pressure, pain in the abdomen and lower extremities, dizziness, and headache. **A:** After intravenous administration of 100 mL of Omnipaque 350, 3D CT-reconstructed volume-rendering image shows significant narrowing of the lower thoracic and abdominal aortic segments, most pronounced at the diaphragmatic hiatus (*arrow*). There is also mild dilatation of proximal renal and mesenteric arteries. **B:** After surgery, which consisted of placement of abdominal aorta graft, 3D CT reconstructed volume-rendering image obtained after intravenous administration of 125 mL of Omnipaque 350 injected at a rate of 4.0 mL/s demonstrates the abdominal aorta graft (*curved arrow*) that extends from the thoracic aorta to the bifurcation. The native abdominal aorta is diffusely narrowed (*arrow*) and shows sclerotic plaques. Visualized branches of the bypass graft include the left renal artery, celiac artery, and superior mesenteric artery, all of which are patent.

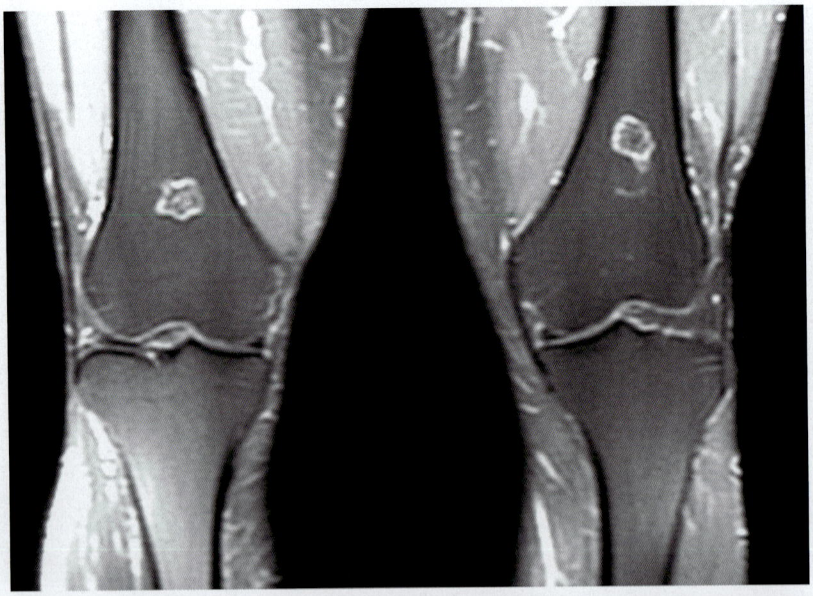

A

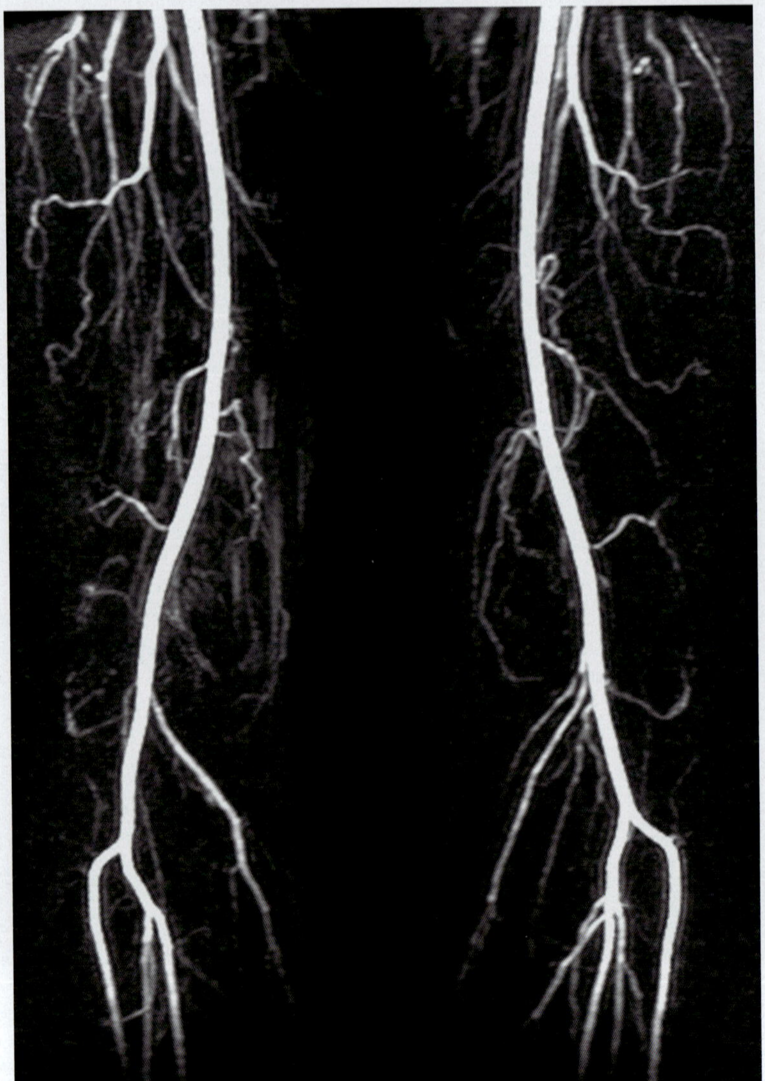

B

Figure 2.34 ■ **MR angiography, normal study.** A 27-year-old woman was diagnosed with mixed connective tissue disease. Because vasculitis and occlusion of femoral artery were also suspected, she underwent magnetic resonance arteriography. Coronal MRI of the knee **(A)** demonstrated medullary bone infarctions in the distal femora; however MRA **(B)** shows no abnormalities of the vessels.

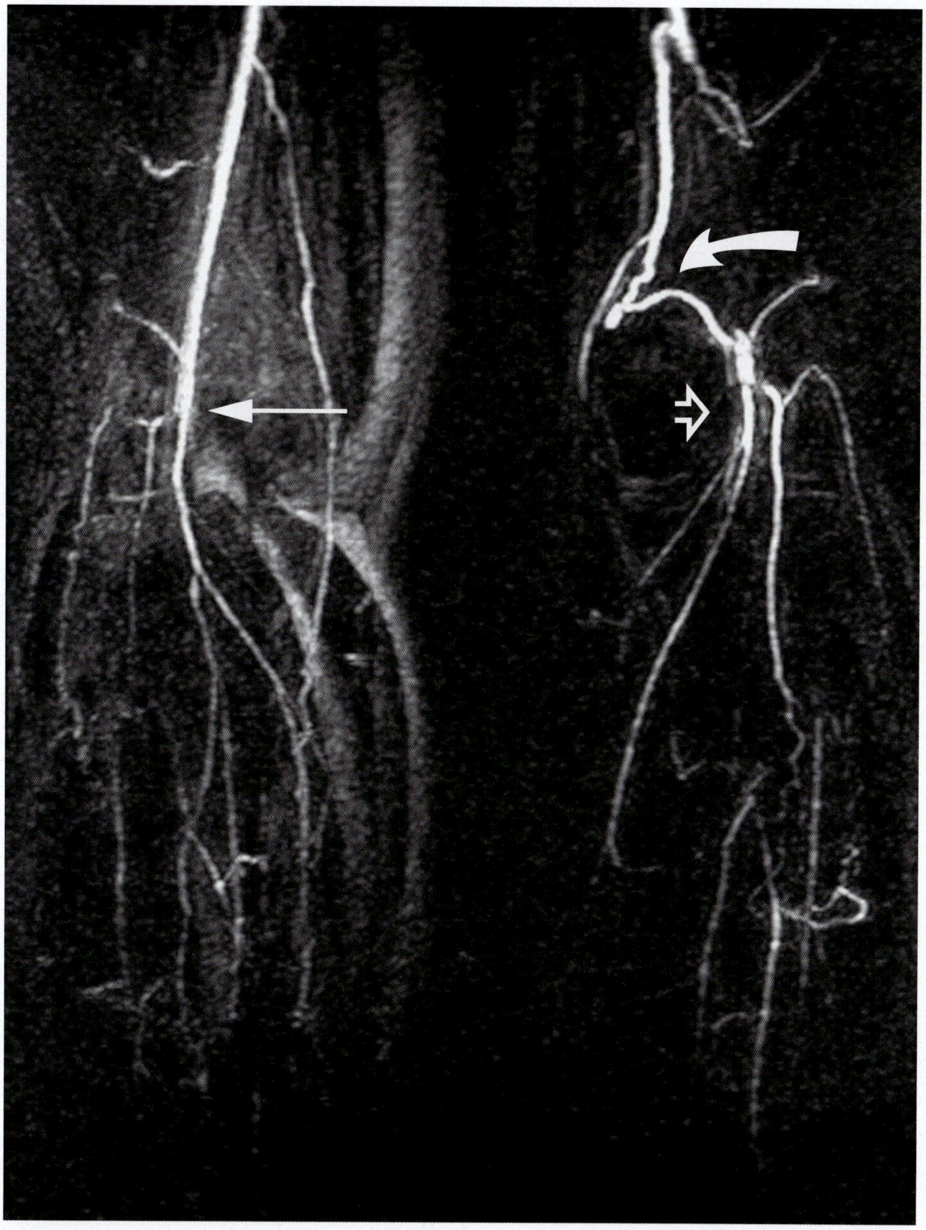

Figure 2.35 ■ **MR angiography, artery occlusion.** A 67-year-old woman with clinically documented rheumatoid arthritis presented with a history of intermittent pain in both lower extremities exaggerating by walking. MRI obtained after intravenous injection of 20 cc of Magnevist gadolinium-based contrast shows significant narrowing of the right popliteal artery (*arrow*) and a complete occlusion of the left popliteal artery (*curved arrow*) with collateral circulation and reconstitution of the short distal segment at the level of popliteal fossa (*open arrow*).

has allowed reduction in exogenous contrast dose without compromising overall image quality. It is an effective modality allowing detection of aneurysms, vessel stenosis, and obstruction; by using the double invasion recovery (DIR) "black blood" technique (by suppressing the signal from flowing blood while maintaining high signal in the surrounding stationary tissues), it can also assess the vessel wall thickness. Conventional arteriography, however, can be used therapeutically by employing embolization with specially designed coils or clot-promoting or endogenously formed clotted material to stop localized areas of hemorrhage, often preventing a major abdominal surgical procedure in an otherwise severely compromised patient. Central vessels occlusion is achieved by detachable balloons, metallic coils, or Gelfoam particles. Conversely, for peripheral and capillary vessels occlusion, Ethibloc, tissue glue and particles with an average size from 500 μm to 750 μm can be employed.

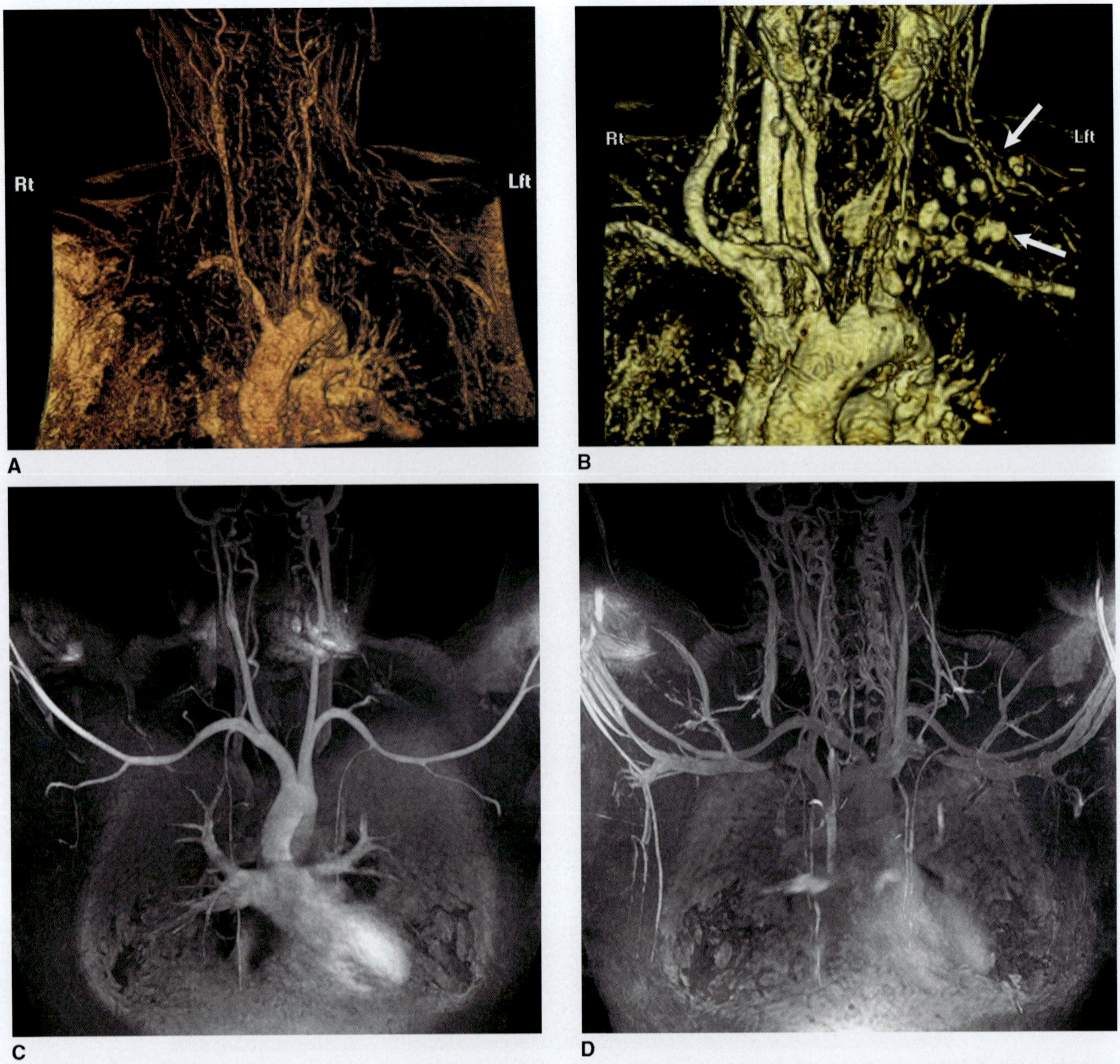

Figure 2.36 ■ **MR angiography of Takayasu arteritis.** After intravenous administration of 20 mL of gadodiamide (a gadolinium-based contrast agent), 3D MR angiography of the chest and neck was performed in a 64-year-old man diagnosed with myelodysplastic syndrome and large vessel arteritis. **A:** In the arterial phase, note the narrowing of the left subclavian and left carotid arteries. **B:** In addition, the mixed arterial and venous phase demonstrates occlusion of the left subclavian, left internal jugular, and left brachiocephalic veins. Note several enlarged neck lymph nodes (*arrows*) representing Hodgkin lymphoma. Normal chest MR angiogram in arterial **(C)** and mixed **(D)** phases is shown for comparison.

MYELOGRAPHY AND CT MYELOGRAPHY

Myelography is still occasionally being used alone (Figs. 2.37 to 2.40) or in conjunction with CT in evaluation of spinal stenosis or disk herniation (Figs. 2.41 and 2.42); however, its role has been significantly diminished with use of CT and magnetic resonance imaging (MRI).

DISKOGRAPHY

Diskography is a radiologic procedure consisting of injection of a contrast material into the nucleus pulposus under fluoroscopic guidance. Although this is a controversial procedure abandoned by many radiologists, under tightly restricted indications and immaculate technique, a diskogram can yield valuable information. Diskography is an

(Continued on page 49)

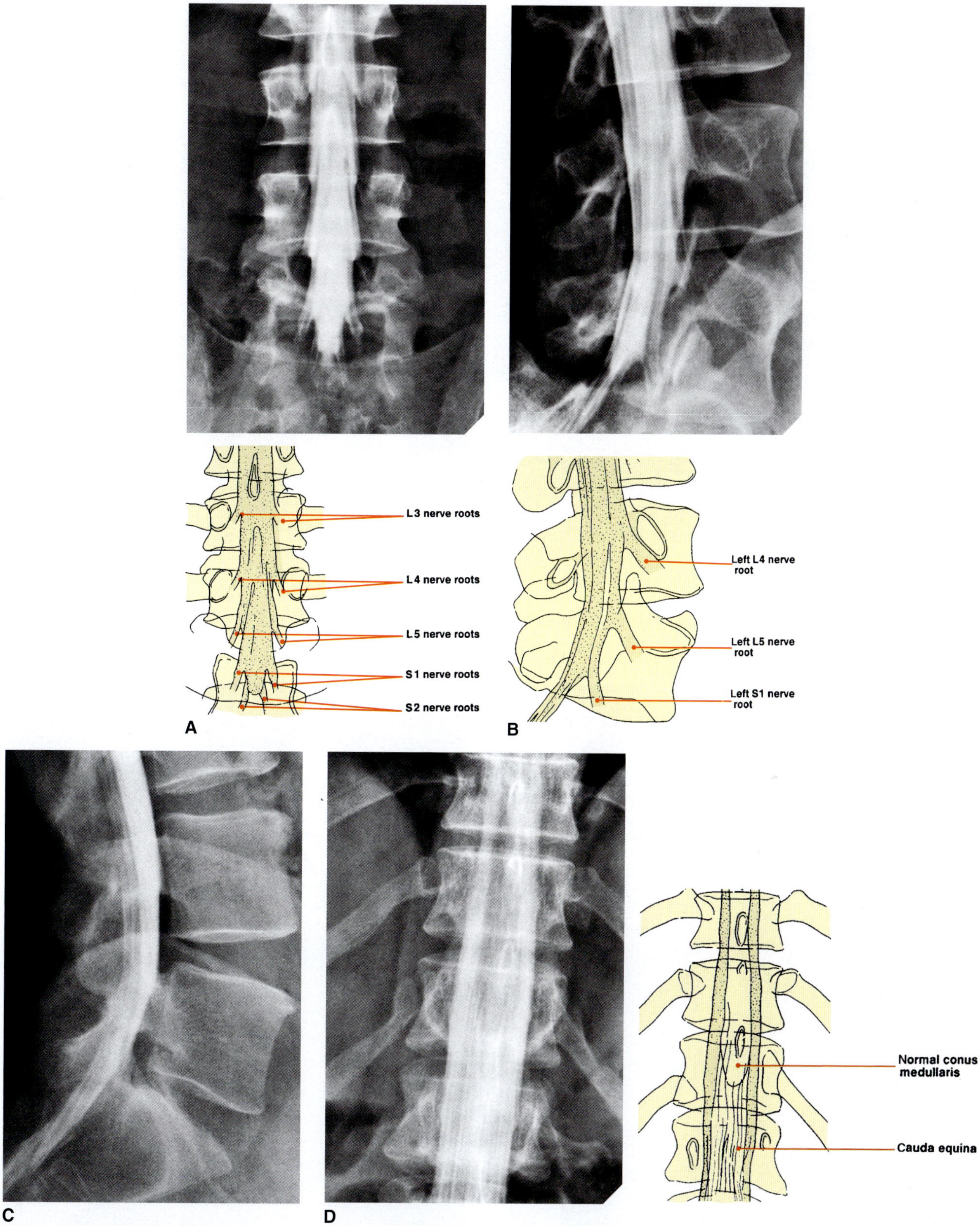

Figure 2.37 ■ Myelography. For myelographic examination of the lumbar spine, the patient is prone on the table. The puncture site, usually at the L3–L4 or L2–L3 level, is marked under fluoroscopic control. A 22-gauge needle is inserted into the subarachnoid space, and free flow of spinal fluid indicates proper placement. Iohexol or iopamidol (15 mL), in a concentration of 180 mg iodine per milliliter, is slowly injected, and films are obtained in the posteroanterior **(A)**, left and right oblique **(B)**, and cross-table lateral **(C)** projections. In these normal studies, contrast is seen outlining the subarachnoid spaces of the thecal sac as well as the cul-de-sac or most caudal part of the subarachnoid space. The nerve roots appear symmetric on both sides of the contrast column. A linear filling defect represents a nerve root in its contrast-filled sleeve. The length of the root pocket may vary from one patient to another, but in each patient, all roots are approximately equal in length. It is imperative during myelographic examination of the lumbar segment to obtain one spot film of the thoracic segment at the level T10–T12 **(D)** because tumors localized in the conus medullaris may mimic the clinical symptoms of a herniated lumbar disk.

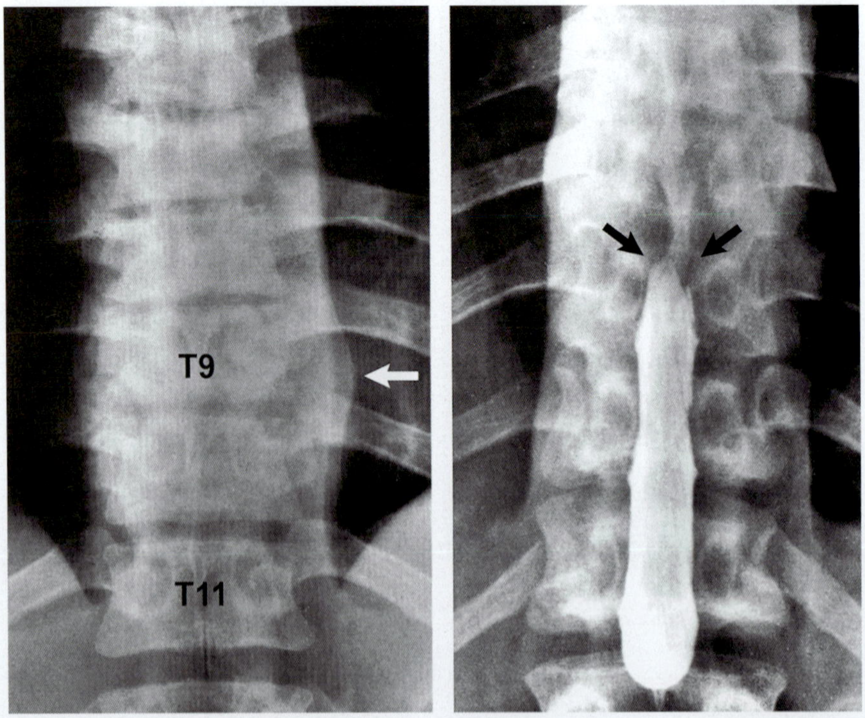

A B

Figure 2.38 ■ **Myelography of disk infection.** A 39-year-old man with a history of pulmonary tuberculosis developed acute neurologic symptoms of spinal cord compression. **A:** Anteroposterior radiograph of the lower thoracic spine shows minimal disk-space narrowing at T9–T10 and a large paraspinal mass (*arrow*). **B:** Myelogram shows complete obstruction of the flow of contrast agent in the subarachnoid space at the level of disk infection (*arrows*).

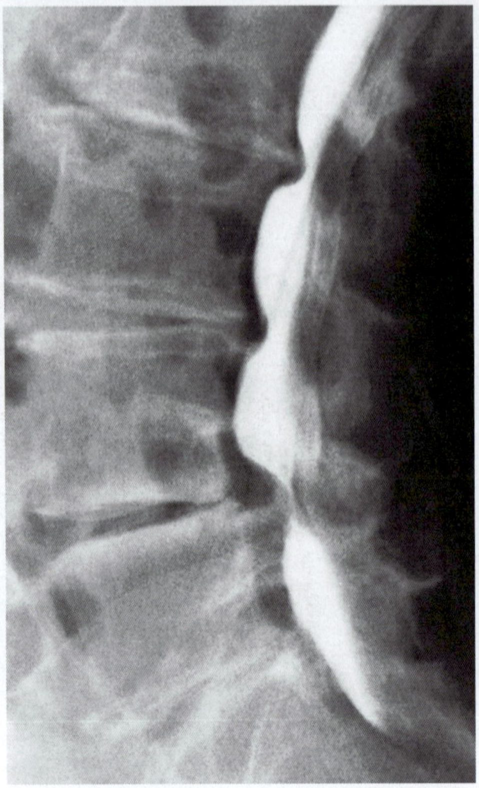

Figure 2.39 ■ **Myelography of spinal stenosis.** Lateral radiograph of the lumbosacral spine obtained after injection of metrizamide into the subarachnoid space shows an "hourglass" configuration of the contrast agent in the thecal sac, a feature characteristic of spinal stenosis. This appearance results from concominent hypertrophy of the facet joints and posterior bulging of the intervertebral disks.

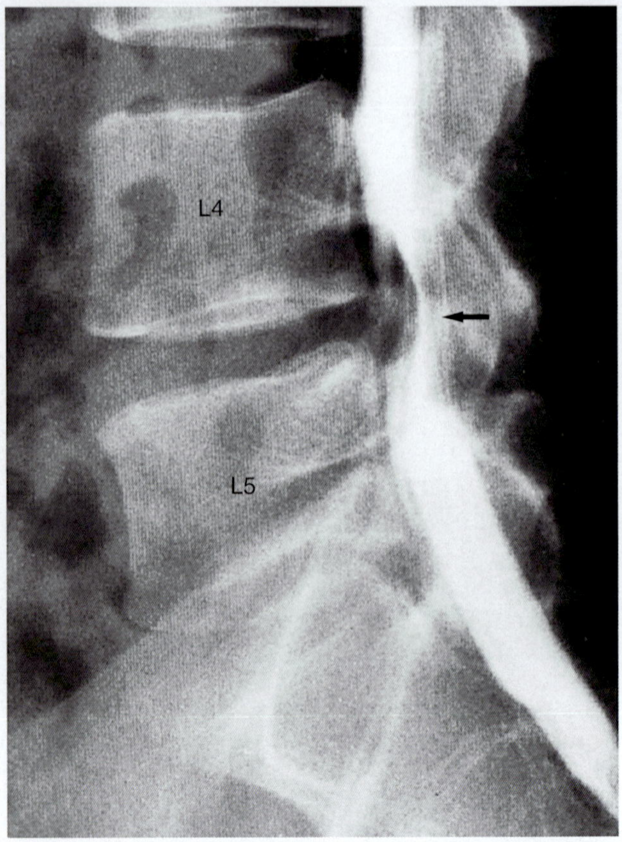

Figure 2.40 ■ **Myelography of disk herniation.** Lateral spot film obtained during myelography in a 38-year-old man demonstrates a large posterior herniation of the intervertebral disk L4–L5 (*arrow*).

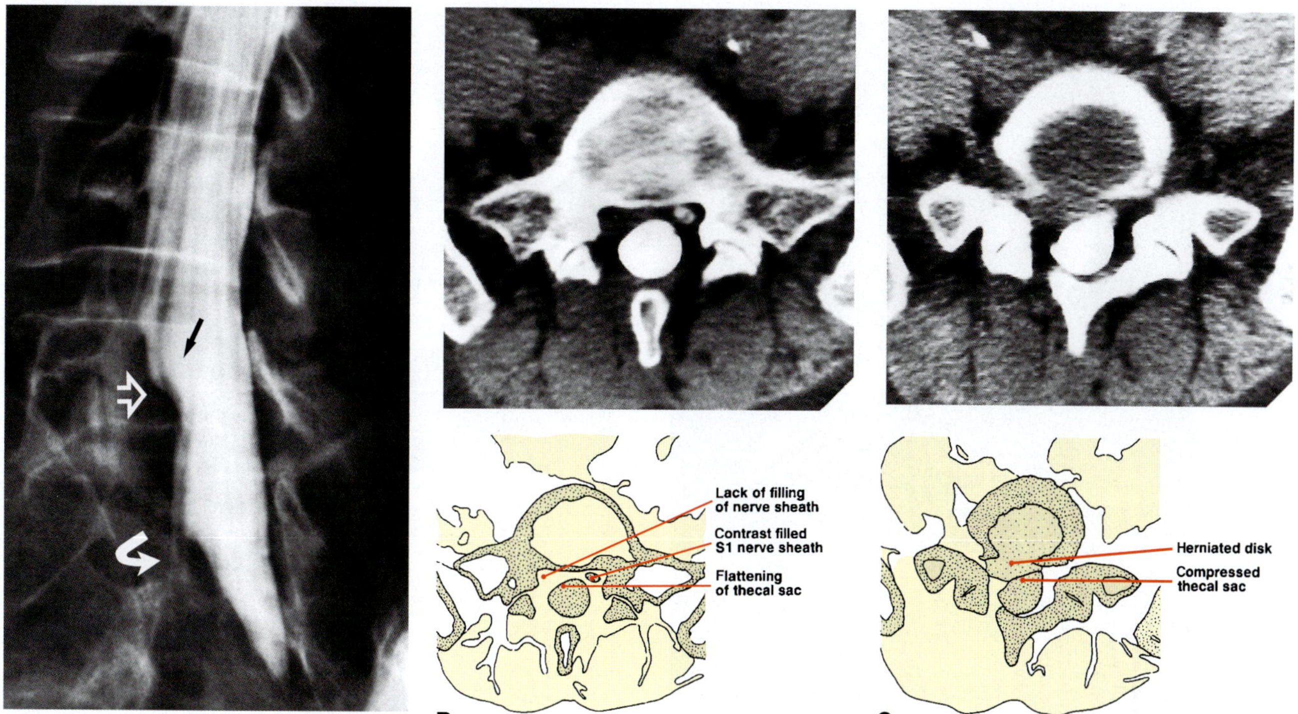

Figure 2.41 ■ **CT myelography of disk herniation.** A 47-year-old man presented with severe back pain radiating to the right buttock and leg. **A:** Spot film in the oblique projection obtained during myelography shows an extradural defect on the right side of the thecal sac at the L5–S1 disk space (*arrow*) involving the right S1 nerve root, which is cut off (*open arrow*). The S2 nerve root is normally outlined (*curved arrow*). **B, C:** CT sections also obtained during myelography demonstrate the lack of opacification of the S1 nerve root on the right side and a large herniation of the L5–S1 disk compressing the thecal sac from the right.

effective aid to determine the source of a patient's low back pain. It is not purely an imaging technique because the symptoms produced during the test (pain during the injection of contrast, known as pain provocation) are considered to have even greater diagnostic value than do the obtained radiographs. This technique should always be combined with CT examination (so-called CT diskography) (Figs. 2.43 and 2.44).

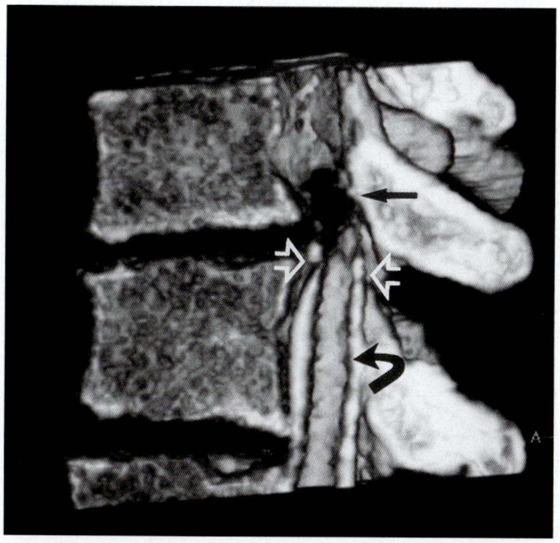

Figure 2.42 ■ **3D CT myelography of disk herniation.** A 3D CT-reconstructed image in maximum intensity projection (MIP) of the lower thoracic spine was obtained after contrast agent was injected into the thecal sac (CT myelography). There is disk herniation at the level of T7–T8 (*arrow*) associated with complete obstruction of contrast flow (*open arrows*). The *curved arrow* points to the spinal cord.

SCINTIGRAPHY (RADIONUCLIDE BONE SCAN)

Scintigraphy is a modality that detects the distribution in the body of a radioactive agent injected into the vascular system. After an intravenous administration of a radiopharmaceutical agent, the patient is placed under a scintillation camera, which detects the distribution of radioactivity in the body by measuring the interaction of gamma rays emitted from the body with sodium iodide crystals in the head of the camera. The photoscans are obtained in multiple projections and may include either the entire body or selected parts. One major advantage of skeletal scintigraphy over all other imaging techniques (excluding positron emission tomography [PET]) is its ability to image the entire skeleton at once (Fig. 2.45). As Johnson remarked, it provides a "metabolic picture," anatomically localizing a lesion by assessing its metabolic activity compared with that of adjacent normal bone. A bone scan can confirm the presence of the disease, demonstrate the distribution of the lesion,

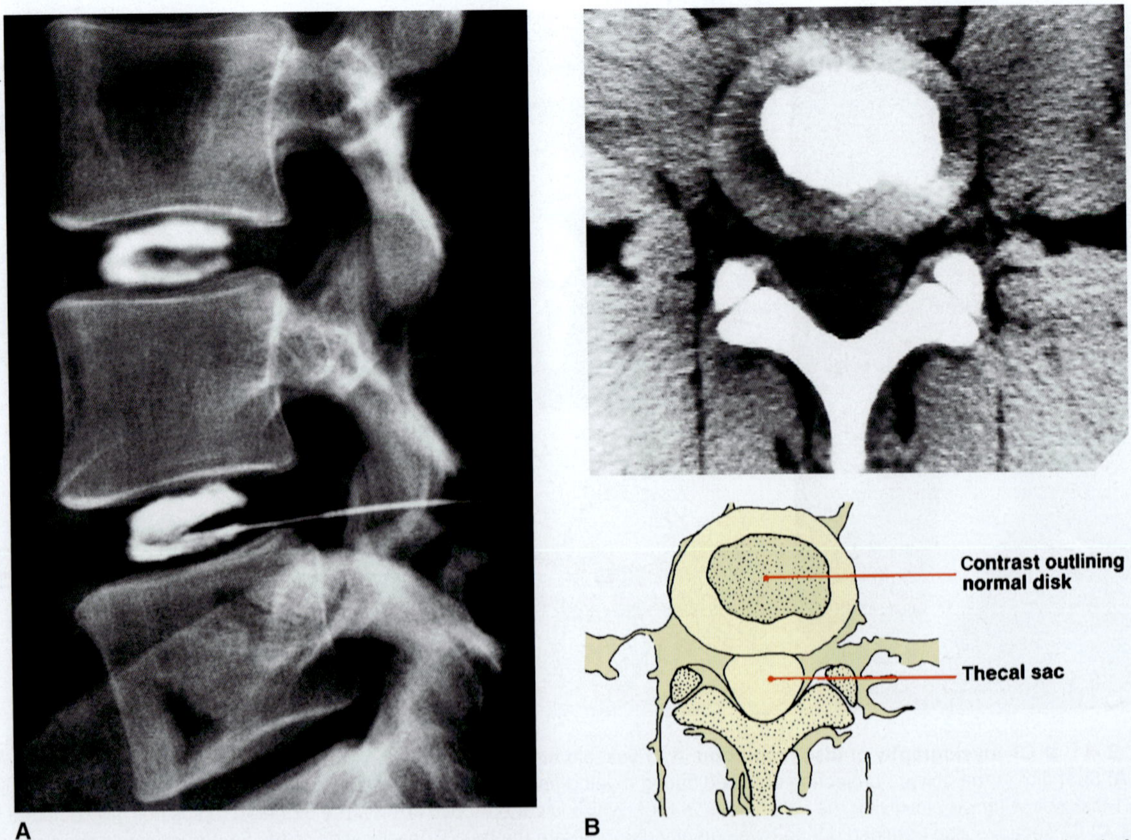

Figure 2.43 ■ **Diskography.** For diskographic examination of the lumbar spine, the patient is prone on the table, and the level of the injection, depending on the indication, is marked. The needle is inserted into the center of the nucleus pulposus, and about 2 mL to 3 mL of metrizamide is injected. **A:** Lateral radiograph of a normal diskogram shows a concentration of contrast agent in the nucleus pulposus outlining the disk; there should be no leak of contrast while the needle is in place. **B:** CT section through the L3–L4 disk space after diskography shows the normal appearance of this structure.

and help to evaluate the activity of the pathologic process. Although it is a very sensitive modality, its specificity is very low. Indications for skeletal scintigraphy include traumatic conditions, tumors, various arthritides, infections, and metabolic bone diseases. The detected abnormality may consist of either decreased uptake of a bone-seeking radiopharmaceutical agent (e.g., in the early stage of osteonecrosis) or increased uptake (e.g., in case of fractures, neoplasms, or arthritis). Some anatomic structures under normal conditions may show increased activity (such as sacroiliac joints or growth plates).

In rheumatology, radionuclide bone scanning is much more commonly used than other techniques, mainly for evaluating the distribution of arthritis in different joints. The radiopharmaceuticals currently in use in bone scanning include organic diphosphonates—ethylene diphosphonate (HEPD) and methylene diphosphonate (MDP)—labeled with 99m technetium (^{99m}Tc), a gamma emitter with a 6-hour half-life; MDP is more commonly used, typically in a dose that provides 15 mCi (555 MBq) of ^{99m}Tc (see later). Its uptake in bone is related to both osteoblastic activity and the regional blood flow. After intravenous injection of the radiopharmaceutical, ~ 50% of the dose localizes in bone, with the remainder circulating freely in the body and eventually excreted by the kidneys. A gamma camera can then be used in a procedure known as a four-phase radionuclide bone scanning. Scintigraphy can determine the distribution of arthritic changes in the skeleton (Figs. 2.46 and 2.47) and at the specific sites (Figs. 2.48 to 2.52), as well as in areas usually not detected by standard radiography like sternomanubrial or temporomandibular joints among others. This technique is also useful in distinguishing infected joint from infected periarticular soft tissues if radiography is not diagnostic and the patient cannot undergo MRI because of contraindications such as the presence of cardiac pacemaker, cerebral aneurysm clips, or claustrophobia. With cellulitis, diffusely increased uptake of the radiopharmaceutical agent is present in the first two phases, but there is no significant increase of uptake in the third or fourth delayed phases (Fig. 2.53). Conversely, osteomyelitis and septic arthritis cause focally increased uptake in all four phases (Fig. 2.54). Radionuclide bone scanning is also an effective modality to discriminate whether the failure of arthroplasty occurred secondary to mechanical loosening of the prosthesis or infection (Figs. 2.55 to 2.60). To distinguish infectious arthritis from other forms of arthritides, indium-111 (^{111}In) labeled white blood cells (WBCs), either alone or in combination with ^{99m}Tc sulfur colloid (also known as indium leukocyte imaging) (Figs. 2.61 and 2.62)

(Continued on page 53)

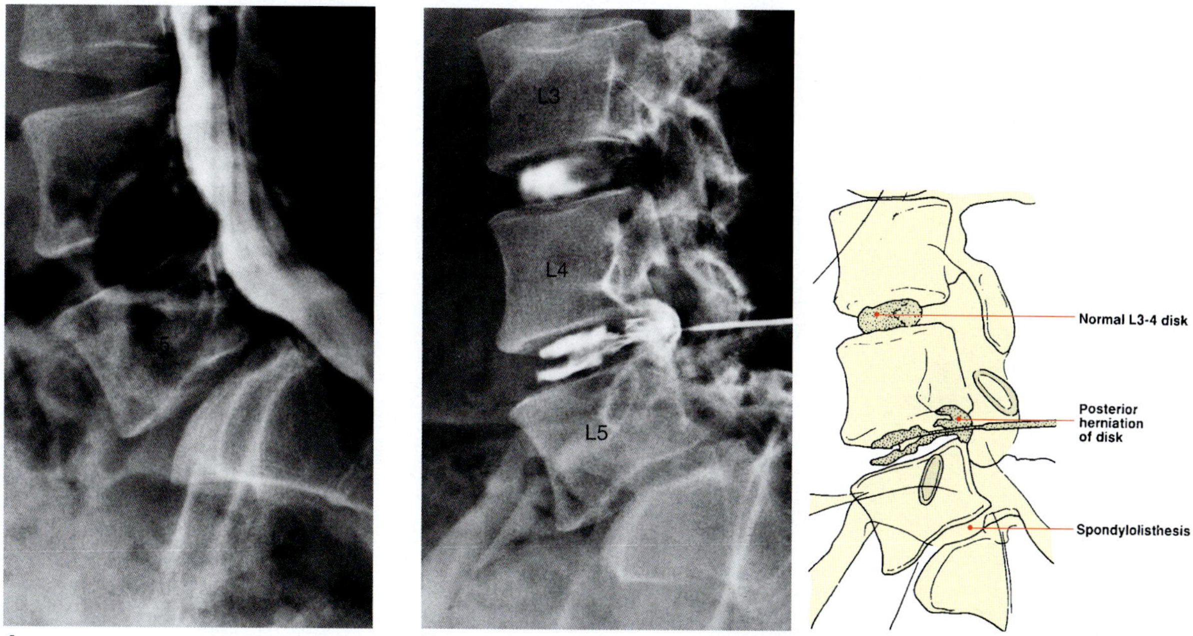

A B

Figure 2.44 ■ **Diskography of disk herniation.** A 30-year-old construction worker strained his lower back at work and was admitted to the hospital with severe sciatic pain. **A:** Lateral radiograph of the lumbar spine obtained during myelographic examination reveals a slight separation of the ventral aspect of the dural sac from the dorsal aspect of L5 due to grade 1 spondylolisthesis at L5–S1 level. In addition there is an extradural pressure defect on the ventral aspect of the dural sac at the level L4–L5, and a much smaller defect at the L3–L4 disk space. **B:** A diskogram using metrizamide contrast agent was performed at the L3–L4 and L4–L5 levels. At L4–L5 there is posterior disk herniation. **C:** Following diskography, axial CT section through the level of L4–L5 confirms posterior herniation of the opacified disk material (*arrow*).

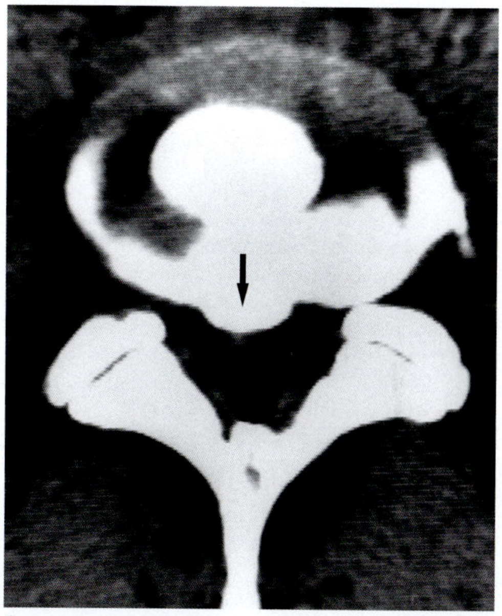

C

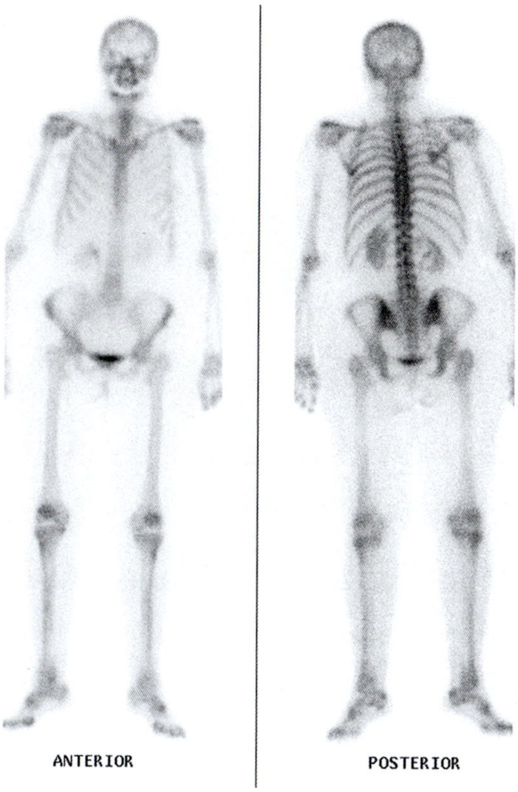

Figure 2.45 ■ **Scintigraphy.** Normal whole body radionuclide bone scan in anterior and posterior projection obtained after intravenous injection of 15 mCi (555 MBq) of ^{99m}Tc-labeled MDP.

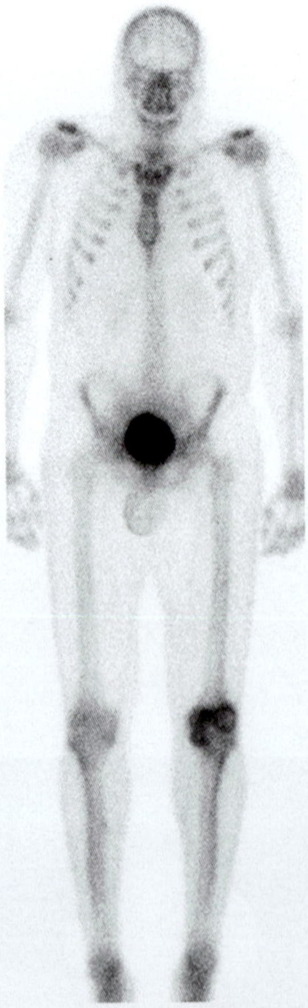

Figure 2.46 ■ Scintigraphy of osteoarthritis. Whole body technetium radionuclide bone scan shows increased uptake of the radiopharmaceutical agent in the left knee, and acromioclavicular and sternoclavicular joints in a patient with osteoarthritis.

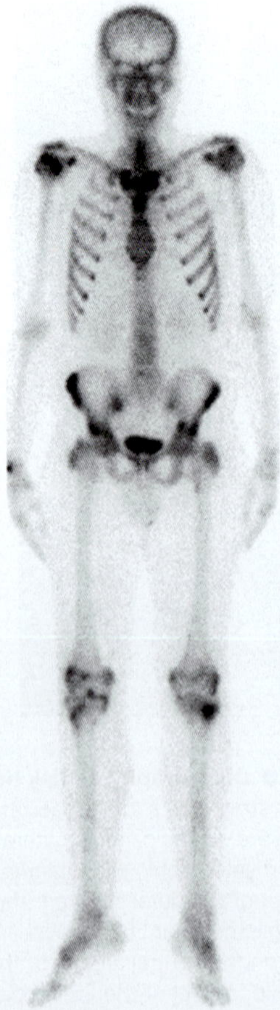

Figure 2.47 ■ Scintigraphy of juvenile seronegative spondyloarthropathy. Scintigraphy using ^{99m}Tc-labeled MDP obtained in an 18-year-old man shows increased uptake of the radiopharmaceutical tracer in sternoclavicular joints, both shoulders, both knees, lower lumbar spine, and sacroiliac joints.

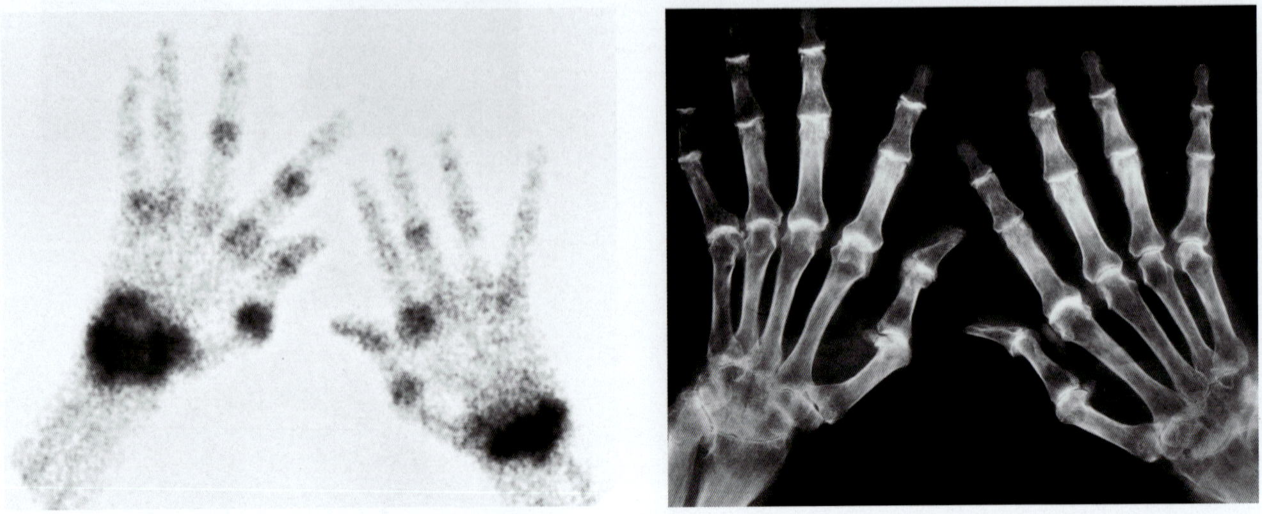

A B

Figure 2.48 ■ Scintigraphy of psoriatic arthritis. A: Radionuclide bone scan obtained 2 hours after the intravenous injection of 15 mCi (555 MBq) of ^{99m}Tc-labeled MDP shows an increased uptake of radiopharmaceutical tracer in several joints of the hand and wrist. **B:** Conventional radiograph of the same patient shows advanced psoriatic arthritis.

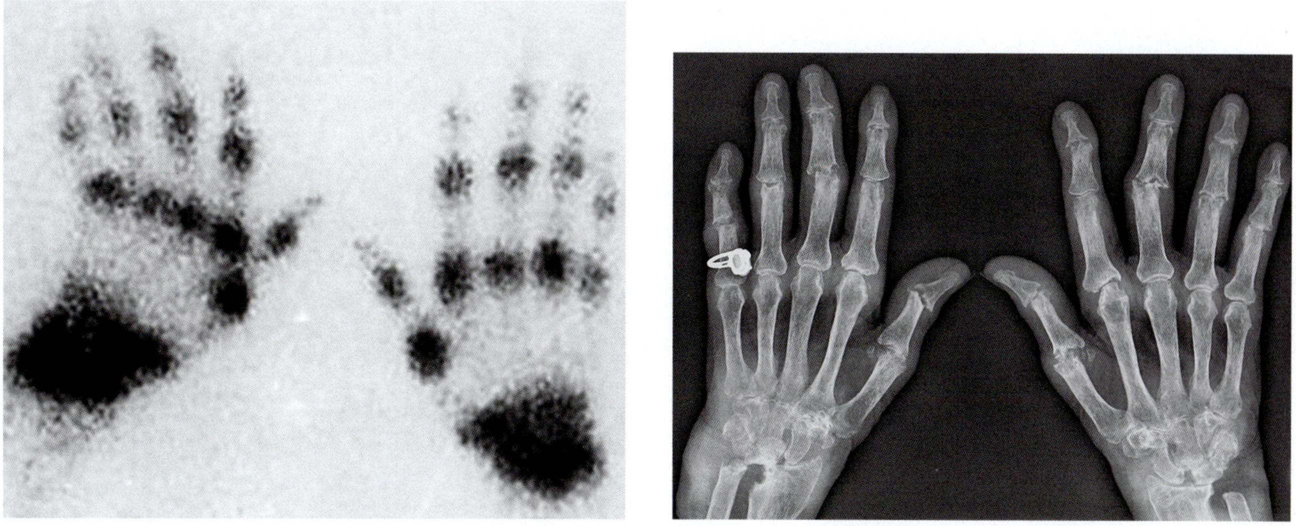

A B

Figure 2.49 ■ Scintigraphy of rheumatoid arthritis. A: Radionuclide bone scan obtained 2 hours after the intravenous injection of 15 mCi (555 MBq) of ^{99m}Tc- labeled MDP shows an increased uptake in several joints of the hand and wrist. **B:** Conventional radiograph of both hands of the same patient shows joints erosions typical of RA.

and ^{57}Ga scans are employed. The use of ^{99m}Tc hexamethylpropylene amine oxime (HMPAO)–labeled WBC for diagnosing infectious processes has also been recently advocated. The kinetics and normal distribution of such leukocytes are similar to those of ^{111}In-labeled leukocytes. The superior resolution and count density of ^{99m}Tc, however, gives this technique an advantage over the use of ^{111}In-labeled WBCs. Another radiopharmaceutical used for detection of infection and inflammation is ^{99m}Tc-labeled interleukin 8 (IL-8). A small protein (8.5 kDa) that belongs to the CXC subfamily of chemokines, IL-8 is a chemotactic cytokine that binds with a high affinity to receptors expressed on neutrophils. More recently, imaging of the joints affected by rheumatoid arthritis was attempted using ^{99m}Tc-labeled specific murine anti-CD4 and nonspecific human immunoglobulin. The rationale to use this radiopharmaceutical agent was the presence of CD4 molecules on T helper cells and macrophages, both abundantly present in inflammatory infiltrates of rheumatoid arthritis. Moreover, some investigators developed a method for imaging inflammatory joints using a monoclonal antibody (1.2B6) against E-selectin, an endothelial cell–specific adhesion molecule. They compared ^{111}In–anti-E-selectin

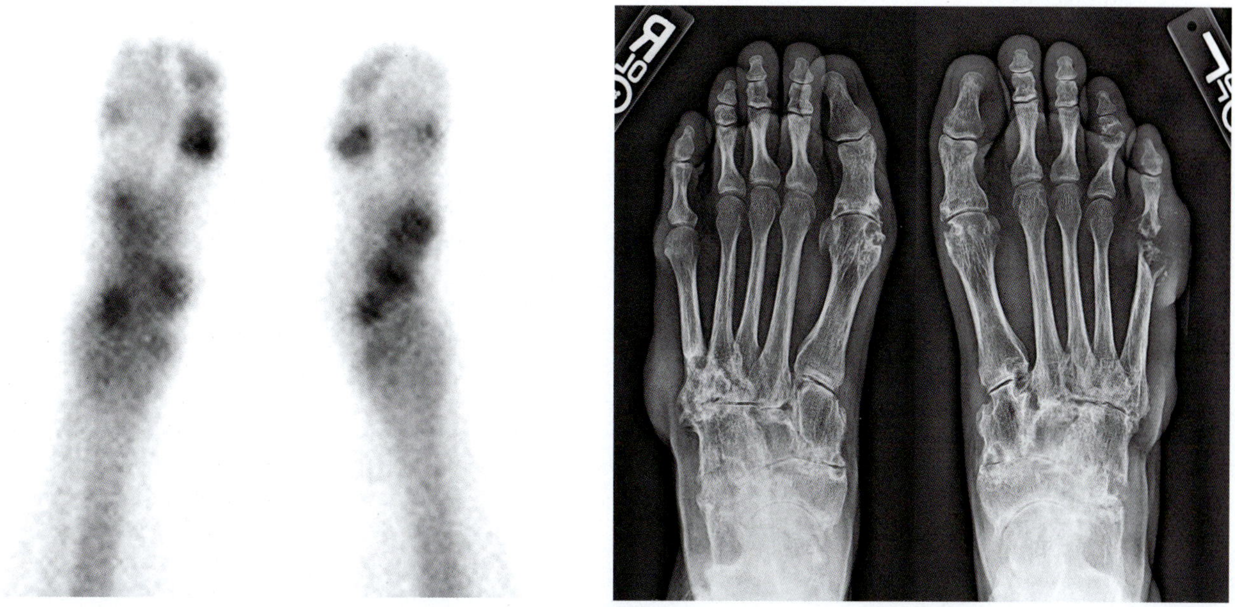

A B

Figure 2.50 ■ Scintigraphy of gouty arthritis. A: Radionuclide bone scan of both feet of a 66-year-old man with clinically documented gouty arthritis, obtained after intravenous injection of 15 mCi (555 MBq) of ^{99m}Tc-labeled MDP, shows several foci of increased uptake of the radiopharmaceutical tracer. **B:** Anteroposterior radiograph of both feet shows characteristic articular and periarticular erosions, some of them associated with soft tissue masses representing gouty tophi.

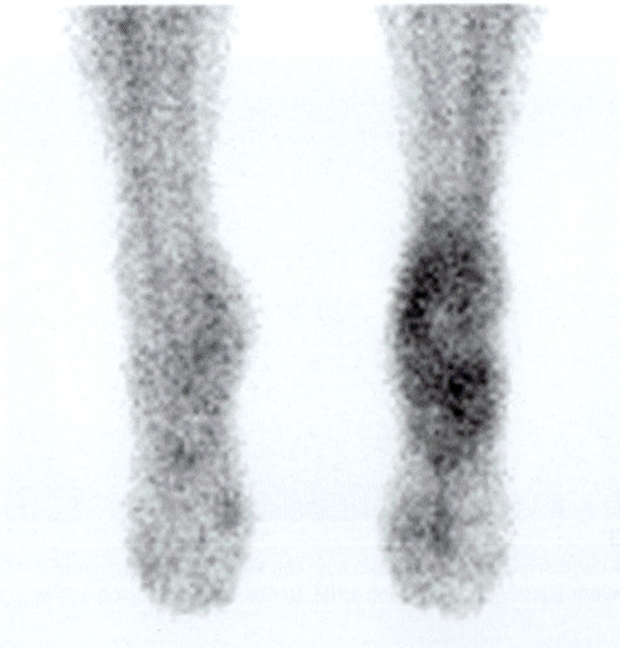

A

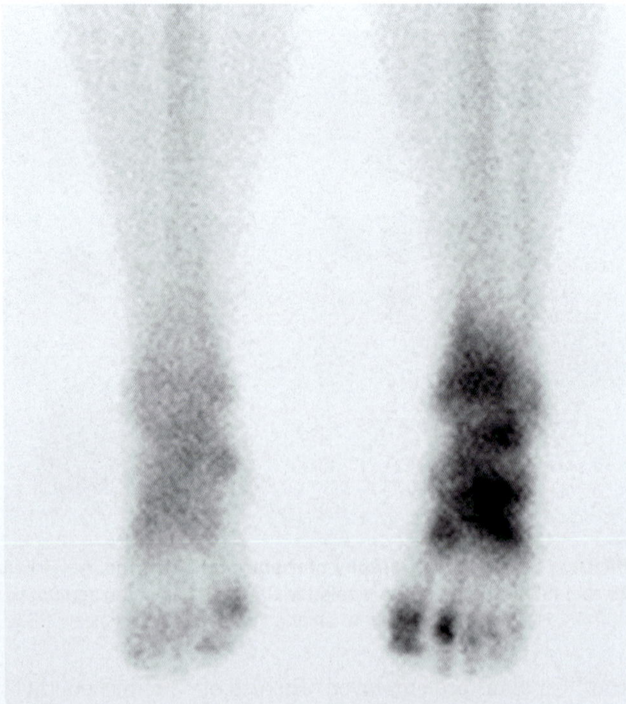

B

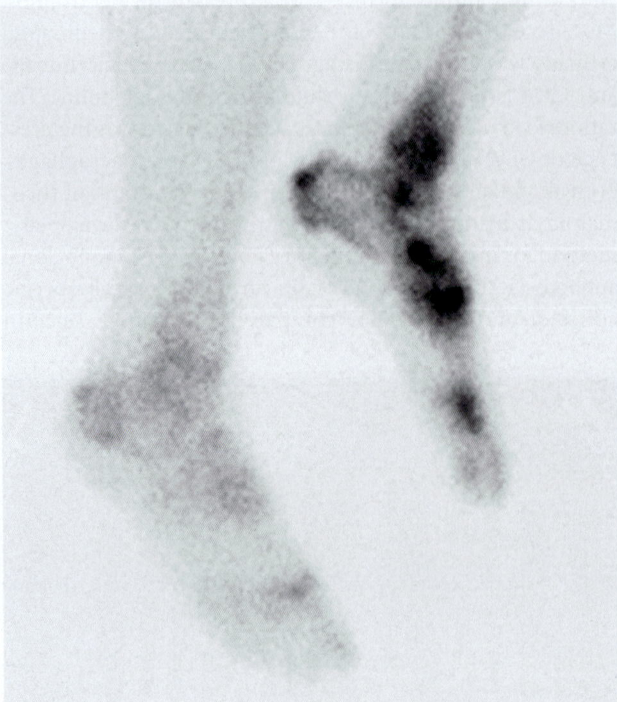

C

Figure 2.51 ■ Scintigraphy of osteoarthritis. A 55-year-old woman developed posttraumatic osteoarthritis in her left foot and ankle. **A:** Technetium blood pool image shows increase activity within the ankle and hindfoot. Frontal **(B)** and lateral **(C)** delayed planar images of both feet show increased uptake of radiotracer at the site of affected joints. The right foot and ankle demonstrate normal uptake.

mAb and ^{99m}Tc-labelled human nonspecific immunoglobulins in the scintigraphic imaging of rheumatoid arthritis, concluding that ^{111}In-1.2B6 is a sensitive method by which to assess RA activity and that targeting is more intense and specific than using ^{99m}Tc human immunoglobulin.

Serial examinations with bone scintigraphy, as Brower and Flemming have pointed out, have also been helpful in evaluating the activity of arthritis at a particular point in time. Such examinations may differentiate active disease from arthritis in remission.

Bone-Seeking Radiopharmaceutical Tracers

Several bone-seeking tracers are available for scintigraphic imaging. Those that are most commonly used are as follows.

Diphosphonates

In recent years, there has been remarkable progress in the development of new gamma-emitting diagnostic agents for radionuclide imaging. The radiopharmaceuticals currently in use in bone scanning include the organic diphosphonates—HEPD and MDP labeled with ^{99m}Tc, a pure gamma-emitter with a 6-hour half-life. MDP is more commonly used, typically in a dose that provides 15 mCi (555 MBq) of ^{99m}Tc. After intravenous injection of the radiopharmaceutical tracer, ~ 50% of the dose localizes in bone. The remainder circulates freely in the body and eventually is excreted by the kidneys. A gamma camera can then be used in a procedure known as *a four-phase isotope bone scan*. The *first phase*, termed the radionuclide angiogram, is the first minute after injection, when the serial images demonstrate radioactive isotope in the major blood vessels. In the *second phase*, the blood pool scan, which lasts from 1 to 3 minutes after injection, isotope is detected in the vascular system and the extracellular spaces in the soft

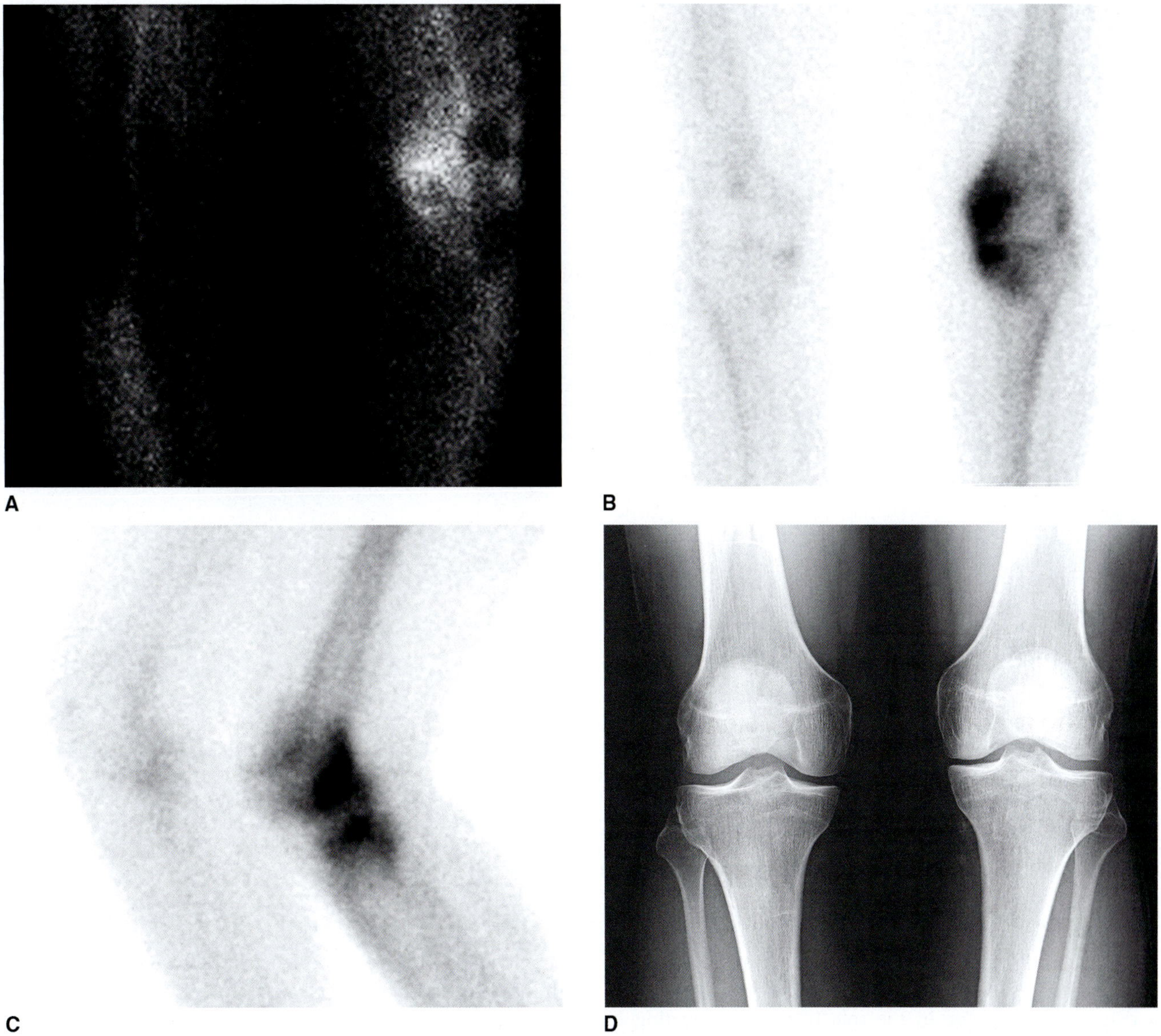

Figure 2.52 ■ **Scintigraphy of osteoarthritis. A:** Technetium blood pool image shows increased activity in the region of the left knee. Delayed planar images in **(B)** frontal and **(C)** lateral projections show increased uptake of the radiopharmaceutical tracer localized to the medial joint compartment of the left knee. The right knee demonstrates normal activity. **D:** Anteroposterior radiograph of both knees confirms osteoarthritis of the medial joint compartment of the left knee.

tissues before being taken up by bone. The *third phase*, or static bone scan, usually occurs 2 to 3 hours after injection and discloses radiopharmaceutical in the bone. This phase may be divided into two stages. In the first stage, the isotope diffuses passively through the bone capillaries. In the second stage, the radionuclide is concentrated in the bone. The most intense localization thus occurs in the first and second phases in areas with increased blood flow, and in the third phase in areas with increased osteogenic activity, increased calcium metabolism, and active bone turnover. The *fourth phase* is a 24-hour static image.

Gallium-67

Gallium-67 (^{67}Ga) citrate scintigraphy is occasionally used to diagnose infectious process in bones and joints. Although the target site of gallium localization is soft tissue, gallium also may localize to some extent in bones, because it is incorporated into the calcium hydroxyapatite crystals as a calcium analogue, and in bone marrow as an iron analogue. Gallium accumulates in regions of infection because of an association with bacterial and cellular debris as well as with leukocytes. Because WBCs migrate to the foci of inflammation and infection, some of the gallium is transported intracellularly to these sites. The sensitivity of ^{67}Ga for abscess detection varies from 75% to 99%. The images are usually obtained 6 and 24 hours following the injection of 5 mCi (185 MBq) of this radiopharmaceutical. These images have been shown to be extremely accurate in following response to therapy of chronic osteomyelitis and infectious arthritis. In particular, changing activity of ^{67}Ga uptake parallels the patient's clinical course in septic arthritis more closely

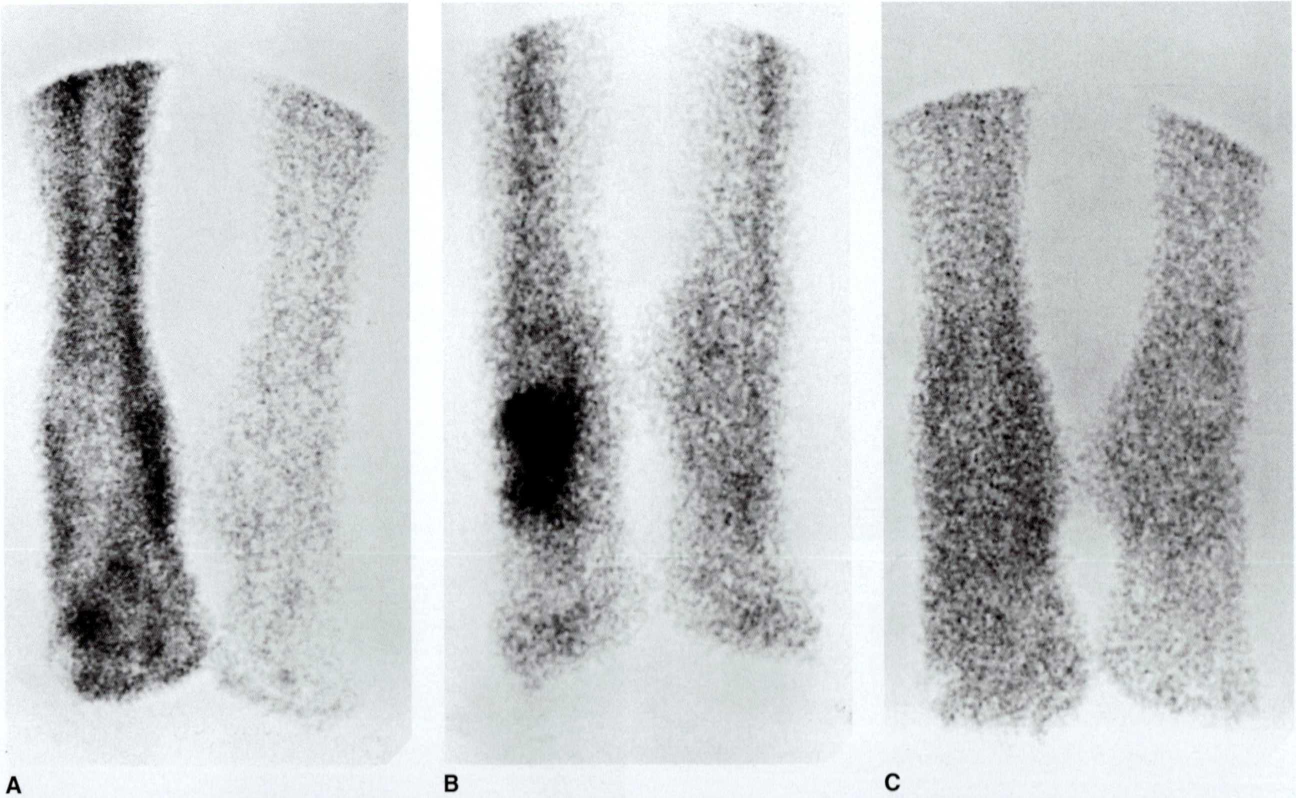

Figure 2.53 ■ **Scintigraphy of soft tissue infection.** A 52-year-old woman with pain in her right ankle had cellulitis around the ankle joint. Although radiographs did not reveal changes in the joint suggestive of infectious arthritis, this possibility could not be ruled out clinically because early changes of infection may not be detected on standard radiographs. A three-phase radionuclide bone scan was performed. **A:** In the first phase, 1 minute after intravenous injection of a 15 mCi (555 MBq) bolus of ^{99}mTc-labeled MDP, there is increased activity in the major vessels of the right leg. **B:** In the second phase, 3 minutes after injection, a blood pool scan demonstrates increased uptake in the area of the infected soft tissues. **C:** In the third phase, 2 hours after injection, almost complete washout of the radiopharmaceutical agent, with no evidence of localization in the bones on both sides of the joint, excludes the diagnosis of infectious arthritis.

than images obtained after injection of technetium-labeled diphosphonates. Over the past decade, there has been a considerable change in the role of gallium imaging of infections. Once the mainstay of radionuclide imaging for infection, gallium scanning has now been supplanted by labeled leukocyte imaging. The ^{67}Ga citrate scan, however, enhances and complements the diagnostic value of the ^{99m}Tc MDP scan. In conjunction with the latter, gallium scintigraphy has been used to improve the specificity of technetium imaging. For example, sequential technetium–gallium imaging is superior to technetium MDP scintigraphy alone in distinguishing cellulitis from osteomyelitis and in precise localization of infectious foci.

Indium

The diagnostic advantage of ^{111}In oxine labeled with blood cells over other bone-seeking radiopharmaceuticals in detecting inflammatory abnormalities in the skeletal system has recently been advocated. Because leukocytes labeled with ^{111}In are not usually incorporated into areas of increased bone turnover, indium imaging presumably reflects inflammatory activity only, and early experience has shown it to be specific in the detection of abscesses and acute infectious processes, including septic arthritis. The sensitivity varies from 75% to 90%, and specificity, as recently reported, is around 91%. False-negative results are often seen in patients with chronic infections in which there was reduced inflow of circulating leukocytes. False-positive results are seen in patients who have an inflammatory process without infection (such as rheumatoid arthritis being mistaken for septic arthritis).

Nanocolloids

Over the past decade, particularly in Europe, very small particles of ^{99m}Tc-labeled colloid of human serum albumin were tried as a bone marrow imaging agent. Approximately 86% of these particles are 30 nm or smaller, and the remainder are between 30 nm and 80 nm. This nanocolloid apparently has sensitivity for the detection of osteomyelitis in the extremities equal to that of indium-labeled leukocytes. Recently, the evaluation of sacroiliitis was attempted using ^{99m}Tc nanocolloid; however, the clinical value of this method has not been yet determined.

(Continued on page 58)

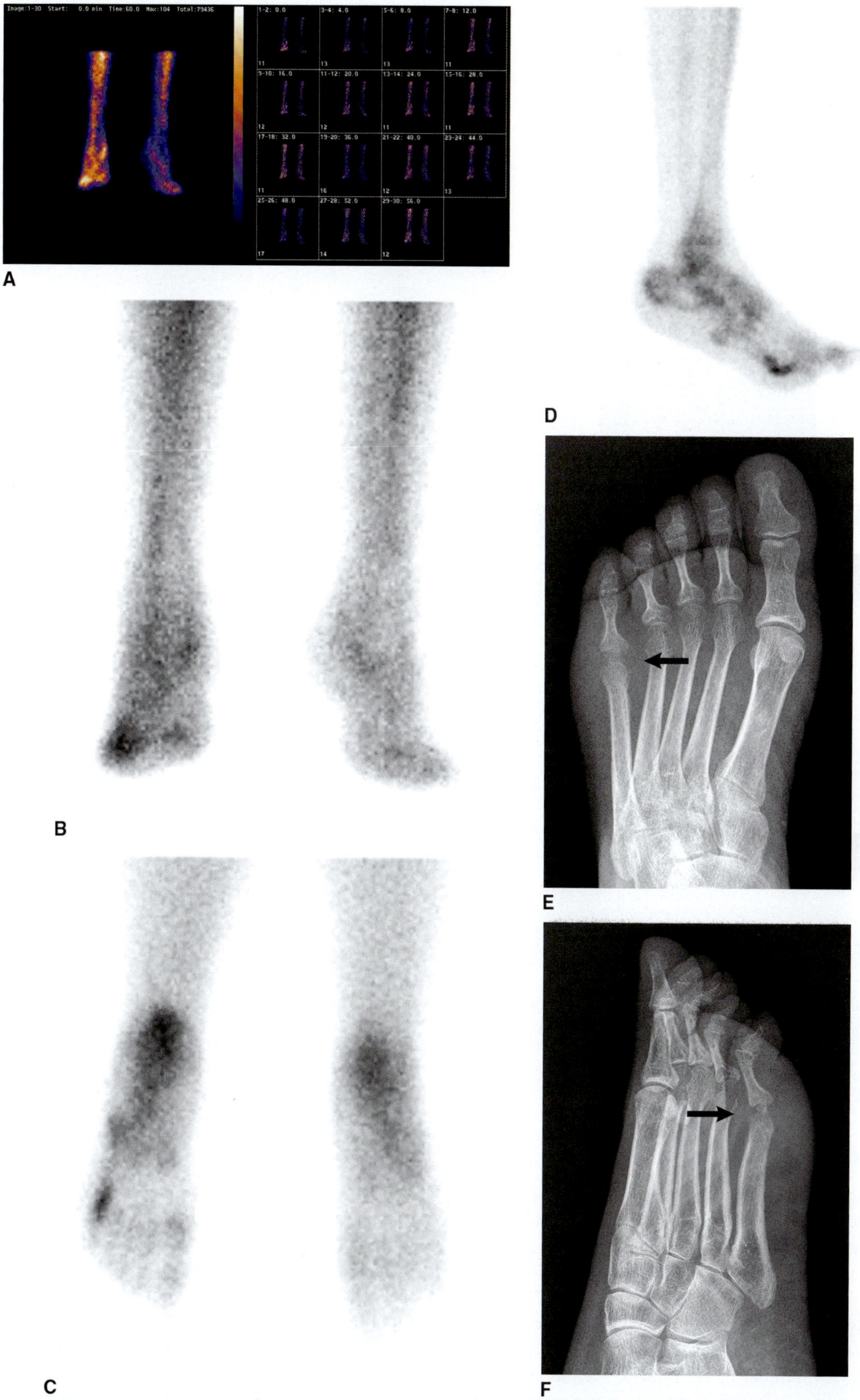

Figure 2.54 ■ **Scintigraphy of joint infection.** After intravenous injection of 25 mCi of ^{99m}Tc-labeled MDP, three-phase skeletal scintigraphy of the right and left foot was performed in a 48-year-old woman with sickle cell anemia, in whom septic arthritis of the 5th metatarsophalangeal joint was clinically suspected. **A:** The anterior radionuclide angiogram shows increased blood flow in the right lower extremity including the ankle and foot. **B:** The blood pool image demonstrates the increased activity of the radiopharmaceutical tracer at the fifth toe, confirmed on the delayed planar images **(C, D)**. Anteroposterior **(E)** and oblique **(F)** radiographs of the right foot show destruction of the fifth metatarsophalangeal joint and a large soft tissue mass (*arrow*). Aspiration/biopsy of the affected area revealed coagulase-negative oxacillin-resistant staphylococci.

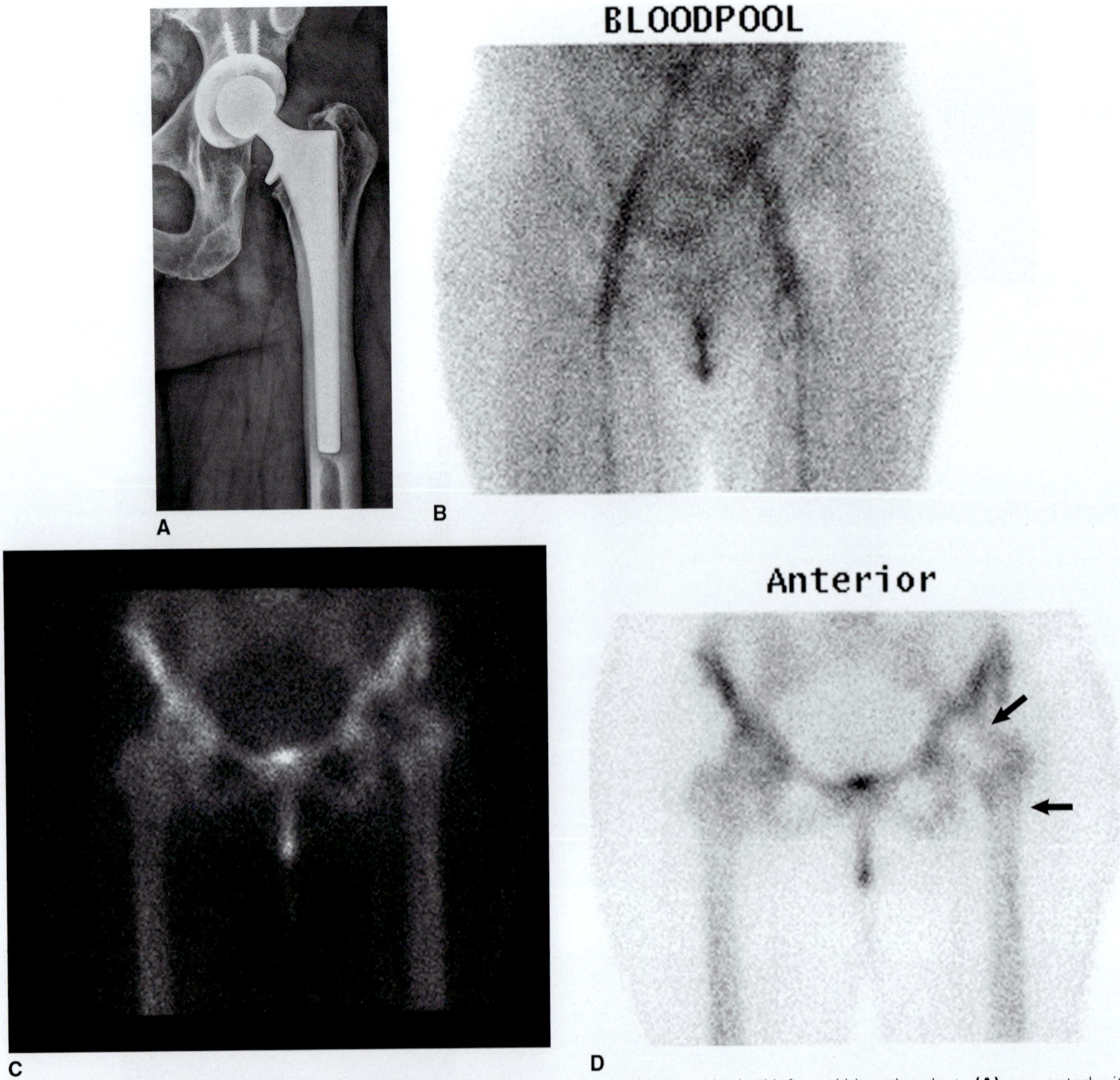

Figure 2.55 ■ **Normal scintigraphy of total hip arthroplasty.** A 47-year-old man who had left total hip arthroplasty **(A)**, presented with pain for a few weeks. Because of the clinical impression of loosening of the prosthesis or infection, radionuclide bone scan was performed. Following the intravenous administration of 24.6 mCi of ^{99m}Tc-labeled MDP, anterior radionuclide angiogram **(B)** of the pelvis shows normal perfusion. **C:** The immediate blood pool image shows normal activity. **D:** The delayed planar image of the pelvis shows normal uptake of the radiopharmaceutical tracer. Metallic photopenic artefact (*arrows*) is a normal finding corresponding to the prosthesis.

Immunoglobulins

Recently, radiolabeled human polyclonal immunoglobulin G (IgG) has been used as an agent for imaging infections. This labeled immunoglobulin is thought to bind to Fc receptors expressed by cells (macrophages, polymorphonuclear leukocytes, and lymphocytes) involved in inflammatory response. In one study of 128 patients, polyclonal IgG yielded a sensitivity of 91% and specificity of 100%. Polyclonal immunoglobulins have a number of advantages, such as availability in kit form and the fact that they do not require in vivo labeling.

Chemotactic Peptides

The same investigators who developed ^{111}In-labeled IgG are also pioneering the use of radiolabeled chemotactic peptides for infection imaging. These are small peptides that are produced by bacteria. They bind to high-affinity receptors on the cell membrane of polymorphonuclear leukocytes and mononuclear phagocytes, stimulating chemotaxis. Rather than using the native peptide, synthetic analogues are created that allow radiolabeling. The small size of ^{111}In-labeled chemotactic peptides allows the component to pass quickly through the vascular walls and enter the site of infection.

(Continued on page 60)

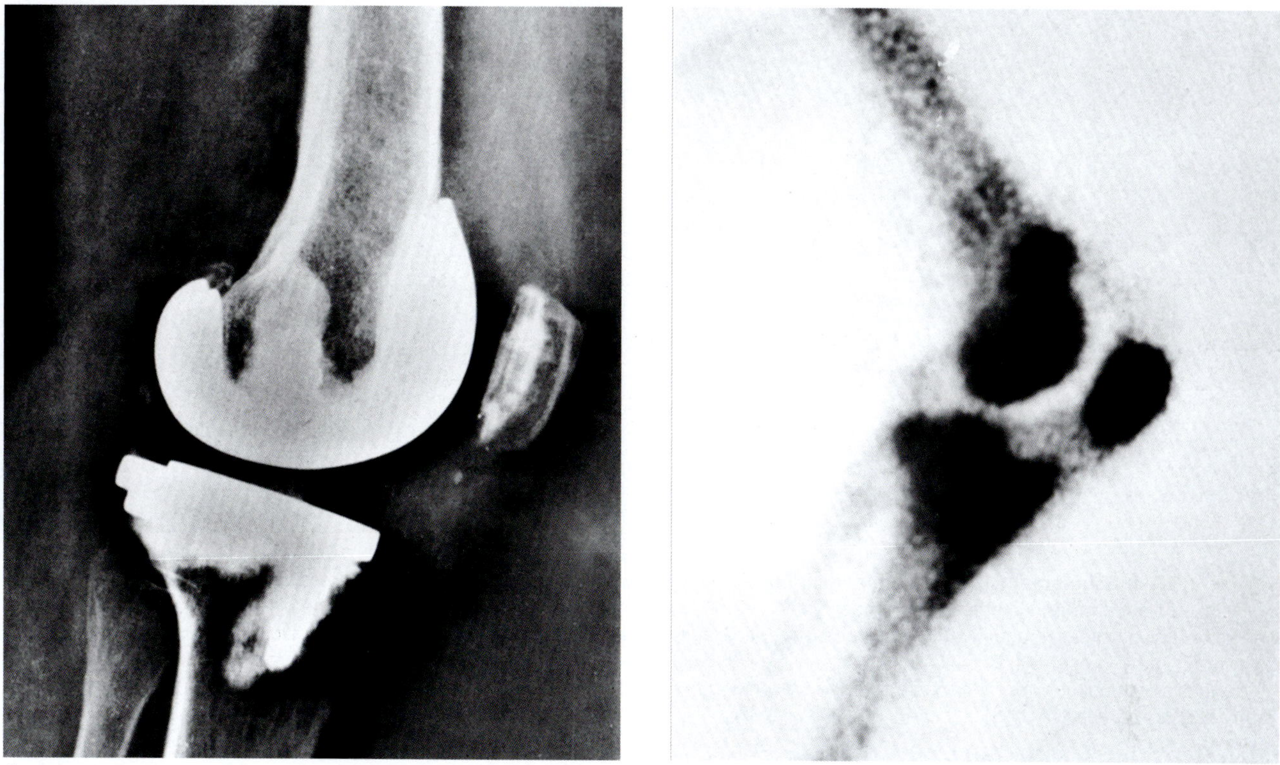

A B

Figure 2.56 ■ Scintigraphy (technetium) of infected arthroplasty. Eighteen months after undergoing total knee arthroplasty, the patient presented with increasing knee pain. **A:** Lateral radiograph of the knee shows status post three-part cemented nonconstrained arthroplasty. Areas of osteolysis at all three components of the prosthesis suggest an infection. **B:** This diagnosis was confirmed by the radionuclide bone scan using ^{99m}Tc-labeled MDP, which shows intense uptake of the radiopharmaceutical tracer around all parts of the knee prosthesis. This is in contrast to simple mechanical loosening of the prosthesis, which would have shown focal increased uptake at the site of maximal movement (commonly at the tibial component). (From Bullough PG. *Atlas of Orthopedic Pathology with Clinical and Radiologic Correlation.* 2nd ed. New York: Gower Medical Publishing; 1992:4.7, Fig. 4.10.)

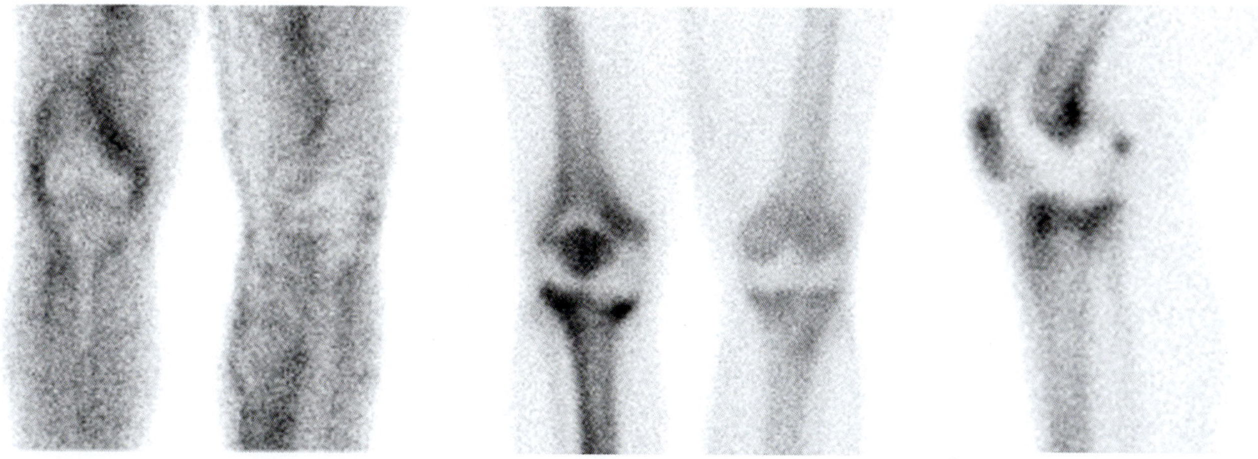

A B C

Figure 2.57 ■ Scintigraphy (technetium) of infected arthroplasty. A 63-year-old man underwent bilateral total knee arthroplasty. A radionuclide bone scan using 25.0 mCi of ^{99m}Tc-labeled MDP was performed to evaluate for possible infection. **A:** Anterior blood pool image of both knees shows increased activity around the right knee prosthesis. The activity around the left knee prosthesis is normal. The anterior planar delayed image of both knees **(B)** and lateral image of the right knee **(C)** show increased uptake of the radiopharmaceutical tracer localized to all three components of the right knee prosthesis. The left knee prosthesis shows no abnormalities. The infection was confirmed by knee joint aspiration followed by fluid analysis and culture.

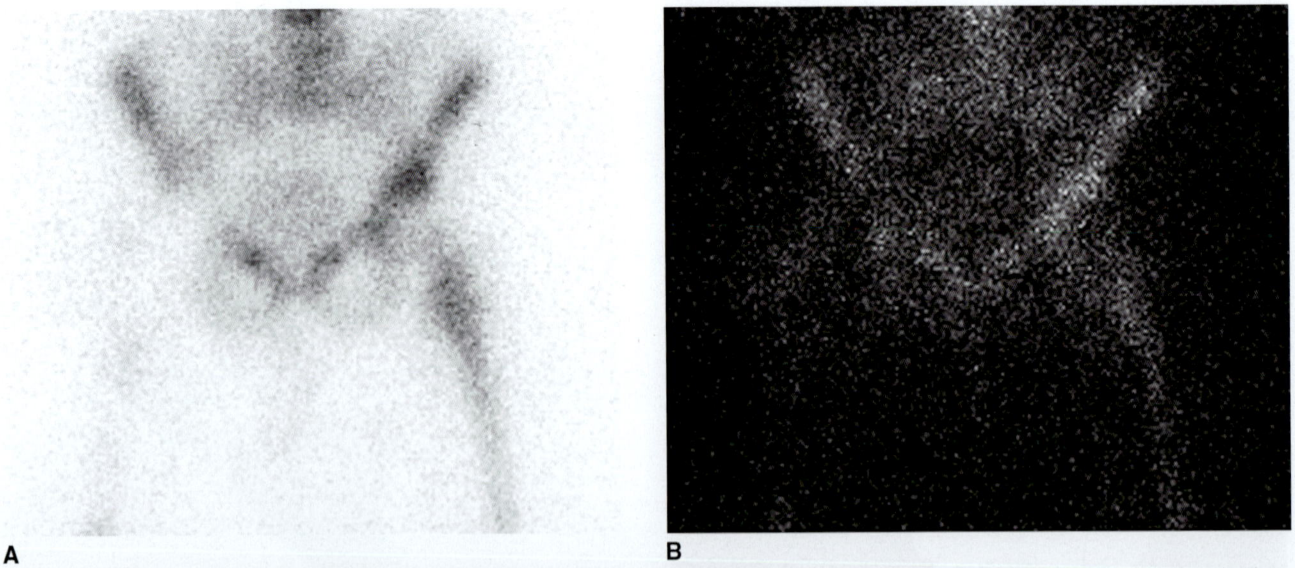

Figure 2.58 ■ Scintigraphy (technetium and indium) of infected arthroplasty. A 59-year-old man had bilateral total hip arthroplasties for advanced osteoarthritis. He presented with fever and severe pain in the left hip. **A:** Delayed image of the planar radionuclide technetium bone scan shows increased uptake of the radiopharmaceutical agent in the region of the left hip prosthesis. Observe normal uptake at the site of the right hip prosthesis. **B:** Indium bone scan using ^{111}In oxine-labeled WBCs shows increased uptake around the left hip prosthesis. The diagnosis of infection was confirmed by fluid aspiration and microbiological examination that revealed methicillin-resistant strain of *Staphylococcus aureus* (MRSA).

Iodine

Iodine-125 (^{125}I) is used in a radionuclide technique known as single-photon absorptiometry (SPA) to determine bone mineral density at peripheral bone sites such as finger and radius. This method measures primarily the density of the cortical bone.

Gadolinium

Gadolinium-153 (^{153}Gd) is a radionuclide source used in a technique known as dual-photon absorptiometry (DPA), which is also used to calculate bone mineral density. This technique permits the measurement of central sites of bone such as the spine and the hip. ^{153}Gd produces photons of two

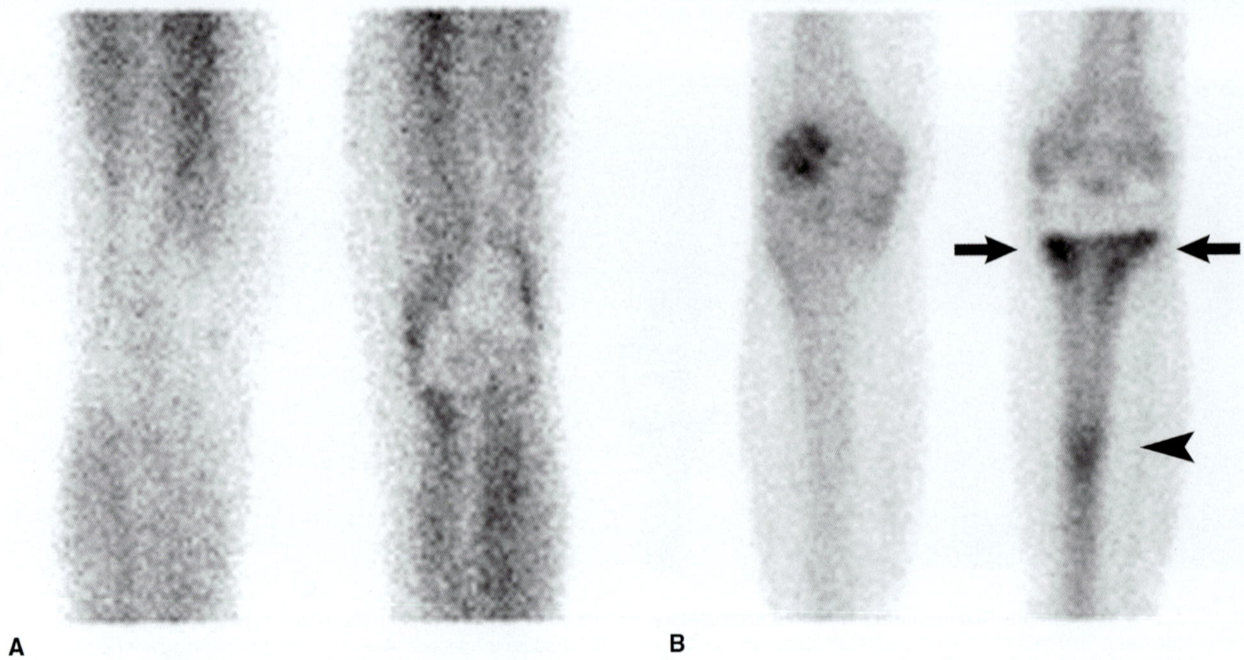

Figure 2.59 ■ Scintigraphy of mechanical loosening of the prosthesis. Twenty-four months after undergoing left total knee arthroplasty, a 58-year-old man presented with discomfort and occasional pain at the site of knee replacement. The radiographs (not shown here) demonstrated no obvious abnormalities. Radionuclide bone scan was performed next. **A:** The blood pool image obtained after intravenous administration of 22.2 mCi of ^{99m}Tc-labeled MDP shows increased activity surrounding the tibial component of the prosthesis. **B:** The planar delayed image shows increased activity of the radiopharmaceutical tracer mostly at the site of the tibial plateau (*arrows*) and at the distal end of the tibial stem (*arrowhead*). The focal increased uptake in the right patella is due to the prior fracture.

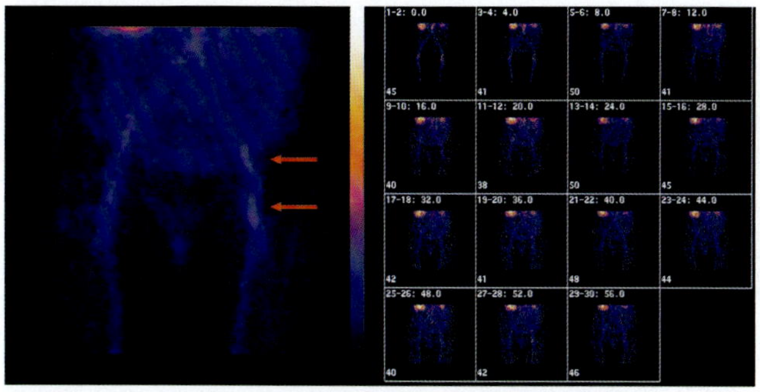

A

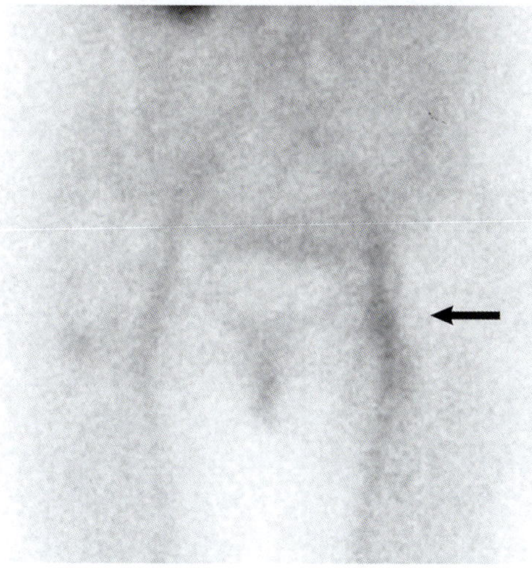

B

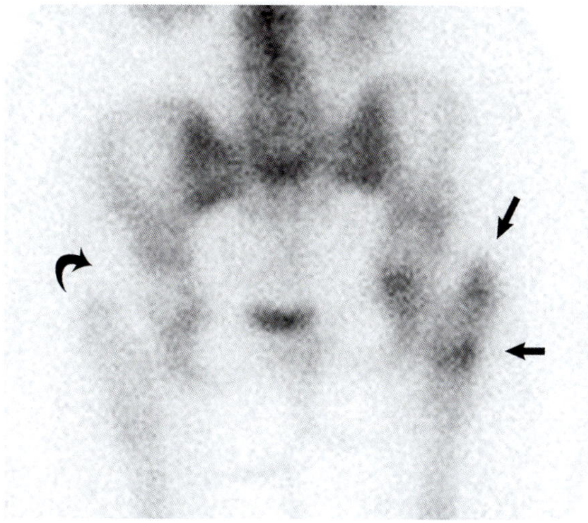

C

Figure 2.60 ■ **Scintigraphy of mechanical loosening of the prosthesis.** A 54-year-old woman underwent bilateral total hip arthroplasties for advanced osteoarthritis. The radionuclide bone scan using 25 mCi of ^{99m}Tc-labeled MDP was performed to evaluate her symptoms referred to the left hip. **A:** Anterior projection of radionuclide angiogram of the pelvis shows increased flow at the level of left proximal femur at the site of femoral component of the prosthesis (*arrows*). **B:** Blood pool image shows increased activity of the radiopharmaceutical tracer in the proximal femur (*arrow*). **C:** Delayed planar image shows concentration of the uptake at the site of femoral component of the prosthesis (*arrows*). Observe a normal activity of the tracer at the site of the uncomplicated right total hip arthroplasty (*curved arrow*).

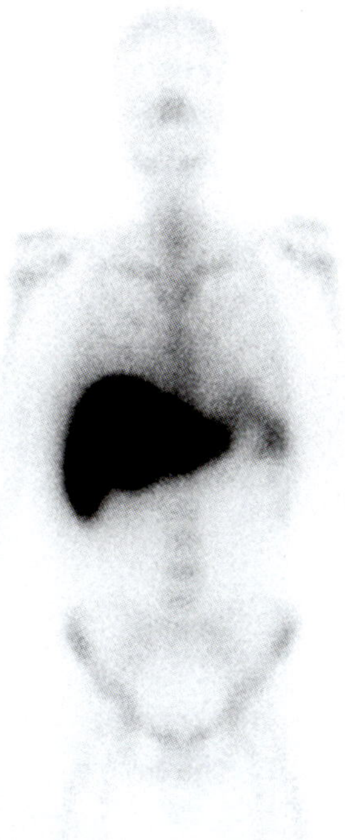

Figure 2.61 ■ **Normal white blood cells (WBC) indium scintigraphy.** The patient's WBCs were withdrawn, labeled with 0.528 mCi of ^{111}In-oxine, and reinjected into the anticubital vein. The following day, 9.5 mCi of ^{99m}Tc-labeled sulfur colloid was injected into the venous system. Delayed whole body imaging was performed using dual-energy Tc-99m and In-111. Normal uptake of radiopharmaceutical agent is seen in the bone marrow. Increased uptake by the liver and spleen is also a normal finding. There are no areas of discordantly increased accumulation of tagged WBCs to suggest infection.

energy levels, and the images are generated on a whole-body rectilinear scanner. The measurements are obtained for compact and trabecular bone.

Single Photon Emission Computed Tomography (SPECT) and SPECT/CT

With the development of single-photon emission tomography (SPET) and single photon emission CT (SPECT), diagnostic precision in evaluating joint abnormalities has increased tremendously. SPECT is defined as tomographic scintigraphy in which computer-generated 3D images of radioactive tracer distribution are produced by detection of single photons from acquired multiple-planar images. Instrumentation efficacy for SPECT is improving with the introduction of multiple crystal detectors, fan beam, and cone beam collimators; the detection of a greater fraction of photons; and improved algorithms. In comparison with scintigraphic planar images, SPECT provides increased contrast resolution using a tomographic mode similar to conventional tomography, which eliminates noise from the tissue outside the plane of imaging (Fig. 2.63). It provides not only qualitative information on the uptake of bone-seeking radiopharmaceuticals but also quantitative data. SPECT images are viewed in the transverse, sagittal, and coronal planes as well as the 3D mapping. The principal benefit of SPECT is the improvement of detection and anatomic localization of a lesion, thus producing a better diagnostic sensitivity. Bone

(Continued on page 63)

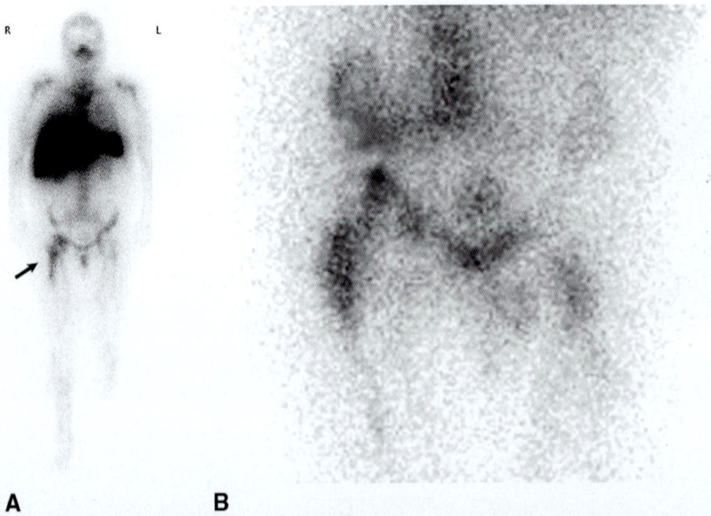

Figure 2.62 ■ **WBC indium scintigraphy of infectious arthritis and osteomyelitis.** A 48-year-old man with streptococcal bacteremia developed acute onset of right hip pain. The patient's WBCs were withdrawn and labeled with 0.548 mCi ^{111}In oxine, and then readministered into the venous system. The following day, 10.2 mCi of ^{99m}Tc-labeled sulfur colloid was injected, and delayed whole body **(A)** and one localized to the pelvis **(B)** images were obtained. Normal uptake of radiopharmaceutical agent is seen in the bone marrow, liver, and spleen. There is abnormal discordantly increased WBC accumulation in the area of the right hip joint and proximal femur (*arrow*), confirming the clinical diagnosis of infectious arthritis and osteomyelitis.

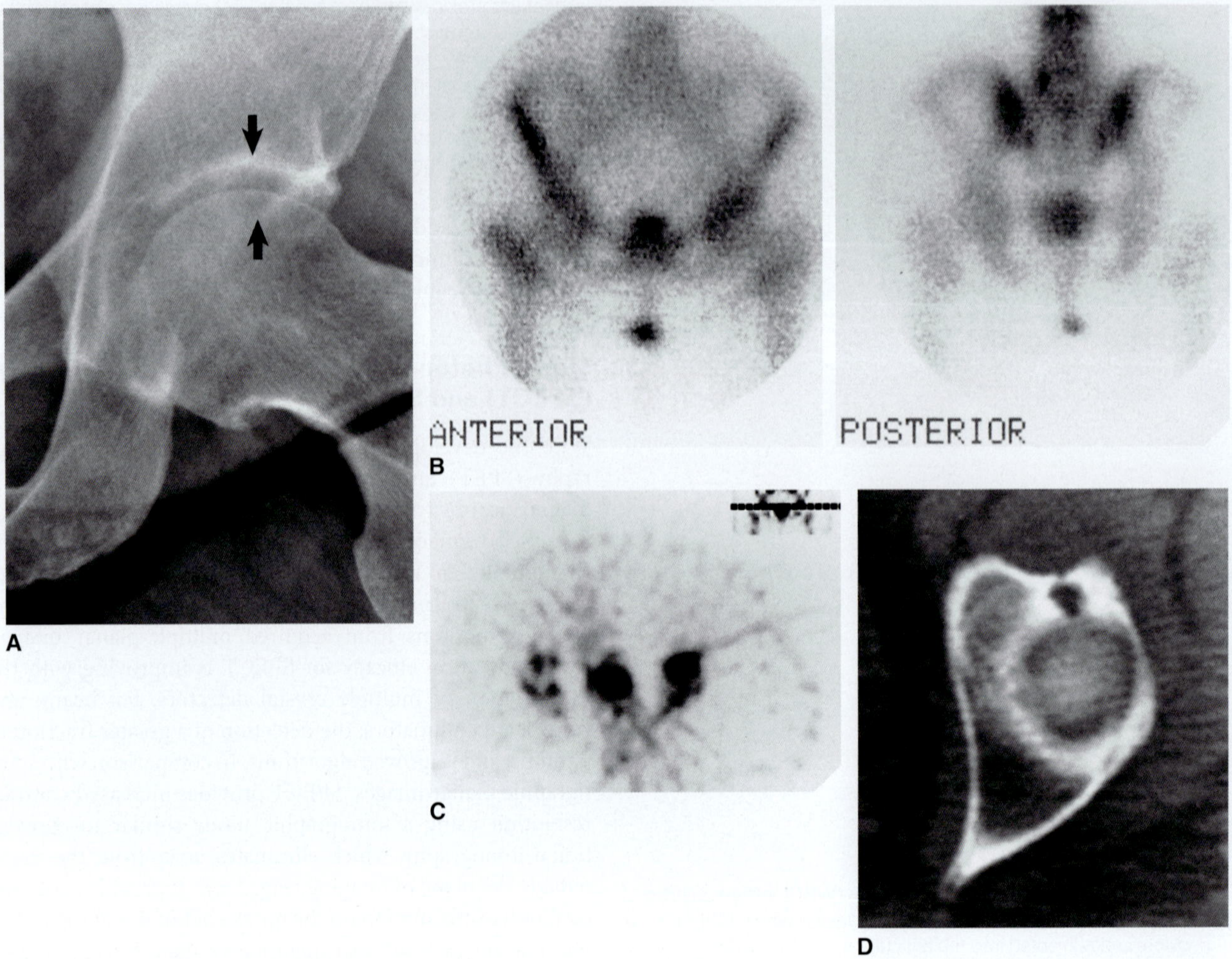

Figure 2.63 ■ **SPECT of osteoarthritis.** A 46-year-old woman presented with left hip pain of several months' duration. **A:** Anteroposterior radiograph of the left hip shows only minimal degenerative changes. A small radiolucent focus in the superior portion of the acetabulum (*arrows*) raised some concerns about the diagnosis. **B:** Conventional radionuclide bone scan in anterior and posterior projections demonstrated a slight increase in the uptake of the tracer localized to the left hip joint. **C:** On the tomographic section of SPECT, at the level of the acetabula (*inset*), there is an area of increased activity localized to the anterosuperior aspect of the left acetabulum and focal areas of activity related to osteophytes of the femoral head. **D:** CT image shows a large degenerative cyst (geode) in the acetabulum in the area corresponding to abnormal uptake of tracer on SPECT section, confirming the diagnosis of osteoarthritis.

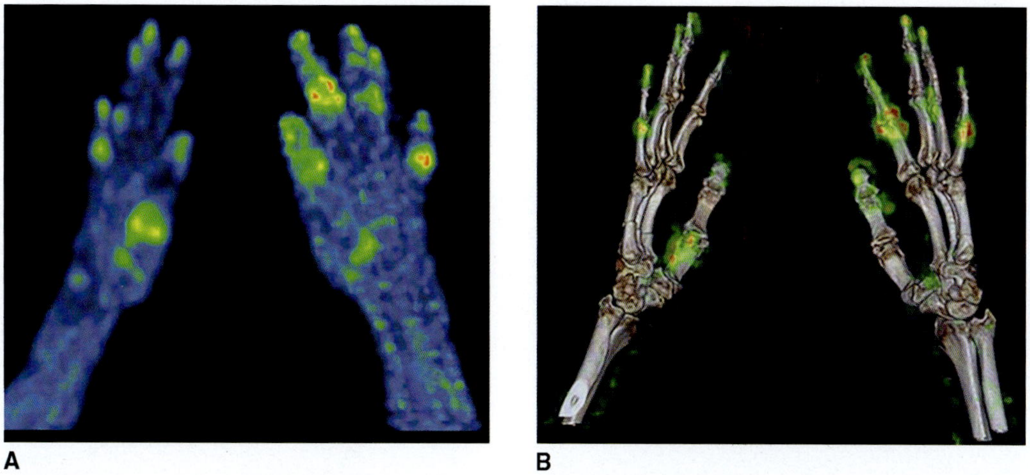

Figure 2.64 ■ **SPECT/CT of rheumatoid arthritis.** Tc-99m-labeled MDP SPECT **(A)** and SPECT/CT 3D-reconstructed image **(B)** shows rheumatoid arthritis involving several joints of both hands.

SPECT has proved particularly useful in the detection of lesions in large and complex anatomic structures, in which it allows the removal of overlying and underlying activity from areas of interest. The widest applications have been found in imaging of the spine, pelvis, knees, and ankles. Recently high-resolution SPECT and SPECT/CT trials have been attempted to detect osseous alterations in early stages of rheumatoid arthritis (Fig. 2.64) and erosive osteoarthritis, as well as in mechanical (Fig. 2.65) and infectious (Fig. 2.66) loosening of the orthopedic implants, with promising results. Integrated SPECT/CT scanners are gaining popularity as hybrid molecular imaging devices that can acquire SPECT and CT images in a single examination. Hybrid SPECT/CT combines the functional imaging capabilities of SPECT with the precise

(Continued on page 65)

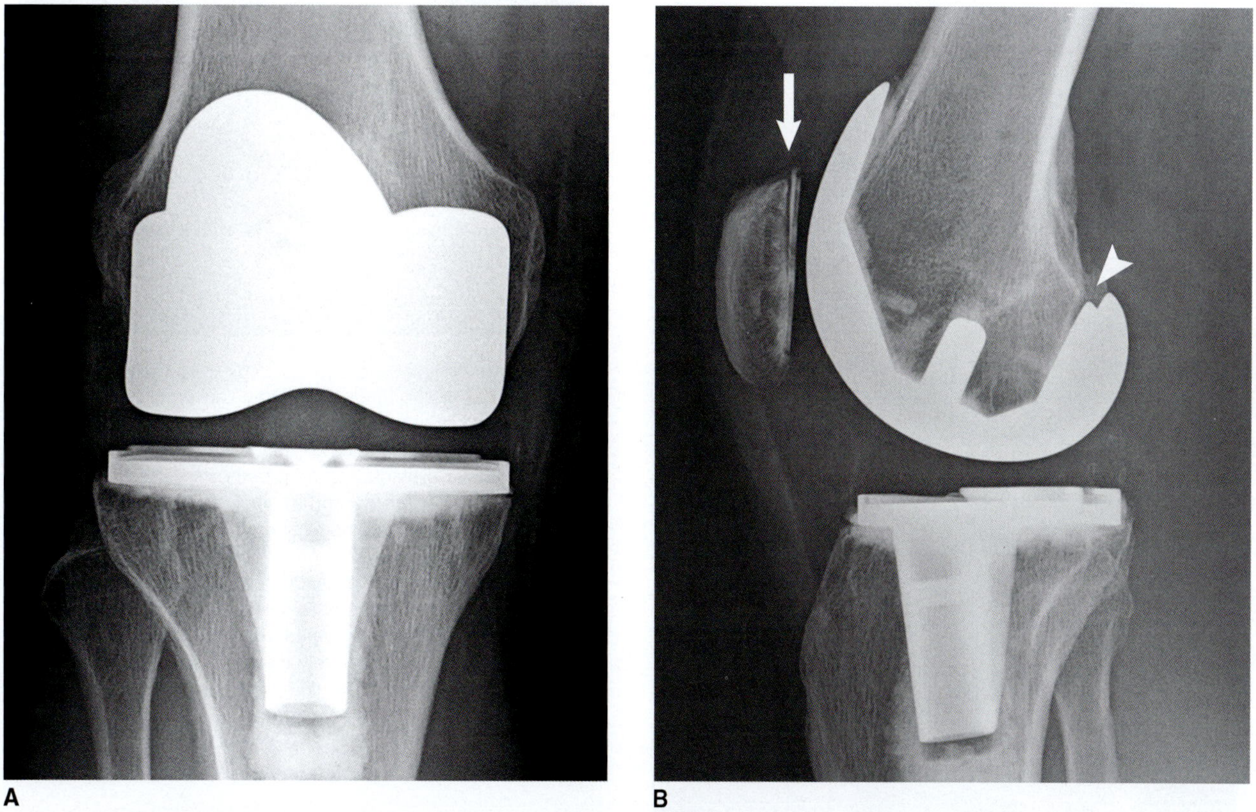

Figure 2.65 ■ **SPECT/CT of mechanical loosening of prosthesis.** A 60-year-old man, who had a three-part cemented nonconstrained total knee arthroplasty for osteoarthritis, presented with knee pain for past few weeks. **A:** Anteroposterior radiograph of the right knee shows no obvious abnormalities of femoral or tibial components. **B:** Lateral radiograph shows a small radiolucent gap at the patellar component (*arrow*), and a similar gap at the posterior bracket of the femoral component (*arrrowhead*), suggesting loosening of the prosthesis.

(Continued)

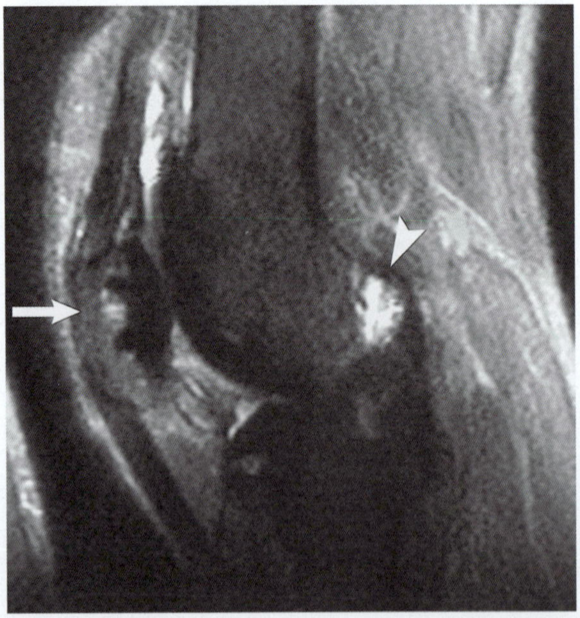

C

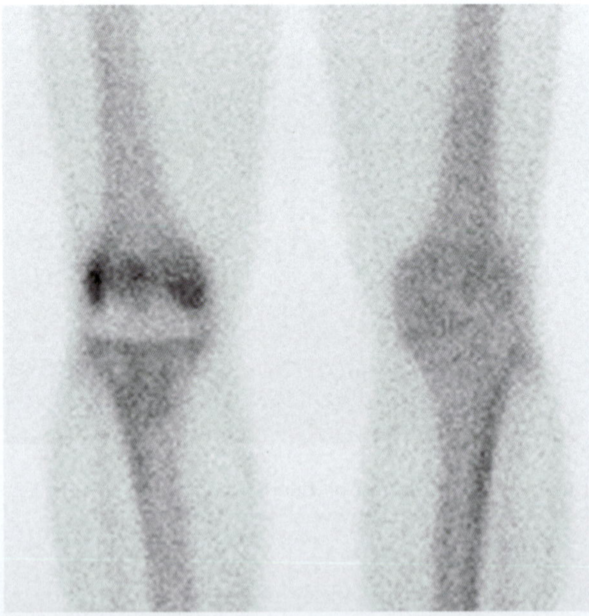

D

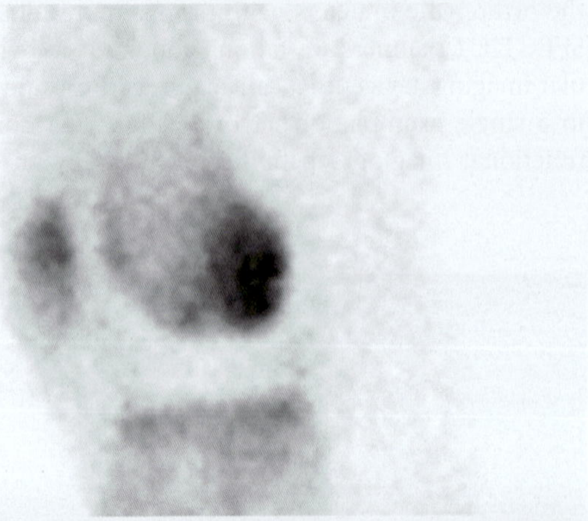

E

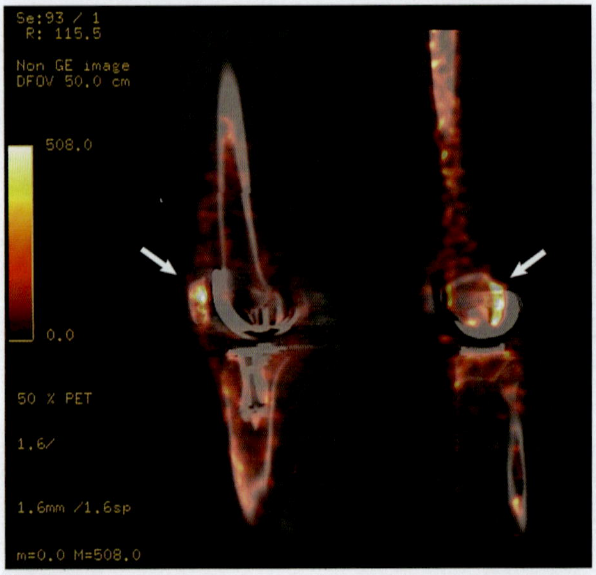

F

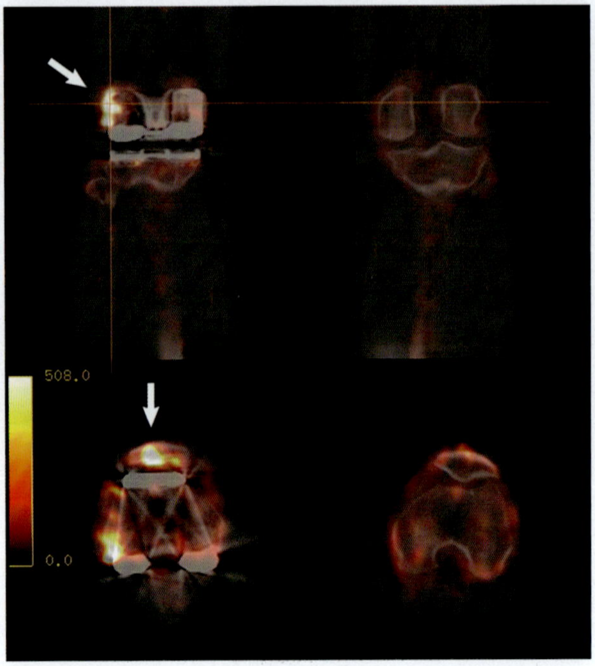

G

Figure 2.65 ■ (*Continued*) **C:** Sagittal inversion recovery (IR) MR image obtained using specialized multiacquisition variable-resonance image combination (MAVRIC) sequence to minimize metallic artifacts around prosthesis shows increased signal at the patellar (*arrow*) and femoral (*arrowhead*) prosthetic components. Radionuclide bone scan in frontal **(D)** and lateral **(E)** projections, obtained after intravenous administration of ^{99m}Tc-labeled MDP, shows increased uptake of radiopharmaceutical tracer at the site of femoral and patellar components. SPECT/CT images in sagittal **(F)** and coronal and axial **(G)** planes show more accurately the sites of loosening at the superior aspect of the patellar component and at posterolateral part of the femoral component (*arrows*).

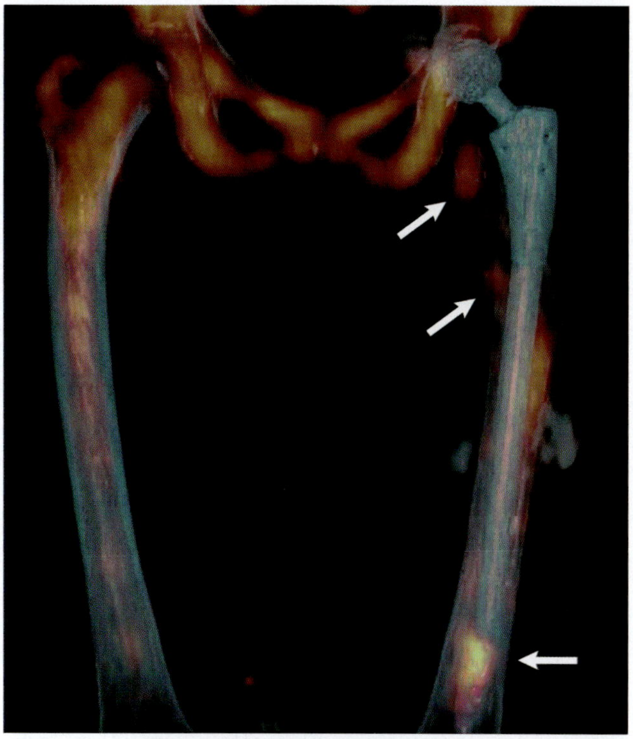

A

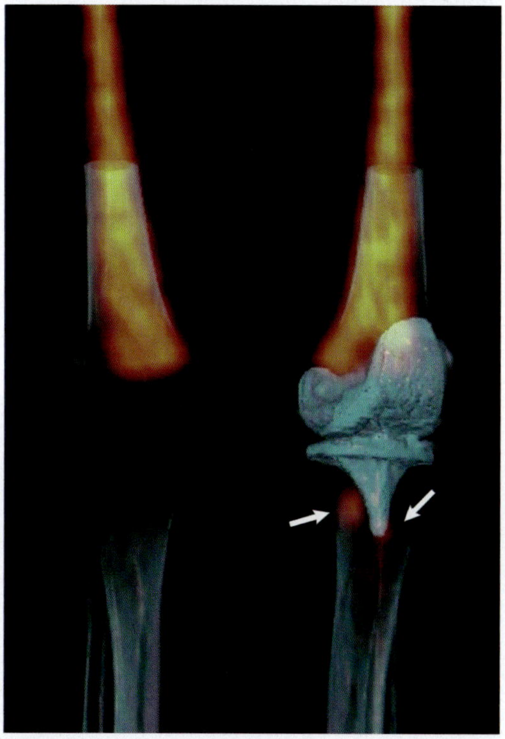

B

anatomic characterization provided by CT, thus improving the sensitivity and specificity of scintigraphic techniques and diagnostic accuracy of morphologic abnormalities. By precisely localizing areas of abnormal radiopharmaceutical tracer uptake coupled with ability to generate 3D images, this technique significantly improves sensitivity and specificity of pathologic findings.

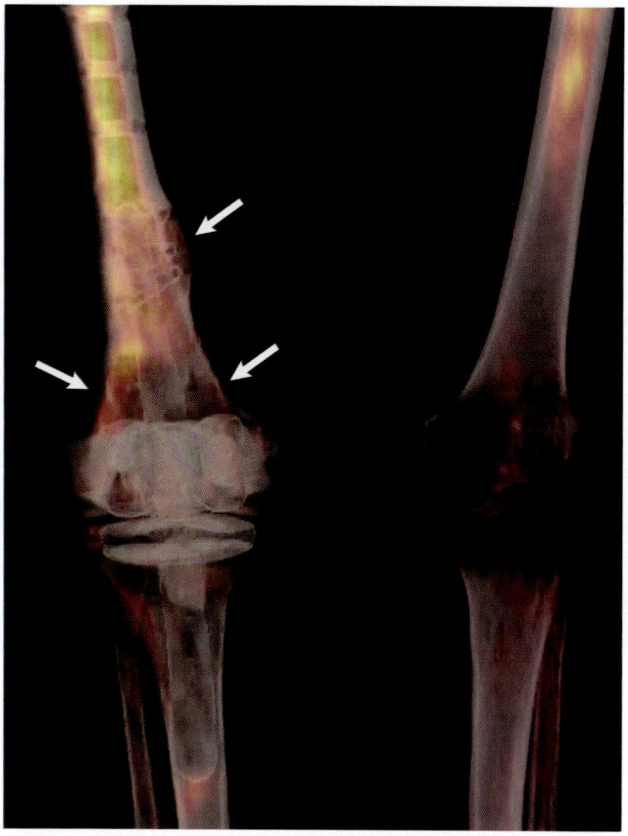

C

Figure 2.66 ■ **SPECT/CT immunoscintigraphy of infected total joint arthroplasties. A:** Imaging performed in an 81-year-old woman using antigranulocyte scintigraphy with ^{99m}Tc-labeled monoclonal antibodies shows increased radioactivity at the site of the distal end of femoral component of the left hip prosthesis, as well as within the medial aspect of the proximal part of the stem (*arrows*). **B:** Imaging using the same radiotracer, performed in a 75-year-old woman, shows increased activity at the site of the tibial component of the left knee prosthesis (*arrows*). **C:** Imaging performed in a 79-year-old woman shows increased activity at the site of the femoral component of the right knee prosthesis (*arrows*).

Positron Emission Tomography (PET), PET/CT, and PET/MRI

PET is a diagnostic imaging technique using molecules labeled with isotopes that emit positrons from their nucleus, which allows the identification of biochemical and physiologic alterations in the body and assesses the level of metabolic activity and perfusion in various organs. The process produces biologic images based on the detection of gamma rays that are emitted by a radioactive substance, such as 18F-labeled 2-fluoro-2-deoxyglucose (^{18}F-FDG). PET differs from other single-photon radionuclide scans in its ability to correct for tissue attenuation signal loss and its relatively uniform spatial resolution. Although one of the main applications of this technique is in oncology, including the detection of primary and metastatic tumors and recurrences of the tumor after treatment, this modality was found to be also

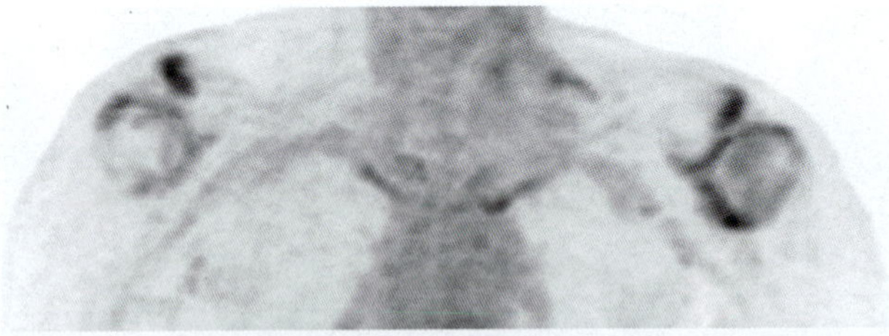

Figure 2.67 ■ 18F-FDG PET of osteoarthritis. Observe increased metabolic activity in both shoulders in this patient with osteoarthritis.

effective in diagnosing and localizing the abnormalities associated with varieties of rheumatologic disorders (Figs. 2.67 and 2.68). Recently, PET in combination with CT (PET/CT) became more frequently used in rheumatology. PET/CT combines in a single gantry system a PET and CT, allowing a sequential acquisition of images derived from both systems at the same time and thus combining them into a single superimposed image. Two- and three-dimensional image reformation may be rendered as a function of a common software and control system. The advantage of this fusion image is clear: the functional images obtained with PET that depicts the spatial distribution of metabolic and biochemical activities in the tissues are precisely correlated with anatomic images obtained with CT (Figs. 2.69 to 2.72). This technique proved to be also effective in monitoring response to treatment (Figs. 2.73 and 2.74).

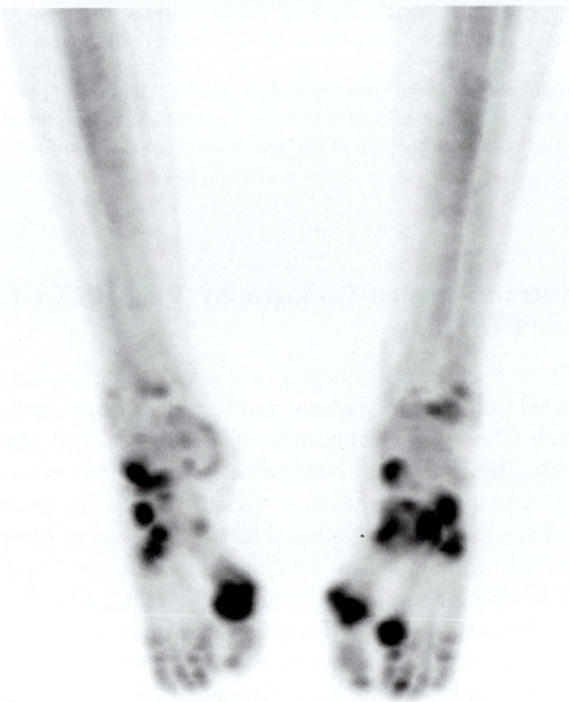

Figure 2.68 ■ 18F-FDG PET of gout. Image of both feet shows several foci of increased metabolic activity at the site of tophaceous gouty arthritis in a 61-year-old man.

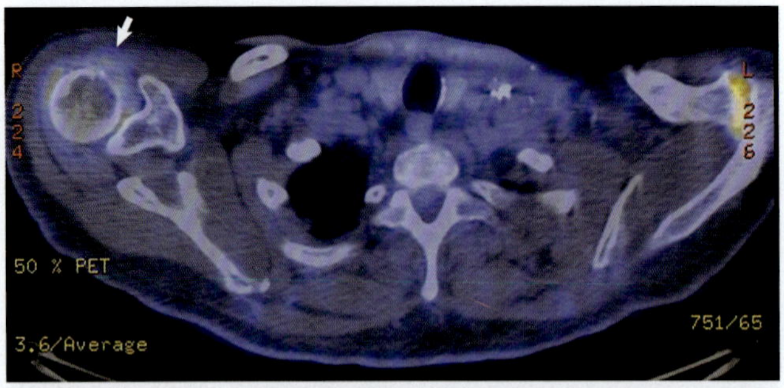

Figure 2.69 ■ 18F-FDG PET/CT of rheumatoid arthritis. A fused PET/CT image of the right shoulder of a 47-year-old woman with clinically proven rheumatoid arthritis shows increased metabolic activity in the joint (*arrow*) consistent with inflammatory synovitis.

PET/MRI is the newest hybrid technology with the capability for instantaneous fusion of anatomic and functional data, which allows integrated scanning for simultaneous PET and MRI. To avoid the interference of magnetic fields on PET performance, the traditional PET detectors based on scintillators coupled with photomultiplier tubes were substituted with the avalanche photodiodes and silicone photomultipliers. This technique combines the strengths of MRI—including the lack of ionizing radiation as well as high-resolution and high-contrast morphologic imaging of osseous structures and soft tissues—with the highest sensitivity of PET and its ability to obtain functional images depicting metabolic and biochemical activity in the tissues, as in PET/CT. The limited clinical applications yielded encouraging results, particularly in the evaluation of the progress of treatment of some of the inflammatory arthritides (Fig. 2.75).

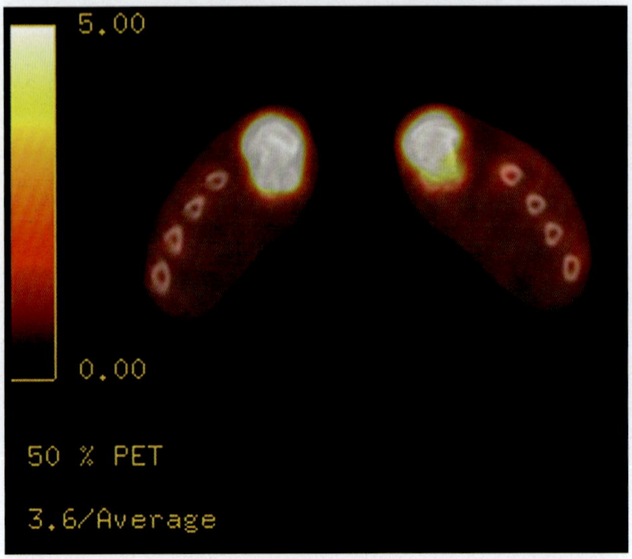

Figure 2.70 ■ 18F-FDG PET/CT of gout. A fused PET/CT axial (short axis) image of both feet of a 49-year-old man shows increased metabolic activity in both first metatarsophalangeal joints.

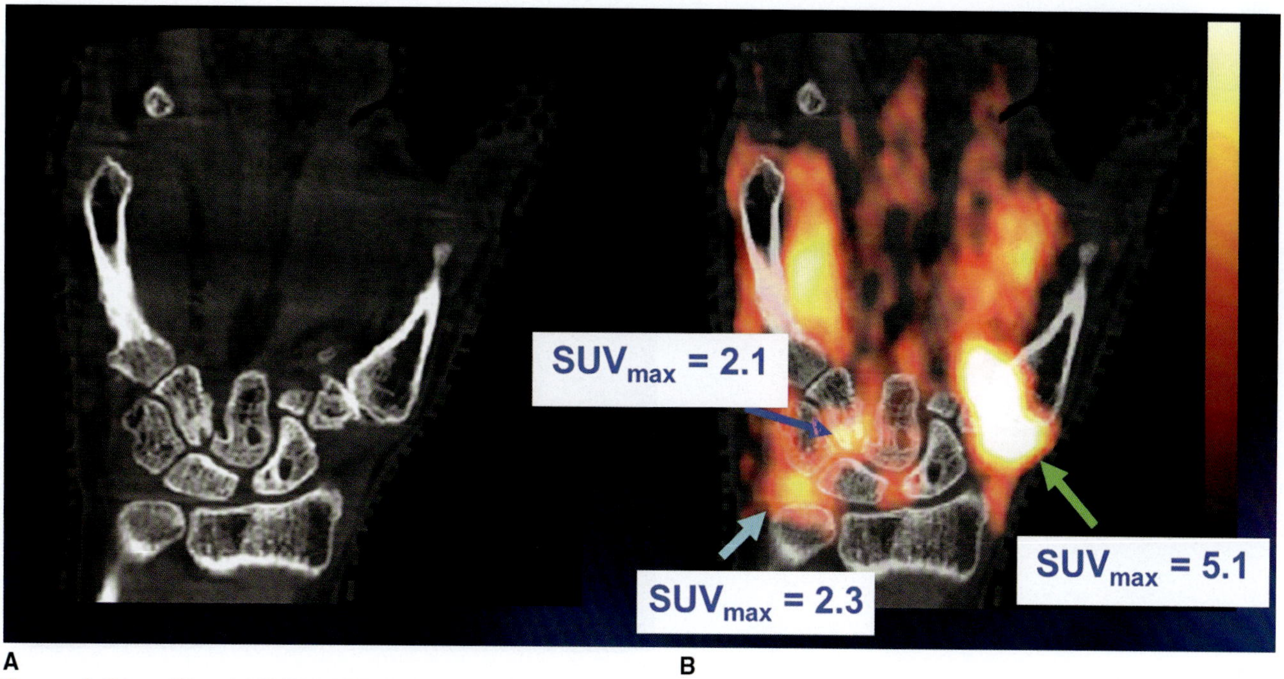

Figure 2.71 ■ **CT and 18F-FDG PET/CT of rheumatoid arthritis and osteoarthritis. A:** Coronal reformatted CT image of the right wrist of a 49-year-old woman with clinically documented rheumatoid arthritis shows erosions of several carpal bones, including the hamate, triquetrum, capitate, and scaphoid. In addition, there is narrowing, subchondral sclerosis, and osteophyte formation of the first carpometacarpal joint typical of osteoarthritis. **B:** Coronal fused PET/CT image shows increased accumulation of the FDG radiotracer (increased metabolic activity) at the sites of active inflammatory synovitis and erosions (*blue* and *turqoise arrows*), and at the site of osteoarthritis (*green arrow*). SUV_{max}, standarized uptake value.

ULTRASOUND (US)

In the past several years US has made an enormous impact in the field of radiology and has become a useful tool in musculoskeletal imaging. It has several inherent advantages. It is relatively inexpensive, allows comparisons with the opposite normal side, uses no ionizing radiation, and can be performed at the bedside as well as in the operating room. It is a noninvasive modality, relying on the interaction of propagated sound waves with tissue interfaces in the body. Whenever the directed pulsing of sound waves encounters an interface between tissues of different acoustic impedance, reflection or refraction occurs. The sound waves reflected back to the US transducer are recorded and converted into images. Various types of US scanning are available. Most modern US equipment displays dynamic information in "real time," similar to information that is provided by fluoroscopy. With real-time US, the images may be obtained in any scan plane by simply moving the transducer. Thus, imaging may include transverse or longitudinal images, and any obliquity can be produced. Modern probe technology and higher frequency transducers of 7.5 MHz to 20.0 MHz that have excellent spatial resolution have extended usefulness of US for evaluation of anatomy and pathology of different joints and periarticular structures (Figs. 2.76 and 2.77). Structures examined by US can be hyperechoic, hypoechoic, or anechoic or may demonstrate mixed echogenicity relative to surrounding tissue. For instance, tendons and ligaments are generally hyperechoic, but a tendon affected by tendinosis is hypoechoic; fluid collections are anechoic, and synovial proliferation (synovitis) can be hyperechoic, isoechoic, or hypoechoic. Ultrasound imaging has been applied to arthritides and enthesopathies, including degenerative and inflammatory joint diseases, particularly in evaluation of early abnormalities seen in rheumatoid arthritis. US can detect crucial manifestations of inflammatory arthritides such as hyperemia, synovitis, tenosynovitis, inflammatory pannus, joint effusion, and erosive changes, even at a very early stage (Figs. 2.78 and 2.79). Joint and tendon pathology is readily demonstrated by US. In particular, tenosynovitis of flexor and extensor tendons of the hand associated with edema, which results in alteration of echogenicity and widening and thickening of the tendons, is an early finding in rheumatoid arthritis and can be effectively displayed on gray-scale imaging as hypo- or isoechoic areas within and around a joint or tendon sheath (Figs. 2.80 and 2.81). US can also identify some of the soft tissue complications of arthritis, such as tendon or ligament rupture or subcutaneous nodules and cyst formation. This modality also helps to differentiate popliteal fossa masses in patients with rheumatoid arthritis, in whom complications of an arthritic process (e.g., popliteal cyst or hypertrophied synovium) may be distinguished from conditions not related to arthritis

(Continued on page 72)

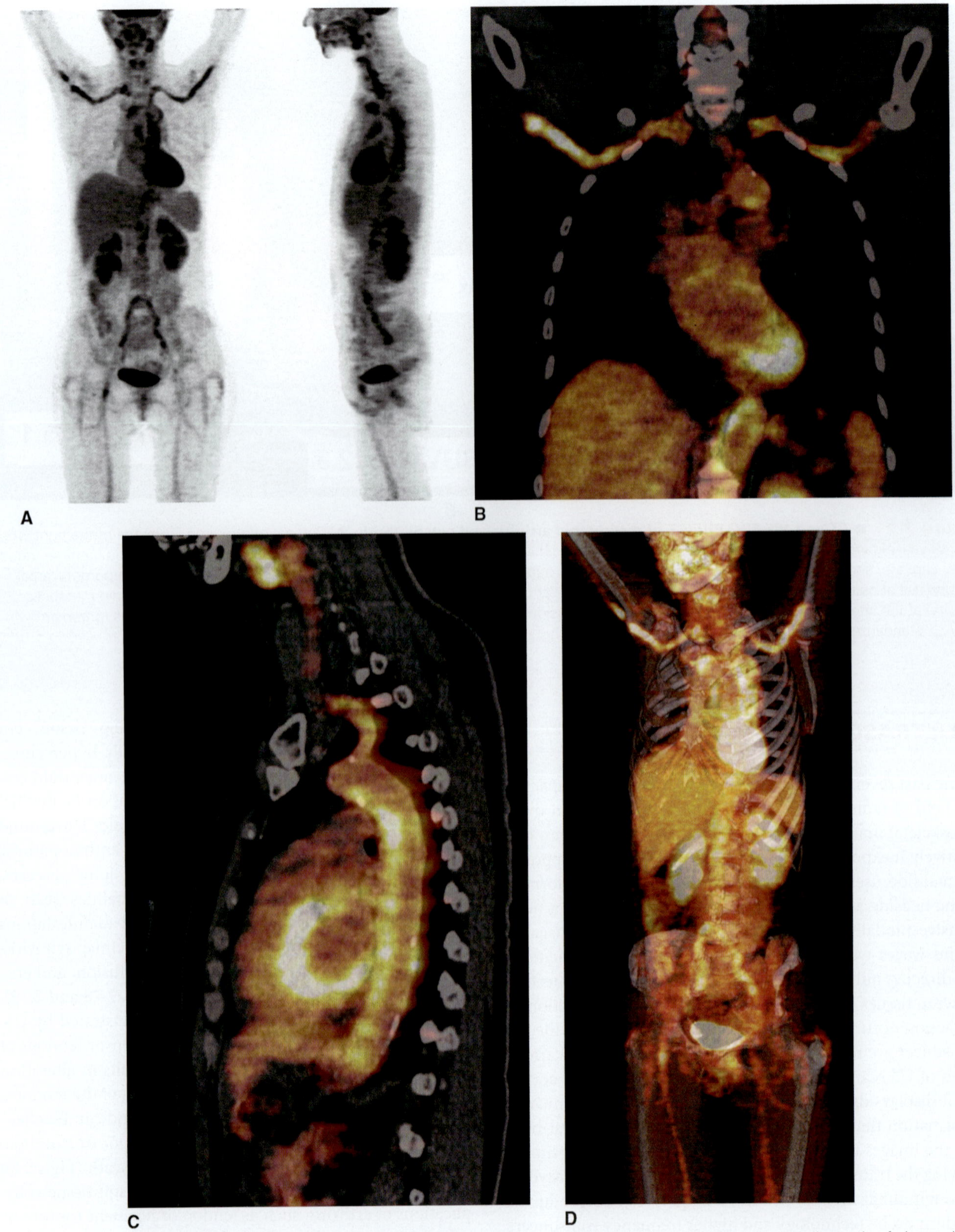

Figure 2.72 ■ **18F-FDG PET and PET/CT of giant cell arteritis.** A 58-year-old woman with clinically suspected diagnosis of giant cell arteritis underwent PET/CT examination. **A:** Frontal and lateral whole body 18F-FDG PET shows increased metabolic activity in the aorta, both subclavian arteries, and common iliac arteries. **B:** Fused PET/CT image demonstrates increased metabolic activity in both subclavian arteries. **C:** Lateral projection shows increased metabolic activity in thoracic aorta. **D:** Fused reconstructed PET/CT image in volume-rendering technique more effectively demonstrates the abnormalities depicted in parts **A–C**.

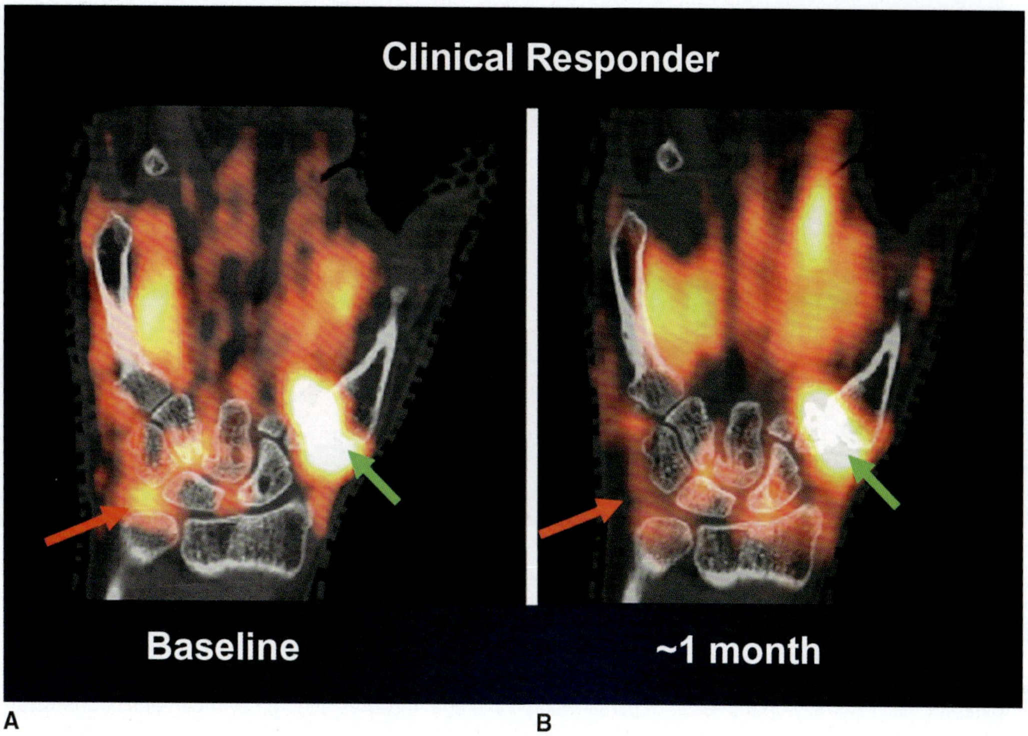

Figure 2.73 ■ 18F-FDG PET/CT evaluation of response of rheumatoid arthritis to treatment. A: Coronal fused PET/CT image of the wrist of a 49-year-old woman with rheumatoid arthritis (same patient as depicted in *Fig. 2.71*) shows increased accumulation of the 18F-FDG radiotracer at sites of multiple osseous erosions including triquetropisiform joint (*red arrow*). There is also increased metabolic activity in the first carpometacarpal joint due to osteoarthritis (*green arrow*). **B:** Coronal PET/CT fused image of the wrist obtained after 1 month of treatment with tumor necrosis factor (TNF)-alpha inhibitor (etanercept) shows significant reduction in signal at the sites of inflammatory arthritis (*red arrow*), suggesting reduced inflammation in the synovium. Note lack of improvement at the site of osteoarthritis (*green arrow*).

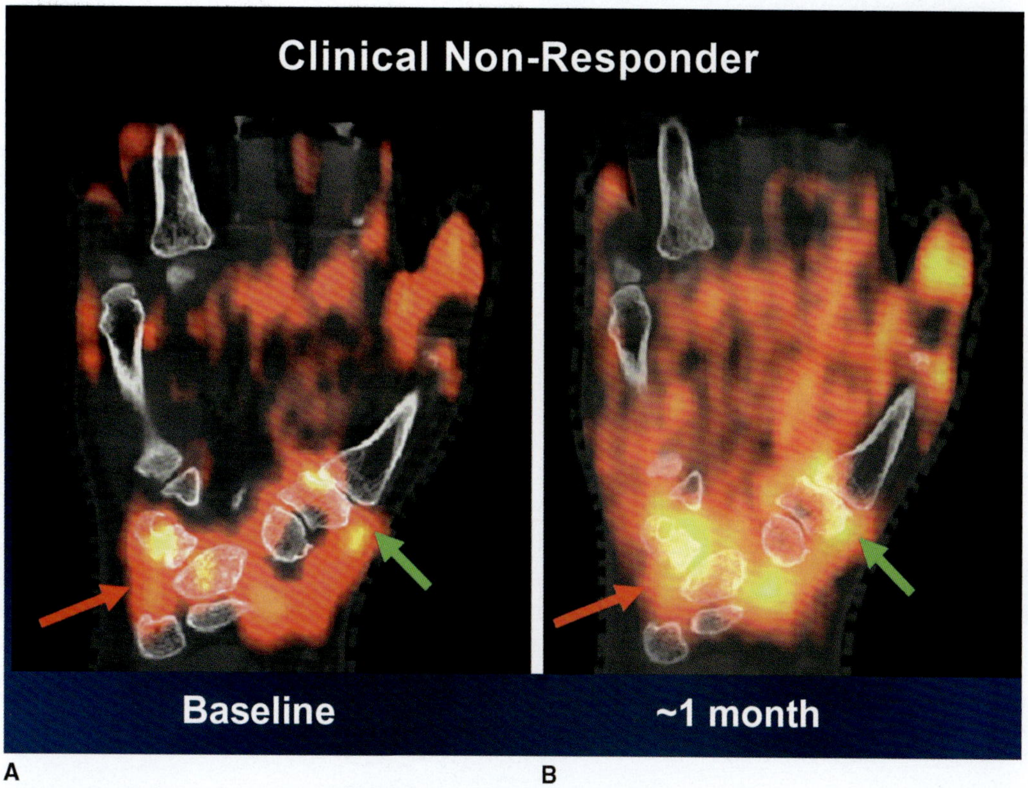

Figure 2.74 ■ 18F-FDG PET/CT evaluation of response of rheumatoid arthritis to treatment. A: Coronal fused PET/CT image of the wrist of 63-year-old woman with rheumatoid arthritis shows high metabolic activity at the sites of synovitis in the carpal joints (*red* and *green arrows*). **B:** Same image obtained after 1 month of treatment with TNF-alpha inhibitor shows further increase in metabolic activity (*red* and *green arrows*) indicating lack of response to therapy.

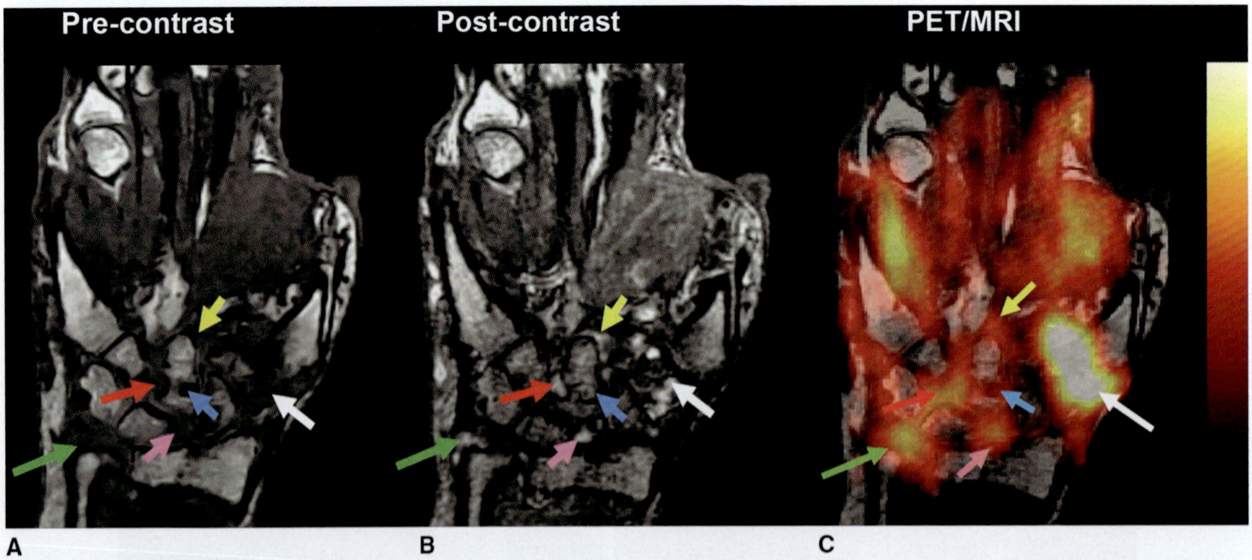

Figure 2.75 ■ **18F-FDG PET/MRI of rheumatoid arthritis and osteoarthritis. A:** Coronal T1-weighted MRI of the left wrist of a 49-year-old woman (same patient as depicted in *Fig. 2.71*) shows erosions of multiple joints (*colored arrows*). The *white arrow* points to osteoarthritis of the first carpometacarpal (CMC) joint. **B:** On the coronal T1-weighted fat-suppressed MR image obtained after intravenous administration of gadolinium, there is increased signal intensity at the site of erosions (*colored arrows*). **C:** Fused PET/MRI image shows increased metabolic activity at the site of erosions (*colored arrows*) and at the site of OA (*white arrow*). The significantly increased activity at the first CMC osteoarthritic joint may be the result of partial volume average, the sites affected by rheumatoid arthritis being smaller in size.

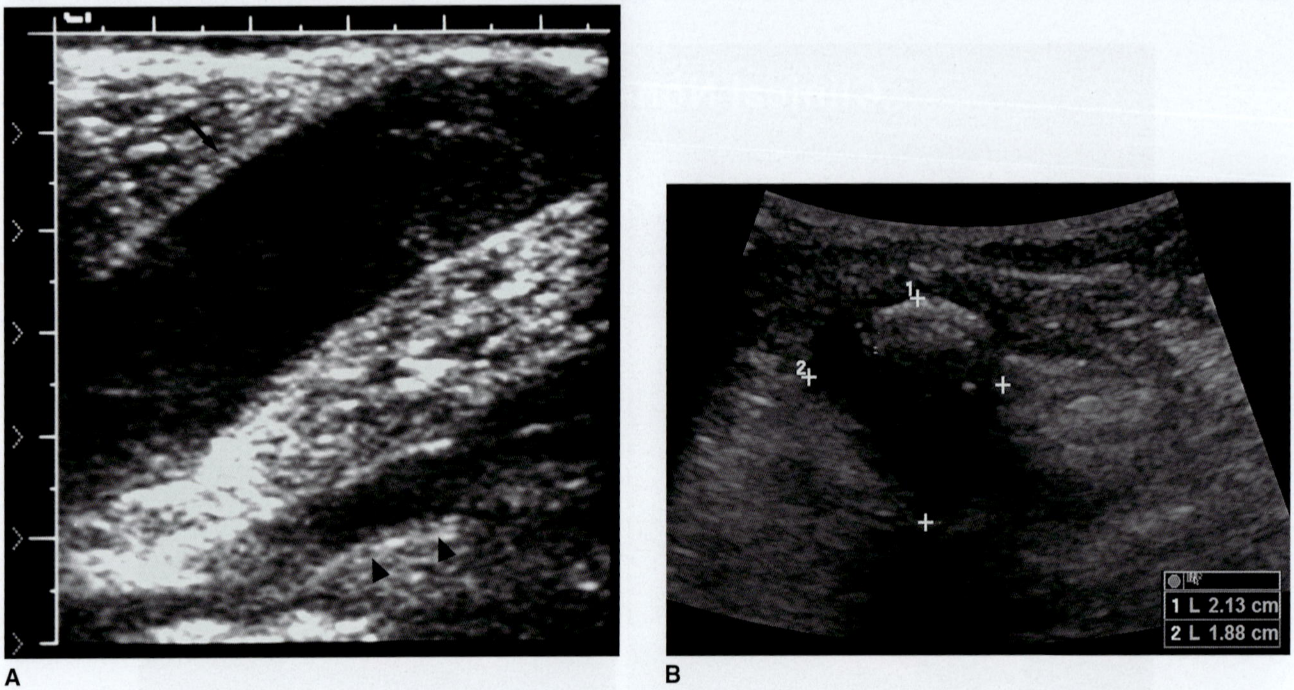

Figure 2.76 ■ **Ultrasound of the popliteal cyst. A:** A 45-year-old woman with clinically documented rheumatoid arthritis presented with pain in the back of the knee radiating to the leg. Clinically, deep vein thrombosis (DVT) was suspected and US was performed. The study was negative for DVT but demonstrated a large fluid-filled Baker cyst (*arrow*). The *arrowheads* point to the patent popliteal vein. **B:** US of the popliteal fossa performed in a 51-year-old woman with osteoarthritis of the left knee shows a Baker cyst.

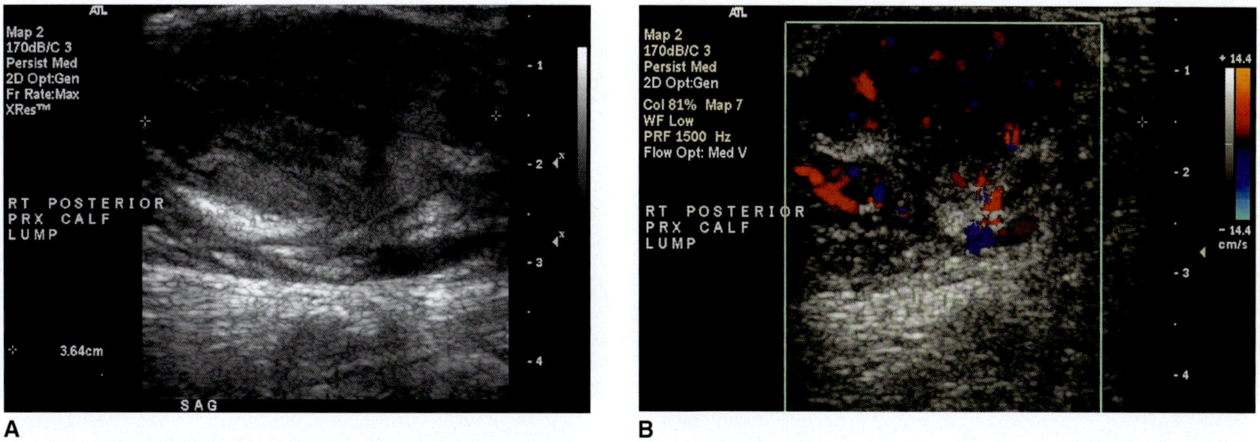

Figure 2.77 ■ **Ultrasound of the ruptured popliteal cyst.** A 41-year-old woman presented with a painful mass in the popliteal region. Color-flow US shows portion of the intact Baker cyst with hyperechoic heterogeneous fluid collection **(A)** and the site of chronic rupture of this cyst **(B)** associated with internal debris, secondary inflammatory changes, and hypervascularity.

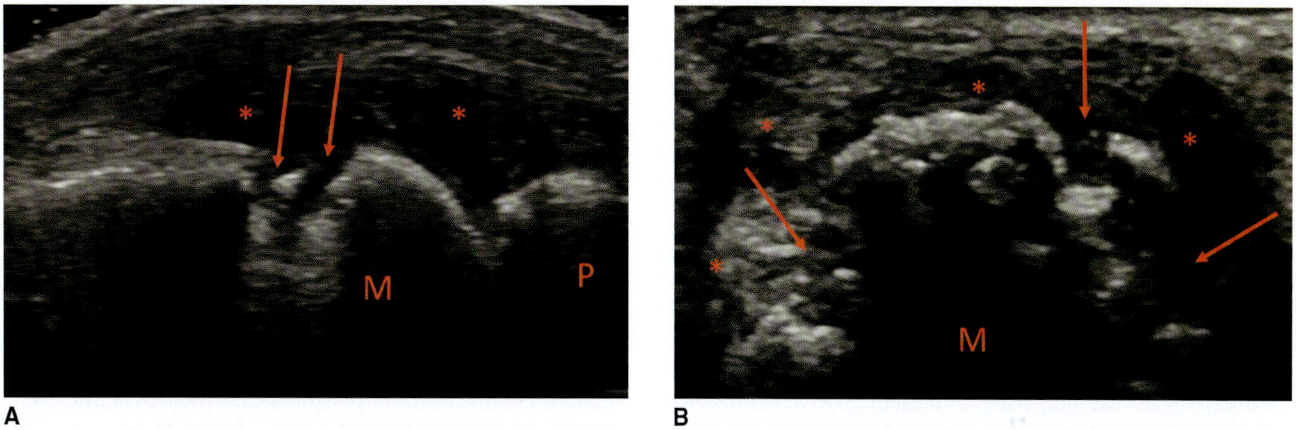

Figure 2.78 ■ **Ultrasound of erosions. A:** Image in the longitudinal plane of the hand in a patient with rheumatoid arthritis demonstrates erosion in the dorsoradial aspect of the second metacarpal head *(arrows)*. M, metacarpal head; P, proximal phalanx of the index finger; asterisks, synovitis and effusion. **B:** Image in the transverse plane of the wrist in another patient with rheumatoid arthritis shows large erosions at the base of the third metacarpal bone (*arrows*) associated with synovitis (*asterisks*). M, 3rd metacarpal bone.

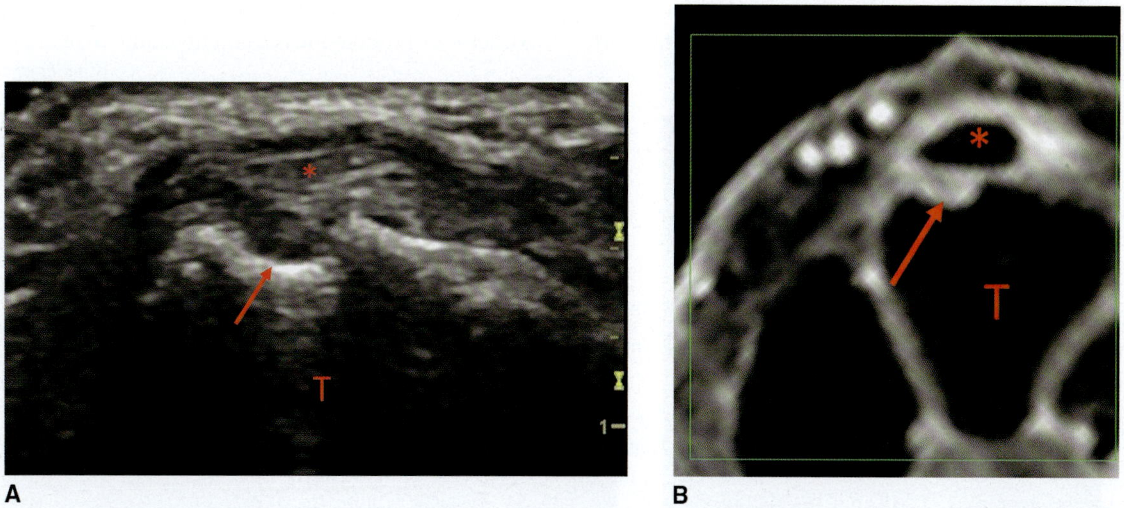

Figure 2.79 ■ **Ultrasound and MRI of erosion.** The US image **(A)** and companion 3D water excitation spoiled gradient-echo (SPGR) MRI **(B)** of the wrist of a patient with rheumatoid arthritis show erosion (*arrow*) in the dorsal aspect of the triquetral bone (T). The extensor carpi ulnaris tendon (*asterisks*) overlies the erosion.

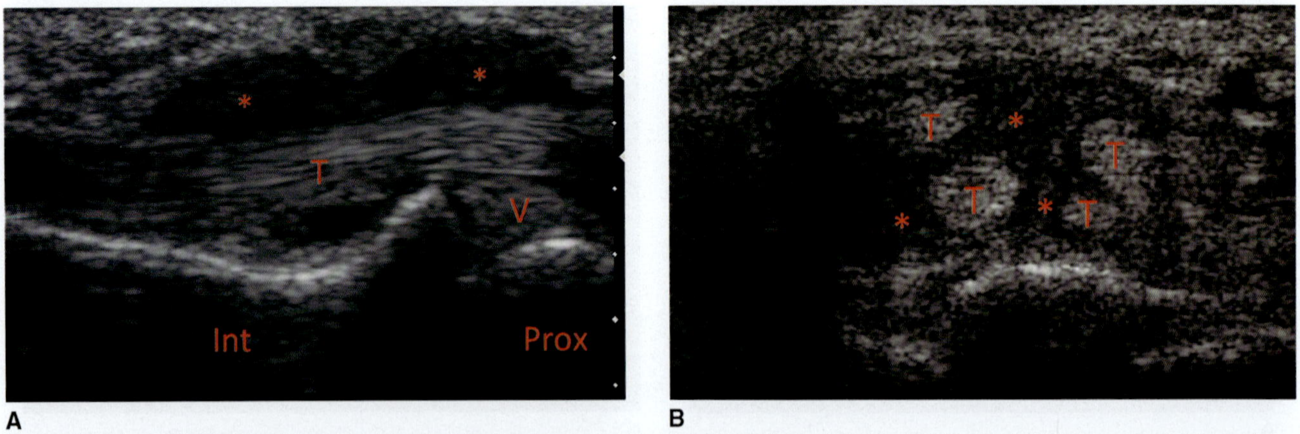

Figure 2.80 ■ **Ultrasound of flexor tenosynovitis. A:** Image in the longitudinal plane at the level of the proximal interphalangeal joint of the index finger of a woman with rheumatoid arthritis shows low reflective synovitis (*asterisks*) surrounding the flexor digitorum profunda tendon (T). Int, intermediate phalanx; Prox, proximal phalangeal head; V, volar plate. **B:** In another patient with rheumatoid arthritis, the synovitis surrounding the flexor tendons within the carpal tunnel is seen as low reflective change around the tendons. T, flexor tendons; asterisks, synovitis.

(e.g., popliteal artery aneurysm) (see Figs. 2.76 and 2.77). It also can demonstrate the presence of foci of hydroxyapatite crystals (calcific tendinopathy) (Fig. 2.82) and chondrocalcinosis (Fig. 2.83).

More recently, US techniques such as Doppler US or color-flow imaging, which expresses speed and direction of blood flow in the vessels in color, have found limited application in musculoskeletal imaging. Color Doppler US is a method in which direction and velocity information is interpreted and encoded into the gray-scale image as a color signal. In this mode the color hue is assigned based on the velocity of the moving reflectors. This modality is used mainly to detect arterial narrowing and deep venous thrombosis, occasionally seen in patients with rheumatoid arthritis (Figs. 2.84 and 2.85), although some investigators have explored the use of power Doppler US in the evaluation of rheumatoid synovitis and some complications of rheumatoid arthritis, such as superimposed infection of the soft tissues (cellulitis) (Fig. 2.86). Doppler flow signal is an excellent marker for disease activity in rheumatoid arthritis. It can directly assess the hyperemic blood flow within the inflammatory joint. One of the advantages of this technique is its ability to serve as a responsive indicator and predictor of therapeutic outcome in rheumatologic disorders. Intensity of Doppler signals decreases significantly with anti–tumor necrotic factor (TNF)-alpha, soluble TNF-alpha receptor etanercept, and corticosteroids treatment. More recently, intravenous microbubble (small, typically 3 μm in diameter gas-filled bubbles with perfluorocarbon or nitrogen gas) contrast agents were introduced to increase the sensitivity of detecting tissue vascularity by power Doppler technique, hence creating an even a stronger potential for monitoring the response to therapy.

The newest development in this area is introduction of 3D (actually, because of added real-time dynamic component, "four-dimensional") US. Three-dimensional US provides functional utility in the evaluation of the joints by adding a craniocaudal projection (revolving spatial image). The important advantage of this technique is not only the acquisition of images in real time but also subsequent reconstruction and viewing at a workstation, allowing further manipulation of the volume image. This permits the extraction of usable measurements and enhancement of the

(Continued on page 75)

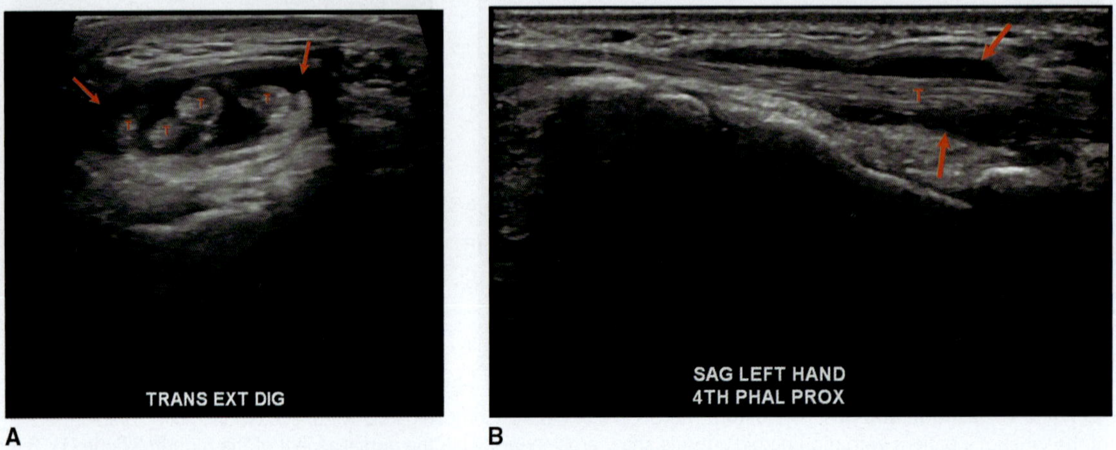

Figure 2.81 ■ **Ultrasound of extensors tenosynovitis. A:** Image in the transverse plane of the left wrist shows fluid (*arrows*) surrounding the thickened extensor tendons (*T*). **B:** Image in the sagittal plane shows lobulated fluid *(arrows)* tracking along the thickened extensor digitorum tendon of the ring finger (*T*).

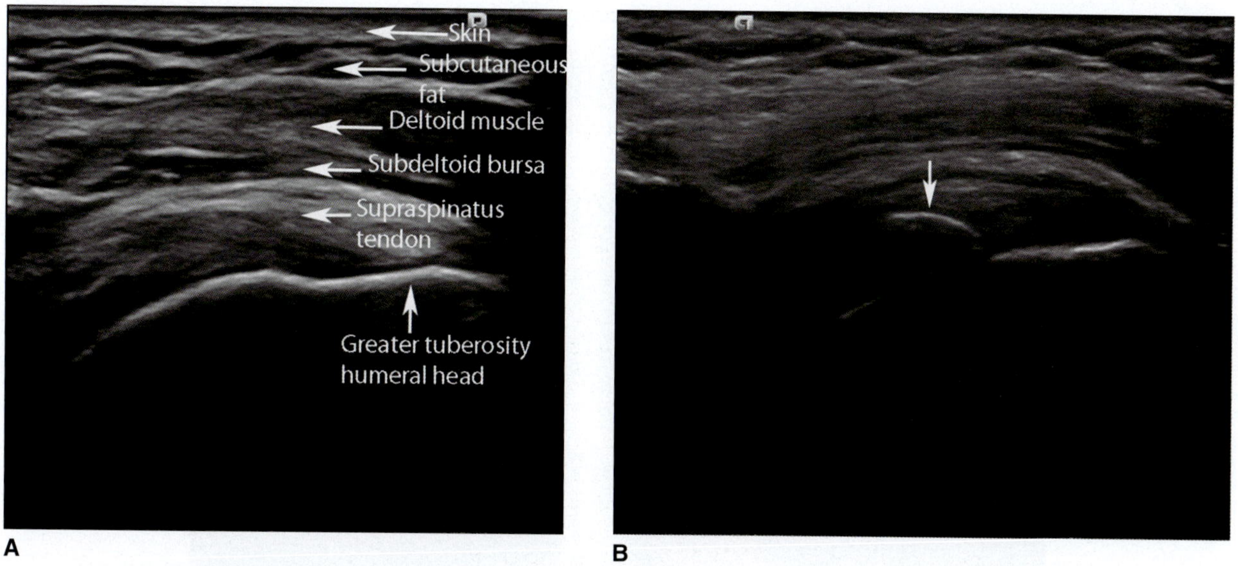

Figure 2.82 ■ Ultrasound of calcific tendinopathy. A: Longitudinal scan over the shoulder shows the anatomic structures including the attachment of the supraspinatus tendon to the greater tuberosity of the humerus. **B:** In another patient, the longitudinal scan shows curvilinear echogenic focus with acoustic shadowing (*arrow*) secondary to intrasubstance deposition of calcium hydroxyapatite crystals within the supraspinatus tendon, consistent with calcific tendinopathy.

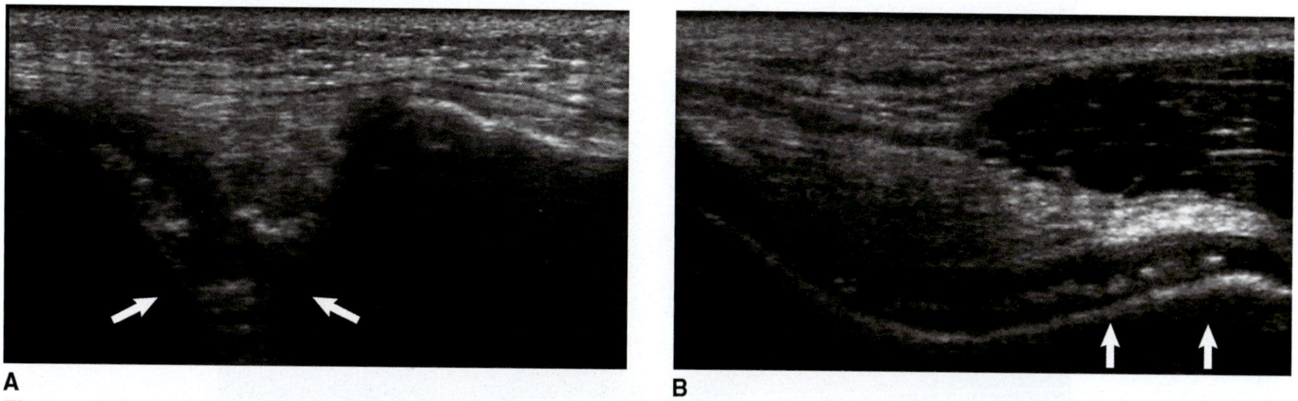

Figure 2.83 ■ Ultrasound of chondrocalcinosis. A: Longitudinal scan over the knee shows calcifications of the medial meniscus (*arrows*). **B:** Transverse scan shows calcifications within the articular cartilage of the medial femoral condyle (*arrows*).

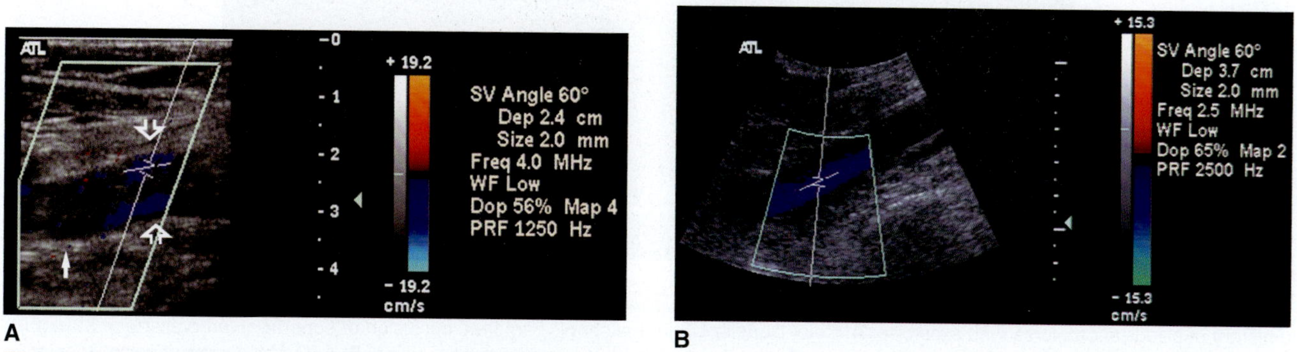

Figure 2.84 ■ Ultrasound of deep vein thrombosis. A 76-year-old man with history of rheumatoid arthritis presented with a chronic pain in the left lower extremity. **A:** Color Doppler image of the popliteal fossa shows hypoechoic area in the popliteal vein (*arrow*) representing an intraluminal thrombus. More proximately noted is diminished blood flow around the blood clot (*arrows*). **B:** A normal color Doppler US image of the opposite (*right*) popliteal fossa is shown for comparison.

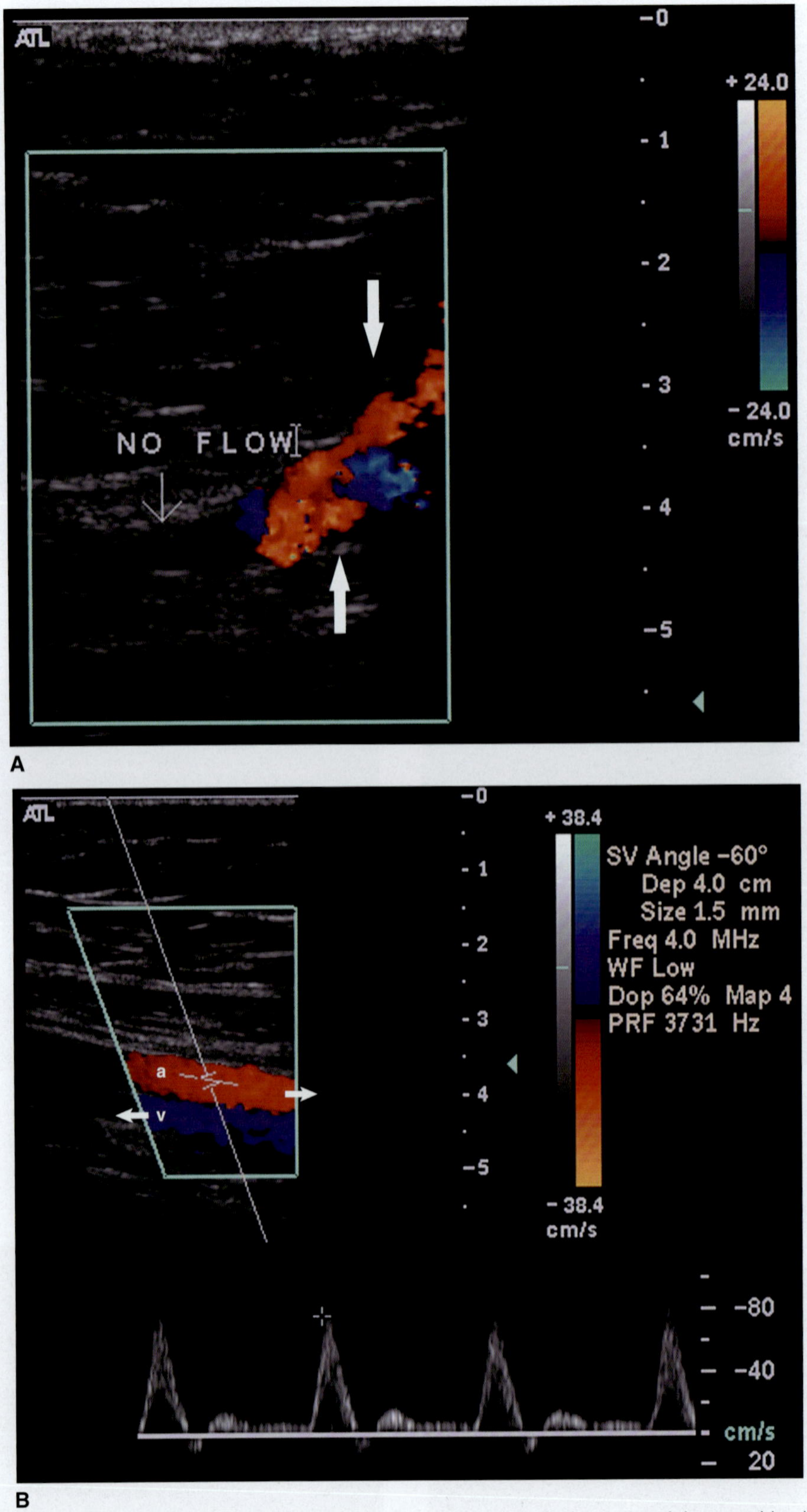

Figure 2.85 ■ **Ultrasound of arterial occlusion.** A 67-year-old woman with clinically documented rheumatoid arthritis presented with a history of claudication worse with excercise. **A:** Color Doppler US image shows complete occlusion of superficial femoral artery. Stream turbulence (*white thick arrows*) is compatible with hemodynamically significant stenosis or occlusion. **B:** A normal color and pulse Doppler image is shown for comparison. The *arrows* indicate the direction the blood flow in a vein (*v*) and artery (*a*).

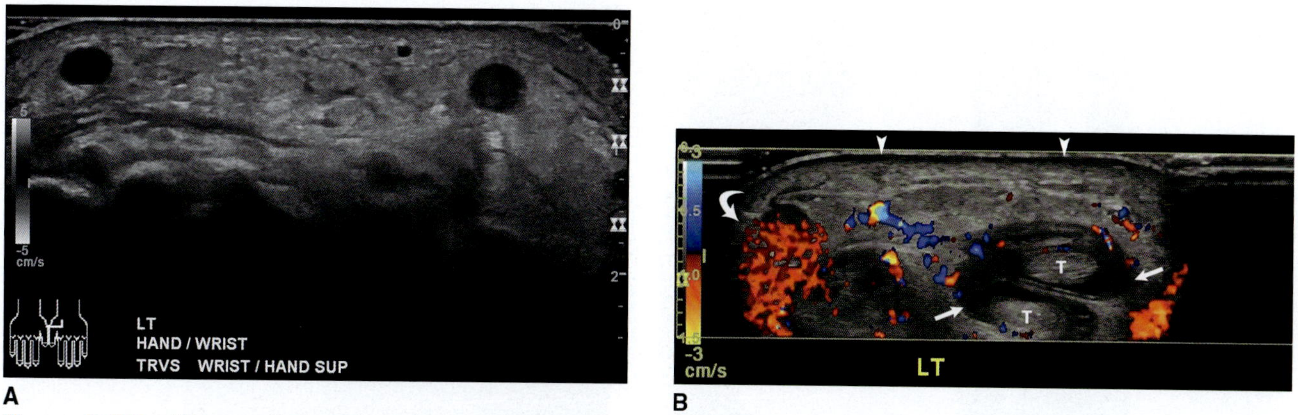

A B

Figure 2.86 ■ Ultrasound of tenosynovitis and cellulitis. Transverse **(A)** gray-scale and **(B)** color-flow US of the left wrist of a 66-year-old woman with rheumatoid arthritis shows subcutaneous edema and increased echogenicity with "cobble-stone" appearance (*arrowheads*) consistent with cellulitis. Note also increased vascularity (*curved arrow*) and thickening of the extensor tendons and synovitis (*arrows*).

anatomic information obtained from the images. Because this technology provides a global perspective, it facilitates defining the extent of tendinopathies, articular erosions, and synovial inflammatory activity.

MAGNETIC RESONANCE IMAGING (MRI)

MRI is based on the re-emission of an absorbed radiofrequency (rf) signal while the patient is in a strong magnetic field. An external magnetic field is usually generated by a magnet with field strength of 0.2 (Tesla) to 3.0 T. The system includes a magnet, rf coils (transmitter and receiver), gradient coils, and computer display unit with digital storage facilities. The detailed physical principles of MRI cannot be discussed here because of space limitation, and only a brief overview is given.

The ability of MRI to image body parts depends on the intrinsic spin of atomic nuclei with an odd number of protons and/or neutrons (e.g., hydrogen), thus generating a magnetic moment. Atomic nuclei of tissues placed within the main magnetic field, from the usual random alignment of their magnetic poles, tend to align along the direction of that field. The application of rf pulses causes the nuclei to absorb energy and induces resonance of particular sets of nuclei, which results in their orientation to the magnetic field. The required frequency of the pulse is determined by the strength of the magnetic field and the particular nucleus undergoing investigation. When the rf field is removed, the energy absorbed during the transition from a high- to low-energy state is subsequently released, and this can be recorded as an electrical signal, which provides data from which digital images are derived. Signal intensity refers to the strength of the radio wave that a tissue emits after excitation. The strength of the radio wave determines the degree of brightness of the imaged structures. A bright (white) area in an image is said to demonstrate high signal intensity, whereas a dark (black) area is said to demonstrate low signal intensity. The intensity of a given tissue is a function of the concentration of hydrogen atoms (protons) resonating within the imaged volume and of the longitudinal and transverse relaxation times, which, in turn, depend on the biophysical state of the tissue's water molecules.

Two relaxation times are described, termed T1 and T2. The T1 relaxation time (longitudinal) is used to describe the return of protons back to equilibrium after the application and removal of the rf pulse. T2 relaxation time (transverse) is used to describe the associated loss of coherence or phase between individual protons immediately after the application of the rf pulse. A variety of rf pulse sequences can be used to enhance the differences in T1 and T2, thus providing the necessary image contrast. The most commonly used sequences are spin echo (SE), inversion recovery (IR), chemical selective suppression (CHESS), and fast scan (FS) technique. SE short repetition time (TR) (800 msec or less) and short echo delay time (TE) (40 msec or less) pulse sequence (or T1) provide good anatomic detail (Fig. 2.87A). Intermediate TR (1,000 msec or more) and short TE (30 msec or less) sequences are known as proton or spin density images. They represent a mixture of T1 and T2 weighting, and although they provide good anatomic details, the tissue contrast is somewhat impaired (Fig. 2.87B). Long TR (2,000 msec or more) and long TE (60 msec or more) pulse sequence (or T2), also known as water-sensitive sequence, provides good contrast, sufficient for the evaluation of pathologic processes (Fig. 2.87C). Occasionally multiplanar gradient recalled (MPGR) sequences are used, which represent fast gradient echo sequences with slice-selective rf pulses. This family of pulse sequences was originally developed to obtain T2-weighted images in less time than with conventional spin echo technique. With low flip angle, long echo time, and long repetition time, they are termed T2*-weighted pulse sequences, and they heighten sensitivity to susceptibility effects (artifactual signal loss at the interface between tissues of widely different magnetic properties, such as metal and soft tissues). T2* weighting is particular effective in depicting paramagnetic deoxyhemoglobin, methemoglobin, and hemosiderin in the tissues, as well as in adequately demonstrating the ligaments, articular cartilage, and fibrocartilaginous structures such as glenoid labrum or knee menisci (Fig. 2.87D).

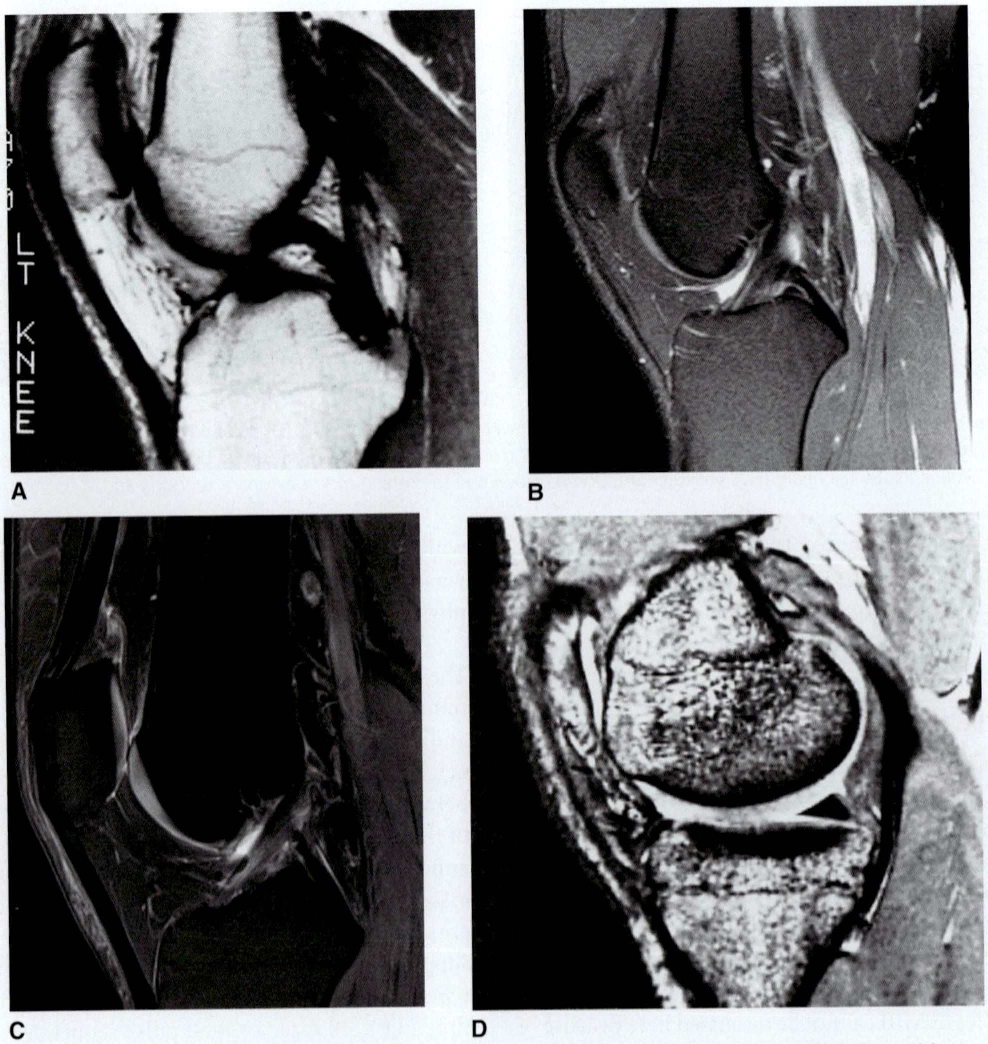

Figure 2.87 ■ Magnetic resonance imaging (MRI) sequences. A: Sagittal SE T1-weighted (TR 600/TE 20 msec) image. **B:** Sagittal PD-weighted fat-suppressed (TR 1500/TE 30 msec) image. **C:** Sagittal T2-weighted (TR 2500/TE 80 msec) image. **D:** Sagittal MPGR T2*-weighted (flip angle 30 degrees, TR 35/TE 15 msec) image. The various anatomic structures of the knee are clearly depicted because of variations in signal intensity of bone, articular cartilage, fibrocartilage, ligaments, muscles, fat, and fluid.

Inversion recovery (IR) sequences can be combined with multiplanar imaging to shorten scan time. With a short inversion time (TI), in the range of 100 to 150 msec, the effects of prolonged T1 and T2 relaxation times are cumulative and the signal from fat is suppressed. This technique, called short tau IR (STIR), has been useful for evaluating musculoskeletal tumors. Fat suppression technique is commonly used in MRI to detect adipose tissue or suppress the signal from fat (Fig. 2.88, see also Fig. 2.87B). There are three methods to achieve this goal: frequency-selective (chemical) fat saturation, inversion recovery imaging, and opposed-phase imaging (Table 2.1). One of the indications for fat suppression is the assessment of small amounts of bone marrow edema in the subchondral bone, often accompanying osteochondral pathology, such as in osteochondritis dissecans or osteonecrosis.

The musculoskeletal system is ideally suited for the evaluation by MRI because different tissues display different signal intensities on T1- and T2-weighted images. The images displayed may have a low signal intensity, intermediate signal intensity, or high signal intensity. Low signal intensity may be subdivided into signal void (black) and signal lower than

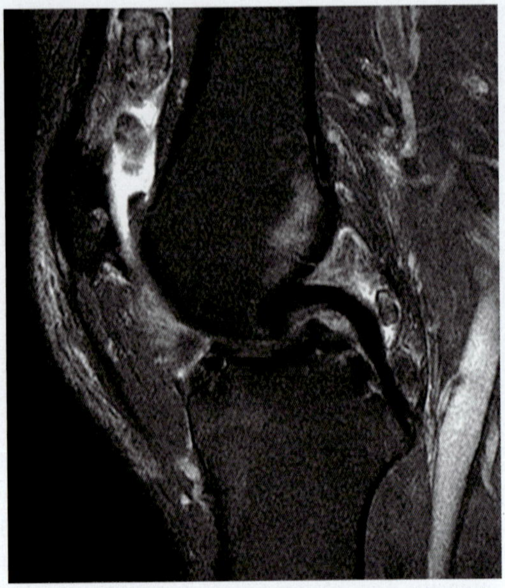

Figure 2.88 ■ MRI fat-suppressed sequence. Sagittal T2-weighted fat-suppressed image of the knee shows several intra-articular osteochondral bodies in this 67-year-old woman with osteoarthritis.

Table 2.1 FAT SUPPRESSION TECHNIQUES

Methods	Advantages	Disadvantages
Frequency-selective (chemical) fat saturation	Lipid specific Signal in nonfat tissue unaffected Excellent imaging of small anatomic detail Can be used with any imaging sequence	Occasionally inadequate fat suppression Water signal may be suppressed Heterogeneities in areas of sharp variations in anatomic structures Increased imaging time
Inversion recovery (STIR)	Excellent contrast resolution Very good for tumor detection Can be used with low-field-strength magnets	Low signal-to-noise ratio Tissue with a short T1 and long T1 may produce the same signal intensity Signal from mucoid tissue, hemorrhage, and proteinaceous fluid may be suppressed
Opposed-phase	Ability to demonstrate small amounts of lipid tissue Simple, fast, and available on every MRI system	Fat signal only partially suppressed Suppresses water signal Difficult to detect small tumors imbedded in fat In postgadolinium studies, contrast material may be undetected

STIR, short time inversion recovery; MRI, magnetic resonance imaging.

that of normal muscle (dark). Intermediate signal intensity may be subdivided into signal equal to that of normal muscle and signal higher than that of muscle but lower than that of subcutaneous fat. High signal intensity may be subdivided into that equal to subcutaneous fat (bright) and signal higher than that of fat (extremely bright). High signal intensity of fat planes and differences in the signal intensities of various anatomic structures allow the separation of the different tissue components including muscles, tendons, ligaments, vessels, nerves, hyaline cartilage, fibrocartilage, cortical bone, and trabecular bone (see Fig. 2.87). For instance, fat and yellow (fatty) bone marrow display high signal intensity on T1-weighted images and intermediate signal on T2-weighted images; hematomas (acute or subacute) display relatively high signal intensity on T1- and T2-weighted sequences. Cortical bone, air, ligaments, tendons, and fibrocartilage display low signal intensity on both T1- and T2-weighted images. Red (hematopoietic) bone marrow displays low signal on T1-weighted images and low-to-intermediate signal on T2 weighting. Fluid displays intermediate signal on T1-weighted images and high signal on T2-weighted images (Table 2.2). Traumatic conditions of the bones and soft tissues are particularly well suited to the

Table 2.2 MAGNETIC RESONANCE IMAGING SIGNAL INTENSITIES OF VARIOUS TISSUES

	Image	
Tissue	T1-Weighted	T2-Weighted
Hematoma, hemorrhage (acute, subacute)	Intermediate/high	High
Hematoma, hemorrhage (chronic)	Low	Low
Fat, fatty marrow	High	Intermediate
Muscle, nerves, hyaline cartilage	Intermediate	Intermediate
Cortical bone, tendons, ligaments, fibrocartilage, scar tissue	Low	Low
Hyaline cartilage	Intermediate	Intermediate
Red (hematopoietic) marrow	Low	Intermediate
Air	Low	Low
Fluid	Intermediate	High
Proteinaceous fluid	High	High
Tumors (generally)	Intermediate to low	High
Lipoma	High	Intermediate
Hemangioma	Intermediate (slightly higher than muscle)	High

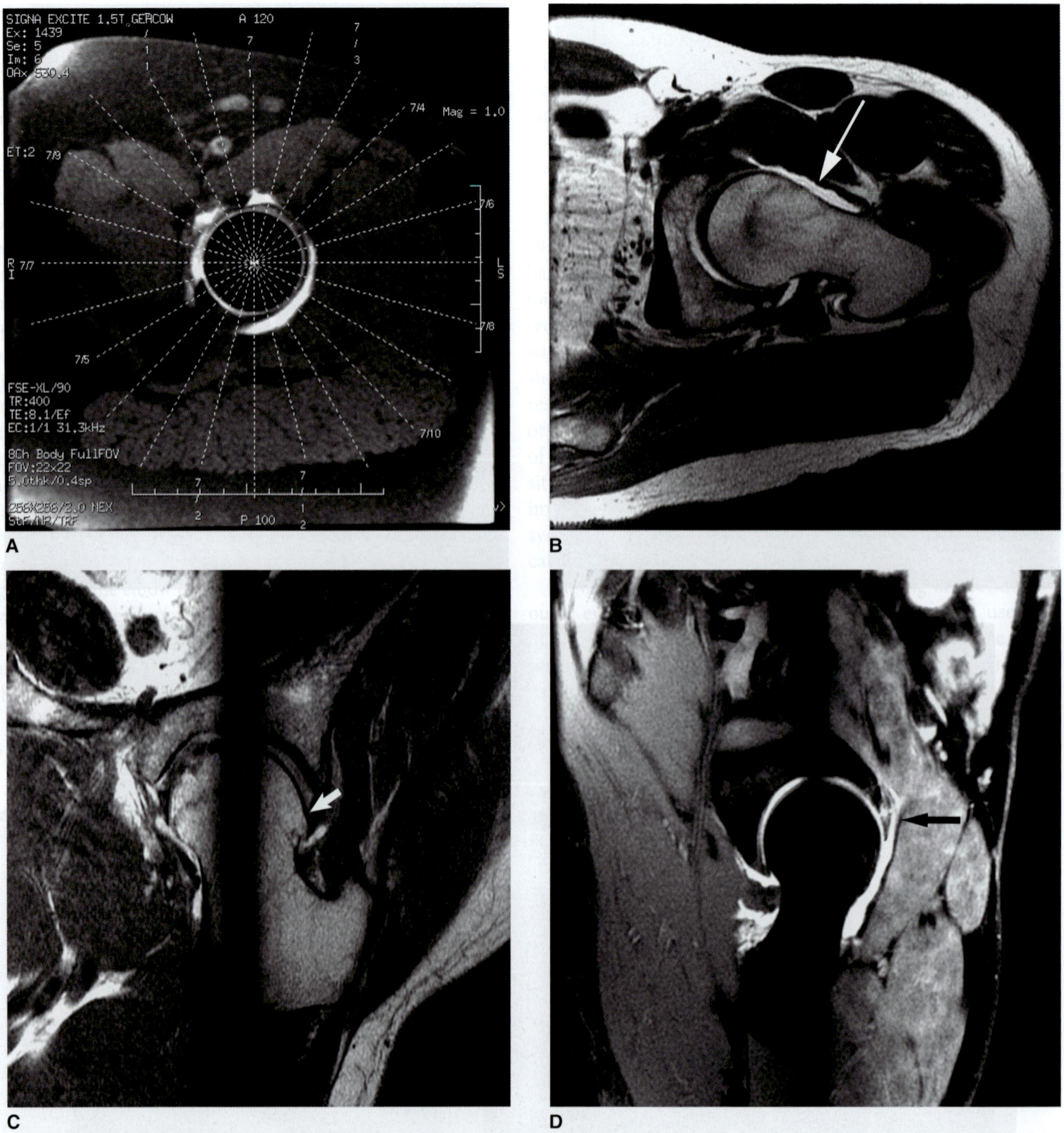

Figure 2.91 ■ **MR arthrography of the femoroacetabular impingement syndrome.** A 28-year-old man presented with a left hip and groin pain for several months. Conventional radiographs (not shown here) were highly suggestive of a cam-type FAI syndrome, confirmed on radial MR arthrography. **A:** Prescription of the radial plane images off the oblique axial en face image of the acetabulum. **B:** Transverse oblique FSE T1-weighted MR image obtained through the center of the femoral neck shows nonspherical shape of the femoral head and excessive bone formation at the anterosuperior aspect of the head/neck junction (*arrow*). **C:** The radial reformatted PD-weighted MR image shows a prominent osteophyte (*arrow*). **D:** Oblique axial PD-weighted fat-suppressed radial image shows a tear of the superior acetabular labrum (*arrow*).

Interest in measuring specific structural and biochemical components of the cartilage has led to such techniques as T2 mapping, ultrashort echo time (UTE) imaging, diffusion-weighted imaging (DWI), T1 in the rotating frame (T1 rho) imaging, and sodium (^{23}Na) MRI. Because sodium-23 atoms are associated with negatively charged glycosaminoglycan (GAG), loss of GAG due to cartilage degeneration results in loss of sodium ions from the tissue. That mechanism provides the basis for the latter technique, which proved to be effective in assessing the loss of proteoglycan (PG) molecules from the cartilage matrix in very early stages of osteoarthritis (Fig. 2.94). A novel approach to the assessment of

(Continued on page 82)

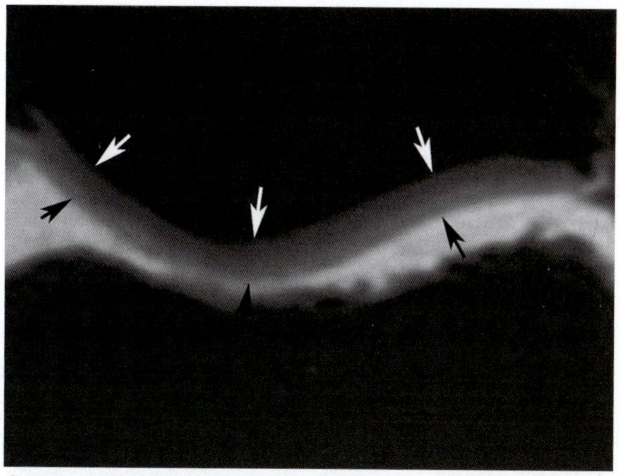

A

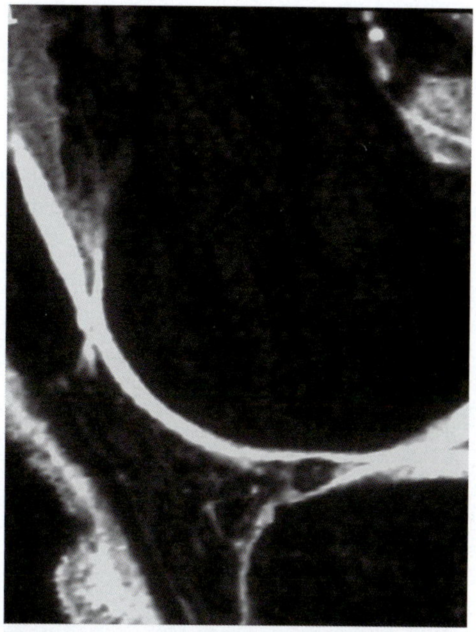

B

Figure 2.92 ■ FLASH MRI of the articular cartilage. **A:** Axial 2D FT FLASH. Note the hyaline articular cartilage of the patella (*arrows*) in contrast with the joint fluid. **B:** Sagittal 3D FT fat-saturated FLASH. Note the contrast between the bright articular cartilage and the adjacent infrapatellar fat, allowing excellent visualization of the articular surface.

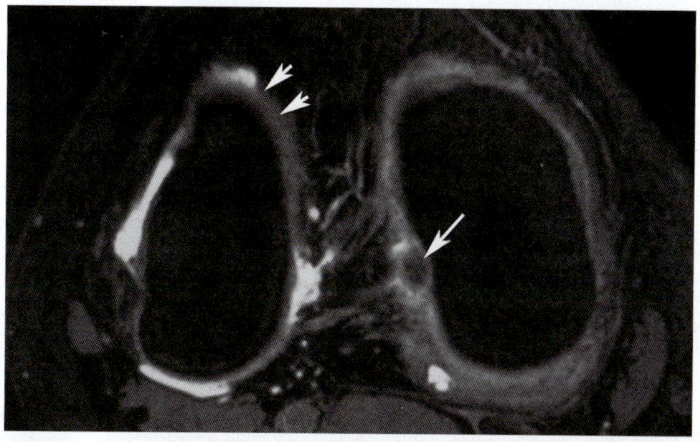

Figure 2.93 ■ DESS MRI of the articular cartilage. Axial DESS pulse sequence demonstrates a displaced fragment of medial meniscus (*long arrow*). Note the contrast between the joint fluid and the articular hyaline cartilage in the lateral femoral condyle (*short arrows*).

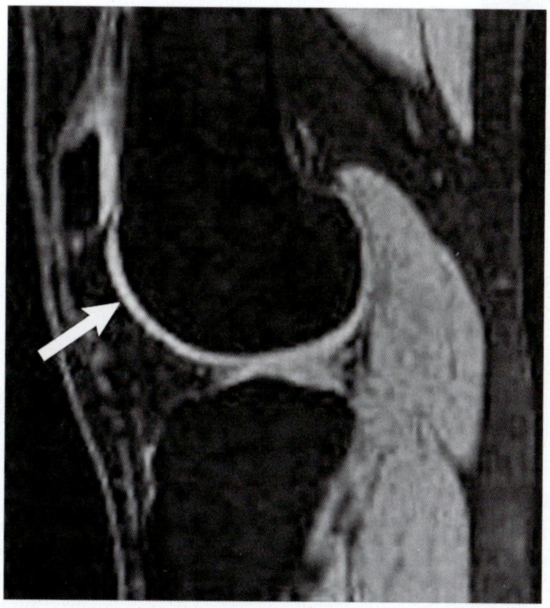

A

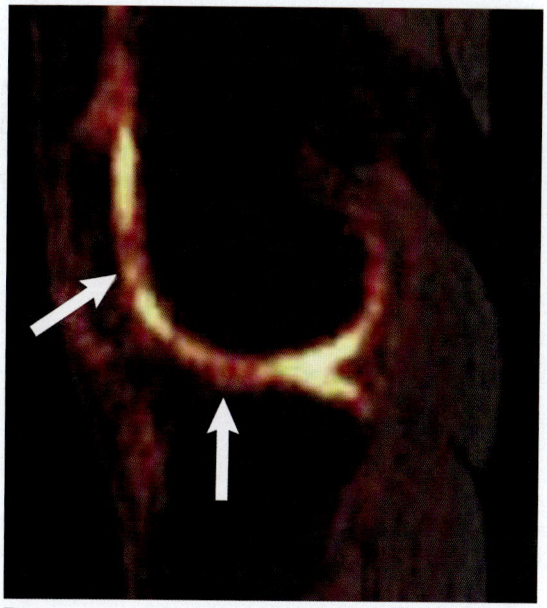

B

Figure 2.94 ■ Sodium-23 MRI of the articular cartilage. **A:** 2D sagittal proton density–weighted fast spin echo (FSE) MR image of the knee shows normal articular cartilage of the distal femur (*arrow*). **B:** Same knee examined with Sodium-23 (^{23}Na) FLASH proton density–weighted MRI demonstrates a focal loss of glycosaminoglycen (GAG) (*arrows*) consistent with early osteoarthritis.

biochemical changes within a morphologically intact cartilage is a contrast agent–based technique known as delayed gadolinium-enhanced MRI of cartilage (dGEMRIC). This technique measures the T1 variations within the cartilage following intravenous administration of negatively charged Gd-DTPA and provides information regarding cartilage glycosaminoglycan content (Fig. 2.95). The newest improvement in the evaluation of articular cartilage of the knee is the introduction of so-called vastly undersampled isotropic projection steady-state free precession (VIPR-SSFP) imaging pulse sequence, which combines a balanced SSFP technique with 3D radial multiplanar image acquisition. In addition to providing important clinical information regarding the cartilage, this technique is also effective in the evaluation of the ligaments, menisci, and osseous structures of the knee in symptomatic patients. Fluctuating equilibrium MR (FEMR)

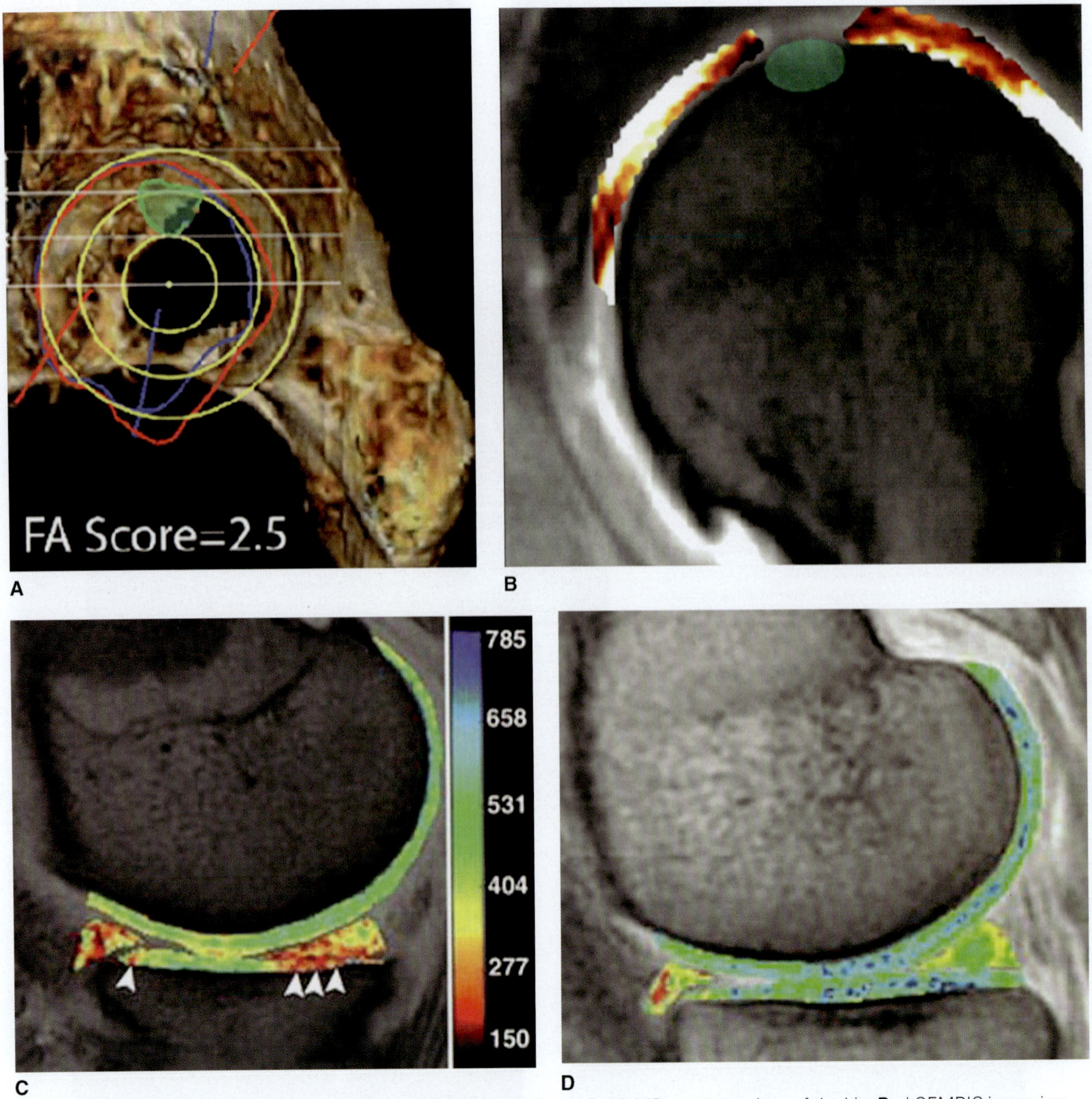

Figure 2.95 ■ **MRI of the articular cartilage—d-GEMRIC technique. A:** 3D MR reconstructions of the hip. **B:** d-GEMRIC image in a patient with hip dysplasia. The 3D reconstructions are generated from MR data obtained during a conventional MRI of the hip. These 3D models are used to assess the osseous morphologic abnormalities that can occur along the surfaces of the acetabulum and femoral head. The d-GEMRIC parametric maps are generated from MR data obtained during intravenous administration of gadolinium contrast. **C:** In another patient, sagittal MR image of the knee using d-GEMRIC technique shows cartilage changes typical of osteoarthritis (*arrowheads*). **D:** Normal appearance of the knee using the same technique is shown for comparison.

is a variant of SSFP, a technique that by rendering a bright fluid signal while preserving cartilage signal is also useful in cartilage imaging. Finally, it is worthy to mention the most recent trials of cartilage imaging using Fourier transform infrared microscopy (FTIR-MS), a method based on the absorption of infrared light by molecules at characteristic frequencies, which yielded very promising results.

As one can see from the previous discussion, MRI of the joints provides excellent contrast between soft tissues and bone. Articular cartilage, fibrocartilage, cortex, and spongy bone can be distinguished from each other by their specific signal intensities. It is an excellent modality for demonstrating the rheumatoid nodules and synovial abnormalities in patients with rheumatoid arthritis. MRI's ability to contrast the synovium-covered joint from other soft tissue structures allows for noninvasive delineation of the degree of synovial hypertrophy that accompanies synovitis, previously demonstrable only by means of arthrography or arthroscopy. Because synovitis is often accompanied by joint effusion, this too can be effectively demonstrated by MRI (Fig. 2.96). In particular, when this technique is combined with intravenous administration of Gd-DTPA, it is highly effective in the differentiation between fluid-filled joints and tendon sheaths from synovitis. Both fluid and intra-articular synovial tissue exhibit intermediate signal intensity on T1-weighted images and a high signal on T2 weighting. However, gadolinium-enhanced T1-weighted images will show high-intensity signal of inflammatory pannus/synovial tissue, whereas fluid will not enhance (Figs. 2.97 and 2.98). MRI is also quite helpful in diagnosing Baker cyst (Fig. 2.99). Occasionally, MRI may provide some additional information on osteoarthritis (Fig. 2.100) and hemophilic arthropathy (Fig. 2.101). With the development of more sophisticated orthopedic methods for cartilage repair in osteoarthritis, such as new articular cartilage replacement techniques including chondrocyte

(Continued on page 87)

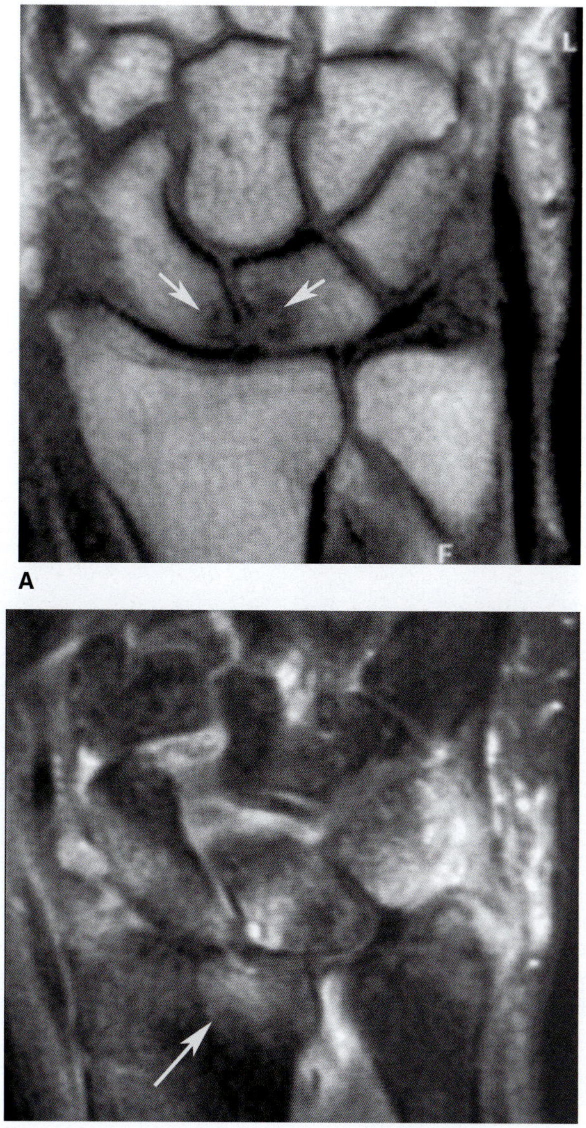

A

B

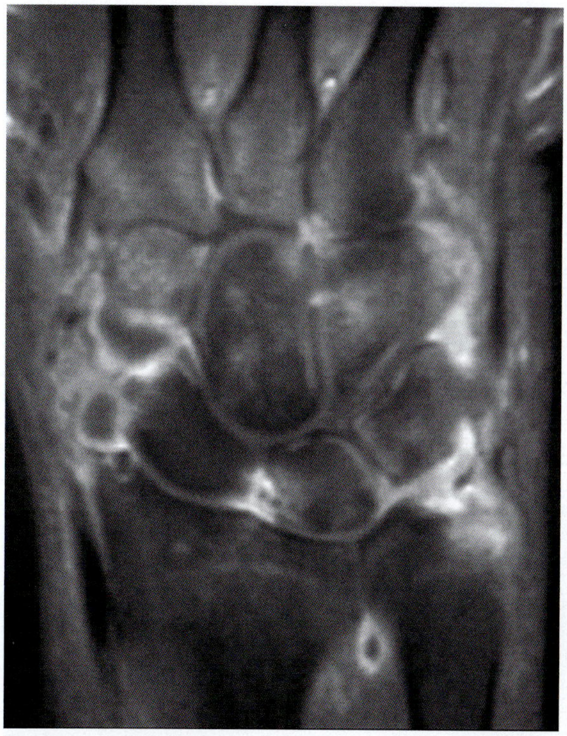

C

Figure 2.96 ■ **MRI of rheumatoid arthritis.** Conventional radiographs (not shown here) showed questionable erosions in the scaphoid and lunate bones. **A:** Coronal T1-weighted MRI confirms the presence of scaphoid and lunate erosions (*arrows*). **B:** Coronal short time inversion recovery (STIR) MRI demonstrates additionally extensive bone marrow edema of the entire proximal carpal row, ulnar styloid process, and distal radius (*arrow*) (pre-erosive edema). **C:** Coronal T1-weighted fat-saturated MRI obtained after intravenous injection of gadolinium demonstrates strong enhancement of the synovium and multiple areas within the carpal bones, proximal metacarpals, and ulnar styloid, the hallmarks of severity and extension of the inflammation.

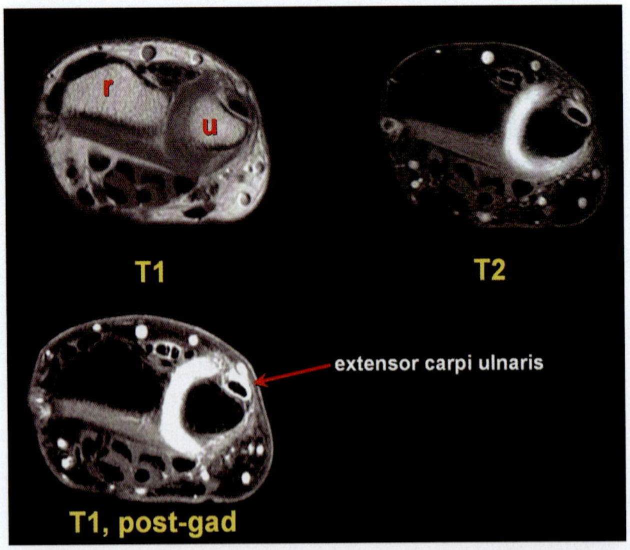

Figure 2.97 ■ MRI of rheumatoid arthritis, depiction of synovitis. Axial T1-weighted, T2-weighted, and contrast-enhanced T1-weighted MR images of the wrist of the 28-year-old woman with clinical diagnosis of rheumatoid arthritis show advantage of post-gadolinium study for diagnosis of synovitis of the distal radioulnar joint and extensor carpi ulnaris tendon. Although the high signal on T2 weighting may indicate either fluid or inflammatory pannus, the marked enhancement on postgadolinium sequences confirms the presence of the latter, because fluid would not enhance. r, radius; u, ulna.

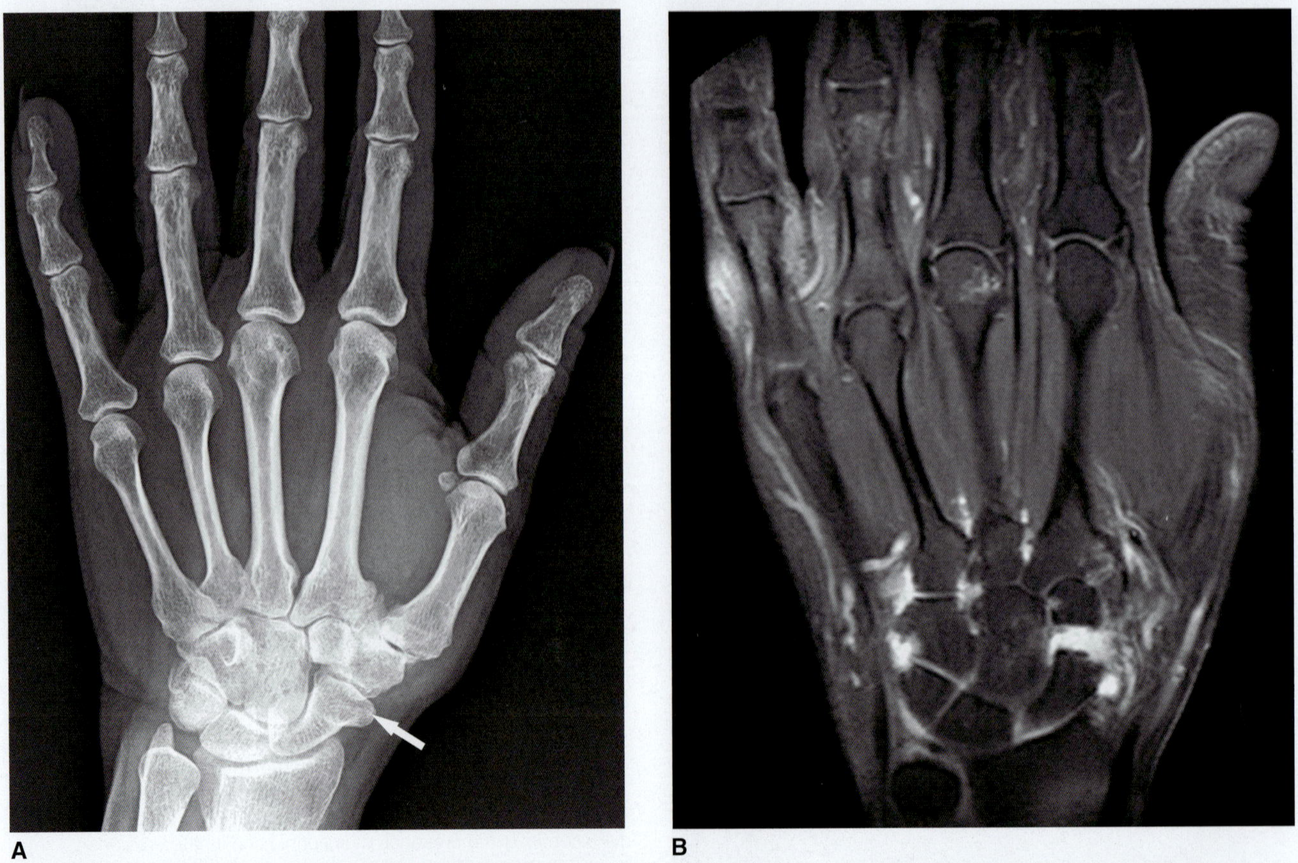

Figure 2.98 ■ MRI of rheumatoid arthritis, depiction of synovitis and erosions. A 42-year-old man with skin lesions clinically diagnosed as psoriasis, presented with 4-month history of pain in the right wrist. **A:** Dorsovolar radiograph shows small cystlike lesion in the distal scaphoid (*arrow*) but no erosions nor other radiographic features of inflammatory arthritis. **B:** Coronal T1-weighted fat-suppressed MRI obtained after intravenous administration of gadolinium shows erosions of the head of the third metacarpal, scaphoid, triquetrum, and hamate bones, and extensive synovitis in the intercarpal articulations, consistent with inflammatory arthritis.

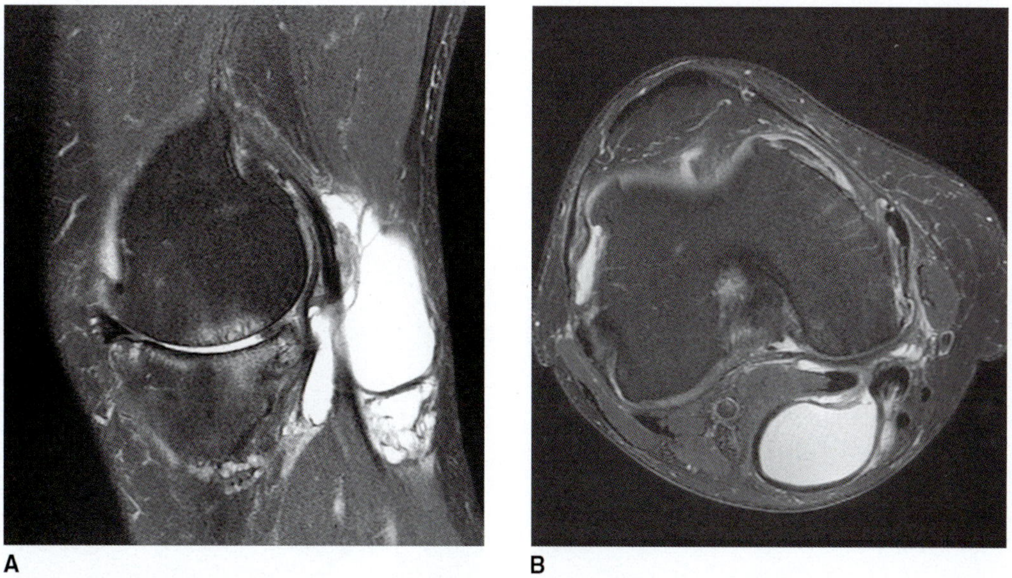

Figure 2.99 ■ **MRI of the Baker cyst.** Sagittal **(A)** and axial **(B)** proton density–weighted fat-suppressed images of the knee of the 60-year-old woman with rheumatoid arthritis demonstrate a large multiloculated and septated popliteal cyst filled with high-intensity fluid. Note also destruction of the articular cartilage of the medial femoral condyle and proximal tibia associated with subchondral erosions.

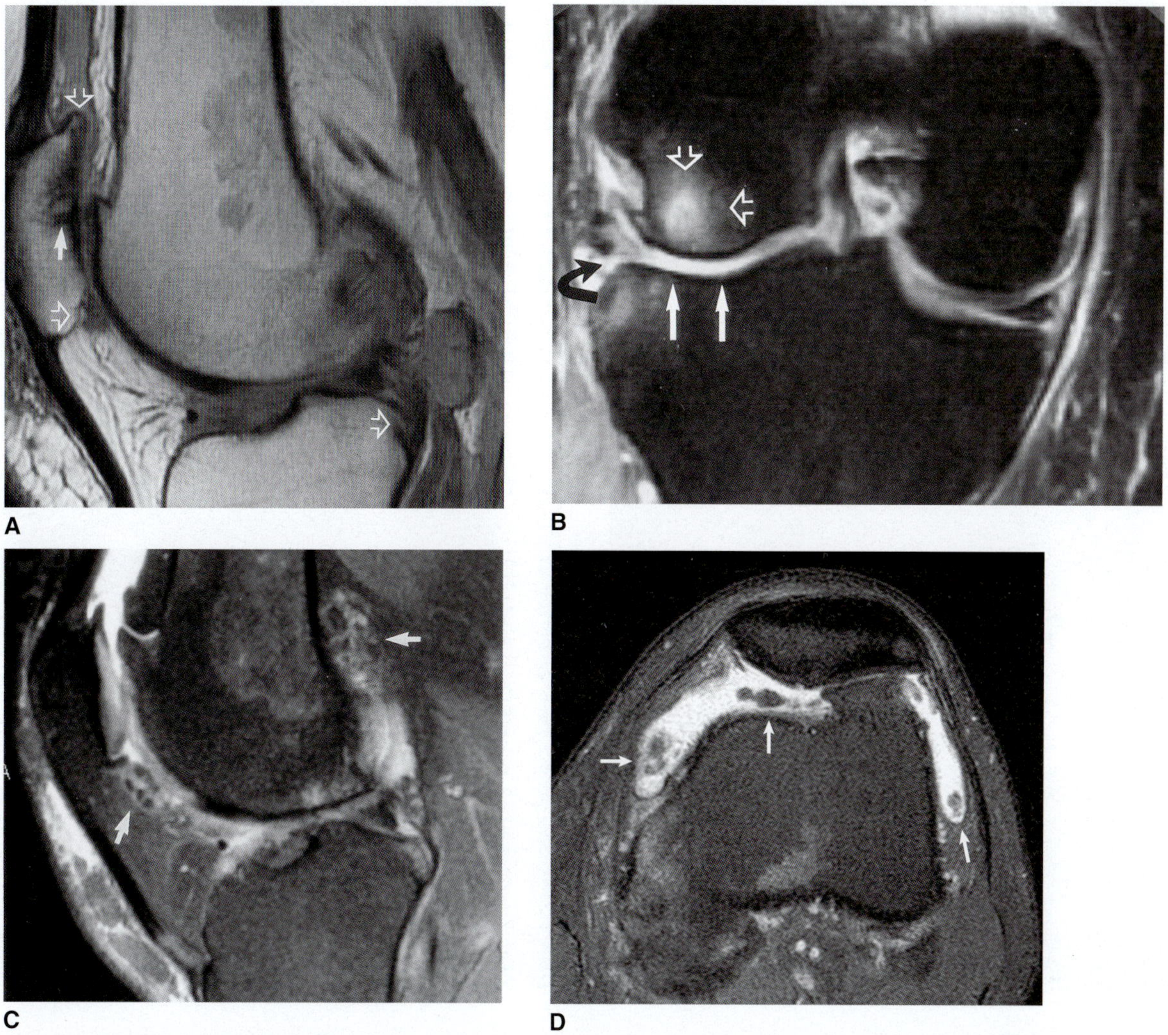

Figure 2.100 ■ **MRI of osteoarthritis. A:** Sagittal proton density–weighted MRI of a 62-year-old woman with osteoarthritis of the right knee shows involvement of the femoropatellar compartment. Note joint space narrowing, subchondral cyst (*arrow*), and osteophytes (*open arrows*). **B:** Coronal T2-weighted fat-suppressed MR image shows complete destruction of articular cartilage of the lateral joint compartment (*arrows*), subchondral edema (*open arrows*), and degenerative tear of the lateral meniscus (*curved arrow*). Sagittal **(C)** and axial **(D)** T2-weighted fat-suppressed MR images of the knee of a 60-year-old man show osteoarthritis complicated by multiple osteochondral bodies (*arrows*).

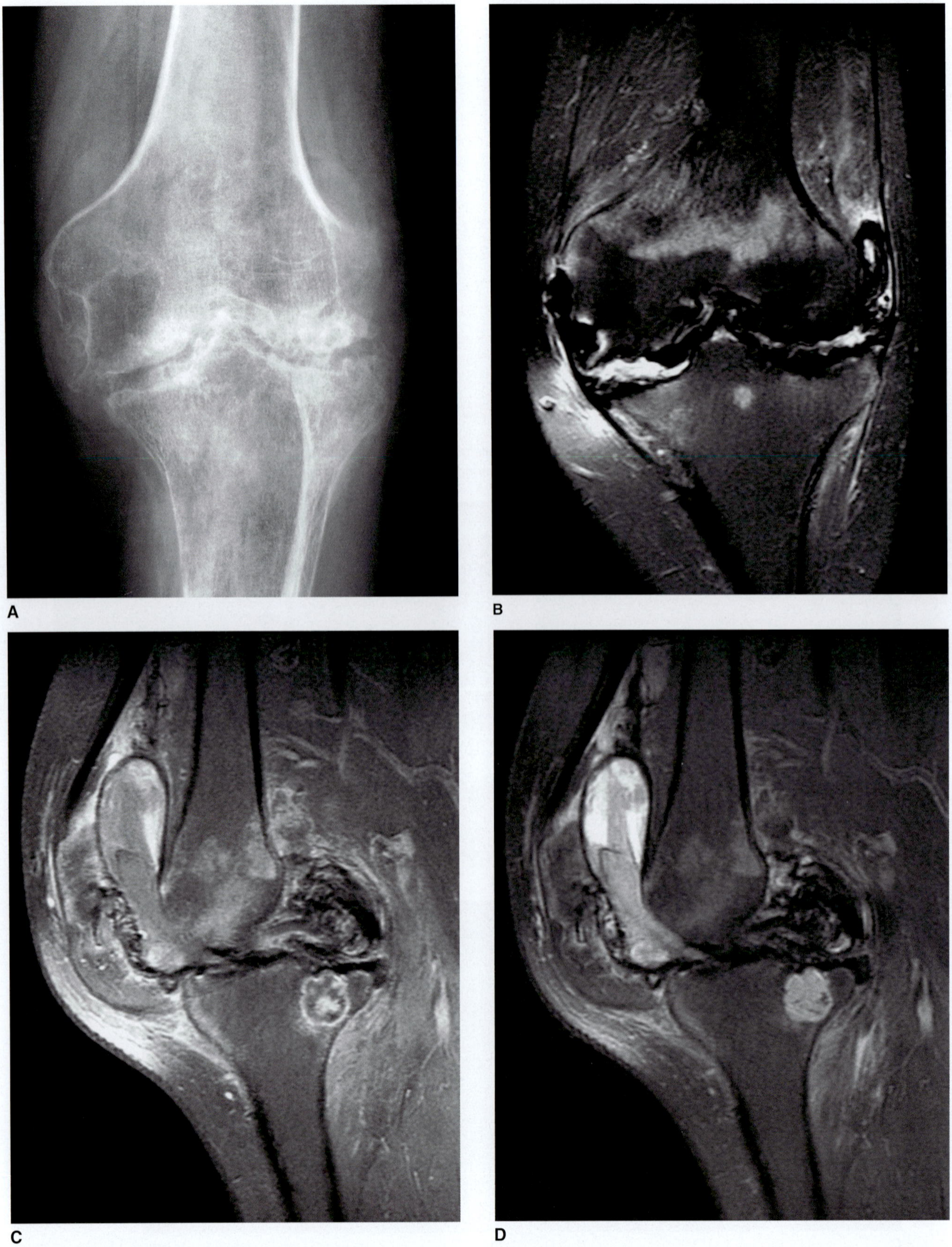

Figure 2.101 ■ **MRI of hemophilic arthropathy.** Anteroposterior radiograph of the left knee **(A)**, coronal proton density–weighted fat-suppressed **(B)**, sagittal T1-weighted contrast-enhanced fat-suppressed **(C)**, and sagittal proton density–weighted fat-suppressed **(D)** MR images of a 34-year-old man show destructive changes of all three joint compartments. Note heterogeneous appearance of bloody effusion in the joint and suprapatellar bursa.

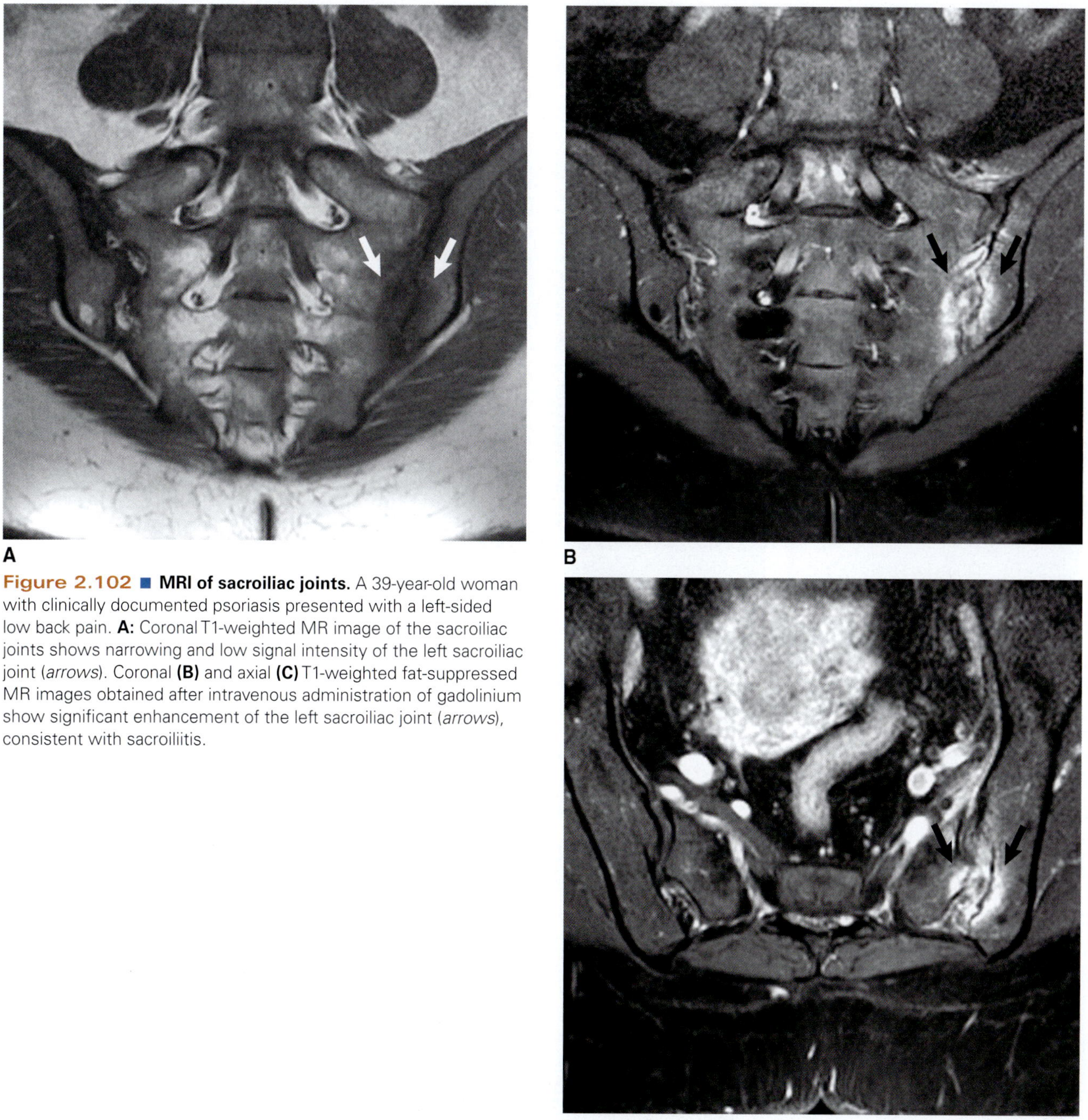

A B C

Figure 2.102 ■ MRI of sacroiliac joints. A 39-year-old woman with clinically documented psoriasis presented with a left-sided low back pain. **A:** Coronal T1-weighted MR image of the sacroiliac joints shows narrowing and low signal intensity of the left sacroiliac joint (*arrows*). Coronal **(B)** and axial **(C)** T1-weighted fat-suppressed MR images obtained after intravenous administration of gadolinium show significant enhancement of the left sacroiliac joint (*arrows*), consistent with sacroiliitis.

transplantation, osteochondral transplantation, and cartilage growth-stimulating factors, optimized MRI of these interventions for diagnosis and treatment planning in osteoarthritis is essential.

Recent investigations of the value of contrast-enhanced MRI with or without subtraction technique proved to be useful for early detection of active sacroiliitis (Fig. 2.102). The most important role of MRI, however, is in the evaluation of the spine (Fig. 2.103). MR images in the sagittal plane are useful for demonstrating hypertrophy of the ligamentum flavum or the vertebral facets, grading the degree of foramina stenosis, and measuring the sagittal diameter of the spinal canal and the spinal cord. MR images in the axial plane facilitate detailed analysis of the facet joints and more accurate measurement of the thickness of the ligamentum flavum and the diameter of the spinal canal. The quality of evaluation of medulla oblongata and spinal cord abnormalities by MRI in the cervical area in patients with rheumatoid arthritis (Fig. 2.104) and of spinal stenosis in patients with advanced degenerative changes of the spine (Fig. 2.105) surpasses that obtained with other modalities. MRI is particularly useful in the examination of patients with pain related to disk disease because it can differentiate normal, degenerated, and herniated disks noninvasively (Figs. 2.106 and 2.107). In fact, MRI can identify the changes of disk degeneration long before conventional radiography or CT can detect them.

(Continued on page 90)

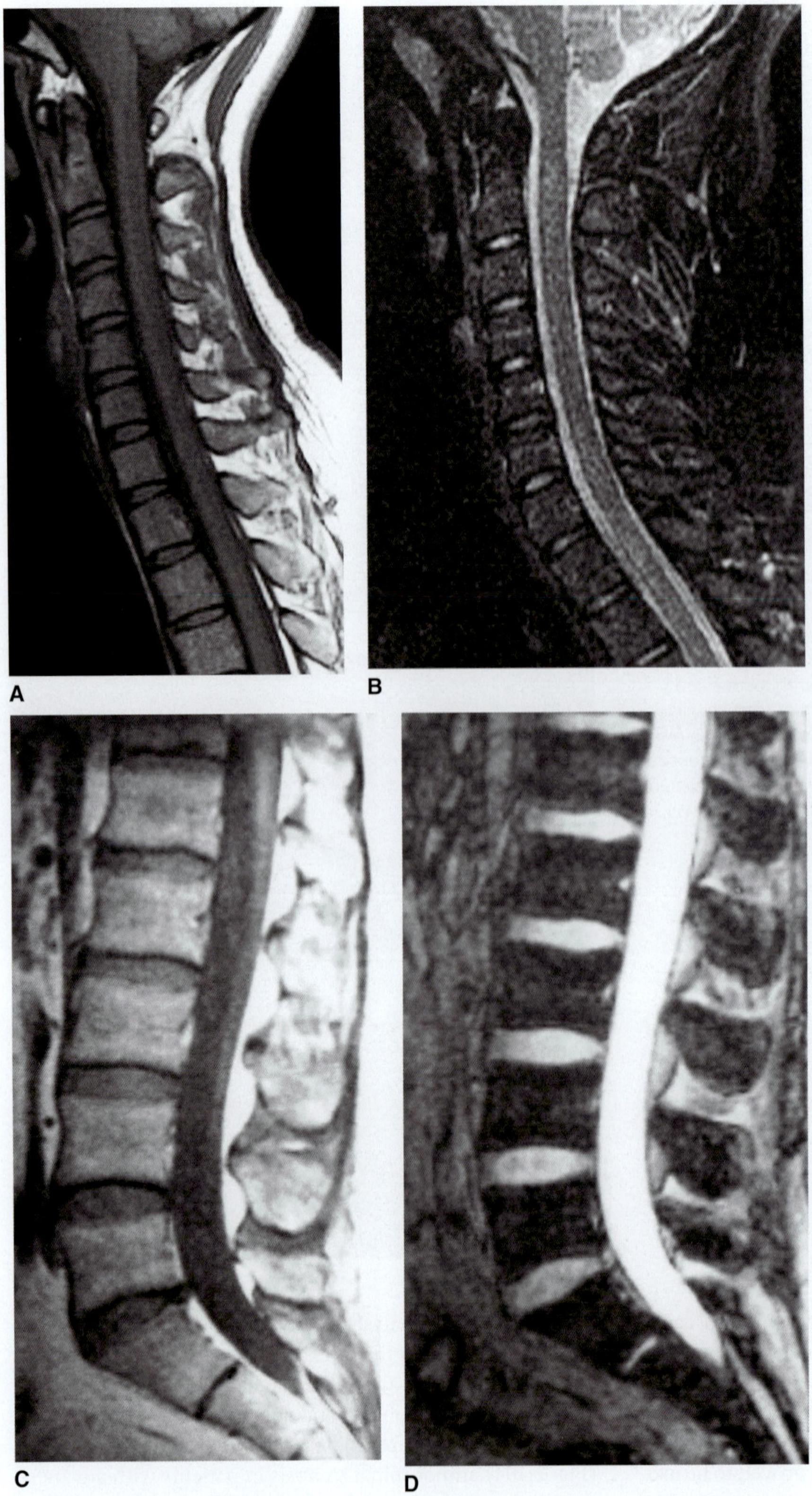

Figure 2.103 ■ **MRI of the normal cervical and lumbar spine. A:** T1-weighted spin echo sagittal midline section of the cervical spine demonstrates anatomic details of the bones and soft tissues. The craniocervical junction is well outlined. The foramen magnum is defined by the fat within the occipital bone and clivus. The anterior and posterior arches of C1 appear as small oval marrow-containing structures at the upper cervical spine. The spinal cord is of an intermediate signal intensity outlined by lower signal of cerebrospinal fluid. The intervertebral disks are imaged with low signal intensity. **B:** Short time inversion recovery (STIR) sagittal image shows vertebral bodies and spinous processes to be of low signal intensity. The high water content of the intervertebral disks produces a very high signal similar to that of cerebrospinal fluid. The cord is imaged as an intermediate–signal intensity structure. **C:** On this spin-echo T1-weighted sagittal midline section (repetition time [TR] 800/echo time [TE] 20 msec) of the lumbar spine, the tip of the conus medullaris is identified at the T12–L1 level, surrounded by low–signal intensity cerebrospinal fluid. Epidural fat is of very high signal intensity. It is most clearly seen posteriorly, but also some fat is present anteriorly at the lumbosacral junction. Intervertebral disks are of an intermediate signal intensity because of their high water content. The low–signal intensity lines along the ventral and dorsal aspects of the vertebral body are related to the anterior and posterior longitudinal ligaments and cortical bone of the vertebral bodies. These ligaments also span and cover the anterior and posterior portions of the disks. The thin black line along the inferior end plate and the bright line at the superior portion of each vertebral body are due to a chemical shift artifact. **D:** Gradient-echo T2-weighted sagittal midline section (MPGR; TR 1000/TE 12 msec, flip angle 22.5 degrees) provides an image with a similar appearance to that of the myelographic technique because of its very high gray-scale contrast. There is clear delineation of the thecal sac filled with high–signal intensity cerebrospinal fluid. The posterior longitudinal ligament and dura are silhouetted against the high water signal of the cerebrospinal fluid and the intervertebral disks. The epidural fat is of intermediate-to-low signal intensity, and the vertebral bodies are of a very low signal intensity. A high signal intensity of the mid posterior cleft in the vertebral bodies is related to the basivertebral veins.

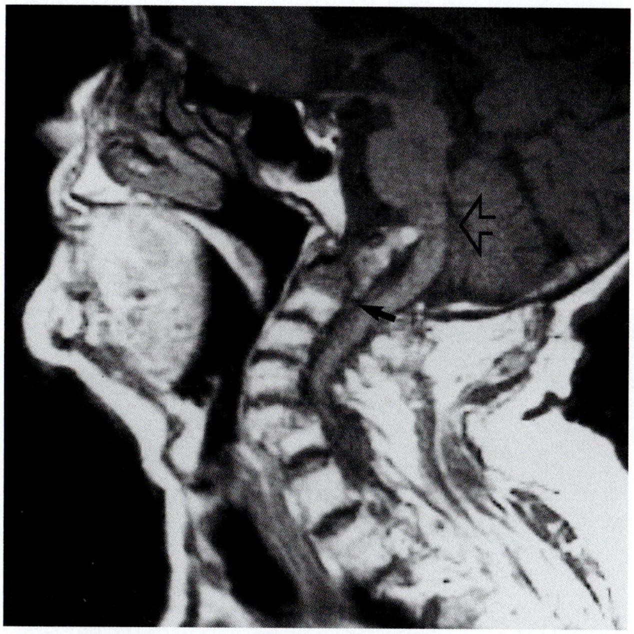

Figure 2.104 ■ **MRI of rheumatoid arthritis of the cervical spine.** A 52-year-old woman with advanced rheumatoid arthritis presented with chronic neck pain, weakness of the upper limbs, numbness in both hands, and occasional dyspnea and cardiac arrhythmia. A sagittal spin echo T1-weighted MR image shows inflammatory pannus eroding odontoid (*arrow*) and cranial settling with cephalad migration of C2 impinging on the medulla oblongata (*open arrow*).

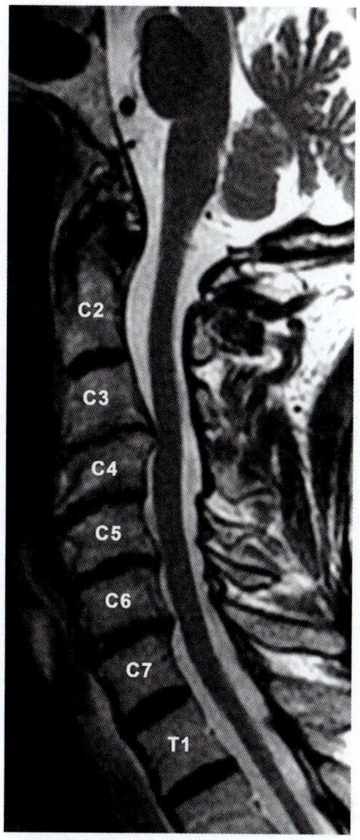

Figure 2.105 ■ **MRI of cervical spinal stenosis.** A 78-year-old woman presented with neck pain accompanied by numbness and weakness of the upper extremities. Sagittal T2-weighted MR image of the cervical spine shows narrowing of the several intervertebral disk spaces associated with bulging of the disks and formation of posterior osteophytes impinging on the ventral aspect of the thecal sac. At C3–C4 level, there is also impingement of the spinal cord.

Figure 2.106 ■ **MRI of lumbar spinal stenosis.** A 67-year-old man presented with low back pain and right-sided radiculopathy. Sagittal T2-weighted MR image shows exaggerated lumbar lordosis, degenerative disk disease at multiple levels associated with posterior bulging, retrospondylolisthesis at T12–L1, L1–L2, L2–L3, and L3–L4 levels, anterolisthesis at L4–L5 level, narrowing of the spinal canal, and compression of the cauda equina nerve roots.

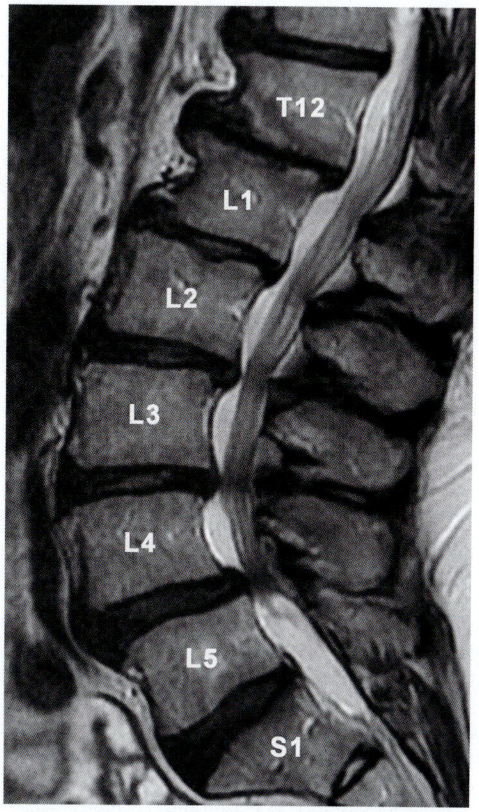

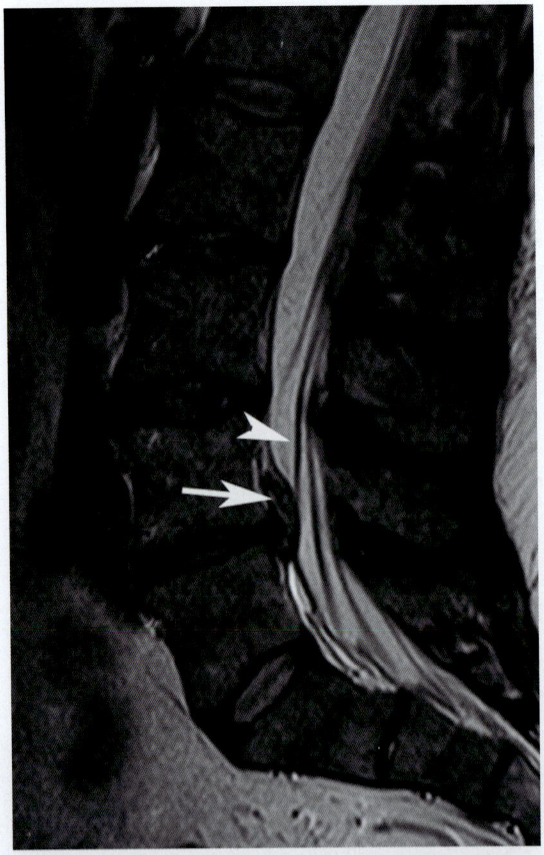

A

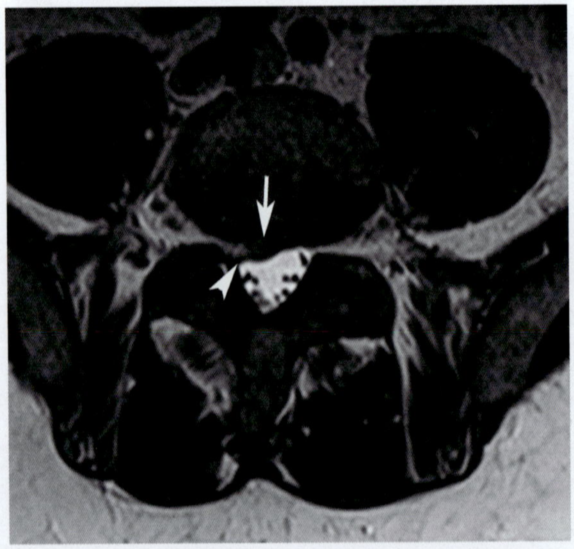

B

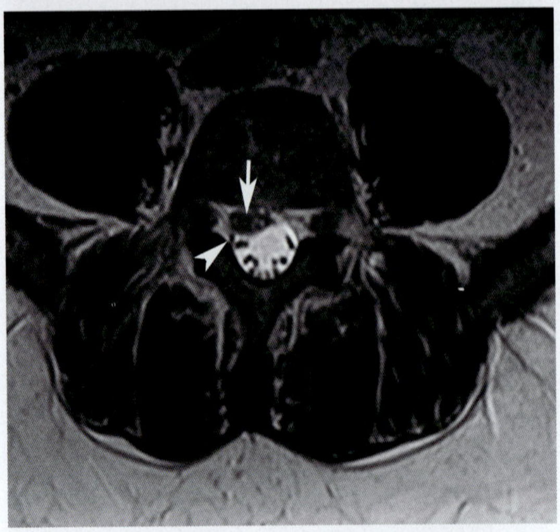

C

Figure 2.107 ■ MRI of intervertebral disk herniation. A 46-year-old man presented with right radiculopathy. **A:** Sagittal T2-weighted MRI demonstrates a central and right paracentral disk herniation of the extrusion type at the L4–L5 level, extending cephalad (*arrow*), with impingement of the right L5 nerve root (*arrowhead*). **B:** Axial T2-weighted MRI at the level of the L4–L5 disk space demonstrates the extruded disk material (*arrow*) and the posterior displacement of the L4 nerve root (*arrowhead*). **C:** Axial T2-weighted MRI above the disk space L4–L5 at the level of the L4 vertebra demonstrates the superiorly displaced disk material (*arrow*) with compression of the thecal sac in the right lateral recess and contacting the L4 nerve root (*arrowhead*).

SUGGESTED READINGS

Algin O, Gokalp G, Baran B, et al. Evaluation of sacroiliitis: contrast-enhanced MRI with subtraction technique. *Skeletal Radiol.* 2009;38:983–988.

Ash Z, Marzo-Ortega H. Ankylosing spondylitis—the changing role of imaging. *Skeletal Radiol.* 2012;41:1031–1034.

Aufdermaur M. Pathogenesis of square bodies in ankylosing spondylitis. *Annals Rheum Dis.* 1989;48:628–631.

Aydin F, Cengiz AK, Gungor F. Tc-99m labeled HMPAO white blood scintigraphy in pediatric patients. *Mol Imaging Radionucl Ther.* 2012;21:13–18.

Bales JG, Wall LB, Stern PJ. Long-term results of Swanson silicone arthroplasty for proximal interphalangeal joint osteoarthritis. *J Hand Surg [Am].* 2014;39:455–461.

Beckers C, Ribbens C, Andre B, et al. Assessment of disease activity in rheumatoid arthritis with (18)F-FDG PET. *J Nucl Med.* 2004;45:956–964.

Belizna C, Subra JF, Henrion D, et al. Large-vessel arteritis and myelodysplastic syndrome: report of two cases. *Eur J Haematol.* 2004;73:128–133.

Bhargava P, He G, Samarghandi A, Delpassand ES. Pictorial review of SPECT/CT imaging application in clinical nuclear medicine. *Am J Nucl Med Mol Imaging.* 2012;2:221–231.

Bianchi S, Martinoli C, Abdelwahab, IF. High-frequency ultrasound examination of the wrist and hand. *Skeletal Radiol.* 1999;28:121–129.

Bierri G, Dietemann J-L. Imaging evaluation of inflammation in the musculoskeletal system: current concepts and perspectives. *Skeletal Radiol.* 2013;42:1347–1359.

Biswal S, Resnick DL, Hoffman JM, Gambhir SS. Molecular imaging: integration of molecular imaging into the musculoskeletal imaging practice. *Radiology.* 2007;244:651–671.

Bleeker-Rovers CP, Rennen HJ, Boerman OC, et al. 99m Tc-labeled interleukin 8 for the scintigraphic detection of infection and inflammation: first clinical evaluation. *J Nucl Med.* 2007;48:337–343.

Blomley MJK, Cooke JC, Unger EC, et al. Microbubble contrast agents: a new era in ultrasound. *British Med J.* 2001;322:1222–1225.

Boutry N, Morel M, Flipo R-M, et al. Early rheumatoid arthritis: a review of MRI and sonographic findings. *Am J Roetgenol.* 2007;189:1502–1509.

Brenner W. 18F-FDG PET in rheumatoid arthritis: there still is a long way to go. *J Nucl Med.* 2004;45:927–929.

Brosseau L, Welch V, Tugwell P, et al. Low level laser therapy for osteoarthritis and rheumatoid arthritis: a metaanalysis. *J Rheumatol.* 2000;27: 1961–1969.

Brower AC, Flemming DJ. *Arthritis in Black & White.* 3rd ed. Philadelphia, PA: Elsevier/Saunders; 2012:1–26.

Bruno MA, Mosher TJ, Gold GE. *Arthritis in Color: Advanced Imaging of Arthritis.* Philadelphia, PA: Saunders/Elsevier; 2009.

Bruno MA, Wakefield RJ. Ultrasound evaluation of rheumatoid arthritis. In: Bruno MA, Mosher TJ, Gold GE, eds. *Arthritis in Color: Advanced Imaging of Arthritis.* Philadelphia, PA: Saunders/Elsevier; 2009:96–122.

Burgkart R, Glaser C, Hyhlik-Durr A, et al. Magnetic resonance imaging-based assessment of cartilage loss in severe osteoarthritis: accuracy, precision, and diagnostic value. *Arthritis Rheum.* 2001;44:2072–2077.

Bybel B, Brunken RC, DiFilippo FP, et al. SPECT/CT imaging: clinical utility of an emerging technology. *Radiographics.* 2008;28:1097–1113.

Chapman PT, Jamar F, Keelan ETM, et al. Use of radiolabeled monoclonal antibody against e-selectin for imaging of endothelial activation in rheumatoid arthritis. *Arthritis Rheum.* 1996;39:1371–1375.

Chaudhari AJ, Bowen SL, Burkett GW, et al. High-resolution 18F-FDG PET with MRI for monitoring response to treatment in rheumatoid arthritis. *Eur J Nucl Med Mol Imaging.* 2010;37:1047.

Chaudhari AJ, Ferrero A, Godinez F, et al. Characterization of an extremity PET/CT system for assessing early response to treatment in human inflammatory arthritis. *J Nucl Med.* 2012;53(Suppl 1):434.

Chavhan GB, Babyn PS, Thomas B, et al. Principles, techniques, and applications of T2*-based MR imaging and its special applications. *Radiographics.* 2009;29:1433–1449.

Chen TS, Crues III JV, Ali M, Troum OM. Magnetic resonance imaging is more sensitive than radiographs in detecting change in size of erosions in rheumatoid arthritis. *J Rheumatol.* 2006;33:1957–1967.

Choi J-A, Gold G. MR imaging of articular cartilage physiology. *Magn Reson Imaging Clin N Am.* 2011;19:249–282.

Cohen MJ, Shyman A, Klein M, et al. Large vessel (Takayasu's) arteritis in a patient with myelodysplastic syndrome: is there a common pathogenesis? *Clin Lymphoma Myeloma Leuk.* 2011;11:60–63.

Crema MD, Roemer FW, Marra MD, et al. Articular cartilage in the knee: current MR imaging techniques and applications in clinical practice and research. *Radiographics.* 2011;31:37–61.

Crema MD, Watts VGJ, Guermazi A, et al. A narrative overview of the current status of MRI of the hip and its relevance for osteoarthritis research—what we know, what has changed and where are we going? *Osteoarthritis Cartilage.* 2017;25:1–13.

Datz FL, Morton KA. New radiopharmaceuticals for detecting infection. *Invest Radiol.* 1993;28:356–365.

Desai MA, Peterson JJ, Warren Garner H, Kransdorf MJ. Clinical utility of dual-energy CT for evaluation of tophaceous gout. *Radiographics.* 2011;31:1365–1375.

Dumarey N, Egrise D, Blocklet D, et al. Imaging infection with 18F-FDG-labeled leucocyte PET/CT: initial experience in 21 patients. *J Nucl Med.* 2006;47:625–632.

Eckstein F, Adam C, Sittek H, et al. Non-invasive determination of cartilage thickness throughout joint surfaces using magnetic resonance imaging. *J Biomech.* 1997;30:285–289.

Erickson SJ. High-resolution imaging of the musculoskeletal system. *Radiology.* 1997; 205:593–618.

Farrant JM, Grainger AJ, O'Connor PJ. Advanced imaging in rheumatoid arthritis. Part 2: erosions. *Skeletal Radiol.* 2007;36:381–389.

Farrant JM, O'Connor PJ, Grainger AJ. Advanced imaging in rheumatoid arthritis. Part 1: synovitis. *Skeletal Radiol.* 2007;36:269–279.

Forrester DM. Imaging of the sacroiliac joints. *Radiol Clin North Am.* 1990;28:1055–1072.

Fowler JR, Baratz ME. Distal Interphalangeal joint arthrodesis. *J Hand Surg [Am].* 2014;39:126–128.

Gersing AS, Solka M, Joseph GB, et al. Progression of cartilage degeneration and clinical symptoms in obese and overweight individuals is dependent on the amount of weight loss: 48-month data from the Osteoarthritis Initiative. *Osteoarthritis Cartilage.* 2016;24:1126–1134.

Goerres GW, Forster A, Uebelhart D, et al. F-18 FDG whole-body PET for the assessment of disease activity in patients with rheumatoid arthritis. *Clin Nucl Med.* 2006;31:386–390.

Gold GE, Chen CA, Koo S, et al. Recent advances in MRI of articular cartilage. *Am J Roentgenol.* 2009;193:628–638.

Gold GE, McCauley TR, Gray ML, Disler DG. What's new in cartilage? *Radiographics.* 2003;23:1227–1242.

Gold GE, Thedens DR, Pauly JM, et al. MR imaging of articular cartilage of the knee: new methods using ultrashort TEs. *Am J Roentgenol.* 1998;170:1223–1226.

Greenspan A. Back to the future – conventional radiography in rheumatology. *J Ultrason.* 2016;16:417–421.

Greenspan A, Norman A. Radial head-capitellum view in elbow trauma [Letter]. *Am J Roentgenol.* 1983;140:1273–1275.

Greenspan A, Norman A. Radial head-capitellum view: an expanded imaging approach to elbow injury. *Radiology.* 1987;164:272–274.

Gu JT, Nouven L, Chaudhari AJ, MacKenzie JD. Molecular characterization of rheumatoid arthritis with magnetic resonance imaging. *Top Magn Reson Imaging.* 2011;22:61–69.

Hartung MP, Grist TM, Francois J. Magnetic resonance angiography: current status and future directions. *J Cardiovasc Mag Res.* 2011;13:19–40.

Huellner MW, Burkert A, Schleich FS, et al. SPECT/CT versus MRI in patients with nonspecific pain of the hand and wrist – a pilot study. *Eur J Nucl Med Mol Imaging.* 2012;39:750–759.

Jamar F, Houssiau FA, Devogelaer JP, Peters AM. Scintigraphy using a technetium 99m-labelled anti-E-selectin Fab fragment in rheumatoid arthritis. *Rheumatology.* 2001;41:53–61.

Jamar F, Chapman PT, Manicourt DH, et al. A comparison between 111In-anti-E-selectin mAb and 99mTc-labelled human non-specific immunoglobulin in radionuclide imaging of rheumatoid arthritis. *Br J Radiol.* 1997;70:473–481.

Kim NR, Choi J-Y, Hong SH, et al. "MR corner sign": value for predicting presence of ankylosing spondylitis. *Am J Roentgenol.* 2008;191:124–128.

Kim S-H, Chung S-K, Bahk Y-W, et al. Whole-body and pinhole bone scintigraphic manifestations of Reiter's syndrome: distribution patterns and early and characteristic signs. *Eur J Nucl Med.* 1999;26:163–170.

Klauser A, Frauscher F, Shirmer M. Value of contrast-enhanced power Doppler ultrasonography (US) of the metacarpophalangeal joints in rheumatoid arthritis. *Eur Radiol.* 2004;14:545–548.

Kubota K, Ito K, Morooka M, et al. FDG PET for rheumatoid arthritis: basic considerations and whole-body PET/CT. *Ann N Y Acad Sci.* 2011;1228:29–38.

Kursunoglu-Brahme S, Riccio T, Weissman MH, et al. Rheumatoid knee: role of gadopentetate-enhanced MR imaging. *Radiology.* 1990;176:831–835.

Lang P, Brem M, Neumann G, et al. Magnetic resonance imaging of articular cartilage. In: Weismann BN, ed. *Imaging of Arthritis and Metabolic Bone Disease.* Philadelphia, PA: Saunders/Elsevier; 2009:49–59.

Li X, Ma CB, Link TM, et al. *In vivo* T1ρ and T2 mapping of articular cartilage in osteoarthritis of the knee using 3T MRI. *Osteoarthritis Cartilage.* 2007;15:789–797.

Link TM, Stahl R, Woeltler K. Cartilage imaging: motivation, techniques, current and future significance. *Eur Radiol.* 2007;17:1135–1146.

Linke R, Kuwert T, Uder M, et al. Skeletal SPECT/CT of the peripheral extremities. *Am J Roentgenol.* 2010;194:329–335.

Lund PJ, Heikal A, Maricic MJ, et al. Ultrasonographic imaging of the hand and wrist in rheumatoid arthritis. *Skeletal Radiol.* 1995;24:591–596.

MacKenzie JD, Yen YF, Mayer D, et al. Detection of inflammatory arthritis by using hyperpolarized 13C-pyruvate with MR imaging and spectroscopy. *Radiology.* 2011;259:414–420.

Marenzana M, Hagen CK, Borges PDN, et al. Synchroton- and laboratory-based X-ray phase-contrast imaging for imaging mouse articular cartilage in the absence of radiopaque contrast agents. *Philos Trans A Math Phys Eng Sci.* 2014;372:20130127 doi: 10.1098/rsta.2013.0127.

McKinney JR, Sussman MS, Moineddin R, et al. Accuracy of magnetic resonance imaging for measuring maturing cartilage: a phantom study. *Clinics (Sao Paulo).* 2016;71:404–411.

Mamisch TC, Tratting S, Quirbac S, et al. Quantitative T2 mapping of knee cartilage: differentiation of healthy control cartilage and cartilage repair tissue in the knee with unloading – initial results. *Radiology.* 2010;254:818–826.

Martins FPP, Gutfilen B, de Souza SAL, et al. Monitoring rheumatoid arthritis synovitis with 99mTc-anti-CD3. *Br J Radiol.* 2008;81:25–29.

Massoud TF, Gambhir SS. Molecular imaging in living subjects: seeing fundamental biological processes in a new light. *Genes Dev.* 2003;17:545–580.

McCauley TR, Disler DG. State of the art. MR imaging of articular cartilage. *Radiology.* 1998;209:629–640.

McGonagle D. The history of erosions in rheumatoid arthritis: are erosions history? *Arthritis Rheum.* 2010;62:312–315.

Mhlanga JC, Carrino JA, Lodge M, et al. 18F-FDG PET of the hands with a dedicated high-resolution PEM system (arthro-PET): correlation with PET/CT, radiography and clinical parameters. *Eur J Nucl Med Mol Imaging.* 2014;41:2337–2345.

Miese F, Scherer A, Ostendorf B, et al. Hybrid 18F-FDG PET-MRI of the hand in rheumatoid arthritis: initial results. *Clin Rheumatol.* 2011;30: 1247–1250.

Moon CH, Kim J-H, Zhao T, Bae KT. Quantitative 23Na MRI of human knee cartilage using dual-tuned 1H/23Na transceiver array radiofrequency coil at 7 tesla. *J Magn Res Imag.* 2013;38:1063–1072.

Mountz JM, Alavi A, Mountz JD. Emerging optical and nuclear medicine imaging methods in rheumatoid arthritis. *Nature Rev Rheum.* 2012;8:719–728.

Oinas J, Rieppo L, Finilla MAJ, et al. Imaging of osteoarthritic human articular cartilage using Fourier Transform Infrared Microspectroscopy combined with multivariate and univariate analysis. *Scientific Reports.* 2016;6:article number 30008, doi:10.1038/srep30008.

Omoumi P, Mercier GA, Lecouvet F, et al. CT arthrography, MR arthrography, PET, and scintigraphy in osteoarthritis. *Radiol Clin N Am.* 2009;47:595–615.

Ostendorf B, Mattes-Gyorgy K, Reichelt DC, et al. Early detection of bony alterations in rheumatoid and erosive arthritis of finger joints with high-resolution single photon emission computed tomography, and differentiation between them. *Skeletal Radiol.* 2010;39:55–61.

Ostergaard M, Dohn UM, Ejbjerg BJ, McQueen FM. Ultrasonography and magnetic resonance imaging in early rheumatoid arthritis: recent advances. *Curr Rheumatol Rep.* 2006;8:378–385.

Ostergaard M, Ejbjerg B, Szkudlarek M. Imaging in early rheumatoid arthritis: roles of magnetic resonance imaging, ultrasonography, conventional radiography and computed tomography. *Best Pract Res Clin Rheumatol.* 2005;19:91–116.

Oudjhane K, Azouz EM, Hughes S, Paquin JD. Computed tomography of the sacroiliac joints in children. *Can Assoc Radiol J.* 1993;44:313–314.

Palestro CJ, Tronco GC, Tomas MD, Rini JN. Combined labeled leukocyte and technetium 99m sulfur colloid bone marrow imaging for diagnosing musculoskeletal infections. *Radiographics.* 2006;26:859–870.

Peterfy CG, Genant HK. Emerging applications of magnetic resonance imaging in the evaluation of articular cartilage. *Radiol Clin North Am.* 1996;34:195–213.

Peterfy CG, Majumdar S, Lang P, et al. MR imaging of the arthritic knee: improved discrimination of cartilage, synovia, and effusion with pulsed saturation transfer and fat-suppressed T1-weighted sequences. *Radiology.* 1994;191: 413–419.

Petscavage J, Ha AS, Chew FS. Arthroplasty of the hand: radiographic outcomes of pyrolytic carbon Interphalangeal and metacarpophalangeal joint replacements. *Am J Roentgenol.* 2011;197:1177–1181.

Put S, Westhovens R, Lahoutte T, Matthys P. Molecular imaging of rheumatoid arthritis: emerging markers, tools, and techniques. *Arthritis Res Ther.* 2014;16:208–221.

Raya JG, Horng A, Dietrich O, et al. Articular cartilage: in vivo diffusion-tensor imaging. *Radiology.* 2012;262:550–559.

Recht MP, Resnick D. MR imaging of articular cartilage: current status and future directions. *Am J Roentgenol.* 1994;163:283–290.

Reynolds PPM, Heron C, Pilcher J, Kiely PDW. Prediction of erosion progression using ultrasound in established rheumatoid arthritis: a 2-year follow-up study. *Skeletal Radiol.* 2009;38:473–478.

Roemer FW, Crema MD, Tratting S, Guermazi A. Advances in imaging of osteoarthritis and cartilage. *Radiology.* 2011;260:332–354.

Rosado-de-Castro PH, Lopes de Souza SA, Alexandre D, et al. Rheumatoid arthritis: nuclear medicine state-of-the-art. *World J Orthop.* 2014;5:312–318.

Rowbotham EL, Grainger AJ. Rheumatoid arthritis: ultrasound versus MRI. *Am J Roentgenol.* 2011;197:541–546.

Schillaci O, Danieli R, Manni C, Simonetti G. Is SPECT/CT with a hybrid camera useful to improve scintigraphic imaging interpretation? *Nucl Med Commun.* 2004;25:705–710.

Schmitt B, Zbyn S, Steizeneder D, et al. Cartilage quality assessment by using glycosaminoglycan chemical exchange saturation transfer and 23Na MR imaging at 7 T. *Radiology.* 2011;260:257–264.

Sebes JI, Nasrallah NS, Rabinowitz JG, Masi AT. The relationship between HLA-B27 positive peripheral arthritis and sacroillitis. *Radiology.* 1978;126: 299–302.

Shapiro EM, Borthakur A, Gougoutas A, Reddy R. ^{23}Na MRI accurately measures fixed charge density in articular cartilage. *Magn Reson Med.* 2002;47:284–291.

Soldatos T, Pezeshk P, Ezzati F, et al. Cross-sectional imaging of adult crystal and inflammatory arthropathies. *Skeletal Radiol.* 2016;45:1173–1191.

Subramanian G, McAfee JG. A new complex of 99m-Tc for skeletal imaging. *Radiology.* 1971;99:192–196.

Suzuki A, Takemura A, Inaba R, et al. Magnetic resonance coronary angiography to evaluate coronary arterial lesions in patients with Kawasaki disease. *Cardiol Young.* 2006;16:563–571.

Szkudlarek M, Court-Payen M, Strandberg C, et al. Contrast-enhanced power Doppler ultrasonography of the metacarpophalangeal joints in rheumatoid arthritis. *Eur Radiol.* 2003;13:163–168.

Tagil M, Geijer M, Abramo A, Kopylov P. Ten years' experience with a pyrocarbon prosthesis replacing the proximal Interphalangeal joint. A prospective clinical and radiographic follow-up. *J Hand Surg Eur Vol.* 2014;39:587–595.

Tehranzadeh J, Ashikyan O, Anavim A, Tramma S. Enhanced MR imaging of tenosynovitis of hand and wrist in inflammatory arthritis. *Skeletal Radiol.* 2006;35:814–822.

Tehranzadeh J, Ashikyan O, Dascalos J. Advanced imaging of early rheumatoid arthritis. *Radiol Clin North Am.* 2004;42:89–107.

Toprak H, Kilic E, Serter A, et al. Ultrasound and Doppler US in evaluation of superficial soft-tissue lesions. *J Clin Imaging Sci.* 2014;4:12.

Trattnig S, Welsch G, Juras V, Zbyn S. Na-23 MR imaging at 7 T after knee matrix-associated autologous chondrocyte transplantation: preliminary results. *Radiology.* 2010;257:175–184.

Van Dyck P, Kenis C, Vanhoenacker FM, et al. Comparison of 1.5- and 3-T MR imaging for evaluating the articular cartilage of the knee. *Knee Surg Sports Traumatol Arthrosc.* 2014;22:1376–1384.

Wang H, Smith RN, Spooner AE, et al. Giant cell aortitis of the ascending aorta without signs or symptoms of systemic vasculitis is associated with elevated risk of distal aortic events. *Arthritis Rheum.* 2012;64: 317–319.

Weber U, Ostergaard M, Lambert RGW, Maksymowych WP. The impact of MRI on the clinical management of inflammatory arthritides. *Skeletal Radiol.* 2011;40:1153–1173.

Weissman BN. *Imaging of Arthritis and Metabolic Bone Disease.* Philadelphia, PA: Saunders/Elsevier; 2009:3–103.

Winalski CS, Palmer WE, Rosenthal DI, Weissman BN. Magnetic resonance imaging of rheumatoid arthritis. *Radiol Clin North Am.* 1996;34:243–258.

Yildiz A, Gungor F, Tuncer T, Karayalcin B. The evaluation of sacroiliitis using 99m Tc-nanocolloid and 99m Tc-MDP scintigraphy. *Nucl Med Comm.* 2001;22:785–794.

Zbyn S, Mlynarik V, Juras V, et al. Sodium MR imaging of articular cartilage pathologies. *Curr Radiol Rep.* 2014;2:41–57.

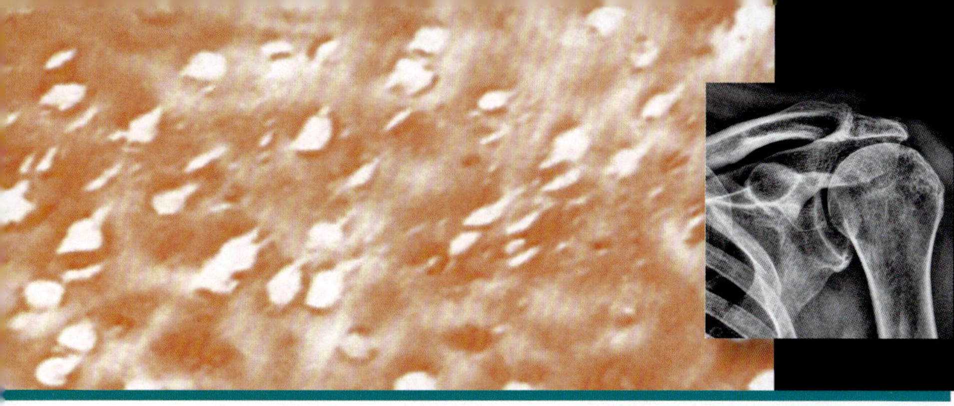

CHAPTER 3

Clinical and Imaging Features of the Arthritides and Arthropathies

CLINICAL FEATURES

The accurate diagnosis of specific arthritis or arthropathy depends on many factors; however, the most important is to understand the patterns of symptoms and the mechanism of disease.

The clinical manifestations and laboratory data, in conjunction with the imaging findings, are of significant help in making the diagnosis of a specific arthritic process. The various arthritides, for example, have different frequencies of occurrence between the genders. Rheumatoid arthritis is much more common in females, and erosive osteoarthritis is seen almost exclusively in middle-aged women. Psoriatic arthritis, reactive arthritis (formerly known as a Reiter syndrome), and gouty arthritis are more common in males. Clinical symptoms are of further assistance. Patients with reactive arthritis, for example, usually present with urethritis, conjunctivitis, and mucocutaneous lesions, and those with psoriatic arthritis may present with swelling of a single finger, the so-called sausage digit (Fig. 3.1; see also Fig. 1.4G) as well as changes in the skin and fingernails (Fig. 3.2; see also Fig. 1.4A–F). Patients with gouty arthritis may exhibit soft tissue masses, representing chronic tophi, on the dorsal aspect of the hands or feet (see Fig. 1.5). Patients with inflammatory arthritis commonly exhibit swollen joints and alignment deformities (Fig. 3.3; see also Figs. 1.2 and 1.3).

Laboratory data are also essential. Gouty arthropathy, for instance, is associated with elevated serum uric acid concentrations, and examination of synovial fluid reveals monosodium urate crystals (see Fig. 1.11). The synovial fluid of patients with calcium pyrophosphate dihydrate (CPPD) crystal deposition disease contains calcium pyrophosphate crystals (see Figs. 1.9 and 1.10). Findings of ragocytes with cytoplasmatic inclusions of ingested aggregated IgG immunoglobulin within the synovial fluid of patients with rheumatoid arthritis can be a significant diagnostic feature (see Fig. 1.7). The detection of autoantibodies is another important aid in the diagnostic workup. Rheumatoid factor (RF) is a typical finding in rheumatoid arthritis. Patients lacking the specific

(Continued on page 95)

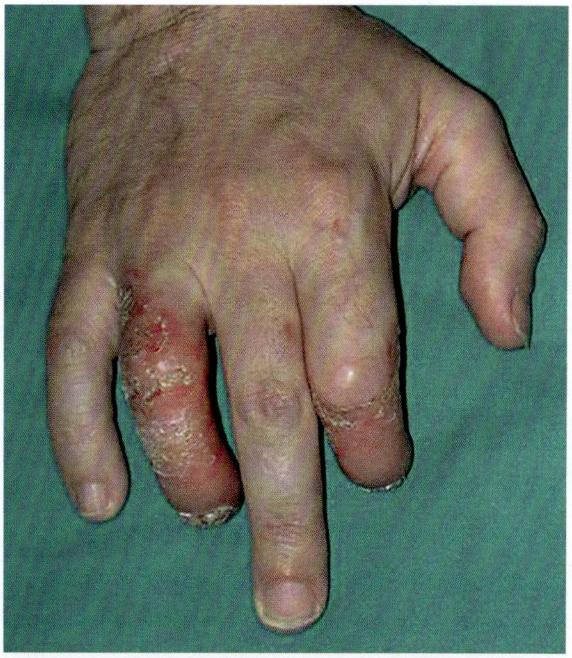

Figure 3.1 ■ **Psoriatic arthritis—sausage digits.** Diffuse swelling of the index and ring fingers represents dactylitis. Observe also typical for psoriasis skin changes.

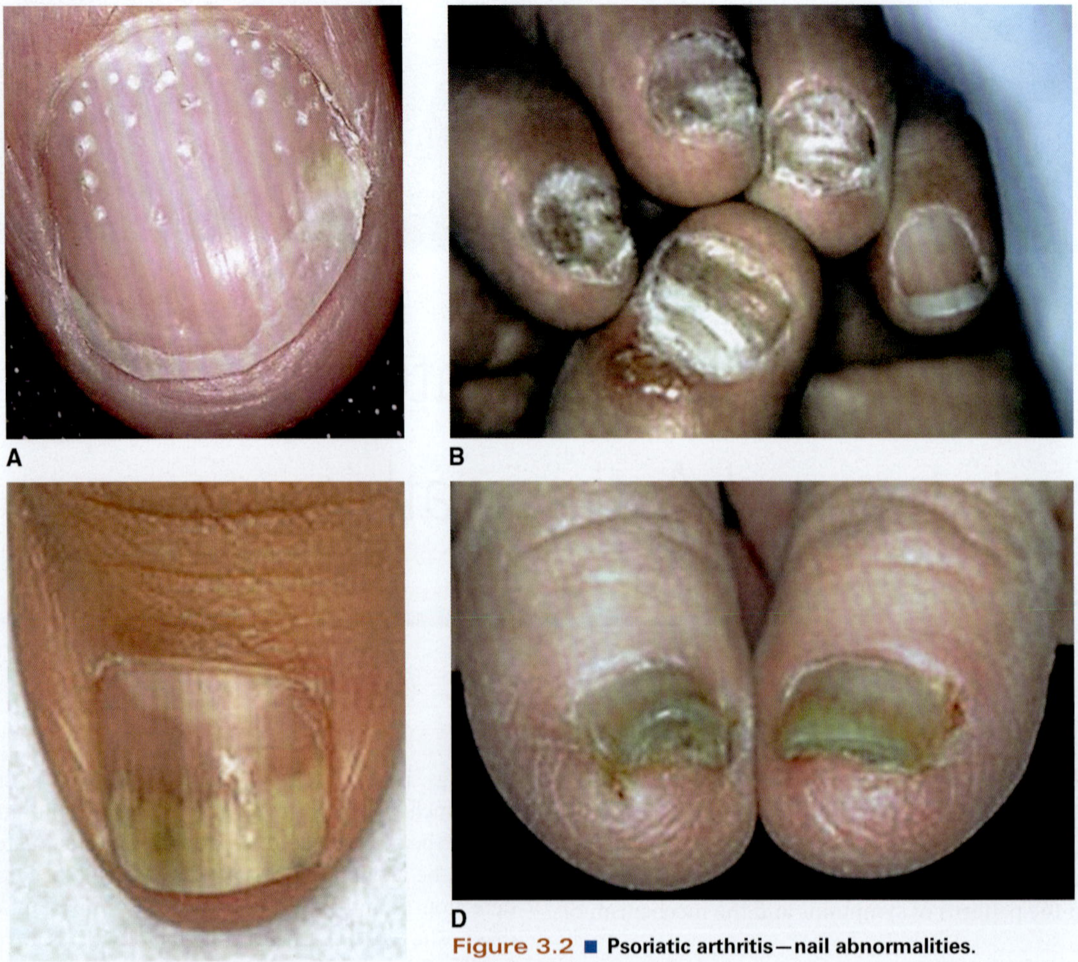

A B C D

Figure 3.2 ■ **Psoriatic arthritis—nail abnormalities.** **A:** Pitting. **B:** Leukonychia. **C:** Splinter hemorrhages. **D:** Subungual hyperkeratosis.

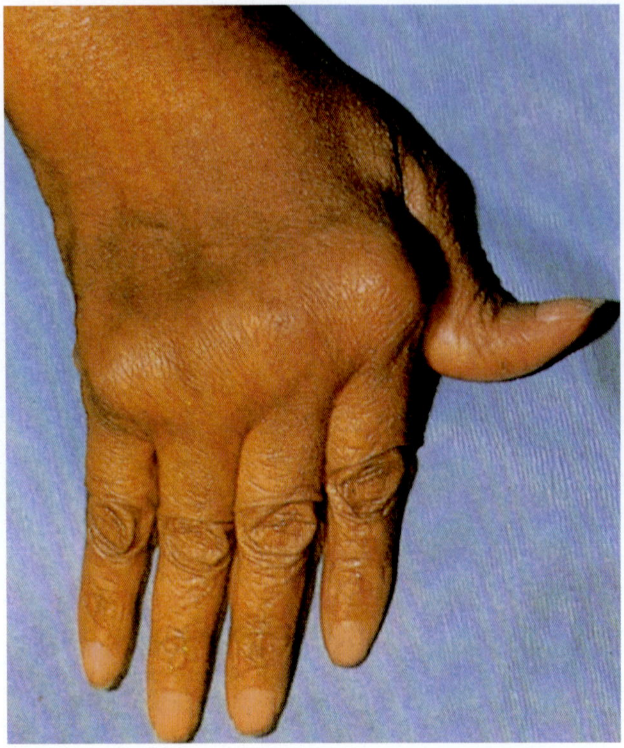

Figure 3.3 ■ **Rheumatoid arthritis—joints malalignments.** Ulnar deviation in the metacarpophalangeal joints is accompanied by swelling. Observe also hyperextension of the thumb, known as a "hitchhiker's thumb" deformity. (From Bullough PG. *Atlas of Orthopedic Pathology with Clinical and Radiologic Correlation.* 2nd ed. New York: Gower Medical Publishing; 1992, Fig. 11.2.)

antibodies represented by RF are said to have "seronegative" arthritis. Anti–cyclic citrullinated peptide antibodies are also specific for RA. Patients with lupus arthritis have a positive lupus erythematosus cell test. The presence of a positive ANA is one of the most important abnormalities detected in patients with SLE, although it may be positive in some other autoimmune conditions. The presence of anti-dsDNA, anti-Sm, and anti-RNP antibodies is another highly specific factor for the diagnosis. Lastly, identification of the antigens of the major histocompatibility complex, particularly human leukocyte–associated antigens HLA-B27 and HLA-DR4, has in recent years become the crucial tests in the diagnosis of arthritic disease. It has been reported that 95% of patients with ankylosing spondylitis, 86% of patients with reactive arthritis, and 60% of patients with psoriatic arthropathy test positively for antigen HLA-B27, whereas a majority of those with rheumatoid arthritis exhibit the HLA-DR4 antigen. This is helpful in differentiating certain types of arthritides, as well as distinguishing psoriatic arthritis from rheumatoid arthritis in cases in which the radiographic presentation of these conditions may be very similar.

IMAGING FEATURES

The true or diarthrodial joint consists of cartilage covering the articular ends of the bones forming the joint (see Fig. 1.18A); the articular capsule, which is reinforced by ligamentous structures; and the joint space, which is lined with synovial membrane and filled with synovial fluid (Fig. 3.4). Because of its physicochemical constitution, articular cartilage absorbs only a minimal amount of x-rays, thus appearing radiolucent on a radiographic film. The radiolucent articular cartilage, together with the joint cavity filled with synovial fluid, creates the so-called radiographic joint space.

The abnormality of the joint in arthritis usually consists of destruction of the articular cartilage, which appears on radiographs as a narrowing of the radiographic joint space, usually accompanied by subchondral erosion; narrowing of the joint is the cardinal sign of arthritis (Fig. 3.5). It should be kept in mind, however, that in some arthritic processes, the joint space may not become narrow, appearing instead slightly expanded. This happens, for example, in the early stages of some arthritides, when joint effusion and ligamentous laxity cause distention of the joint with fluid, but the articular cartilage has not yet been destroyed. It may also be seen in rare instances when granulation pannus erodes the subchondral bone without destroying the articular cartilage (Fig. 3.6).

Other radiographic signs specific to different types of arthritis include periarticular soft tissue swelling, periarticular osteoporosis, and, in the more advanced stages of some arthritides, complete destruction of the joint with subluxation or dislocation and ankylosis (joint fusion) (Fig. 3.7).

The radiographic presentation of arthritis depends on the type and stage of the disease, as well as the site of the original insult characteristic for the various forms of arthritis or arthropathy (Fig. 3.8)—whether it is the articular cartilage, as in osteoarthritis (Fig. 3.9); the synovial membrane, as in inflammatory arthritis (Fig. 3.10); the synovial membrane, subchondral bone, and periarticular soft tissues, as in infectious arthritis (Fig. 3.11); or the synovial membrane, articular cartilage, subchondral bone, and periarticular soft tissues, as in some metabolic arthropathies (Fig. 3.12).

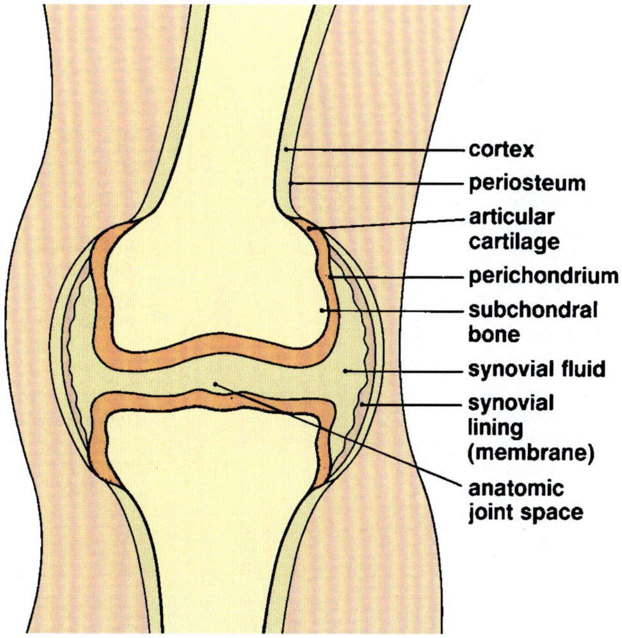

Figure 3.4 ■ The constituent structures of a synovial (diarthrodial) joint.

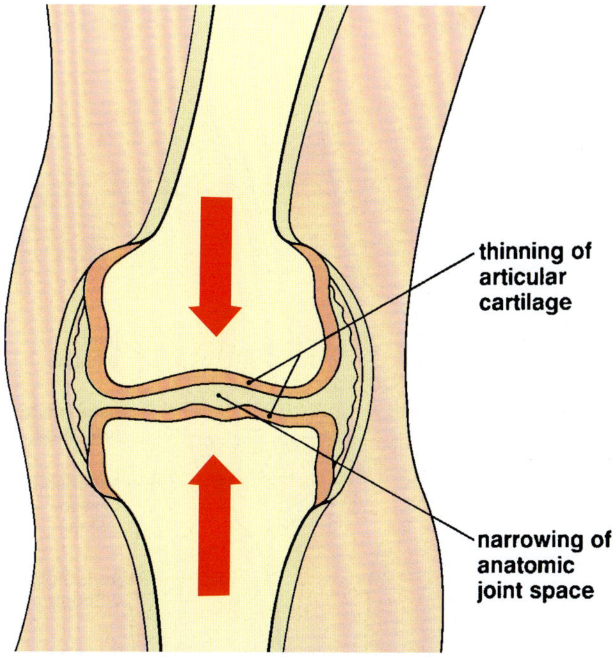

Figure 3.5 ■ Narrowing of the joint space. The cardinal sign of an arthritic process is narrowing of the radiographic joint space. Thinning of the articular cartilage reduces the space mechanically.

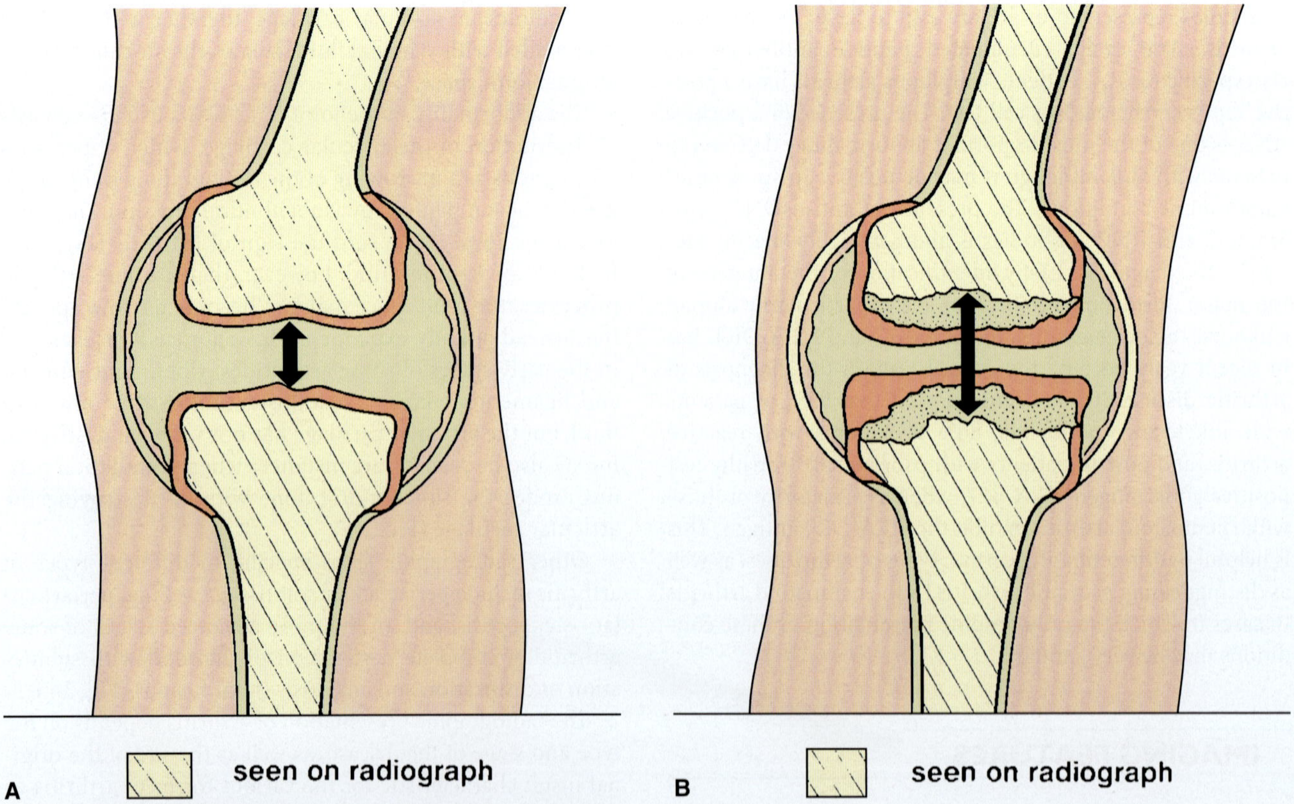

Figure 3.6 ■ A and B: Variations in the width of the joint space.

The radiographic diagnosis of arthritis, as Resnick observed, is based on the evaluation of two fundamental parameters: the *morphology* of the articular lesion and its *distribution* in the skeleton. If these findings are combined with the history, physical examination, and relevant laboratory data in a given case, then the accuracy of the diagnosis is markedly improved.

Morphology of the Articular Lesion

The various arthritides and arthropathies exhibit morphologically distinct features, as observed radiographically in the large (Fig. 3.13) and small (Fig. 3.14) joints. In the degenerative form of the disease known as osteoarthritis (osteoarthrosis), thinning of the articular cartilage results in localized narrowing of the joint space; there is also

(Continued on page 99)

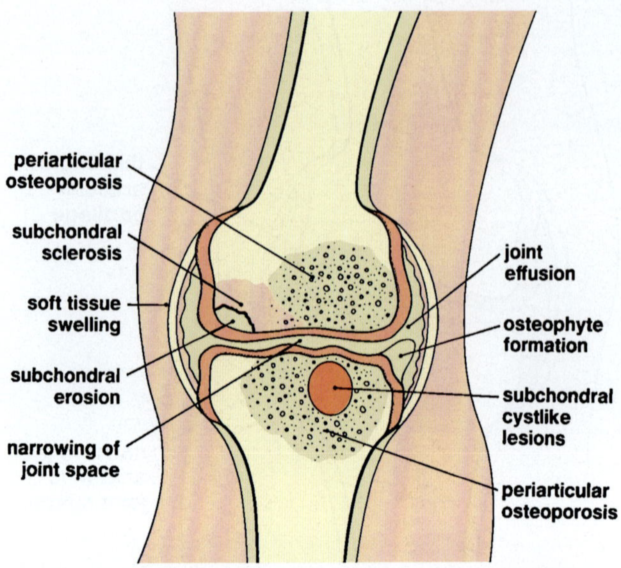

Figure 3.7 ■ Radiographic features of various arthritides. Summary representation of radiographic features seen in the arthritides. Not all of these features are seen in every type of arthritis.

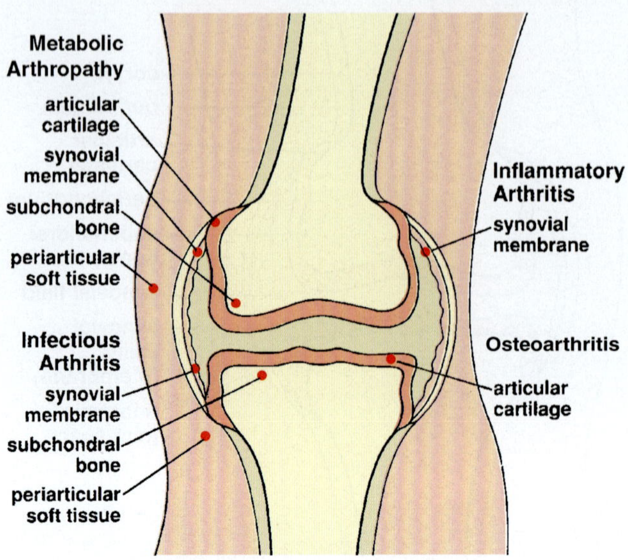

Figure 3.8 ■ Target sites of various arthritides and arthropathies.

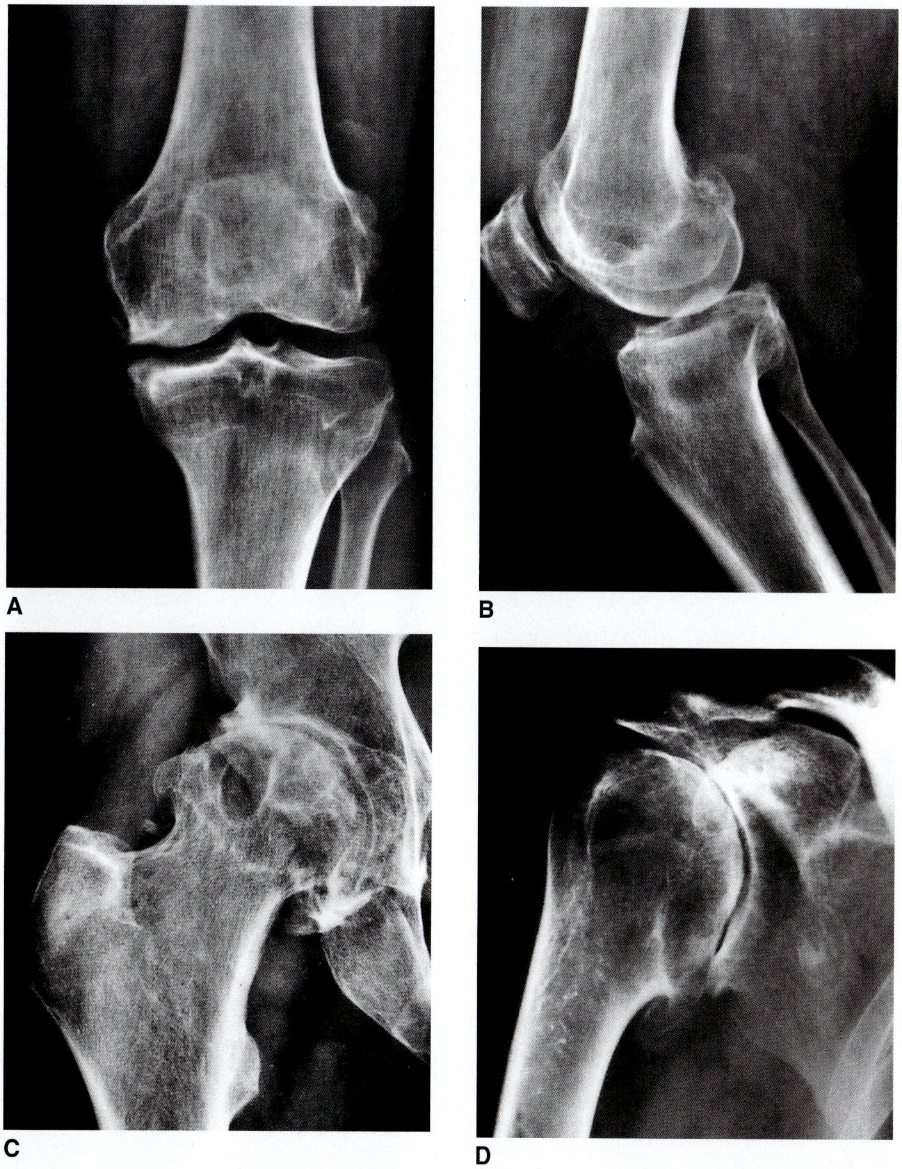

Figure 3.9 ■ Osteoarthritis. A 58-year-old woman presented with a history of pain in the left knee. **A:** Anteroposterior radiograph of the knee demonstrates narrowing of the medial femorotibial joint compartment and marginal osteophytes arising from both the medial and lateral femoral condyles—findings typical of osteoarthritis (degenerative joint disease). **B:** Lateral radiograph demonstrates, in addition, osteophytes at the anterior and posterior aspects of the articular end of the tibia, which are not appreciated on the anteroposterior projection. Involvement of the femoropatellar joint compartment and the presence of synovitis, represented by suprapatellar joint effusion, are also well demonstrated. **C:** Conventional radiograph of the hip demonstrates the typical morphologic changes seen in degenerative joint disease (osteoarthritis): focal narrowing of the joint space (here at the weight-bearing segment), subchondral sclerosis, cystlike lesions, and marginal osteophytes. Note the lack of osteoporosis. **D:** Anteroposterior radiograph of the right shoulder of a 58-year-old man shows the typical features of osteoarthritis, including joint space narrowing, subchondral sclerosis, and osteophyte formation.

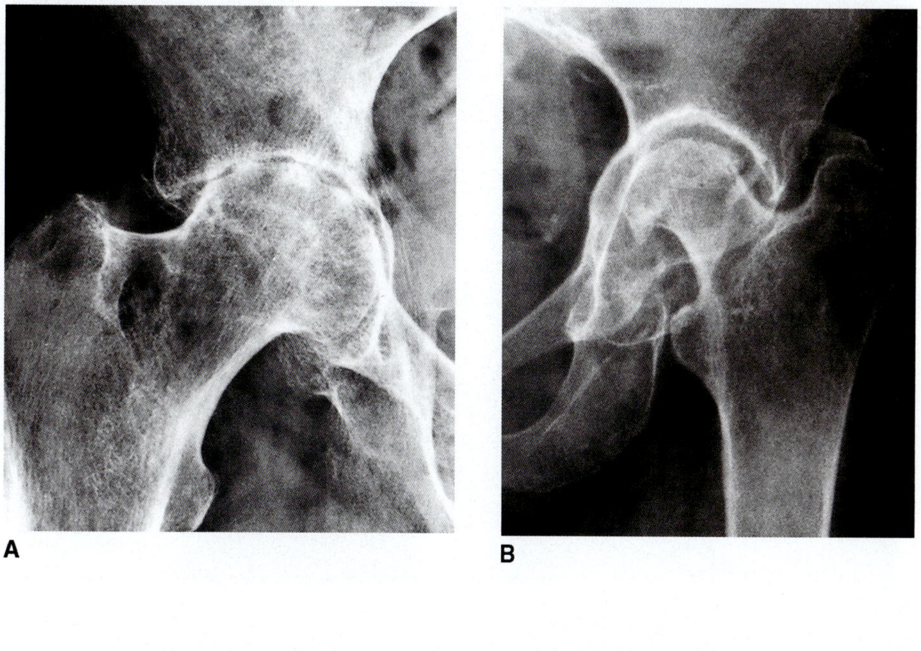

Figure 3.10 ■ Rheumatoid arthritis. A: Inflammatory arthritis, seen here in the hip, is marked by diffuse, uniform narrowing of the joint space, axial migration of the femoral head, marginal and central subchondral erosions, and severe periarticular osteoporosis. Note the almost total absence of reactive subchondral sclerosis and the lack of osteophyte formation. **B:** Anteroposterior radiograph of the left hip of a 59-year-old woman with advanced rheumatoid polyarthritis demonstrates the typical erosions of the femoral head and acetabulum. Note the lack of osteophytosis and the only very minimal reactive sclerosis.

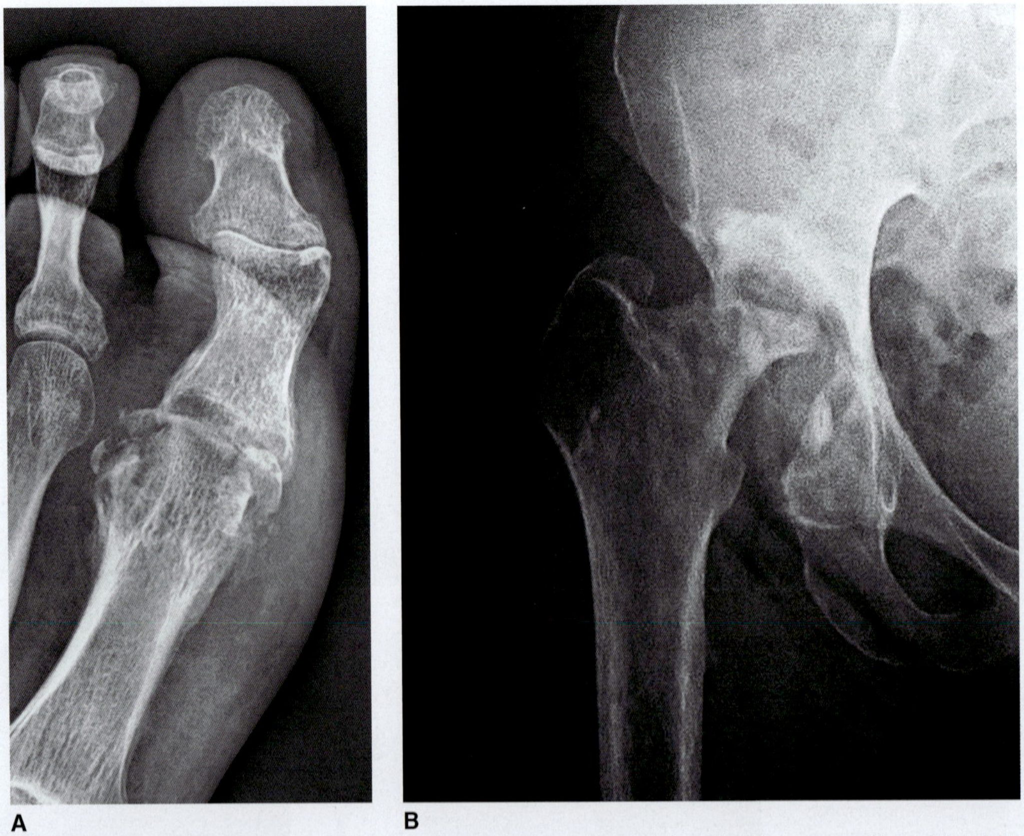

Figure 3.11 ■ **Infectious arthritis. A:** A 48-year-old diabetic man presented with pain and soft tissue swelling of the right big toe for the past 3 months. Anteroposterior radiograph shows destruction of the first metatarsophalangeal joint associated with soft tissue swelling and edema typical for septic arthritis. **B:** In another patient, a 45-year-old HIV-positive man, who presented with a history of right hip joint pain for several months, anteroposterior radiograph shows extensive destruction of the right femoral head and neck and right acetabulum consistent with septic arthritis. Hip joint aspiration and culture revealed methicillin-resistant *Staphylococcus aureus* (MRSA) infection.

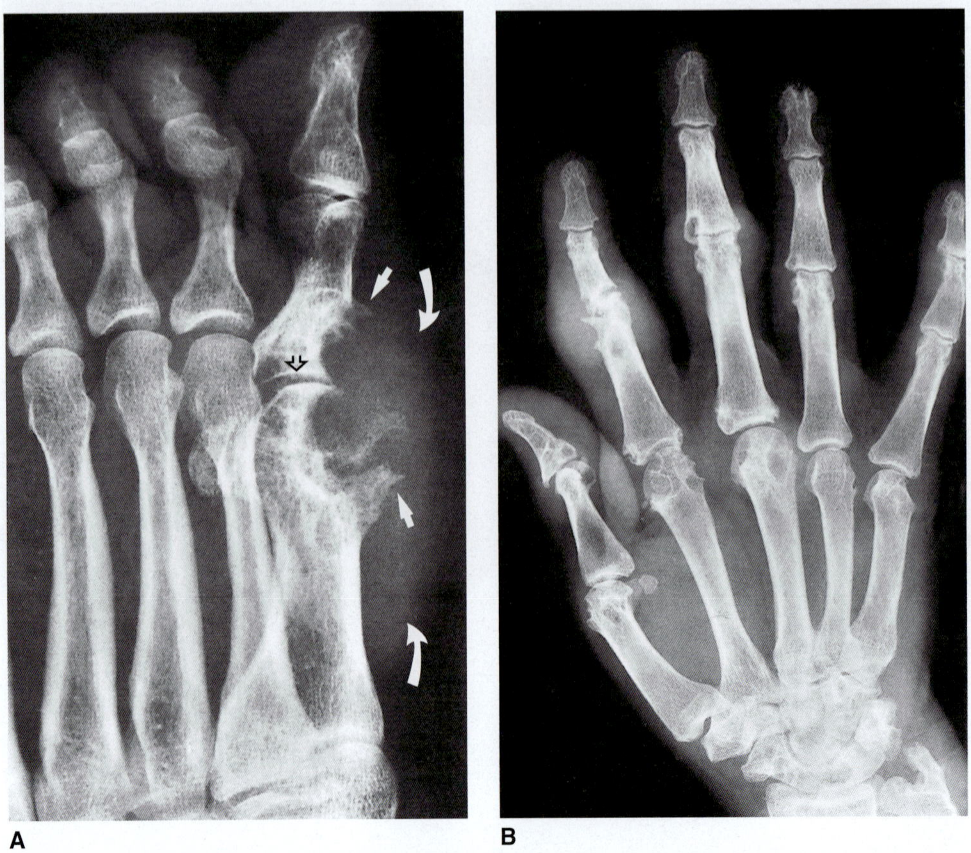

Figure 3.12 ■ **Metabolic arthropathy (gout). A:** Asymmetric periarticular erosions that spare part of the joint are typical of gouty arthritis, seen here involving the first metatarsophalangeal joint of the right foot. Note the characteristic overhanging edge at the site of erosion (*arrows*) and the soft tissue mass representing a tophus (*curved arrows*); osteophytes and osteoporosis are absent, and the joint is partially preserved (*open arrow*). **B:** The asymmetric marginal erosions affecting various articulations in the hand of a 38-year-old man with tophaceous gout are characteristic of a metabolic process involving the subchondral bone. Note the preservation of part of the joint and the location of several erosions at some distance from the joint space.

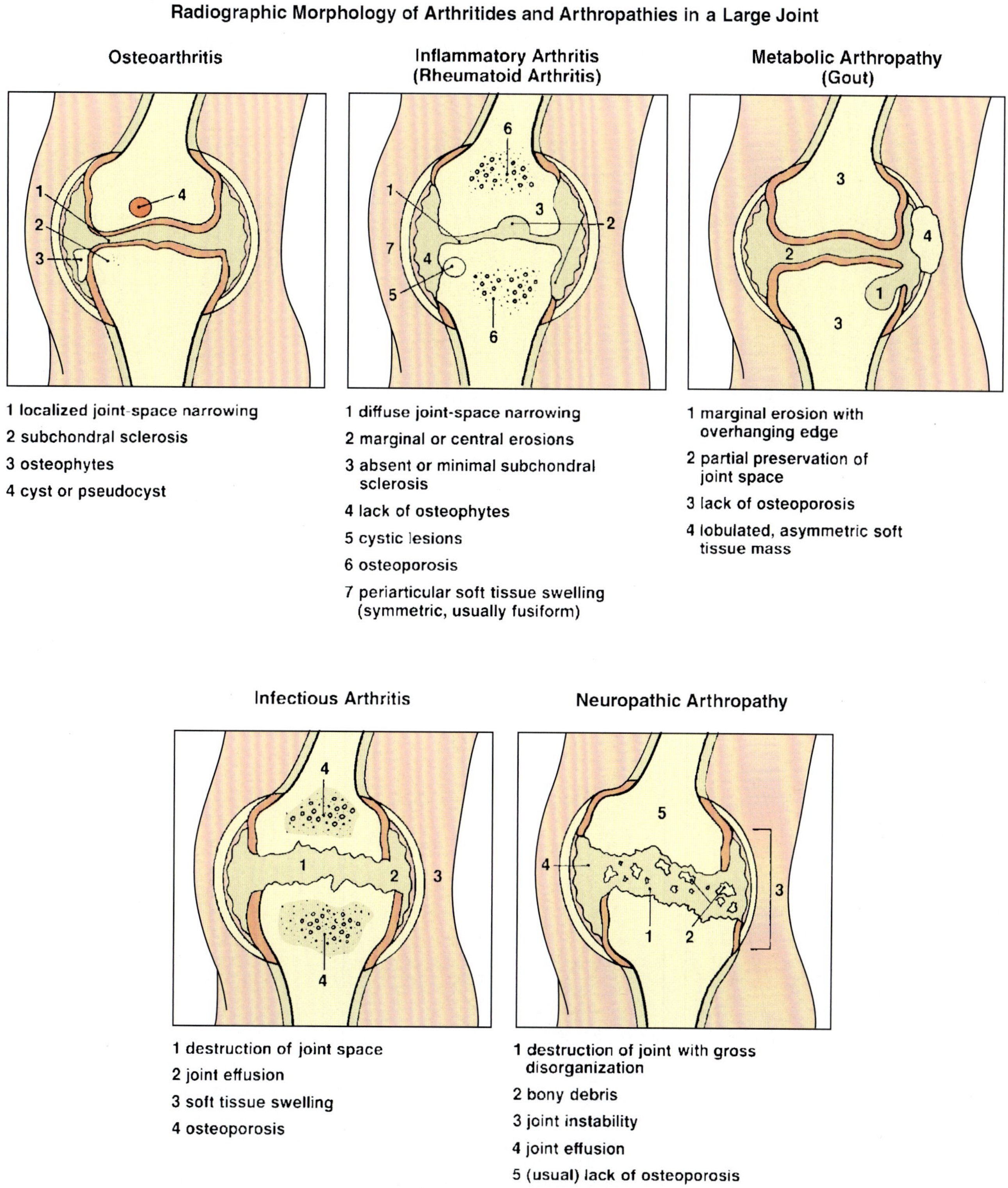

Figure 3.13 ■ **Morphologic features distinguishing the various arthritides and arthropathies in a large joint.**

subchondral sclerosis and osteophyte and cyst formation, but generally osteoporosis is absent (Fig. 3.15). Erosive osteoarthritis is characterized by central articular erosions and marginal proliferation of bone assuming the so-called gull-wing deformity (Fig. 3.16). Inflammatory arthritides, such as rheumatoid arthritis, are characterized by a diffuse, usually multicompartmental narrowing of the joint space associated with marginal or central erosions, periarticular osteoporosis, and symmetric periarticular soft tissue swelling; subchondral sclerosis is minimal or absent,

(Continued on page 102)

Radiographic Morphology of Arthritides and Arthropathies in the Hand

Osteoarthritis

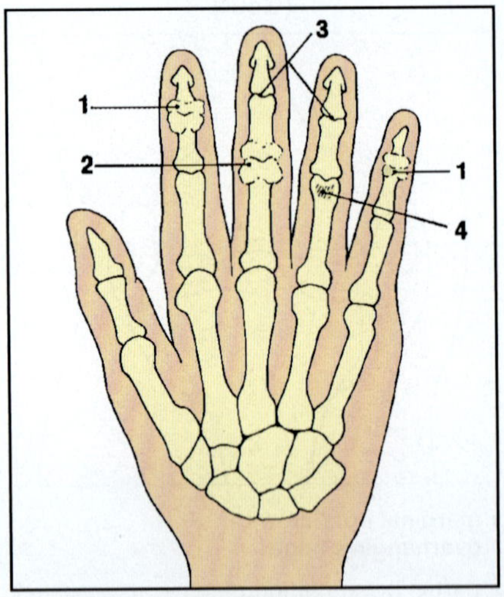

1 Heberden nodes
2 Bouchard nodes
3 joint space narrowing
4 subchondral sclerosis

Erosive Osteoarthritis

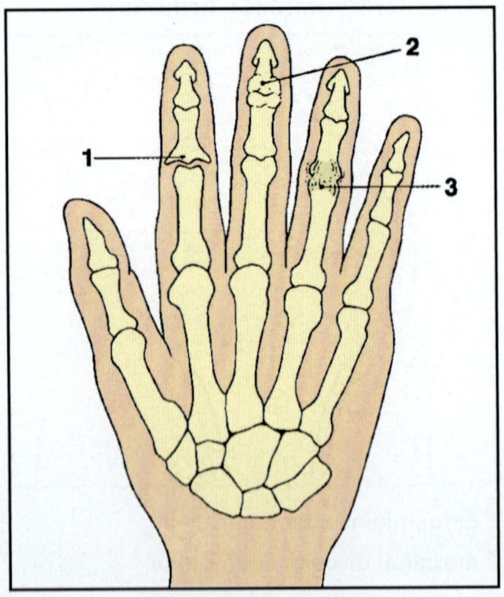

1 gull-wing erosion
2 Heberden nodes (occasionally)
3 interphalangeal ankylosis

Rheumatoid Arthritis

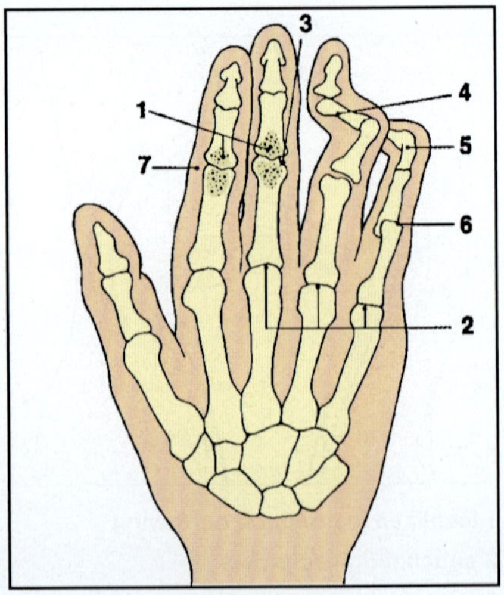

1 periarticular osteoporosis
2 joint space narrowing
3 marginal erosions
4 boutonniére deformity
5 swan-neck deformity
6 subluxations and dislocations
7 soft tissue swelling (symmetric, fusiform)

Gouty Arthropathy

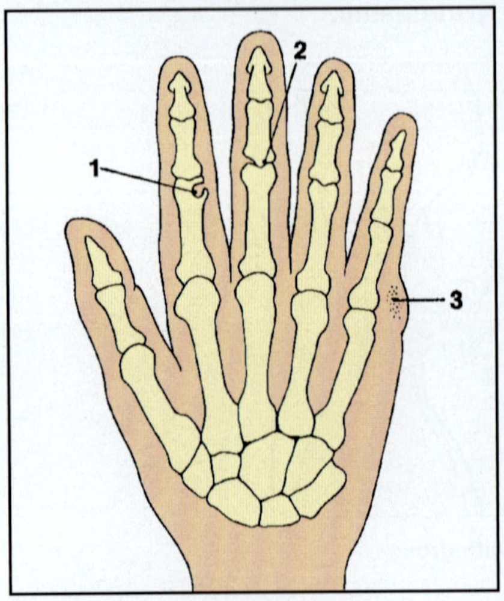

1 asymmetric erosion with overhanging edge
2 partial preservation of joint space
3 asymmetric soft tissue swelling with or without calcifications (tophus) (usually at dorsal aspect)

Psoriatic Arthritis

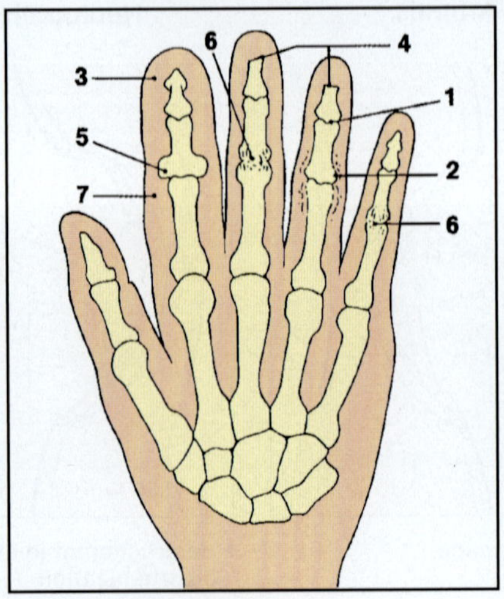

1 joint space narrowing
2 fluffy periostitis
3 "sausage digit" (soft tissue swelling of single digit)
4 erosion of terminal tufts
5 "mouse-ear" type of articular erosion
6 interphalangeal ankylosis
7 soft tissue swelling

Lupus Arthropathy

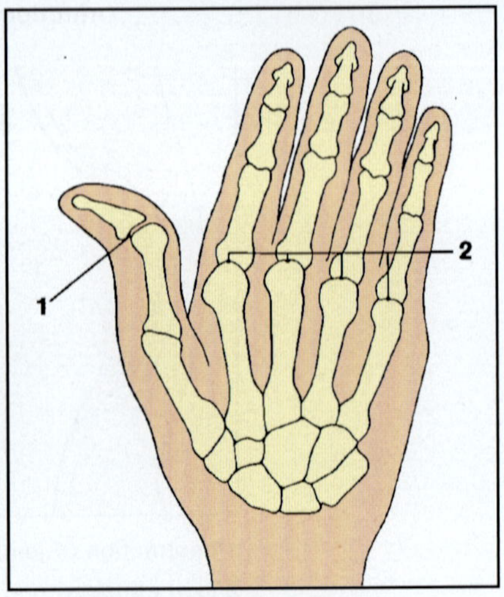

1 hitchhiker's thumb deformity
2 flexible deformities (subluxations)

Figure 3.14 ■ Morphologic features distinguishing the various arthritides and arthropathies in the small joints of the hand.

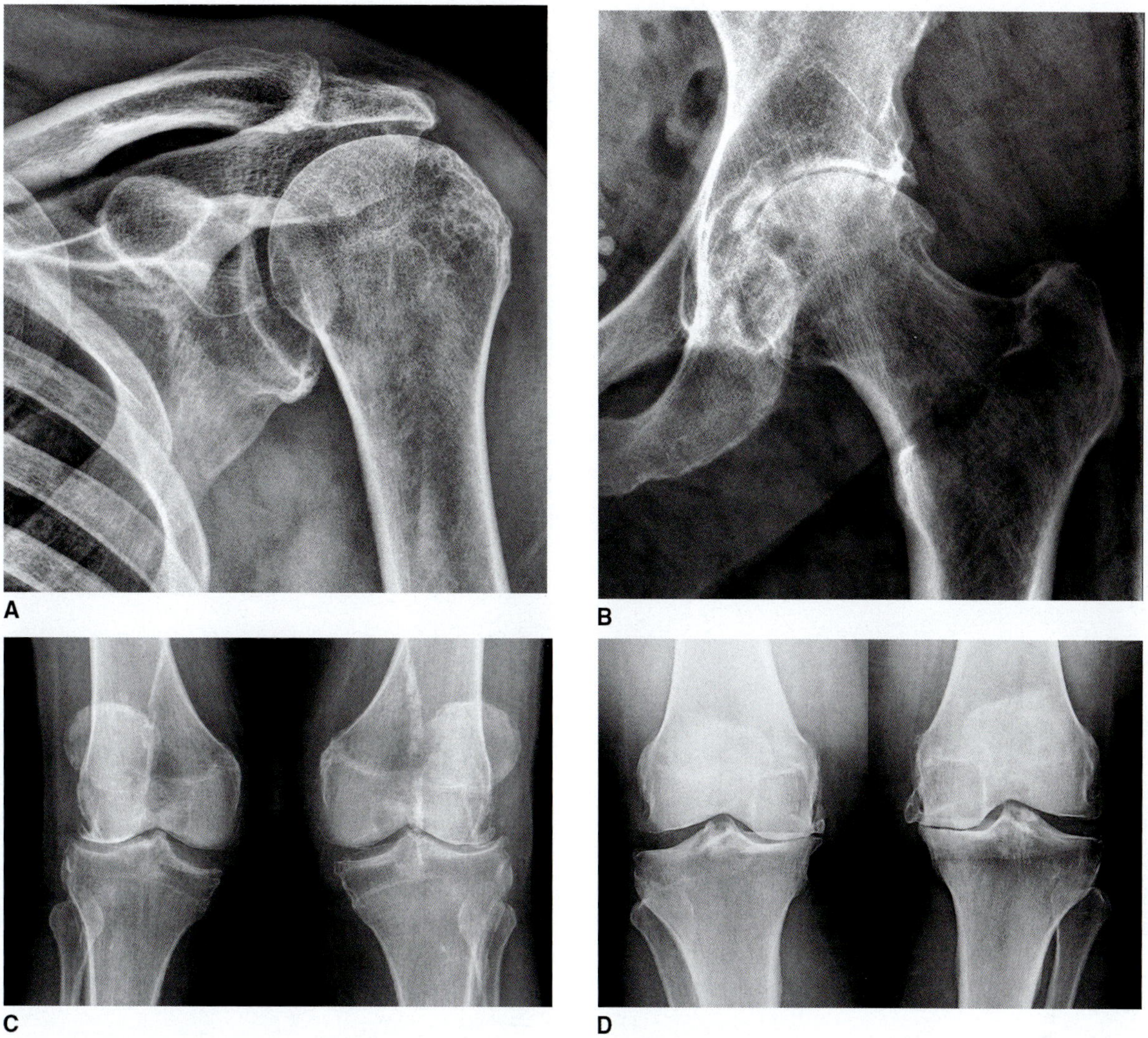

Figure 3.15 ■ **Osteoarthritis. A:** Anteroposterior radiograph of the left shoulder of a 79-year-old man shows narrowing of the glenohumeral and acromioclavicular joints associated with subchondral sclerosis and osteophyte formation. **B:** Anteroposterior radiograph of the left hip of a 70-year-old woman shows significant narrowing and subchondral sclerosis of the hip joint and osteophytes arising from the acetabulum and femoral head. **C:** Anteroposterior weight-bearing radiograph of both knees of an 80-year-old woman shows prominent osteophytosis and narrowing of the lateral joint compartments resulting in valgus deformity. **D:** Anteroposterior weight-bearing radiograph of both knee of a 77-year-old man shows prominent osteophytosis and narrowing of the medial joint compartments resulting in varus deformity.

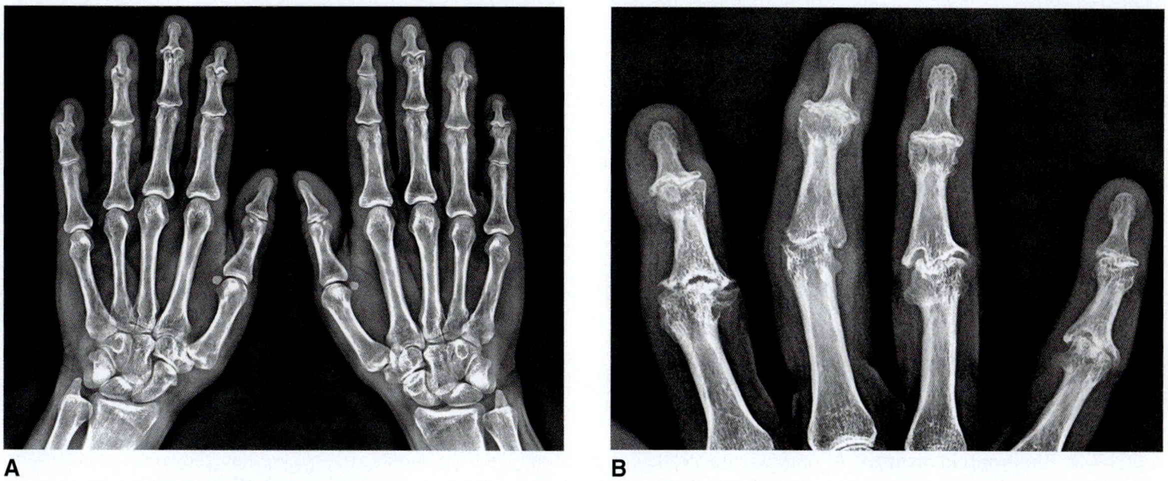

Figure 3.16 ■ **Erosive osteoarthritis. A:** Dorsovolar radiograph of both hands of a 59-year-old woman who presented with long history of joint pains shows erosions of the distal interphalangeal joints with typical "gull-wing" configuration due to central erosions and peripheral osseous proliferation. **B:** In another patient, a 63-year-old woman, the characteristic gull-wing erosions are present in the proximal and distal interphalangeal joints.

and formation of osteophytes is lacking (Fig. 3.17). In a metabolic arthropathy such as gout, well-defined osseous (articular or periarticular) erosions, displaying a so-called overhanging edge, are usually associated with preservation of part of the joint space and localized, asymmetric soft tissue nodules; osteophyte formation and osteoporosis are absent (Fig. 3.18). Infectious arthritis is characterized by the complete destruction of both articular ends of the bones forming the joint; all communicating joint compartments are invariably involved, with diffuse osteoporosis, joint effusion, and periarticular soft tissue swelling (Fig. 3.19). Neuropathic arthropathy is marked

(Continued on page 104)

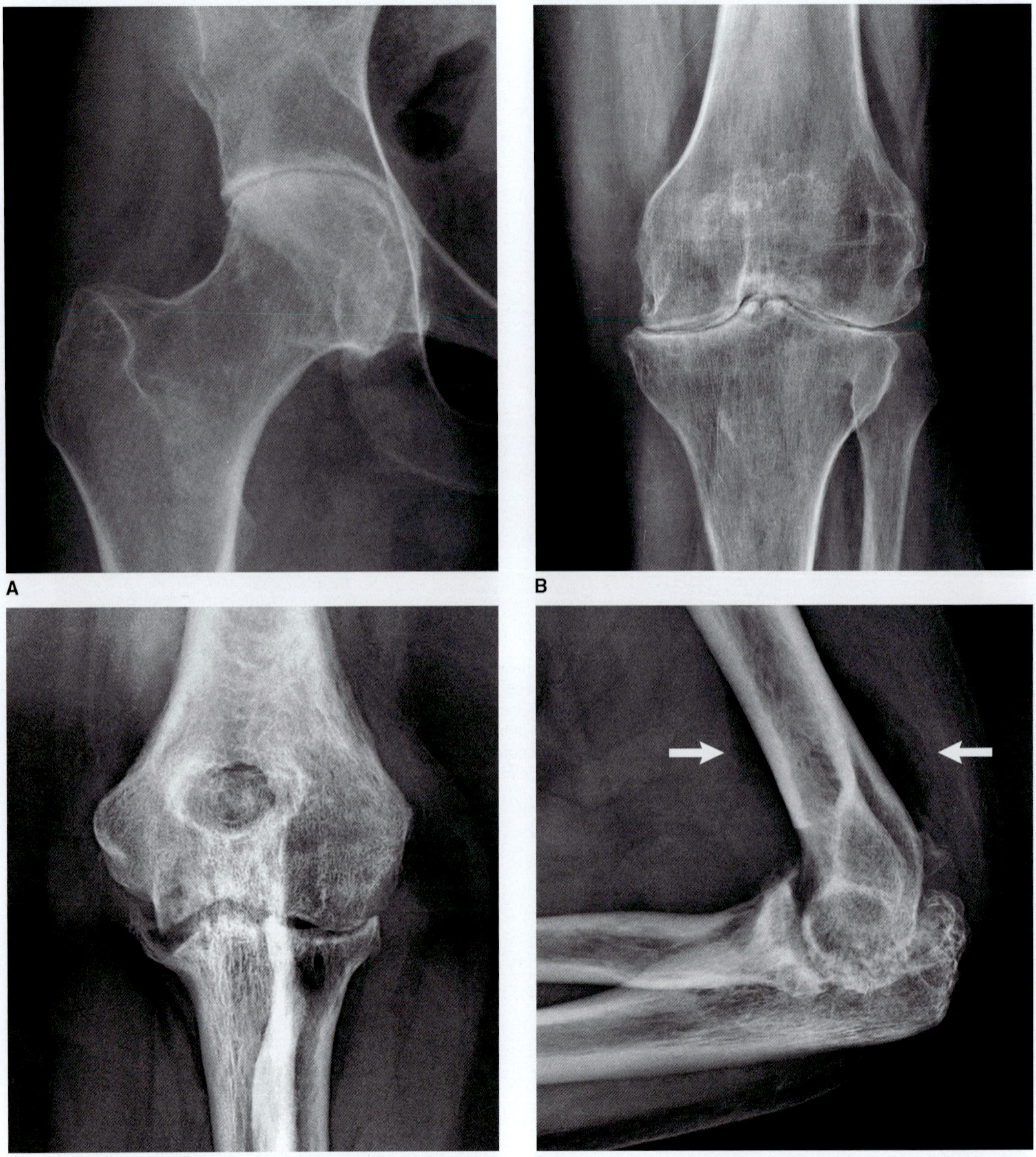

A B C D

Figure 3.17 ■ Rheumatoid arthritis. A: Anteroposterior radiograph of the right hip of a 42-year-old woman shows concentric narrowing of the joint space and axial migration of the femoral head. **B:** Anteroposterior radiograph of the left knee of a 63-year-old woman shows diffuse narrowing of the medial and lateral joint compartments. Observe periarticular osteoporosis and almost complete lack of osteophytes and subchondral sclerosis. Anteroposterior **(C)** and lateral **(D)** radiographs of the elbow of a 50-year-old woman show periarticular osteoporosis and erosions of the elbow joint compartments. Note also a positive anterior and posterior fat-pad sign (*arrows*) indicative of joint effusion.

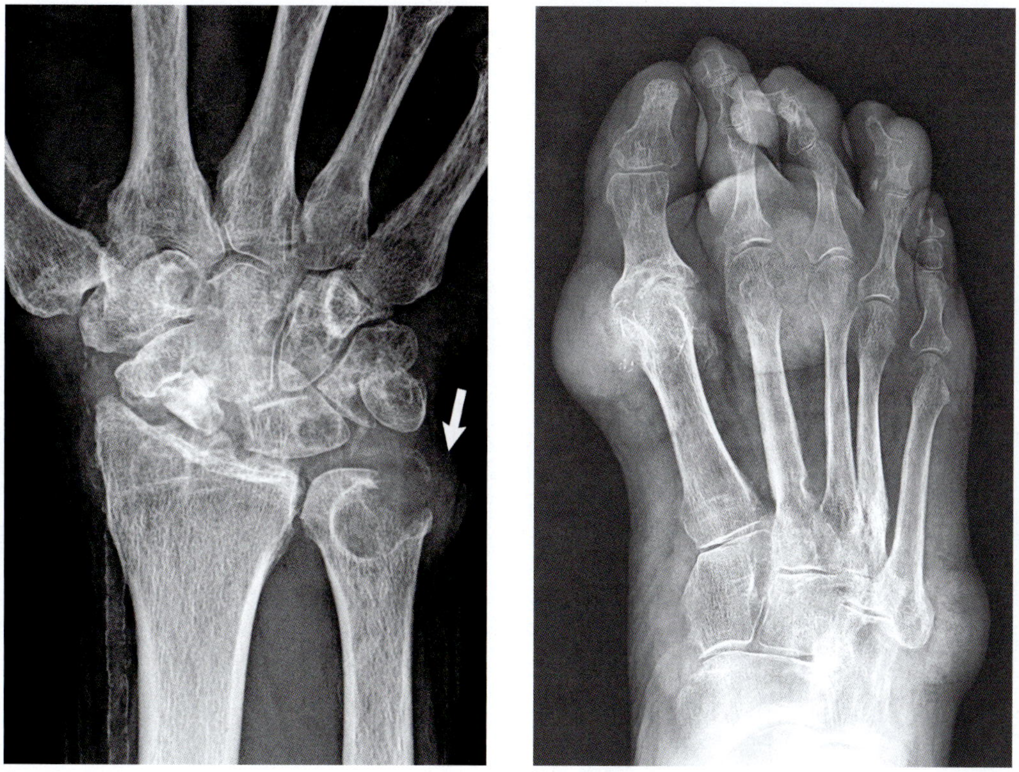

A B

Figure 3.18 ■ **Gouty arthropathy. A:** Dorsovolar radiograph of the left wrist of a 72-year-old man shows several erosions of the carpal bones and large erosion with characteristic overhanging edges of the distal ulna associated with a tophus (*arrow*). **B:** Anteroposterior radiograph of the left foot of a 61-year-old man shows typical periarticular erosions of the tarsometatarsal joints as well as the second, fourth, and fifth metatarsophalangeal joints. In addition, there are articular erosions of the first metatarsophalangeal and distal interphalangeal joint of the fourth toe. Note numerous dense soft tissue masses representing gouty tophi.

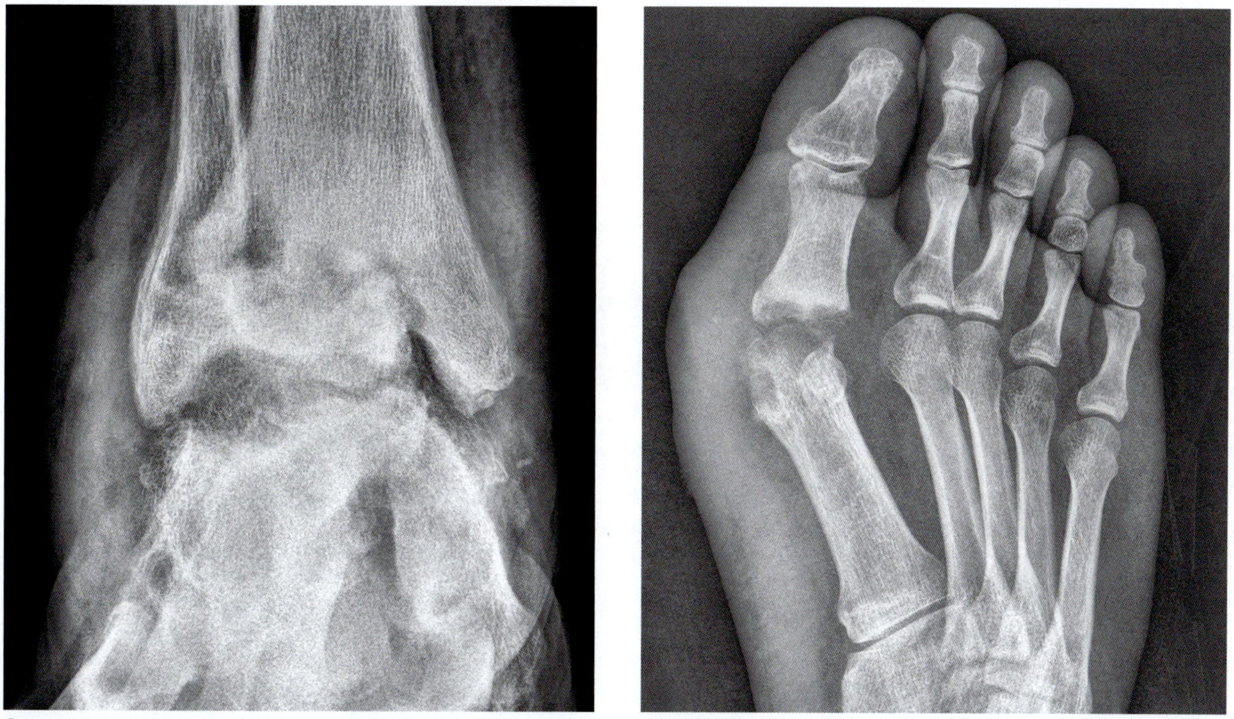

A B

Figure 3.19 ■ **Infectious arthritis. A:** Anteroposterior radiograph of the right ankle of a 63-year-old man shows complete destruction of the articular cartilage and adjacent subchondral bone of the distal tibia and talus, associated with diffuse soft tissue swelling and edema. **B:** Dorsoplantar radiograph of the left foot of a 26-year-old man shows destruction of the first metatarsophalangeal joint associated with large soft tissue swelling exhibiting foci of air.

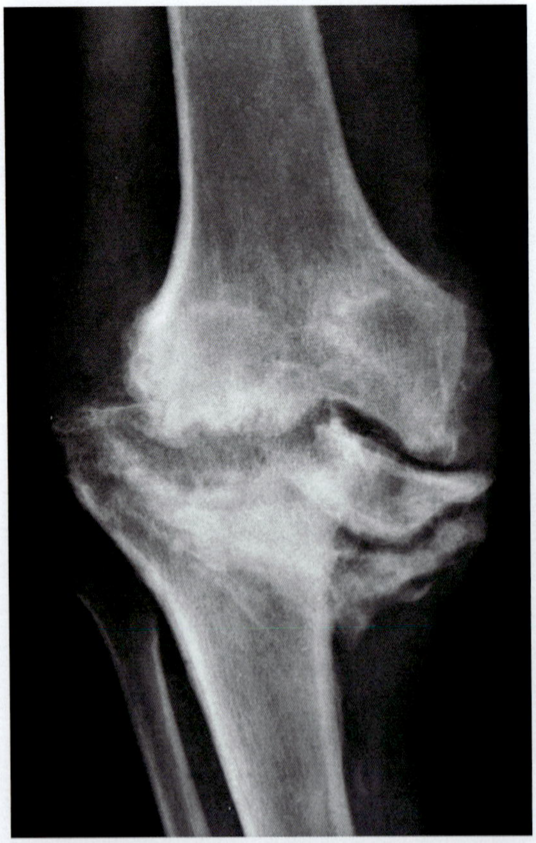

Figure 3.20 ■ **Neuropathic arthropathy.** The neuropathic joint is morphologically identified by gross articular disorganization, multiple bony debris, and joint effusion, as seen here in the knee. Note the lack of osteoporosis. The amount of destruction evident in this case results in severe joint instability.

by destruction of the articular surfaces, which leaves bony debris, and a substantial joint effusion; osteoporosis is usually lacking. Depending on the amount of destruction, varying degrees of joint instability are present (Fig. 3.20).

Analysis of the morphologic features of an arthritic lesion at certain sites other than the diarthrodial joints may be of further assistance in differentiating the various arthritides and reaching a correct diagnosis. Two such sites that are frequently affected are the heel and the spine. In the heel (Fig. 3.21), degenerative changes are usually manifested by a traction osteophyte (enthesophyte) at the posterior and plantar aspects of the calcaneus (Fig. 3.22A). Rheumatoid arthritis produces erosive changes in the area of the retrocalcaneal bursa secondary to inflammatory rheumatoid bursitis (Fig. 3.22B). Psoriatic arthritis (Fig. 3.22C), reactive arthritis (Fig. 3.22D), and ankylosing spondylitis all produce a characteristic "fluffy" periostitis that results in a broad-based osteophyte at the site of attachment of the fascia plantaris on the plantar aspect of the calcaneus, associated with erosions of the plantar surface and the posterior aspect of this bone.

Similarly, the morphology of arthritic lesions in the spine offers important indications of the disease process at work (Fig. 3.23). Among the inflammatory arthritides, for instance, rheumatoid arthritis causes a characteristic erosion of the odontoid process (Fig. 3.24). Moreover, as a result of inflammatory pannus and erosion of the transverse ligament between the anterior arch of the atlas and C2, there may be subluxation in the atlantoaxial joint. This is usually manifested by an increase to more than

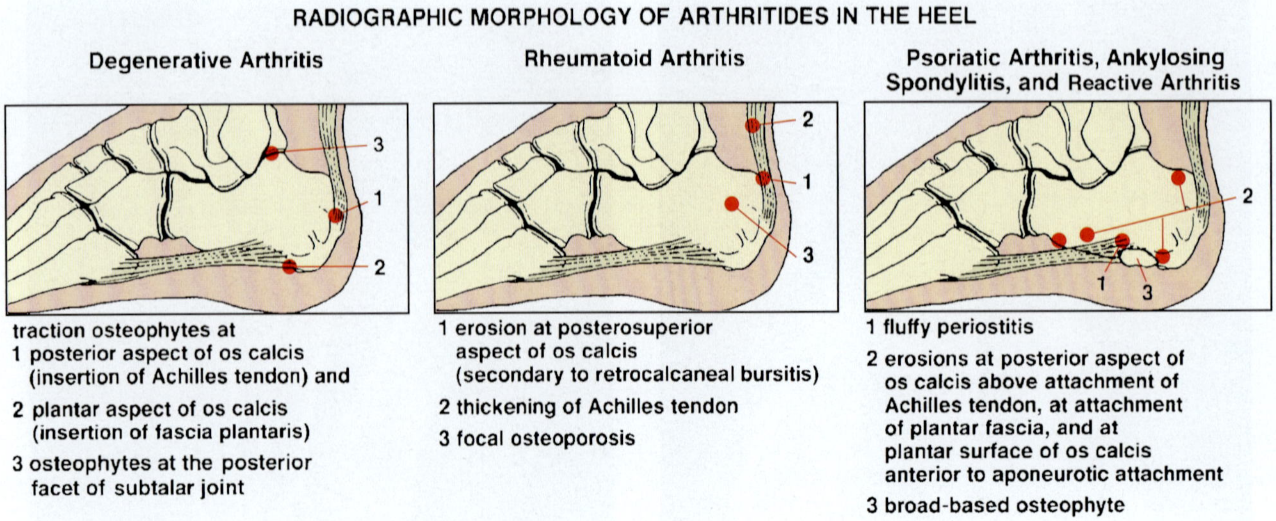

Figure 3.21 ■ **Arthritic changes in the heel.** Morphologic features distinguishing the various arthritides as manifest in arthritic lesions at the heel.

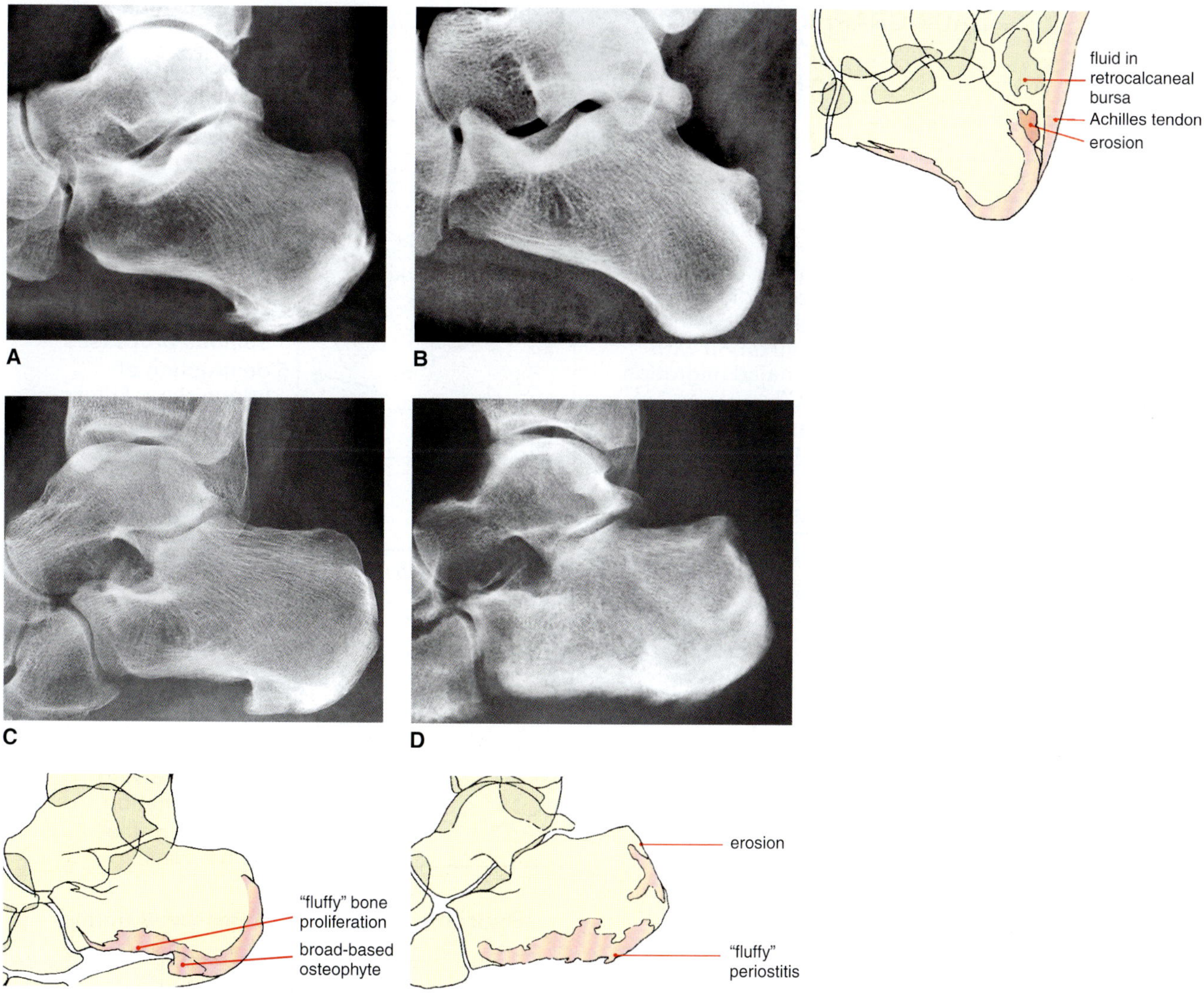

Figure 3.22 ■ Arthritic changes in the heel. The morphology of arthritic lesions in the heel can be helpful in differentiating the various arthritides. **A:** In the degenerative variant, traction osteophytes (enthesophytes) are evident at the insertions of the Achilles tendon and fascia plantaris on the posterior and plantar aspects of the os calcis. **B:** Rheumatoid arthritis typically exhibits retrocalcaneal bursitis and erosion of the posterosuperior aspect of the os calcis at the site of the bursa. Note the fluid-filled retrocalcaneal bursa projecting into the triangular-shaped fat pad anterior to the Achilles tendon. **C:** The calcaneus in psoriatic arthritis characteristically shows a coarse, broad-based osteophyte arising from the plantar aspect of the bone at the insertion of the fascia plantaris. Note the "fluffy" outline and bone proliferation along the plantar aspect of the os calcis. **D:** In this case of reactive arthritis, there is erosion of the posterior aspect of the os calcis, bone sclerosis, and a "fluffy" periostitis along its plantar aspect.

3 mm in the distance between the arch of the atlas and the dens, as demonstrated on a lateral view of the cervical spine in flexion (Fig. 3.25; see also Fig. 2.17). Erosions of the apophyseal joints of the cervical spine, sometimes leading to fusion, are frequently seen in juvenile idiopathic arthritis, formerly known as juvenile rheumatoid arthritis (Fig. 3.26).

Arthritic lesions involving other segments of the spine also exhibit distinguishing features that help in differentiating the disease process. Degenerative changes may manifest in the cervical, thoracic, or lumbar spine by the appearance of marginal osteophytes, narrowing and sclerosis of the apophyseal joints, and narrowing of the disk spaces (Fig. 3.27). In ankylosing spondylitis, in the early stages of the disease, there is a characteristic "squaring" of the vertebral bodies associated with sclerotic changes at the anterior aspect at the site of anterior longitudinal ligament due to osteitis (anterior spondylitis) and secondary reactive bone formation, as well as small erosions at the corners of the vertebral bodies, at the site of attachment of the annulus fibrosus to the vertebral endplate, surrounded by reactive sclerosis and osseous proliferation, so-called shiny corners or Romanus lesion (Fig. 3.28A). This

(Continued on page 109)

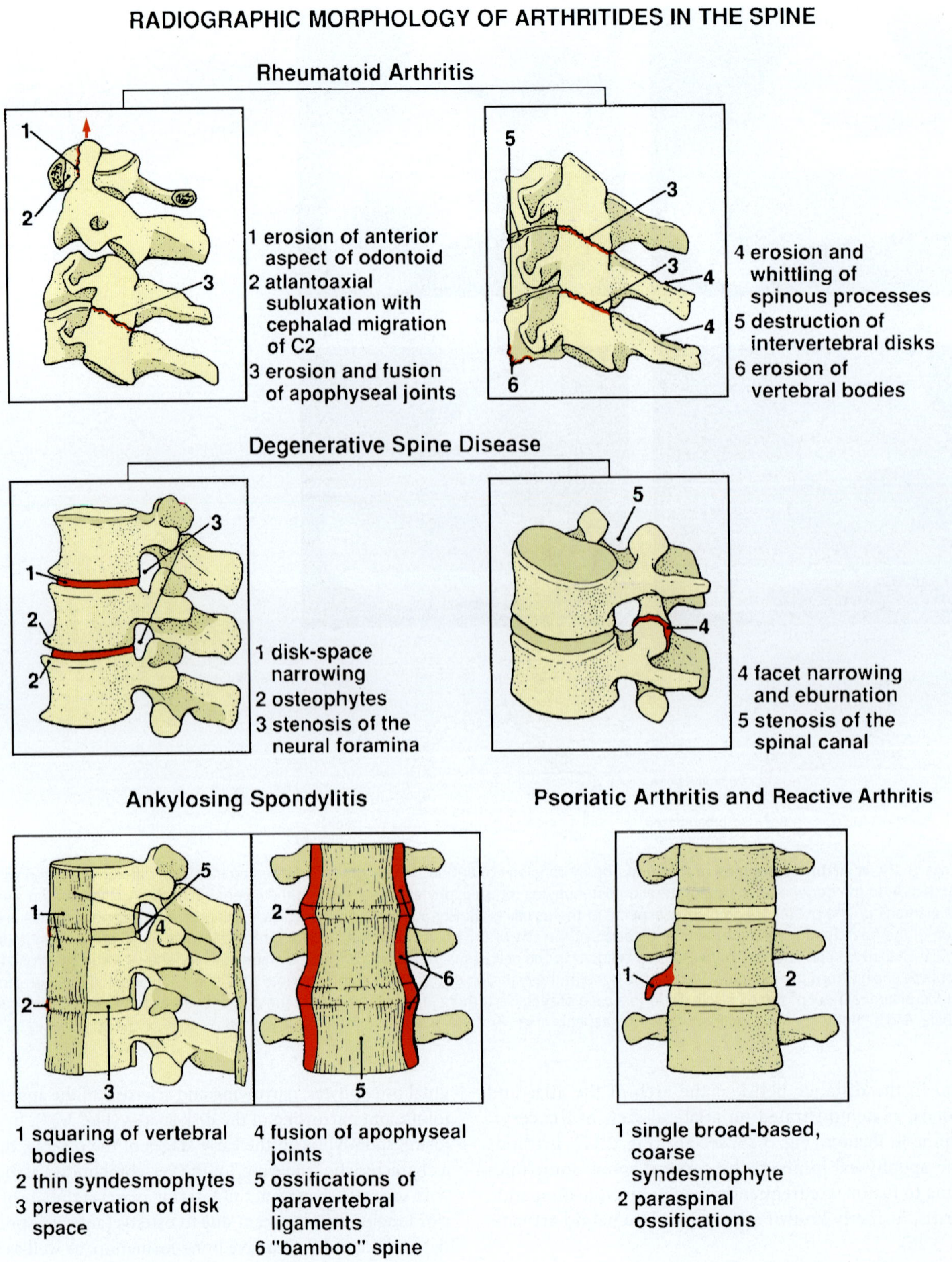

Figure 3.23 ■ **Arthritides of the spine.** Morphologic features distinguishing the various arthritides as manifested in the spine.

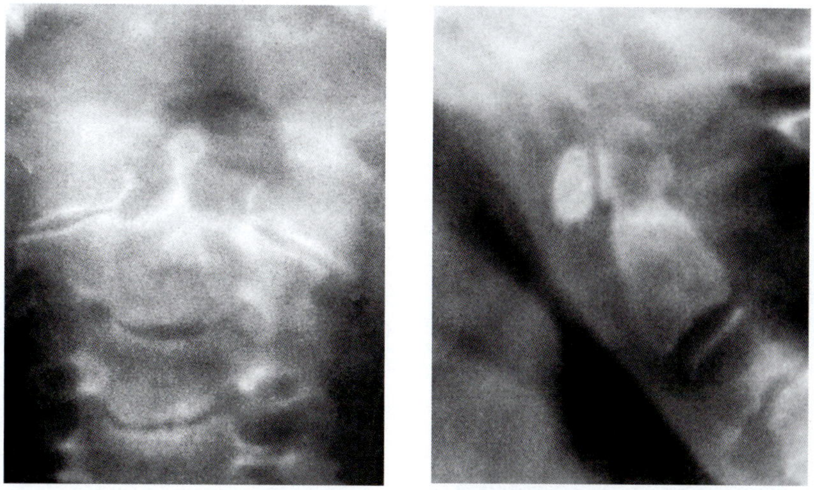

A B

Figure 3.24 ■ **Rheumatoid arthritis of the cervical spine.** Anteroposterior **(A)** and lateral **(B)** trispiral tomograms of the cervical spine in a 55-year-old woman with a 15-year history of rheumatoid arthritis show erosion of the odontoid process typical for this condition.

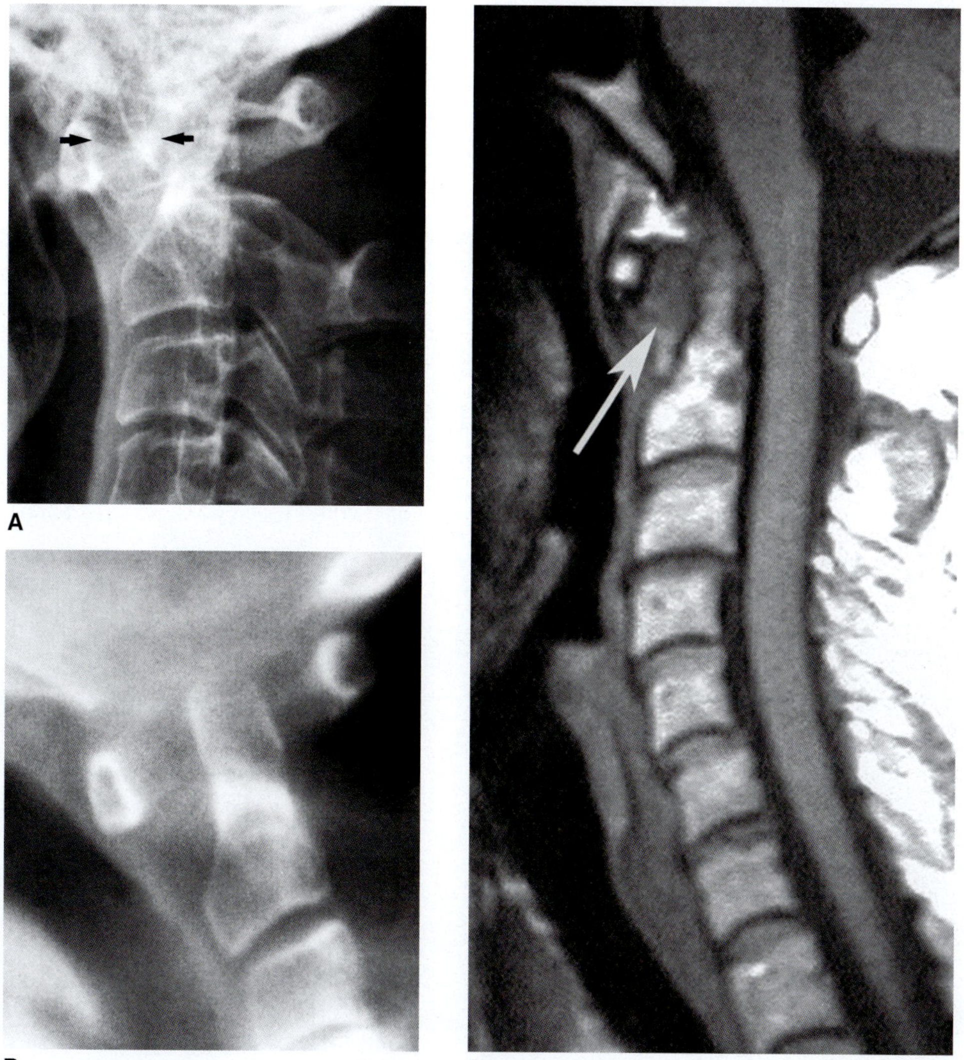

A B C

Figure 3.25 ■ **Rheumatoid arthritis of the cervical spine. A:** Lateral radiograph of the cervical spine in flexion in a 68-year-old woman with a long history of rheumatoid arthritis shows a marked increase in the distance between the anterior arch of the atlas and the odontoid process (*arrows*), measuring 12 mm; normally, it should not exceed 3 mm. **B:** Trispiral tomogram demonstrates the atlantoaxial subluxation more clearly. **C:** Sagittal T1-weighted MRI of the cervical spine in another patient with rheumatoid arthritis demonstrates increased space between the anterior arch of C1 and the odontoid process, which is eroded. Note the low–signal intensity inflammatory pannus (*arrow*).

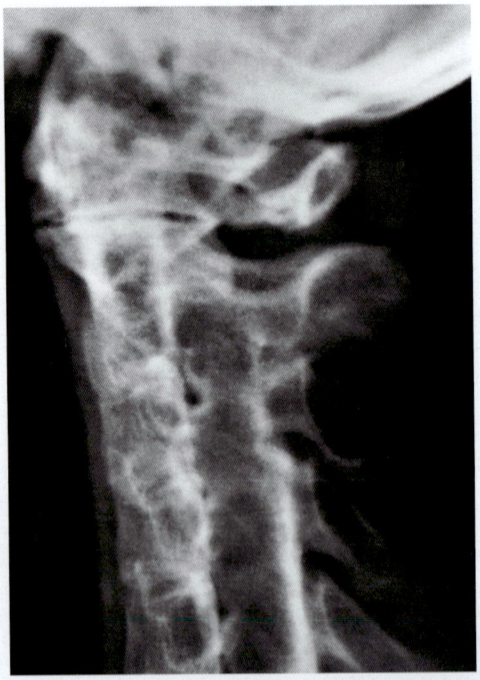

Figure 3.26 ■ Juvenile idiopathic arthritis. Lateral radiograph of the cervical spine in a 34-year-old woman with juvenile idiopathic arthritis since age 20 shows the typical involvement of the apophyseal joints. In this case, there is complete fusion of the joints.

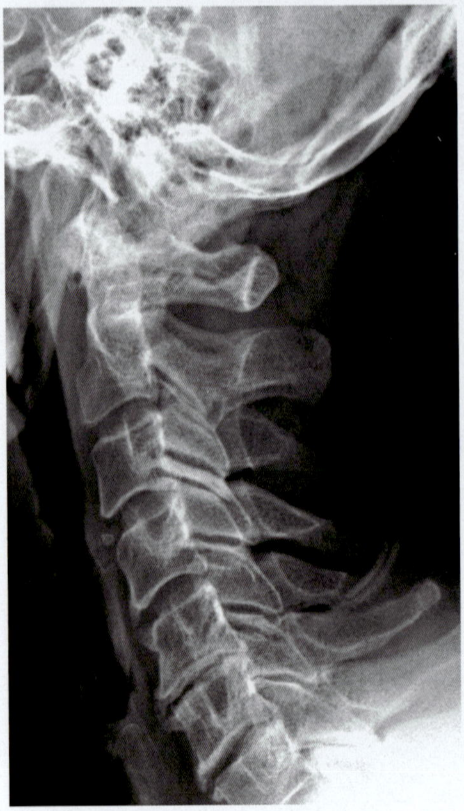

A

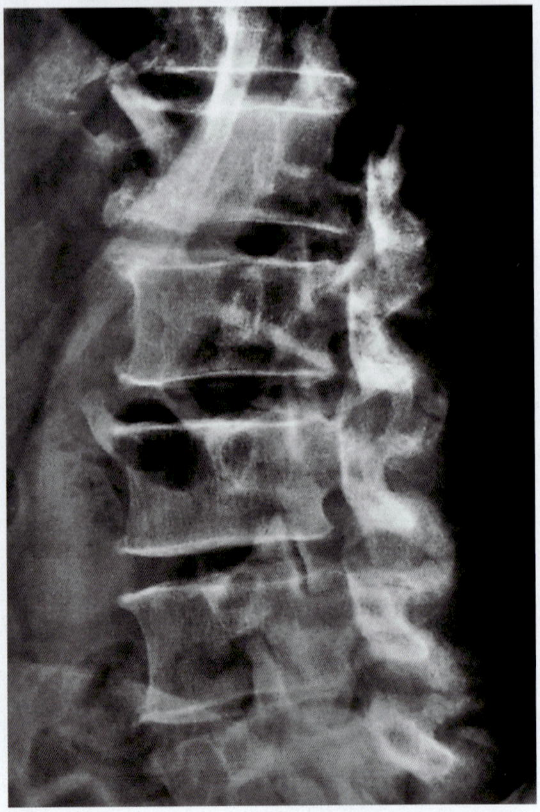

B

Figure 3.27 ■ Degenerative spine disease. A: Lateral radiograph of the cervical spine of a 66-year-old man shows narrowing of the several disk spaces of the lower segment, osteophyte formation from the anterior and posterior aspects of the vertebral bodies, and narrowing and eburnation of the facet joints. **B:** Oblique radiograph of the lumbar spine in a 72-year-old woman shows narrowing and eburnation of the articular margins of the facet joints, osteophytosis, and narrowing of the intervertebral disk spaces—a combination of the effects of true facet joint arthritis, spondylosis deformans, and degenerative disk disease.

follows the formation of delicate syndesmophytes arising from the anterior aspects of the vertebral bodies (Fig. 3.28B, C), which differ morphologically from degenerative osteophytes. In the later stages of this condition, inflammation and fusion of the apophyseal joints lead to the appearance of what has been called "bamboo" spine; the sacroiliac joints are also invariably affected (Fig. 3.29). In psoriasis and reactive arthritis, one can occasionally see a single, coarse osteophyte/syndesmophyte in the lumbar spine, frequently bridging adjacent vertebral bodies, as well as paravertebral ossifications; there are also associated inflammatory changes in the sacroiliac joints (Fig. 3.30).

(Continued on page 111)

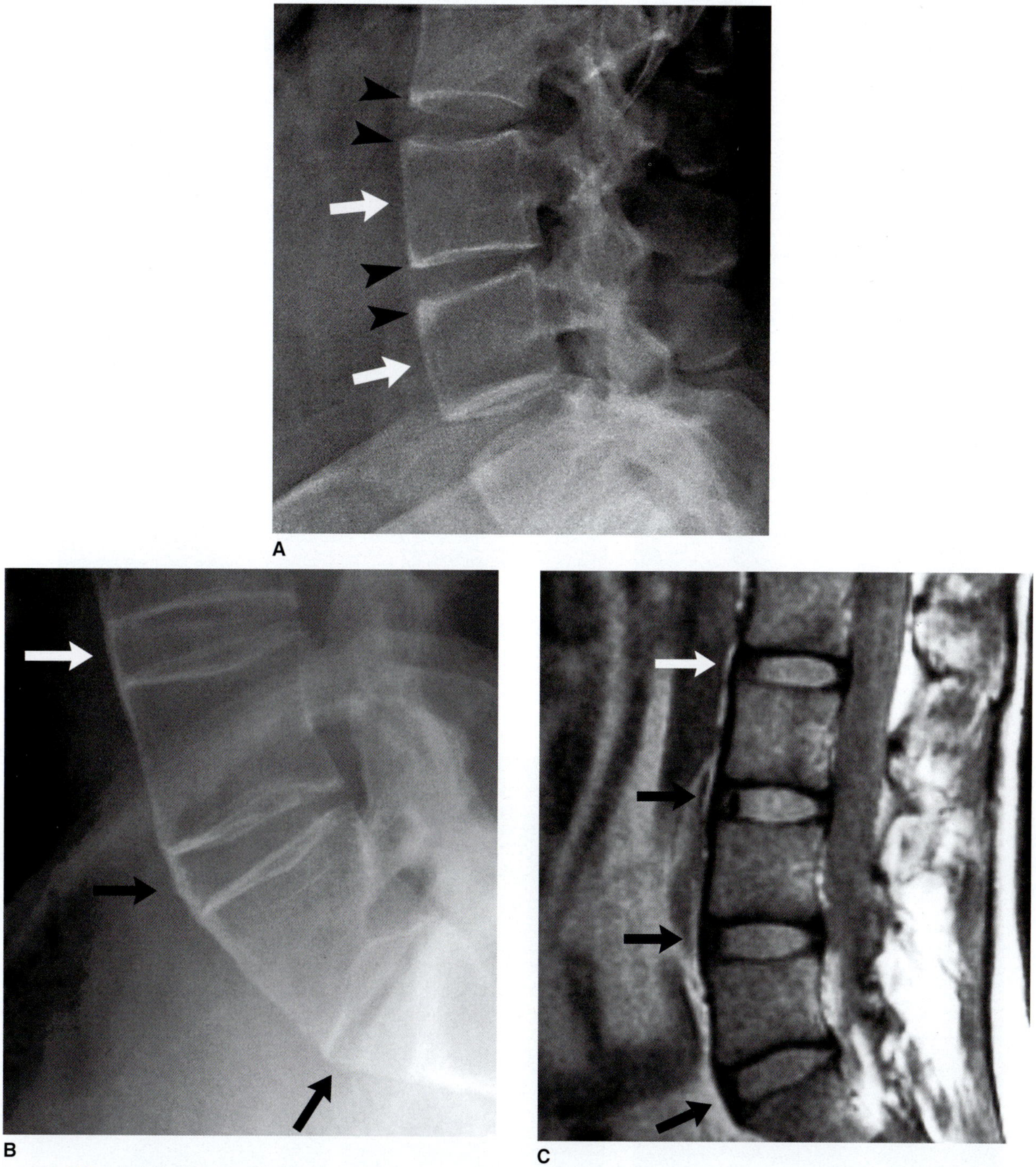

Figure 3.28 ■ **Ankylosing spondylitis. A:** A lateral radiograph of the lower lumbar spine of a 33-year-old man shows early inflammatory changes manifesting by so-called shiny corners (Romanus lesion) (*arrowheads*) and squaring of the vertebral bodies (*arrows*). Lateral radiograph **(B)** and sagittal T1-weighted MR image **(C)** of the lumbar spine show characteristic delicate, vertically oriented syndesmophytes (*arrows*).

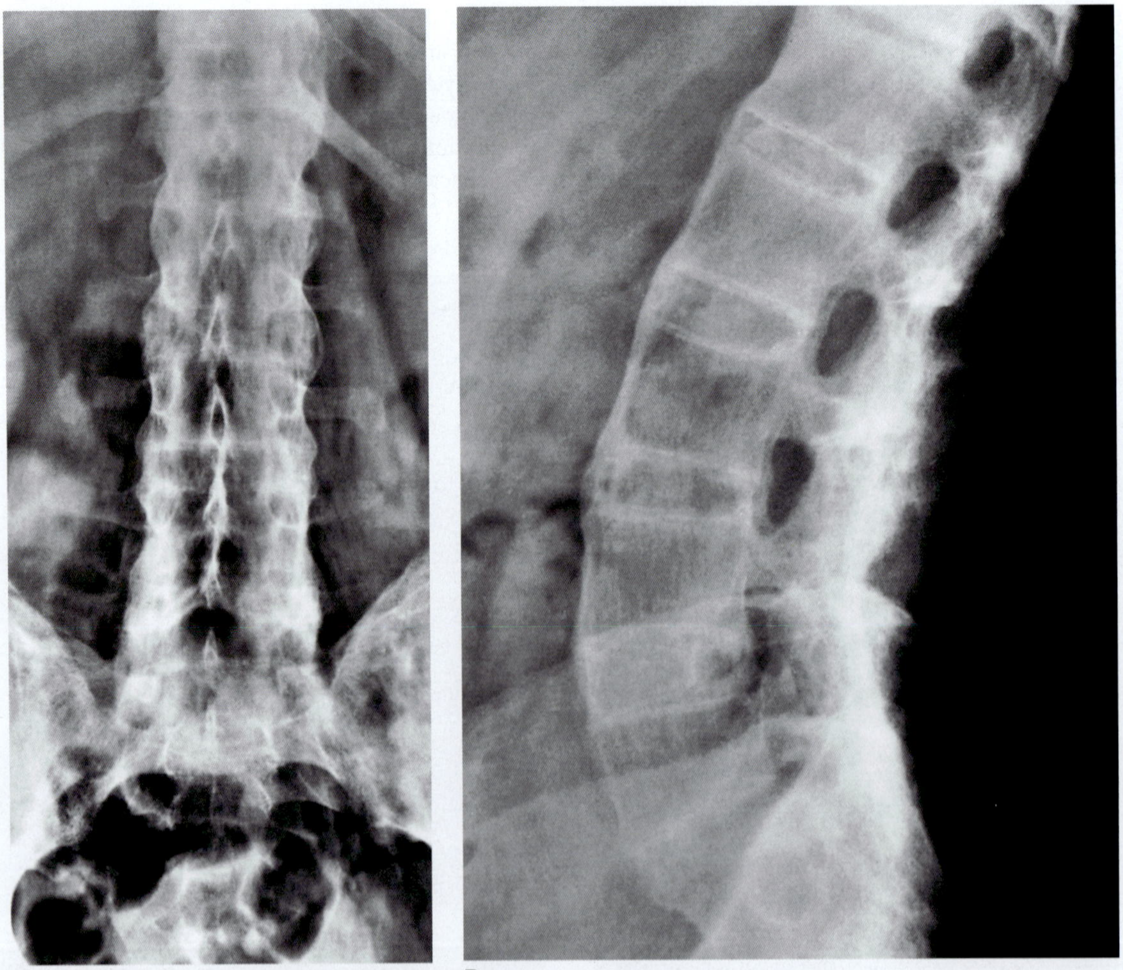

A B

Figure 3.29 ■ **Ankylosing spondylitis.** Anteroposterior **(A)** and lateral **(B)** radiographs of the lumbar spine in a 31-year-old man with advanced ankylosing spondylitis demonstrate the typical appearance of "bamboo spine" secondary to inflammation, ossification, and fusion of the apophyseal joints associated with ossification of the anterior and posterior longitudinal ligaments, as well as the supraspinous and interspinous ligaments. Note also the fusion of the sacroiliac joints.

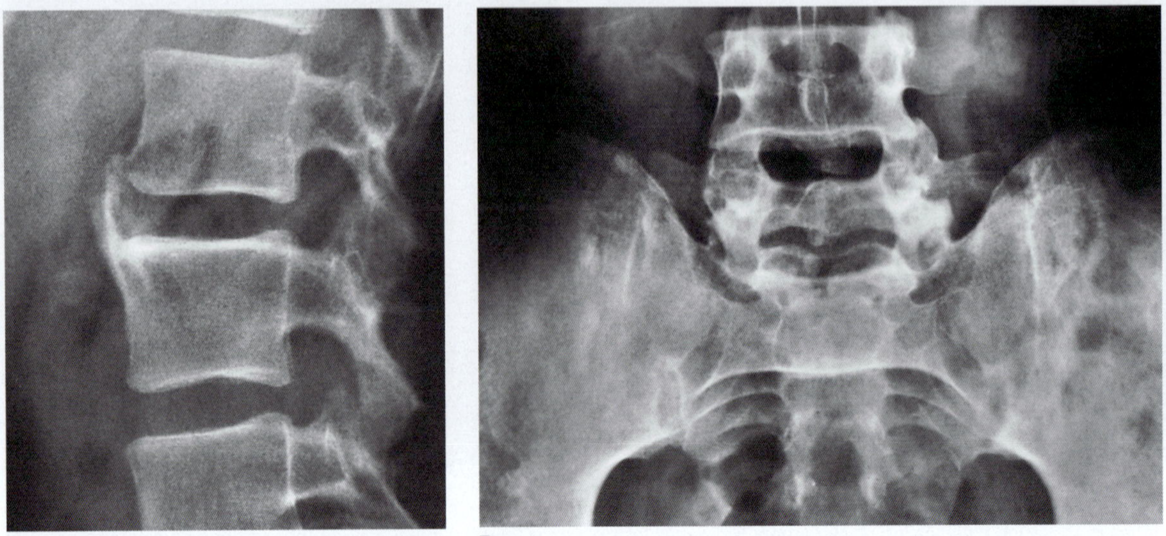

A B

Figure 3.30 ■ **Reactive arthritis. A:** Lateral radiograph of the lumbar spine in a 27-year-old man shows a single, coarse osteophyte/syndesmophyte bridging the bodies of L1 and L2. **B:** Anteroposterior radiograph of the lumbosacral segment shows the effects of the inflammatory process on the sacroiliac joints (sacroiliitis).

Distribution of the Articular Lesion

Distribution of the lesions in the skeleton varies with the type of arthritis (Fig. 3.31). Osteoarthritis tends to have a characteristic distribution in the skeletal system. Typically, the large joints such as the hip and knee and the small joints of the hand and wrist are involved, whereas the shoulder, elbow, and ankle are spared. Inflammatory arthritides, however, have different sites of predilection in the skeleton, depending on the specific variant of the disease. Rheumatoid arthritis, for example, involves most of the large joints such as the hip, knee, elbows, and shoulders, and small joints of the hands and feet. In the cervical spine, the C1–C2 articulation and the apophyseal joints are frequently affected. Juvenile idiopathic arthritis, previously known as juvenile rheumatoid arthritis, has a similar pattern of distribution, except that the distal interphalangeal joints of the hand may also be affected. Psoriatic arthritis, in contrast to rheumatoid arthritis, has a predilection for the distal interphalangeal joints, as well as the sacroiliac joints, resembling reactive arthritis in this respect. Erosive osteoarthritis, which some investigators consider a variant of osteoarthritis, others a variant of rheumatoid arthritis, and still others a distinct form of arthritis, has a tendency to affect the proximal and distal interphalangeal joints of the hand.

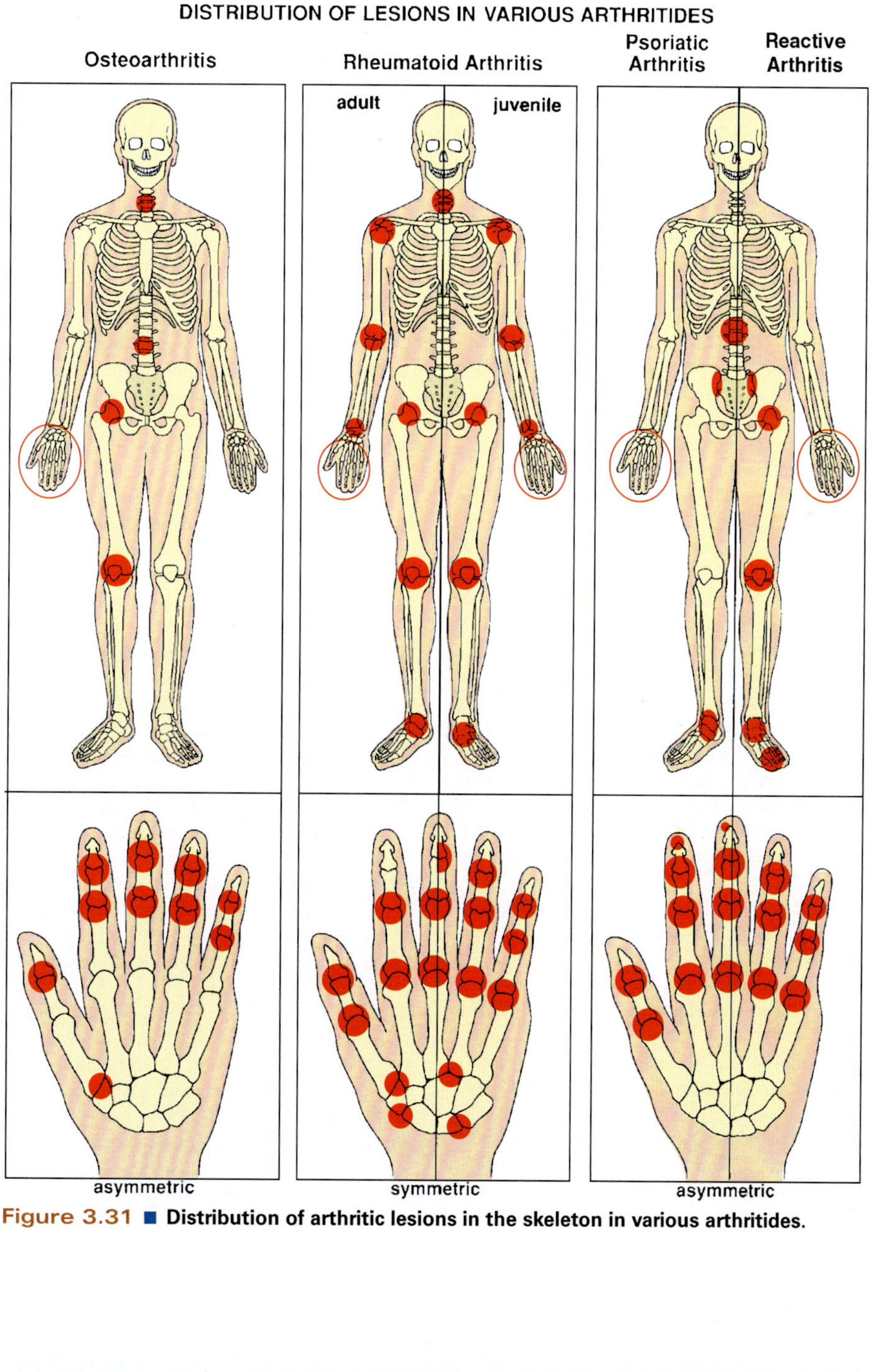

Figure 3.31 ■ **Distribution of arthritic lesions in the skeleton in various arthritides.**

SUGGESTED READINGS

Alcala JMF, Douat D, Pinheiro DL, et al. Radiographic changes of the cervical spine in rheumatoid arthritis. *Rev Brasil Rheumatol (English Ed).* 2013;53:388–393.

Alexander C. Use of a binary search pattern and discriminator analysis in the radiologic diagnosis of arthritis. *Semin Arthritis Rheum.* 1986;16:104–117.

Alexander CJ. Heberden's and Bouchard's nodes. *Ann Rheum Dis.* 1999;58:675–678.

Anandarajah AP, Ritchlin CT. The diagnosis and treatment of early psoriatic arthritis. *Nat Rev Rheumatol.* 2009;5:634–641.

Bathon JM, Martin RW, Fleischmann RM, et al. A comparison of etanercept and methotrexate in patients with early rheumatoid arthritis. *N Engl J Med.* 2000;343:1586–1593.

Belhorn LR, Hess EV. Erosive osteoarthritis. *Semin Arthritis Rheum.* 1993;22:298–306.

Bongartz T, Sutton AJ, Sweeting MJ, et al. Anti-TNF antibody therapy in rheumatoid arthritis and the risk of serious infections and malignancies. *JAMA.* 2005;295:2275–2285.

Bresnihan B, Newmark R, Robbins S, et al. Effects of anakinra monotherapy on joint damage in patients with rheumatoid arthritis. Extension of a 24-week randomized, placebo-controlled trial. *J Rheumatol.* 2004;31: 1103–1111.

Brower AC, Allman RM. Pencil pointing: a vascular pattern of deossification. *Radiographics.* 1983;3:315–325.

Brower AC, Kransdorf MJ. Evaluation of disorders of the sacroiliac joint. *Appl Radiol.* 1992;21:31–43.

Buckland-Wright JC, Walker SR. Incidence and size of erosions in the wrist and hand of rheumatoid patients: a quantitative microfocal radiographic study. *Ann Rheum Dis.* 1987;46:463–467.

Carter JD. Reactive arthritis: defined etiologies, emerging pathophysiology, and unresolved treatment. *Infect Dis Clin North Am.* 2006;20:827–847.

Carter JD, Espinoza LR, Inman RD, et al. Combination antibiotics as a treatment for chronic *Chlamydia*-induced reactive arthritis: a double-blind, placebo-controlled, prospective trial. *Arthritis Rheum.* 2010;62:1298–1307.

Carter JD, Hudson AP. Reactive arthritis: clinical aspects and medical management. *Rheum Dis Clin North Am.* 2009;35:21–44.

Castelino M, Barton A. Genetic susceptibility factors for psoriatic arthritis. *Curr Opin Rheumatol.* 2010;22:152–156.

Choi HK, Burns LC, Shojania K, et al. Dual energy CT in gout: a prospective validation study. *Ann Rheum Dis.* 2012;71:1466–1471.

Cicuttini FM, Baker J, Hart DJ, Spector TD. Relation between Heberden's nodes and distal interphalangeal joint osteophytes and their role as markers of generalised disease. *Ann Rheum Dis.* 1998;57:246–248.

Cobby M, Cushnaghan J, Creamer P, Dieppe P, et al. Erosive osteoarthritis: is it a separate disease entity? *Clin Radiol.* 1990;42:258–263.

Cohen SB, Moreland LW, Cush JJ, et al. A multicentre, double blind, randomized, placebo controlled trial of anakinra (Kineret), a recombinant interleukin 1 receptor antagonist, in patients with rheumatoid arthritis treated with background methotrexate. *Ann Rheum Dis.* 2004;63:1062–1068.

Colmegna I, Cuchacovich R, Espinoza LR. HLA-B27-associated reactive arthritis: pathogenetic and clinical considerations. *Clin Microbiol Rev.* 2004;17:348–369.

Cushnaghan J, Dieppe P. Study of 500 patients with limb joint osteoarthritis. I. Analysis by age, sex, and distribution of symptomatic joint sites. *Ann Rheum Dis.* 1991;50:8–13.

Edwards JC, Szczepanski L, Szechinski J, et al. Efficacy of B-cell targeted therapy with rituximab in patients with rheumatoid arthritis. *N Engl J Med.* 2004;350:2572–2581.

El-Khoury GY, Larson RK, Kathol MH, et al. Seronegative and seropositive rheumatoid arthritis: radiographic differences. *Radiology.* 1988;168: 517–520.

Emery P, Fleischmann R, Filipowicz-Sosnowska A, et al. The efficacy and safety of rituximab in patients with active rheumatoid arthritis despite methotrexate treatment: results of a phase IIb randomized, double-blind, placebo-controlled, dose-ranging trial. *Arthritis Rheum.* 2006;54:1390–1400.

Ernst ME, Fravel MA. Febuxostat: a selective xanthine-oxidase/xanthine dehydrogenase inhibitor for management of hyperuricemia in adult with gout. *Clin Ther.* 2009;31:2503–2518.

Fitzgerald O, Winchester R. Psoriatic arthritis: from pathogenesis to therapy. *Ann Rheum Dis.* 2006;65:1373–1378.

Genovese MC, Becker JC, Schiff M, et al. Abatacept for rheumatoid arthritis refractory to tumor necrosis factor alpha inhibition. *N Engl J Med.* 2005;353:1114–1123.

Goldring SR. Periarticular bone changes in rheumatoid arthritis: pathophysiological implications and clinical utility. *Ann Rheum Dis.* 2009;68: 297–299.

Gottlieb A, Menter A, Mendelsohn A, et al. Ustekinubab, a human interleukin 12/23 monoclonal antibody, for psoriatic arthritis: randomized, double-blind, placebo-controlled, cross-over trial. *Lancet.* 2009;373:633–640.

Greenspan A. Erosive osteoarthritis. *Semin Musculoskelet Radiol.* 2003;7: 155–159.

Hajialilo M, Kolahi S, Khabaazi A, Farzin H. The cervical spine involvement in rheumatoid arthritis. *Internet J Rheumatol.* 2012;7:1–6.

Hoffman GS. Polyarthritis: the differential diagnosis of rheumatoid arthritis. *Semin Arthritis Rheum.* 1978;8:115–141.

Jacobson JA, Girish G, Jiang Y, Resnick D. Radiographic evaluation of arthritis: inflammatory conditions. *Radiology.* 2008;248:378–389.

Jacobson JA, Girish G, Jiang Y, Sabb BJ. Radiographic evaluation of arthritis: degenerative joint disease and variations. *Radiology.* 2008;248:737–747.

Kapasi OA, Ruby LK, Calney K. The psoriatic hand. *J Hand Surg Am.* 1982;7A:492–497.

Keat A. Reiter's syndrome and reactive arthritis in perspective. *N Engl J Med.* 1983;309:1606–1615.

Khalkhali I, Stadalnik RC, Wiesner KB, Shapiro RF. Bone imaging of the heel in Reiter's syndrome. *AJR Am J Roentgenol.* 1979;132:110–112.

Klecker R, Weissman BN. Imaging features of psoriatic arthritis and Reiter's syndrome. *Semin Musculoskelet Radiol.* 2003;7:115–126.

Leandro MJ, Cambridge G, Ehrenstein MR, et al. Reconstitution of peripheral blood B cells after depletion with rituximab in patients with rheumatoid arthritis. *Arthritis Rheum.* 2006;54:613–620.

Malik A, Schumacher HR, Dinella JE, Clayburne GM. Clinical diagnostic criteria for gout: comparison with the gold standard of synovial fluid crystal analysis. *J Clin Rheumatol.* 2009;15:22–24.

Martel W, Braunstein EM, Borlaza G, et al. Radiologic features of Reiter disease. *Radiology.* 1979;132:1–10.

McGonagle D, Benjamin M, Tan AL. The pathogenesis of psoriatic arthritis and associated nail disease: not autoimmune after all? *Curr Opin Rheumatol.* 2009;21:340–347.

Mease PJ. Psoriatic arthritis: update on pathophysiology, assessment and management. *Ann Rheum Dis.* 2011;70(Suppl 1):i77–84.

Narvaez JA, Narvaez J, Serrallonga M, et al. Cervical spine involvement in rheumatoid arthritis: correlation between neurological manifestations and magnetic resonance imaging findings. *Rheumatology.* 2008;47: 1814–1819.

Navallas M, Ares J, Beltran B, et al. Sacroiliitis associated with axial spondyloarthropathy: new concepts and latest trends. *Radiographics.* 2013;33: 933–956.

O'Dell J, Haire CE, Erikson N, et al. Treatment of rheumatoid arthritis with methotrexate alone, sulfasalazine, and hydroxychloroquine, or a combination of all three medications. *N Engl J Med.* 1996;334:1287–1291.

Patton JT. Differential diagnosis of inflammatory spondylitis. *Skeletal Radiol.* 1976;1:77–85.

Perez-Ruiz F, Dalbeth N, Urresola A, et al. Imaging of gout: findings and utility. *Arthritis Res Ther.* 2009;11:232–239.

Rees F, Doherty S, Hui M, et al. Distribution of finger nodes and their association with underlying radiographic features of osteoarthritis. *Arthritis Care Res.* 2012;64:533–538.

Ritchlin CT, Kavanaugh A, Gladman DD, et al. Treatment recommendations for psoriatic arthritis. *Ann Rheum Dis.* 2009;68:1387–1394.

Rothschild BM. Distinguishing erosive osteoarthritis and calcium pyrophosphate deposition disease. *World J Orthop.* 2013;4:29–31.

Sankowski AJ, Lebkowska UM, Cwikla J, et al. Psoriatic arthritis. *Pol J Radiol.* 2013;78:7–17.

Schoellnast H, Deutschmann HA, Hermann J, et al. Psoriatic arthritis and rheumatoid arthritis: findings in contrast-enhanced MRI. *AJR Am J Roentgenol.* 2006;187:351–357.

Siddle HJ, Hensor EMA, Hodgson RJ, et al. Anatomical location of erosions at the metatarsophalangeal joints in patients with rheumatoid arthritis. *Rheumatology.* 2014;53:932–936.

Soriano ER, Rosa J. Update on the treatment of peripheral arthritis in psoriatic arthritis. *Curr Rheumatol Rep.* 2009;11:270–277.

Stecher RM. Heberden's nodes: the clinical characteristic of osteo-arthritis of the fingers. *Ann Rheum Dis.* 1948;7:1–8.

Strauss EJ, Alfonso D, Baidwan G, Di Cesare PE. Orthopedic manifestations and management of psoriatic arthritis. *Am J Orthop.* 2008;37:138–147.

Tan AL, Tanner SF, Conaghan PG, et al. Role of metacarpophalangeal joint anatomic factors in the distribution of synovitis and bone erosion in early rheumatoid arthritis. *Arthritis Rheum.* 2003;48:1214–1222.

Terkeltaub R. Update on gout: new therapeutic strategies and options. *Nat Rev Rheumatol.* 2010;6:30–38.

Weinblatt ME, Polisson R, Blotner SD, et al. The effects of drug therapy on radiographic progression of rheumatoid arthritis. Results of a 36-week randomized trial comparing methotrexate and auranofin. *Arthritis Rheum.* 1993;36:613–619.

Weissman BN. Imaging techniques in rheumatoid arthritis. *J Rheumatol Suppl.* 1994;42:14–19.

Wolf F, Michaud K. Lymphoma in rheumatoid arthritis: the effect of methotrexate and anti-tumor necrosis factor therapy in 18,572 patients. *Arthritis Rheum.* 2004;50:1740–1751.

Wortman RL, Schumacher HR Jr. Monosodium urate deposition arthropathy part I: review of the stages and diagnosis of gout. *Adv Stud Med.* 2005;5:133–138.

Wortmann RL, Schumacher HR Jr. Monosodium urate deposition arthropathy part II: treatment and long term management of patients with gout. *Adv Stud Med.* 2005;5:183–196.

CHAPTER 4

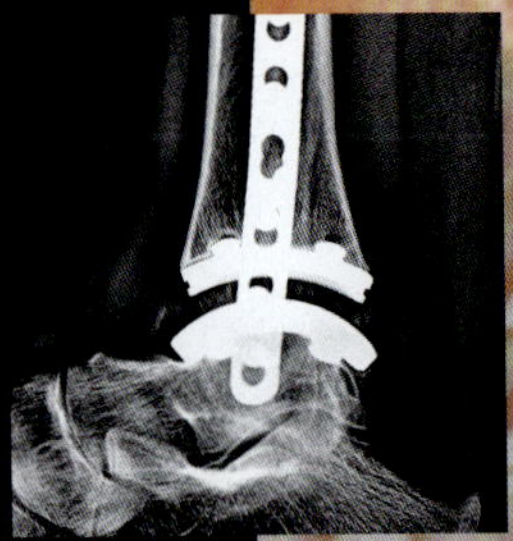

Treatment of the Arthritides and Arthropathies

MEDICAL TREATMENT

The treatment of rheumatologic diseases has undergone a revolution in the past decade. In the past, the paradigm for the management of inflammatory arthritides, such as ***rheumatoid arthritis***, ***psoriatic arthritis***, and ***ankylosing spondylitis***, was to treat with nonsteroidal anti-inflammatory drugs (NSAIDs), followed by increasing use of more potent medication; this was often called a pyramid scheme. However, this is no longer the case. The current dogma is to treat patients early and aggressively with disease-modifying drugs and, in particular, to include the use of the biologic drugs such as agents that inhibit tumor necrosis factor (TNF), IL-6, or CD20-bearing B cells. Discussion of these therapies is beyond the scope of this textbook, but it is important to note that the biologic drugs have a significant potential to modify disease, reduce the systemic manifestations, and slow the progression of destructive changes in the joints. They do, however, carry significant side effects and must be monitored on a regular basis. For this reason, we recommend that the use of such drugs be done by rheumatologist and not by family practitioners or internists, unless a rheumatologist concurrently follows the patient. Interestingly, this is likewise the case for patients with ***gout***. In the past, treatment consisted of anti-inflammatory drugs and often the use of allopurinol. However, a whole variety of new drugs have been introduced that modulate different levels of uric acid metabolism, and here again, our recommendation is that such usage should be done by rheumatologists. Treatment for ***CPPD crystal deposition*** disease associated with ***pseudogout syndrome*** is essentially the same as for gout, including oral administration of colchicine. Unfortunately, the treatment model has not significantly changed for ***systemic lupus erythematosus (SLE)***, in which there have been no significant improvements in drugs or drug protocols for more than a decade. Although there are agents that block B-cell activation and have been approved for SLE, they are, for the most part, disappointing. The treatment of first choice for ***reactive arthritis*** consists of NSAIDs, such as ibuprofen. Systemic glucocorticoids or intra-articular injections of steroids can also be beneficial. Because reactive arthritis is associated with infection caused by *Shigella*, *Salmonella*, *Campylobacter*, *Yersinia*, or *Chlamydia trachomatis*, appropriate antibiotic treatment should be administered if infection is active.

Finally, we note that despite intensive efforts at understanding cartilage repair and new bone formation, the treatment of ***osteoarthritis*** has remained unchanged. The major handicap is a late diagnosis of the disease, because majority of the patients present to the medical facilities with the already advanced, nondiagnosed osteoarthritis lasted for years. There are already pathologic changes in cartilage water content and an age-related influence of normal tissue repair. These factors are superimposed, among others, on influence of obesity, prior injury, and poor conditioning. Most patients with osteoarthritis can be managed through nonpharmacological and pharmacological therapy. The former includes education, weight management, bracing, and appropriate exercise with goal to delay the progression of the disease, alleviate symptoms, and improve function. Nutritional supplements such as glucosamine and chondroitin sulfate may be beneficial for some patients. Occasionally, therapeutic ultrasound and pulsed electromagnetic field therapy proved to be helpful. The pharmacological therapy includes nonnarcotic analgesics such as acetaminophen and nonsteroidal anti-inflammatory drugs. The use of opiates is strongly discouraged. Some patients benefit from intra-articular injections of corticosteroids or hyaluronan, particularly for osteoarthritis of the knee. The latter drug produces symptomatic relief through one or more of a large number of mechanisms. It decreases the sensitivity of pain fibers, enhances proteoglycan synthesis by chondrocytes, reduces quantities and activity of proinflammatory mediators and matrix metalloproteinases, and alters the behavior of immune system cells.

The bottom line and importance of these paradigms and treatments are that the improvements in the care of patients with rheumatoid arthritis, psoriatic arthritis, and ankylosing spondylitis have been nothing less than earth shattering, but carry with them an enormous price tag, the potential for drug toxicity, and the recommendation that only rheumatologists prescribe and follow the use of such medications. Clearly the diagnosis becomes essential, and to this end, this textbook that focuses on imaging will provide this important link.

RADIOTHERAPY

Radiotherapy was used in the past in several rheumatologic disorders in an attempt to relieve symptoms of inflammation. In particular, radiotherapy for ankylosing spondylitis was used extensively in the 1950s. With the recognition of significant long-term complications from high doses of radiation, including the development of pulmonary fibrosis, leukemias, lymphomas, osteosarcomas, and other malignant tumors, this approach has generally been abandoned. More recently, radiosynovectomy that involves an intra-articular injection of small radioactive articles became a well-established therapy for arthritic disorders to treat synovitis. Intra-articular radiotherapy using yttrium 90 (Y90) was attempted in patients with rheumatoid arthritis. Some investigators reported promising results after radiation synovectomy for inflamed small joints of the hands injecting under fluoroscopic or sonographic guidance erbium-169 (169Er) citrate colloid. The other radiopharmaceutical used for this purpose included rhenium 186 (186Re) sulfur colloid, lutetium 177 (177Lu)-labeled hydroxyapatite particles, colloidal chromium phosphate (32P), and radioactive colloid gold (198Au). In selected patients with systemic lupus erythematosus and with rheumatoid arthritis, the use of the total lymphoid irradiation as a localized means of immune suppression (TLI) has been studied. In Europe, teleradiotherapy of inflamed joints in the patients with rheumatoid arthritis has been tried, using a 20 MeV linear accelerator delivering a total dose of 20 Gy, without however significant results.

ORTHOPEDIC TREATMENT

Similar modalities as for diagnosis are used for monitoring the results of medical and surgical treatment of arthritis. Because the most effective treatment, particularly when large joints are involved, entails corrective and reconstructive procedures such as femoral or tibial osteotomy or total joint replacement of the hip, knee, ankle, shoulder, or elbow, the orthopedic surgeon follows the postsurgical progress of the patient with sequential radiographic examinations. In osteoarthritis of the hip, the corrective procedures most often performed are varus or valgus osteotomies of the proximal femur to improve the congruence of the articular surfaces and redistribute the stress forces over different areas of the joint. Similarly, a high tibial osteotomy is performed to correct severe varus or valgus deformities in osteoarthritis of the knee, particularly in cases of unicompartmental involvement (Fig. 4.1). The radiographic techniques used in monitoring the outcome of these procedures, which in fact represent

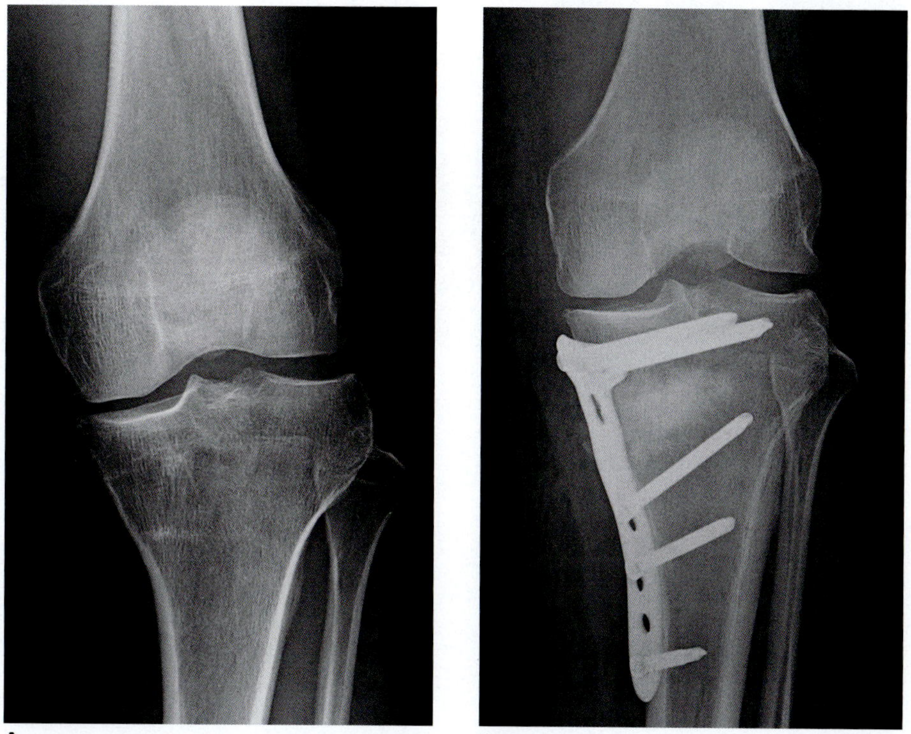

A B

Figure 4.1 ■ Corrective high tibial valgus osteotomy. A: A 37-year-old man presented with osteoarthritis affecting the medial joint compartment of the left knee, which resulted in varus deformity. **B:** To alleviate the symptoms, a proximal tibia wedge valgus osteotomy with reamed intramedullary autograft was performed. Note correction of varus deformity after surgery.

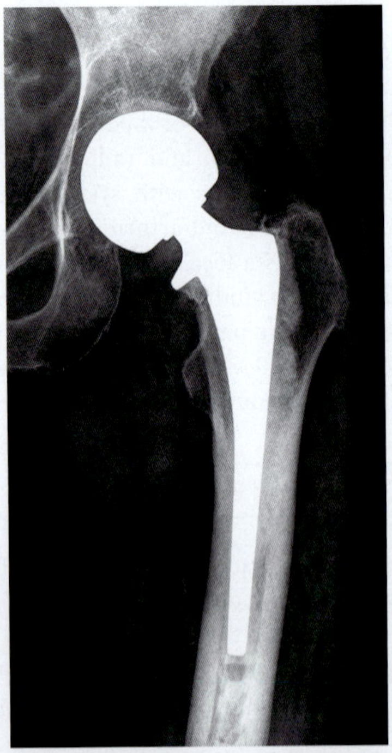

Figure 4.2 ■ Hemiarthroplasty of the hip joint. Anteroposterior radiograph of the left hip of a 61-year-old woman, who was diagnosed with advanced osteonecrosis of the femoral head, shows status post hemiarthroplasty using bipolar type of the prosthesis. The cemented stem of the prosthesis is in neutral position within the femoral shaft.

iatrogenic surgical fractures, are similar to those used in evaluating traumatic fractures. As in traumatic fractures, the radiologist also pays attention to similar features, such as bone union, nonunion, or delayed union.

In patients in whom ***total hip arthroplasties*** were performed, radiographic scrutiny is also essential. At present, two basic types of hip arthroplasty are used in orthopedic practice: bipolar hip hemiarthroplasty and total hip arthroplasty. The first type is used mainly for patients with fracture of the femoral head and neck and those with advanced femoral head osteonecrosis.

Bipolar prosthesis has a metallic cup the size of the resected femoral head filled with polyethylene, providing an articular cavity to accommodate the metallic femoral head attached to the stem (Fig. 4.2). The principle of this type of construction is that the motion between the metallic femoral head and the inner polyethylene insert reduces the wear of the native acetabulum. Total hip arthroplasty is commonly used in patients with advanced arthritis of the hip joint. The modern systems are modular, meaning that the femoral stem, head, acetabular shell, and liner consist of separate pieces. The prosthetic components, commonly composed of cobalt–chrome alloy or titanium (femoral stem) and metal or ceramic (femoral head), are usually cemented to the bone with polymethylmethacrylate (PMMA) (Fig. 4.3), although cementless fixation is now gaining popularity. The latter

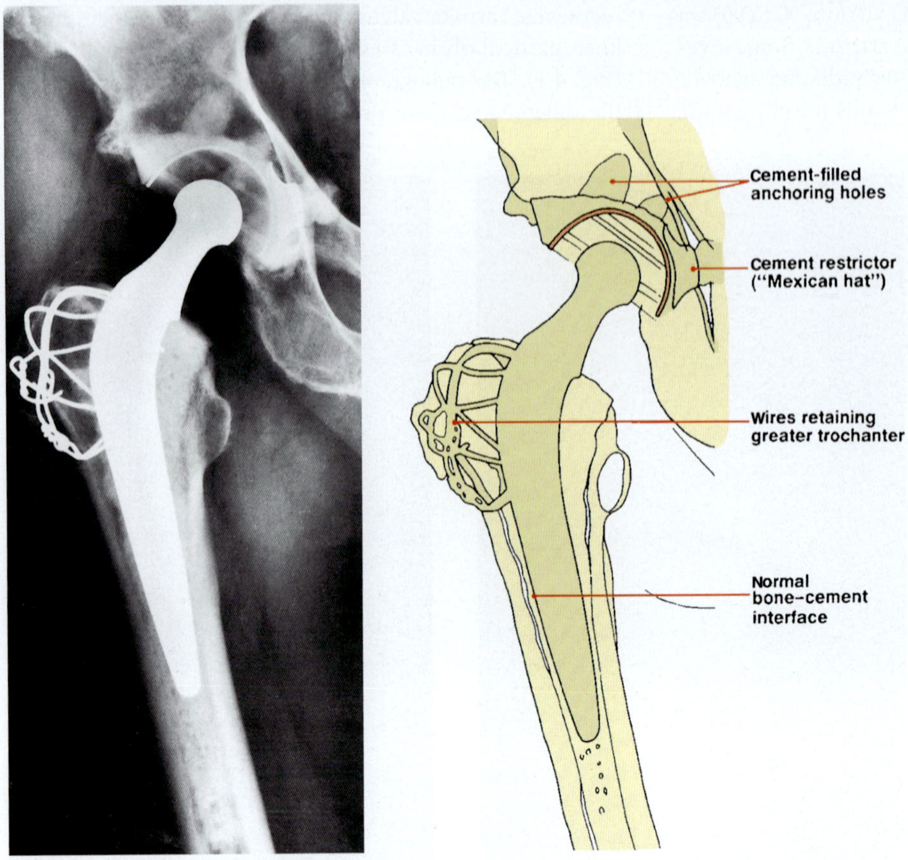

Figure 4.3 ■ Cemented total hip arthroplasty. A 69-year-old man underwent total hip replacement because of advanced osteoarthritis. The Charnley low-friction total hip prosthesis was inserted. On the anteroposterior radiograph of the right hip, one can evaluate all the parts of the prosthesis. Note that the acetabular component is oriented ~45 degrees to the horizontal plane and is cemented to the bone with methylmethacrylate previously impregnated with barium sulfate to make it visible radiographically. A wire-mesh cement restrictor ("Mexican hat") prevents significant leakage of methylmethacrylate into the pelvis. The stem of the prosthesis is in the neutral position in the medullary canal of the femur. Note the extent of cement below the distal end of the prosthesis, for secure anchoring. Metallic wires for improved stability have reattached the greater trochanter, which was osteotomized to facilitate exposure of the joint. Note the normal appearance of the bone–cement interface.

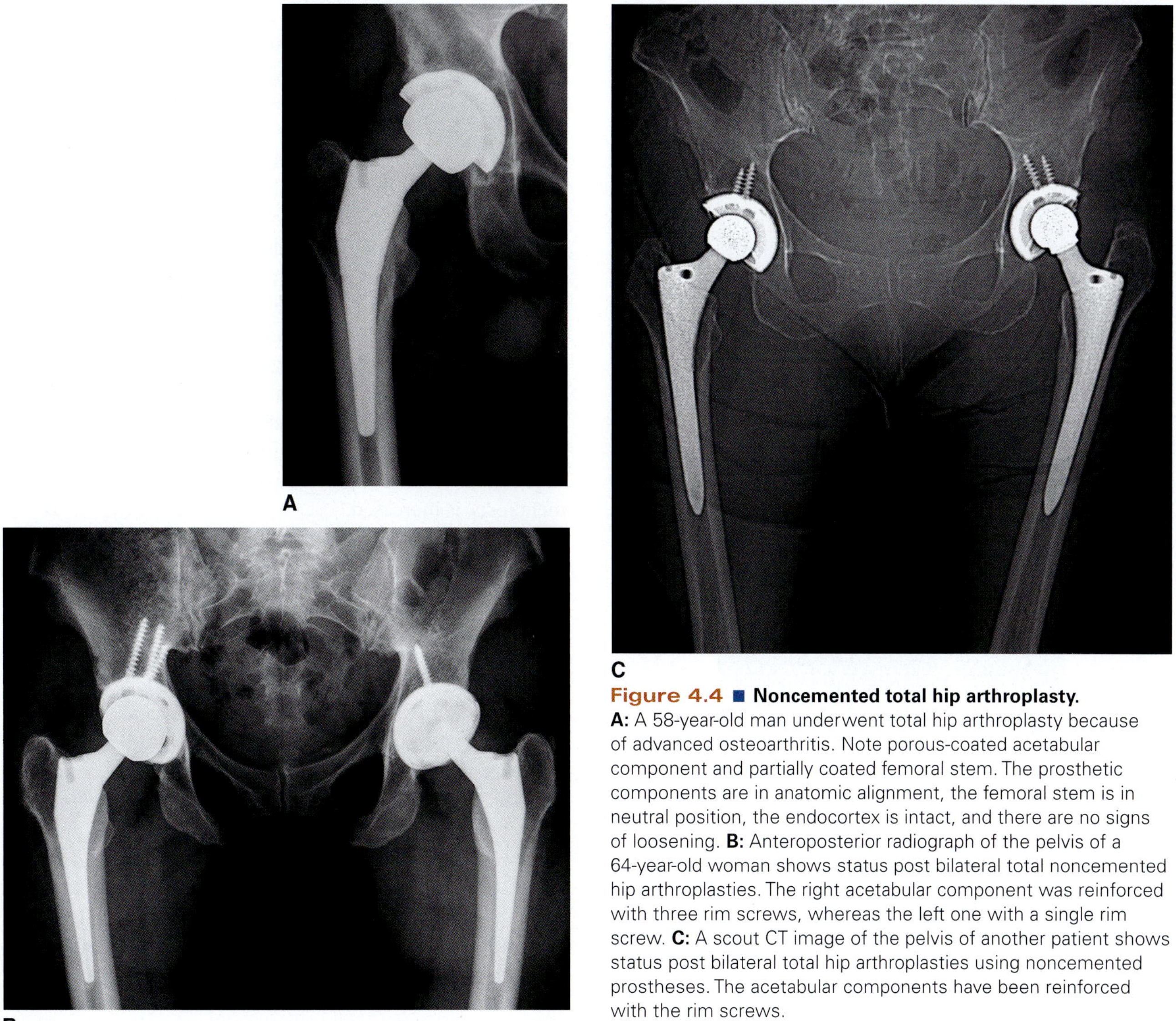

A

B

C

Figure 4.4 ■ Noncemented total hip arthroplasty. **A:** A 58-year-old man underwent total hip arthroplasty because of advanced osteoarthritis. Note porous-coated acetabular component and partially coated femoral stem. The prosthetic components are in anatomic alignment, the femoral stem is in neutral position, the endocortex is intact, and there are no signs of loosening. **B:** Anteroposterior radiograph of the pelvis of a 64-year-old woman shows status post bilateral total noncemented hip arthroplasties. The right acetabular component was reinforced with three rim screws, whereas the left one with a single rim screw. **C:** A scout CT image of the pelvis of another patient shows status post bilateral total hip arthroplasties using noncemented prostheses. The acetabular components have been reinforced with the rim screws.

technique is based on the use of a rough or porous surface on the prosthetic parts that enables ingrowth of the bone. A bioactive coating (i.e., hydroxyapatite) can also be used for the same purpose. Acetabular components, which contain a polyethylene liner with or without metal backing, usually have a porous coating over the entire surface of the cup, whereas femoral components can be either partially or fully coated (Fig. 4.4A). Cementless acetabular components are sometimes reinforced with the rim screws or spikes (Fig. 4.4B). Occasionally, so-called hybrid arthroplasties are performed with cementless acetabular and cemented femoral components (Fig. 4.5).

Alternative to conventional total hip arthroplasty, especially in younger patients, metal-on-metal (MOM) hip resurfacing arthroplasty (HRA) has been advocated (Fig. 4.6). There are different types of this prosthesis, but most of them are made from high carbon cobalt–chromium alloys and consist of a femoral component, which can be cemented or noncemented, and an uncemented acetabular component, which achieves primary fixation through press-fit and circumferential fins. The acetabular components are coated using various methods and material providing a bone ingrowth surface at the implant–bone interface to achieve maximum stability. The advantage of this type of arthroplasty include the durability of the prosthetic components, low volumetric wear rate, an increased level of inherent stability using large heads with reduced rate of dislocation, preservation of metaphyseal and diaphyseal bone stock, optimization of stress transfer to the proximal femur, optimal range of movement, and improved biomechanics of the hip joint. The disadvantage of this type of hip arthroplasty is shedding metal particles leading to periprosthetic osteolysis and metallosis with formation of pseudotumors (see text below).

After total hip replacement using *cemented components*, it is important to evaluate the position of the prosthesis, with particular reference to the degree of inclination of the acetabular component, the position of the stem of the prosthesis (whether it is in valgus, varus, or the neutral position), and

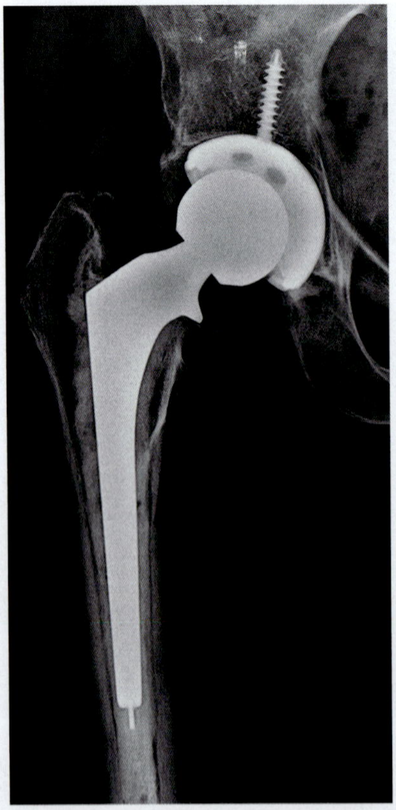

Figure 4.5 ■ Hybrid total hip arthroplasty. Anteroposterior radiograph of the right hip of a 66-year-old woman shows a hybrid type of total hip prosthesis. Note that the femoral stem of the prosthesis has been cemented in a neutral position within the femoral shaft and the acetabular component has been reinforced with a single rim screw.

the status of the separated and rejoined greater trochanter, among other features (see Fig. 4.3). Equally important is the evaluation of cement–bone interface to detect the radiolucent area suggestive of prosthesis loosening (see Fig. 4.22). It is important to remember that at the cement–bone interface, a thin fibrous layer may form as response to focal necrosis of osseous tissue because of the heat of the cement polymerization. This radiolucent zone is usually not wider than 2 mm and becomes stable by 2 years after arthroplasty. After total hip arthroplasty using *noncemented components* (see Fig. 4.4), radiologic evaluation should focus on the interface between the prosthesis and the bone to detect areas of bone resorption (focal osteolysis) associated with endosteal scalloping that may indicate loosening of the prosthesis. Additional abnormalities to look for are progressive subsidence, migration, or tilt of the components. With HRA, there is well-documented risk of femoral neck fracture. Groin pain may occur secondary to impingement of the femoral neck on the acetabular component resulting in femoral neck scalloping. Because the implant consists of a metal-on-metal articulation made from cast cobalt–chromium alloys, the incidents of production of wear particles, and hence the occurrence of metallosis, is increased.

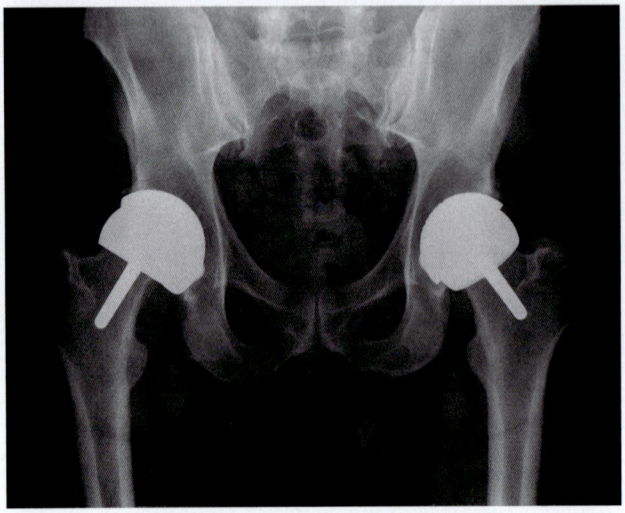

Figure 4.6 ■ Total hip resurfacing arthroplasty. A 42-year-old man with osteoarthritis of both hip joints underwent metal-on-metal total resurfacing hip arthroplasties.

Although two-compartmental and unicompartmental knee arthroplasties are occasionally performed, the most common type is a ***total knee arthroplasty***. This procedure combines resurfacing the femoral, tibial, and patellar articular surfaces by using metal and polyethylene bearing surfaces. The major prosthesis categories include posterior cruciate ligament-retaining, posterior cruciate ligament-substituting or stabilized, unlinked constrained or varus–valgus constrained, and rotating-hinge knee implants. Femoral and tibial components can be either cemented, noncemented, or anchored with the screws. A patellar component invariably consists of high-density polyethylene, which can be metal-backed. Modern three-part (three-compartmental) condylar cemented nonconstrained arthroplasty is performed using metal femoral component, which resurfaces both condyles and the trochlear notch, and a tibial component, which consists of a metal-backed polyethylene tray that articulates with the femoral component (Fig. 4.7). Some tibial components may contain a locking-mechanism clip that locks the tibial polyethylene tray into the tibial base plate. Occasionally, femoral and tibial components can include varying length stems that supplement prosthesis fixation, and tibial component may be augmented with prominent pegs for additional stability. Fully constrained rotating-hinge total knee arthroplasty is usually performed for revision of failed nonconstrained knee arthroplasty and in patients with ligament deficiency, severe bone loss, or severe knee joint instability (Fig. 4.8). This type of implant allows the flexion–extension movement combined with rotation of the femur on the tibial component or with rotation of the tibial polyethylene liner on the metal tibial tray, thus allowing a more physiologic range of motion and reducing the stress transfer to the bone–prosthesis interface compared with the old fixed-hinge models. After a total knee arthroplasty with a condylar type of prosthesis, it is important to evaluate the position of the tibial component relative to the tibial shaft, as well as the axial alignment and the status of the methylmethacrylate fixation

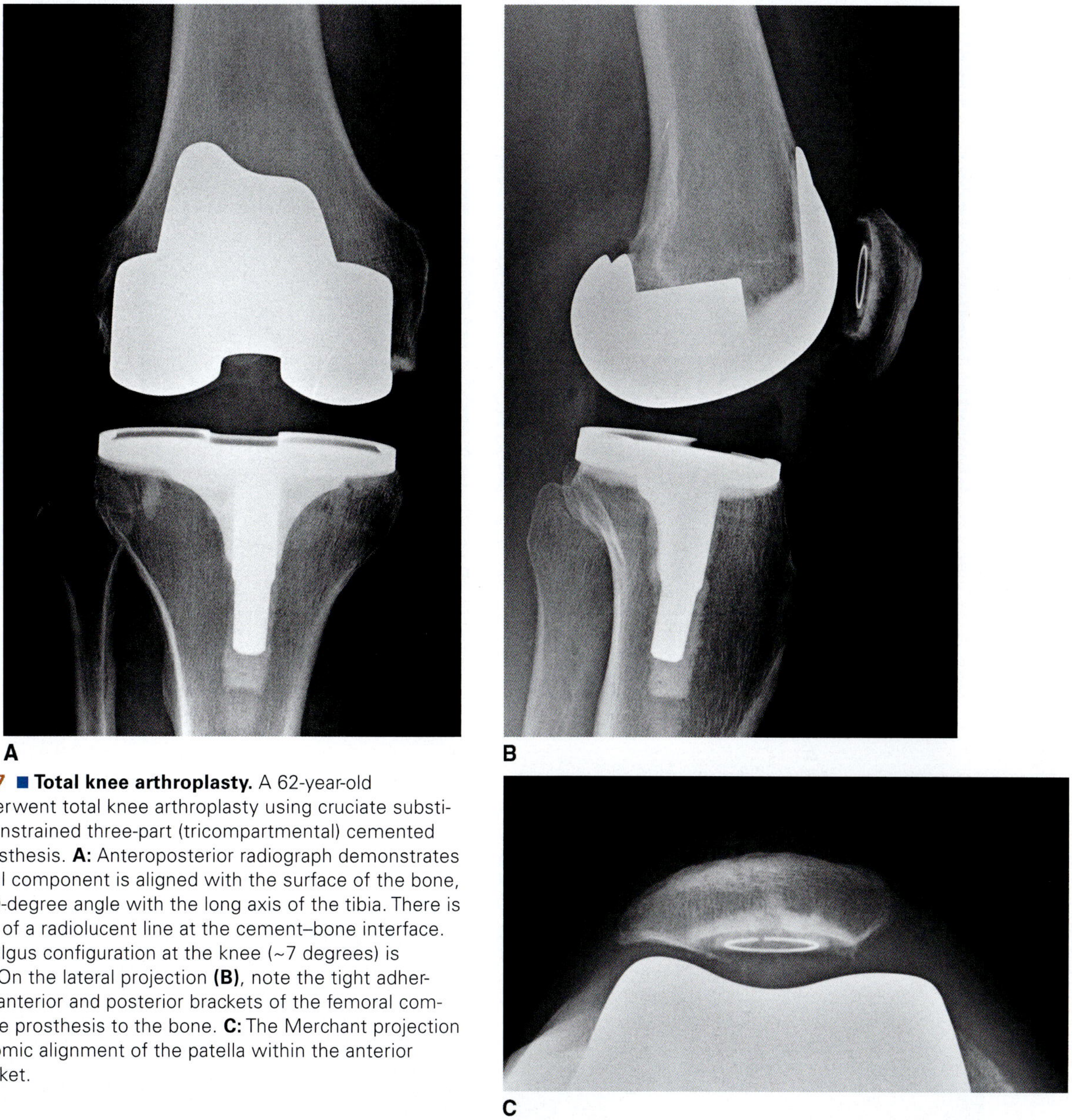

Figure 4.7 ■ **Total knee arthroplasty.** A 62-year-old woman underwent total knee arthroplasty using cruciate substituting nonconstrained three-part (tricompartmental) cemented condylar prosthesis. **A:** Anteroposterior radiograph demonstrates that the tibial component is aligned with the surface of the bone, forming a 90-degree angle with the long axis of the tibia. There is no evidence of a radiolucent line at the cement–bone interface. The slight valgus configuration at the knee (~7 degrees) is acceptable. On the lateral projection **(B)**, note the tight adherence of the anterior and posterior brackets of the femoral component of the prosthesis to the bone. **C:** The Merchant projection shows anatomic alignment of the patella within the anterior femoral bracket.

of the components (see Fig. 4.7). The tibial component should be aligned perpendicular to the long axis of the tibia on the anteroposterior view of the knee and perpendicular or in slight (up to 6 degrees) flexion on the lateral view. The anterior bracket (flange) of the femoral component should be flushed with the anterior femoral cortex.

Unicompartmental arthroplasty is performed for isolated unicompartmental osteoarthritis, usually in the medial or lateral compartment (Fig. 4.9), although patellofemoral unicompartmental arthroplasty is also occasionally performed (Fig. 4.10).

Total ankle arthroplasty devices incorporate two basic designs: three-component (mobile-bearing) and two-component (fixed-bearing) types. Three-component types are characterized by separate tibial and talar components separated by a fully conforming mobile polyethylene spacer. Two-component types have only a single partially conforming articulation between the tibial and talar components, with the polyethylene spacer fixed to the tibial component. Recently, third-generation ankle implants became increasingly favored over first- and second-generation prostheses, which were cemented and constrained, hence leading to a higher failure rates. The most popular among the third-generation implants is the INBONE prosthesis, a fixed-bearing design with a modular system for both the tibial and talar components (Fig. 4.11A, B). Another popular implant

(Continued on page 121)

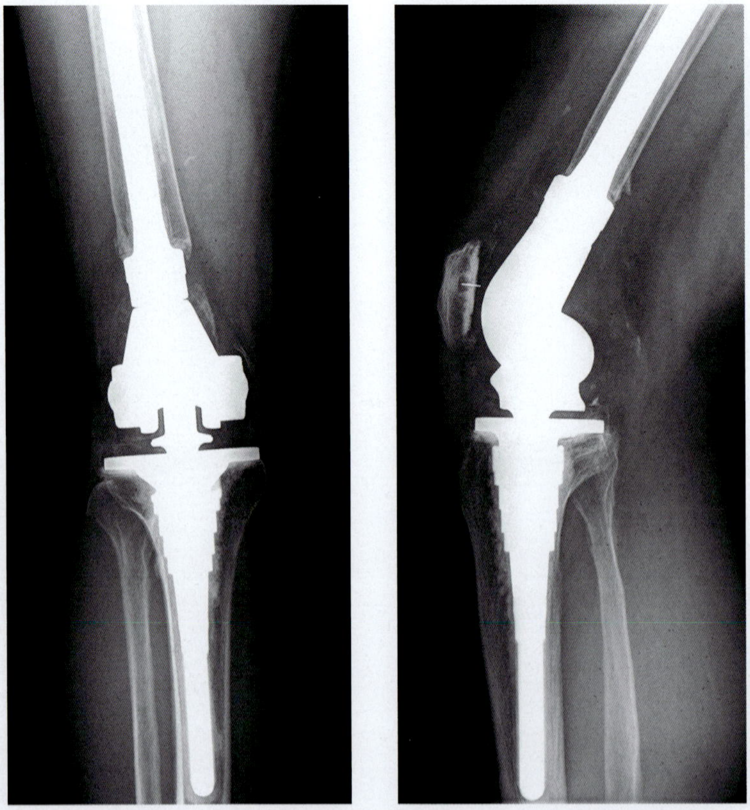

A B

Figure 4.8 ■ Total hinged knee arthroplasty. A 74-year-old man presented with two failed total nonconstrained knee arthroplasties performed in the past for advanced osteoarthritis. In the third attempt, the three-part constrained hinge prosthesis was implanted, as seen here on anteroposterior **(A)** and lateral **(B)** radiographs.

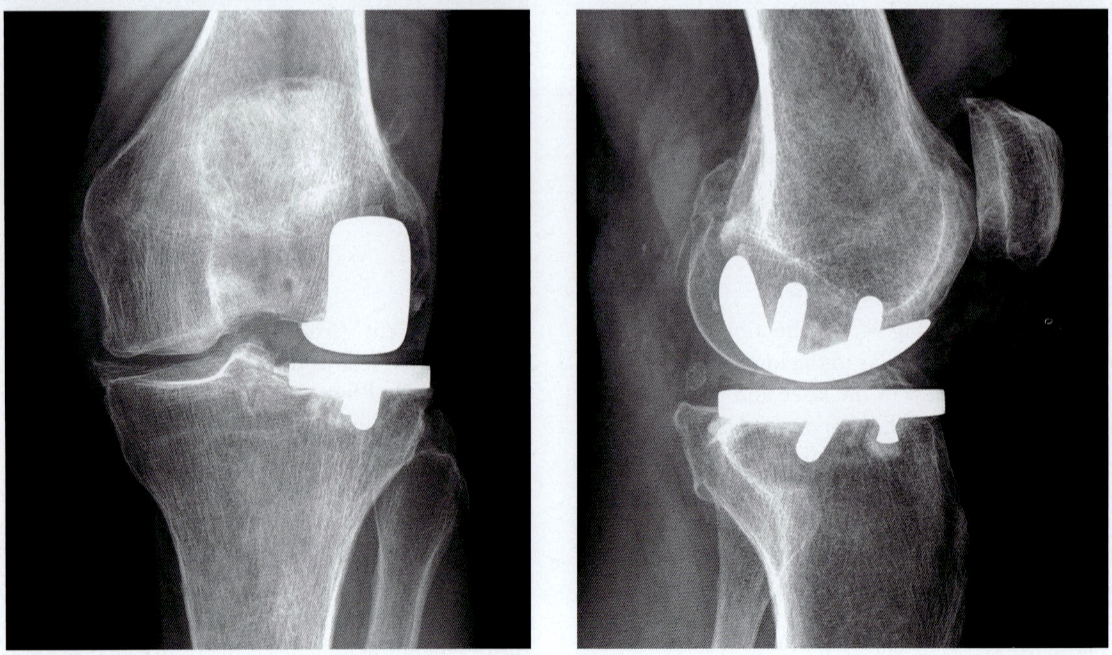

A B

Figure 4.9 ■ Unicompartmental knee arthroplasty. Anteroposterior **(A)** and lateral **(B)** radiographs of the left knee of a 73-year-old man, who, because of advanced osteoarthritis of the lateral joint compartment but relative good preservation of the medial and femoropatellar compartments, underwent a unicompartmental knee arthroplasty, show anatomic alignment of the prosthetic components.

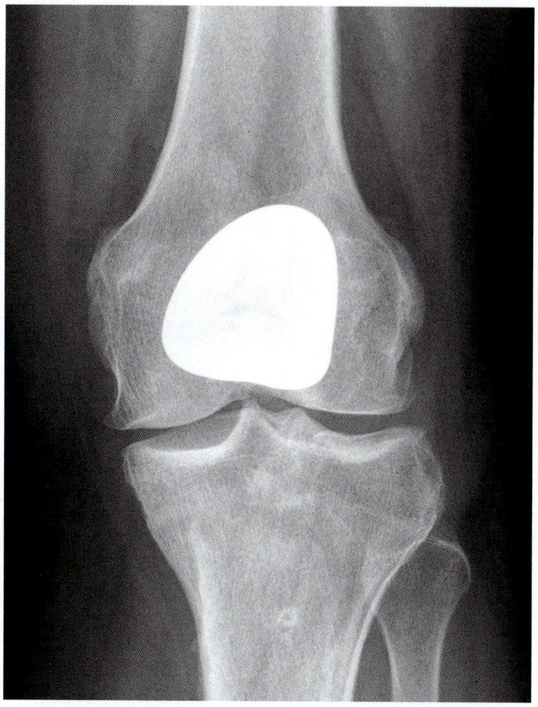

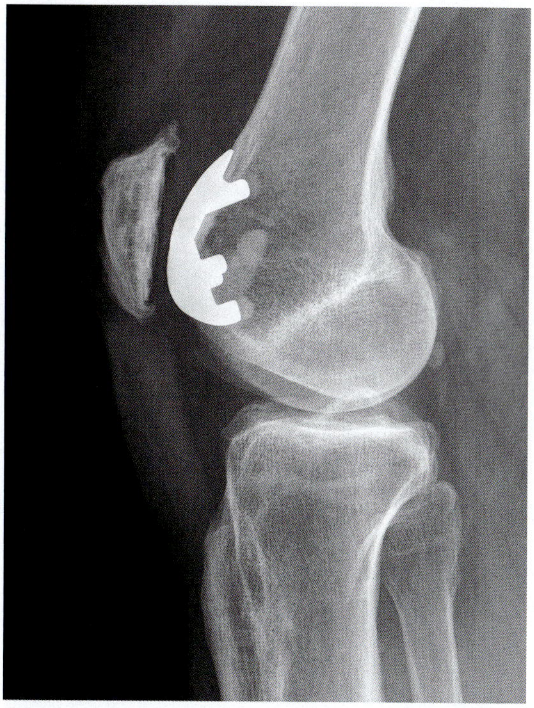

A B

Figure 4.10 ■ **Unicompartmental knee arthroplasty.** Anteroposterior **(A)** and lateral **(B)** radiographs of the left knee show femoropatellar unicompartmental arthroplasty.

is a Zimmer third-generation trabecular metal prosthesis (Fig. 4.11C, D). After total ankle arthroplasty, in addition to assessing the position and alignment of the prosthetic parts, attention should be paid to the possible subsidence of the talar component, which should not exceed 5 mm, best evaluated on the lateral view of the ankle. Furthermore, syndesmotic fusion (if performed) and status of adjacent osseous structures should be evaluated.

After a ***total shoulder arthroplasty***, whether conventional (Fig. 4.12) or the one using reverse (Delta or Aequalis) shoulder prosthesis (Fig. 4.13), alignment of the prosthetic components and metal–cement and cement–bone interface must be evaluated. Reverse shoulder arthroplasty makes use of a semiconstrained prosthesis that comprises a humeral component, lateralized polyethylene insert, glenosphere, and metaglene, consisting of a base plate that is secured by locking and nonlocking screws to the native glenoid. The humeral component consists of a metal stem that is monoblock or modular and a cup-shaped proximal portion. All humeral components are cemented. With the reverse shoulder arthroplasty, radiologic evaluation should include the position of the glenosphere, which should be flush with the glenoid, and the humeral component that should be centered on the glenosphere proximally and centered within the humeral shaft distally. In addition, the position of the anchoring screws within the scapula, relationship of the humeral component to the scapula, and status of supporting bone should be evaluated. In particular, the inferior border of the glenoid should be examined for erosions and heterotopic ossifications and one should look for unique for this prosthesis complication such as notching of the inferior scapula by the humeral component, and acromial stress fractures.

There are three basic types of ***total elbow arthroplasty***: nonconstrained or resurfacing elbow arthroplasty, semiconstrained elbow arthroplasty, and constrained elbow arthroplasty (Fig. 4.14). In the first type, the prosthesis consists of two separate metal components, humeral and ulnar, which articulate by a high-density polyethylene component. The major complication with this implant is subluxation and dislocation. The semiconstrained prosthesis consists of titanium or cobalt–chromium ulnar and humeral stems that are linked by a pin and bushing, which consists of a polyethylene ring in between the metal components to reduce friction. Constrained elbow prosthesis consists of rigid hinges, constructed with either metal-on-metal or metal and high-density polyethylene parts connected through either a bushing or a separate polyethylene piece that links the humeral and ulnar components. The radial head is commonly resected proximally to the annular ligament. Radiologic evaluation focuses on emerging complications, such as heterotopic ossifications, perihardware lucency indicative of loosening (the humeral component is more prone to this complication), periprosthetic fracture, subluxation or dislocation of the prosthesis, wear and breakdown of bushing, and hardware fracture.

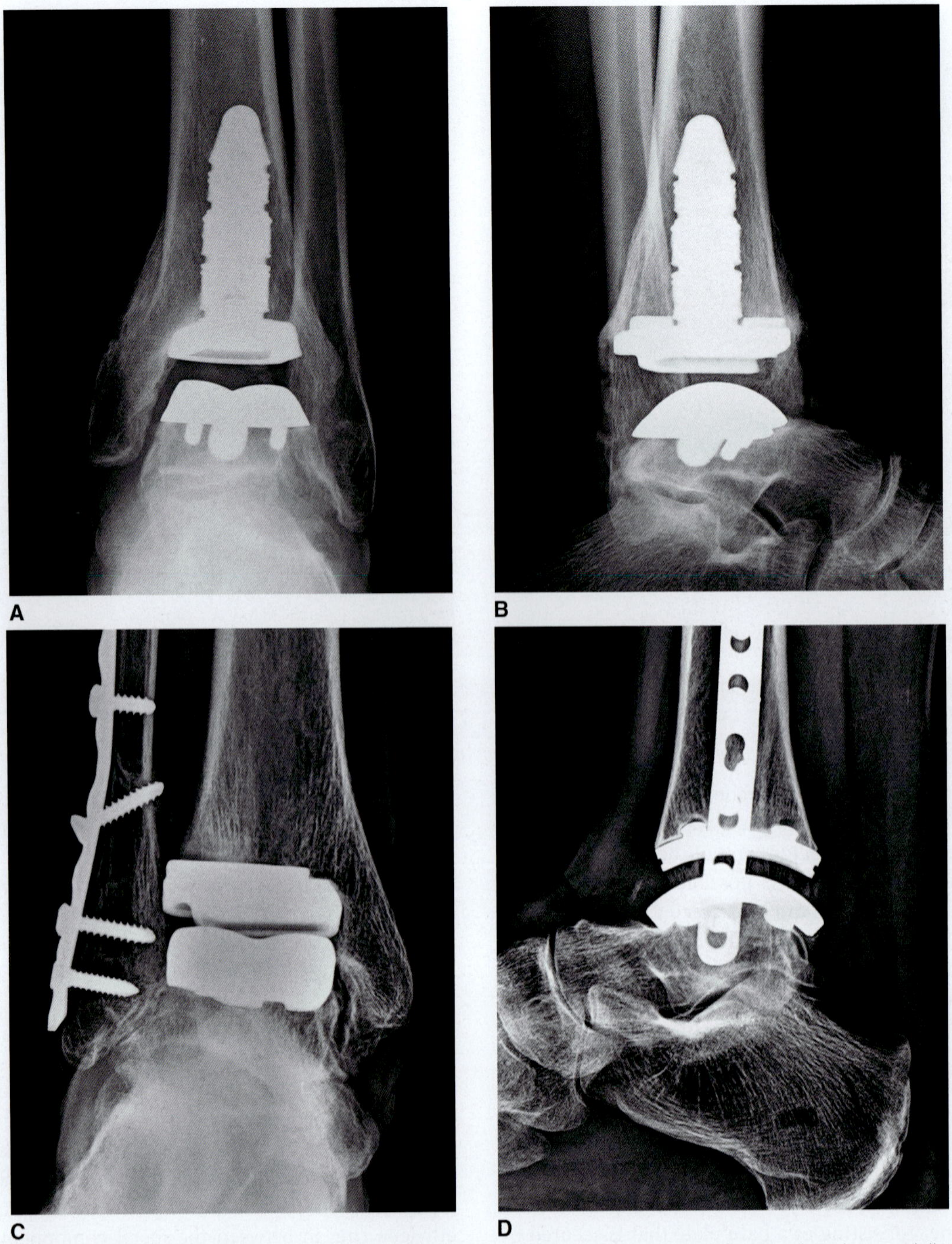

Figure 4.11 ■ **Total ankle arthroplasty.** Anteroposterior **(A)** and lateral **(B)** radiographs of the left ankle show intramedullary fixation total INBONE ankle prosthesis. The noncemented prosthetic components made from a titanium alloy and incorporating a cobalt–chrome polyethylene articulation are porous coated for bone ingrowth. Anteroposterior **(C)** and lateral **(D)** radiographs of the right ankle of another patient show a third-generation Zimmer trabecular metal total ankle prosthesis. Note status post fibular osteotomy with a side plate and screws fixation.

In the hands and feet, occasionally, either hemiarthroplasties or total joint arthroplasties are performed for osteoarthritis and rheumatoid arthritis using either metal (Figs. 4.15 and 4.16) or silastic (elastomere–rubber, or silicone-polymer) type of prostheses (Figs. 4.17 and 4.18). These implants provide instant stability with excellent pain relief, leading to improve range of motion and function. The complications of silastic prostheses include fractures (see Fig. 4.34), subluxations, dislocations, loosening of the implants, infection (see Fig. 4.36), silicone synovitis (see Figs. 4.34 and 4.35 and text below), and silicon lymphadenopathy.

(Continued on page 126)

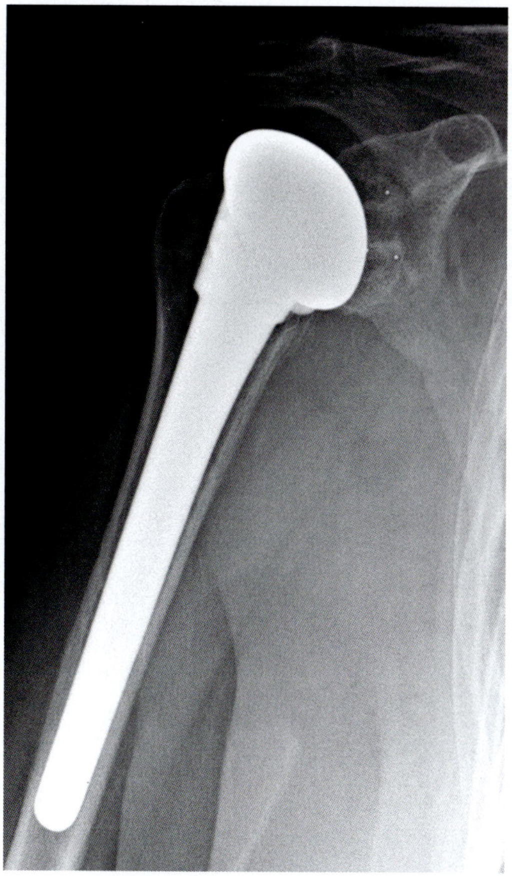

Figure 4.12 ■ **Total shoulder arthroplasty.** Anteroposterior radiograph of the right shoulder shows total shoulder arthroplasty with a conventional prosthesis in anatomic alignment.

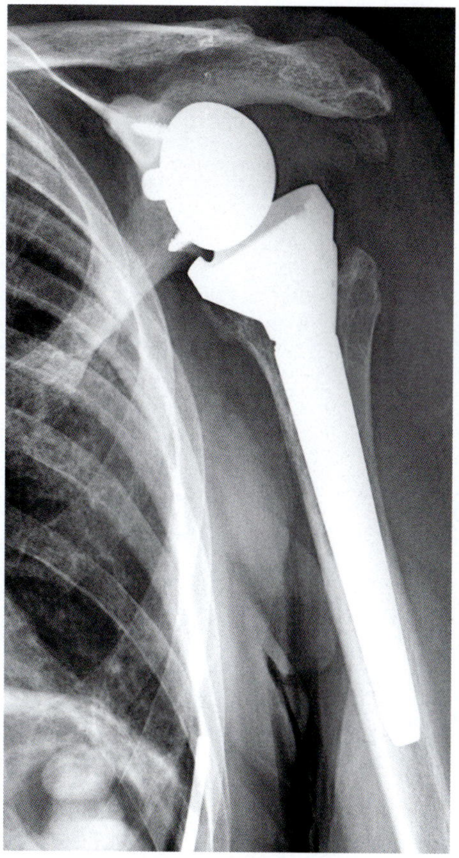

Figure 4.13 ■ **Total reversed shoulder arthroplasty.** Anteroposterior radiograph of the left shoulder shows total shoulder arthroplasty with a Delta reverse shoulder system in anatomic alignment.

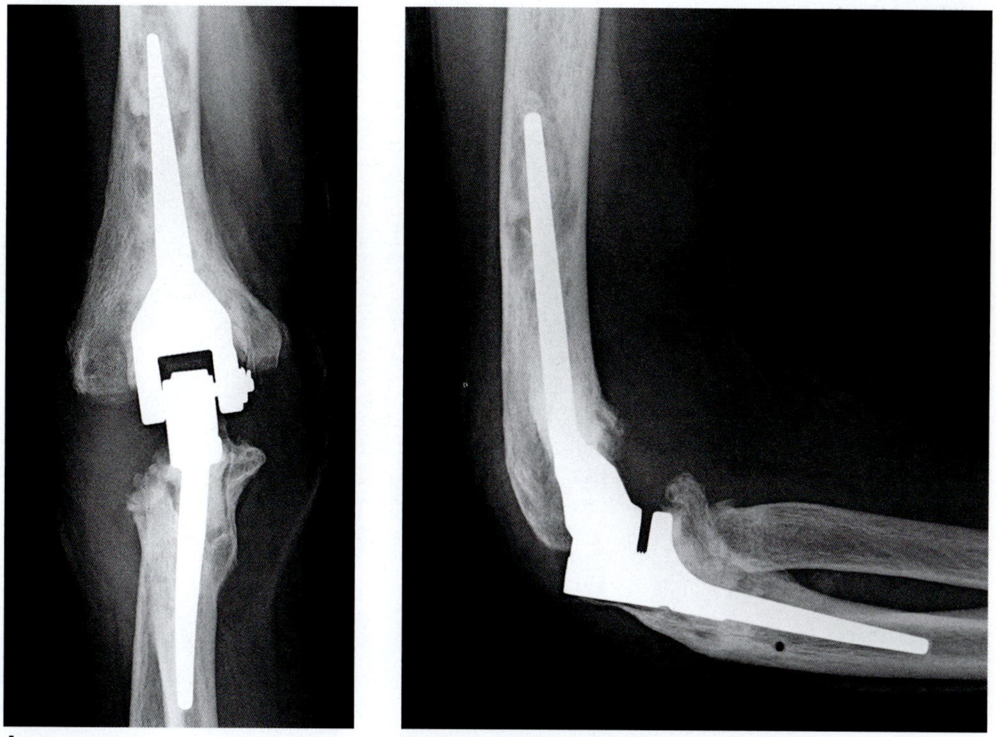

A B

Figure 4.14 ■ **Total elbow arthroplasty.** Anteroposterior **(A)** and lateral **(B)** radiographs of the right elbow of a 72-year-old woman show total hinged elbow prosthesis. Note that the radial head has been resected.

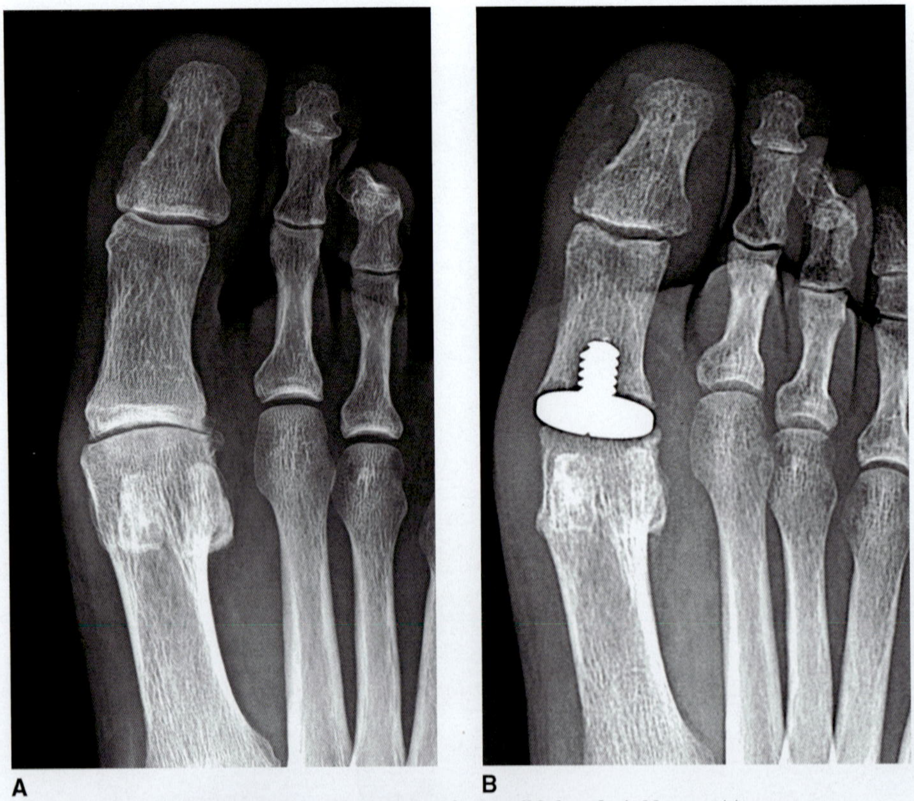

Figure 4.15 ■ **Metallic hemiarthroplasty of a small joint. A:** A 62-year-old woman presented with osteoarthritis at the first metatarsophalangeal joint. **B:** Hemiarthroplasty was performed using metallic prosthesis implanted into the proximal phalanx.

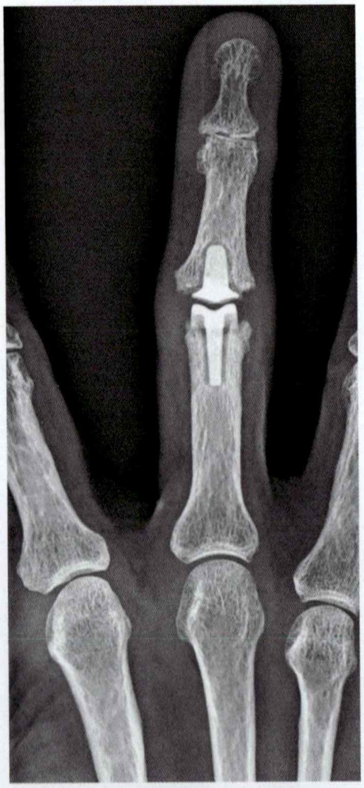

Figure 4.16 ■ **Metallic arthroplasty of a small joint.** A 48-year-old man underwent noncemented metallic arthroplasty of the proximal interphalangeal joint of the middle finger for posttraumatic arthritis.

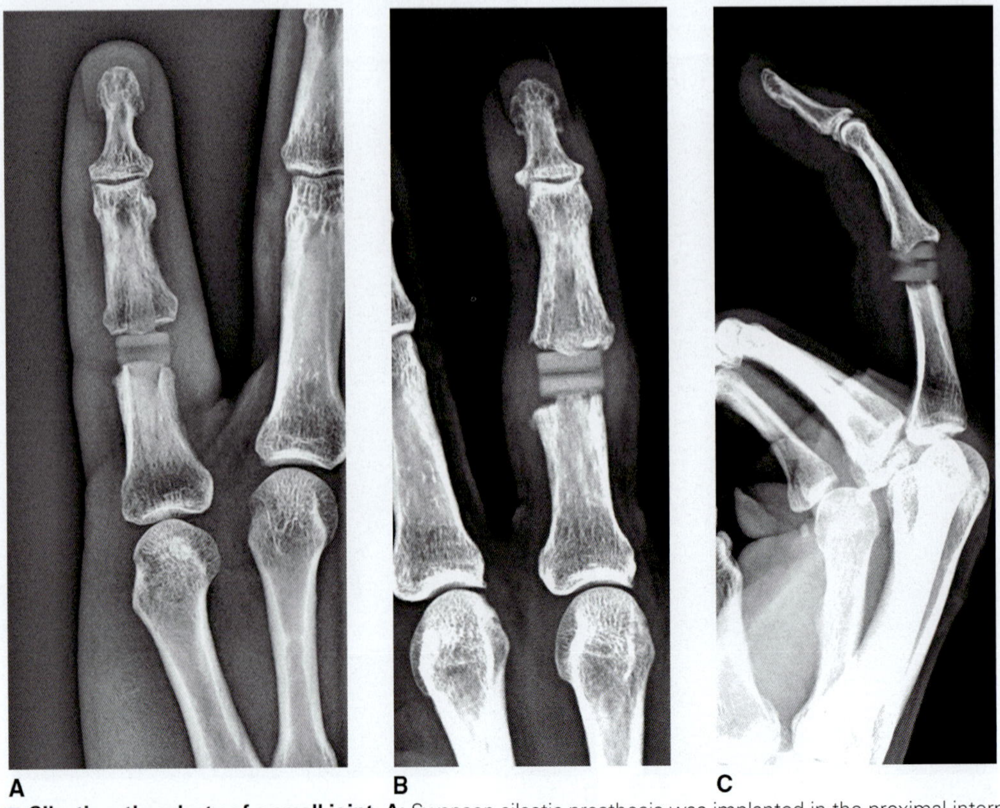

Figure 4.17 ■ **Silastic arthroplasty of a small joint. A:** Swanson silastic prosthesis was implanted in the proximal interphalangeal joint of the small finger of this 39-year-old woman with posttraumatic arthritis. Anteroposterior **(B)** and lateral **(C)** radiographs of the index finger of another patient show status post silastic arthroplasty.

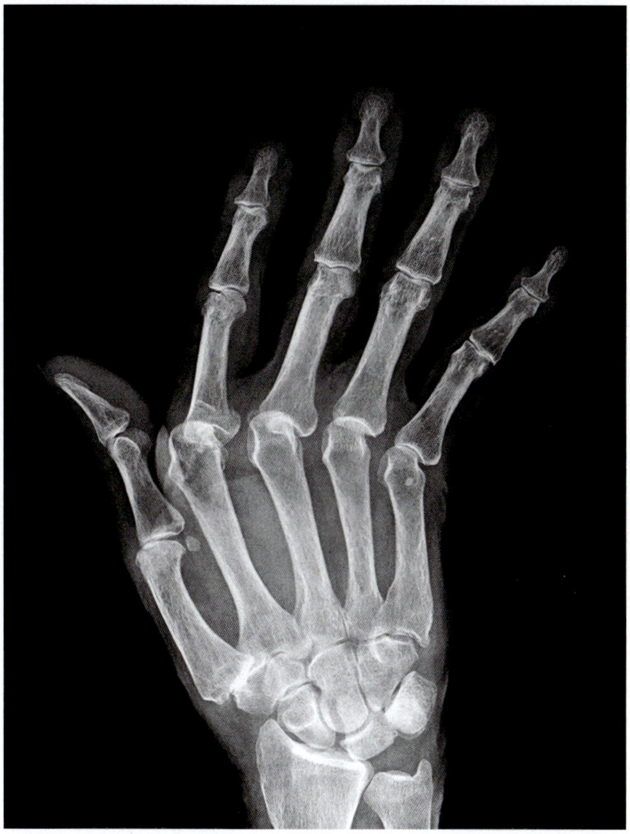

A

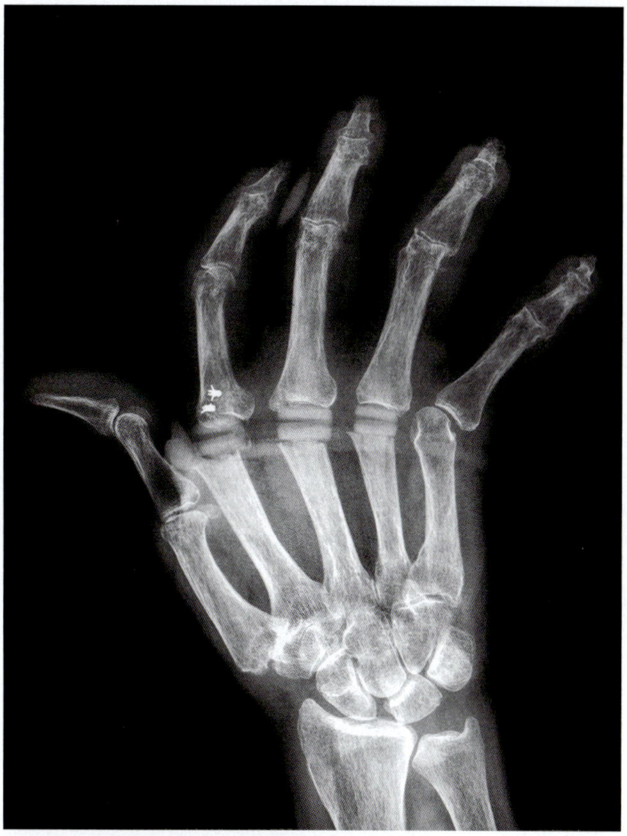

B

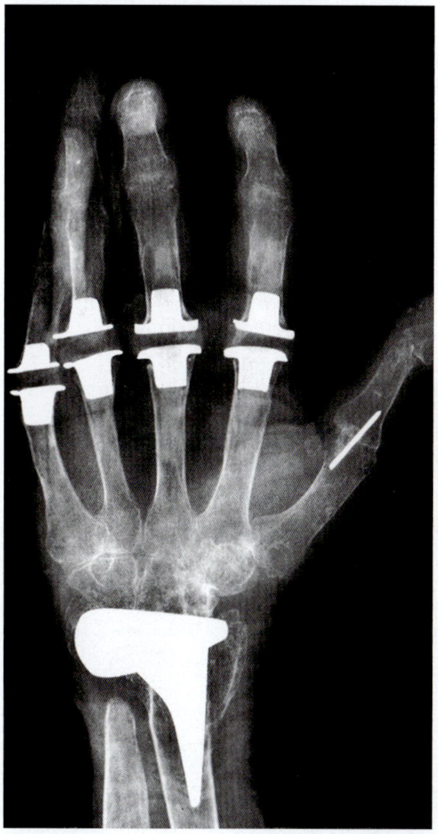

C

Figure 4.18 ■ **Silastic arthroplasty of the small joints.** **A:** A 68-year-old man was diagnosed with CPPD crystal deposition disease affecting second, third, and fourth metacarpophalangeal joints. **B:** Swanson silicone implants were used to replace the affected joints. **C:** In another patient, a woman with advanced juvenile idiopathic arthritis, silastic flexible hinge (two-stem) prostheses with circumferential titanium grommets were implanted in the second to fifth metacarpophalangeal joints. Note in addition the radiocarpal prosthesis and fusion of the first metacarpophalangeal joint.

COMPLICATIONS OF SURGICAL TREATMENT

As important as evaluating the outcome of the surgical treatment of arthritic disease is monitoring the complications that may arise from such treatment, especially those after osteotomies and joint replacement procedures. These complications, among others, include thrombophlebitis, hematomas, heterotopic bone formation, the intrapelvic leakage of acrylic cement, infection, loosening, subluxation or dislocation of a prosthesis, and fracture of a prosthesis.

Venous Thrombosis and Thrombophlebitis

A rather frequent complication in the immediate postoperative period, particularly in patients with previous circulatory problems, thrombophlebitis is related to venous stasis and the lack of movement of the surgically treated extremity; sudden pain and swelling of the leg are common clinical findings. The venous soleal plexus in the calf is the most common site of thrombus formation. Radiologically, this complication can be detected by venography (Fig. 4.19), radionuclide scanning, or US. On radionuclide scan, an increased gamma count rate in an area of the lower extremities following intravenous administration of ^{125}I-labeled fibrinogen suggests adherence of the tracer to a developing clot. US can detect venous thrombosis using compression technique. Lack of compressibility of a vein is thought to be the single most reliable finding in differentiating between thrombosed and normal veins. Other criteria useful in detection of vein thrombosis are the presence of echogenic intraluminal material and enlargement of the vein.

Hematoma

The formation of a hematoma is a common complication of surgery for arthritic disease. However, it usually subsides within a short time, unless it is associated with infection. This complication can be easily detected with MRI.

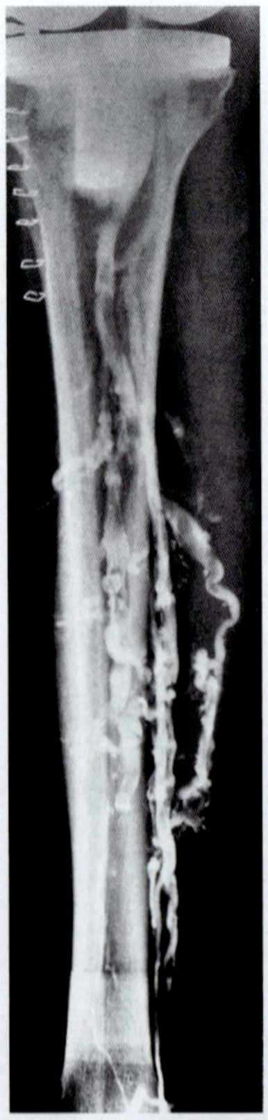

Figure 4.19 ■ Venous thrombosis. A 67-year-old woman with rheumatoid arthritis, who recently underwent total knee arthroplasty, presented with pain and swelling of the left leg. A venogram shows multiple thrombi in the soleal venous plexus of the lower extremity.

Leakage of Acrylic Cement

Intrapelvic leakage of methylmethacrylate may lead to vascular and neurologic damage, visceral necrosis, and urinary tract disorders, as a result of the heat of polymerization of the acrylic cement (Fig. 4.20). To prevent an accidental leak, a wire-mesh restrictor ("Mexican hat") is applied around the acetabular anchoring holes of the prosthesis (see Fig. 4.3).

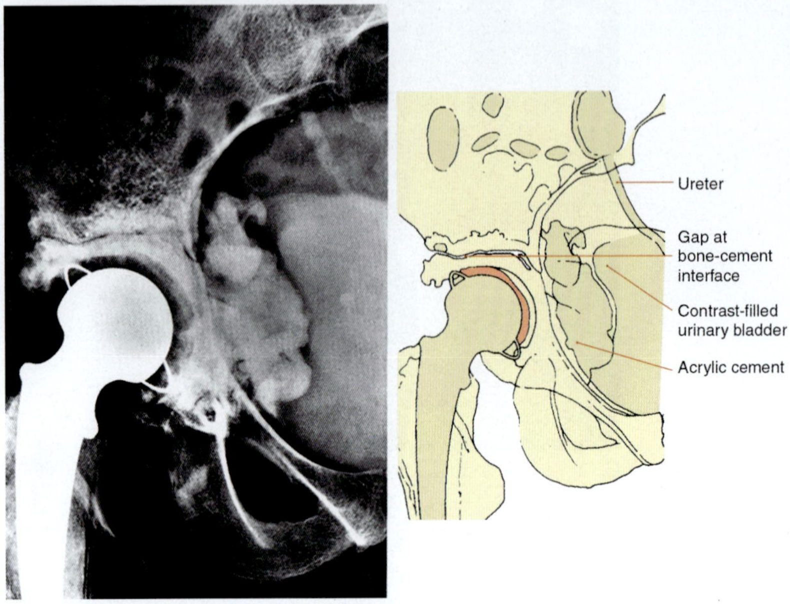

Figure 4.20 ■ Intrapelvic leakage of the cement. A 46-year-old woman, who underwent total hip arthroplasty, presented with right hip pain and intermittent symptoms from the urinary tract. An intravenous urogram shows a large mass of acrylic cement compressing the right wall of the urinary bladder.

Heterotopic Bone Formation

This is a relatively common complication of surgery for arthritic disease in the hip. It occurs when primitive mesenchymal cells in the surrounding soft tissues are transformed into osteoblastic cells, which form mature lamellar bone. It typically occurs around the femoral neck of the prosthesis and adjacent to the greater trochanter. The amount of new bone that forms in the adjacent soft tissues varies: if extensive, it may interfere with function of the hip joint. Conventional radiography (Fig. 4.21) and occasionally CT are sufficient to evaluate this complication.

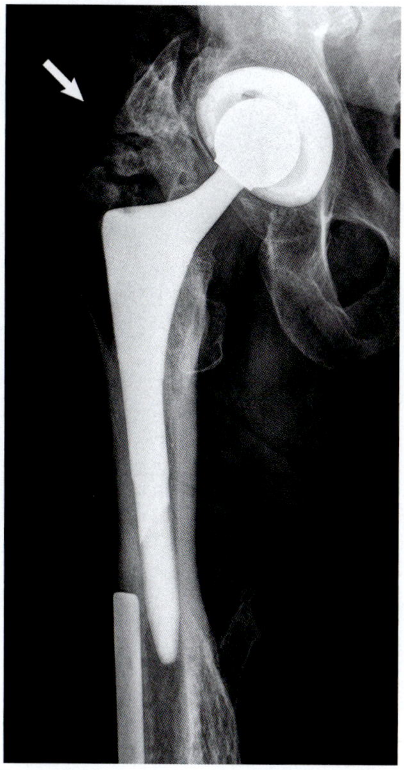

Figure 4.21 ■ Heterotopic bone formation. Anteroposterior radiograph of the right hip of a 58-year-old man who underwent a total hip arthroplasty for osteoarthritis shows one of the complications of this procedure—heterotopic bone formation (*arrow*).

Infection

Although infection may occur at any time postoperatively, it is usually observed shortly after the joint replacement procedure. Clinically, it is manifested by pain, elevation of temperature, and discharge from the wound. The radiographic findings in cases of infection include soft tissue swelling, rarefaction of bone, and, occasionally, a periosteal reaction. Scintigraphy using either ^{99m}Tc-labeled MDP (see Figs. 2.56 and 2.57) or ^{111}In-oxine–labeled white blood cells (see Fig. 2.58) has been reported to be very useful in these circumstances. More recently, SPECT/CT imaging also effectively demonstrated this complication (see Fig. 2.66).

Loosening of Prosthesis

Infection after a joint replacement procedure may result in loosening of prosthesis, but loosening may also be seen as a late complication resulting from mechanical factors. The standard radiographic projections are usually sufficient to reveal this development (Figs. 4.22 to 4.26). In cemented prosthesis, the circumferential radiolucent gap at the

(Continued on page 129)

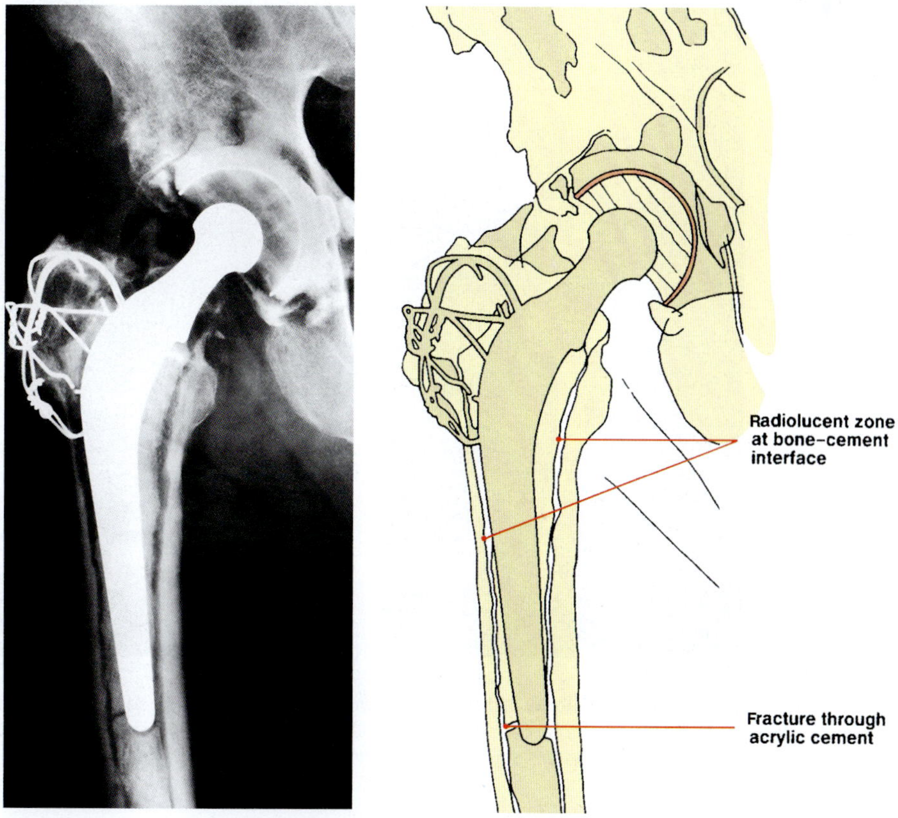

Figure 4.22 ■ Loosening of the hip prosthesis. Anteroposterior radiograph of the right hip of a 69-year-old woman shows a wide radiolucent zone at the bone–cement interface characteristic of loosening of Charnley hip prosthesis. Note the fracture through the acrylic cement at the distal segment of the prosthetic stem.

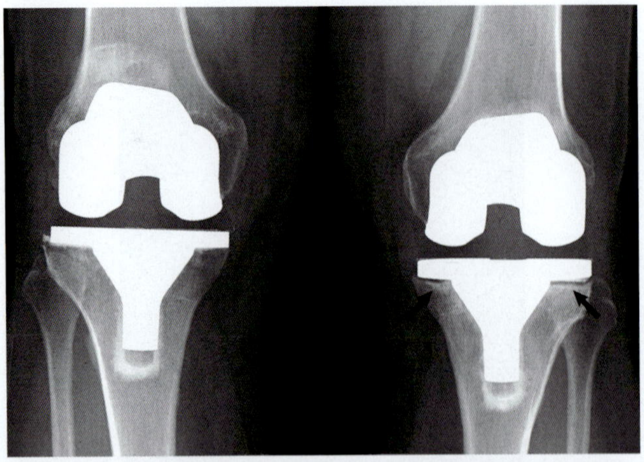

Figure 4.23 ■ Loosening of the tibial component of knee prosthesis. Anteroposterior radiograph of both knees of a 67-year-old man who underwent bilateral total knee arthroplasties for osteoarthritis shows loosening of the tibial component of the left prosthesis (*arrows*).

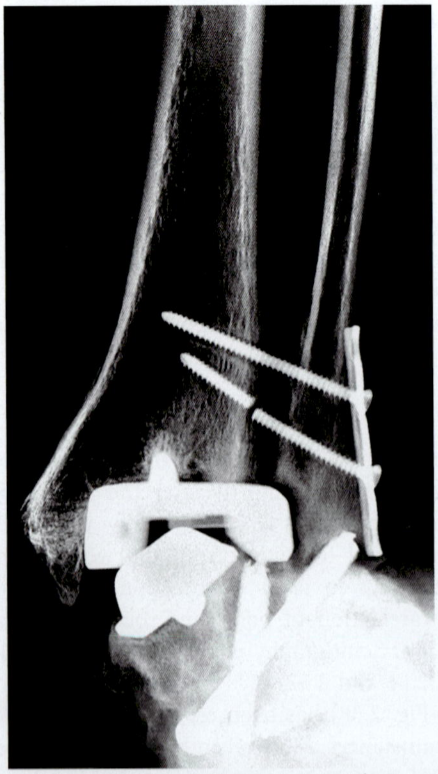

Figure 4.24 ■ Failure of total ankle arthroplasty. Oblique radiograph of the left ankle shows a failure of total ankle arthroplasty after placement of semiconstrained Agility prosthesis. Note malalignment of the tibial and talar parts of the prosthesis and a break of the distal syndesmotic screw.

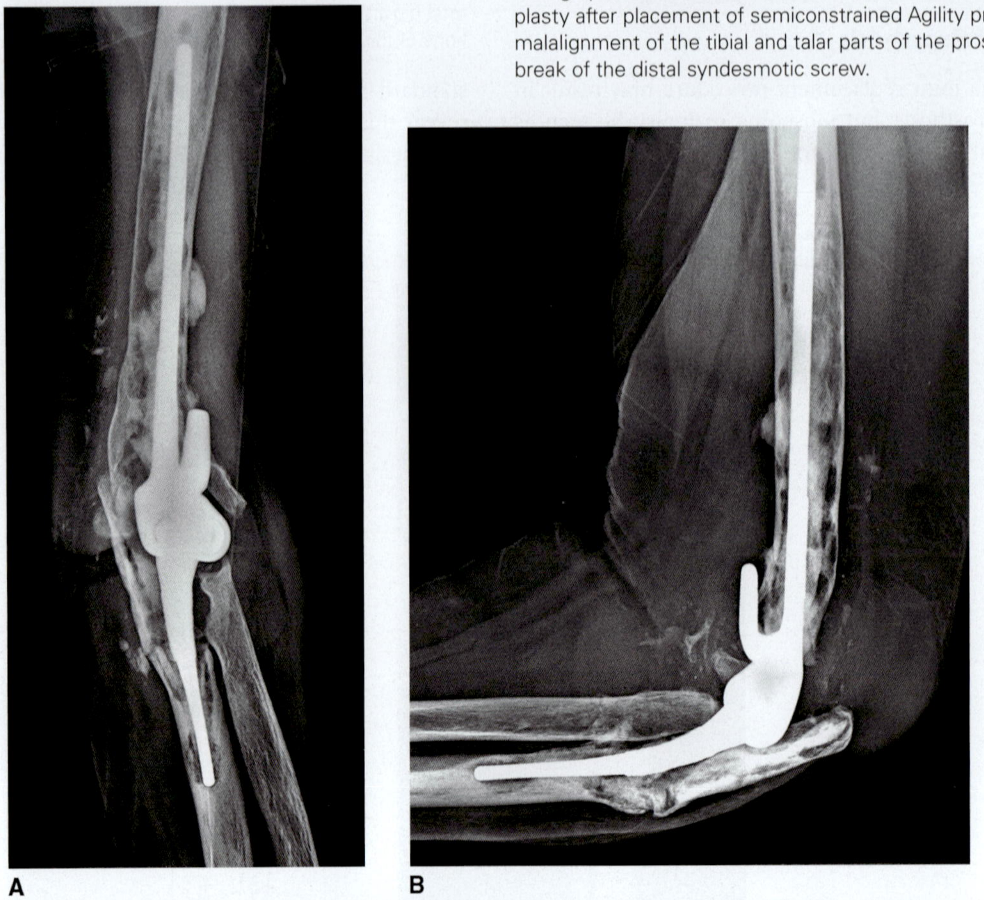

Figure 4.25 ■ Failure of total elbow arthroplasty. Oblique **(A)** and lateral **(B)** radiographs of the left elbow of a 58-year-old woman with rheumatoid arthritis show failure of total cemented semiconstrained elbow arthroplasty. Note focal bone resorption at the tip of the ulnar prosthetic component, periprosthetic fracture of the proximal ulna, and a gap at the cement–bone interface of humeral prosthetic component.

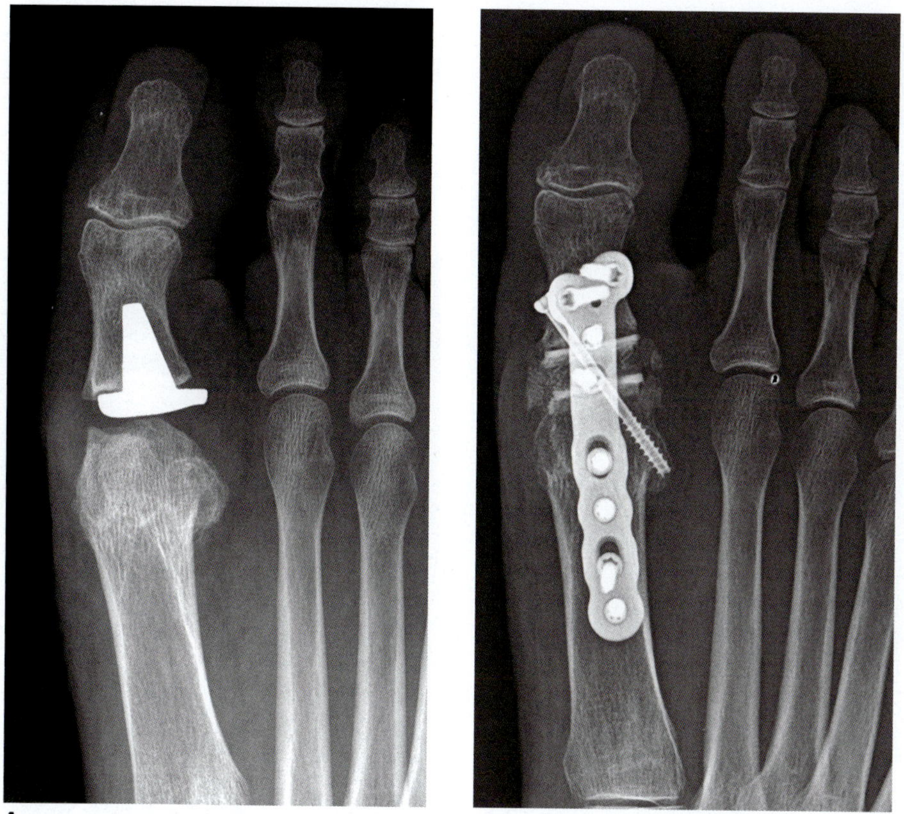

A B

Figure 4.26 ■ **Failure of hemiarthroplasty.** Subluxation and loosening of the hemiarthroplasty of the first metatarsophalangeal joint **(A)** were corrected by arthrodesis **(B)** achieved by placement of the bone graft and metallic plate and screw fixation.

cement–bone interface 2 mm or wider suggests loosening of the implant. The more effective technique for demonstrating loosening of prosthesis, however, is arthrography. The subtraction technique is commonly used to demonstrate the cardinal sign of loosening—the extension of contrast agent into the gap that develops at the interface of the bone and acrylic cement (Fig. 4.27). At times, when even arthrography is inconclusive, traction applied on the examined hip by pulling on the leg can be helpful in demonstrating occult loosening of prosthesis. A radionuclide bone scan may occasionally be helpful in differentiating infectious loosening from the mechanical loosening (see Figs. 2.56 to 2.60). Foci of increased activity, representing accumulation of radioisotope, are consistent with mechanical loosening, whereas diffuse increased activity indicates infection.

Subluxation and Dislocation of Prosthesis

This complication is easily diagnosed on conventional radiography: on the anteroposterior view of the hip (Fig. 4.28A, B), anteroposterior view of the shoulder (Fig. 2.28D), or lateral view of the knee (Fig. 4.28C).

Fracture of Prosthesis

Similarly to the subluxations and dislocations, this rare complication is also effectively demonstrated on conventional radiography (Fig. 4.29).

Prosthetic Component Wear

Most commonly this complication is related to the wear of a polyethylene lining of the acetabular cup of the hip prosthesis on the superolateral side. It is recognized on the radiography by asymmetric position of the prosthetic head within the acetabular component (Fig. 4.30). After total knee arthroplasty, similar complication may occur. The smallest polyethylene wear particles induce a cytokine-mediated, intra-articular inflammatory reaction, referred to as "particle disease" (see below), which may result in polyethylene wear-induced synovitis. This complication shows on MRI synovial thickening associated with dense synovial proliferation and debris with low-to-intermediate signal intensity (similar to that of skeletal muscle), and variable amounts of interspersed fluid and joint distention.

(Continued on page 133)

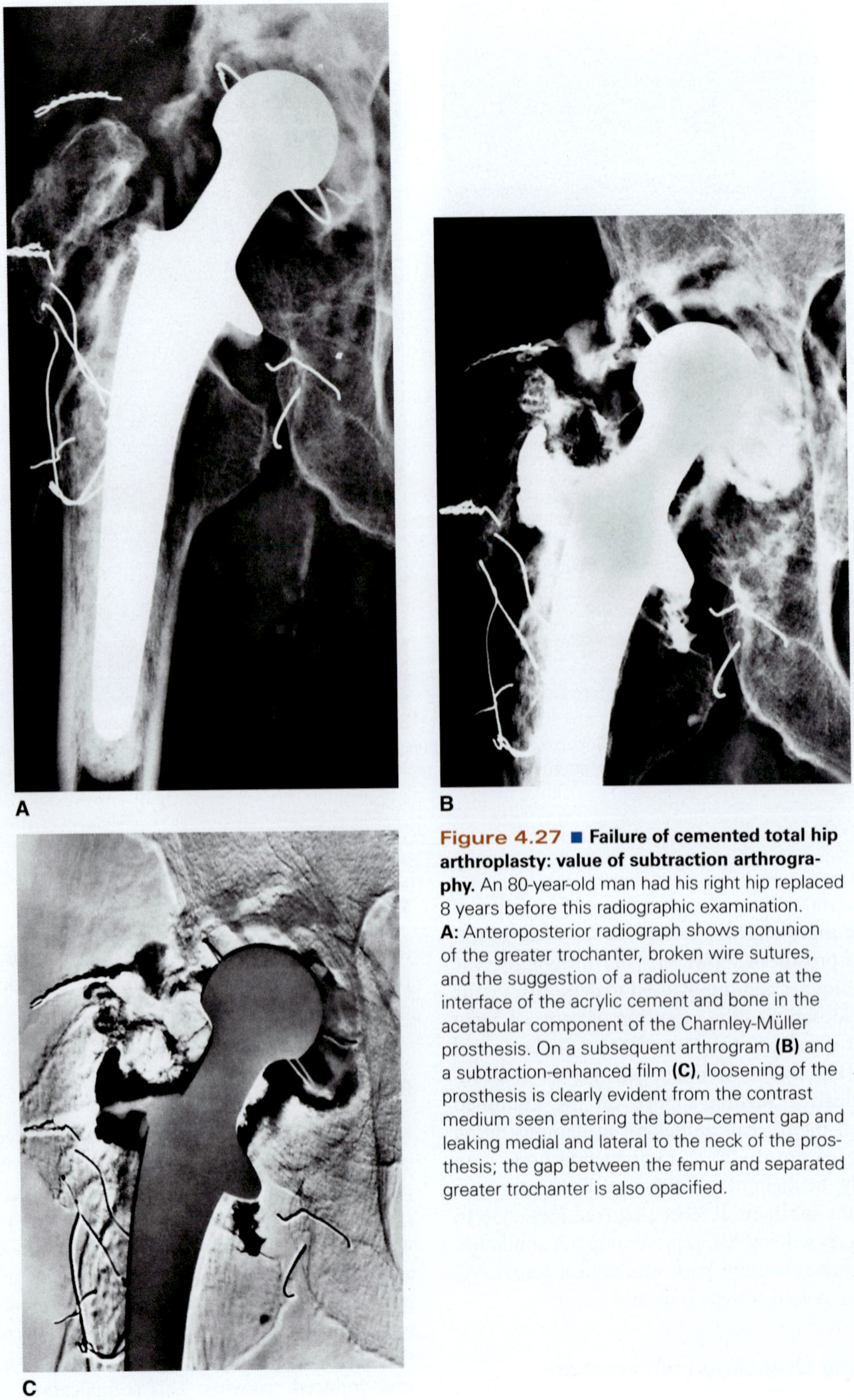

Figure 4.27 ■ **Failure of cemented total hip arthroplasty: value of subtraction arthrography.** An 80-year-old man had his right hip replaced 8 years before this radiographic examination. **A:** Anteroposterior radiograph shows nonunion of the greater trochanter, broken wire sutures, and the suggestion of a radiolucent zone at the interface of the acrylic cement and bone in the acetabular component of the Charnley-Müller prosthesis. On a subsequent arthrogram **(B)** and a subtraction-enhanced film **(C)**, loosening of the prosthesis is clearly evident from the contrast medium seen entering the bone–cement gap and leaking medial and lateral to the neck of the prosthesis; the gap between the femur and separated greater trochanter is also opacified.

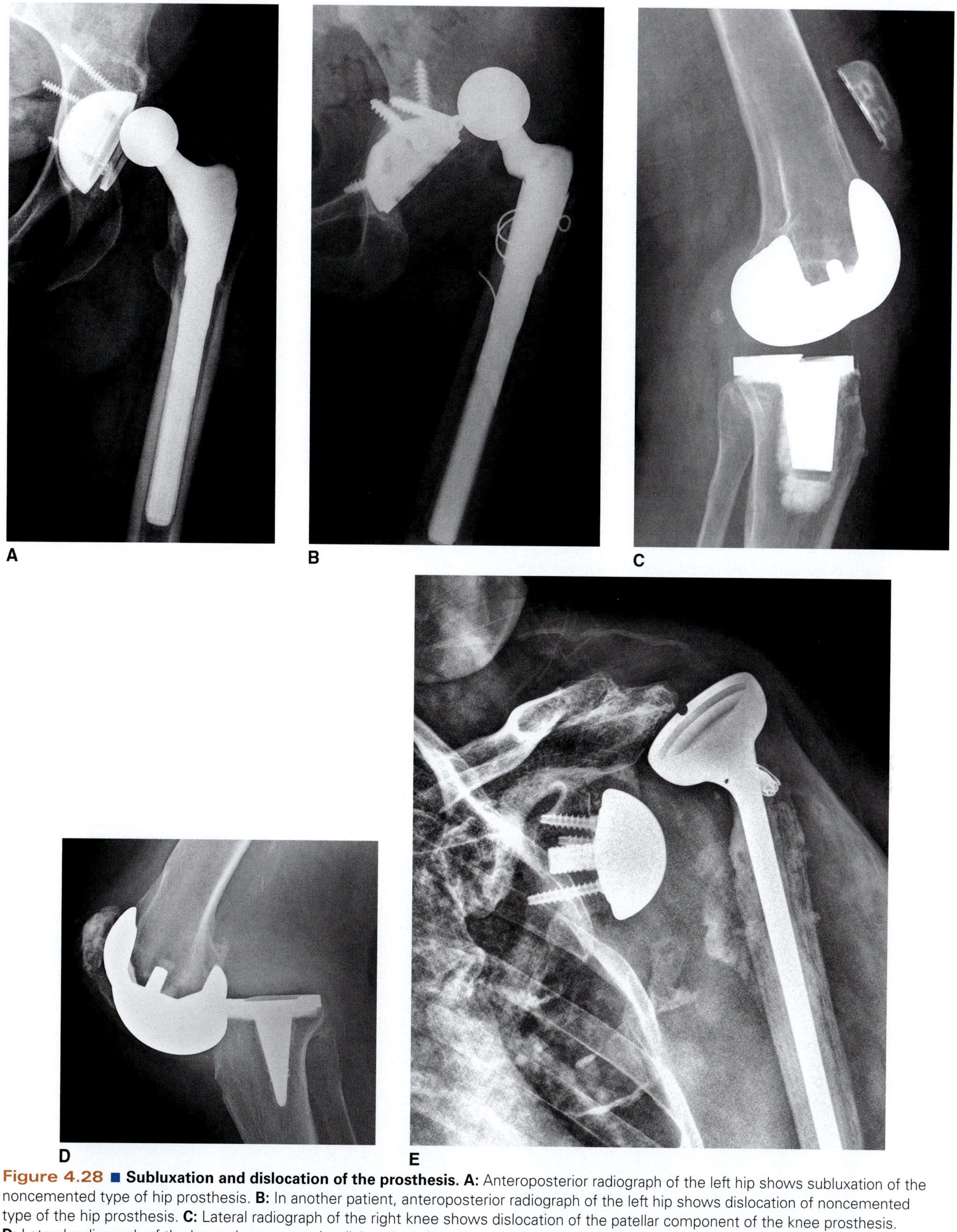

Figure 4.28 ■ **Subluxation and dislocation of the prosthesis. A:** Anteroposterior radiograph of the left hip shows subluxation of the noncemented type of hip prosthesis. **B:** In another patient, anteroposterior radiograph of the left hip shows dislocation of noncemented type of the hip prosthesis. **C:** Lateral radiograph of the right knee shows dislocation of the patellar component of the knee prosthesis. **D:** Lateral radiograph of the knee shows posterior dislocation of the three-part cemented cruciate-retaining nonconstrained prosthesis. **E:** Anteroposterior radiograph of the left shoulder shows dislocation of the reverse type of shoulder prosthesis.

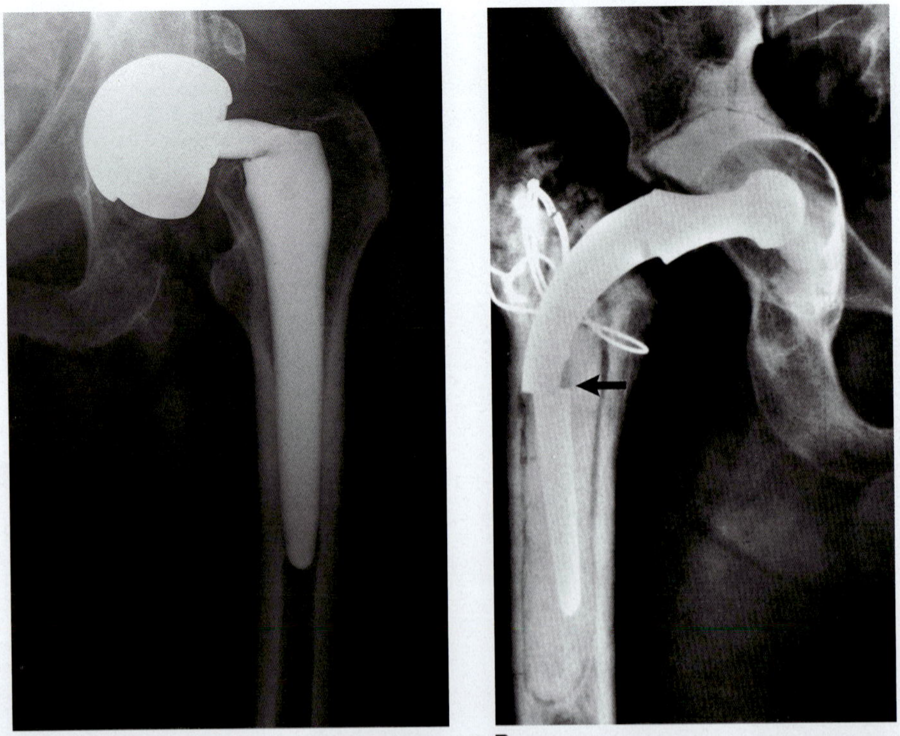

A B

Figure 4.29 ■ **Fracture of the prosthesis. A:** Anteroposterior radiograph of the left hip shows a fracture of the hip prosthesis at the junction of the neck of the prosthesis and femoral component. **B:** Anteroposterior radiograph of the right hip in another patient shows a fracture of the stem of the cemented prosthesis (*arrow*). In addition, note the break of the wires retaining the previously osteotomized greater trochanter, and a radiolucent gap at the cement–bone interface of the femoral and acetabular components, diagnostic of loosening of the prosthesis.

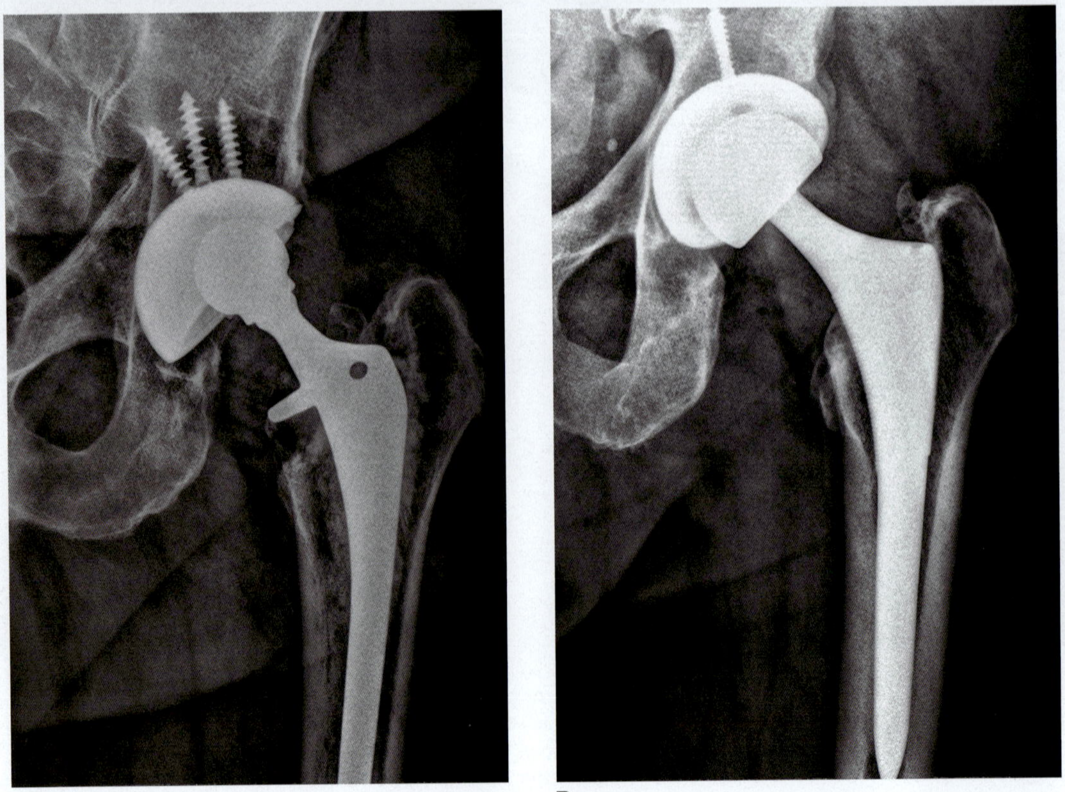

A B

Figure 4.30 ■ **Complication of total hip arthroplasty—polyethylene wear.** A 72-year-old man presented with hip pain after left total hip arthroplasty performed 4 years prior to the current admission. **A:** Anteroposterior radiograph of the hip shows eccentric position of the prosthetic femoral head within the acetabular cup secondary to the wear of polyethylene lining. Note in addition bone resorption at the site of the acetabular rim screws. **B:** Normal symmetric position of the prosthetic femoral head within the acetabular cup and proper alignment is shown for comparison.

Particle Disease (Metallosis)

This complication, also known as particle inclusion disease, giant cell granulomatosis, or aggressive granulomatosis, is the result of inflammation and osteolysis secondary to shedding of micron- and submicron-size portions of the prosthesis. It is a histiocytic response (release of cytokines) that occurs as a result of macrophage reaction to any of the components that are shed of the surface of the prosthesis. It commonly occurs from 1 to 5 years after implantation of cementless prostheses. It has been reported in the setting of total hip, total shoulder, total knee, and unicompartmental knee arthroplasties. It may occur secondary to wear in metal-on-metal arthroplasties or in arthroplasties with a polyethylene component because of abnormal contact between metal surfaces following erosion or displacement of the polyethylene. The rate of metallosis complication depends upon the material used—titanium components are more likely to cause this complication than cobalt–chromium components. The patient may be asymptomatic until substantial loss of bone, at which time he or she may experience pain and limitation of motion. Radiography is usual diagnostic, demonstrating fluffy increased densities in the periprosthetic soft tissues ("cloud sign"), radiolucency at the metal–bone interface, endosteal scalloping without reactive sclerosis, or large focal defects. At times, metallic particles are seen in the vicinity of the prosthesis (Figs. 4.31 and 4.32).

Loosening of Silicon Prosthesis, Silicone Synovitis, and Infection

Mechanical loosening of the silicon prosthesis is best evaluated by CT (Fig. 4.33). Silicone synovitis, which represents the tissue response to the shedding of silicone particles from the implants that are damaged by shear and compressive forces, is a more serious complication. The radiographic findings include nodular soft tissue swelling and well-defined subchondral lytic defects and osseous erosions, as well as deformity or fracture of the prosthesis (Figs. 4.34 and 4.35). Infection of silastic implant is best evaluated with MRI. In addition to multiple small hypointense particles in the vicinity of the implants, this modality shows intermediate-to-mild hyperintensity osseous lesions on proton- and T2-weighted sequences. These signal intensities

(Continued on page 136)

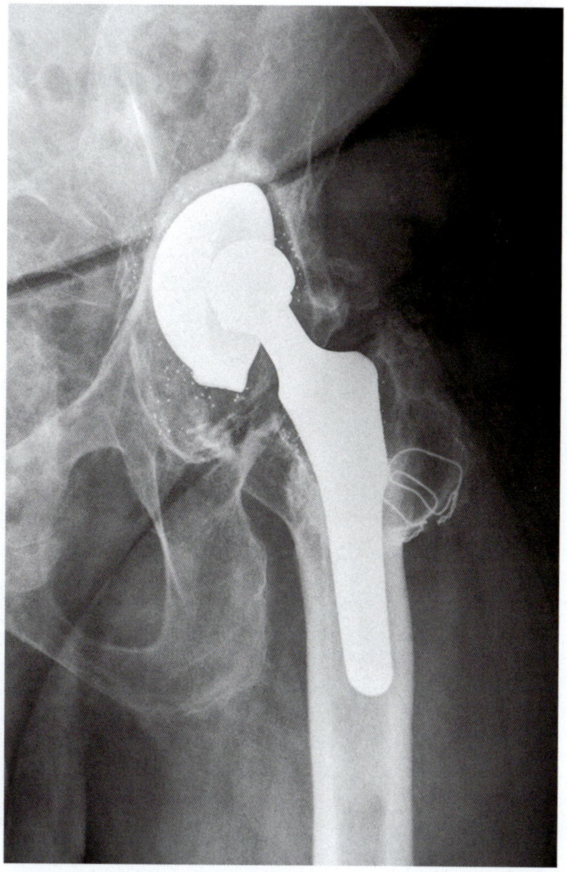

Figure 4.31 ■ Particle disease (metallosis). A 60-year-old man had total noncemented hip arthroplasty performed 5 years prior to this examination. There is extensive bone destruction surrounding the acetabular component of the prosthesis, which represents giant cell granulomatosis. Note also numerous metallic particles in the vicinity of the prosthesis.

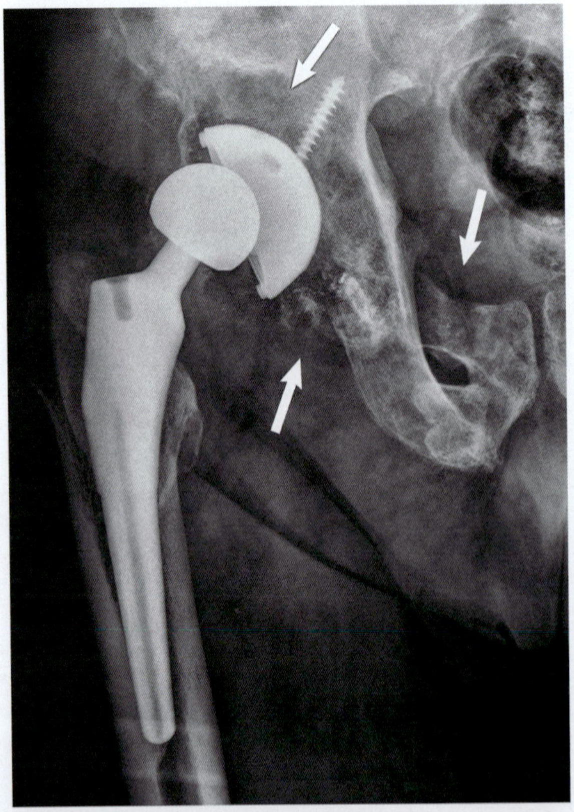

A

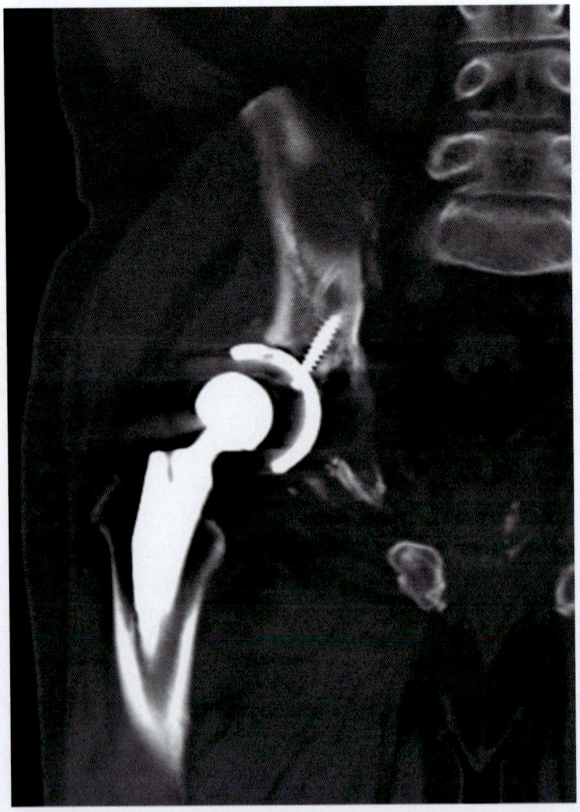

B

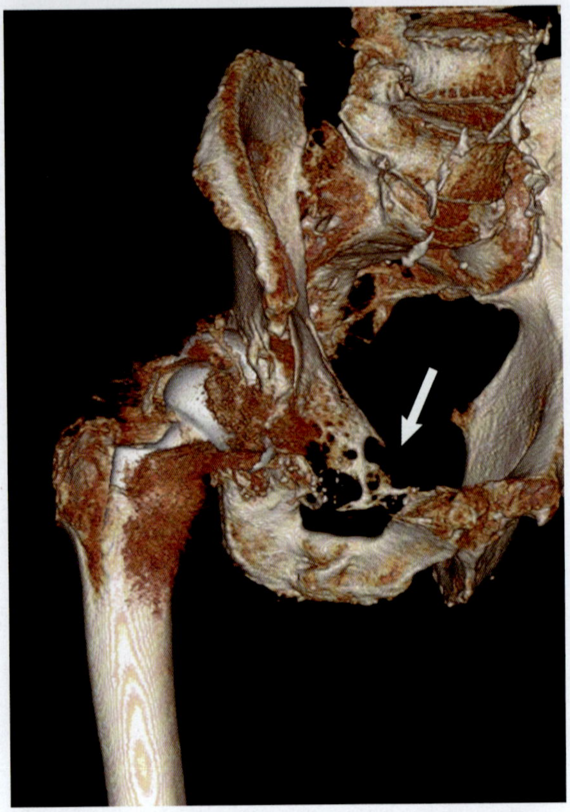

C

Figure 4.32 ■ **Particle disease (metallosis).** A 61-year-old woman presented with severe pain at the site of right total hip arthroplasty. **A:** Anteroposterior radiograph of the right hip shows subluxation of noncemented hip prosthesis. In addition, note destructive changes of the bone at the site of the acetabular component and in the pubic and ischial bones (*arrows*). Coronal reformatted CT image **(B)** and 3D-reconstructed CT image **(C)** demonstrate the bone destruction more accurately. Particularly, the destruction of the pubic bone is well depicted (*arrow*).

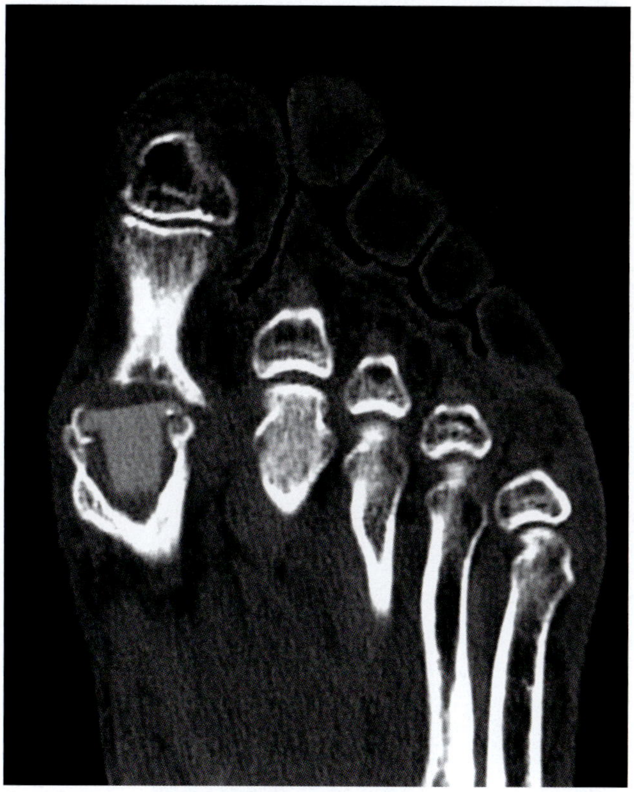

A

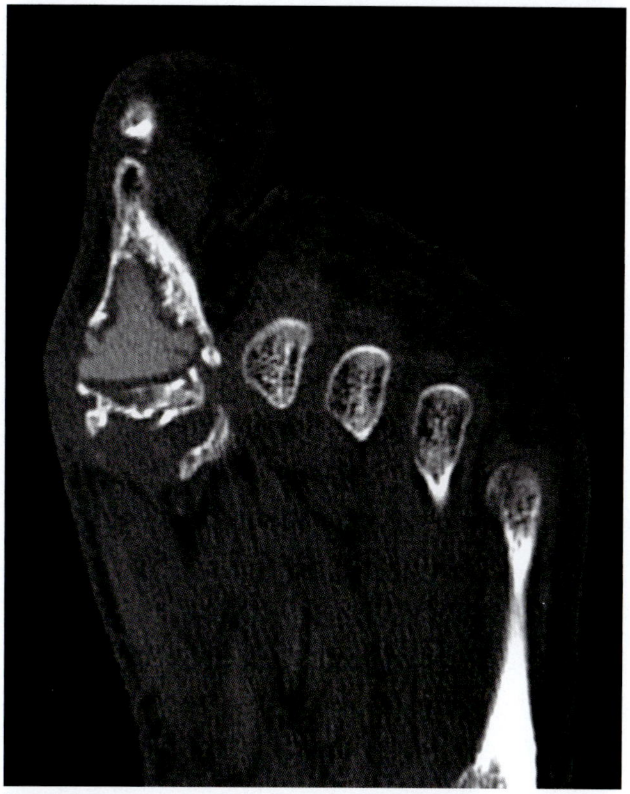

B

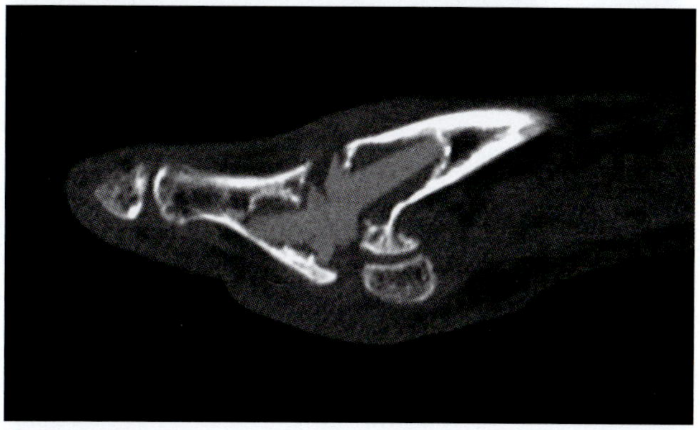

C

Figure 4.33 ■ **Failure of silastic prosthesis.** Coronal reformatted CT images of the left foot of a patient who underwent silastic arthroplasty of the first metatarsophalangeal joint demonstrate a wide gap separating the metatarsal **(A)** and the phalangeal **(B)** part of the prosthesis from bone. **C:** Reformatted sagittal CT image of the great toe shows the loosening of the prosthesis more clearly.

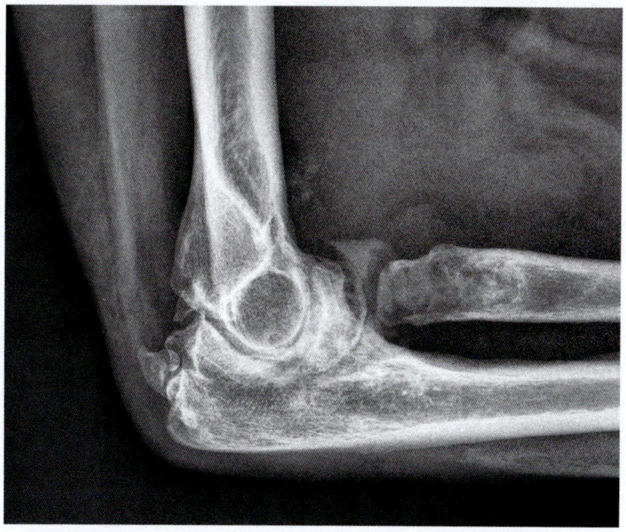

Figure 4.34 ■ **Silicone synovitis.** A 67-year-old woman with posttraumatic osteoarthritis of the right elbow had resection of the radial head and replacement with silastic radial head prosthesis. A lateral radiograph of the elbow shows fracture of the implant, erosive changes in the proximal radius and capitellum, and elbow joint effusion with silicone debris, all features consistent with silicone synovitis. Note also osteoarthritis of the ulna–trochlear joint compartment and heterotopic ossifications around the olecranon.

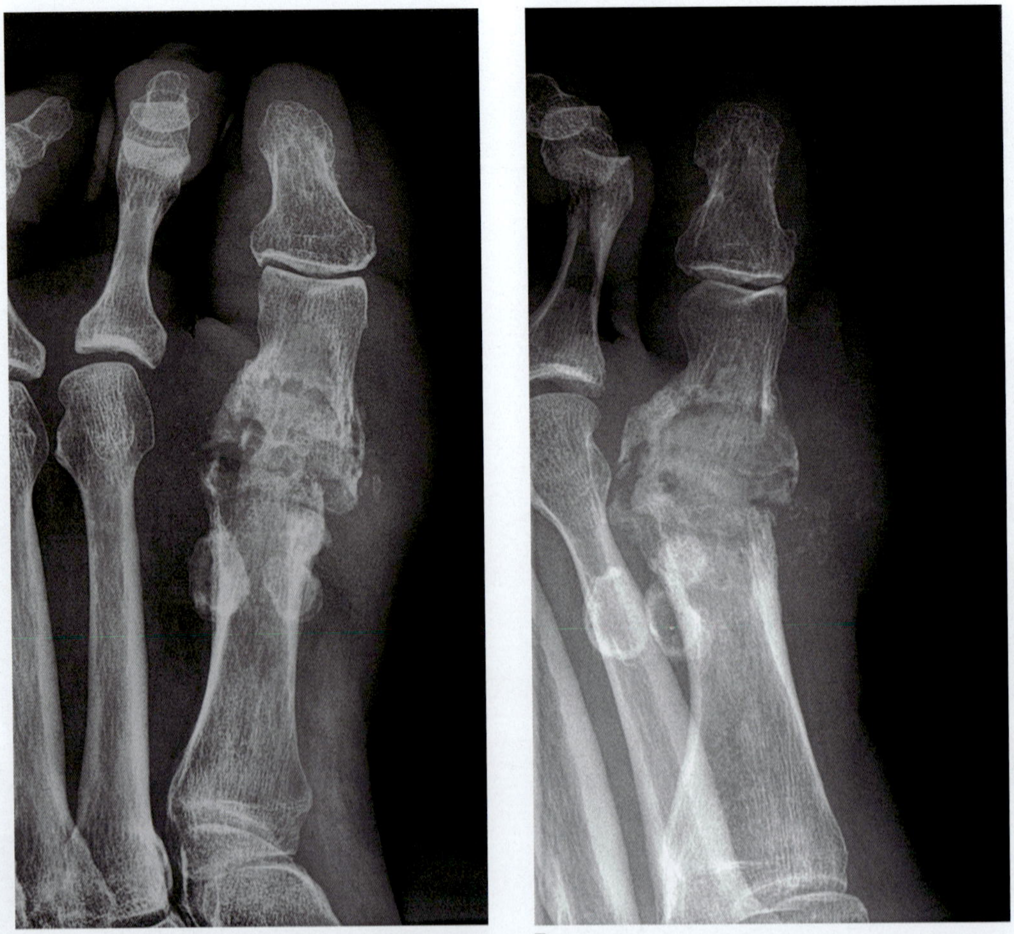

A B

Figure 4.35 ■ **Silicone synovitis.** A 72-year-old woman who underwent first metatarsophalangeal joint arthroplasty presented with pain and swelling of the great toe. Anteroposterior **(A)** and oblique **(B)** radiographs of the great toe show fragmentation of the prosthesis, silastic debris, osseous erosions, and a large soft tissue swelling, typical findings of silicone synovitis.

characteristics are consistent with the presence of inflammatory and fibrous tissue (Fig. 4.36).

Arthrofibrosis

This is a complication following knee arthroplasty characterized by chronic pain, global capsular contraction, and progressive loss of range of motion and may lead to complete joint stiffness. Arthrofibrosis is caused by the formation of dense fibrous tissue along the synovial lining of the entire joint because of excessive fibroplasia with resulting adhesions and impairment of the extensor mechanism of the knee.

Patellar Clunk Syndrome

This is a complication of total knee arthroplasty at the site of patellofemoral prosthetic components that manifests by a locking sensation or impaired motion during flexion and extension of the knee prosthesis. At physical examination, an audible clunking noise occurs during knee extension. This syndrome is caused by formation of focal fibrous tissue at the junction of the superior pole of the patella and quadriceps tendon, occurring usually about a year after joint replacement. One of the mechanisms of this complication is the entrance of the fibrous tissue into the intercondylar notch with knee flexion, and its displacement with knee extension, resulting in audible clunk.

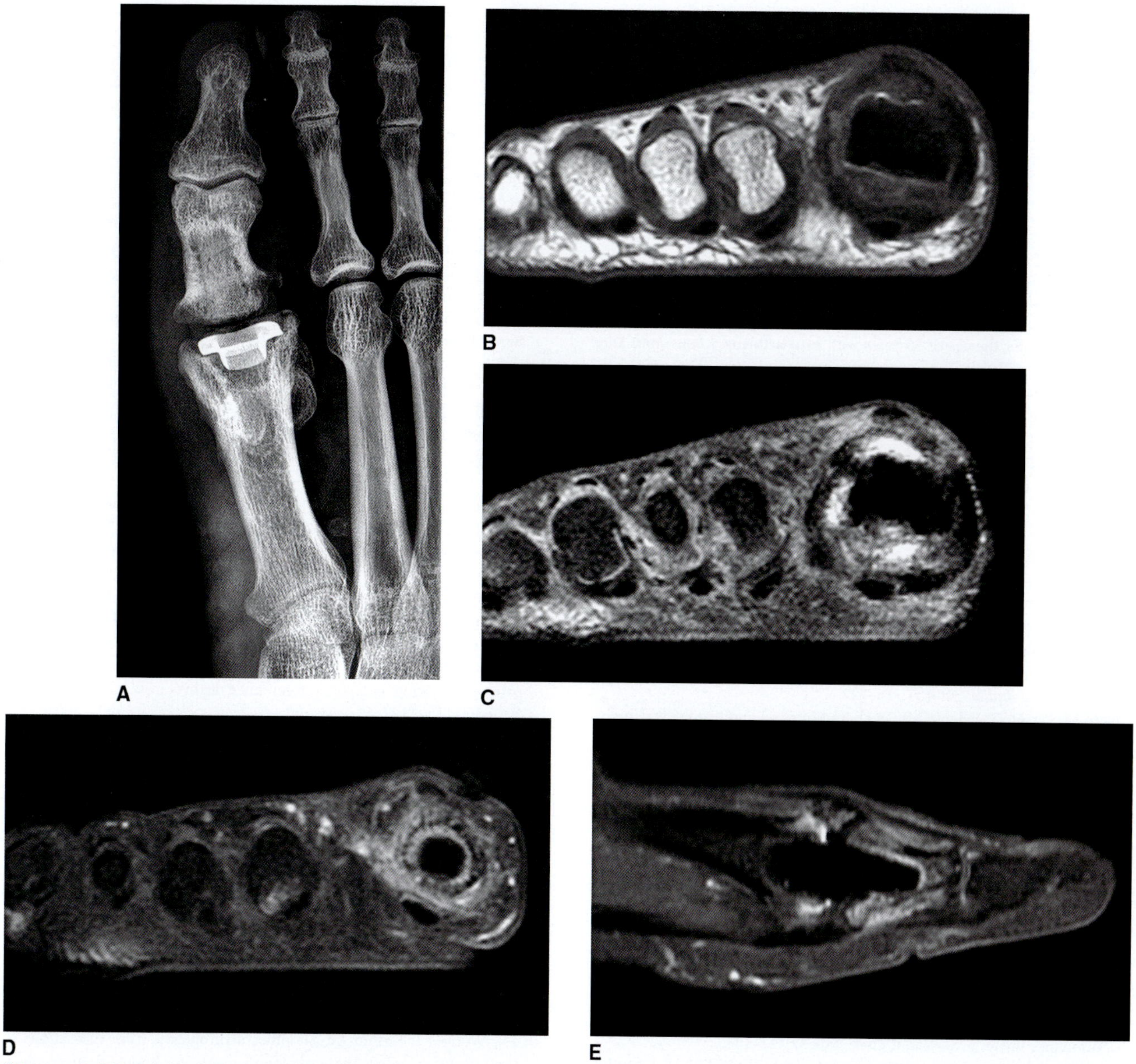

Figure 4.36 ■ **Infection of silastic prosthesis. A:** Anteroposterior radiograph of the great toe of the left foot shows status post first metatarsophalangeal arthroplasty using Swanson silicone device with circumferential titanium grommet. There is soft tissue swelling surrounding the prosthesis. In addition, there is radiolucent zone surrounding the prosthetic stems. **B:** Axial (short-axis) T1-weighted MR image through the metatarsal heads shows low-intensity implant in place. **C:** Axial STIR MR image shows high-signal edema surrounding the implant. Axial **(D)** and sagittal **(E)** T1-weighted fat-suppressed MR images obtained after intravenous administration of gadolinium show enhancement of the bone and soft tissue surrounding the distal portion of the prosthesis.

SUGGESTED READINGS

Allen AM, Ward WG, Pope TL Jr. Imaging of the total knee arthroplasty. *Radiol Clin North Am.* 1995;33:289–303.

Amstutz HC, Beaule PE, Dorey FJ, et al. Metal-on-metal hybrid surface arthroplasty: two to six-year follow-up study. *J Bone Joint Surg Am.* 2004;86:28–39.

Anderson LS, Staple TW. Arthrography of total hip replacement using substraction technique. *Radiology.* 1973;109:470–472.

Atkinson RE, Smith RJ. Silicone synovitis following silicone implant arthroplasty. *Hand Clin.* 1986;2:291–299.

Bai XS, Petscavage-Thomas JM, Ha AS. Total elbow arthroplasty: a radiographic outcome study. *Skeletal Radiol.* 2016;45:789–794.

Barrack RL. Evolution of the rotating hinge for complex total knee arthroplasty. *Clin Orthop Relat Res.* 2001;392:292–299.

Barrack RL, Tanzer M, Kattapuram SV, et al. The value of contrast arthrography in assessing loosening of symptomatic uncemented total hip components. *Skeletal Radiol.* 1994;23:37–41.

Bauer TW, Parvizi J, Kobayashi N, et al. Diagnosis of periprosthetic infection. *J Bone Joint Surg Am.* 2006;88A:869–882.

Bauer TW, Schils, J. The pathology of total joint arthroplasty. I. Mechanisms of implant fixation. *Skeletal Radiol.* 1999;28:423–432.

Beight JL, Yao B, Hozack WJ, et al. The patellar "clunk" syndrome after posterior stabilized total knee arthroplasty. *Clin Orthop Relat Res.* 1994;299:139–142.

Bestic JM, Peterson JJ, DeOrio JK, et al. Postoperative evaluation of the total ankle arthroplasty. *AJR Am J Roentgenol.* 2008;190:1112–1123.

Bong MR, Di Cesare PE. Stiffness after total knee arthroplasty. *J Am Acad Orthop Surg.* 2004;12:164–171.

Boubaker A, Delaloye AB, Blanc CH, et al. Immunoscintigraphy with anti-granulocyte monoclonal antibodies for the diagnosis of septic loosening of hip prosthesis. *Eur J Nucl Med.* 1995;22:139–147.

Chan M-K, Chowchuen P, Workman T, et al. Silicone synovitis: MR imaging in five patients. *Skeletal Radiol.* 1998;27:13–17.

Chang EY, McAnally JL, Van Horne JR, et al. Metal-on-metal total hip arthroplasty: do symptoms correlate with MR imaging findings? *Radiology.* 2012;265:848–857.

Choi S-J, Koch KM, Hargreaves BA, et al. Metal artifact reduction with MAVRIC at 3-T MRI in patients with hip arthroplasty. *AJR Am J Roentgenol.* 2015;204:140–147.

Conti SF, Wong YS. Complications of total ankle replacement. *Clin Orthop.* 2001;391:105–114.

Daniel J, Pynsent PB, McMinn DJ. Metal-on-metal resurfacing of the hip in patients under the age of 55 years with osteoarthritis. *J Bone Joint Surg Br.* 2004;86:177–184.

Datir A, Xing M, Kakarala A, et al. Radiographic evaluation of INBONE total ankle arthroplasty: a retrospective analysis of 30 cases. *Skeletal Radiol.* 2013;42:1693–1701.

Drozdovskii B, Ikonnikov A, Krylov VV. Radiosynoviorthese in the treatment of patients with rheumatoid arthritis. *Med Radiol (Mosk).* 1990;35:6–9.

Drummond J, Tran P, Fary C. Metal-on-metal hip arthroplasty: a review of adverse reactions and patient management. *J Funct Biomater.* 2015;6:486–499.

Easley ME, Vertullo CJ, Urban WC, et al. Total ankle arthroplasty. *J Am Acad Orthop Surg.* 2002;10:157–167.

Fang CSJ, Gibbons CLMH, Athanasau NA. The imaging spectrum of peri-articular inflammatory masses following metal-on-metal hip resurfacing. *Skeletal Radiol.* 2008;37:715–722.

Favero M, Perino G, Valente ML, et al. Radiological and histological analysis of two replaced interphalangeal joints with active subchondral bone resorption in erosive osteoarthritis: a novel mechanism? *Skeletal Radiol.* 2017;46:385–391.

Fritz J, Lurie B, Potter, HG. MR imaging of knee arthroplasty implants. *Radiographics.* 2015;35:1483–1501.

Galli M, Leone A, Tamburrelli FC, et al. Periprosthetic mineralization changes around femoral stems: a prospective 12-month study with DEXA. *Skeletal Radiol.* 2008;37:723–729.

Gallo J, Kaminek P, Ticha V, et al. Particle disease. A comprehensive theory of periprosthetic osteolysis: a review. *Biomed Pap Med Fac Univ Palacky Olomouc Czech Repub.* 2002;146:21–28.

Gaspersic N, Sersa I, Jevtic V, et al. Monitoring ankylosing spondylitis therapy by dynamic contrast-enhanced and diffusion-weighted magnetic resonance imaging. *Skeletal Radiol.* 2008;37:123–131.

Gee R, Munk PL, Keogh C, et al. Radiography of the PROSTALAC (prosthesis with antibiotic-loaded acrylic cement) orthopedic implant. *AJR Am J Roentgenol.* 2003;180:1701–1706.

Giza E, Sullivan M, Ocel D, et al. First metatarsophalangeal hemiarthroplasty for hallux rigidus. *Int Orthop.* 2010;34:1193–1198.

Grammont PM, Baulot E. Delta shoulder prosthesis for rotator cuff rupture. *Orthopedics.* 1993;16:65–68.

Granberry WM, Noble PC, Bishop JO, et al. Use of a hinged silicone prosthesis for replacement arthroplasty of the first metatarsophalangeal joint. *J Bone Joint Surg Am.* 1991;73:1453–1459.

Graninger, M, Handl-Zeller L, Hohenberg G, et al. Teleradiotherapy of joints in rheumatoid arthritis: lack of efficacy. *Ann Rheum Dis.* 2005;64:138–140.

Gratz S, Reize P, Pfestroff A, Hoffken H. Intact versus fragmented 99m Tc-monoclonal antibody imaging of infection in patients with septically loosened total knee arthroplasty. *J Int Med Res.* 2012;40: 1335–1342.

Greenspan A, Norman A. Gross hematuria: a complication of intrapelvic cement intrusion in total hip replacement. *AJR Am J Roentgenol.* 1978;130:327–329.

Griffith HJ, Burke J, Bonfiglio TA. Granulomatous pseudotumors in total joint replacement. *Skeletal Radiol.* 1987;16:146–152.

Griffith HJ, Lovelock JE, Evarts M, et al. The radiology of total hip replacement. *Skeletal Radiol.* 1984;12:1–11.

Griffiths HJ, Priest D, Kushner D. Total hip replacement and other orthopedic hip procedures. *Radiol Clin North Am.* 1995;33:267–287.

Harris WH. Osteolysis and particle disease in hip replacement. A review. *Acta Orthop Scand.* 1994;65:113–123.

Heffernan EJ, Alkabaidan FO, Nielsen TO, et al. The imaging appearances of metallosis. *Skeletal Radiol.* 2008;37:59–62.

Heilpern GN, Shah NN, Fordyce MJ. Birmingham hip resurfacing arthroplasty: a series of 110 consecutive hips with a minimum five-year clinical and radiological follow-up. *J Bone Joint Surg Br.* 2008;90: 1137–1142.

Helito CP, Buarque de Gusmao CV, Angelini FJ, et al. Severe metallosis following total knee arthroplasty: a case report and review of radiographic signs. *Skeletal Radiol.* 2014;43:1169–1173.

Heyse TJ, Figiel J, Hahnlein U, et al. MRI after unicondylar knee arthroplasty: the preserved compartments. *Knee.* 2012;19:923–926.

Hunter TB, Yoshino MT, Dzioba RB, et al. Medical devices of the head, neck, and spine. *Radiographics.* 2004;24:257–285.

Johnstone BR. Proximal interphalangeal joint surface replacement arthroplasty. *Hand Surg.* 2001;6:1–11.

Kamishima T, Tanimura K, Shimizu M, et al. Monitoring anti-interleukin 6 receptor antibody treatment for rheumatoid arthritis by quantitative magnetic resonance imaging of the hand and power Doppler ultrasonography of the finger. *Skeletal Radiol.* 2011;40:745–755.

Karavida N, Notopoulos A. Radiation synovectomy: an effective alternative treatment for inflamed small joints. *Hippokratia.* 2010;14:22–27.

Kenan S, Kahn L, Haramati N, Kenan S. A rare case of pseudotumor formation associated with methyl methacrylate hypersensitivity in a patient following cemented total knee arthroplasty. *Skeletal Radiol.* 2016;45:1115–1122.

Kinahan PE, Fletcher JW. PET/CT standardized uptake values (SUVs) in clinical practice and assessing response to therapy. *Semin Ultrasound CT MR.* 2010;31:496–505.

Knut L. Radiosynovectomy in the therapeutic management of arthritis. *World J Nucl Med.* 2015;14:10–15.

Kresnik E, Mikosch P, Gallowitsch HJ. Clinical outcome of radiosynoviorthesis: a meta-analysis including 2190 treated joints. *Nucl Med Commun.* 2002;23:683–688.

Kurosaka M, Yoshiya S, Mizuno K, et al. Maximizing flexion after total knee arthroplasty: the need and pitfalls. *J Arthroplasty.* 2002;17:59–62.

Lee M-J, Kim S, Lee S-A, et al. Overcoming artifacts from metallic orthopedic implants at high-field-strength MR imaging and multidetector CT. *Radiographics.* 2007;27:791–803.

Lin DJ, Wong TT, Kazam JK. Shoulder arthroplasty, from indications to complications: what the radiologist needs to know. *Radiographics.* 2016;36:192–208.

Little CP, Graham AJ, Karatzas G, et al. Outcomes of total elbow arthroplasty for rheumatoid arthritis: comparative study of three implants. *J Bone Joint Surg Am.* 2005;87:2439–2448.

Manaster BJ. Total hip arthroplasty: radiographic evaluation. *Radiographics.* 1996;16:645–660.

Matsushita I, Morita Y, Geyo R, et al. Severe bone defects and reduced mineralization caused by massive metallosis after total knee arthroplasty: histopathologic and bone morphometric findings. *Mod Rheumatol.* 2007;17:507–510.

Mayo-Smith W, Rosenthal DI, Rosenberg AE, et al. Case report 816. Rapid acceleration of osteolysis from cemented total hip replacement. *Skeletal Radiol.* 1993;22:619–621.

McFarland EG, Sanguanjit P, Tasaki A, et al. The reverse shoulder prosthesis: a review of imaging features and complications. *Skeletal Radiol.* 2006;35:488–496.

McGovern TE, Muscal JT. Radiographic evaluation of periprosthetic metallosis after total knee arthroplasty. *J South Orthop Assoc.* 2002;11: 18–24.

Morgan H, Battista V, Leopold SS. Constraint in primary total knee arthroplasty. *J Am Acad Orthop Surg.* 2005;13:515–524.

Morgan S, Ng A, Clough T. The long-term outcome of silastic implant arthroplasty of the first metatarsophalangeal joint: a retrospective analysis of one hundred and eight feet. *Int Orthop.* 2012;36:1865–1869.

Mulcahy H, Chew FS. Current concepts of hip arthroplasty for radiologists: Part 1, features and radiographic assessment. *AJR Am J Roentgenol.* 2012;199:559–569.

Mulcahy H, Chew FS. Current concepts of hip arthroplasty for radiologists: Part 2, revisions and complications. *AJR Am J Roentgenol.* 2012;199:570–580.

Nikac V, Blazar P, Earp B, Weissman BN. Radiographic and surgical considerations in arthritis surgery of the hand. *Skeletal Radiol.* 2017;46:591–604.

Peimer CA, MedigeJ, Eckert BS, et al. Reactive synovitis after silicone arthroplasty. *J Hand Surg Am.* 1986;11:624–638.

Petscavage JM, Ha AS, Chew FS. Radiologic review of total elbow, radial head, and capitellar resurfacing arthroplasty. *Radiographics.* 2012;32:129–149.

Rahman L, Hall-Craggs M, Muirhead-Allwood SK. Radiology of the resurfaced hip. *Skeletal Radiol.* 2011;40:819–830.

Roberts CC, Ekelund AL, Renfree KJ, et al. Radiologic assessment of reverse shoulder arthroplasty. *Radiographics.* 2007;27:223–235.

Rodriguez JA, Bhende H, Ranawat CS. Total condylar knee replacement: a 20-year followup study. *Clin Orthop Relat Res.* 2001;388:10–17.

Rutherford EE, Tarplett LJ, Davies EM, et al. Lumbar spine fusion and stabilization: hardware, techniques, and imaging appearances. *Radiographics.* 2007;27:1737–1749.

Salvati EA, Ghelman B, McLaren T, Wilson PD Jr. Subtraction technique in arthrography for loosening of total hip replacement fixed with radiopaque cement. *Clin Orthop.* 1974;101:105–109.

Sanchis-Alfonso V. Severe metallosis after unicompartmental knee arthroplasty. *Knee Surg Sports Traumatol Arthrosc.* 2007;15:361–364.

Schmalzried T, Jasty M, Harris W. Periprosthetic bone loss in total hip arthroplasty: polyethylene wear debris and the concept of effective joint space. *J Bone Joint Surg Am.* 1992;74:849–863.

Sharma L. Osteoarthritis treatment. In: Klippel JH, Stone JH, Crofford LJ, White PH, eds. *Primer on the Rheumatic Diseases.* 13th ed. New York: Springer; 2008:235–240.

Sierakowski A, Zweifel C, Sirotakova M, et al. Joint replacement in 131 painful osteoarthritic and post-traumatic distal interphalangeal joints. *J Hand Surg Eur Vol.* 2011;37E:304–309.

Silverman EJ, Ashley B, Sheth NP. Metal-on-metal total hip arthroplasty: is there still a role in 2016? *Curr Rev Musculoskelet Med.* 2016;9:93–96.

Slone RM, Heare MM, Vander Griend RA, et al. Orthopedic fixation devices. *Radiographics.* 1991;11:823–847.

Slone RM, MacMillan M, Montgomery WJ. Spinal fixation. Part 1. Principles, basic hardware, and fixation techniques for the cervical spine. *Radiographics.* 1993;13:341–356.

Slone RM, MacMillan M, Montgomery WJ. Spinal fixation. Part 3. Complications of spinal instrumentation. *Radiographics.* 1993;13:797–816.

Song Z, Borgwardt L, Holby N, et al. Prosthesis infection after orthopedic joint replacement: the possible role of bacterial biofilms. *Orthop Rev (Pavia).* 2013;5:e14.

Stillwater L, Memauri B, Ratanshi I, et al. Radiographic interpretation of carpometacarpal arthroplasty: correlation between radiographic loosening and clinical outcome. *Skeletal Radiol.* 2017;46:1057–1062.

Sutter R, Hodek R, Fucentese SF, et al. Total knee arthroplasty MRI featuring slice-encoding for metal artifact correction: reduction of artifacts for STIR and proton density-weighted sequences. *AJR Am J Roentgenol.* 2013;201:1315–1324.

Swan JS, Braunstein EM, Wellman HN, et al. Contrast and nuclear arthrography in loosening of the uncemented hip prosthesis. *Skeletal Radiol.* 1991;20:15–19.

Swanson A, Lumsden R, Swanson G. Silicone implant arthroplasty of the great toe: a review of single stem and flexible hinge implant. *Clin Orthop.* 1979;142:30–42.

Talbot BS, Weinberg EP. MR imaging with metal-suppression sequences for evaluation of total joint arthroplasty. *Radiographics.* 2016;36:209–225.

Taljanovic MS, Jones MD, Hunter TB, et al. Joint arthroplasties and prostheses. *Radiographics.* 2003;23:1295–1314.

Van der Lugt JC, Rozing PM. Systematic review of primary total elbow prosthesis used for the rheumatoid elbow. *Clin Rheumatol.* 2004;23:291–298.

Woodruff MJ, Cohen AP, Bradley JG. Arthroplasty of the shoulder in rheumatoid arthritis with rotator cuff dysfunction. *Int Orthop.* 2003;27:7–10.

Xing D, Ma XL, Ma JX, et al. Use of anti-granulocyte scintigraphy with 99mTc-labeled monoclonal antibodies for the diagnosis of periprosthetic infection in patients after total joint arthroplasty: a diagnostic meta-analysis. *PLoS One.* 2013;8(7):e69857. http://dx.doi.org/10.1371/journal.pone.0069857

PART II

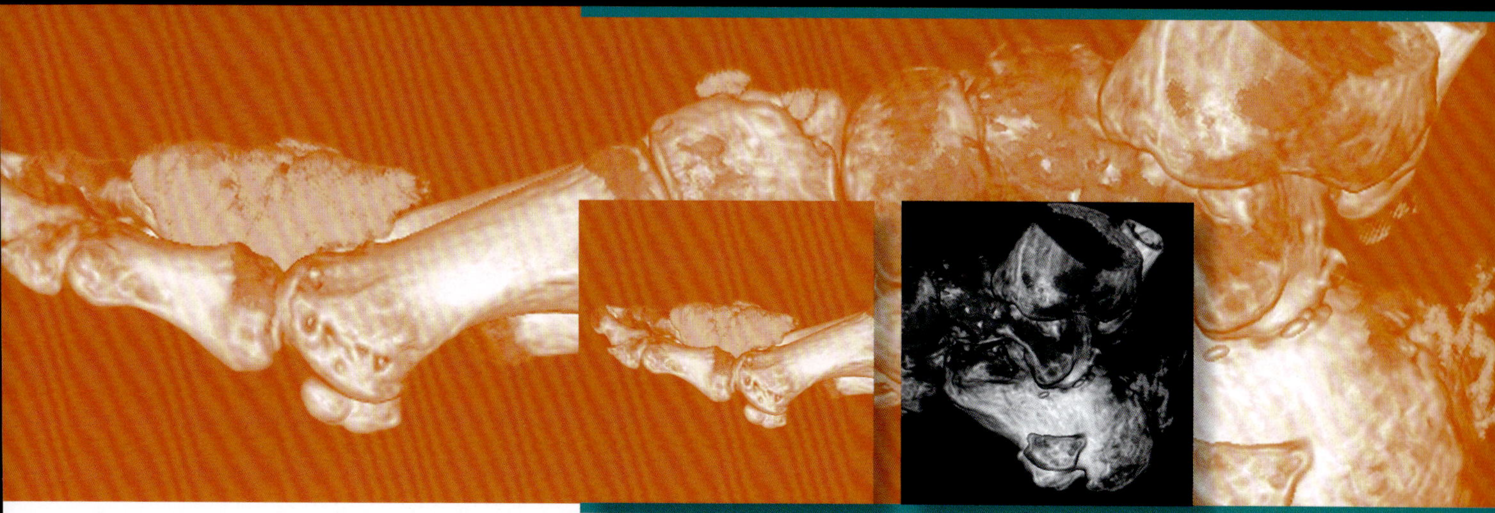

The Most Common Arthritides and Arthropathies

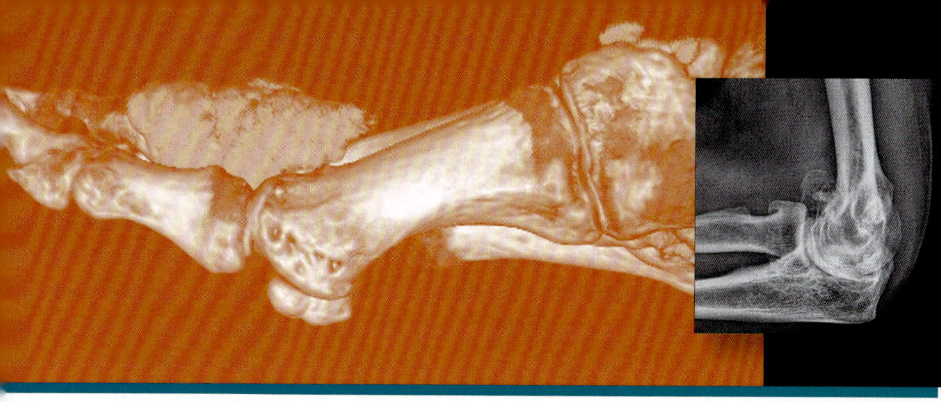

CHAPTER 5

Degenerative Joint Diseases

OSTEOARTHRITIS (OA)

Degenerative joint disease (osteoarthritis, osteoarthrosis) is the most common form of arthritis and represents a heterogeneous group of joint abnormalities with similar clinical, pathologic, and imaging features. Symptomatic OA is defined by the American College of Rheumatology as a group of conditions that lead to joint symptoms and signs, which are associated with the defective integrity of articular cartilage, in addition to related changes in the underlying bone at the joint margins. In 1994, at a meeting of the World Health Organization (WHO) and the American Academy of Orthopedic Surgery, a definition of osteoarthritis was proposed as follows: "OA is the result of both mechanical and biologic events that destabilize the normal coupling of degradation and synthesis of articular cartilage and subchondral bone. Although it may be initiated by multiple factors including genetic, developmental, metabolic, and traumatic, OA involves all of the tissues of the diarthrodial joint. Ultimately, OA is manifested by morphologic, biochemical, molecular, and biomechanical changes in both cells and matrix that leads to softening, fibrillation, ulceration and loss of articular cartilage, sclerosis and eburnation of subchondral bone, osteophytes, and subchondral cysts. When clinically evident, OA is characterized by joint pain, tenderness, limitation of movement, crepitus, occasional effusion, and variable degrees of local inflammation." In its primary (idiopathic) form, OA affects individuals aged 50 years and older; in its secondary form, however, osteoarthritis may be seen in a much younger age group. Patients in the latter group have clearly defined underlying conditions leading to the development of degenerative joint disease (see Fig. 1.1).

Some authorities postulate that there are two types of primary degenerative joint disease. The first form is apparently closely related to the aging process ("wear and tear") and represents not a true arthritis but a senescent process of the joint. It characteristically shows limited destruction of the cartilage, slow progression, lack of significant joint deformity, and no restriction of joint function. This process is not affected by gender or race. It is in reality a manifestation of aging and can be seen in virtually every species, from old fish to old people. The second type, a true osteoarthritis, is unrelated to the aging process, although it shows an increased prevalence with age. Genetic factors have been found to be strong determination of this form of osteoarthritis. The nature of the genetic influence, however, is partially speculative and may involve a structural defect (i.e., collagen), alterations in cartilage or bone metabolism, or alternatively a genetic influence on known environmental risk factors such as obesity, sports, and trauma. Several studies have implicated linkages to osteoarthritis on chromosomes 2q, 9q, 11q, and 16p, among others. Implicated genes include VDR, AGC1, IGF-1, ER alpha, TGF beta, cartilage matrix protein (CRTM), cartilage link protein (CRTL), and collagens II, IX, and XI. Most recent studies also suggested that mutations in the gene *GDF5*, also known as *cartilage-derived morphogenetic protein 1*, could be linked with etiology of osteoarthritis of the hip and knee. Some investigators suggested that osteoarthritis in some families might be caused by the mutations in the type II collagen gene *COL2A1*, which encodes a protein expressed almost exclusively in cartilage. This mutation weakens the matrix and leads to premature degeneration of the cartilage. Marked by progressive destruction of the articular cartilage and reparative processes such as osteophyte formation and subchondral sclerosis, true osteoarthritis progresses rapidly, leading to significant joint deformity. This form may be related to genetic factors, as well as to gender, race, and obesity. It has been shown that osteoarthritis tends to affect women more commonly than men, particularly in the proximal and distal interphalangeal joints and the first carpometacarpal joints. In the population older than 65 years, osteoarthritis affects Caucasians more commonly than African Americans. Obesity is associated with a higher incidence of osteoarthritis in the knees, which may be related to an excessive weight-bearing load on these joints.

Generally, in osteoarthritis, the large diarthrodial joints such as the hip or knee and the small joints such as the interphalangeal joints of the hand are most often affected; the spine, however, is just as frequently involved in the degenerative process (Fig. 5.1). The shoulder, elbow, wrist, and ankle are unusual sites for primary osteoarthritis, and if degenerative changes are encountered in these locations, secondary arthritis should be considered. It should be kept in mind, however, that evidence exists for an association between degenerative arthritis in unusual sites and certain occupations. Even primary osteoarthritic changes may develop more rapidly, for example, in the lumbar spine, knees, and elbows of coal miners and in the wrists, elbows, and shoulders of pneumatic drill operators. Degenerative changes are also commonly seen in the ankles and feet of ballet dancers and in the femoropatellar joints of bicyclists.

Ordinarily, osteoarthritis manifests clinically by two cardinal symptoms: joint pain exacerbated by activity and usually short-lasting joints stiffness. Some other symptoms include focal swelling of the joints, cracking of the joints, locking of the joints, and difficulty with daily activities.

An overview of the clinical and imaging hallmarks of degenerative joint disease is presented in Table 5.1.

(Continued on page 146)

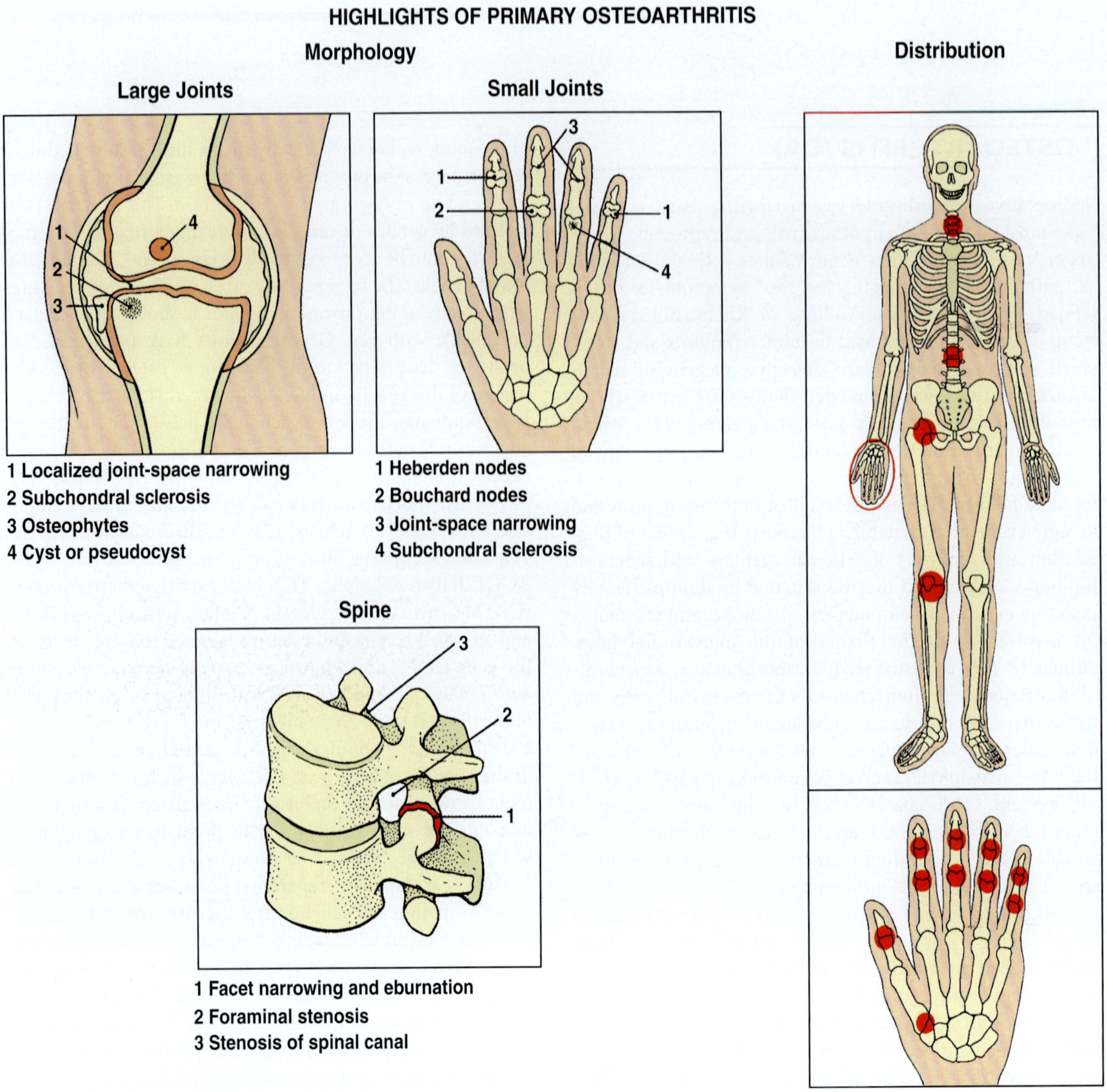

Figure 5.1 ■ **Highlights of the morphology and distribution of arthritic lesions in primary osteoarthritis.**

Table 5.1 CLINICAL AND IMAGING HALLMARKS OF DEGENERATIVE JOINT DISEASE

Type of Arthritis	Site	Crucial Abnormalities	Technique[a]/Projection
Primary osteoarthritis (F > M; >50 years)	Hand	Degenerative changes in: Proximal interphalangeal joints (Bouchard nodes) Distal interphalangeal joints (Heberden nodes)	Dorsovolar view
	Hip	Narrowing of joint space Subchondral sclerosis Marginal osteophytes Cysts and pseudocysts Superolateral subluxation	Anteroposterior view
	Knee	Same changes as in hip Varus or valgus deformity Degenerative changes in Femoropatellar compartment Patella (tooth sign)	Anteroposterior view Weight-bearing anteroposterior view Lateral view Axial view of patella
	Spine	Degenerative disk disease Narrowing of disk space Degenerative spondylolisthesis Osteophytosis Spondylosis deformans Degenerative changes in apophyseal joints Foraminal stenosis Spinal stenosis	 Lateral view Lateral flexion/extension views Anteroposterior and lateral views Anteroposterior and lateral views Oblique views (cervical, lumbar) CT, myelogram, MRI
Secondary osteoarthritis Posttraumatic	Hip Knee Shoulder, elbow, wrist, ankle (unusual sites)	Similar changes to those in primary osteoarthritis History of previous trauma Younger age	Standard views
FAI syndrome	Hips	Bone formation at the head/neck junction Acetabular crossover sign	MRI/MRa
Slipped capital femoral epiphysis	Hips	Herndon hump Narrowing of joint space Osteophytosis	Anteroposterior and frog lateral views
Congenital hip dislocation (F > M)	Hips	Signs of acetabular hypoplasia	Anteroposterior and frog lateral views
Perthes disease (M > F)	Hip	Unilateral or bilateral Osteonecrosis of femoral head Coxa magna Lateral subluxation	Anteroposterior and frog lateral views
Inflammatory arthritis	Hip Knee	Medial and axial migration of femoral head Periarticular osteoporosis Limited osteophytosis	Standard views
Osteonecrosis	Hip Shoulder	Increased bone density Joint space usually preserved or only slightly narrowed Crescent sign	Anteroposterior views (hip, shoulder) Grashey view (shoulder) Frog lateral view (hip)
Paget disease (>40 years)	Hips, knees, shoulders	Coarse trabeculations Thickening of cortex	Standard views of affected joints Radionuclide bone scan
Multiple epiphyseal dysplasia	Epiphyses of long bones	Dysplastic changes Narrowing of joint space Osteophytes	Standard views of affected joints
Hemochromatosis	Hands	Degenerative changes in second and third metacarpophalangeal joints with beak-like osteophytes Chondrocalcinosis	Dorsovolar view
Acromegaly	Large joints	Joint spaces widened or only slightly narrowed	Standard views of affected joint
	Hands	Enlargement of terminal tufts Beaklike osteophytes in heads of metacarpals	Dorsovolar view

[a]Radionuclide bone scan is used to determine the distribution of arthritic lesions in the skeleton.
CT, computed tomography; F, female; FAI, femoroacetabular impingement; M, male; MRa, magnetic resonance arthrography; MRI, magnetic resonance imaging.

OSTEOARTHRITIS OF THE LARGE JOINTS

The hip and knee joints are the most common sites of osteoarthritis. The severity of radiographic changes does not always correlate with the clinical symptoms, which may vary from stiffness and pain to severe deformities and limitation of joint function.

Osteoarthritis of the Hip

Clinical Features

Commonly, the patient presents with a history of gradual onset of slowly worsening hip pain, localized primarily in the groin, aggravated by movement in the joint, and by weight bearing. This is accompanied by decreasing range of motion. The patient is limping and has difficulty to walk normally, particularly going up and down the stairs. Not infrequently, the patient may experience pain in the knee. This phenomenon occurs because branches of the obturator nerve innervate both the knee and the hip joints.

Pathology

Some of the pathologic features of osteoarthritis were already outlined in Chapter 1. Generally, the disease is described as occurring in two stages: loss of articular cartilage, followed by reparative process in adjacent bone and cartilage in an attempt to remodel the joint. Gross specimens of resected osteoarthritic femoral head show alterations in the shape of the articular surface and damaged cartilage. In the weight-bearing areas, the cartilage may be entirely absent, and the subchondral bone has a dense, polished, marble-like appearance, termed eburnation (see Figs. 1.20A and 1.21). Cystic-like defects, known as geodes, may be found, filled either with thick fluid or with loose fibromyxoid tissue (see Fig. 1.25). In the non–weight-bearing areas and around its margins, osteophytes develop (Fig. 5.2, see also Fig. 1.20B). As the articular cartilage is progressively destroyed, the underlying subchondral bone is subjected to increasingly localized overload, leading to pressure necrosis (Fig. 5.3). This superficial necrosis is, however, different from primary avascular necrosis (osteonecrosis) that has distinct etiology and pathogenesis (see Chapter 11).

Histopathology shows hypertrophy and hyperplasia of the synoviocytes. Also present are areas of fibrillation, and increase in the ratio of water to the proteoglycan in the cartilage matrix leads to cartilage softening (chondromalacia) (see Fig. 1.22B), followed by formation of the fissures on the cartilaginous surface (see Fig. 1.23). Extension of the hyperplastic synovium (pannus) into the articular surface of the hip joint is a common finding (Fig. 5.4). In deeper sections, at the cartilage–subchondral bone junction, there is often present marked irregularity and duplication of the tidemark (see Fig. 1.24). In the more advanced stages, subchondral sclerosis predominates due to accelerated bone turnover and apposition of small strips of new bone through the process of increased endochondral ossification and osteoblastic deposition (see Fig. 1.25C).

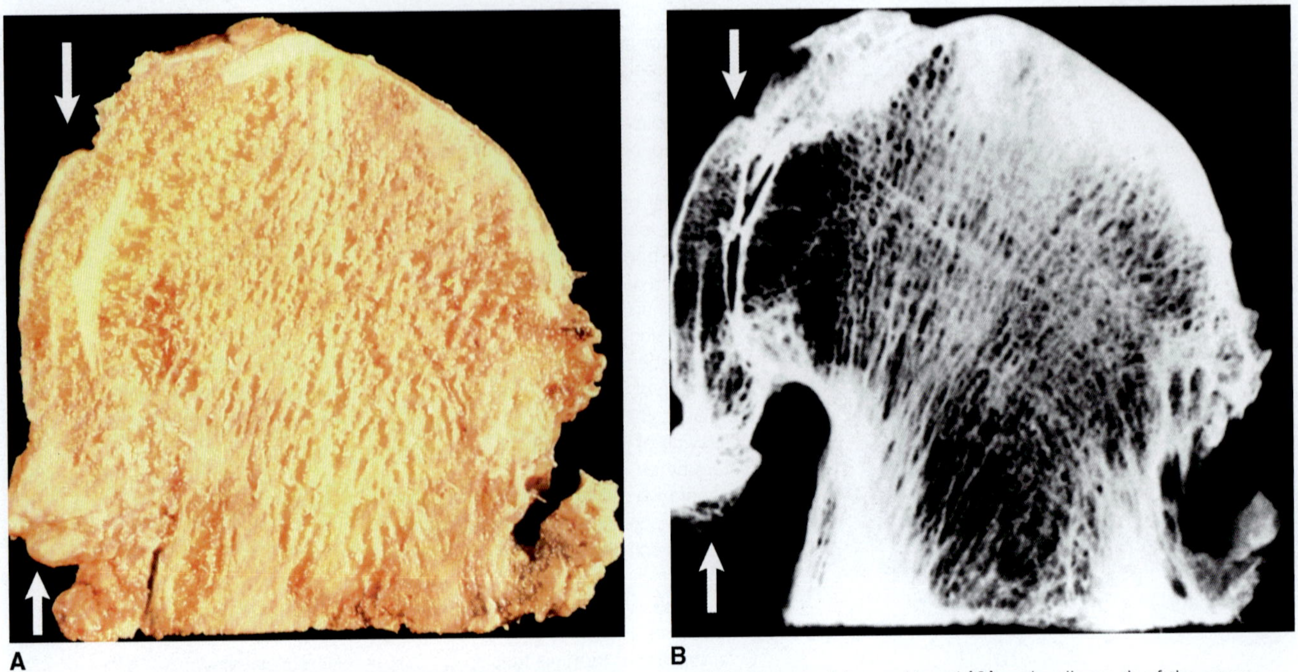

Figure 5.2 ■ Pathology of osteoarthritis of hip joint. Coronal section of the resected femoral head **(A)** and radiograph of the gross specimen **(B)** show a large flat osteophyte extending from the medial aspect to the region of fovea (*arrows*). (Modified from Bullough PG. *Atlas of Orthopedic Pathology with Clinical and Radiologic Correlation.* 2nd ed. New York, NY: Gower Medical Publishing; 1992, Figs. 10.11 and 10.12, p. 10.5.)

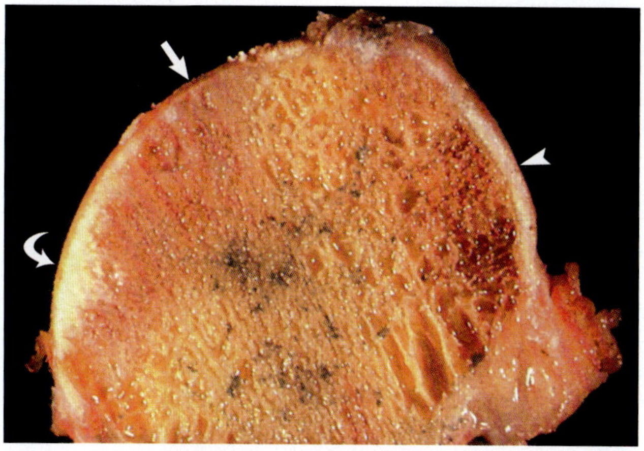

Figure 5.3 ■ Pathology of osteoarthritis of hip joint. Coronal section of the osteoarthritic femoral head shows subchondral bone partially denuded of articular cartilage (*arrow*). Some articular cartilage remains intact (*arrowhead*). Observe in the exposed subchondral bone focal bone marrow necrosis (*yellow area*) because of localized overloading (*curved arrow*). (Modified from Bullough PG. *Atlas of Orthopedic Pathology with Clinical and Radiologic Correlation.* 2nd ed. New York, NY: Gower Medical Publishing; 1992, Fig. 9.31.)

Imaging Features

There are four cardinal imaging features of degenerative joint disease in the hip:

1. Narrowing of the joint space as a result of thinning of the articular cartilage.
2. Subchondral sclerosis (eburnation) caused by reparative processes (remodeling).
3. Osteophyte formation (osteophytosis) as a result of reparative processes in sites not subjected to stress (so-called *low-stress areas*), which are usually marginal (peripheral) in distribution.
4. Cyst or pseudocyst formation resulting from bone contusions that lead to microfractures and intrusion of synovial fluid into the altered spongy bone; in the acetabulum, these subchondral cystlike lesions are referred to as *Eggers cysts.*

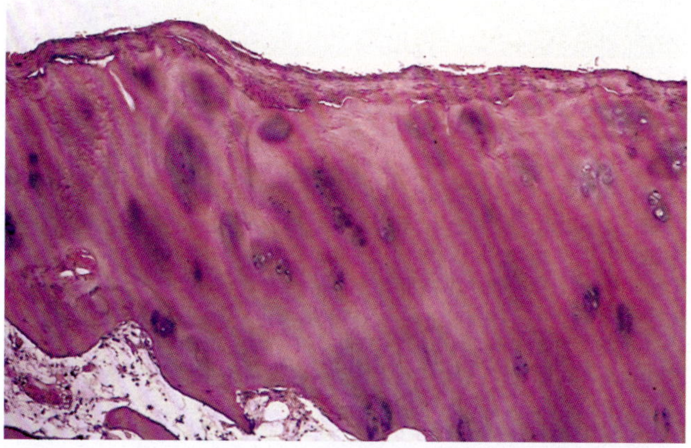

Figure 5.4 ■ Histopathology of osteoarthritis of hip joint. Photomicrograph of a portion of the articular cartilage of a femoral head shows a fibrous pannus extending over the articular surface (H&E, original magnification ×4). (From Bullough PG. *Atlas of Orthopedic Pathology with Clinical and Radiologic Correlation.* 2nd ed. New York, NY: Gower Medical Publishing; 1992, Fig. 9.43, p. 9.17.)

These hallmarks of degenerative joint disease can be readily demonstrated on the standard radiographs of the hip (Fig. 5.5). Computed tomography (CT) (Figs. 5.6, 5.7, and 5.8B) and magnetic resonance imaging (MRI) (Figs. 5.8C and 5.9) may further delineate the characteristic features of osteoarthritis.

As articular cartilage is destroyed and reparative changes develop, evidence emerges of a change in the relation of the femoral head with respect to the acetabulum, known as *migration.* Generally, three patterns of femoral head migration can be observed: superior, which may be either superolateral or superomedial; medial; and axial (Fig. 5.10). The most common pattern is superolateral migration; the medial pattern is less common, whereas axial migration is only exceptionally seen. It should be kept in mind, however, that in inflammatory arthritis of the hip, such as rheumatoid arthritis, in which a previous axial migration of the femoral head is commonly associated with acetabular protrusio, degenerative changes might develop as a complication of the inflammatory process. Thus, one may see secondary osteoarthritis with axial migration (Fig. 5.11).

The osteoarthritis of the hip joint is typically characterized by the presence of osteophytes, which are commonly the most prominent imaging feature of the disease and represent the reparative response to joint destruction. Osteophytes are of two types: peripheral, which arise at the osseous–chondral junction of the femoral neck and head at the sites of capsular attachments, formed through the process of intramembranous ossification, and surface, central osteophytes, occasionally referred to as "surface bumps" because they produce a lumpy and irregular contour to the femoral head, which develop at low-pressure areas at the perimeter of the pressure zones, formed by the process of endochondral bone formation. Similar hypertrophic changes occur on the inferior–posterior wall of the acetabulum. Osteophytes do not develop in the weight-bearing areas because these segments are subjected to constant mechanical abrasions.

Degenerative "cysts" are one of the imaging hallmarks of osteoarthritis, although only some of these structures on histopathologic examination exhibit character of a true cystic lesion. More often, these are solid foci of fibrous or cartilaginous metaplasia; therefore, the term pseudocysts, cystlike lesions, or geodes is probably more accurate. They are usually small, circular, or piriform in shape and confined to subarticular area of sclerotic bone within the segment of high pressure. Larger lesion may also develop deeper in the femoral head and acetabulum. In some cases, a communication channel from the neck of the lesion into the joint cavity can be identified (see Fig. 1.25B).

Postel Coxarthropathy

Occasionally, the degenerative process in the hip may run a more rapid course. In a matter of weeks, a traditionally

(Continued on page 152)

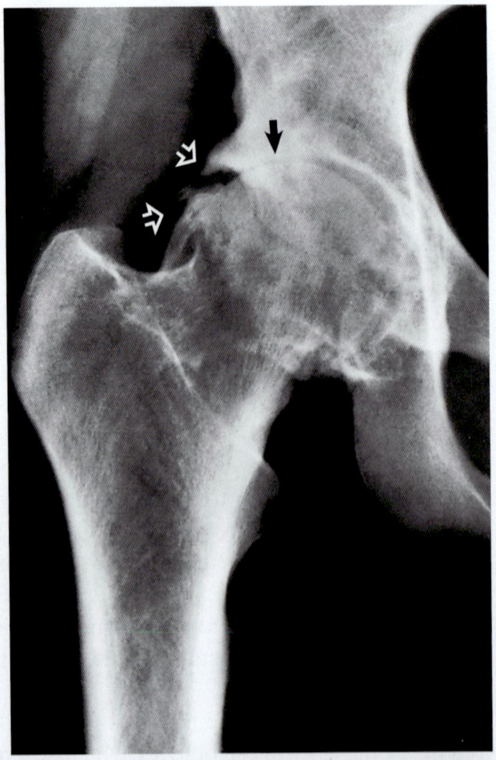

A

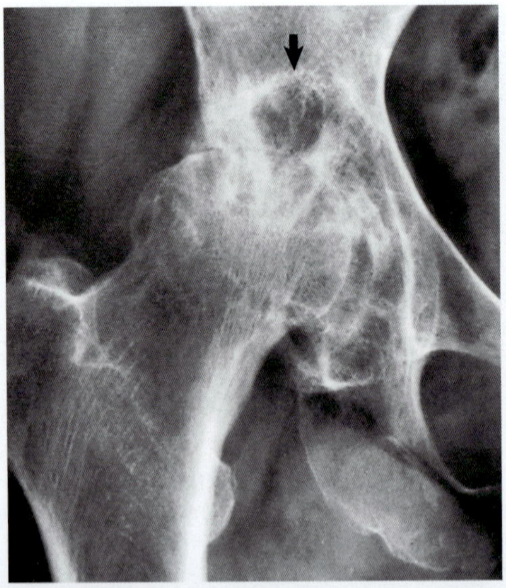

B

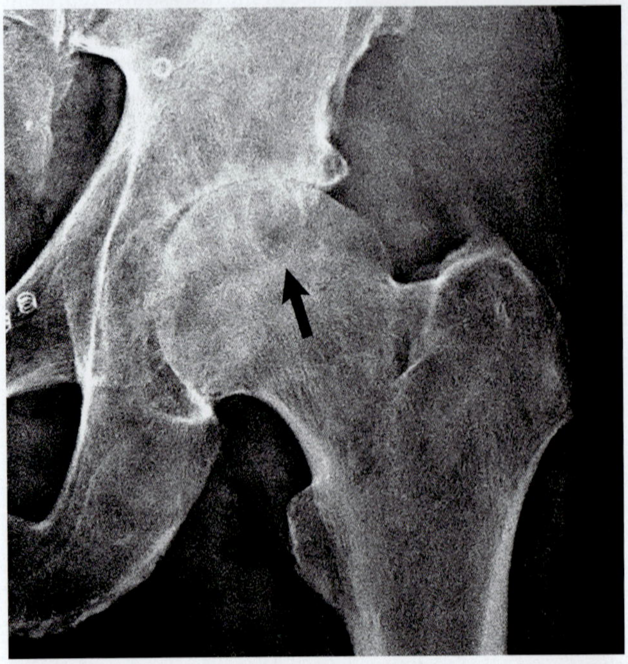

C

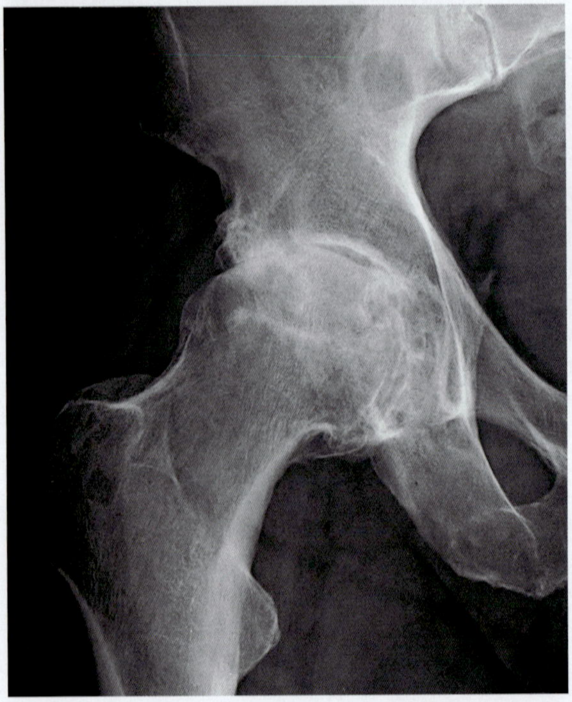

D

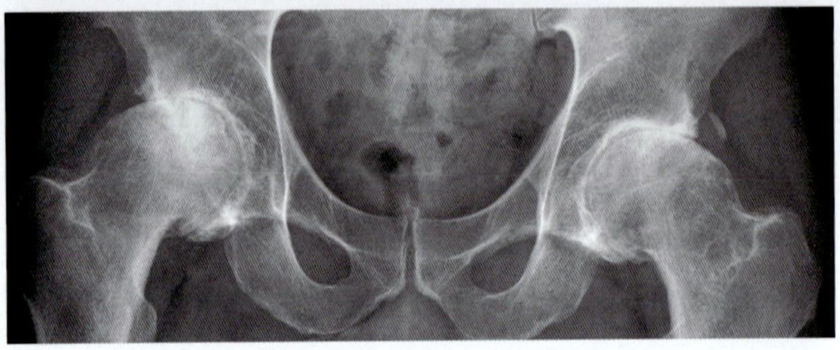

E

Figure 5.5 ■ **Osteoarthritis of the hip joint. A:** A 51-year-old woman presented with a history of right hip pain for the past 10 years and no previous history suggesting predisposing factors for osteoarthritis. Anteroposterior radiograph of the hip demonstrates the radiographic hallmarks of osteoarthritis: narrowing of the joint space, particularly at the weight-bearing segment (*arrow*), formation of marginal osteophytes (*open arrows*), and subchondral sclerosis. Note the lack of osteoporosis. **B:** In another patient, a 65-year-old woman, observe in addition to joint space narrowing, subchondral sclerosis, and osteophytosis, formation of a typical Egger cyst in the acetabulum (*arrow*). **C:** Anteroposterior radiograph of the left hip of a 76-year-old man shows narrowing of the joint space mainly at the weigh-bearing segment, subchondral sclerosis, and geode within the femoral head (*arrow*). **D:** Conventional radiograph of the right hip joint of a 63-year-old woman with a long history of osteoarthritis demonstrates the classic features of this condition: joint space narrowing, subchondral sclerosis, and osteophytosis. **E:** Anteroposterior radiograph shows advanced osteoarthritis of both hip joints in this 70-year-old man.

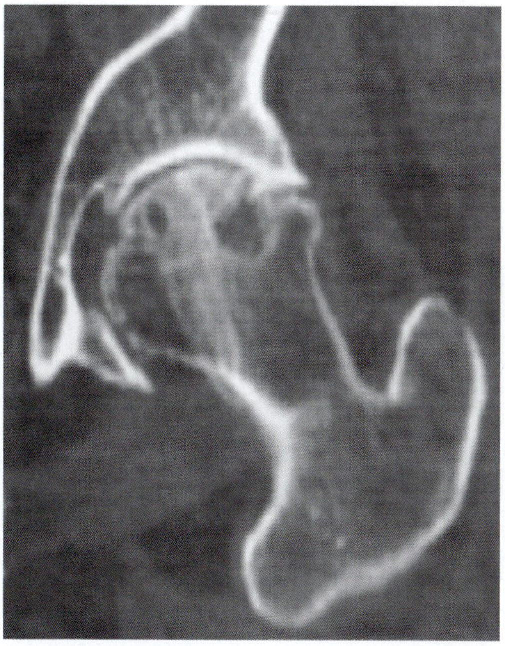

A

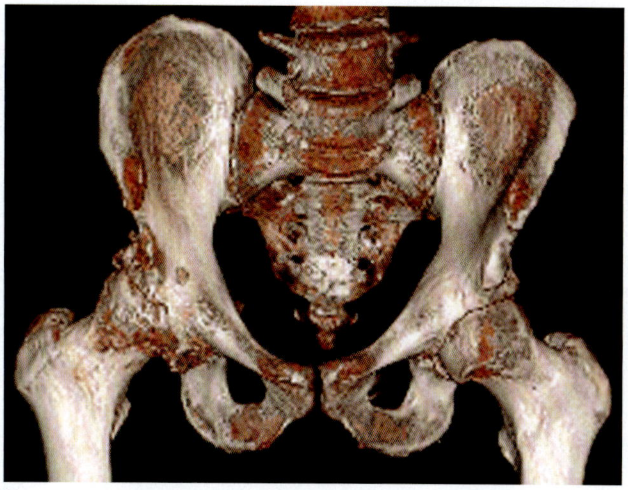

B

Figure 5.6 ■ **CT of osteoarthritis of the hip joint. A:** Coronal reformatted image shows diminution of the joint space, osteophytes, and subchondral cysts in the femoral head. **B:** In another patient, a 69-year-old man, 3D-reconstructed CT image of the pelvis shows advanced osteoarthritis of the right hip joint and moderate OA of the left hip joint.

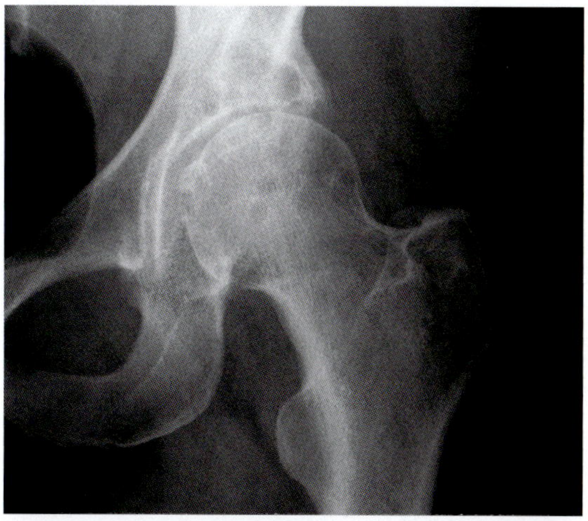

A

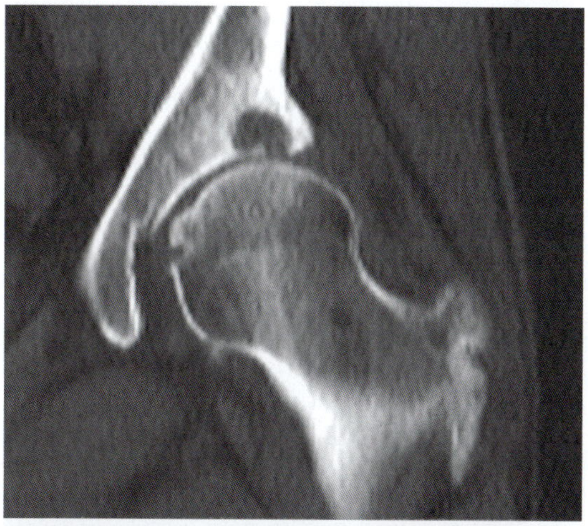

B

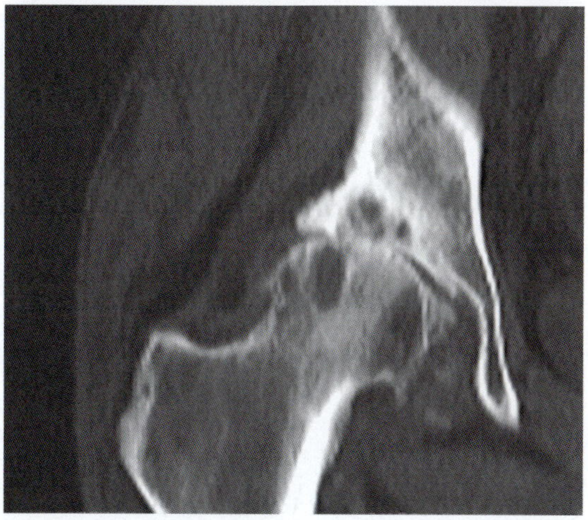

C

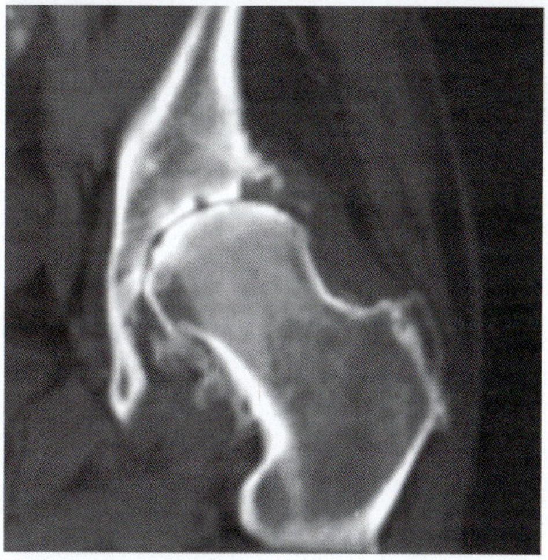

D

Figure 5.7 ■ **CT of osteoarthritis of the hip joint. A:** Anteroposterior radiograph of the left hip of a 66-year-old woman shows narrowing of the joint space, subchondral sclerosis, and cystic-like lesion in the acetabulum, better demonstrated on the coronal reformatted CT image **(B)**. In another patient, a 71-year-old woman, coronal reformatted CT image of the right hip joint **(C)** shows geodes in the femoral head and acetabulum. **D:** Coronal reformatted CT image of the left hip joint of a 55-year-old woman shows narrowing of the joint space, subchondral sclerosis, and osteophytosis.

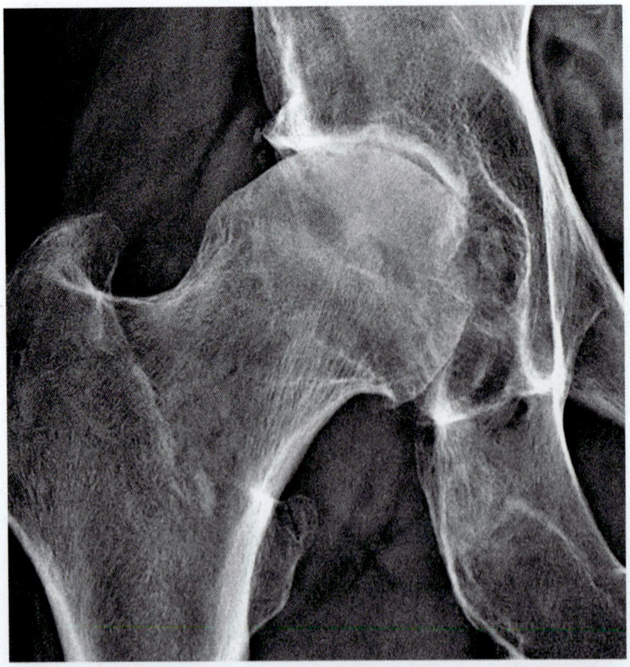

A

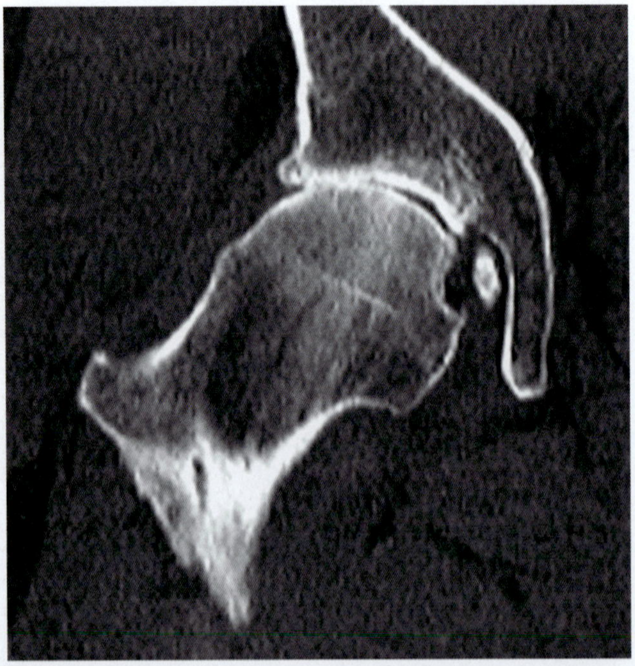

B

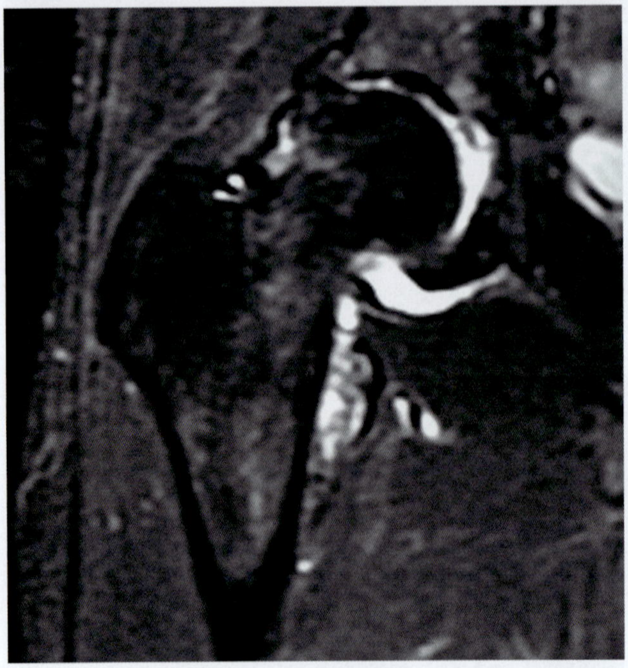

C

Figure 5.8 ■ CT and MRI of osteoarthritis of the hip joint. A 57-year-old man presented with history of pain in the right groin and "locking" and "clicking" in the hip joint. **A:** Conventional radiograph shows advanced osteoarthritis of the hip joint. There is suggestion of an osteochondral body in the medial joint compartment, better demonstrated on the coronal reformatted CT image **(B)**. **C:** Coronal T2-weighted fat-suppressed MR image shows in addition a large joint effusion.

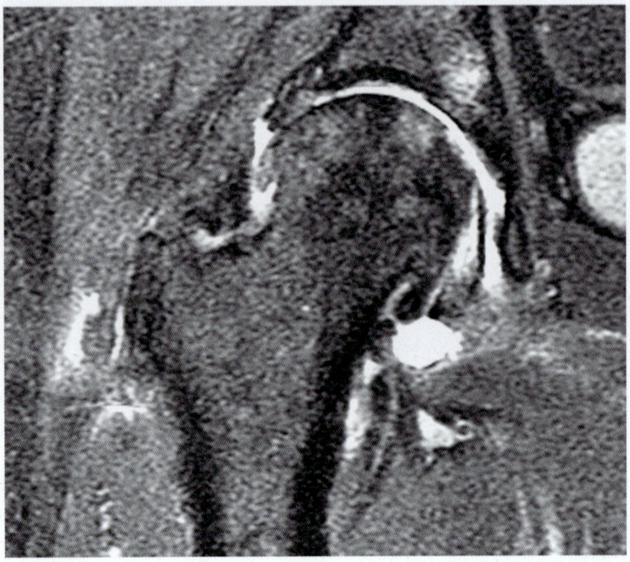

Figure 5.9 ■ MRI of osteoarthritis of the hip. Coronal proton density-weighted fat-suppressed MR image of the right hip of a 68-year-old woman shows joint space narrowing, subchondral sclerosis and bone marrow edema, osteophytes arising from the femoral head and acetabulum, and joint effusion.

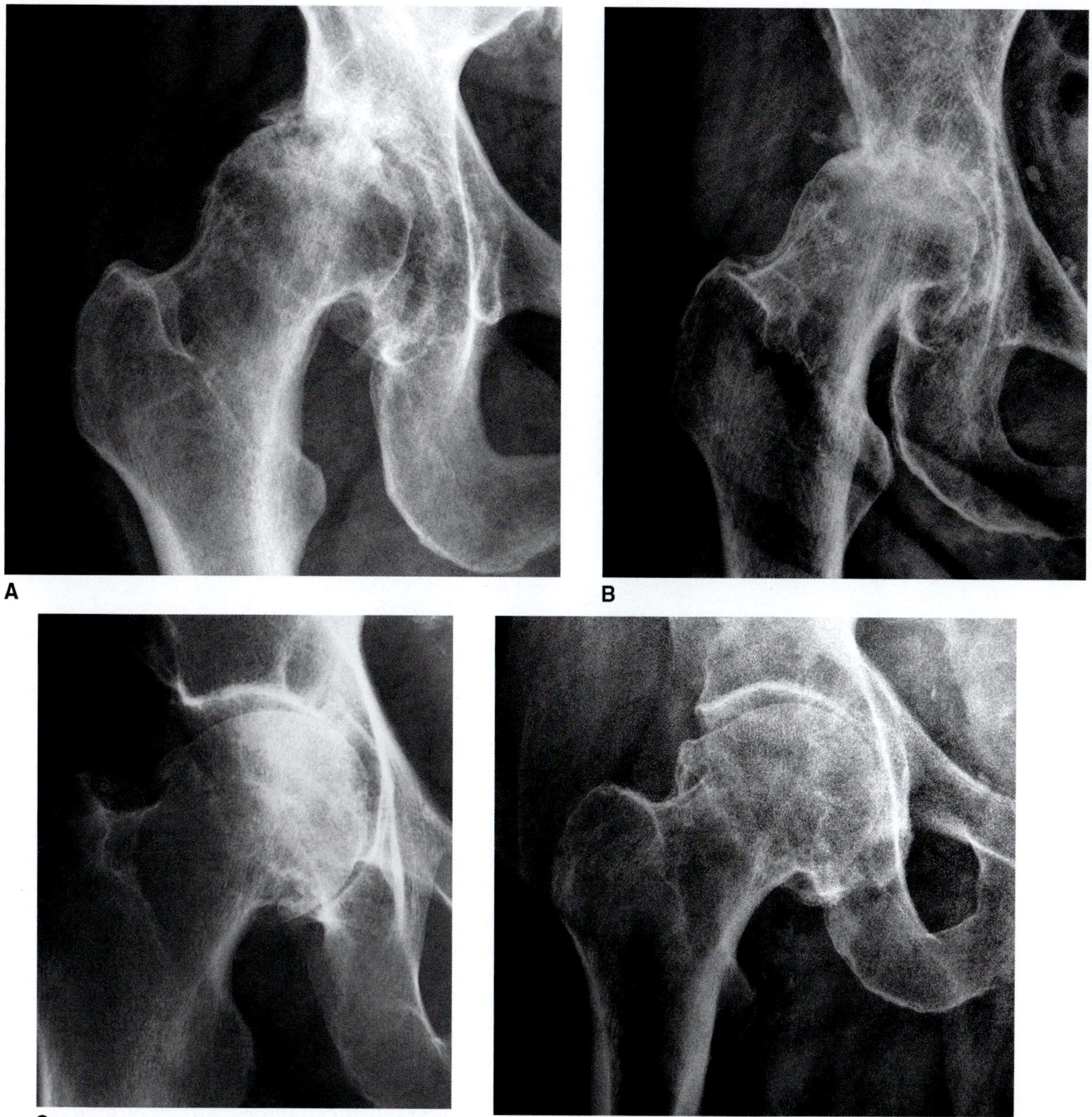

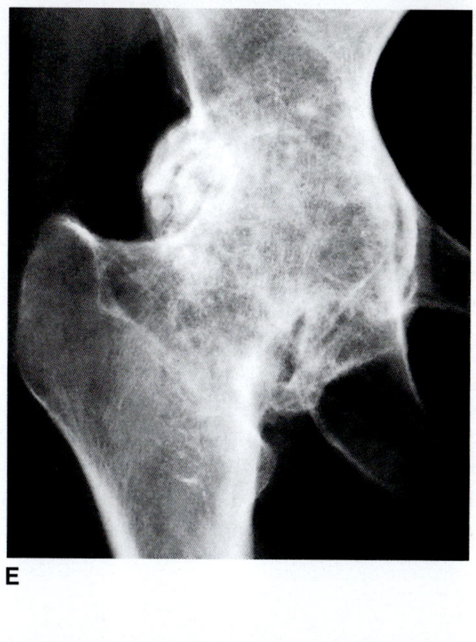

Figure 5.10 ■ Migration of the femoral head.
A: Superolateral migration of the femoral head is present in this 59-year-old woman with advanced osteoarthritis of the right hip joint. **B:** Another example of superolateral migration of the femoral head in an 80-year-old man. **C:** Medial migration of the femoral head is apparent in this 48-year-old woman with osteoarthritis of the right hip. **D:** Another example of medial migration of the femoral head in a 70-year-old man. **E:** Axial migration of the femoral head is evident in this 57-year-old woman who was suspected of having inflammatory arthritis. Clinical and laboratory investigations, however, led to a diagnosis of idiopathic osteoarthritis, which was confirmed on histopathologic examination after total hip replacement.

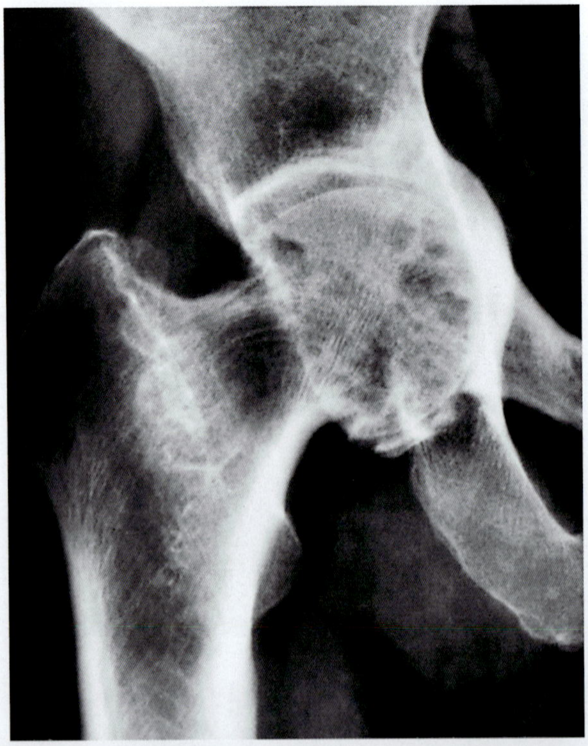

Figure 5.11 ■ Rheumatoid arthritis with superimposed secondary osteoarthritis. Anteroposterior radiograph of the right hip of a 42-year-old woman with a known history of long-standing rheumatoid arthritis shows the typical changes of inflammatory arthritis, including axial migration of the femoral head and acetabular protrusio. Superimposition of secondary osteoarthritis is evident in subchondral sclerosis and formation of marginal osteophytes.

slowly progressive osteoarthritis of the hip is converted into the rapidly progressive, aggressively destructive disease that completely destroys the hip joint. In some of the patients, the major portion of the femoral head may completely disappear. The acetabulum became concentrically enlarged. The pain in the hip is typically disabling and unrelenting. This destructive arthrosis of the hip joint is known as *Postel coxarthropathy*, a condition characterized by rapid chondrolysis that may quickly lead to complete destruction of the hip joint. Originally described by Lequesne, and also by Postel and Kerboull in 1970, this unique hip disorder occurs predominantly in women, with age of onset at 60 to 70 years. In all cases, a rapid clinical course of hip pain is the consistent common symptom. The histologic findings are those of conventional osteoarthritis with severe degenerative changes in the articular cartilage. However, osteophyte formation is absent or minimal. Hypervascularity in the subchondral bone is a common finding. The bone trabeculae are either abnormally thickened or abnormally thinned. Occasionally, one can observe foci of fibrosis, interstitial edema and hemorrhage in the marrow spaces, focal marrow fat fibrosis, and focal areas of bone resorption. The precise pathogenesis of this condition remains unclear, although direct drug toxicity and the analgesic effects of nonsteroidal anti-inflammatory drugs have been implicated. Some investigators have suggested that intra-articular deposition of hydroxyapatite crystals might lead to joint destruction. Others have proposed subchondral bone ischemia, cell necrosis, and insufficiency fracture of the femoral head as a cause of this arthritis. Some investigators demonstrated elevated levels of interleukin-6 (IL-6) and interleukin-1 beta (IL-1β) in the joint fluid as well as elevated secretion of matrix metalloproteinases by fibroblasts from the synovium and subchondral cysts. Because of the rapidity of the process, the radiographic presentation of this condition is marked by very little, if any, reparative changes, mimicking infectious or neuropathic arthritis (Charcot joint) (Figs. 5.12 to 5.14). More recently, Boutry and colleagues reported magnetic resonance imaging (MRI) findings of this form of osteoarthritis. These included joint effusion, a bone marrow edema-like pattern in the femoral head, neck, and acetabulum; femoral head flattening; and cystlike subchondral defects (Fig. 5.15).

Secondary Osteoarthritis

Secondary OA is often seen in the hip joint in patients with predisposing conditions such as previous trauma (Figs. 5.16 and 5.17), slipped capital femoral epiphysis (Fig. 5.18), congenital hip dysplasia/dislocation (Fig. 5.19), osteonecrosis (Fig. 5.20), Paget disease (Fig. 5.21), infectious arthritis (Fig. 5.22), inflammatory arthritides (Figs. 5.23 and 5.24), and femoroacetabular impingement (FAI) syndrome (see text and figures in the next paragraph). The radiographic findings are the same as those described for primary osteoarthritis, but the features of the underlying process also can often be detected. Although the standard radiographic views are usually sufficient for demonstrating these changes, CT, arthrography, or MRI may at times be needed for a more accurate assessment of the status of the articular cartilage.

Femoroacetabular Impingement Syndrome

FAI results from incongruity of the femoral head and acetabulum and is one of the leading causes of precocious osteoarthritis of the hip joint. Two types of FAI have been described based on the predominance of anatomic abnormalities affecting either femoral head or acetabulum. In *cam type*, the nonspherical shape of the femoral head secondary to excessive bone formation at the junction of head and neck results in abutment against the acetabular rim. In *pincer type*, because of deep acetabulum (coxa profunda), acetabular protrusio, or acetabular retroversion, acetabular "overcoverage" of the femoral head limits the range of motion in the hip joint and leads to abnormal stresses on acetabular rim. In both types of FAI, the abnormal mechanism results in damage of the acetabular labrum, thus promoting secondary osteoarthritis. The diagnosis of FAI is based on (a) the patient's clinical history of chronic pain; (b) physical examination revealing reduced range of motion in the hip

(Continued on page 154)

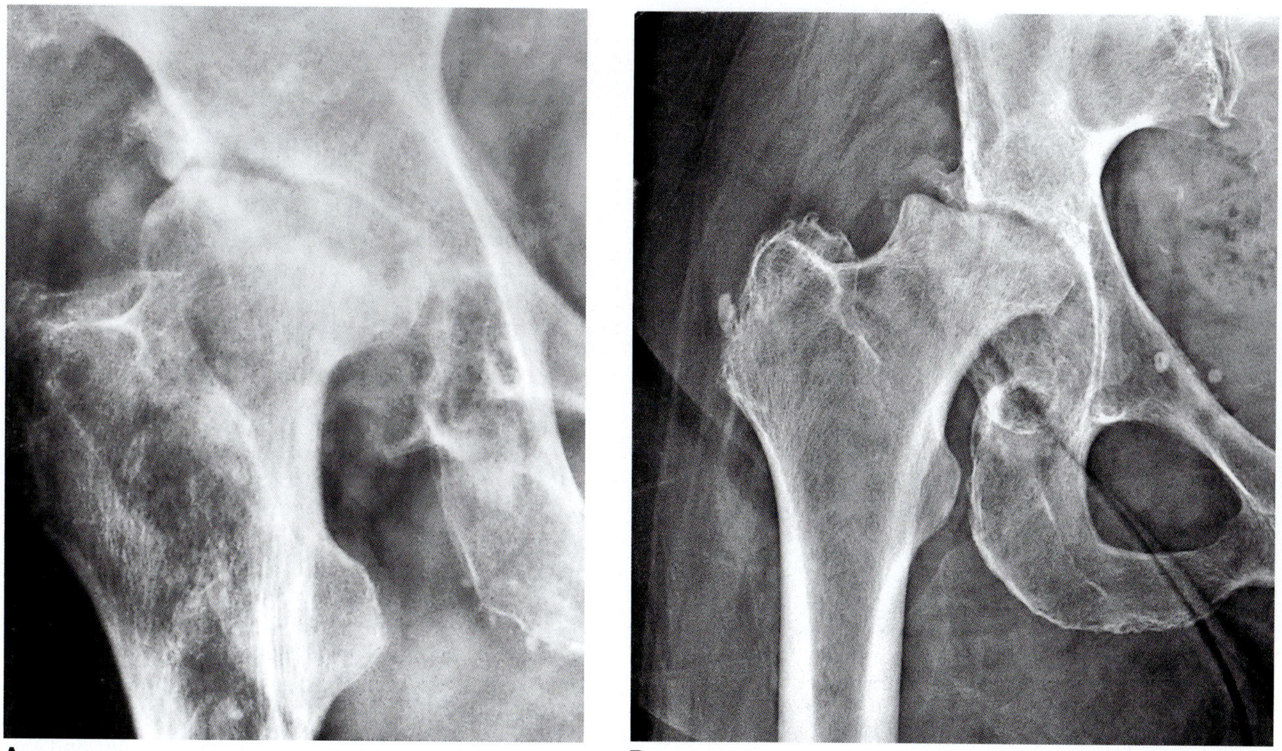

A B

Figure 5.12 ■ **Postel coxarthropathy. A:** Anteroposterior radiograph of the right hip of a 72-year-old man who had pain in the hip for 4 months shows the typical appearance of this arthrosis, which often mimics Charcot joint or infectious arthritis. Note the destruction of the articular portion of the femoral head, which is flattened and laterally subluxed. There is eccentric depression of the lateral articular surface. The same destructive process has led to widening of the acetabulum. **B:** Similar deformity of the right hip joint is seen in this 69-year-old woman. Note relative absence of osteophytes.

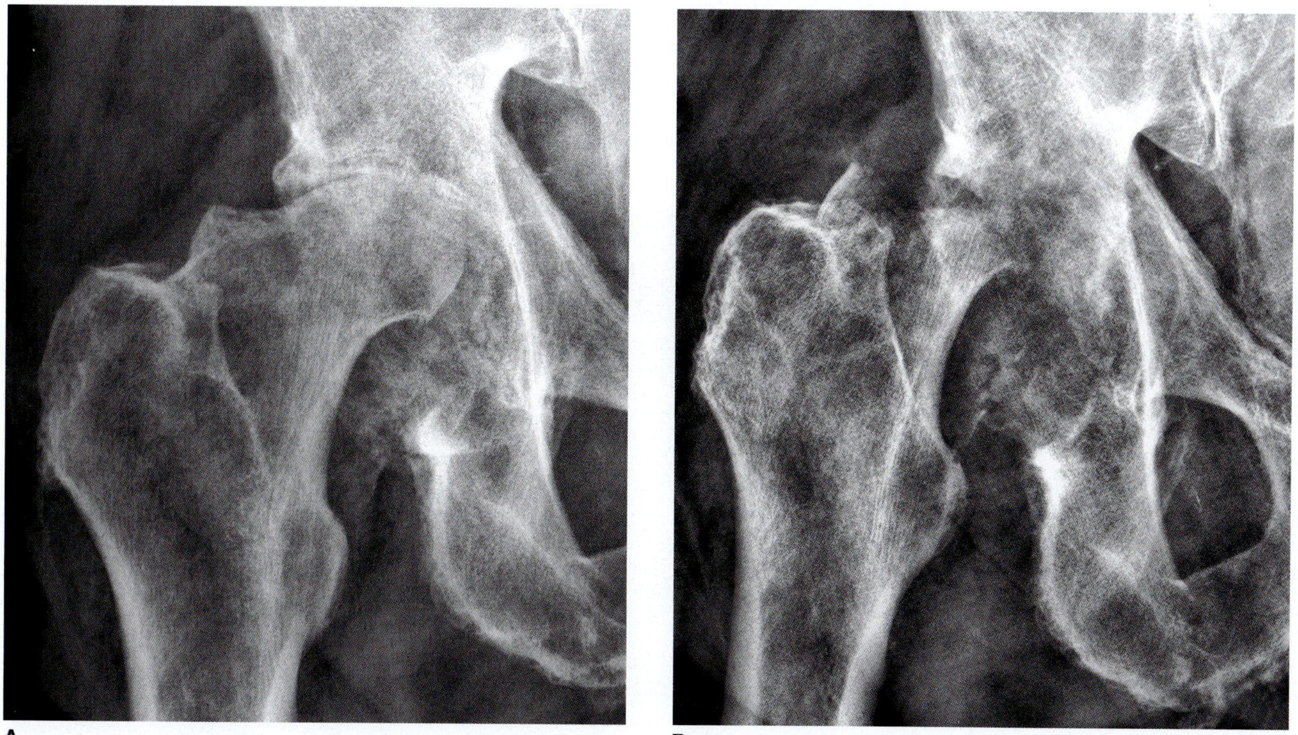

A B

Figure 5.13 ■ **Postel coxarthropathy. A:** Osteoarthritis of the right hip joint in this 61-year-old woman markedly progressed in a very short time as seen on the radiograph obtained 5 months later **(B)**.

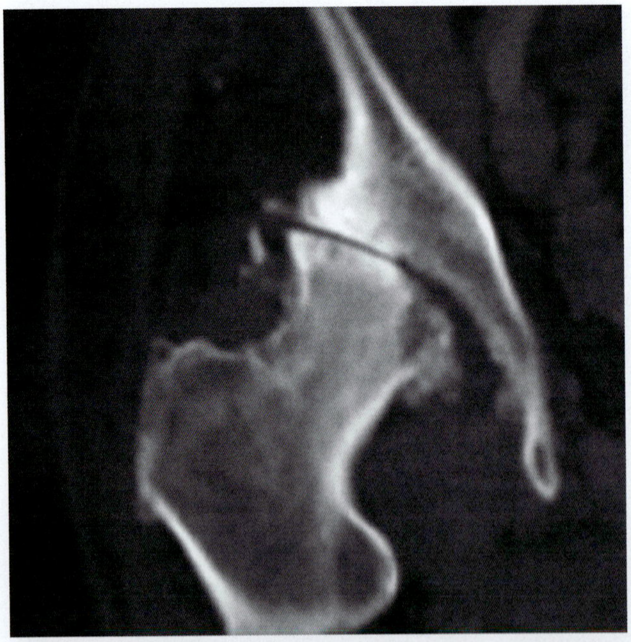

Figure 5.14 ■ CT of Postel coxarthropathy. Coronal reformatted CT image of the right hip shows characteristic features of this destructive arthritis: marked deformity of the femoral head with flattening of the subchondral segment assuming hatchet-like appearance, widening of the acetabulum, and relatively only mild reactive changes.

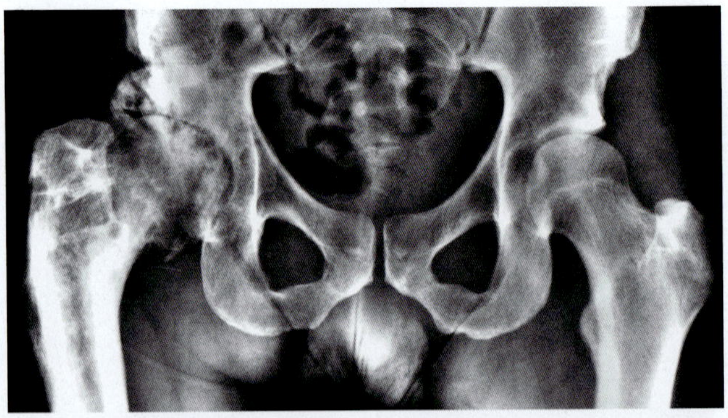

Figure 5.16 ■ Posttraumatic osteoarthritis. Anteroposterior radiograph of the pelvis of a 40-year-old man, who 7 years prior to this examination sustained a complex fracture of the right proximal femur and acetabulum, shows a deformity of the femoral head and neck associated with narrowing of the hip joint space, subchondral sclerosis, and osteophyte formation. Note the completely normal left hip joint.

joint, particularly flexion and internal rotation; and (c) imaging findings on conventional radiography, CT, and MRI. In cam type, conventional radiography demonstrates excessive bone formation at the femoral head/neck junction with loss of normal anatomic "waist" at this site (Fig. 5.25A), occasionally resembling the smooth hand grip of some pistols ("pistol grip deformity" or a "cam effect") (Fig. 5.25B); an os acetabulum, which more likely represents an osseous metaplasia of the cartilaginous labrum or a fragment of damaged acetabular rim; and a radiolucent lesion at the head/neck junction, formerly called *synovial herniation pit*, and now designated as fibroosseous lesion. CT shows these abnormalities even better (Fig. 5.26). MR arthrography (MRa), particularly the radial reformatted images, in addition to the findings listed previously, clearly demonstrates abnormalities of the fibrocartilaginous labrum at the anterosuperior portion of the acetabulum (Fig. 5.27; see also Fig. 2.91). In pincer type, particularly in case of acetabular retroversion, conventional radiograph shows "crossover" sign, when more lateral projection of anterior acetabulum, which normally should project medially to the posterior acetabulum, "crosses" the

(Continued on page 158)

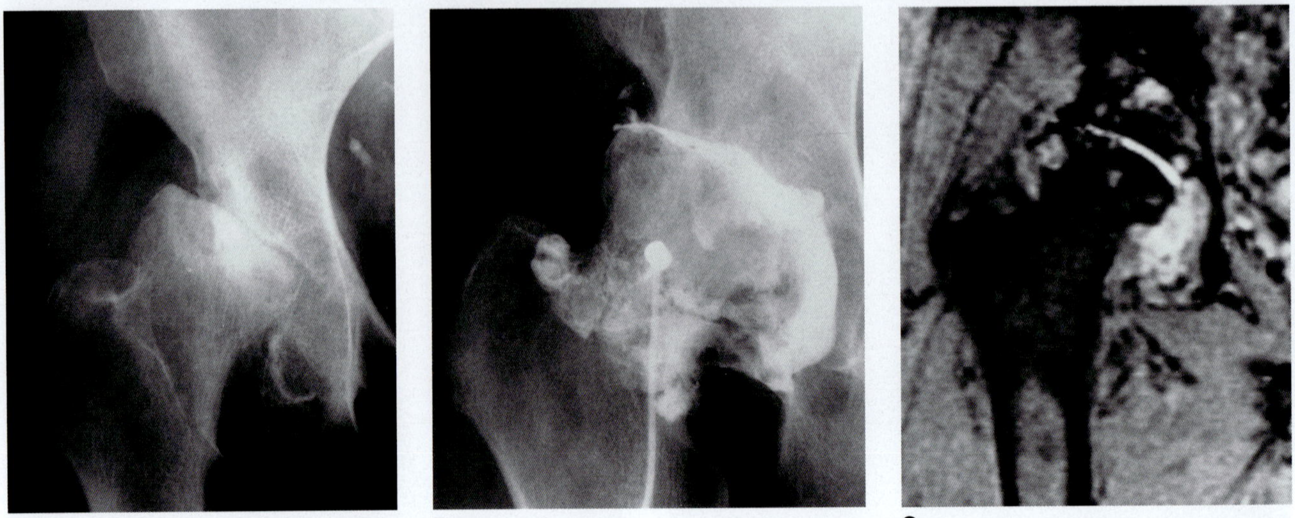

A B C

Figure 5.15 ■ Arthrography and MRI of Postel coxarthropathy. A: Anteroposterior radiograph of the right hip of a 44-year-old man shows destructive changes of the femoral head and acetabulum. **B:** Aspiration arthrogram, which was performed to rule out infection, shows hypertrophic synovitis. **C:** Gradient echo T2*-weighted MRI shows joint effusion, hypertrophied synovium, and subchondral cysts in the acetabulum and femoral head.

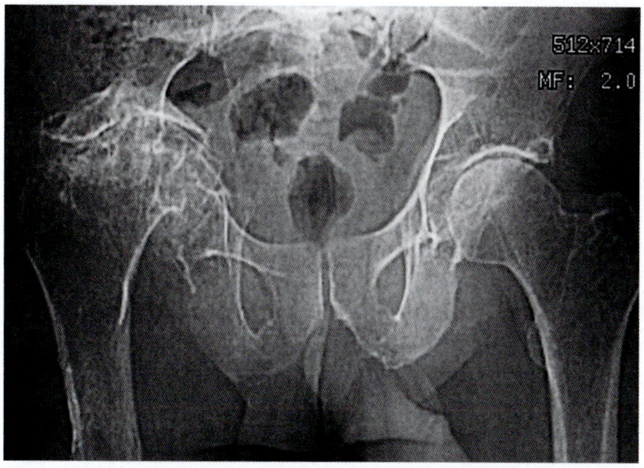

A

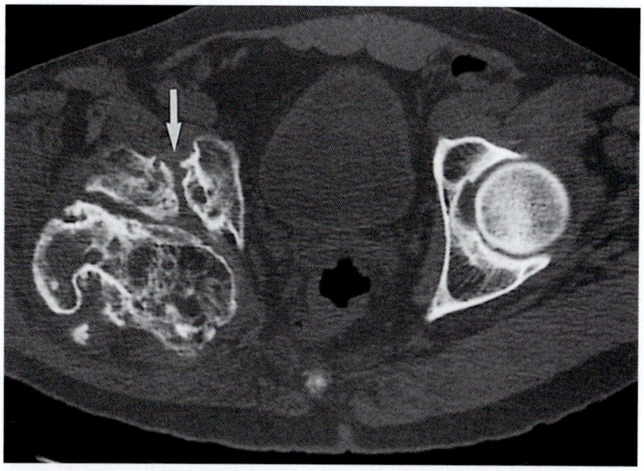

B

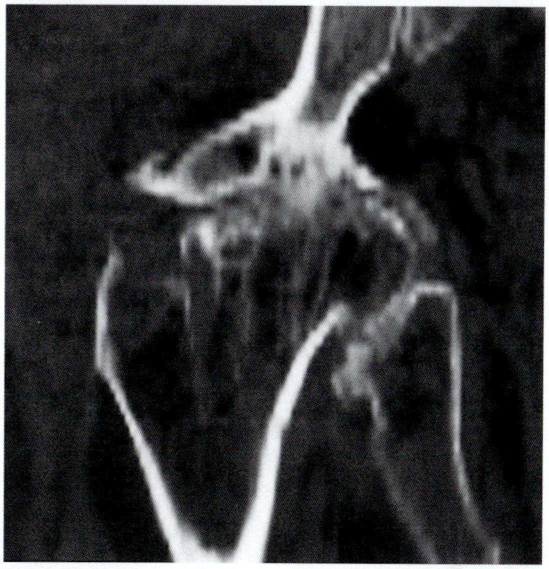

C

Figure 5.17 ■ **CT of posttraumatic osteoarthritis.** A 64-year-old man, who in the past sustained complex right acetabular and femoral fractures, developed secondary osteoarthritis. **A:** Preliminary scout CT image shows posttraumatic deformity of the acetabulum and femoral head associated with acetabular protrusio. **B:** Axial CT section through both hips shows osteoarthritic changes of the right femoral head and ununited fracture of the anterior column (*arrow*). **C:** Coronal reformatted image demonstrates significant narrowing of the joint space, deformity of the femoral head, and periarticular sclerosis. All CT features are consistent with posttraumatic osteoarthritis.

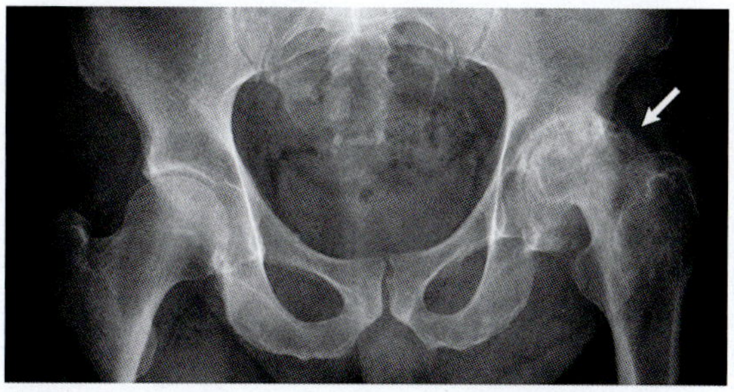

A

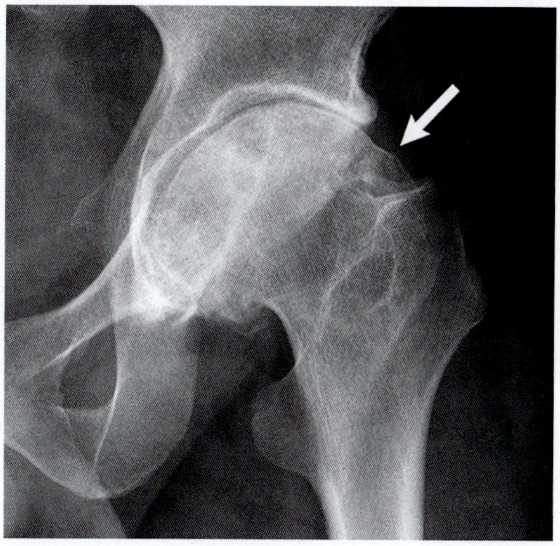

B

Figure 5.18 ■ **Secondary osteoarthritis because of slipped capital femoral epiphysis (SCFE).** **A:** Anteroposterior radiograph of the pelvis of a 40-year-old man with history of SCFE shows osteoarthritic changes of the left hip joint. Note osseous remodeling at the junction of the femoral head and neck, a hallmark of this condition, known as a Herndon hump (*arrow*). **B:** In another patient, a 24-year-old woman with OA of the left hip joint, observe a characteristic Herndon hump (*arrow*) pointing to SCFE as the underlying cause of arthritis.

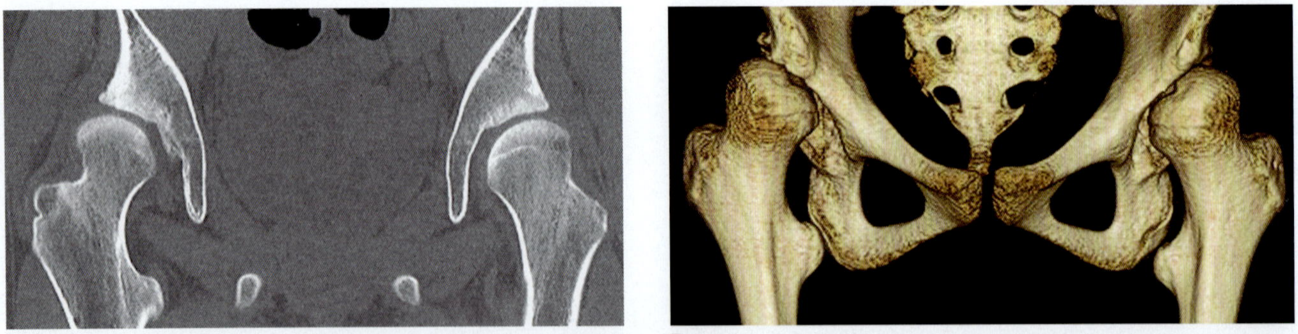

A B

Figure 5.19 ■ Secondary osteoarthritis because of developmental dysplasia of the hips (DDH). Coronal reformatted **(A)** and 3D reconstructed with surface-rendering algorithm **(B)** CT images of the hips of a 30-year-old woman with history of bilateral congenital hip dislocation show dysplastic changes of both hip joints. There is evidence of secondary osteoarthritis manifested by narrowing of the joint spaces, subchondral sclerosis at the site of femoral heads and acetabula, and formation of small marginal osteophytes at the periphery of both acetabula.

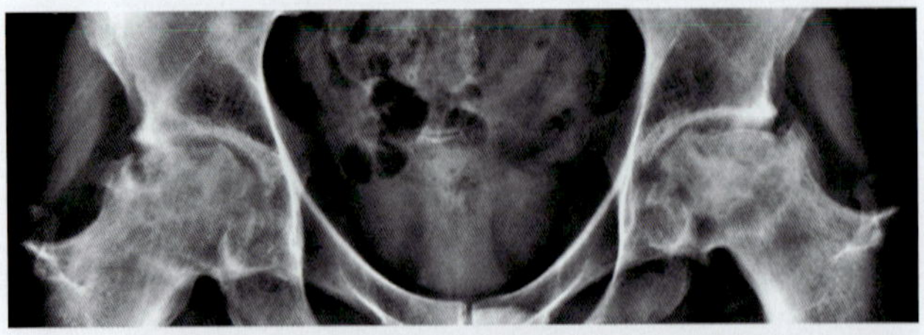

Figure 5.20 ■ Secondary osteoarthritis because of osteonecrosis. A 48-year-old man, a chronic alcoholic, developed osteonecrosis of both femoral heads, marked by increased bone density and subchondral collapse. Secondary osteoarthritis is distinguished by narrowing of the joint space, marginal osteophytosis, and subchondral cyst formation.

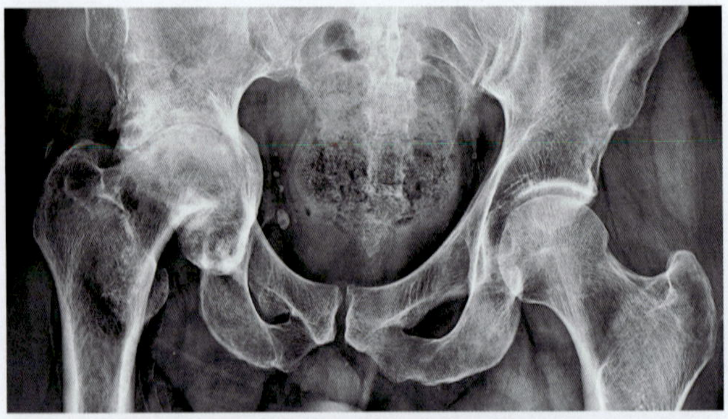

Figure 5.22 ■ Secondary osteoarthritis because of joint infection. Anteroposterior radiograph of the pelvis of a 49-year-old man with history of septic arthritis of the right hip joint and acetabular osteomyelitis shows deformity of the acetabulum, subchondral sclerosis, and significant narrowing of the joint space. Note unremarkable left hip joint.

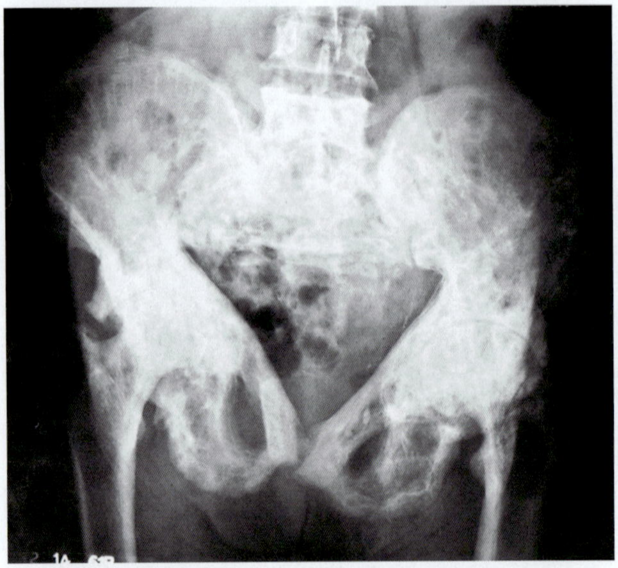

A

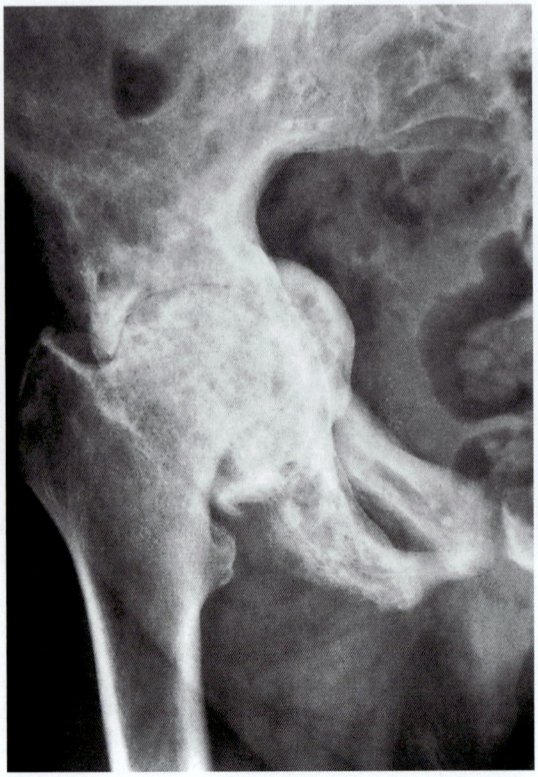

B

Figure 5.21 ■ Secondary osteoarthritis because of Paget disease. A: Radiograph of the pelvis of an 80-year-old woman shows cool phase of Paget disease affecting pelvic bones and both femora. Note advanced osteoarthritis of both hip joints with almost complete obliteration of the joint spaces. **B:** In another patient, a 75-year-old woman with long-standing polyostotic Paget disease, anteroposterior radiograph of the right hip demonstrates advanced osteoarthritis associated with acetabular protrusio.

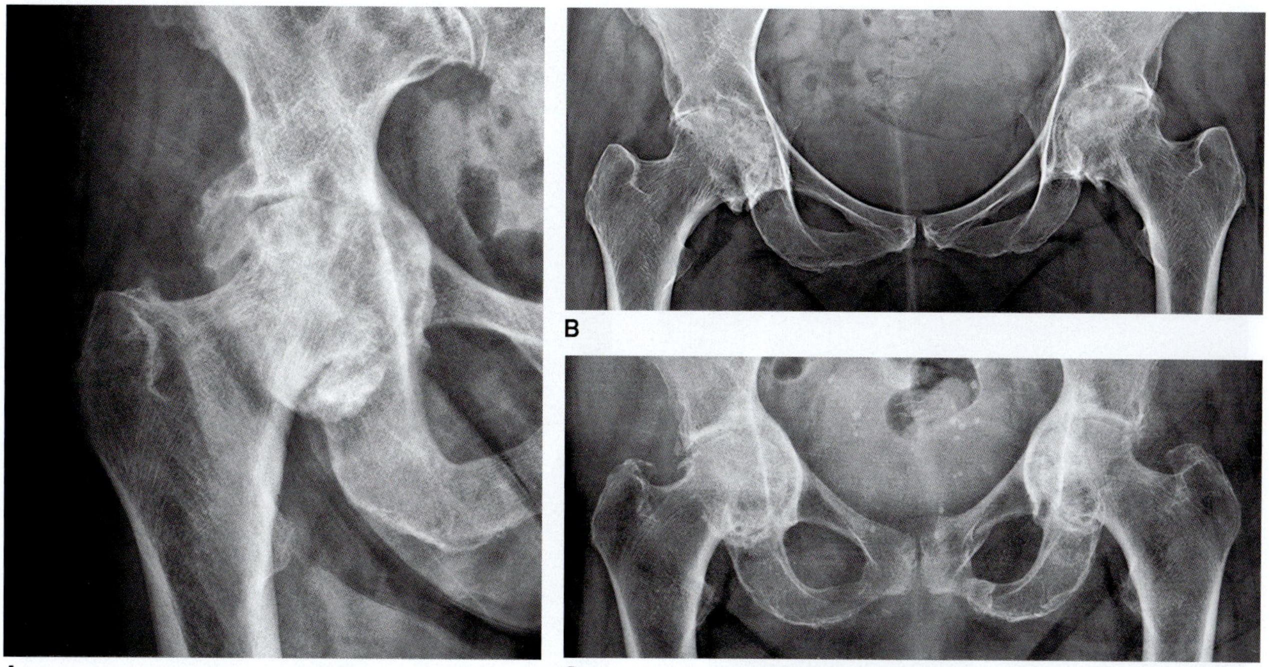

A B C

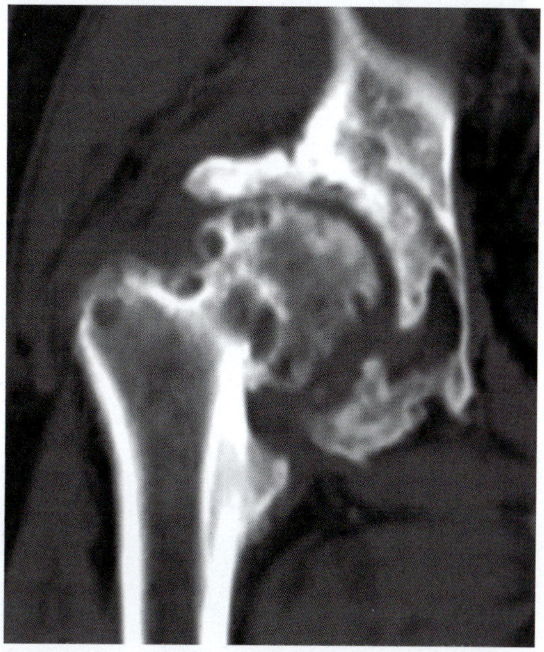

D

Figure 5.23 ■ **Secondary osteoarthritis because of inflammatory arthritis (RA). A:** Radiograph of the right hip of a 60-year-old woman shows concentric narrowing of the joint space and acetabular protrusio, features of inflammatory arthritis. Superimposed are features of osteoarthritis comprising sclerotic changes of the femoral head and acetabulum and osteophytosis. **B:** In another patient, a 38-year-old woman with bilateral hip rheumatoid arthritis, observe typical features of inflammatory arthritis and secondary osteoarthritic changes manifesting mainly by formation of prominent osteophytes. **C:** Similar example of secondary osteoarthritis superimposed on rheumatoid arthritis affecting both hip joints is seen in an 81-year-old woman. **D:** Coronal reformatted CT image of the right hip of a 40-year-old woman with rheumatoid arthritis shows subchondral and osseous erosions of the femoral head and acetabulum and superimposed secondary osteoarthritic changes in form of subchondral sclerosis of the acetabulum and osteophyte formation.

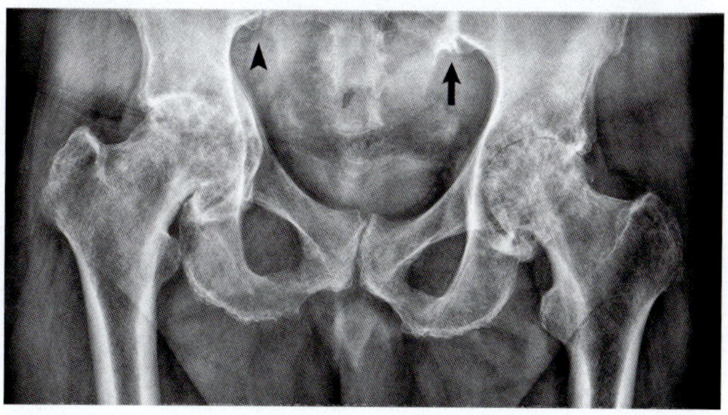

Figure 5.24 ■ **Secondary osteoarthritis because of inflammatory arthritis (psoriasis).** Radiograph of the pelvis of a 64-year-old man with clinically documented psoriasis shows characteristic for inflammatory arthritis concentric narrowing of the hip joints and axial migration of the femoral heads. In addition note the changes of superimposed secondary osteoarthritis marked by subchondral sclerosis, osteophytosis, and cyst formation in the left acetabulum and in the right femoral head. The patient also developed left-sided sacroiliitis (*arrow*). The *arrowhead* points to unaffected right sacroiliac joint.

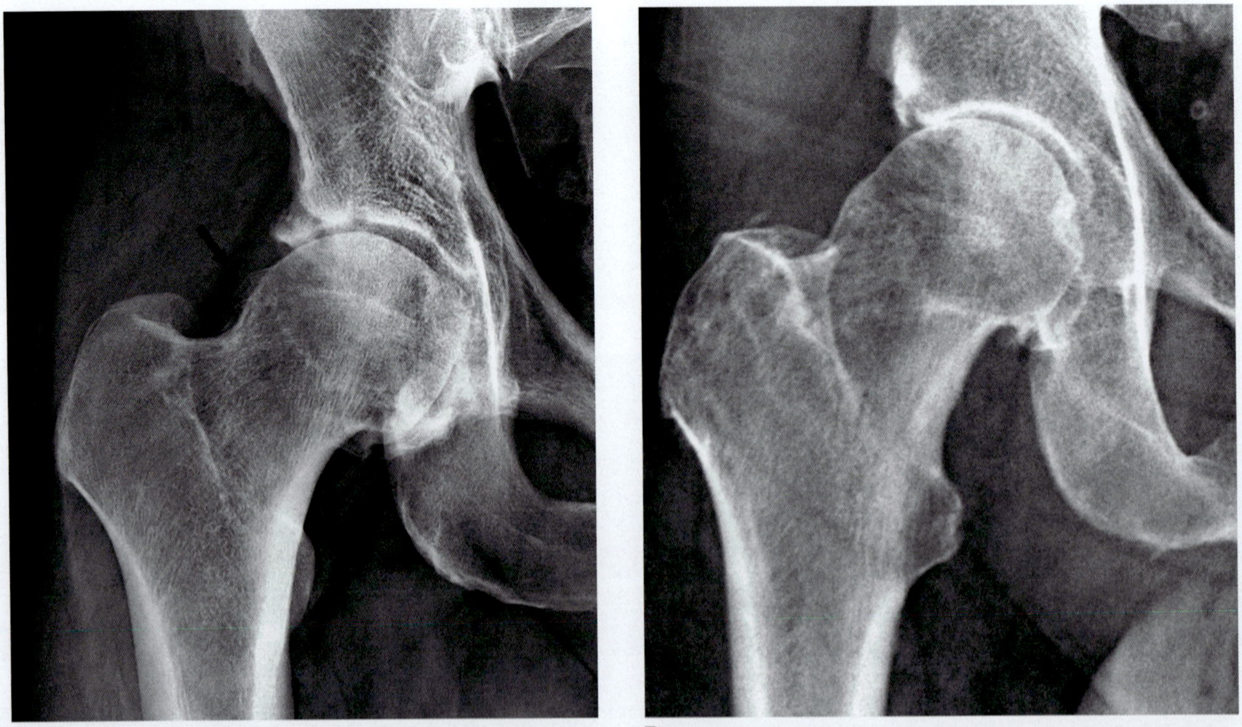

A B

Figure 5.25 ■ **Cam type of FAI. A:** Anteroposterior radiograph of the right hip of a 39-year-old woman shows excessive bone buildup at the femoral head/neck junction (*arrow*). Note secondary osteoarthritis of the hip joint. **B:** In another patient, a 41-year-old man, tubular appearance of the proximal right femur and the osseous prominence at the femoral head/neck junction assumed a "pistol grip" deformity. Also evident is osteoarthritis of the hip joint.

posterior acetabular outline (Fig. 5.28). MRI demonstrates acetabular version and depth of the femoral head coverage (Fig. 5.29). To determine the sphericity of the femoral head and the prominence of the anterior femoral head/neck junction, the alpha angle is calculated on the oblique axial CT or oblique axial MR images (Fig. 5.30). Radial reformatted MR images are of particular value in this respect because they allow optimal visualization of the anterosuperior region of the femoral head/neck junction, where the most significant changes in the alpha angle occur (see Fig. 5.27). The normal alpha angle should not exceed 50 degrees. The larger the alpha angle, the more pronounced is nonspherical shape of the femoral head, and the greater is predisposition for anterior FAI.

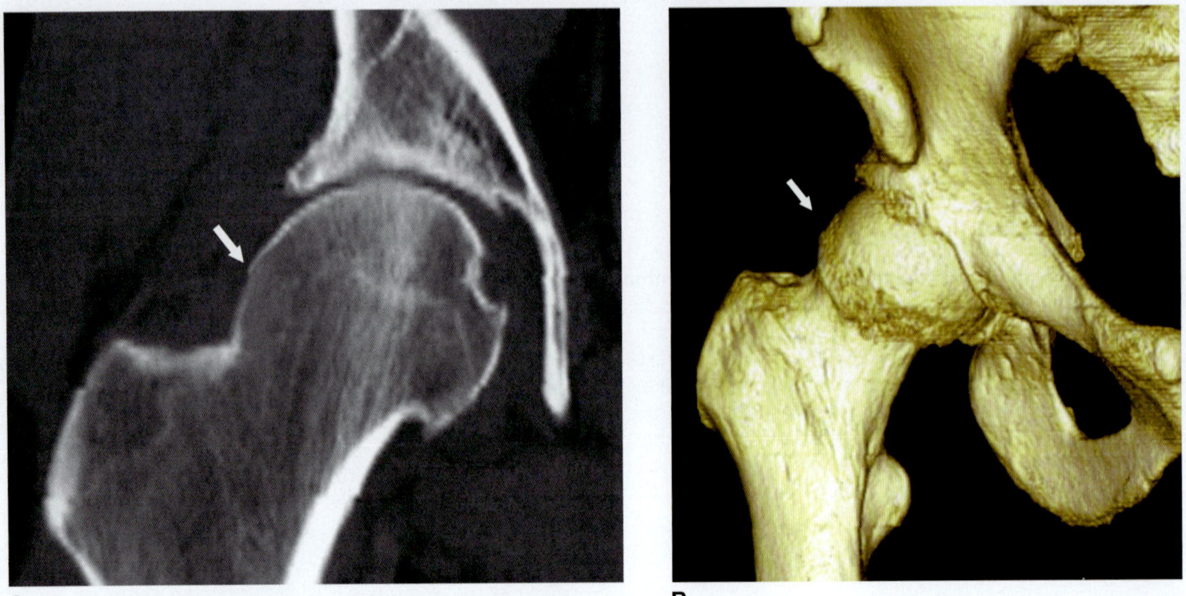

A B

Figure 5.26 ■ **CT of cam type FAI.** Coronal reformatted **(A)** and 3D-reconstructed **(B)** CT image in shaded surface display in a 34-year-old man show bone accretion at the femoral head/neck junction (*arrows*).

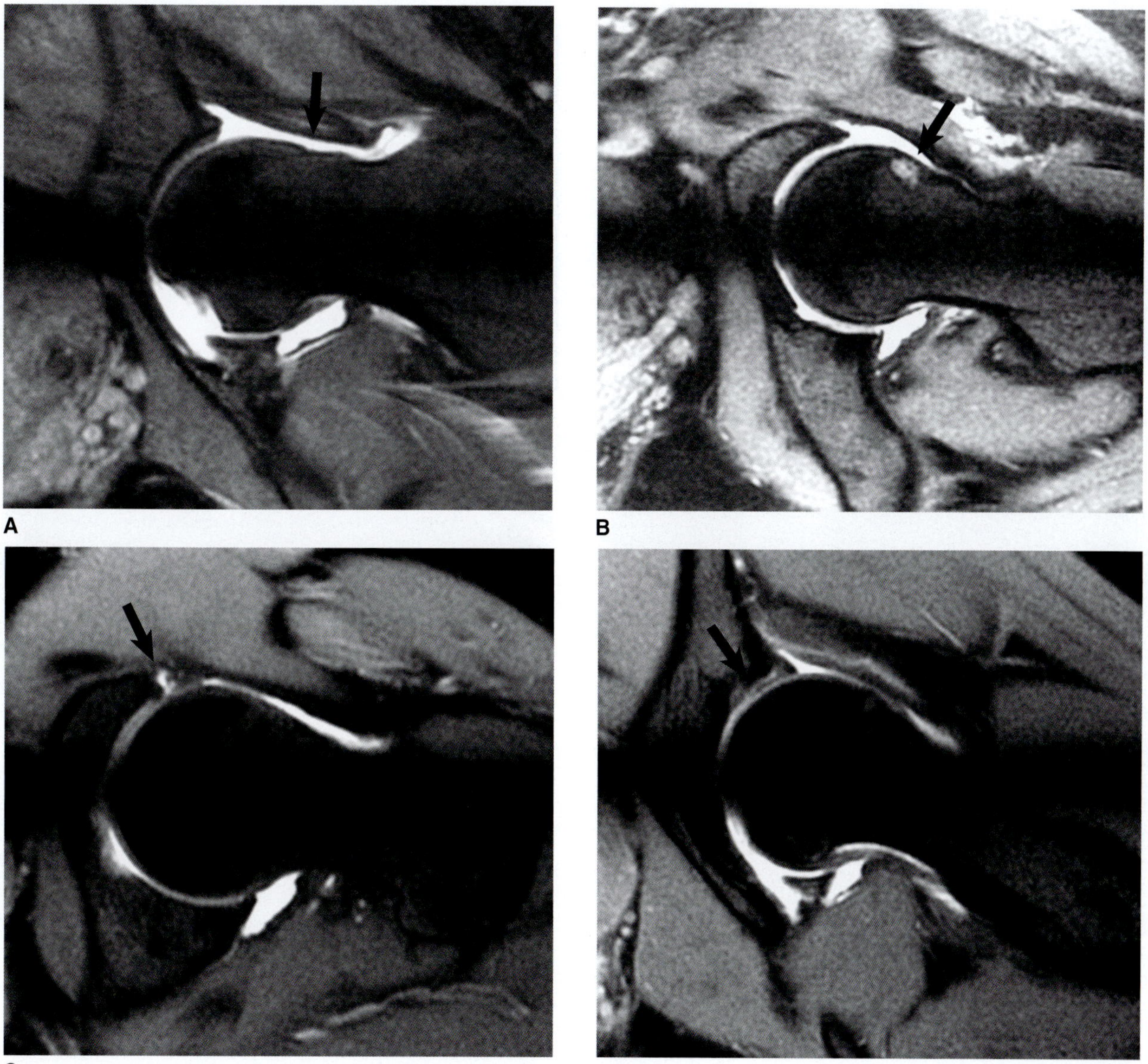

Figure 5.27 ■ **MR arthrography of cam type FAI.** Radial reconstructed MRa images of the hip joint show various characteristic features of this abnormality. **A:** In a 34-year-old woman—a decreased femoral head/neck offset associated with hypertrophic ossification (*arrow*). **B:** In a 32-year-old woman—a fibroosseous lesion at the anterosuperior aspect of the femoral head/neck junction (*arrow*). **C:** In a 38-year-old man—a tear of the superior anterior cartilaginous labrum (*arrow*). **D:** In a 30-year-old woman—a delamination injury to the acetabular labrum (*arrow*).

Treatment of FAI and OA of the Hip Joint

In very early stages of FAI, open or arthroscopic trimming of acetabular rim and/or femoral head may be attempted. In younger patients, labral and acetabular repair and/or osteoplasty with reshaping of femoral head/neck junction contributed to satisfactory results. Occasionally, intertrochanteric flexion–valgus osteotomy may also relieve the clinical symptoms. Periacetabular osteotomy is an effective way to reorient the acetabulum in young adults with symptomatic FAI because of acetabular retroversion. Advanced osteoarthritis, whether primary or secondary, is usually treated surgically by total hip arthroplasty using, among the various types available, either a cemented or a noncemented hip prosthesis. The reader is referred to Chapter 4 for more detailed discussion of management. Nevertheless, we strongly recommend the orthopedic surgeon guidance related to expected outcome and possible complications of treatment.

Osteoarthritis of the Knee

Clinical Features

The symptoms are similar to those experienced by the patients with hip osteoarthritis: swelling around the knee joint, crepitus and joint locking, restricted range of motion, short-lasting morning stiffness, and pain that increases with activity and is relieved by rest. Some patients may experience sleep-disrupting pain at night. As the arthritis is progressing,

(Continued on page 161)

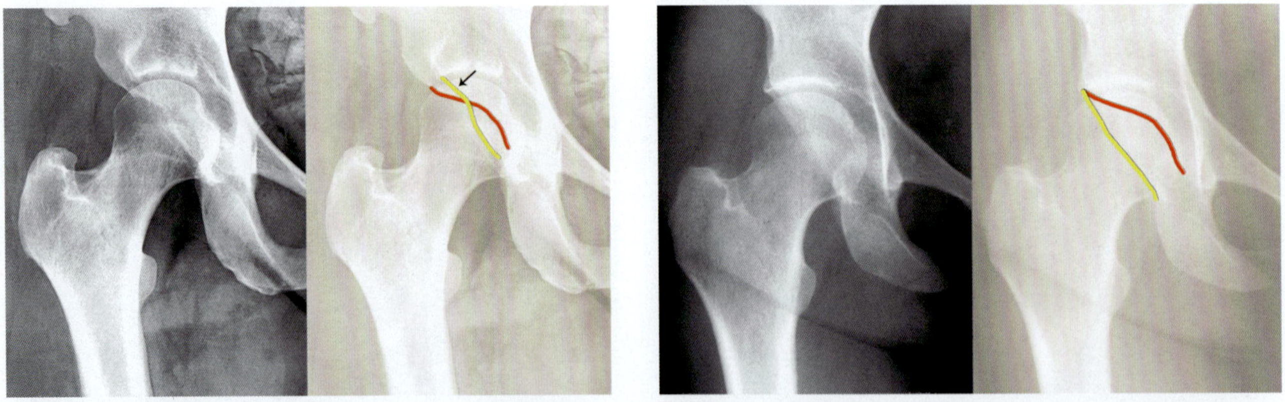

A B

Figure 5.28 ■ Pincer type FAI. A: Anteroposterior radiograph of the left hip in a 29-year-old woman shows a crossover sign. Note that the posterior acetabular rim outline (*yellow line*) projects medially (*arrow*) in relation to the anterior acetabular rim (*red line*), indicative of acetabular retroversion. **B:** In a normal hip joint, the posterior acetabular rim outline projects laterally to the anterior acetabular rim.

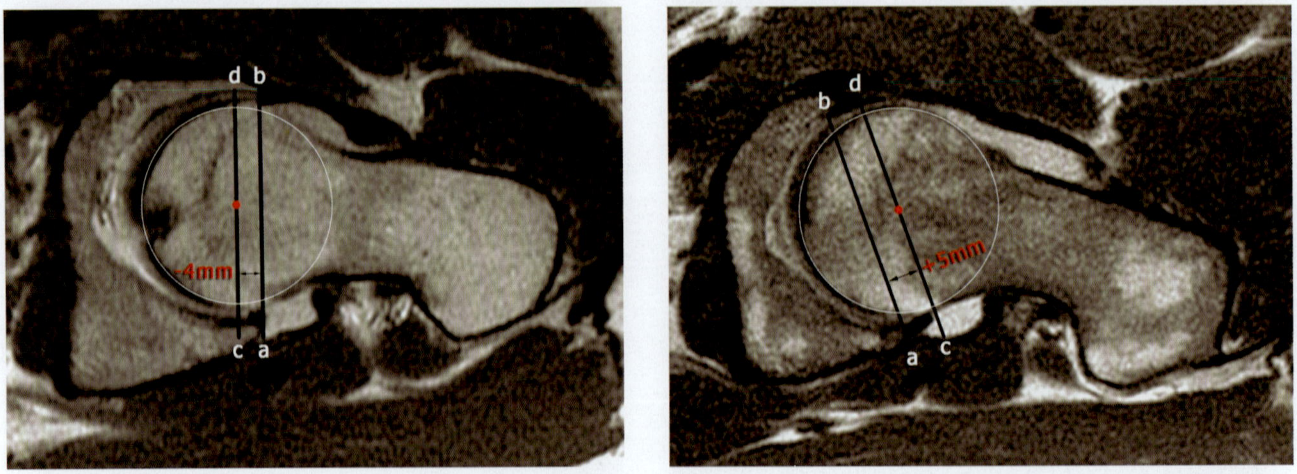

A B

Figure 5.29 ■ MRI of pincer FAI. A: Axial oblique T1-weighted MR image shows deeply seated femoral head secondary to acetabular retroversion. Acetabular depth can be quantified by drawing a line (*ab*) connecting the posterior and anterior acetabular rims and a parallel line (*cd*) that passes through the center of the femoral head (*red dot*). The distance between these two lines defines the acetabular depth, with the value being positive (+) if the center of the femoral head projects lateral to the line connecting the acetabular rims. Negative values (−) indicate deep seating of the femoral head within the acetabulum. **B:** Axial oblique MR image of normal hip joint is shown for comparison.

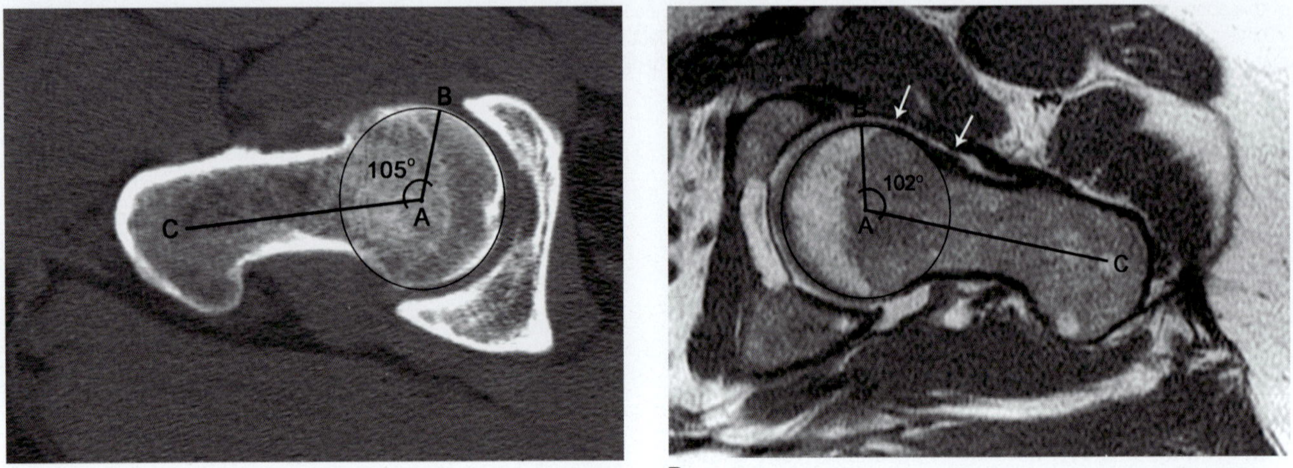

A B

Figure 5.30 ■ Femoroacetabular impingement—calculation of alpha angle. The alpha angle is formed by the intersection of two lines: line *AB*, drawn from the center of the femoral head (*A*) to the point where peripheral osseous contour of the anterior femoral head intersects the extrapolated circle of the femoral head (*B*), and the second line *AC*, drawn from the center of the femoral head (*A*) through the longitudinal axis of the femoral neck (*C*). Normal alpha angle should not exceed 50 degrees. **A:** Alpha angle calculated on the oblique axial CT image of the right hip in a patient with cam FAI. **B:** Alpha angle calculated on the oblique axial MR image of the left hip in a patient with cam FAI. The *arrows* point to excessive bone formation at the anterosuperior aspect of the femoral head/neck junction.

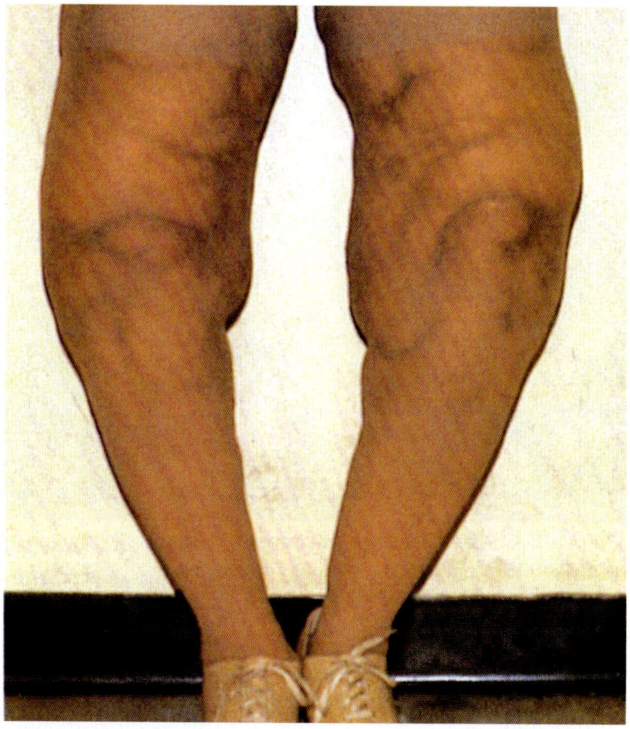

Figure 5.31 ■ Knee deformities. Patient with advanced osteoarthritis of the knee joints affecting predominantly the medial compartments developed varus deformities.

gross deformities of the knees are become obvious, such as valgus or varus configuration (Fig. 5.31).

Pathology

The pathologic findings are very similar to those described for osteoarthritis of the hip. In the early stages, focal abnormalities are seen in the articular cartilage. Starting in the superficial layers, there is loss of proteoglycan, associated with flaking and surface cracking (Fig. 5.32), followed by formation of fissures (see Fig. 1.23) and focal necrosis (see Fig. 5.3). In the later stages, the exposed subchondral bone exhibits characteristic eburnation (Fig. 5.33). Separated fragments of intra-articular osteophytes and fragments of fibrocartilage and hyaline cartilage remain free in the joint cavity as loose intra-articular bodies. Proliferation of cartilaginous cells may occur on the surface of these loose bodies, and consequently, they grow larger (Fig. 5.34). Sometimes, these chondral bodies may reattach to the synovial membrane (Fig. 5.35A) in which case they are invaded by blood vessels, and through the process of endochondral ossification, they become osteochondral bodies (Figs. 5.35B and 5.36).

Imaging Features

The knee is a complex joint comprising three major compartments—the medial femorotibial, the lateral femorotibial, and the femoropatellar—and each of which may be affected by degenerative changes. One of the hallmarks of OA of the knee is narrowing of the joint space. Narrowing can be expressed in both quantitative and semiquantitative terms. Ahlback proposed that narrowing, as a sign of cartilage loss, should be considered if the minimum joint space width is <3 mm and measured on the anteroposterior weight-bearing radiographs with the knee extended and with the x-ray beam parallel to the tibial condyles. Most investigators have accepted this limit. Less frequently used are the semiquantitative parts of the Ahlback's definition, stating that joint

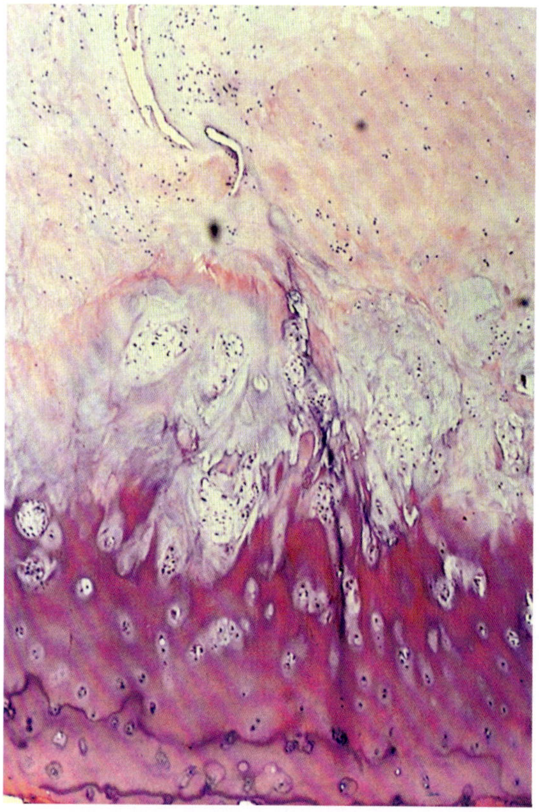

Figure 5.32 ■ Histopathology of osteoarthritis of the knee joint. Photomicrograph of the articular surface of the tibial plateau shows a crack extending deep into the cartilage with focal degenerative changes in the surrounding tissue (H&E, original magnification ×4). (From Bullough PG. *Atlas of Orthopedic Pathology with Clinical and Radiologic Correlation.* 2nd ed. New York, NY: Gower Medical Publishing; 1992, Fig. 9.15.)

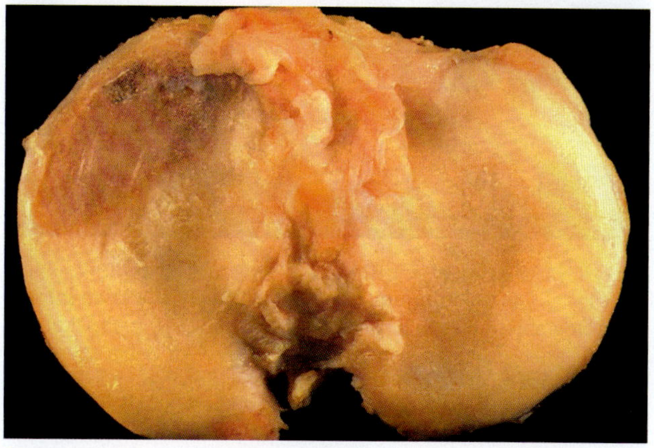

Figure 5.33 ■ Pathology of osteoarthritis of the knee joint. Specimen of the tibial plateau shows cartilage erosion with exposed subchondral bone.

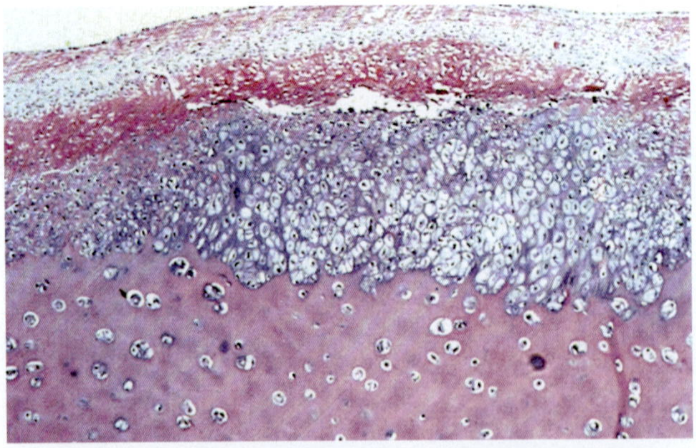

Figure 5.34 ■ Histopathology of osteoarthritis of the knee joint. Proliferation of immature cellular cartilage on the surface of a loose body; the original cartilage is seen in the lower part of the picture (H&E, original magnification ×4). (From Bullough PG. *Atlas of Orthopedic Pathology with Clinical and Radiologic Correlation.* 2nd ed. New York, NY: Gower Medical Publishing; 1992, Fig. 9.36.)

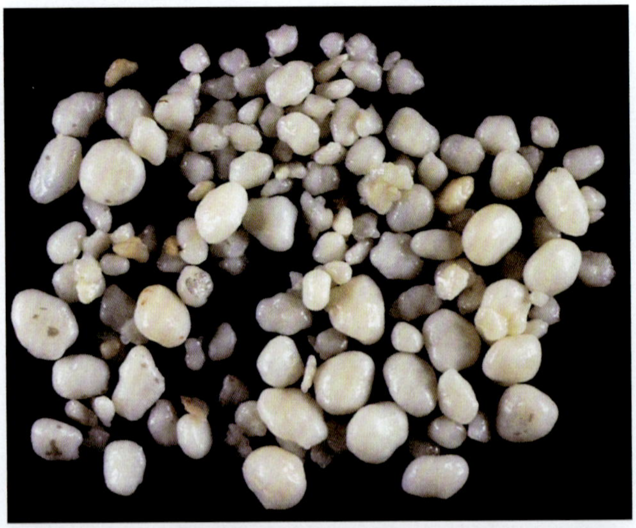

Figure 5.36 ■ Osteochondral bodies. Photograph of multiple osteochondral bodies removed from the osteoarthritic knee joint. In contrast to the intra-articular bodies of primary synovial (osteo) chondromatosis, they are different in sizes. (From Bullough PG. *Atlas of Orthopedic Pathology with Clinical and Radiologic Correlation.* 2nd ed. New York, NY: Gower Medical Publishing; 1992, Fig. 9.40.)

space is narrowed when (1) it is narrower than half the width of the articular space in the same articulation of the other knee and (2) it is decreased in weight bearing as compared with non–weight-bearing position.

As Bennett and associates reported, the pathogenesis of osteoarthritis in the knee joint begins on the surface of the articular cartilage. A loss of articular cartilage accounts for the narrowing of the joint space. If weight bearing continues in an impaired joint, abnormalities develop not only in the cartilage but also in the subchondral bone, menisci, and synovium. Detritic fragments loosen from the joint surface and are discharge to the joint cavity. Shards of bone and cartilage are embedded in the synovial membrane, resulting in so-called detritic synovitis. Attrition of the menisci parallels the deterioration of the articular cartilage. The free edge of the meniscus becomes frayed and wavy, and meniscus may calcify. The imaging features of these changes are similar to those seen in osteoarthritis of the hip, including narrowing of the joint space (usually one or two compartments), subchondral sclerosis, osteophytosis, and subchondral cyst (or pseudocyst) formation. These detritic cystlike lesions, however, are not as common as in the hip joint, and when they do occur, they may be small and often obscured by subchondral sclerosis. Osteophytes are always marginal to the segment of weight bearing and are more pronounced when joint narrowing is advanced. The tibial spines became prominent and broadened, and small osteophytes may form on them as well ("peaking" of the tibial spines). In advanced osteoarthritis, a "vacuum sign" may be seen within the joint space. The standard weight-bearing anteroposterior and lateral projections of the knee are sufficient to demonstrate osteoarthritic process (Figs. 5.37 and 5.38). If the medial joint compartment is affected, the knee may assume a varus configuration,

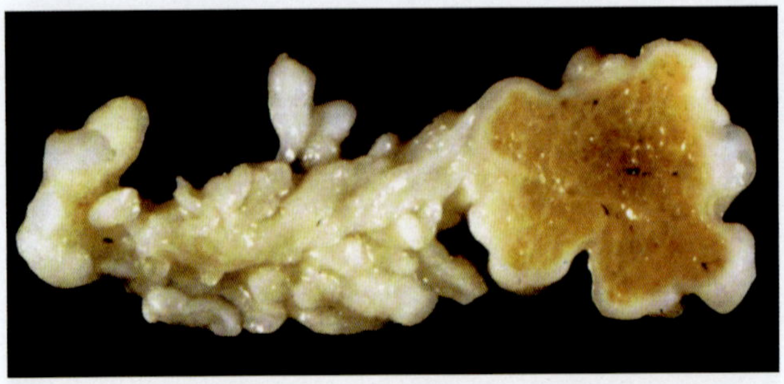

A

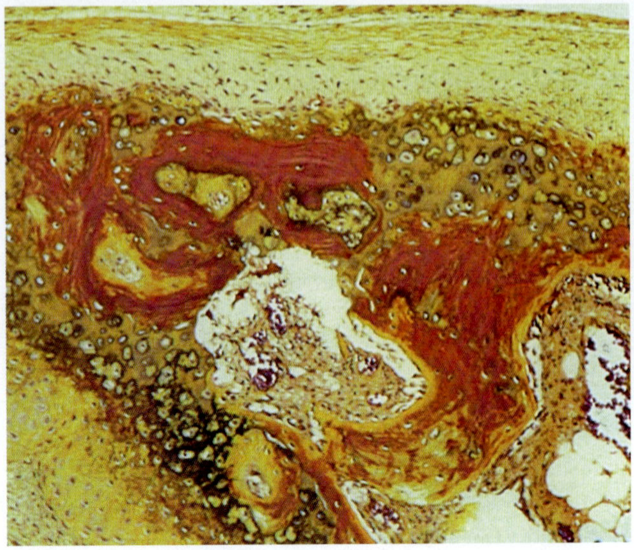

B

Figure 5.35 ■ Pathology of osteoarthritis of the knee joint. **A:** Photograph of bisected specimen of a loose body (*right*) that has become attached to the synovium (*left*). Observe a viable osseous center, which has resulted from vascular invasion and endochondral ossification of loose cartilaginous body. **B:** Photomicrograph of a portion of the same loose body demonstrates formation of the osseous core by the process of endochondral ossification (H&E, original magnification ×10). (From Bullough PG. *Atlas of Orthopedic Pathology with Clinical and Radiologic Correlation.* 2nd ed. New York, NY: Gower Medical Publishing; 1992, Fig. 9.39.)

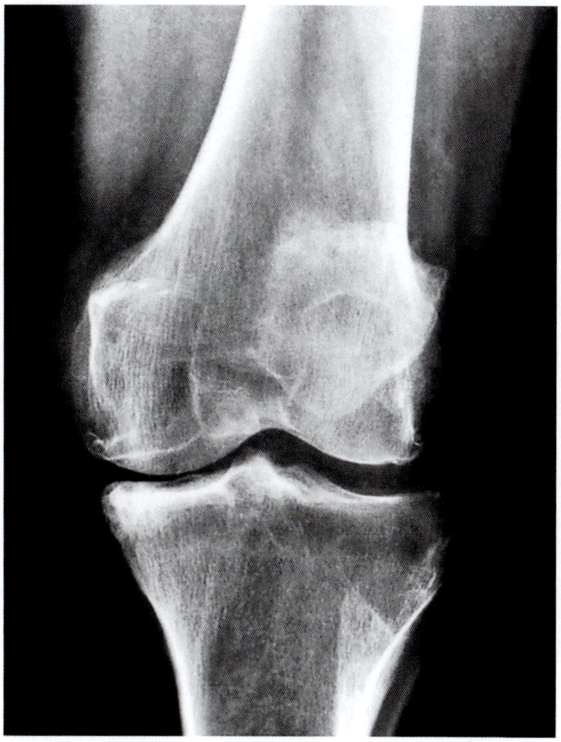

A

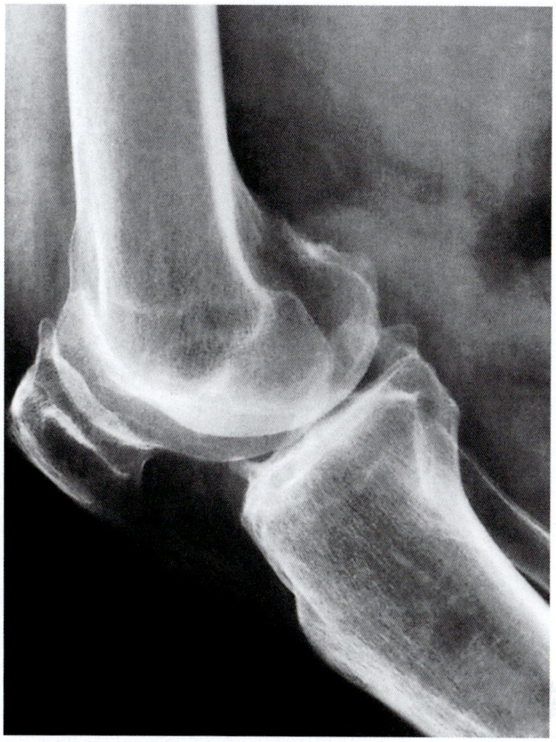

B

Figure 5.37 ■ **Osteoarthritis of the knee joint.** Anteroposterior **(A)** and lateral **(B)** radiographs of the knee of a 57-year-old woman demonstrate narrowing of the medial femorotibial and femoropatellar compartments, subchondral sclerosis, and osteophytosis, which are the typical features of osteoarthritis. Note that osteophytes that were not obvious on the frontal projection are much better demonstrated on the lateral radiograph.

which is best demonstrated on the weight-bearing anteroposterior view (Fig. 5.39A). Involvement of the lateral compartment may lead to a valgus configuration (Fig. 5.39B). CT including three-dimensional (3D)-reconstructed CT images (Fig. 5.40) and MRI (Fig. 5.41) may provide additional information as to the status of osteoarthritic process.

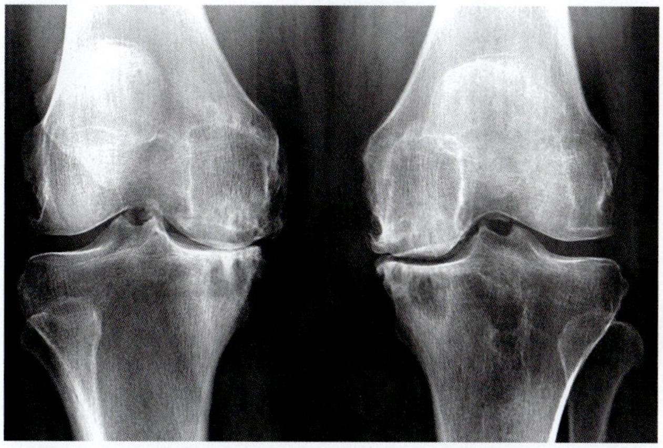

Figure 5.38 ■ **Osteoarthritis of the knee joints.** Anteroposterior weight-bearing radiograph of both knees of a 70-year-old woman shows narrowing of the medial femorotibial joint compartments, more severely affecting the right knee, subchondral sclerosis, osteophyte formation, and subchondral cysts in the proximal tibiae. The lateral joint compartments are only slightly affected.

The femoropatellar joint compartment is also commonly involved in primary osteoarthritis. The lateral radiograph of the knee and axial view of the patella are the most effective means of visualizing degenerative changes of the femoropatellar compartment (Fig. 5.42). In 1957, J.H Kellgren and J.S. Lawrence proposed a scoring system to assess the severity of knee OA on the conventional radiographs, which was in 1961 accepted by World Health Organization (WHO). Based on this classification, *grade 0* was assigned if there were no radiographic features of OA; *grade 1*—if there was minimal joint space narrowing present on the anteroposterior weight-bearing radiographs and osteophyte formation; *grade 2*—if there was definite osteophyte formation with possible joint space narrowing; *grade 3*—if there were multiple osteophytes present associated with definite joint space narrowing, subchondral sclerosis, and possible bone deformity; and *grade 4*—if there were large osteophytes, marked joint space narrowing, severe subchondral sclerosis, and definite bone deformity. More recently, P.R Kornaat and associates have developed a knee osteoarthritis scoring system (KOSS) based on the presence or absence the following features on MRI: cartilaginous lesions, osteophytes, subchondral cysts, bone marrow edema, joint effusion, synovitis, Baker cyst, and meniscal abnormalities.

A frequent complication of osteoarthritis of the knee is the formation of osteochondral bodies, which can be

(Continued on page 166)

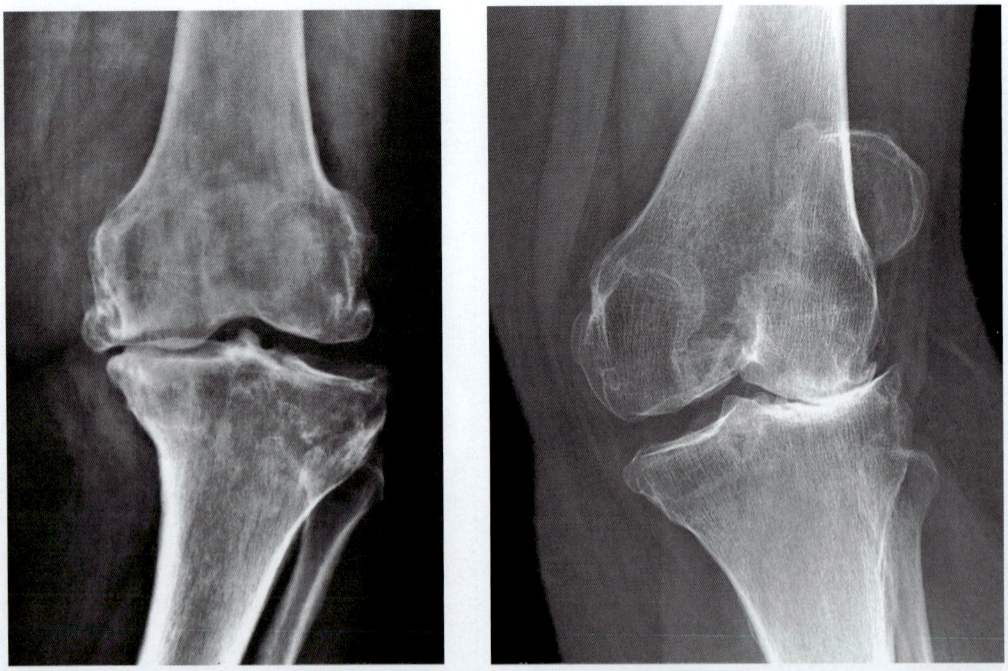

A B

Figure 5.39 ■ Osteoarthritis of the knee joint. A: Weight-bearing anteroposterior radiograph of the knee of a 58-year-old woman demonstrates advanced osteoarthritis of the medial femorotibial joint compartment, which has led to a varus configuration of the joint. **B:** Involvement of the lateral femorotibial joint compartment in advanced osteoarthritis as seen on this weight-bearing anteroposterior radiograph of another patient has resulted in a valgus configuration.

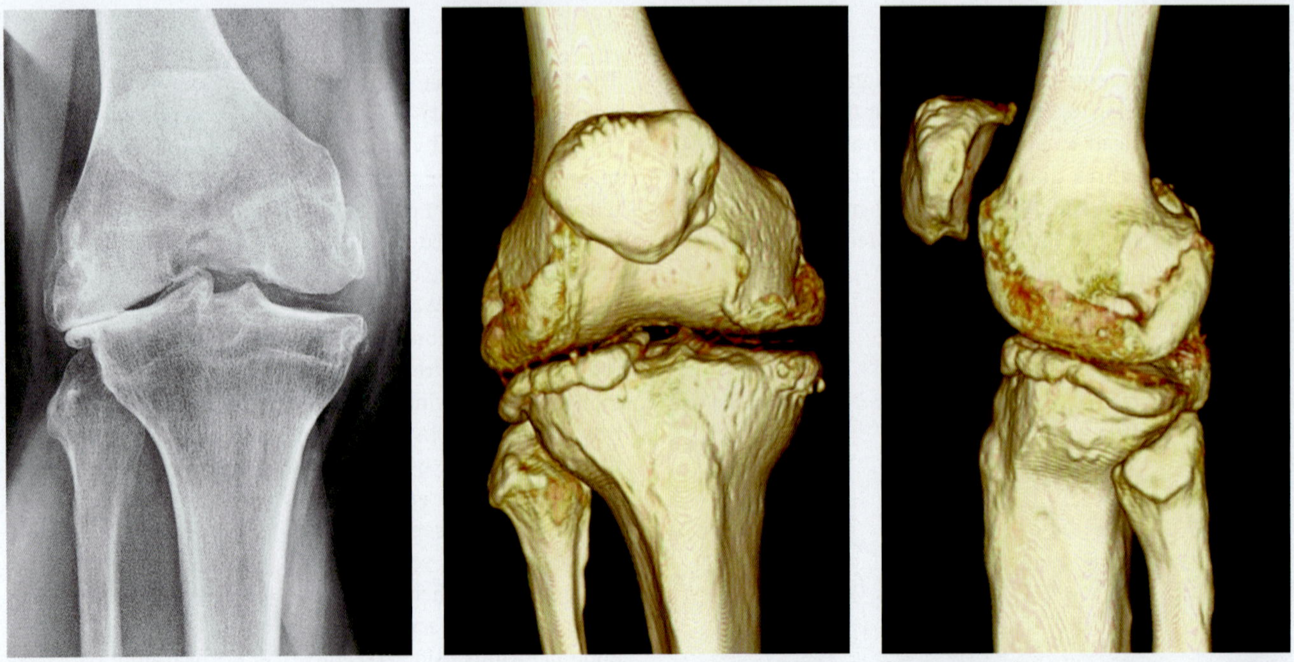

A B C

Figure 5.40 ■ 3D CT of osteoarthritis of the knee joint. A: Radiograph of the right knee of a 58-year-old man shows advanced osteoarthritis. **B, C:** 3D-reconstructed CT images in shaded surface display demonstrate advanced three-compartmental osteoarthritis.

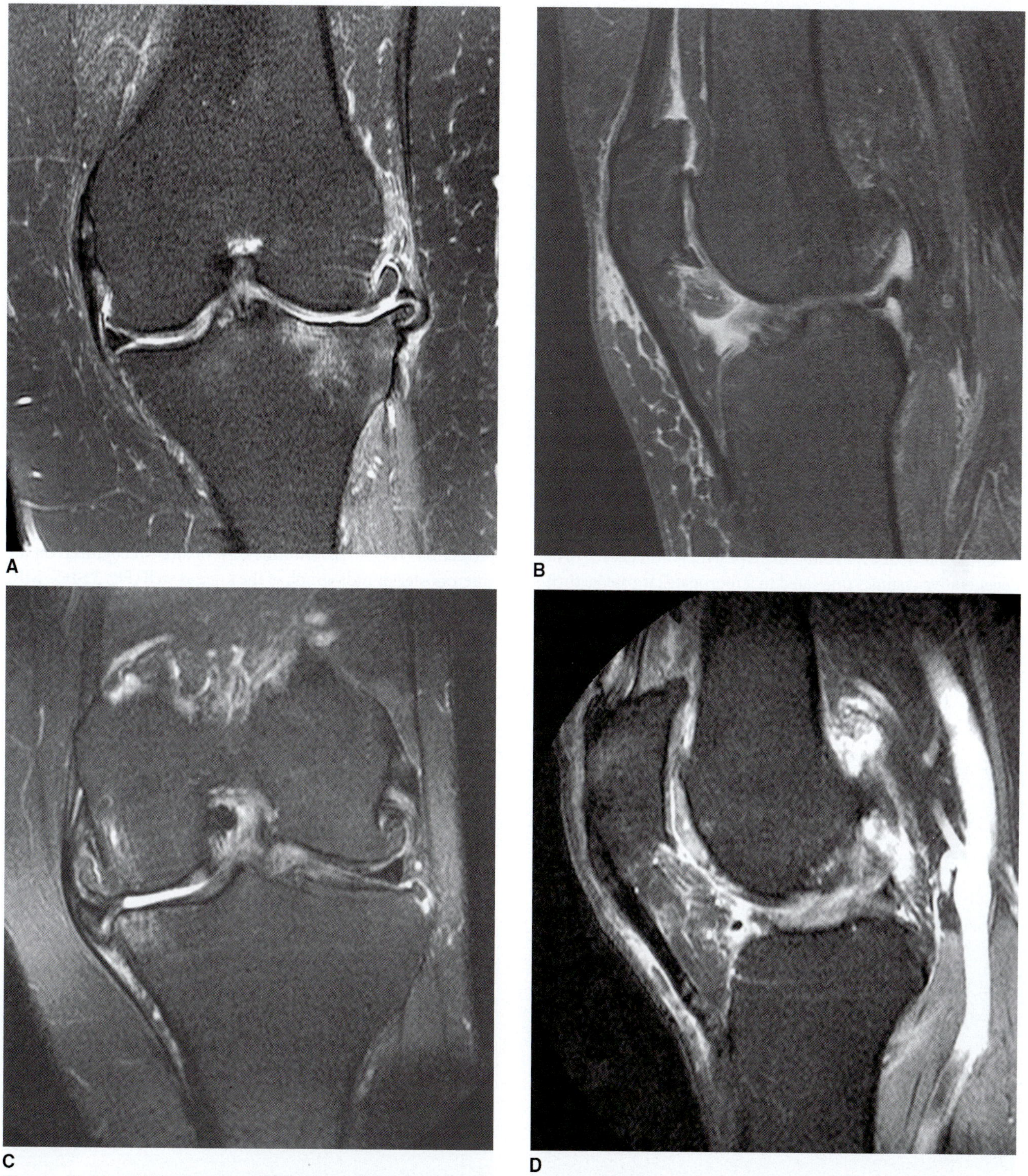

Figure 5.41 ■ **MRI of osteoarthritis of the knee joint.** Coronal **(A)** and sagittal **(B)** proton density-weighted fat-suppressed MR images of the left knee of a 74-year-old woman show prominent osteophytes at the lateral joint compartment as well as at the inferior pole of the patella. There is a marked thinning of the articular cartilage of the lateral femoral condyle, with a focal full-thickness cartilage defect, and complete loss of articular cartilage of the lateral tibial plateau associated with subchondral bone marrow edema. In addition, there is a degenerative tear of the lateral meniscus. Coronal proton density-weighted fat-suppressed **(C)** and sagittal fast spin-echo (FSE) proton density-weighted fat-suppressed **(D)** MR images of the left knee of a 51-year-old woman show complete loss of articular cartilage of the medial femoral condyle and medial tibial plateau associated with subchondral bone marrow edema. There is degenerative tear of the medial meniscus, which is also medially extruded. The anterior cruciate ligament demonstrates degenerative tear, and there is diffuse nodular synovial thickening.

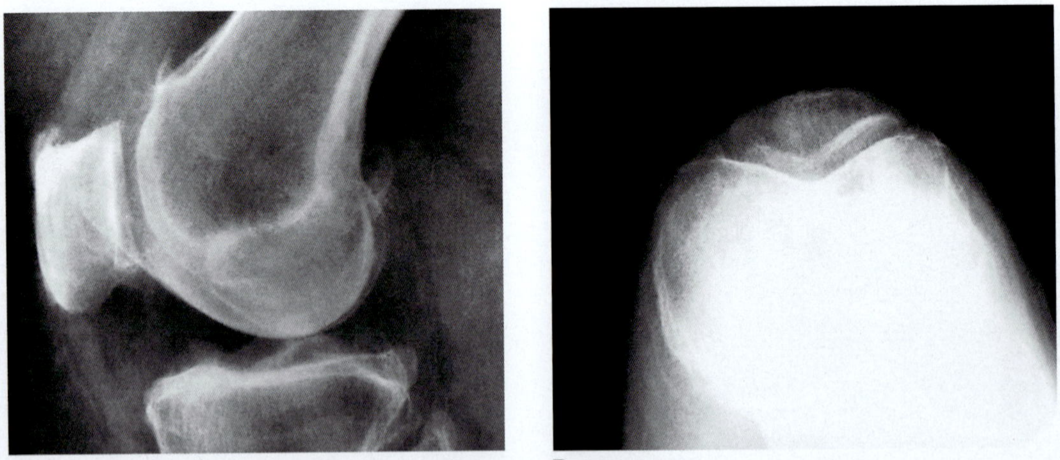

A B

Figure 5.42 ■ Femoropatellar osteoarthritis. Lateral radiograph of the knee **(A)** and axial radiograph of the patella **(B)** of a 72-year-old woman demonstrate narrowing of the femoropatellar joint compartment and osteophytes formation.

demonstrated on the standard projections of the knee (Figs. 5.43 to 5.46). MRI may also be effective in this respect (Figs. 5.47 to 5.50).

Often, particularly in individuals past their fifth decade of life, degenerative changes unrelated to femoropatellar osteoarthritis are seen at the insertion of the quadriceps tendon into the base of the patella. These changes are manifest as vertical ridges resembling teeth on an axial view of the patella and have been designated by Greenspan and colleagues as the "tooth" sign (Fig. 5.51A). The dentate structures represent an enthesopathy probably related to stress at the attachment of the quadriceps apparatus, and their nature is clearly demonstrated on the lateral projection (Fig. 5.51B). At times, they can be recognized on the anteroposterior radiograph of the knee as well (Fig. 5.51C). MRI also effectively demonstrates these changes (Fig. 5.52).

As in the hip joint, one may encounter secondary osteoarthritis in the knee. One of the most common predisposing factors is previous trauma or surgery.

(Continued on page 170)

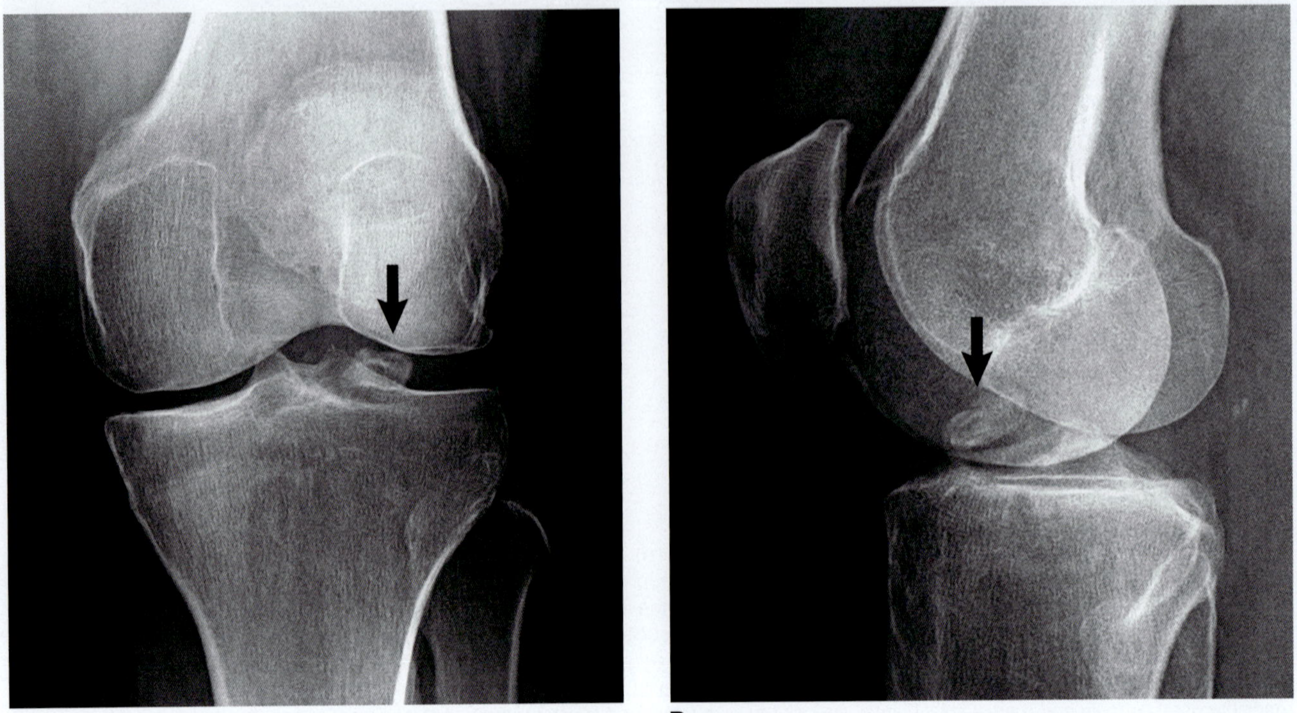

A B

Figure 5.43 ■ Osteoarthritis of the knee complicated by osteochondral body. Anteroposterior **(A)** and lateral **(B)** radiograph of the left knee of a 50-year-old woman shows osteoarthritic changes affecting all three joint compartments, complicated by the presence of an osteochondral body (*arrow*).

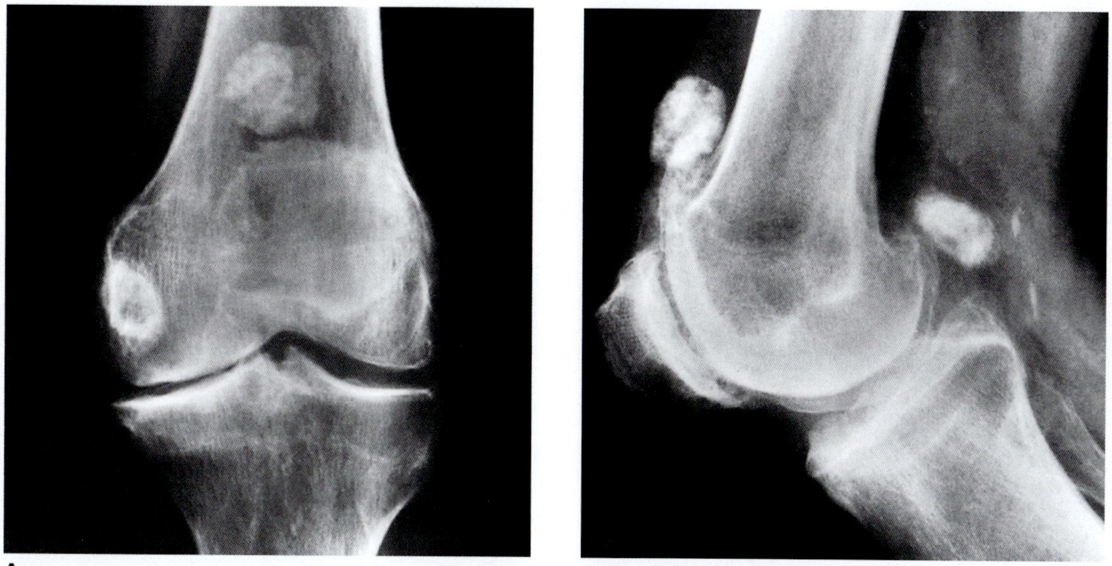

A B

Figure 5.44 ■ **Osteoarthritis of the knee complicated by osteochondral bodies.** Anteroposterior **(A)** and lateral **(B)** radiographs of the left knee of a 66-year-old man with advanced osteoarthritis demonstrate predominant involvement of the medial femorotibial and femoropatellar joint compartments, with formation of two large osteochondral bodies.

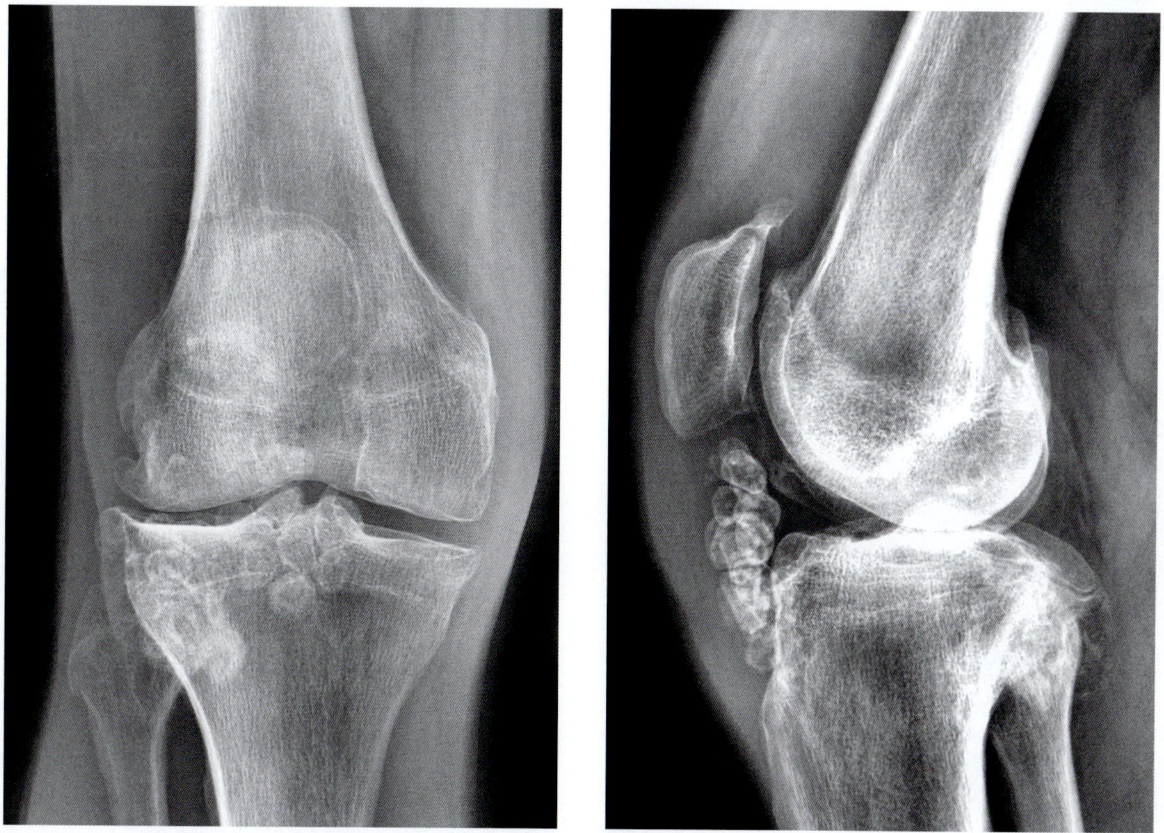

A B

Figure 5.45 ■ **Osteoarthritis of the knee complicated by osteochondral bodies.** Anteroposterior **(A)** and lateral **(B)** radiographs of the right knee show osteoarthritis complicated by numerous osteochondral bodies.

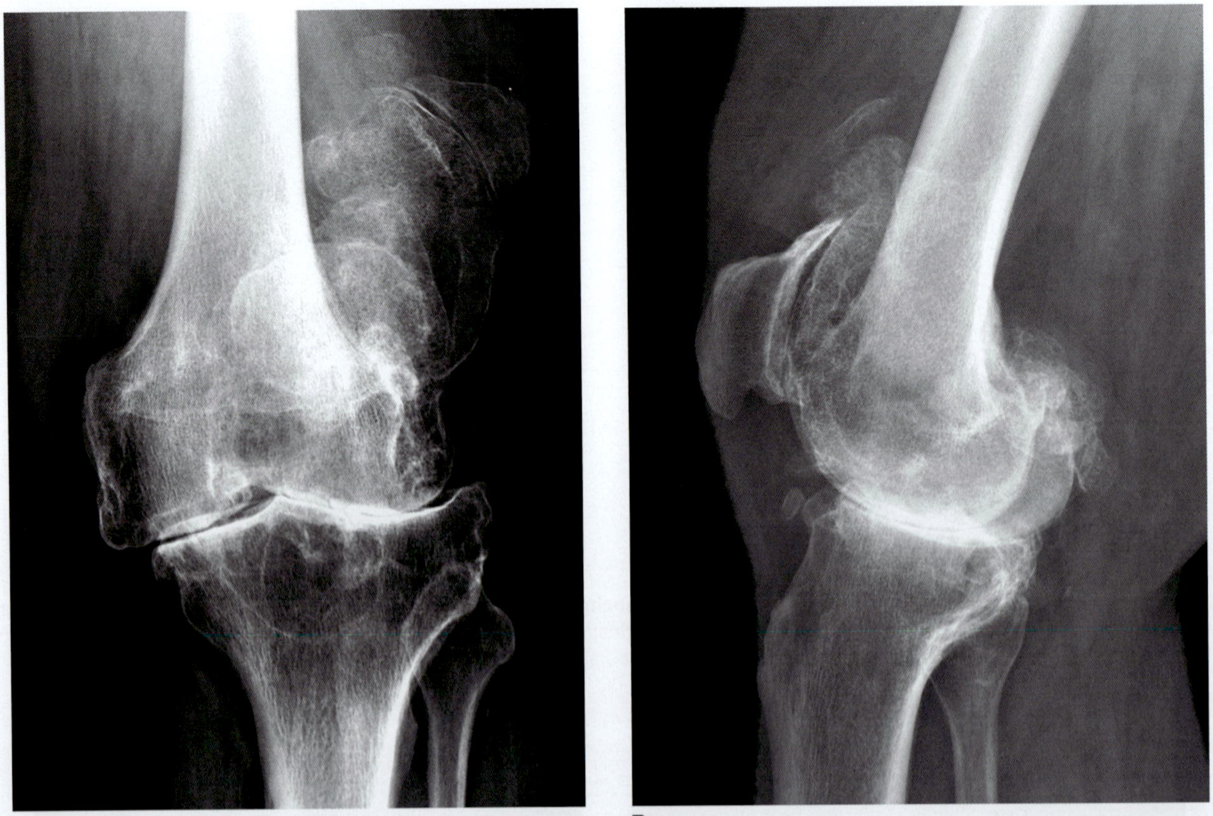

A B

Figure 5.46 ■ Osteoarthritis of the knee complicated by osteochondral bodies. Anteroposterior **(A)** and lateral **(B)** radiographs of the left knee of a 75-year-old man shows advanced tricompartmental osteoarthritis complicated by lateral subluxation and formation of numerous intra-articular osteochondral bodies.

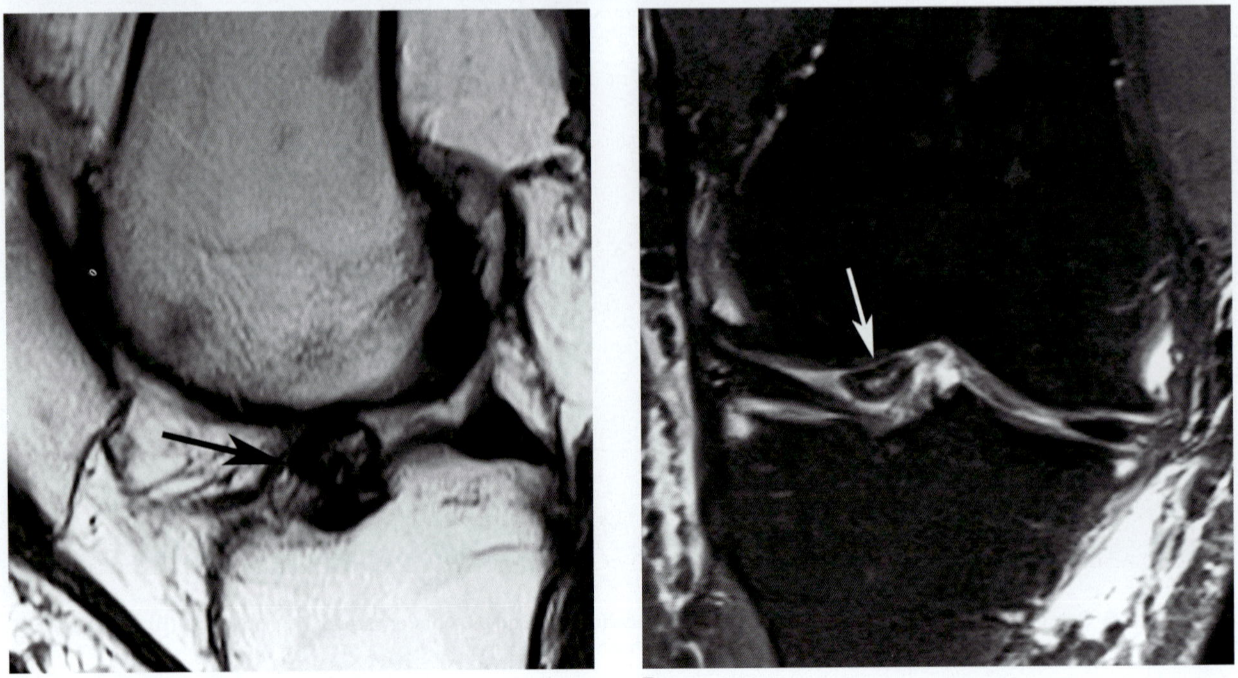

A B

Figure 5.47 ■ MRI of osteochondral body. T1-weighted sagittal **(A)** and T2-weighted coronal **(B)** MR images of the knee show a low-signal intensity osteocartilaginous loose body in the anterior joint space (*arrows*).

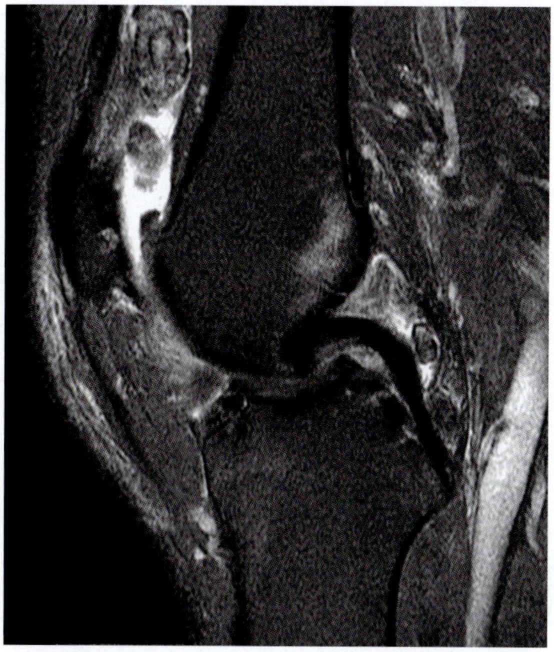

Figure 5.48 ■ MRI of osteochondral bodies. Sagittal T2-weighted fat-suppressed MR image of the knee shows several intra-articular osteochondral bodies in this 67-year-old woman with osteoarthritis.

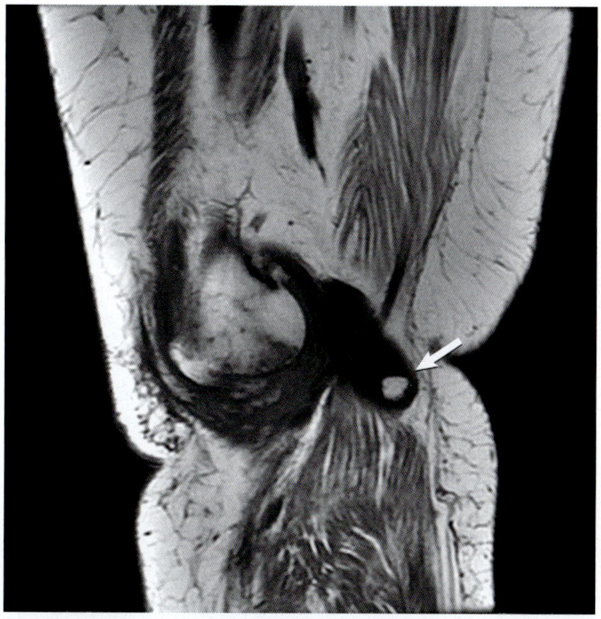

A

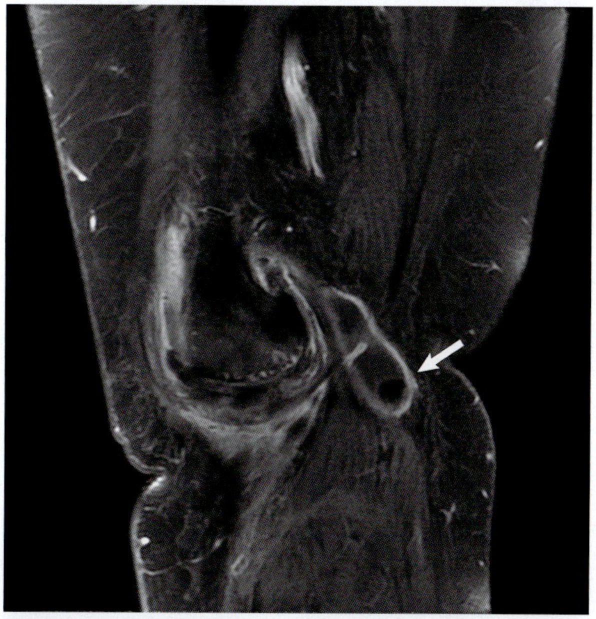

B

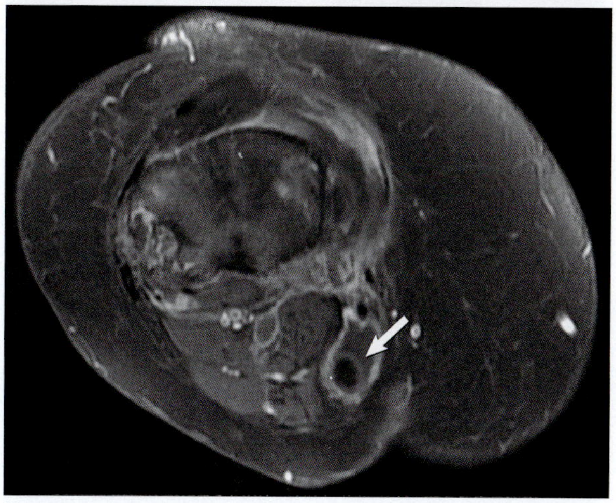

C

Figure 5.49 ■ Baker cyst with osteochondral body. Sagittal T1-weighted **(A)** and sagittal **(B)** and axial **(C)** T1-weighted fat-suppressed MR images of the knee obtained after intravenous administration of gadolinium show an osteochondral body within a popliteal cyst (*arrow*).

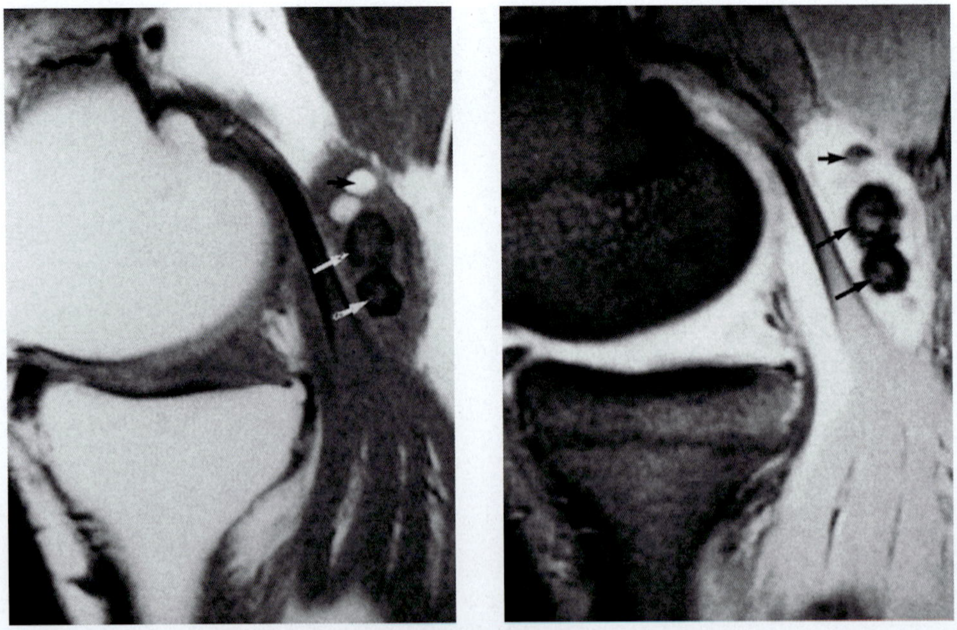

A B

Figure 5.50 ■ **Baker cyst with osteochondral bodies.** Sagittal T1-weighted **(A)** and sagittal T2*-weighted **(B)** MR images show multiple osteochondral loose bodies (*arrows*) in a popliteal (Baker) cyst adjacent to the medial head of gastrocnemius muscle. (From Stoller DW. *MRI in Orthopaedics and Sports Medicine.* Philadelphia, PA: JB Lippincott; 1993.)

Osteoarthritis of Other Large Joints

Other large joints such as the shoulder (Figs. 5.53 and 5.54), elbow (Fig. 5.55), and ankle (Fig. 5.56) can be affected by osteoarthritis, but involvement of these sites in the idiopathic form of the disease is much less common than involvement of the hip or knee. In fact, with evidence of degenerative changes in such sites, one must consider the possibility of secondary rather than idiopathic osteoarthritis (see Table 5.1).

(Continued on page 173)

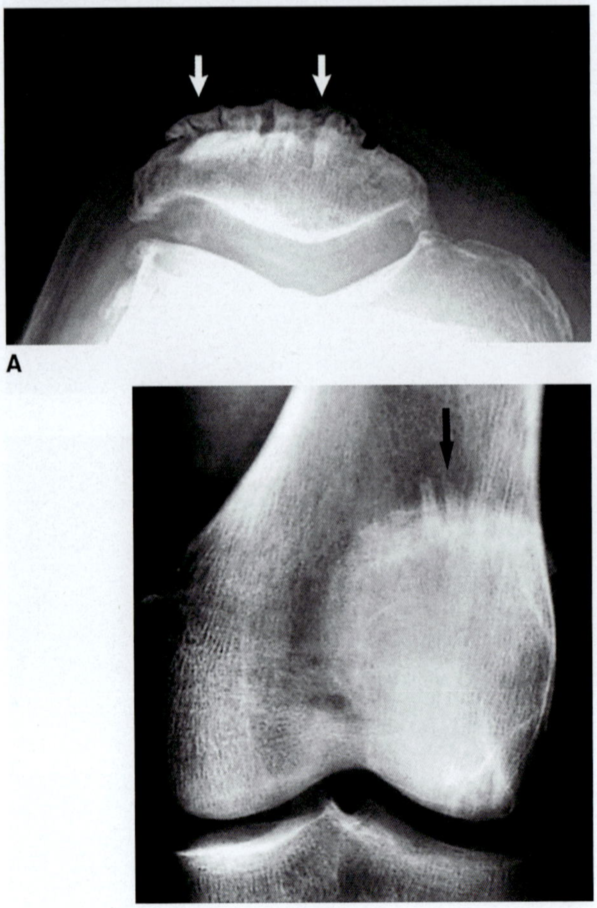

A

C

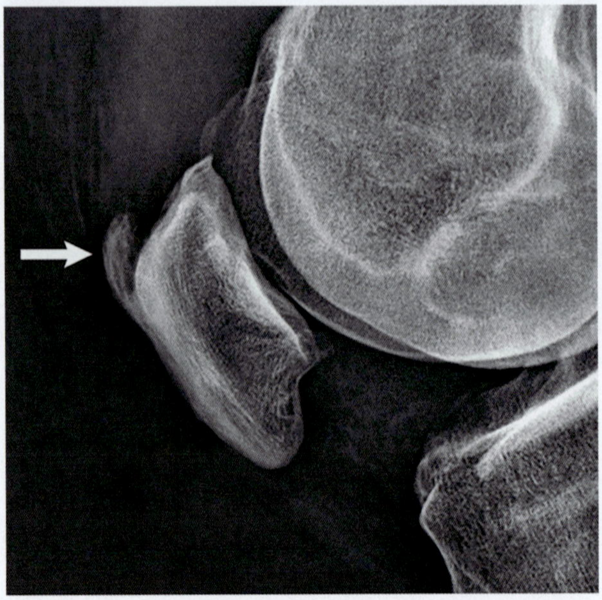

B

Figure 5.51 ■ **Patellar enthesopathy. A:** Axial view of the patella demonstrates dentate structures (*arrows*)—the tooth sign, which represent degenerative ossifications (enthesopathy) at the insertion of the quadriceps tendon into the base of patella (*arrow*), as seen on the lateral view **(B)** in this 55-year-old man. **C:** Occasionally, the tooth sign can also be demonstrated on the anteroposterior projection of the knee (*arrow*), seen here in a 54-year-old woman.

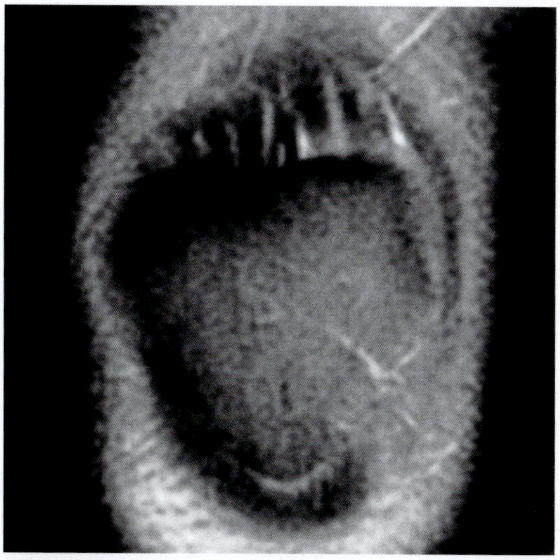

A

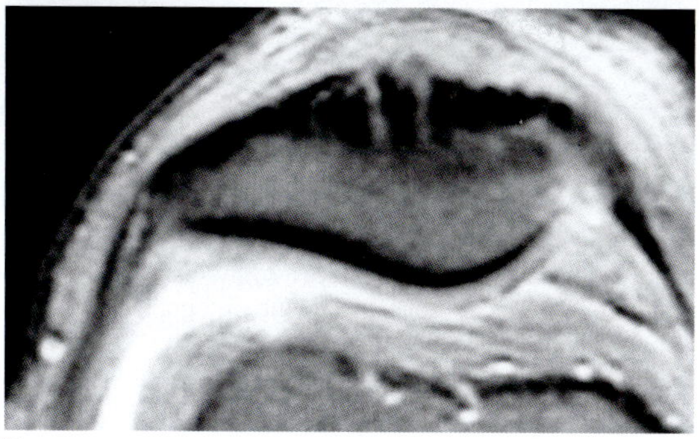

B

Figure 5.52 ■ **MRI of patellar enthesopathy.** Coronal T1-weighted **(A)** and axial T2-weighted **(B)** MR images show tooth sign of the patella.

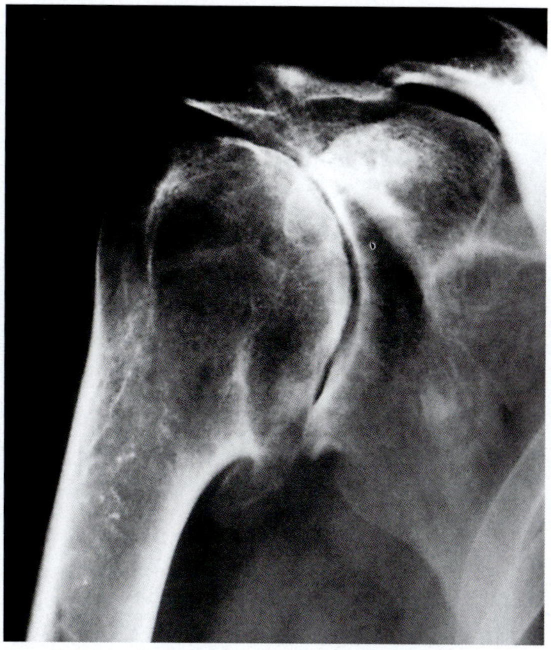

Figure 5.53 ■ **Osteoarthritis of the shoulder joint.** Anteroposterior radiograph of the right shoulder of a 58-year-old man shows the typical features of osteoarthritis; both shoulders were affected. The patient had no history of trauma or other underlying condition to suggest the secondary osteoarthritis.

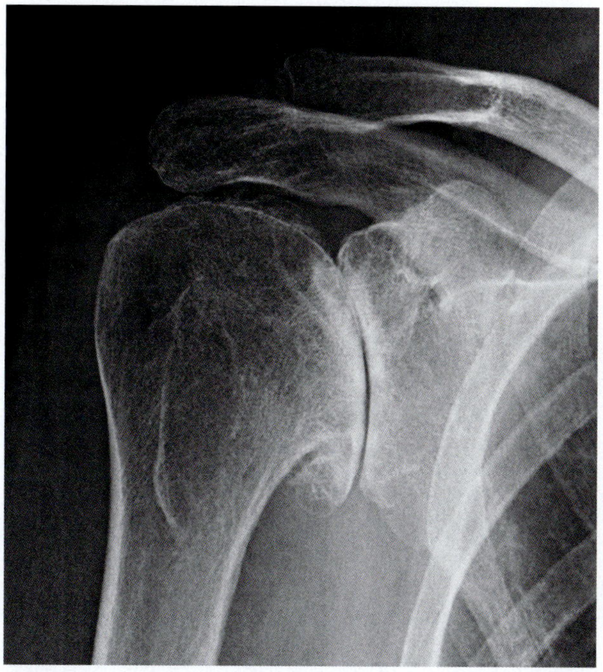

A

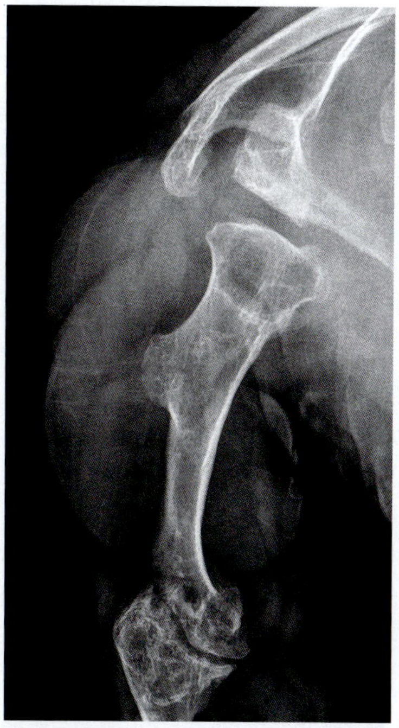

B

Figure 5.54 ■ **Secondary osteoarthritis of the shoulder joint. A:** This 70-year-old man presented with history of several dislocations in the right shoulder joint. Note advanced osteoarthritis of the glenohumeral joint. **B:** Radiograph of the right arm of a 30-year-old woman diagnosed with Morquio-Brailsford disease, a form of mucopolysaccharidosis, in addition to osteoporosis, hypoplasia, and deformities of the bones, demonstrates also osteoarthritis of the shoulder and elbow joints.

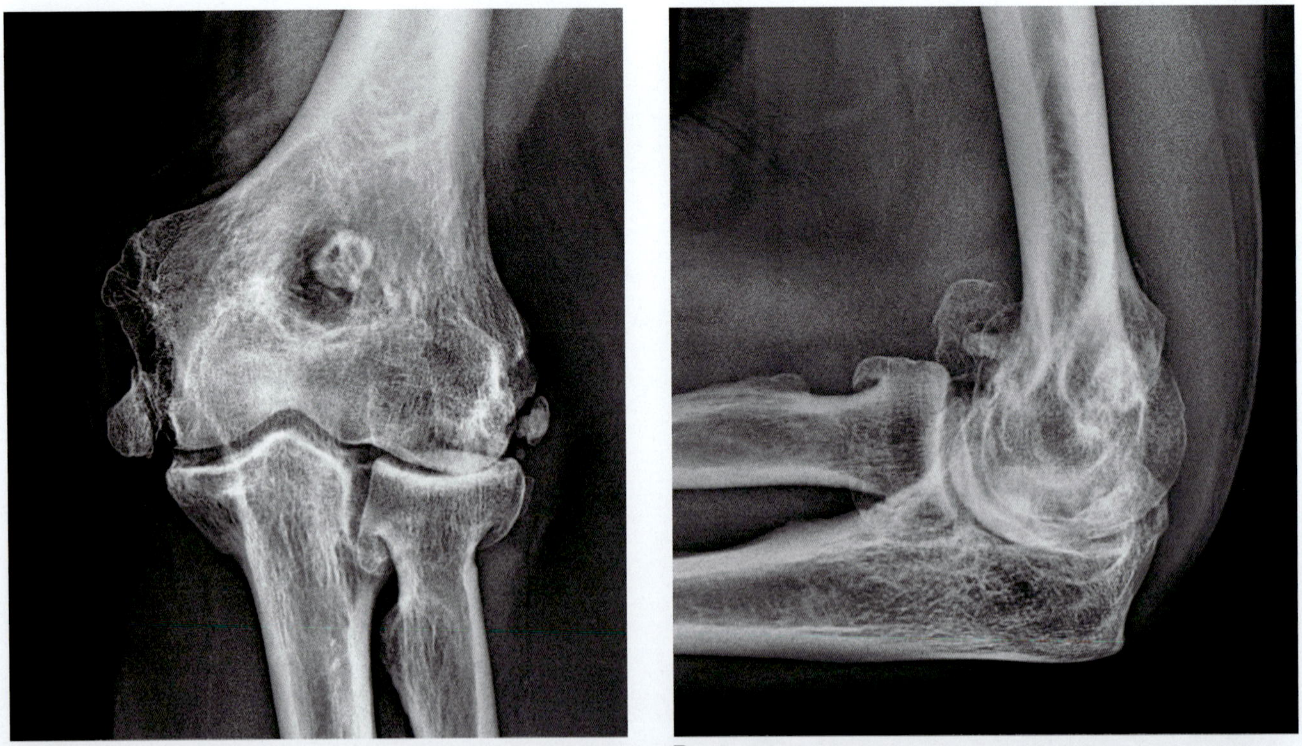

A B

Figure 5.55 ■ **Secondary osteoarthritis of the elbow joint.** Anteroposterior **(A)** and lateral **(B)** radiographs of the elbow joint of a 57-year-old man with history of several prior elbow joint dislocations demonstrate osteoarthritis complicated by the presence of osteochondral bodies.

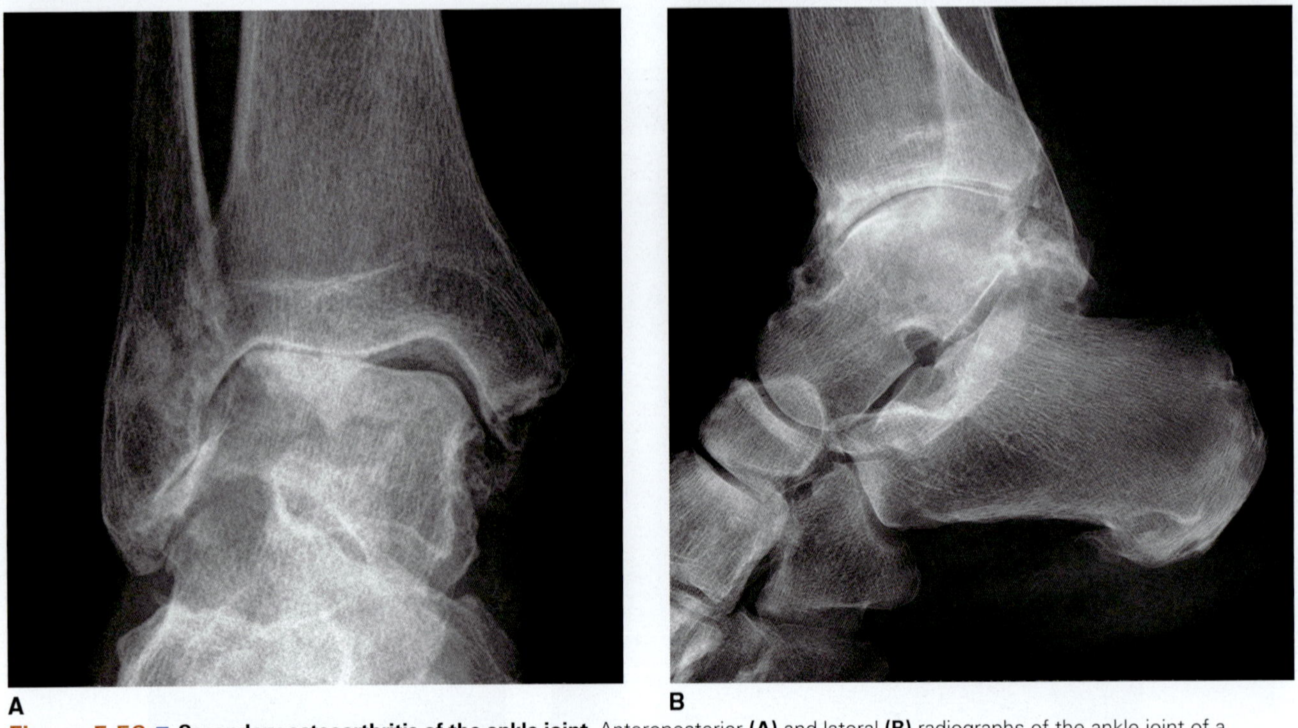

A B

Figure 5.56 ■ **Secondary osteoarthritis of the ankle joint.** Anteroposterior **(A)** and lateral **(B)** radiographs of the ankle joint of a 55-year-old man show posttraumatic osteoarthritis.

OSTEOARTHRITIS OF THE SMALL JOINTS

Primary Osteoarthritis of the Hand

The most commonly affected small joints are those of the hand, particularly the proximal and distal interphalangeal and the first carpometacarpal articulations (see Figs. 3.14 and 5.1). In the distal interphalangeal joints, if hypertrophic phenomena supervene and osteophytes are prominent, these deformities are known as *Heberden nodes*. Similar deformities in the proximal interphalangeal joints are called *Bouchard nodes* (Fig. 5.57). Physical examination commonly will show prominence and swelling of these joints (Fig. 5.58) and tenderness on palpation. If the degenerative changes involve the first carpometacarpal joint (Fig. 5.59), occasionally, they may result in an odd deformation of the thumb (Fig. 5.60). The midcarpal articulations may also be affected, particularly the scaphotrapeziotrapezoid (STT) joint (Figs. 5.61 and 5.62).

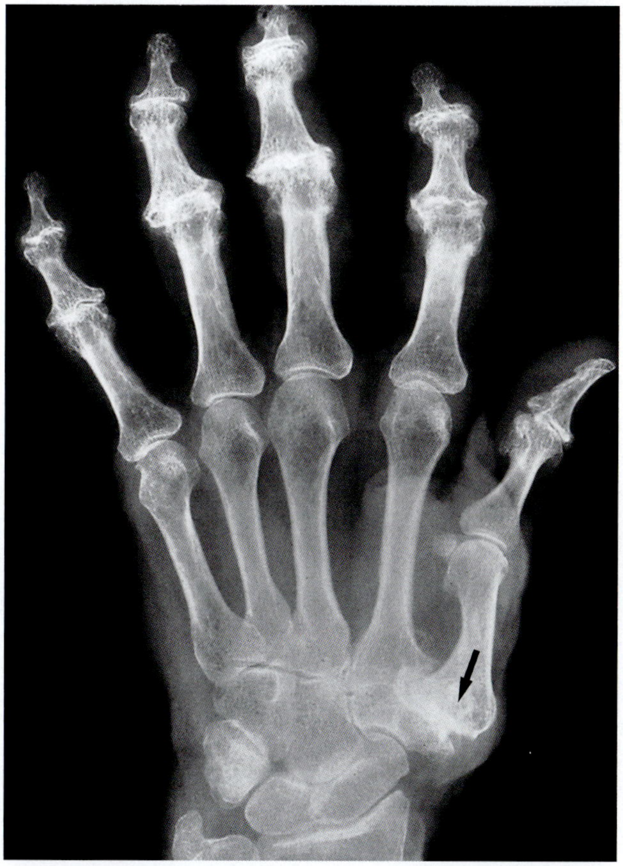

Figure 5.57 ■ Interphalangeal osteoarthritis. Dorsovolar radiograph of right hand of a 74-year-old woman shows degenerative changes in the distal interphalangeal joints, manifested by Heberden nodes, and in the proximal interphalangeal joints, manifested by Bouchard nodes. Note also degenerative changes in the first carpometacarpal joint (*arrow*).

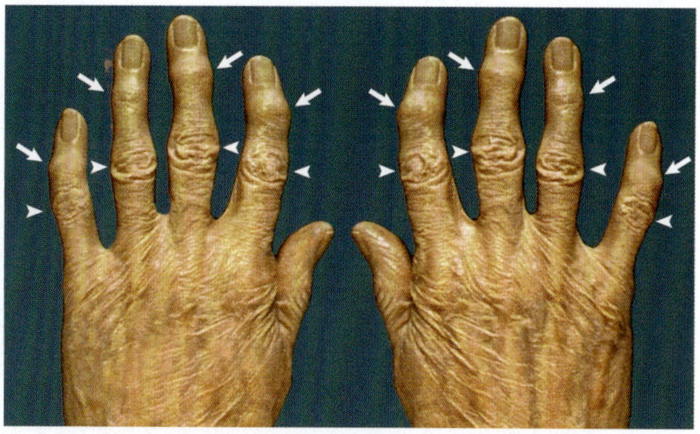

Figure 5.58 ■ Heberden and Bouchard nodes. Clinical photograph of the hands of a 62-year-old woman with interphalangeal osteoarthritis shows prominence of the proximal (*arrowheads*) and distal (*arrows*) interphalangeal joints.

Secondary Osteoarthritis of the Hand

The most characteristic secondary osteoarthritic changes in the small joints may be observed in *acromegaly*. Although the degenerative process in acromegaly also affects large joints such as the hip, knee, shoulder, and the spine, the hand displays the most typical features of this condition. These include soft tissue prominence and enlargement of the terminal tufts and the bases of the terminal phalanges; there may also be widening of some articular spaces and narrowing of others; beaklike osteophytes at the heads of the metacarpals are a prominent feature (Fig. 5.63). Degenerative changes in acromegaly are the result of hypertrophy of articular cartilage, which is not properly nourished by synovial fluid because of its abnormal thickness.

Commonly associated with the development of secondary osteoarthritis in the small joints, *hemochromatosis* (iron storage disease) is a rare disorder characterized by iron deposition in internal organs, articular cartilage, and synovium. Some investigators believe that the arthropathy seen in this condition differs from typical degenerative joint disease and warrants classification in the group of metabolic arthritides (see Chapter 7). In the hand, the second and third metacarpophalangeal joints

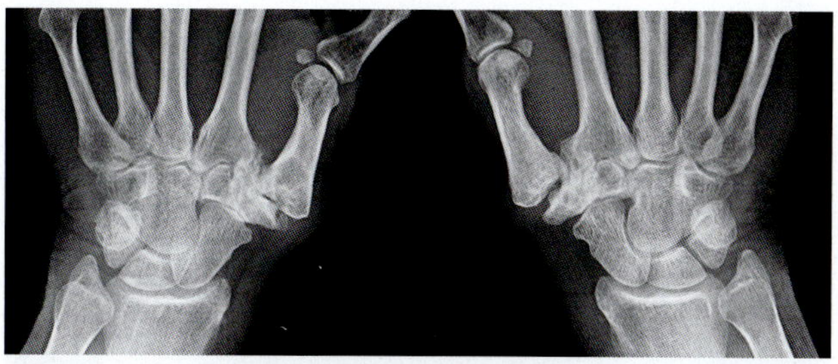

Figure 5.59 ■ Osteoarthritis of the first carpometacarpal joints. Dorsovolar radiograph of both wrists of a 55-year-old woman shows joint space narrowing, subchondral sclerosis, subchondral cysts, and osteophytes at both first carpometacarpal joints.

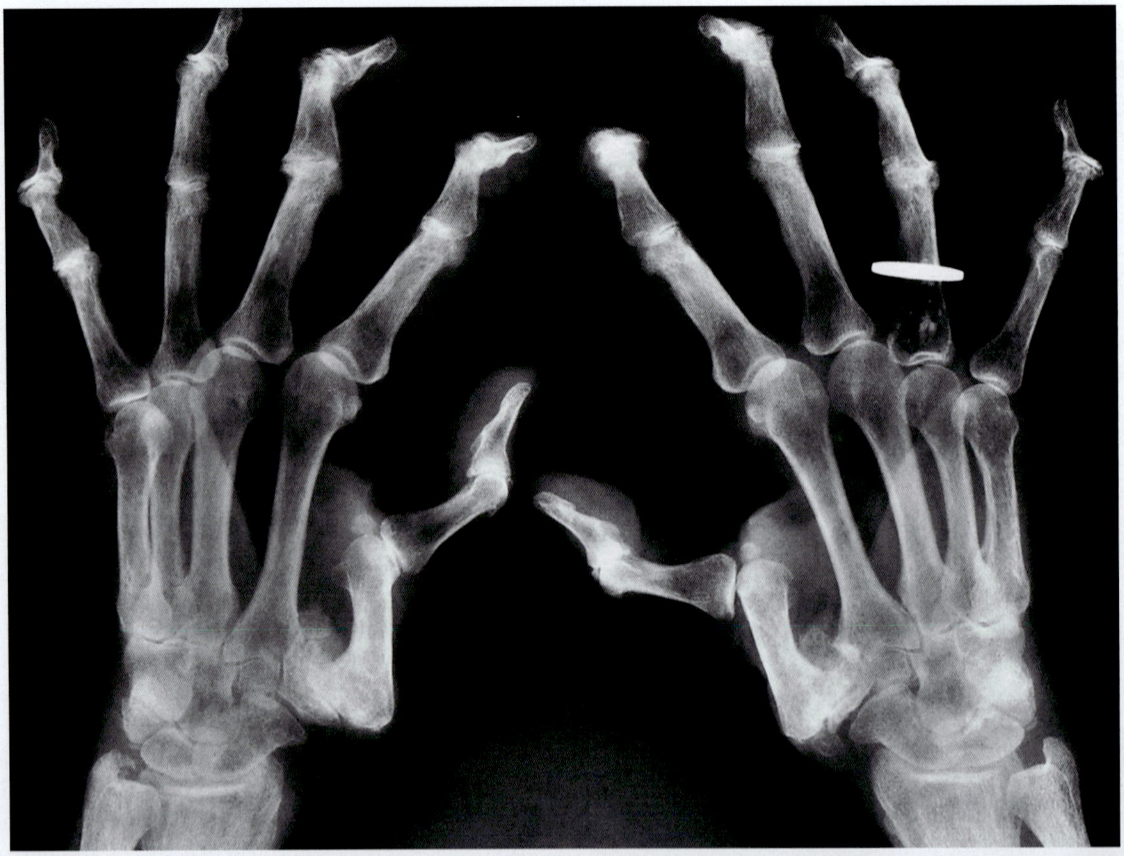

Figure 5.60 ■ Interphalangeal and carpometacarpal osteoarthritis. Dorsovolar radiograph of both hands of a 52-year-old woman in addition to the typical Heberden and Bouchard nodes shows deformative changes at the first carpometacarpal articulations, resulting in an odd configuration of both thumbs.

are characteristically affected (Fig. 5.64), although other small joints such as the interphalangeal and carpal articulations may be involved. Degenerative changes may also be seen at the shoulders, knees, hips, and ankles. Loss of the articular space, eburnation, subchondral cyst formation, and osteophytosis are the most prominent radiographic features of hemochromatosis. The changes may occasionally mimic those seen in calcium pyrophosphate dihydrate (CPPD) deposition disease and rheumatoid arthritis.

Osteoarthritis of the Foot

In the foot, the most commonly affected articulation is the metatarsophalangeal joint of the great toe. This condition is known as *hallux rigidus* or *hallux limitus* (Figs. 5.65 and 5.66). Occasionally, osteoarthritic changes affecting other foot articulations can be encountered (Fig. 5.67).

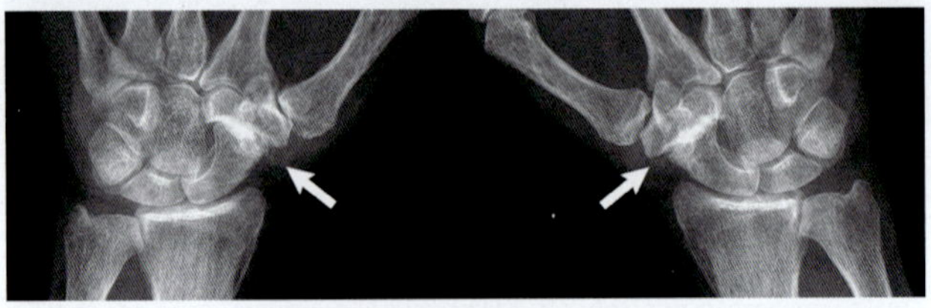

Figure 5.61 ■ STT osteoarthritis. Dorsovolar radiograph of both wrists of a 48-year-old woman shows narrowing and subchondral sclerosis of the scaphotrapeziotrapezoid joints (*arrows*).

DEGENERATIVE DISEASES OF THE SPINE

Degenerative changes may involve the spine at the following sites:

1. The synovial joints—atlantoaxial, apophyseal, uncovertebral (Luschka), costovertebral, and sacroiliac—leading to *osteoarthritis* of these structures
2. The intervertebral disks, leading to the condition known as *degenerative disk disease*
3. The vertebral bodies and annulus fibrosus, leading to the condition known as *spondylosis deformans*
4. The fibrous articulations, ligaments, or sites of ligament attachment to the bone (entheses), leading to the condition known as *diffuse idiopathic skeletal hyperostosis* (DISH)

Frequently, all four conditions coexist in the same patient.

(Continued on page 178)

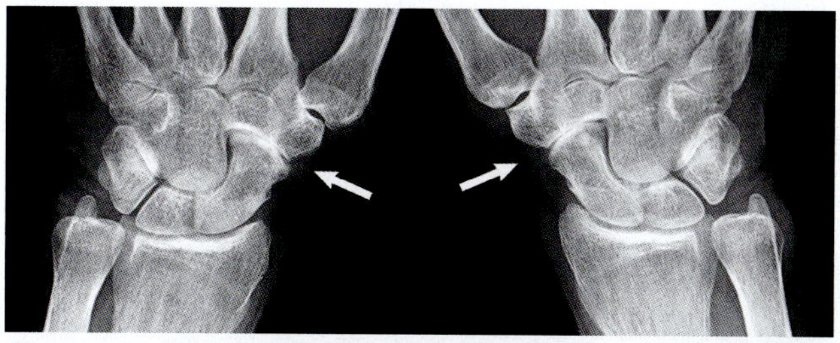

A

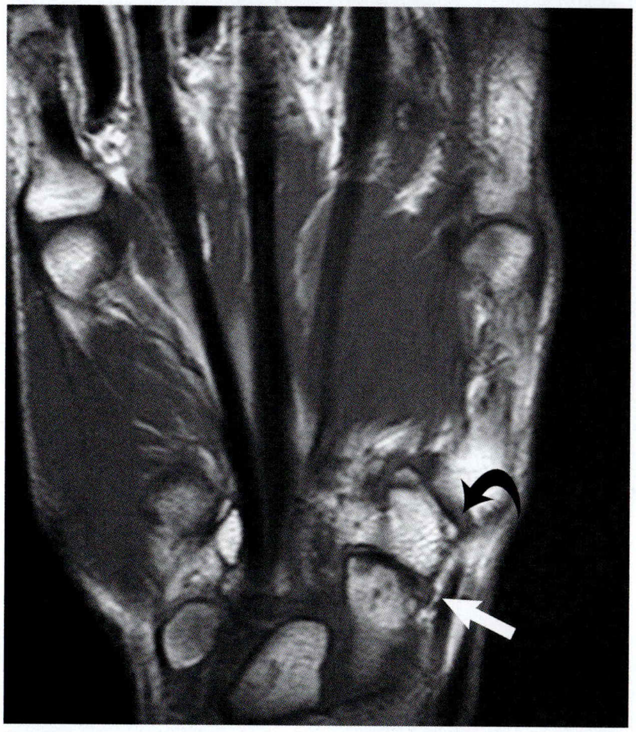

B

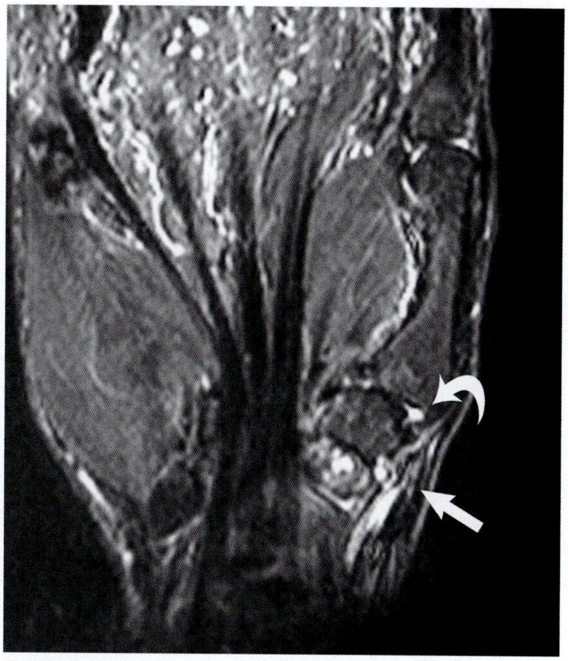

C

Figure 5.62 ■ **MRI of STT osteoarthritis. A:** Frontal radiograph of both wrists of a 63-year-old woman shows narrowing and sclerosis of right and left scaphotrapeziotrapezoid joints (*arrows*). **B:** Coronal T1-weighted MR image of the right wrist shows subchondral sclerosis of the distal pole of the scaphoid bone associated with formation of small subchondral cystic lesions (*arrow*). Minimal narrowing of the first carpometacarpal joint is also present (*curved arrow*). **C:** Coronal T2-weighted MR image shows high signal intensity of fluid-filled cystic lesions and soft tissue edema at the site of STT joint (*arrow*). Early osteoarthritic changes of the first carpometacarpal joint, not so obvious on the radiography, are also present (*curved arrow*).

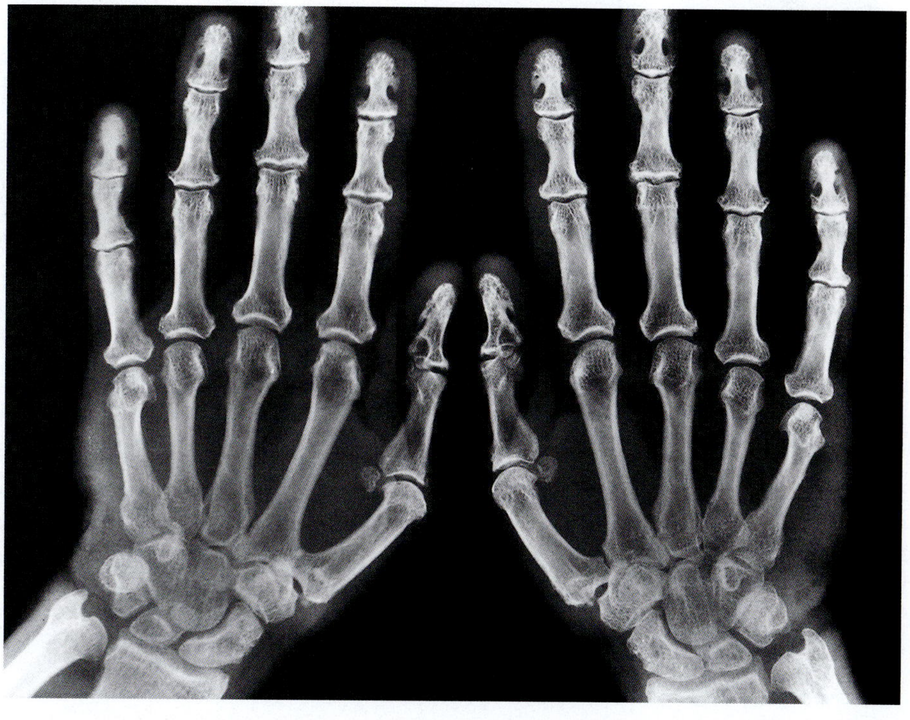

Figure 5.63 ■ **Acromegalic osteoarthritis.** Dorsovolar radiograph of both hands of a 42-year-old man shows widening of some and narrowing of other joint spaces, enlargement of the distal tufts and the bases of terminal phalanges, and beaklike osteophytes affecting particularly the heads of the metacarpals. Note the soft tissue prominence and the large sesamoid bones at the first metacarpophalangeal joints. The sesamoid index (derived by multiplying the vertical and horizontal diameters of the sesamoid bone) is 48 in this patient; normally, it should not exceed 20 to 25.

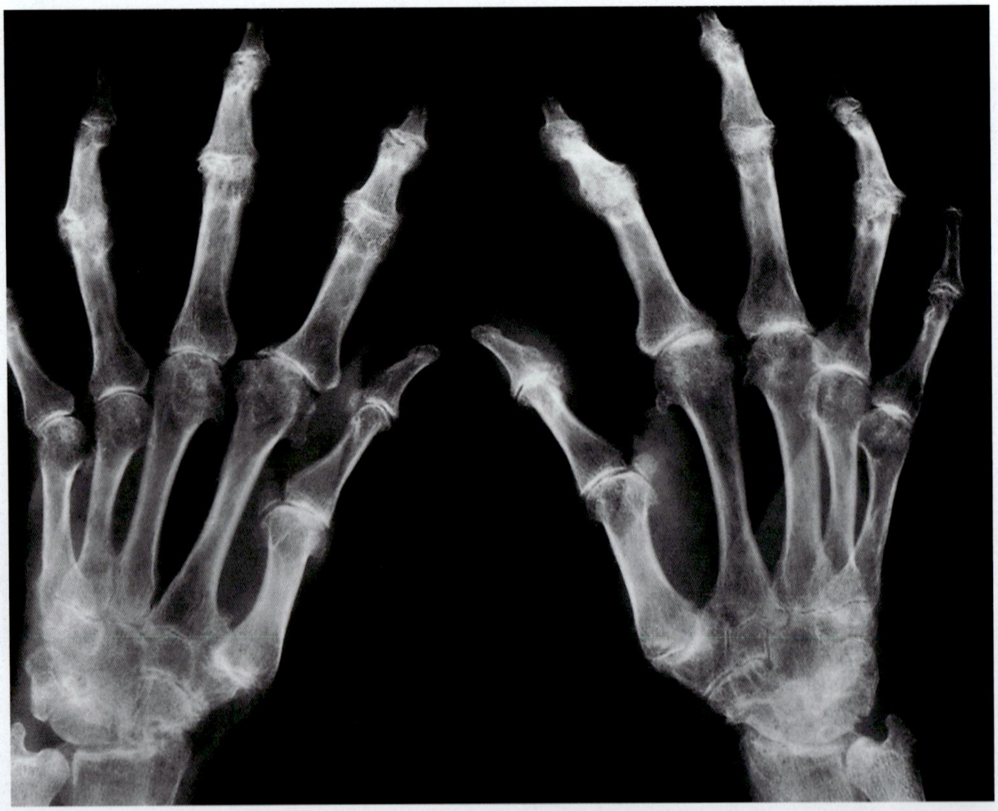

Figure 5.64 ■ Hemochromatosis arthropathy. Oblique radiographs of both hands of a 53-year-old woman show beaklike osteophytes arising from the heads of the second and third metacarpals on the radial aspect of both hands. The interphalangeal, metacarpophalangeal, and carpal articulations are also affected.

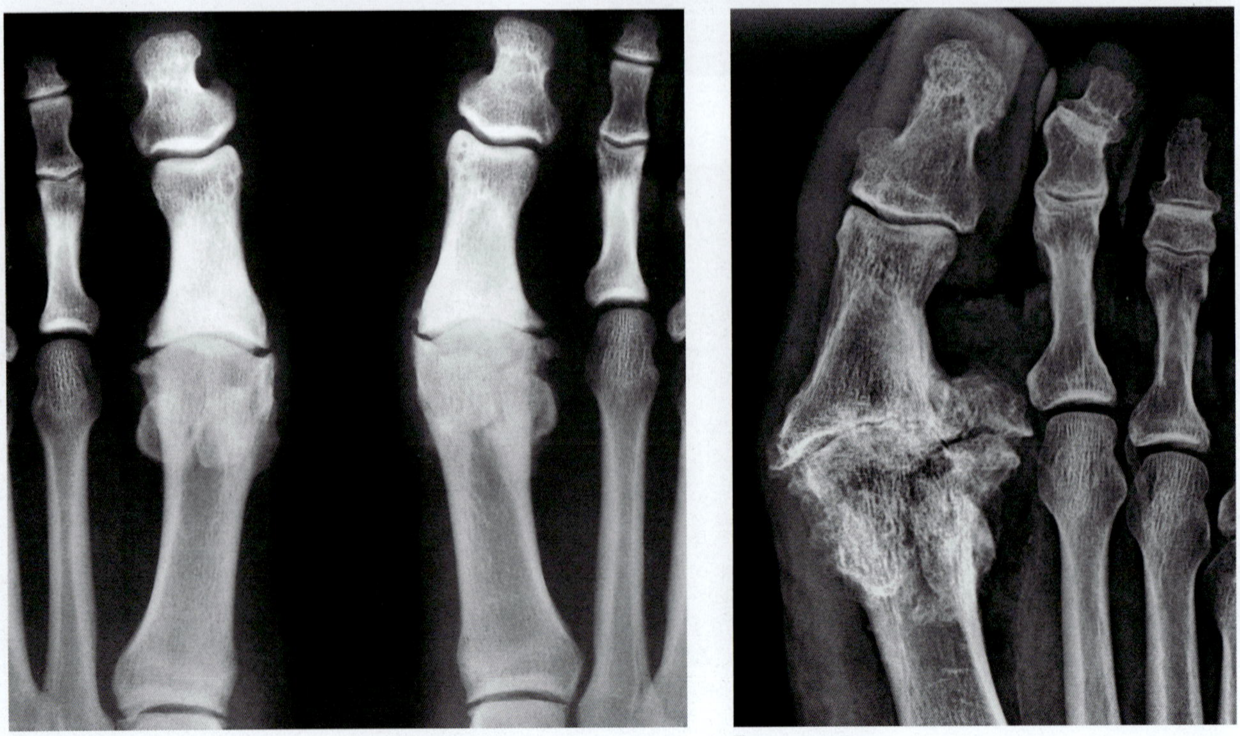

A B

Figure 5.65 ■ Hallux rigidus. A: Dorsoplantar radiograph of the great and second toes of the feet of a 33-year-old man shows osteoarthritis of the first metatarsophalangeal joints, which are known as *hallux rigidus* (*hallux limitus*). Note the narrowing of the joint space, subchondral sclerosis, and marginal osteophytes. **B:** More advanced osteoarthritis of the first metatarsophalangeal joint is seen in this 72-year-old woman.

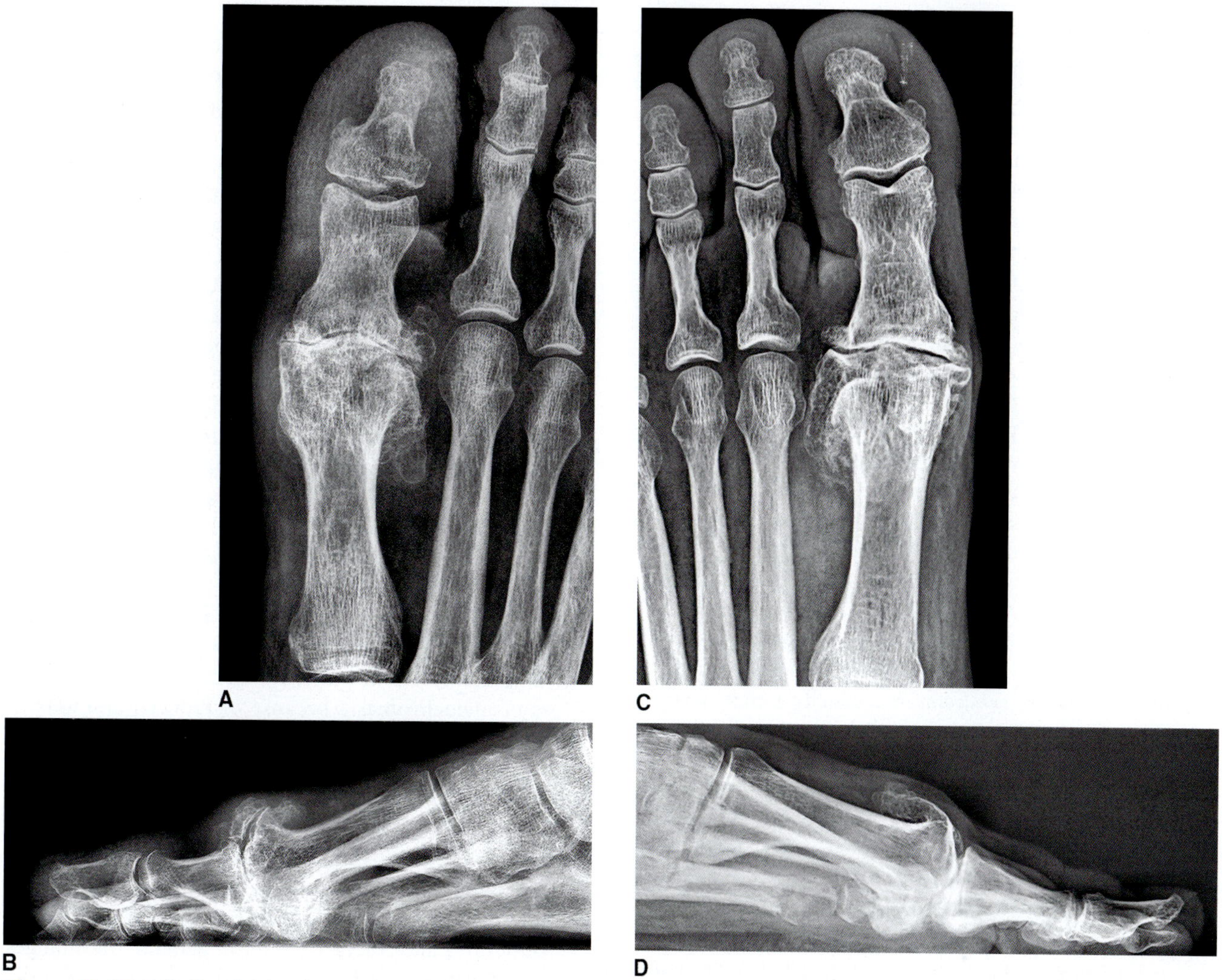

Figure 5.66 ■ **Hallux rigidus.** Anteroposterior **(A)** and lateral **(B)** radiographs of the right great toe of an 80-year-old man show severe narrowing of the first metatarsophalangeal joint associated with subchondral sclerosis and formation of prominent osteophytes. Anteroposterior **(C)** and lateral **(D)** radiographs of the left great toe of a 69-year-old man demonstrate advanced osteoarthritis of the fist metatarsophalangeal joint. Observe on the lateral view a very prominent dorsal osteophyte.

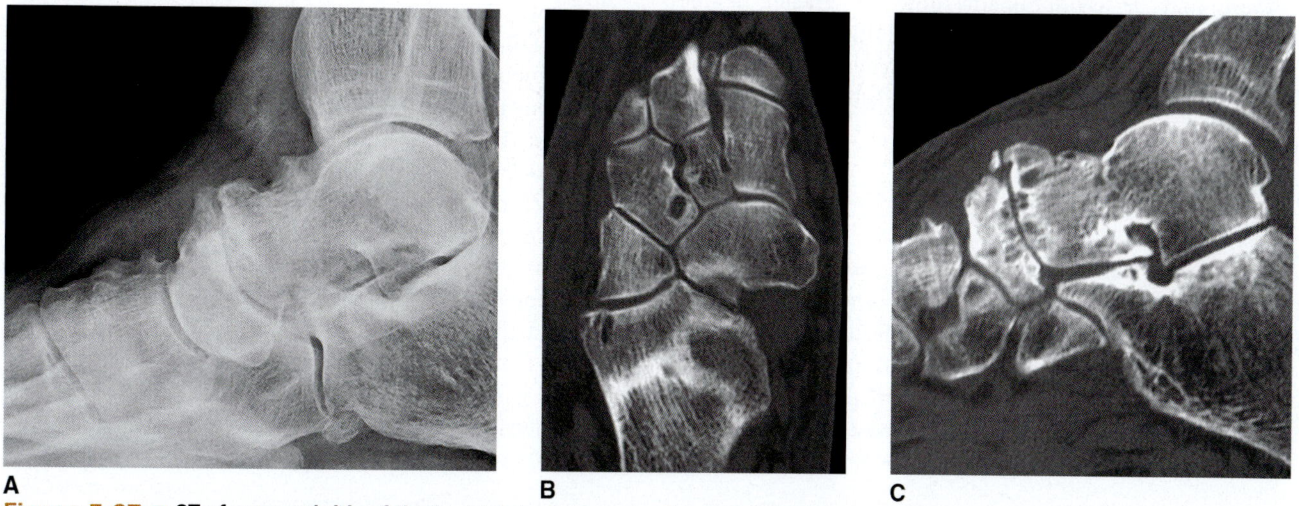

Figure 5.67 ■ **CT of osteoarthritis of the foot joints. A:** Lateral radiograph of the right foot of a 60-year-old man shows narrowing of the talonavicular joint and formation of dorsal osteophytes. Coronal **(B)** and sagittal **(C)** reformatted CT images show in addition subchondral sclerosis and cystlike lesions at the talonavicular, calcaneocuboid, naviculocuneiform, and subtalar joints.

Clinical Features

Patients with *cervical facet joints arthropathy* may complain of neck stiffness and pain, usually more severe during head and neck movements. In patients with *lumbar facet joints osteoarthritis*, the pain may radiate to the posterior thigh and could be exacerbated by bending. Those patients with *degenerative disk disease* experience pain related to activity while twisting, bending, or lifting heavy objects. The symptoms may flare up at time and then return to a low-grade pain level. Some patients become symptomatic when sitting for a long time. Occasionally, back pain may be associated with leg weakness, numbness, or tingling. Assuming reclining position may alleviate the symptoms. The causes of back pain are not completely understood, but include the following: ingrowths of nociceptive nerves into the intervertebral disk, nerve root compression by protruding diskal tissue and osteophytes, sensitization of the nerve roots by tumor necrosis factor alpha produced by protruding intervertebral disk tissue, and local nerve root ischemia. *Intervertebral disk herniation* is associated with radiculopathy and pain in the buttocks, legs, and feet. Commonly, the patients will experience sciatic pain. Patients with *DISH syndrome* are usually either asymptomatic or the pain is minimal, although generalized stiffness is a common complaint and there may be moderate limitation of spine motion. Posture is generally unaffected, although occasionally some patients may develop kyphosis. If the cervical spine is severely affected, the patient may complain of dysphagia. The complications of degenerative spine disease, such as spinal stenosis or spondylolisthesis bring more severe symptoms. The clinical hallmark of *spinal stenosis* is pseudoclaudication (so-called neurogenic claudication). Patient complains of pain and discomfort associated with weakness and paresthesias in the buttocks, thighs, and legs. The gait may become unsteady. Standing or walking induces the symptoms that are relieved by sitting, squatting, or flexing forward. Minimal *spondylolisthesis* may be asymptomatic; however, greater degree of vertebral displacement may result in low back pain with or without radiation into the leg, associated with signs of nerve root impingement, or even cauda equina syndrome.

Pathology

Facet joint arthritis results from the excessive load (combination of applied compression and torsion forces) on these anatomic structures. The morphologic features are identical to those seen in arthritis of other diarthrodial joints, namely, capsular laxity, synovitis, cartilage fibrillation followed by cartilage loss and eburnation of the exposed bone, and formation of marginal osteophytes.

In *degenerative disk disease*, the pathologic changes occur as a result of the disruption of the vertebral end plates. Evidence of degeneration of these structures is seen as microfractures at the bone–cartilage interface, advancing of calcification into the cartilage from the bone surface, and invasion of blood vessels from the subchondral bone into the cartilaginous end plate, with subsequent endochondral ossification. With disruption of the end plate, the disk components show a rapid progress of degeneration manifested by focal necrosis, fissuring, calcification, and tearing of annulus fibrosus. The fibrous tissue is replacing normal disk tissue, including the nucleus pulposus. Large horizontal clefts develop in the central part of the disk containing nitrogen gas, which is seen on the radiography as radiolucent areas termed vacuum phenomenon. As disk degeneration progresses, there is subsequent narrowing of the disk space, followed by new bone formation at the junction of the annulus fibrosus and the vertebral body. Ossification of the cartilaginous end plate also contributes to disk space narrowing (Fig. 5.68).

Histopathologic features are characterized by variety of alternations in the nucleus pulposus, annulus fibrosus, and the vertebral end plate. In nucleus pulposus, there is loss of metachromasia because of reduced amounts of aggrecan and a reduction in the heavily sulfated glycosaminoglycan side chains. Mucoid material is replaced by fibrous tissue. Slits propagate from the nucleus pulposus into the annulus fibrosus. In the annulus fibrosus, blood vessels grow inward from the vasculature of the outer part of annulus. Microscopic tears appear, followed by fibrocartilaginous metaplasia. In the vertebral end plates noted are microfractures and fracture repair. In general, the changes in the end plates are very similar to those occurring in the articular cartilage of diarthrodial joints in osteoarthritis.

Tears in the periphery of the annulus fibrosus where the collagen bundles attach to the vertebral bodies by Sharpey fibers initiate the pathologic process of *spondylosis deformans*. This is followed by anterior and anterolateral protrusio/herniation of disk tissue. Once displacement has occurred, dissection of the anterior longitudinal ligament from its osseous attachment by the displaced disk permits extension of the disk tissue along the anterior aspect of vertebral body. Continuous tearing in these areas stimulates the development of bony outgrowths, termed osteophytes, along the anterior and lateral aspects of the vertebral body (Fig. 5.69).

Diffuse idiopathic skeletal hyperostosis (DISH), also known as ankylosing hyperostosis, occurs as a result of ligamentous ossification without significant disk disease or facet arthropathy, leading to ankylosis of the vertebral column. Pathologic features include ligamentous calcification and ossification with periosteal new bone formation at the anterior vertebral surface, linked to "armor plating" (Fig. 5.70).

(Continued on page 181)

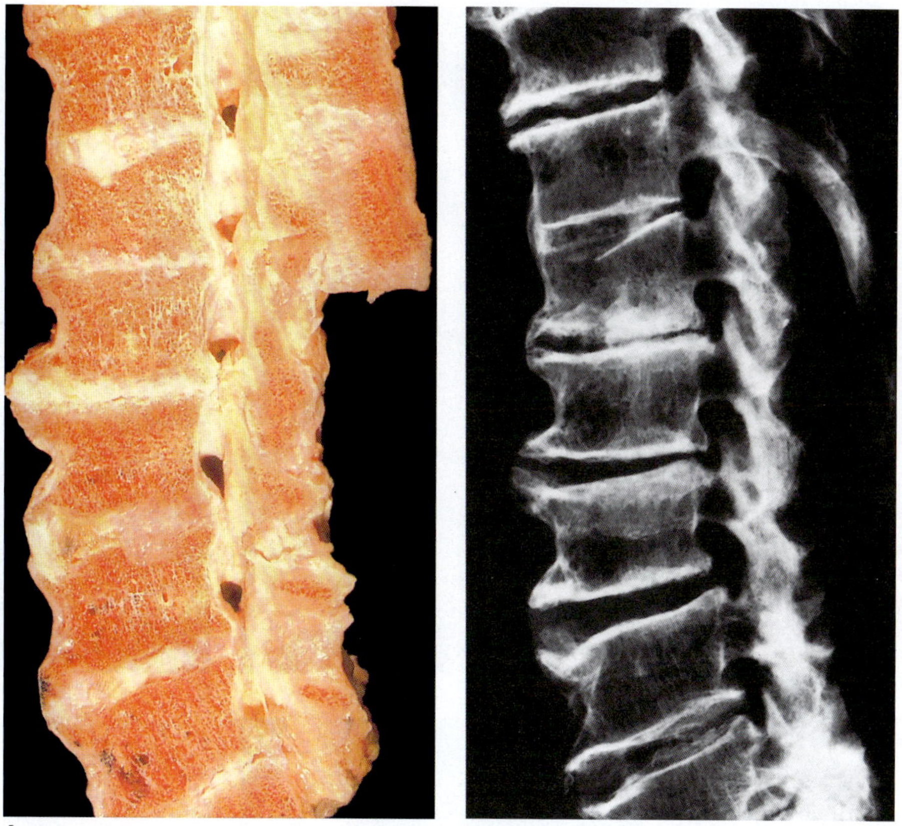

A B

Figure 5.68 ■ **Pathology of the degenerative disk disease.** Sagittal section of the thoracolumbar spine **(A)** and specimen radiograph **(B)** show several degenerative disks. Note narrowing of the disk spaces, end-plate sclerosis, and formation of the anterior osteophytes. (Reprinted from Bullough PG, Boachie-Adjei O. *Atlas of Spinal Diseases*. Philadelphia, PA: JB Lippincott Company; Gower Medical Publishing; 1988; Fig. 7.20, p. 83.)

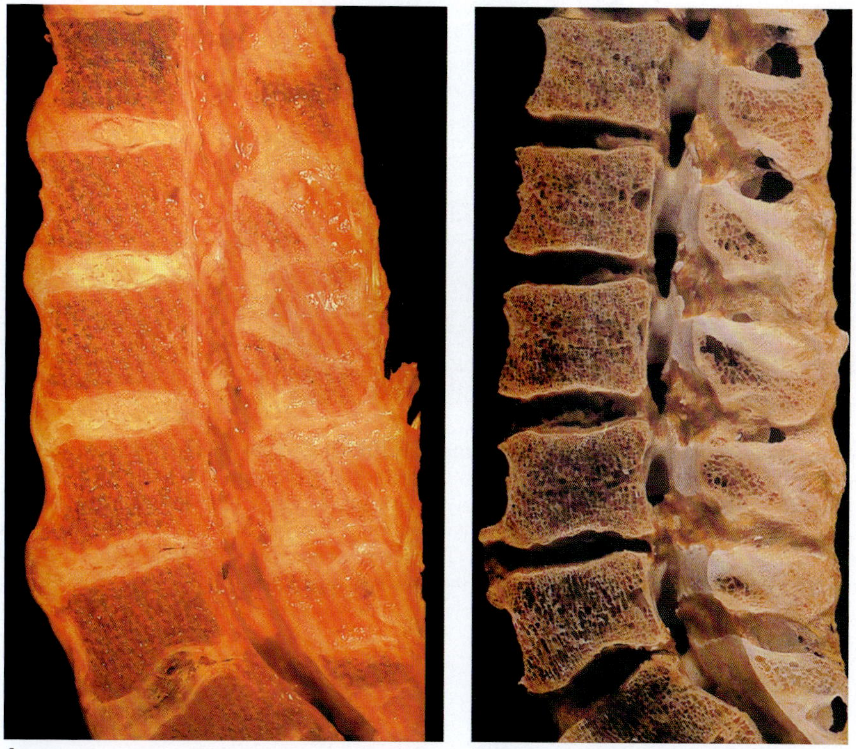

A B

Figure 5.69 ■ **Pathology of spondylosis deformans.** Sagittal section of the lumbar spine **(A)** and macerated specimen **(B)** show anterior protrusio of several intervertebral disks causing bulging of the annulus fibrosus and anterior longitudinal ligament. There is narrowing of the disk space L4–L5 associated with formation of anterior osteophytes, but remaining disk spaces are relatively normal. (Reprinted from Bullough PG, Boachie-Adjei O. *Atlas of Spinal Diseases*. Philadelphia, PA: JB Lippincott Company; Gower Medical Publishing; 1988; Fig. 5.7, p. 60.)

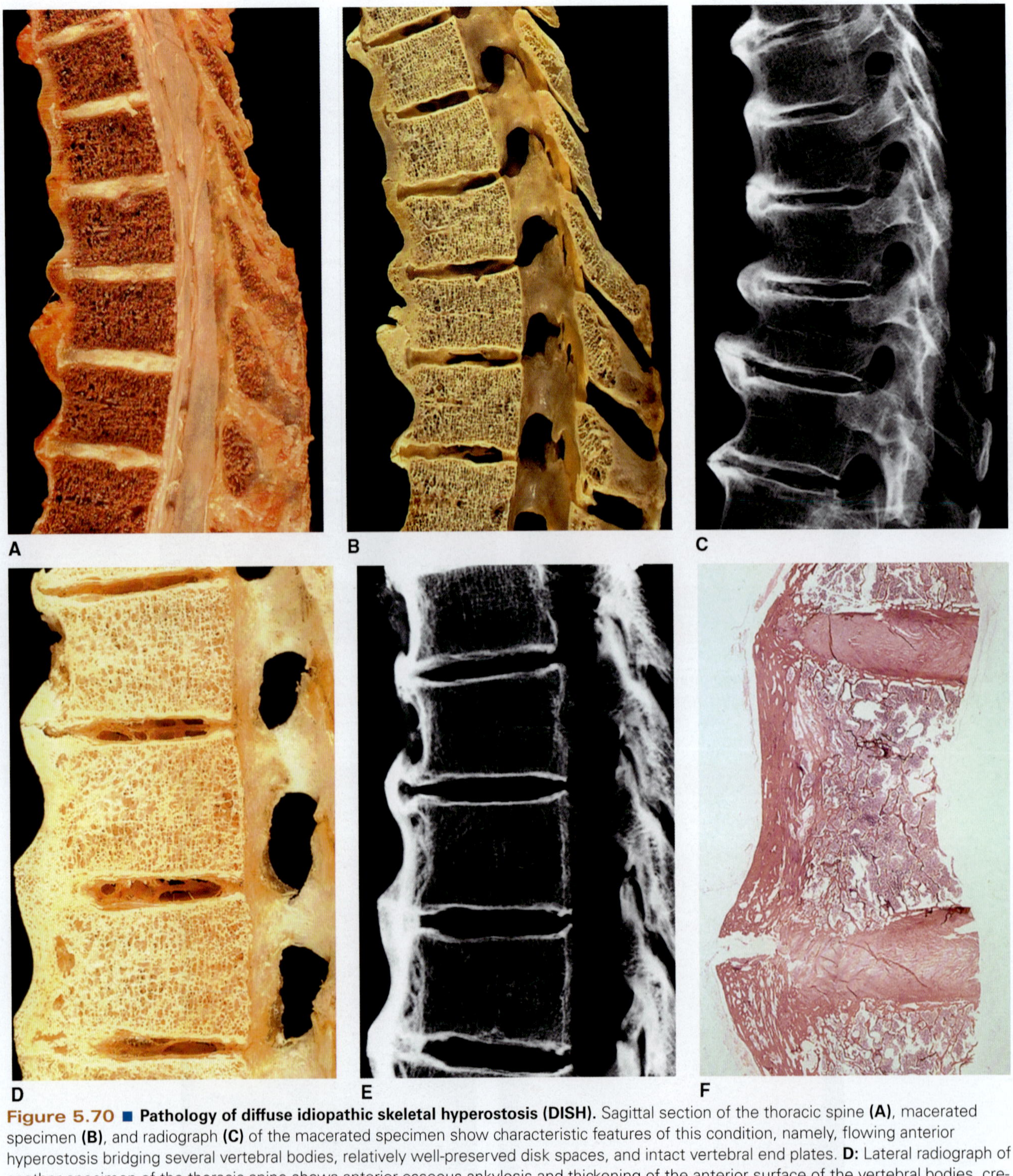

Figure 5.70 ■ Pathology of diffuse idiopathic skeletal hyperostosis (DISH). Sagittal section of the thoracic spine **(A)**, macerated specimen **(B)**, and radiograph **(C)** of the macerated specimen show characteristic features of this condition, namely, flowing anterior hyperostosis bridging several vertebral bodies, relatively well-preserved disk spaces, and intact vertebral end plates. **D:** Lateral radiograph of another specimen of the thoracic spine shows anterior osseous ankylosis and thickening of the anterior surface of the vertebral bodies, creating "armor plate" appearance. The disk spaces are preserved. **E:** On the sagittal section of the specimen, observe ossifications confined to the anterior longitudinal ligament. **F:** A photomicrograph shows the details of anterior flowing hyperostosis. (Reprinted from Bullough PG, Boachie-Adjei O. *Atlas of Spinal Diseases*. Philadelphia, PA: JB Lippincott Company; Gower Medical Publishing; 1988; Fig. 9.33, p. 114.)

Osteoarthritis of the Synovial Joints

Degenerative changes of the vertebral facet joints are very common, particularly in the mid- and lower cervical and the lower lumbar segments. As in the other synovial joints, the characteristic radiographic features include diminution of the joint space, eburnation of subchondral bone, and osteophyte formation, all of which are most easily demonstrated on the oblique projection of the spine (Fig. 5.71). In the cervical spine, osteophytes on the posterior aspect of a vertebral body may encroach on the neural foramina or the thecal sac, causing various neurologic symptoms. In addition to the standard oblique views (Fig. 5.72), conventional tomography (in the past) (Fig. 5.73A) or at the present time CT (Fig. 5.73B) or MRI (Fig. 5.73C,D) may demonstrate these changes (Fig. 5.73). Anterior osteophytes, however, are as a rule asymptomatic unless they are unusually prominent. Involvement of the apophyseal joints may exhibit a "vacuum phenomenon" (Fig. 5.74), which in fact represents gas in the joint. This finding is almost pathognomonic for a degenerative process.

As in other diarthrodial joints, degenerative changes of the sacroiliac joints are manifested by narrowing of the joint space, subchondral sclerosis, and osteophytosis (Fig. 5.75). Occasionally, vacuum phenomenon may be present (Fig. 5.76). It is important to note in the evaluation of the sacroiliac joints that only the lower half of the radiographic sacroiliac joint space is lined by synovium; the upper portion is a syndesmotic joint (Fig. 5.77).

Degenerative Disk Disease

The radiographic findings of degenerative disk disease include disk space narrowing and osteophytosis at the marginal borders of the adjacent vertebral bodies. The vacuum phenomenon in the disk space is common (Fig. 5.78). These radiolucent collections of gas, principally nitrogen, are related to the negative pressure created by abnormally altered joint

(Continued on page 184)

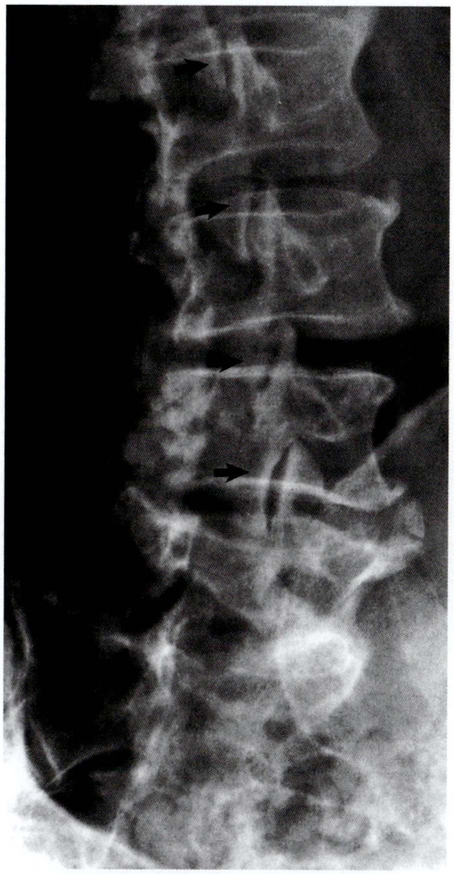

Figure 5.71 ■ Osteoarthritis of the facet joints. Oblique radiograph of the lumbar spine in a 68-year-old man demonstrates advanced osteoarthritis of the facet joints. Narrowing of the joint spaces, eburnation of the articular margins, and small osteophytes (*arrows*) are similar to the changes seen in osteoarthritis of the large synovial joints.

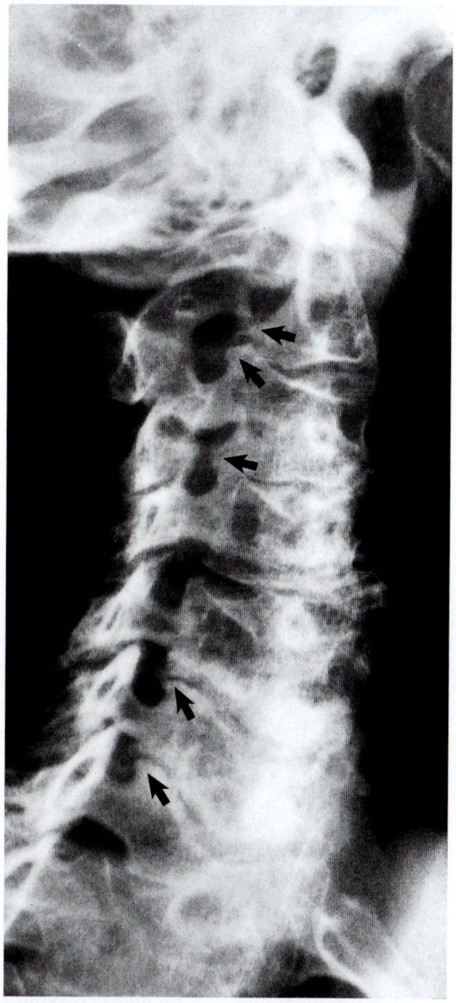

Figure 5.72 ■ Encroachment of the neural foramina. Oblique radiograph of the cervical spine in a 72-year-old woman who reported neck pain radiating to both shoulders reveals multiple posterior osteophytes encroaching on numerous neural foramina (*arrows*).

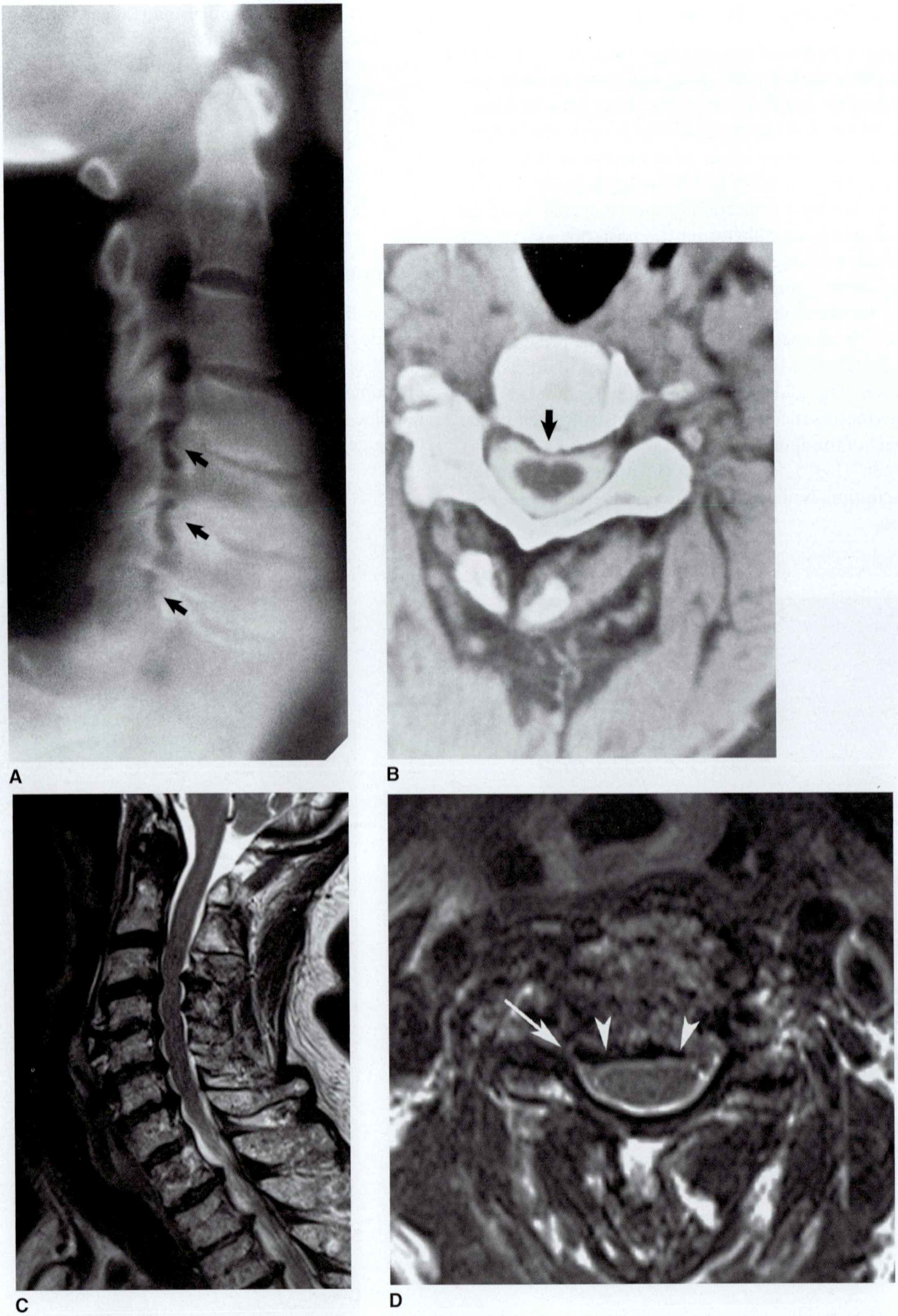

Figure 5.73 ■ **Encroachment of the neural foramina and the thecal sac. A:** Conventional lateral tomogram of the cervical spine in a 56-year-old man demonstrates encroachment of the neural foramina by posterior osteophytes (*arrows*). **B:** CT section at the level of C3 obtained during myelography demonstrates a large posterior osteophyte impinging on the thecal sac and compressing the subarachnoid space filled with contrast agent (*arrow*). **C:** Sagittal T2-weighted MRI in 73-year-old man demonstrates multilevel degenerative disk disease with anterior and posterior osteophytes impinging on the thecal sac. Note the deformity of the ventral aspect of the cord at C3–C4, C4–C5, and C6–C7. **D:** Axial T2-weighted MRI at C4–C5 level demonstrates the posterior osteophytes deforming the ventral aspect of the cord (*arrowheads*) and the narrowing of the right neural foramen (*arrow*).

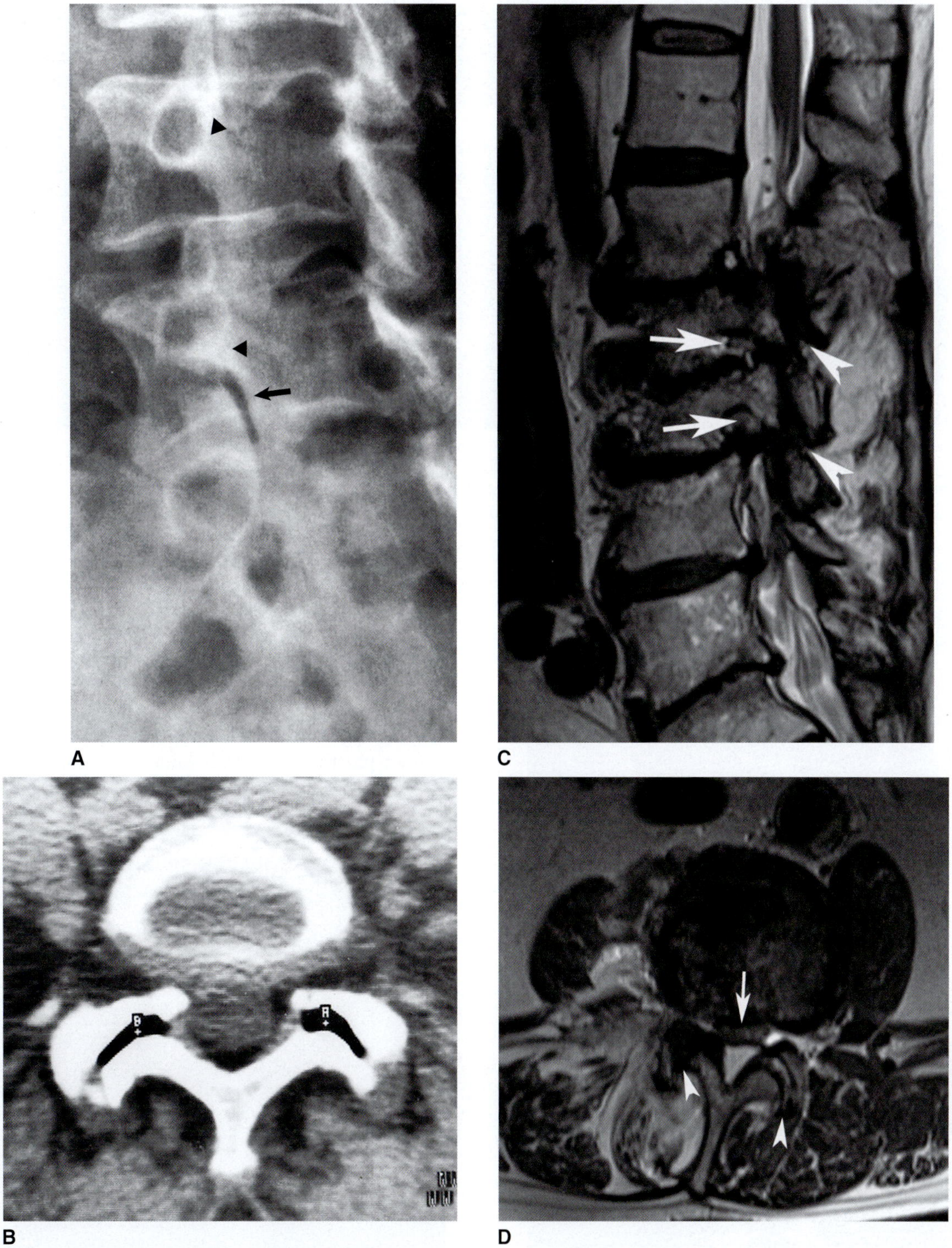

Figure 5.74 ■ **Osteoarthritis of the apophyseal joints. A:** Oblique radiograph of the lumbosacral spine in a 56-year-old man demonstrates a vacuum phenomenon of the facet joint L5–S1 (*arrow*) and eburnation of the subarticular bone (*arrowheads*). **B:** CT section through both facets clearly demonstrates the presence of gas, as confirmed by the Hounsfield values. These units are related to the attenuation coefficient for various tissues in the body and represent absorption values directly related to tissue density. Note also the hypertrophic spur arising from the right facet and encroaching on the spinal canal. **C:** Sagittal T2-weighted MRI in an 84-year-old woman with scoliosis demonstrates advanced degenerative disk disease with severe facet arthrosis (*arrowheads*) associated with stenosis of the neural foramen and impingement of the exiting nerve roots (*arrows*). **D:** Axial T2-weighted MR image demonstrates an annular bulge with bilateral facet arthrosis (*arrowheads*), severe stenosis of the thecal sac associated with clumping of the nerve roots (*arrow*), and bilateral foraminal stenosis, more prominent on the right.

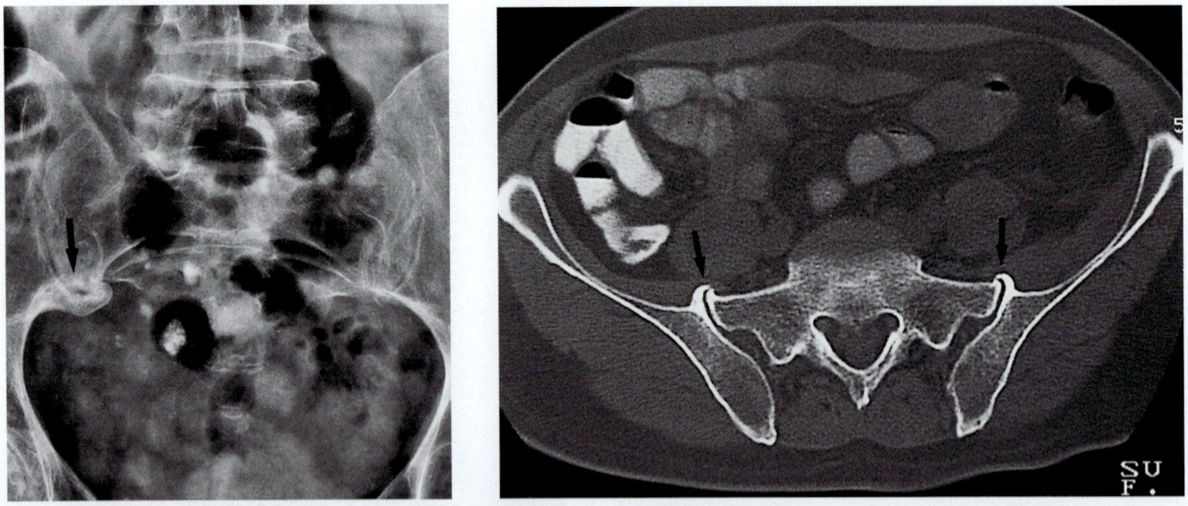

A B

Figure 5.75 ■ Osteoarthritis of the sacroiliac joints. A: Degenerative changes in the sacroiliac joints, seen here affecting predominantly the right sacroiliac joint (*arrow*) in an 82-year-old woman, are manifested by narrowing of the joint space and osteophytosis. **B:** In another patient, a 68-year-old man, osteoarthritis of both sacroiliac joints (*arrows*) is demonstrated on axial CT image.

or disk spaces. Degenerative disk disease, in combination with degenerative changes in the apophyseal joints, may lead to degenerative spondylolisthesis (see Fig. 5.78). Recently, a destructive diskovertebral degenerative disease of the lumbar spine has been reported, similar to rapidly progressing coxarthropathy (see previous text), characterized by vertebral malalignment, severe disk resorption, intervertebral vacuum phenomenon, and "bone sand" formation secondary to vertebral fragmentation.

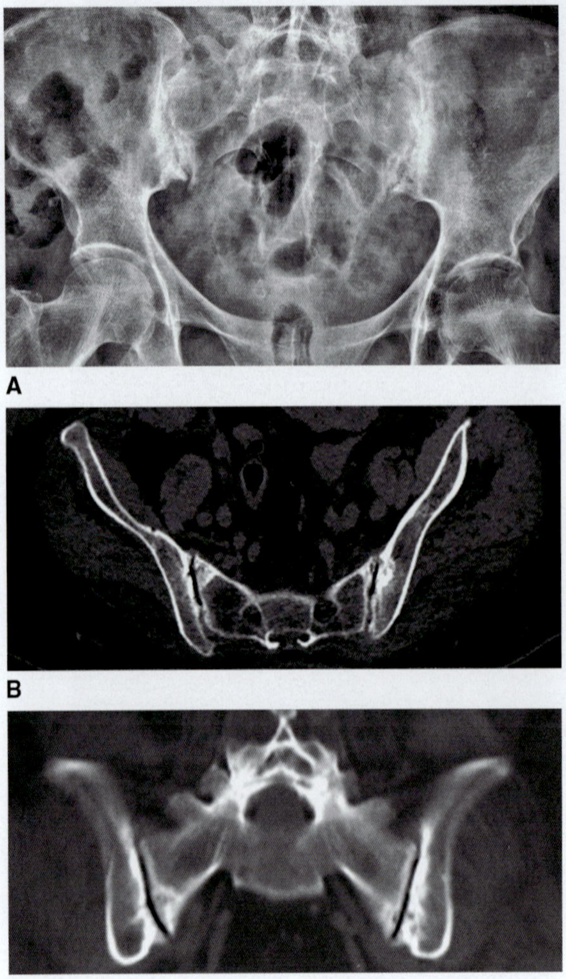

A B C

Figure 5.76 ■ Osteoarthritis of the sacroiliac joints.
A: Anteroposterior radiograph of the pelvis of a 70-year-old woman shows narrowing and sclerosis of both sacroiliac joints associated with formation of marginal osteophytes. Axial **(B)** and coronal **(C)** reformatted CT images show in addition small subchondral cysts and vacuum phenomenon.

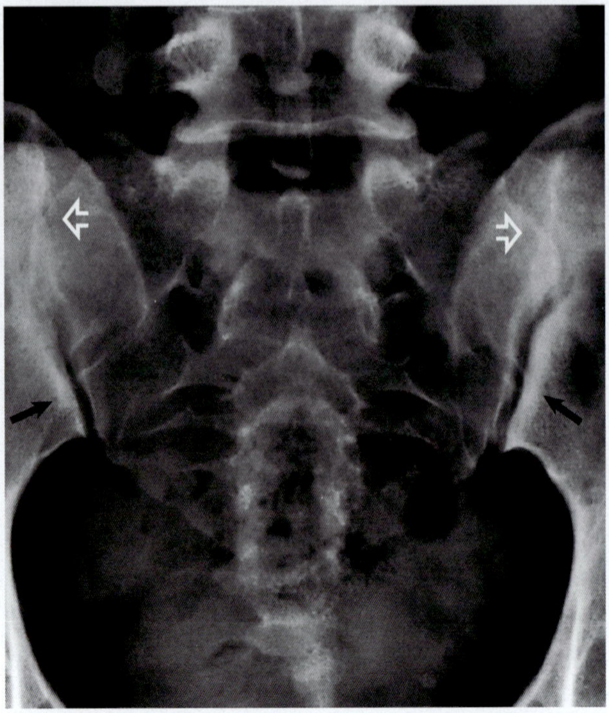

Figure 5.77 ■ Sacroiliac joints. The true diarthrodial portion of the sacroiliac joint comprises only approximately 50% of the radiographic joint space (*arrows*). The upper part is a syndesmotic joint (*open arrows*).

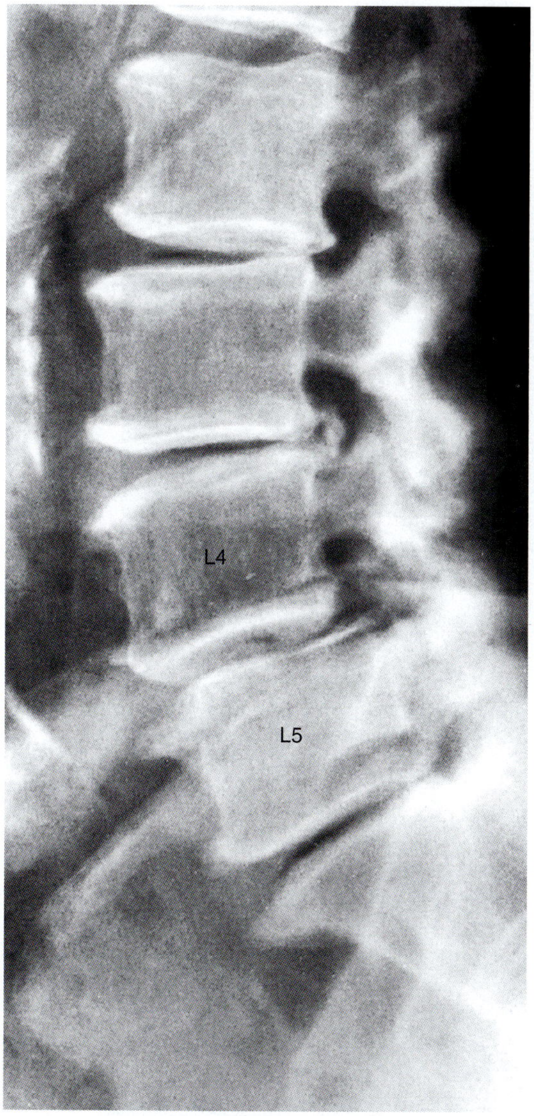

Figure 5.78 ■ Degenerative disk disease. Lateral radiograph of the lumbosacral spine in a 66-year-old woman demonstrates advanced degenerative disk disease at multiple levels. Note the radiolucent collections of gas in several disks (the vacuum phenomenon) as well as the narrowing of the disk spaces and marginal osteophytes. Grade 1 degenerative spondylolisthesis is seen at the L4–L5 level.

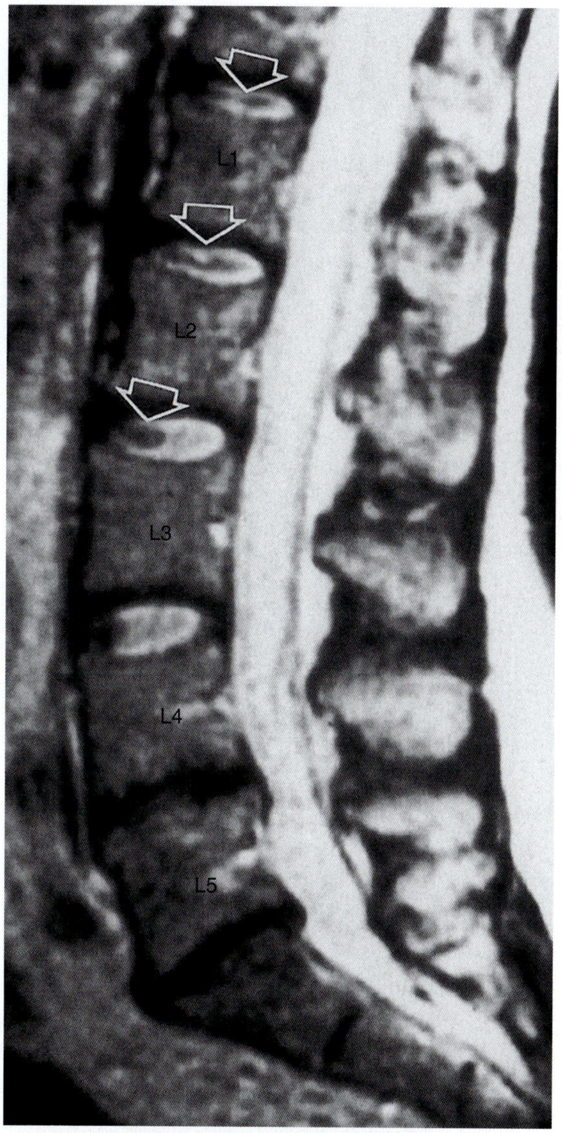

Figure 5.79 ■ MRI of degenerative disk disease. Sagittal T2-weighted MR image shows early degenerative changes in the T12–L1, L1–L2, and L2–L3 intervertebral disks (*open arrows*), more advanced process in the L3–L4 disk, and severe degenerative disk disease at L4–L5 and L5–S1. At the latter levels, markedly decreased intervertebral spaces and low signal intensity of degenerated disks are seen. (From Bloem JL, Sartoris DJ, eds. *MRI and CT of the Musculoskeletal System. A Text-Atlas.* Baltimore, MD: Williams & Wilkins; 1992.)

MRI is highly effective in demonstrating changes of disk degeneration. Decrease in the water content results in a decreased signal intensity of the nucleus pulposus on T2-weighted images (Fig. 5.79). Frequently, additional characteristic alterations are seen in the end plates of the vertebral bodies adjacent to the degenerative disk. These abnormalities consist of a focal decreased signal intensity of the marrow on T1-weighted images and increased signal on T2- or T2*-weighted images (Fig. 5.80). According to Modic, these alterations represent subchondral vascularized fibrous tissue associated with end plate fissuring and disruption (type I). These changes may progress to fatty marrow end-plate conversion (type II) (Fig. 5.81) and later to sclerosis (type III).

Spondylosis Deformans

Spondylosis deformans is a degenerative condition marked by the formation of anterior and lateral osteophytes as a result of anterior and anterolateral disk herniation (Fig. 5.82). The condition occurs more frequently in men, particularly those over 60 years of age. It is also related to occupation: more extensive involvement of the spine is seen in patients who do heavy physical labor. As Schmorl and other investigators have pointed out, the initiating factors in the development of this condition are abnormalities in the peripheral fibers of the annulus fibrosus that result

(Continued on page 188)

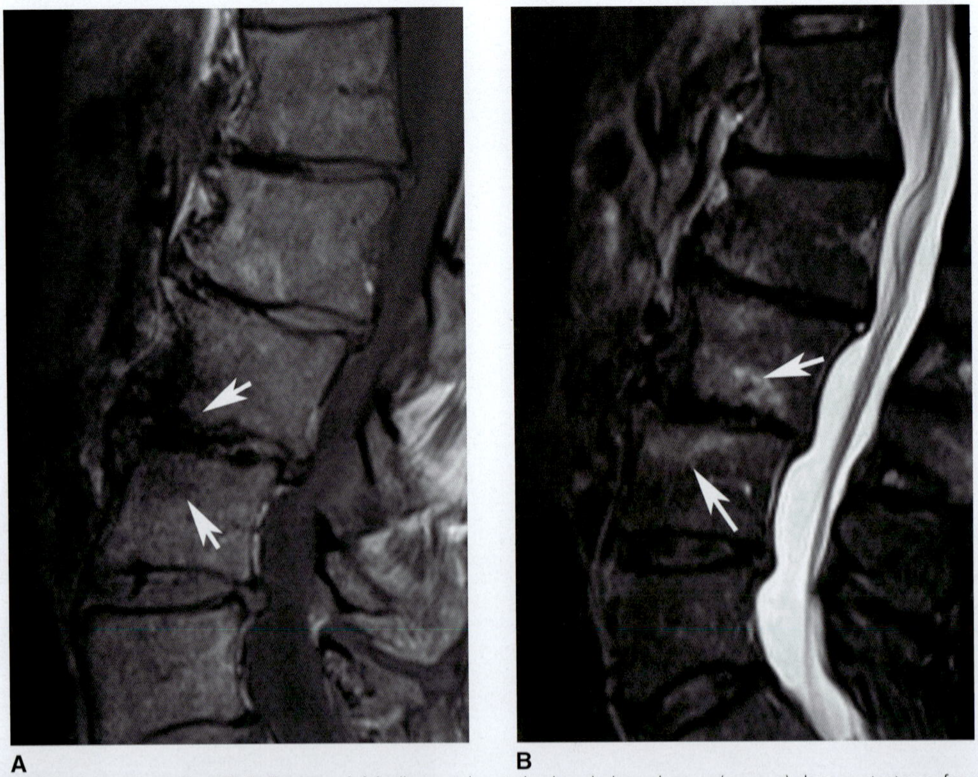

Figure 5.80 ■ **MRI of degenerative disk disease.** A Modic type I vertebral end-plate change (*arrows*) demonstrates a focus of low signal intensity in subchondral marrow on T1-weighted sagittal MR image **(A)** and high signal intensity on short time inversion recovery (STIR) imaging **(B)**.

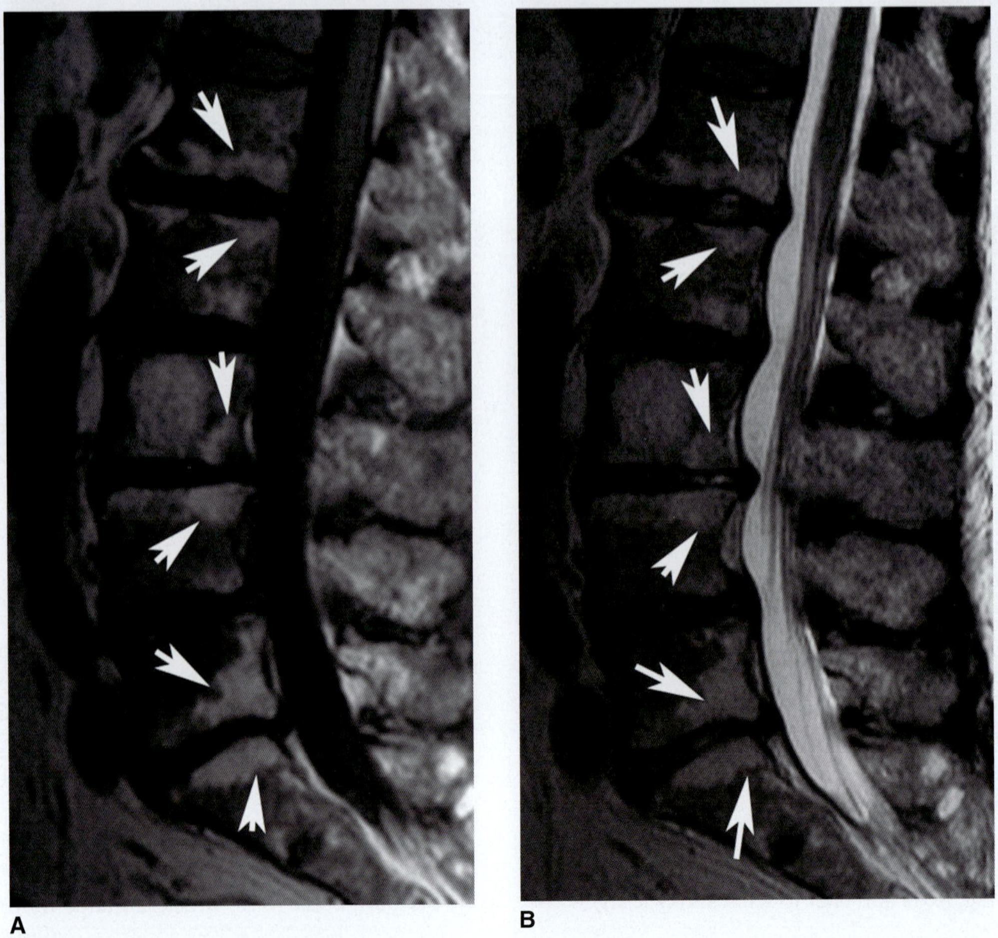

Figure 5.81 ■ **MRI of degenerative disk disease.** Modic type II end-plate changes in degenerative disk disease consisting of focal areas of yellow marrow conversion (*arrows*) are seen on sagittal T1-weighted **(A)** and sagittal T2-weighted **(B)** MR images.

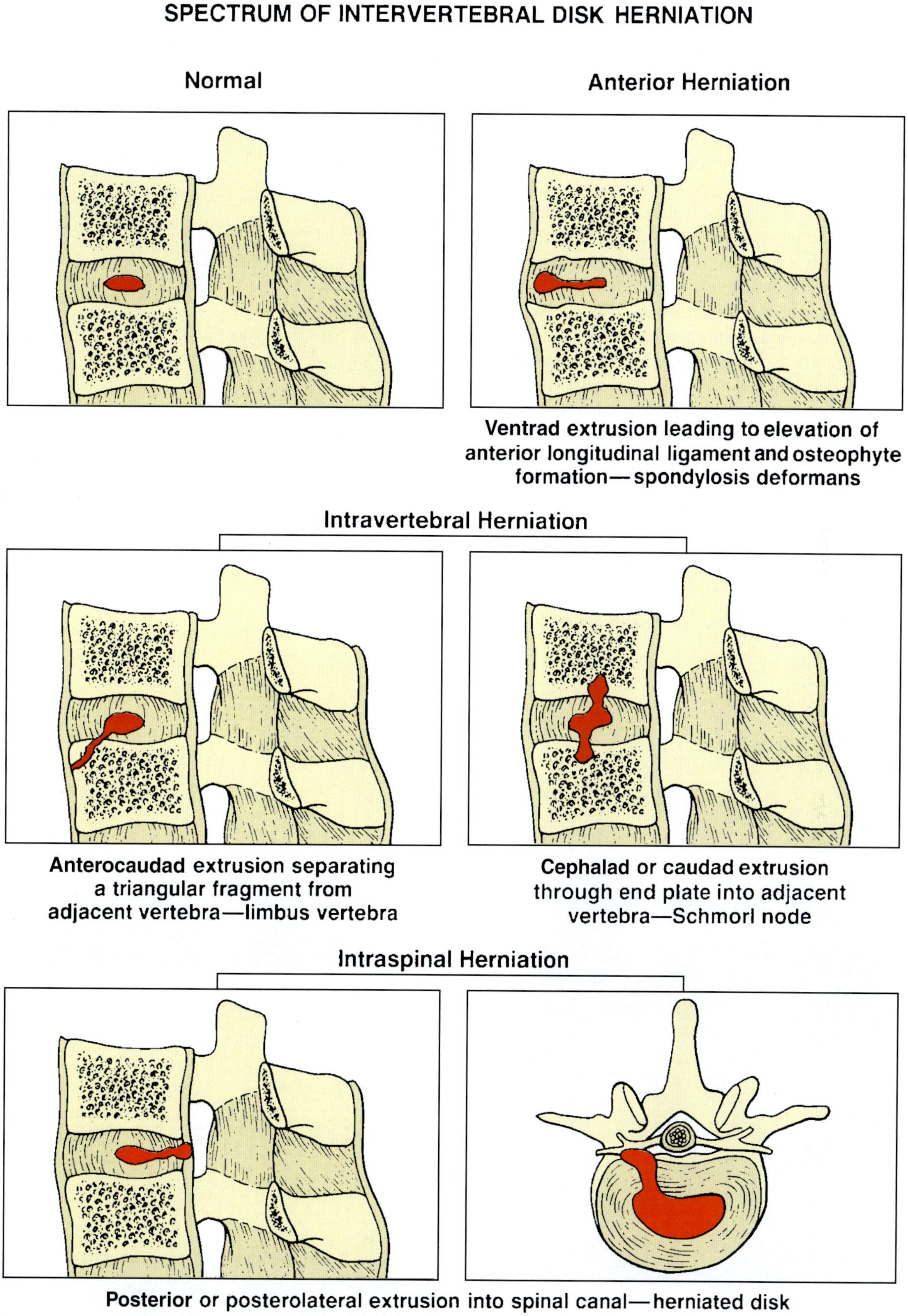

Figure 5.82 ■ **The spectrum of intervertebral disk herniation.**

in weakening of the anchorage of the intervertebral disk to the vertebral body at the site where Sharpey fibers attach to the vertebral rim. Tearing of the fibers weakens the annulus fibrosus. The restraints on the nucleus pulposus are lost, and the disk protrudes forward. Further stress lifts the anterior longitudinal ligament from the vertebral body, and a buttress of periosteal new bone fills the area of separation. The osteophytes enlarge in horizontal direction and occasionally curve to bridge the intervertebral disk space. Unlike degenerative disk disease, the intervertebral spaces in spondylosis deformans are relatively well preserved, with the primary radiographic feature being extensive osteophytosis (Figs. 5.83 and 5.84). Osteophytes at the posterior aspect of the vertebral bodies are more common in the cervical region and less frequent in the thoracic or lumbar segments. These osteophytes must be differentiated from the delicate syndesmophytes of ankylosing spondylitis, from the large characteristically asymmetric bone excrescences that are seen in psoriatic arthritis and reactive arthritis involving the lateral aspect of vertebral bodies, and from the flowing, usually anterior, hyperostosis of the DISH syndrome.

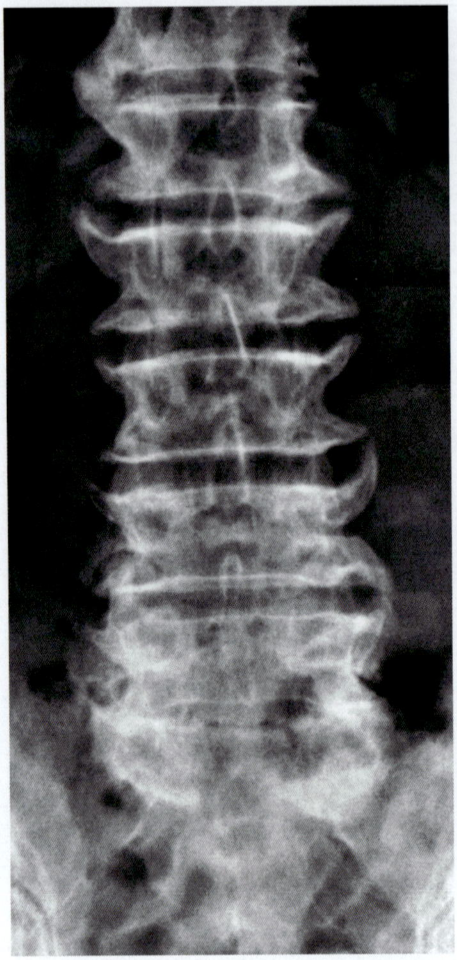

Figure 5.83 ■ **Spondylosis deformans.** Anteroposterior radiograph of the lumbosacral spine in a 68-year-old woman exhibits the typical changes of spondylosis deformans. Note the extensive osteophytosis and relatively well-preserved intervertebral disk spaces.

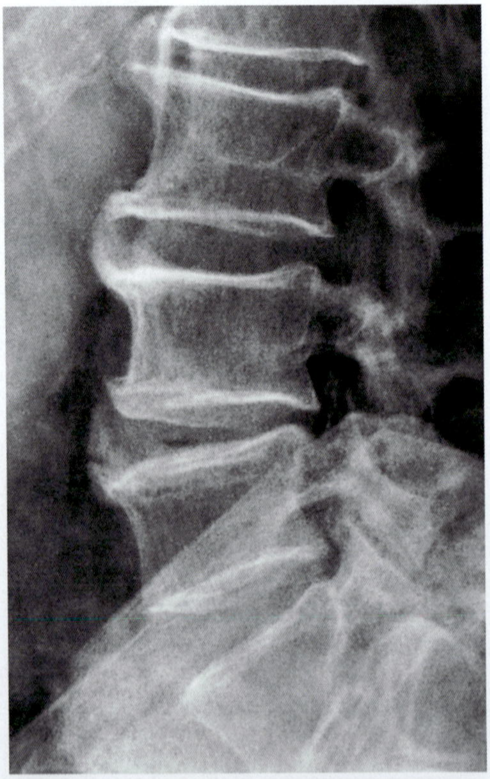

A

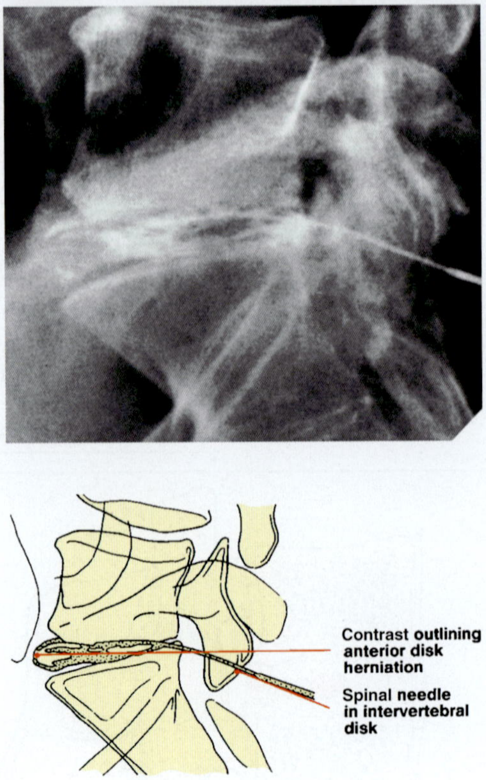

B

Figure 5.84 ■ **Spondylosis deformans. A:** Lateral radiograph of the lumbar spine shows a late stage of spondylosis deformans at the L2–L3, L3–L4, and L4–L5 levels characterized by large osteophytes on the anterior aspect of adjacent vertebral bodies as a result of anterior disk herniation. **B:** Anterior disk herniation can also be identified on diskography by contrast agent outlining the extruded disk material as seen here at L5–S1 level.

Diffuse Idiopathic Skeletal Hyperostosis (DISH)

DISH, a noninflammatory spondyloarthropathy, originally described by Forestier and popularized by Utsinger and Resnick, is characterized by flowing ossification (hyperostosis) along the anterior aspect of the vertebral bodies extending across the disk spaces. A layer of laminated reactive new bone is deposited in apposition to the anterior cortex of the vertebral body, but is usually separated from it by a narrow clear zone. As the condition becomes more advanced, thick hyperostotic, lumpy masses flow continuously over the anterior surface of the spine. Grossly, the appearance is that of a candle wax dripping down the anterior aspect of the spine, similar to melorheostosis. It is also associated with hyperostosis at the sites of tendon and ligament attachments to the bone, ligament ossification, and osteophytosis involving the axial and appendicular skeleton. Calcifications and ossifications may occur near the capsule of the hip joints and ligamentous attachments to the iliac crest, and "whiskering" is seen of the ischial tuberosities. In the knee, ossifications at the insertion of quadriceps tendon into the superior pole of the patella, and in the foot, at the insertion of Achilles tendon and fascia plantaris into the calcaneus are common. In the elbow, ossifications at the triceps tendon insertion to the olecranon are present. A lateral radiograph of the spine best demonstrates characteristic features of DISH. As in spondylosis deformans, the disk spaces and facet joints are usually well preserved (Figs. 5.85 and 5.86). It is important to distinguish this condition from the apparently similar "bamboo spine" seen in ankylosing spondylitis (see Figs. 6.71 and 6.72). In addition to spinal abnormalities, there are commonly associated extraspinal manifestations of this condition in form of extensive enthesopathy.

Complications of Degenerative Disease of the Spine

Degenerative Spondylolisthesis

One of the most common complications of degenerative disease of the spine, degenerative spondylolisthesis results from degenerative changes in the disk and apophyseal joints (Fig. 5.87). In this condition, there is anterior displacement of a vertebra onto the one below, which usually is easily recognized on the lateral view of the spine by the spinous process sign (Figs. 5.88 and 5.89). However, on occasion, the displacement may not be obvious on the standard lateral film, and radiographs must be obtained while the patient maximally extends and flexes the spine (Fig. 5.90). As Milgram pointed out, the stress applied by forward and backward motion of the spine discloses instability (spondylolisthesis), which may be overlooked on other projections.

Degenerative spondylolisthesis occurs in approximately 4% of patients with degenerative disk disease and affects women more frequently than men. It has a predilection for the L4–L5 spinal level. This predilection has been attributed to developmental or acquired alterations in the neural arch that lead to instability and abnormal stress. The stress applied to the vertebra may result in decompensation of the ligaments, hypermobility, instability, and osteoarthritis of adjacent apophyseal joints.

(Continued on page 191)

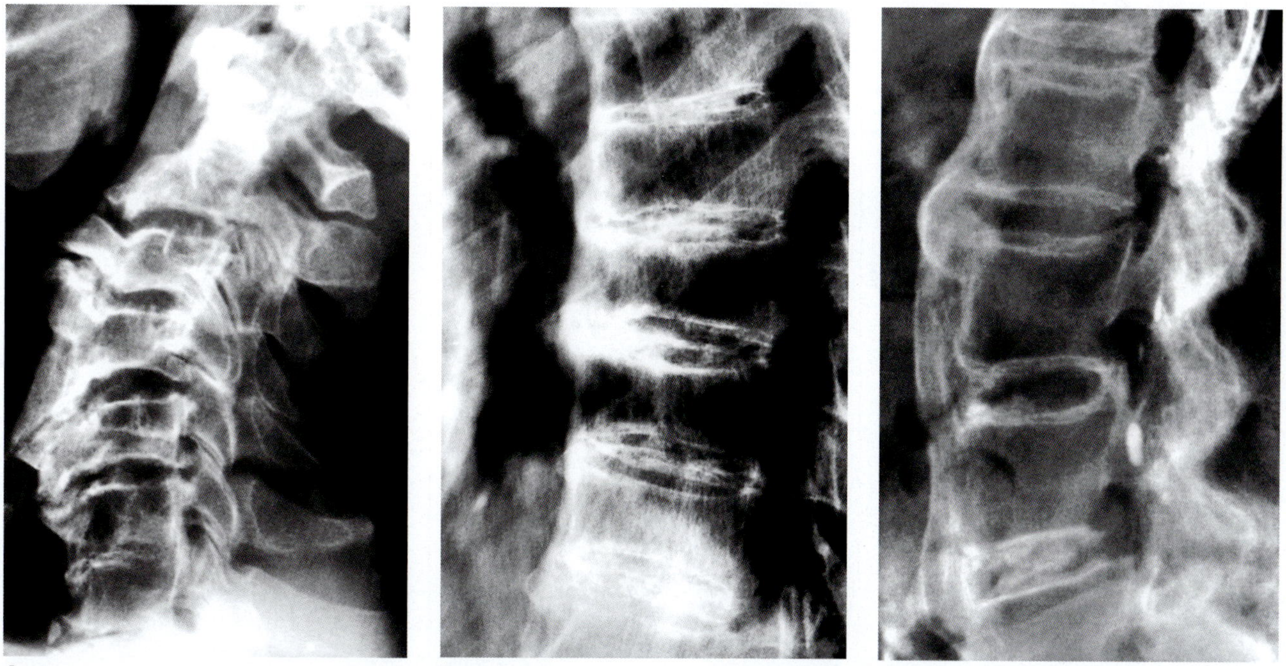

A B C

Figure 5.85 ■ Diffuse idiopathic skeletal hyperostosis. Lateral radiographs of the cervical **(A)**, thoracic **(B)**, and lumbar **(C)** spine in a 72-year-old man with Forestier disease (DISH) show the characteristic flowing hyperostosis extending across the vertebral disk spaces, which are relatively well preserved.

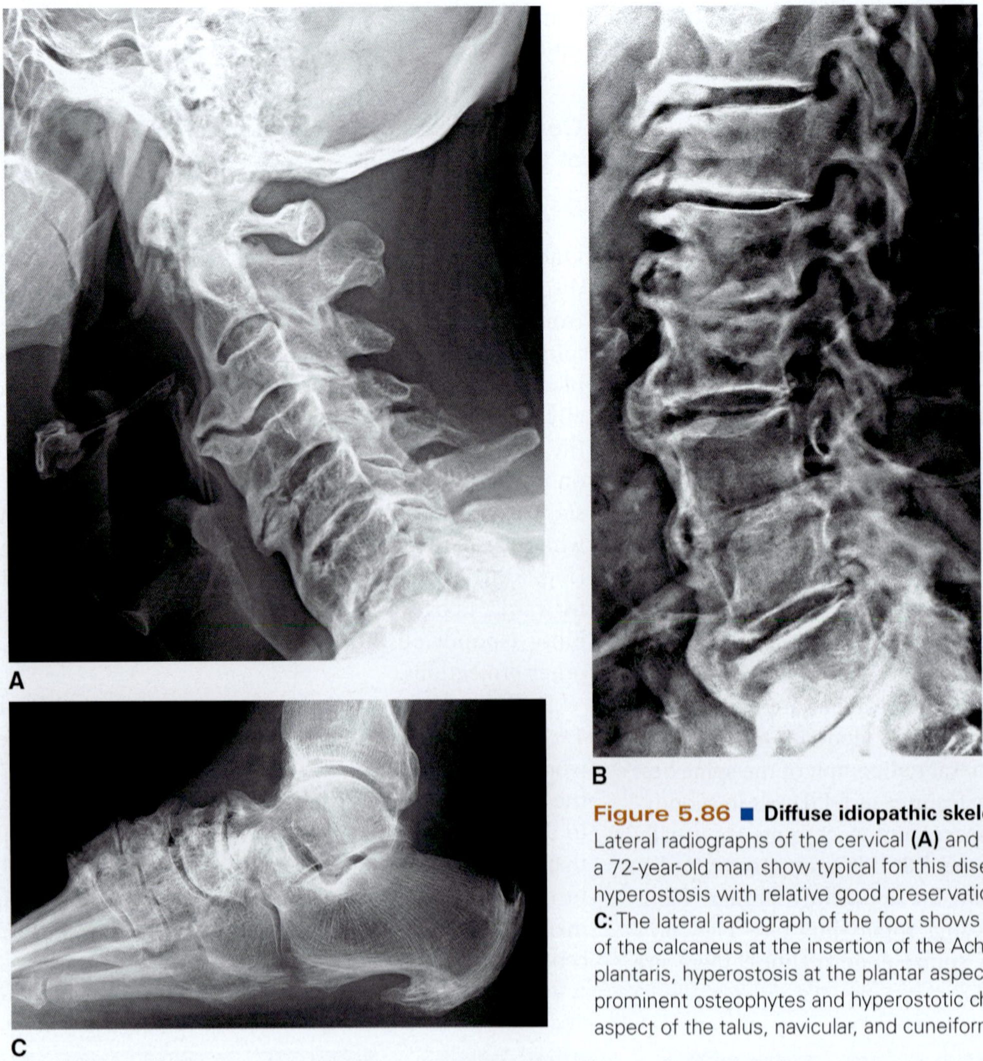

Figure 5.86 ■ Diffuse idiopathic skeletal hyperostosis. Lateral radiographs of the cervical **(A)** and lumbar **(B)** spine of a 72-year-old man show typical for this disease anterior flowing hyperostosis with relative good preservation of the disk spaces. **C:** The lateral radiograph of the foot shows prominent enthesopathy of the calcaneus at the insertion of the Achilles tendon and fascia plantaris, hyperostosis at the plantar aspect of the calcaneus, and prominent osteophytes and hyperostotic changes on the dorsal aspect of the talus, navicular, and cuneiform bones.

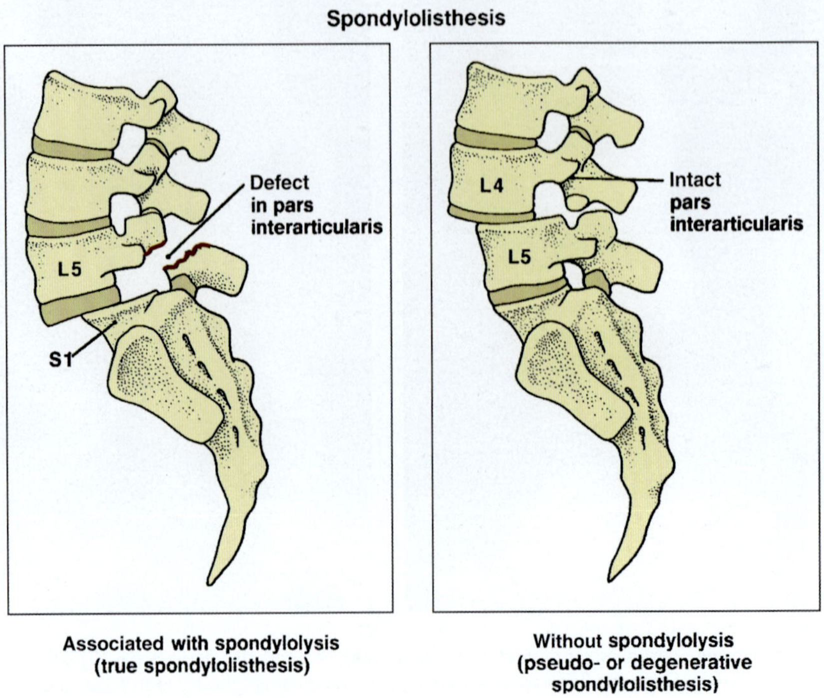

Figure 5.87 ■ Types of spondylolisthesis. Spondylolisthesis may occur in association with spondylolysis (defect in the part interarticularis) or as a complication of degenerative disk disease and facet arthropathy (so-called pseudospondylolisthesis or degenerative spondylolisthesis).

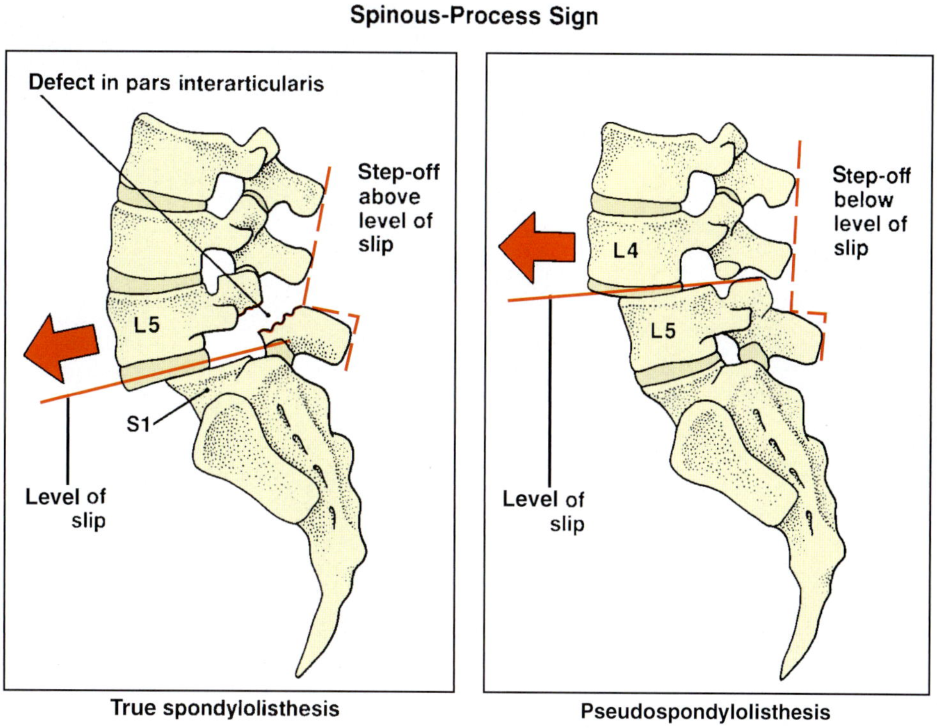

Figure 5.88 ■ The spinous process sign. The spinous process sign can help differentiate true spondylolisthesis associated with the defect in pars interarticularis from degenerative spondylolisthesis (pseudospondylolisthesis) by the presence of a step-off in the spinous processes above the level of vertebral slip in the former and below that level in the latter (*red arrows* indicate direction of slip).

Radiographic findings of degenerative spondylolisthesis include osteoarthritic changes of the facet joints (joint narrowing, marginal eburnation, and osteophyte formation), anterior slippage of the superior vertebra on the inferior vertebra, and, in many instances, intervertebral vacuum phenomenon (see Figs. 5.78 and 5.91B). Invariably, the affected intervertebral disk space is narrowed. CT may also effectively demonstrate this complication (Fig. 5.91).

(Continued on page 193)

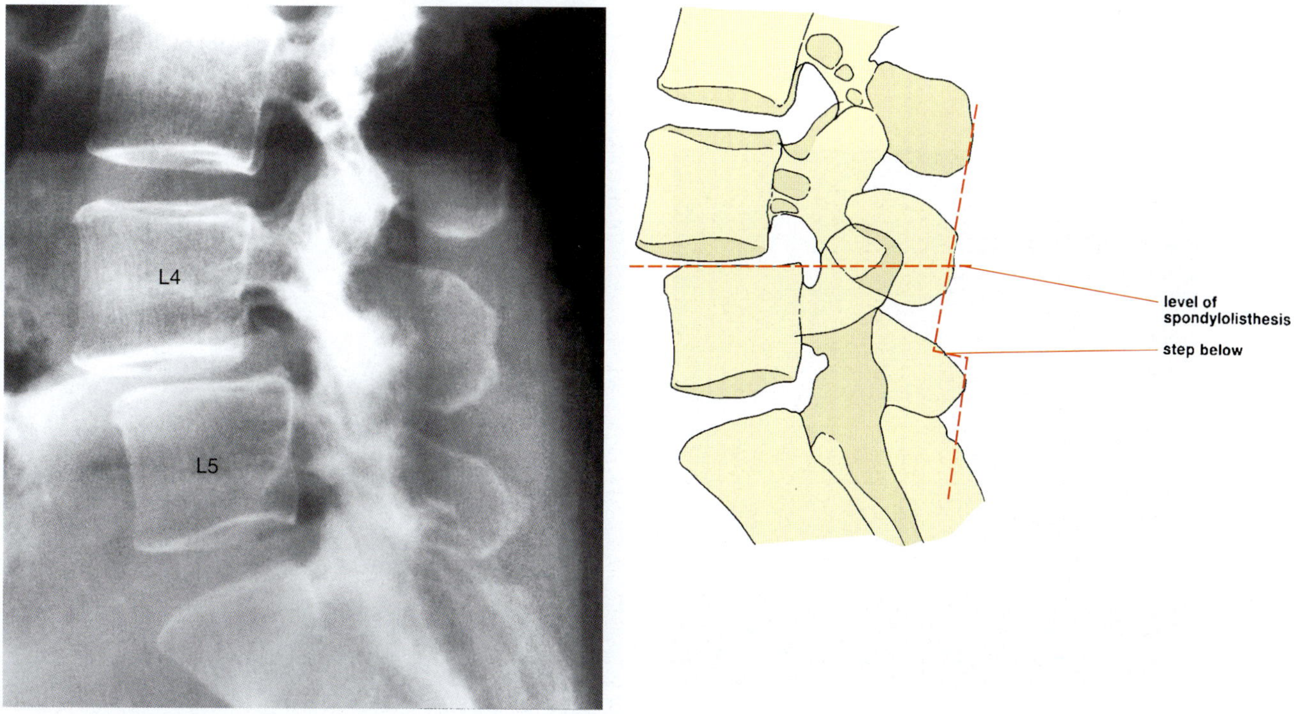

Figure 5.89 ■ Degenerative spondylolisthesis. A 55-year-old woman with degenerative disk disease at L4–L5 and degenerative facet arthritis developed spondylolisthesis, a common complication of this condition. Lateral radiograph of the lumbosacral spine is sufficient to differentiate this condition from spondylolisthesis associated with spondylolysis by the appearance of a step-off of the spinous process at the vertebra below the involved intervertebral space.

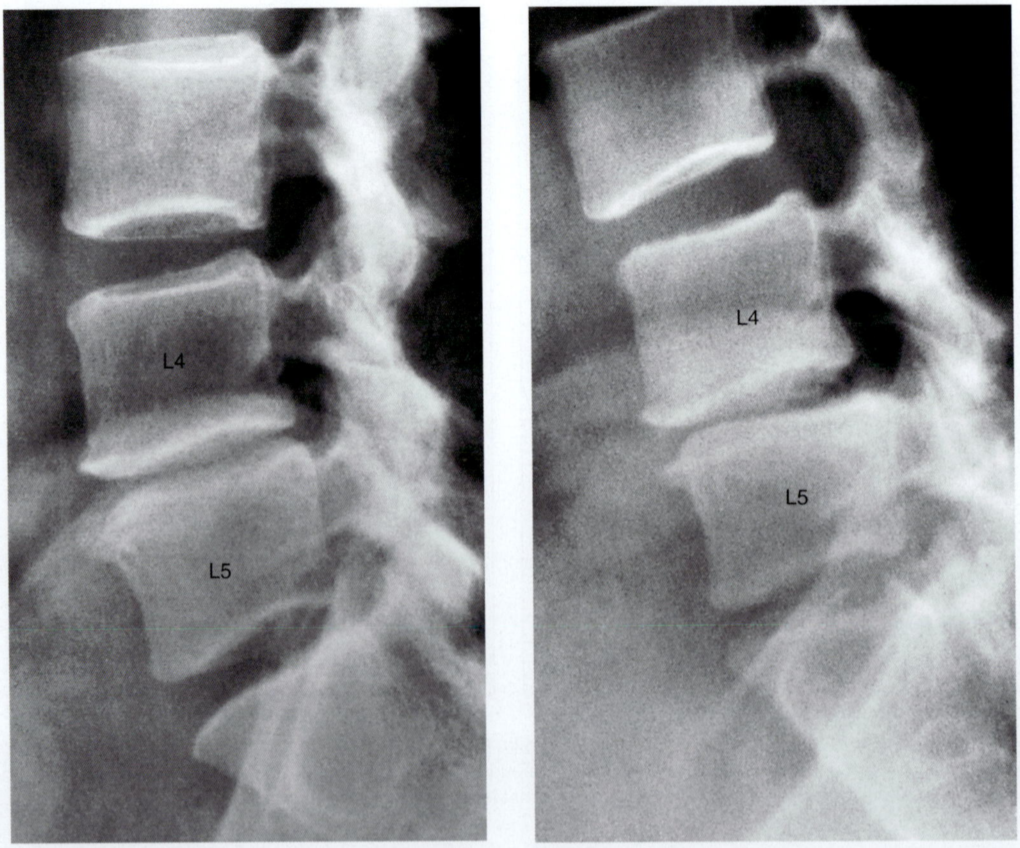

A B

Figure 5.90 ■ Degenerative spondylolisthesis. A 50-year-old man presented with chronic low back pain. **A:** Standard lateral radiograph of the lumbosacral spine in the neutral position shows narrowing of the L4–L5 disk space, indicating degenerative disk disease. There is no evidence of vertebral list. **B:** Lateral radiograph in flexion, however, demonstrates grade 1 spondylolisthesis at L4–L5.

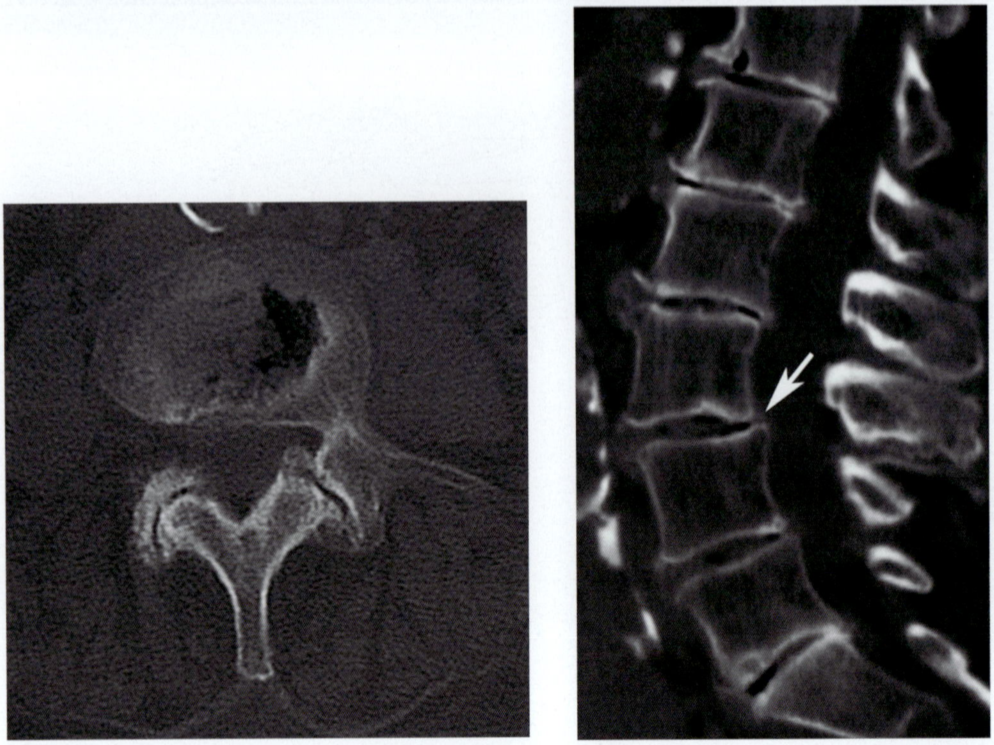

A B

Figure 5.91 ■ CT of degenerative spondylolisthesis and spinal stenosis. **A:** Axial CT of a 70-year-old woman with chronic low back pain shows degenerative disk disease with vacuum phenomenon and bilateral facet arthrosis. **B:** Sagittal CT demonstrates multilevel degenerative disk disease with vacuum phenomenon and degenerative spondylolisthesis at L3–L4 (*arrow*).

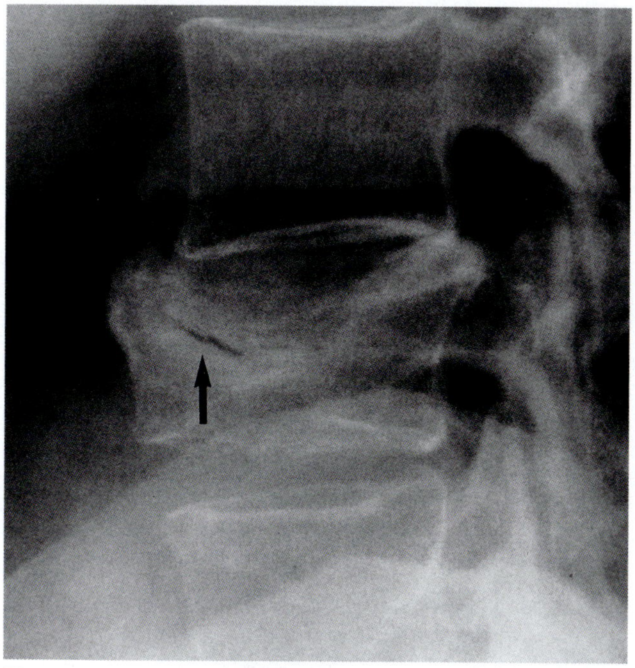

Figure 5.92 ■ Kümmell disease. Lateral radiograph of the lumbar spine shows posttraumatic collapse of the vertebral body of L4 associated with intravertebral vacuum cleft sign (*arrow*).

The intervertebral vacuum phenomenon associated with degenerative disk disease should not be confused with the intravertebral vacuum cleft sign. This sign appears on radiographs as a transverse, linear, or semilunar radiolucency located within the vertebral body. According to recent reports, this sign represents gas (principally nitrogen) in the fracture line of the vertebral body. Although the pathogenesis of this process is not completely clear, the sign is most suggestive of ischemic necrosis of bone. This phenomenon has been also reported in association with Kümmell disease, a delayed posttraumatic collapse of the vertebral body (Fig. 5.92).

Spinal Stenosis

Spinal stenosis is a much more severe complication of degenerative disease of the spine. In its acquired form, it results from hypertrophy of the structures surrounding the spinal canal, such as the pedicles, laminae, articular processes, and posterior aspect of the vertebral bodies as well as the ligamentum flavum. These alternations usually are apparent on conventional radiography; however, spinal stenosis can be better demonstrated by ancillary techniques. Spinal stenosis can be demonstrated by myelography, which can show the impingement of the thecal sac by hypertrophic changes of the posterior parts of the vertebral body and bulging disks, but CT best delineates its details (Fig. 5.93). MRI is also an effective modality in this respect (Fig. 5.94).

Spinal stenosis in the lumbar segment can be divided into three groups on the basis of its anatomic location: stenosis of the spinal canal, stenosis of the subarticular or lateral recesses, and stenosis of the neural foramina.

The causes of stenosis of the central canal are related to hypertrophic changes of osteoarthritis of the apophyseal joints, thickening of the ligamentum flavum, and osteophytes arising from the vertebral bodies. Bone hypertrophy at the site of the facet joints is a major cause of stenosis of the subarticular or lateral recesses, leading to encroachment on the neural elements in this region. The stenosis of the neural foramina is caused by hypertrophic changes and osteophytosis involving the vertebral body and articular process. Moreover, degenerative spondylolisthesis may be associated with distortion of the intervertebral foramen and may lead to compromise of the exiting nerve.

NEUROPATHIC ARTHROPATHY

This acute or chronic destructive arthritis, also known as *Charcot joint*, is grouped with other degenerative joint diseases because it exhibits manifestations similar to those seen in other forms of osteoarthritis—destruction of articular cartilage, subchondral sclerosis, and marginal osteophytosis—but in the most severe form. In the advanced stages of the disease, the joint cartilage is destroyed, and subchondral sclerosis is pronounced. Osteophytes become fragmented, and shards of cartilage and bone debris are discharged into the joint space. This arthropathy usually affects adults over 40 years of age, men more commonly than women. Most frequently it affects the weight-bearing joints of the lower limbs. It manifests as a chronic progressive joint destruction as a consequence of nerve dysfunction around weight-bearing joints. The prime cause is loss of or marked reduction in sensitivity to pain. The patients present with joint swelling and deformity, but without associated pain. In 1868, a French neurologist Jean-Martin Charcot described this condition in association with tabes dorsalis. Neuropathic arthropathy comprises a spectrum of destructive processes in the joint associated with neurosensory deficit. Pathognomonic for neuropathic joints are fragmentation of the bone and cartilage, which are discharged as debris into the joint; chronic synovitis with accumulation of varying amounts of fluid in the joint; and joint instability manifested by subluxation and dislocation (Fig. 5.95). Pathologically, the synovium of affected joint shows the features of osteoarthritis; however, there is usually a considerable amount of hemosiderin deposition. The synovial fluid also resembles that of osteoarthritis. The striking feature is the presence of large amount of debris consisting of fragments of bone and cartilage showing giant cells and foreign body type of macrophage reaction. Underlying conditions leading to neuropathic joint include, among others, diabetes mellitus, syphilis, leprosy, syringomyelia, congenital

(Continued on page 195)

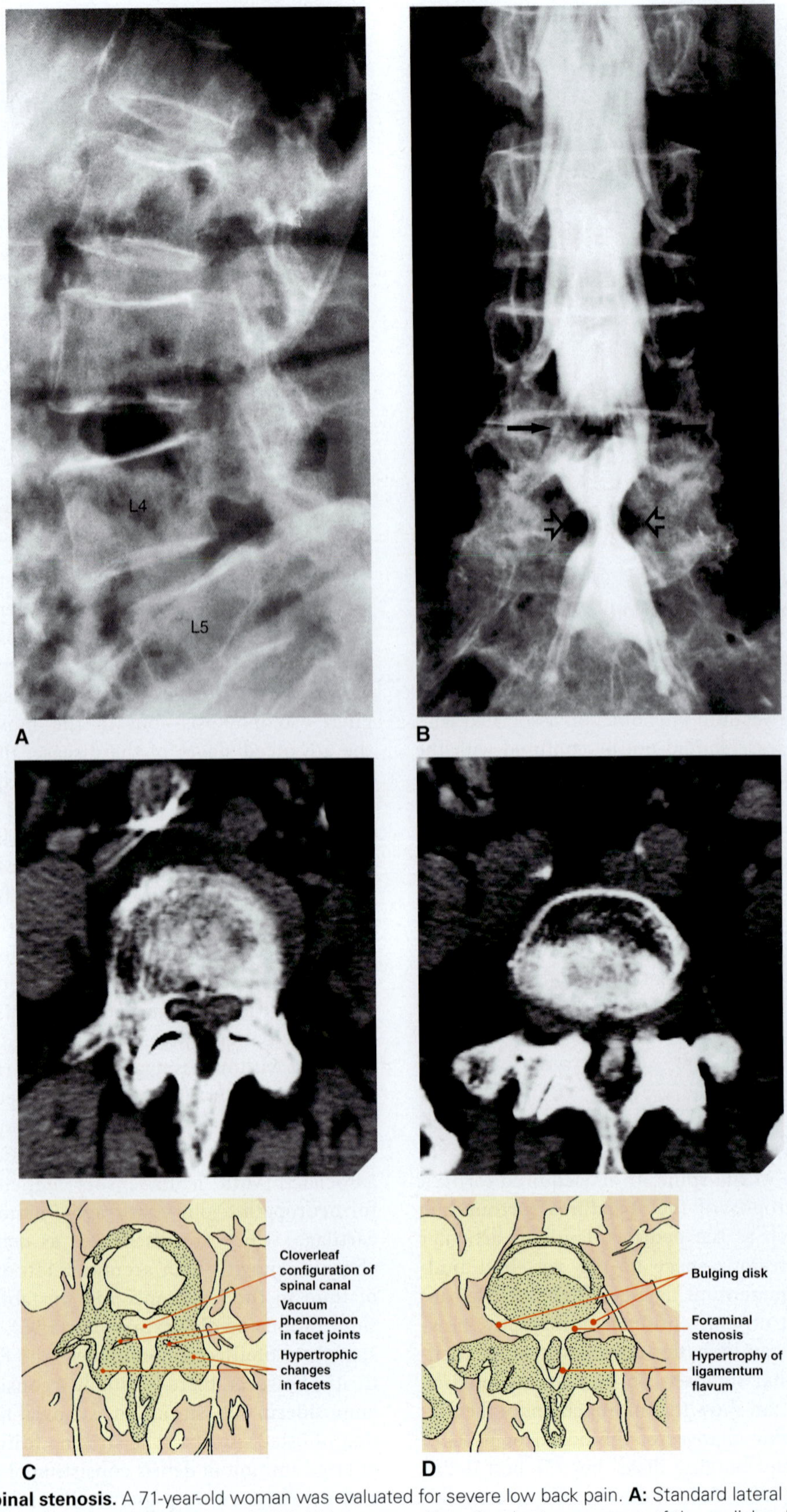

Figure 5.93 ■ **Spinal stenosis.** A 71-year-old woman was evaluated for severe low back pain. **A:** Standard lateral radiograph of the lumbar spine shows degenerative spondylolisthesis at the L4–L5 interspace. Note the short appearance of the pedicles. **B:** Myelogram in the anteroposterior projection also discloses segmental narrowing of the thecal sac; the upper defect is related to spondylolisthesis (*arrows*), the lower to spinal stenosis (*open arrows*). **C, D:** Axial CT images demonstrate the details of the abnormalities—severe spinal and foraminal stenosis, hypertrophy of the ligamenta flava, and posterior bulging of the intervertebral disk. Note the cloverleaf configuration of the spinal canal secondary to marked hypertrophy of the facet joints. The vacuum phenomenon in the apophyseal joints is well demonstrated.

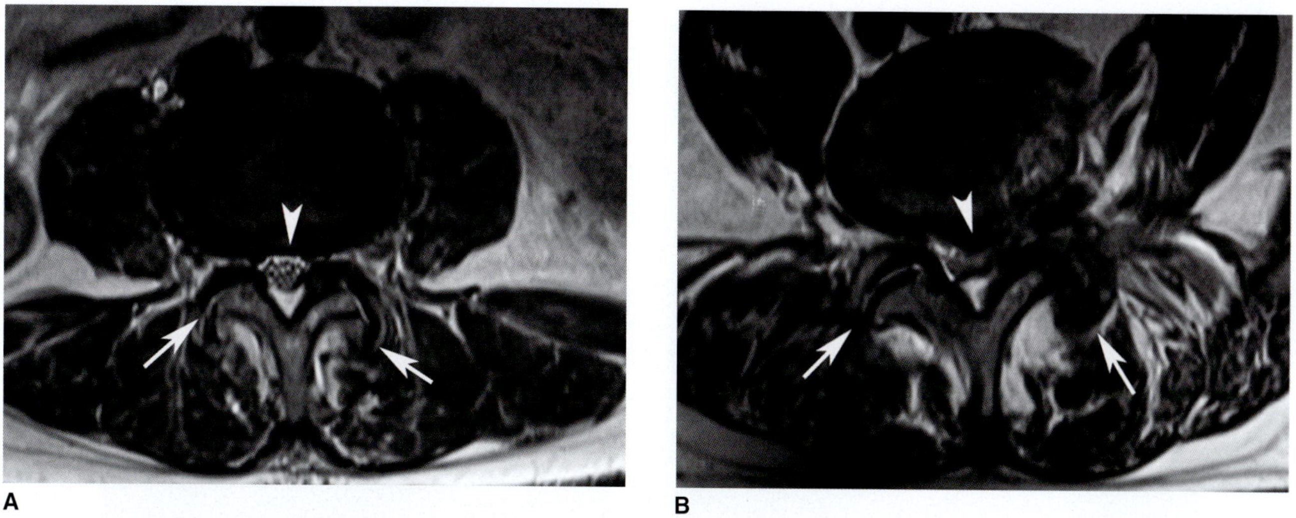

Figure 5.94 ■ MRI of spinal stenosis. A: Moderate spinal canal and thecal sac stenosis in a 45-year-old man. Degenerative changes of the facet joints (*arrows*) and disk bulging (*arrowhead*) contributed to central canal stenosis at the L4–L5 disk level, as demonstrated here on T2-weighted axial MR image. Note the clumping of the nerve roots within the thecal sac. **B:** Severe spinal canal stenosis in an 86-year-old woman. Axial T2-weighted MRI demonstrates almost complete collapse of the thecal sac at L4–L5 level because of a combination of annular bulge with a central disk herniation (*arrowhead*) and severe facet arthrosis (*arrows*).

indifference to pain, and spina bifida with meningomyelocele (Table 5.2). In diabetic patients, the condition has a greater predilection for the joints of the foot and ankle (Fig. 5.96); in patients with syringomyelia, joints of the upper extremities are more commonly affected (Fig. 5.97). The eponym *Charcot joint* was originally reserved for neuropathic joint in syphilitic patients with tabes dorsalis (Fig. 5.98). Currently, this term applies to any joint displaying features of neuropathic arthropathy, regardless of the causative factor.

(Continued on page 197)

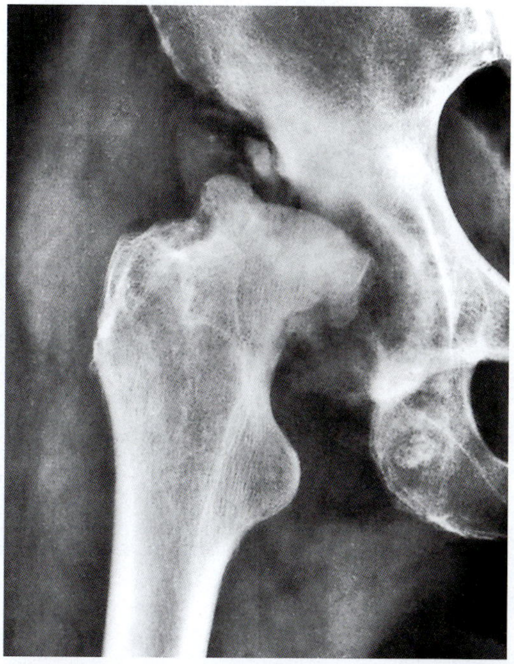

Figure 5.95 ■ Neuropathic joint. Anteroposterior radiograph of the right hip of a 57-year-old woman with neurosyphilis (tabes dorsalis) shows the typical features of neuropathic (Charcot) joint. There is complete disorganization of the joint, fragmentation, and subluxation. The absence of osteoporosis is a characteristic feature of the neuropathic joint. This condition represents the most severe manifestation of degenerative joint disease.

Table 5.2 CAUSES OF NEUROPATHIC ARTHROPATHY

Alcoholism
Amyloidosis
Charcot–Marie–Tooth disease
Congenital indifference to pain
Diabetes mellitus
Extrinsic compression of the spinal cord
Familial dysautonomia (Riley–Day syndrome)
Meningomyelocele
Multiple sclerosis
Peripheral nerve tumors
Pernicious anemia
Poliomyelitis
Spinal cord tumors
Steroids (systemic or intra-articular)
Syringomyelia
Tabes dorsalis (syphilis)
Uremia

Modified from Jones EA, Manaster BJ, May DA, Disler DG. Neuropathic osteoarthropathy: diagnostic dilemmas and differential diagnosis. *Radiographics.* 2000;20:S279–S293.

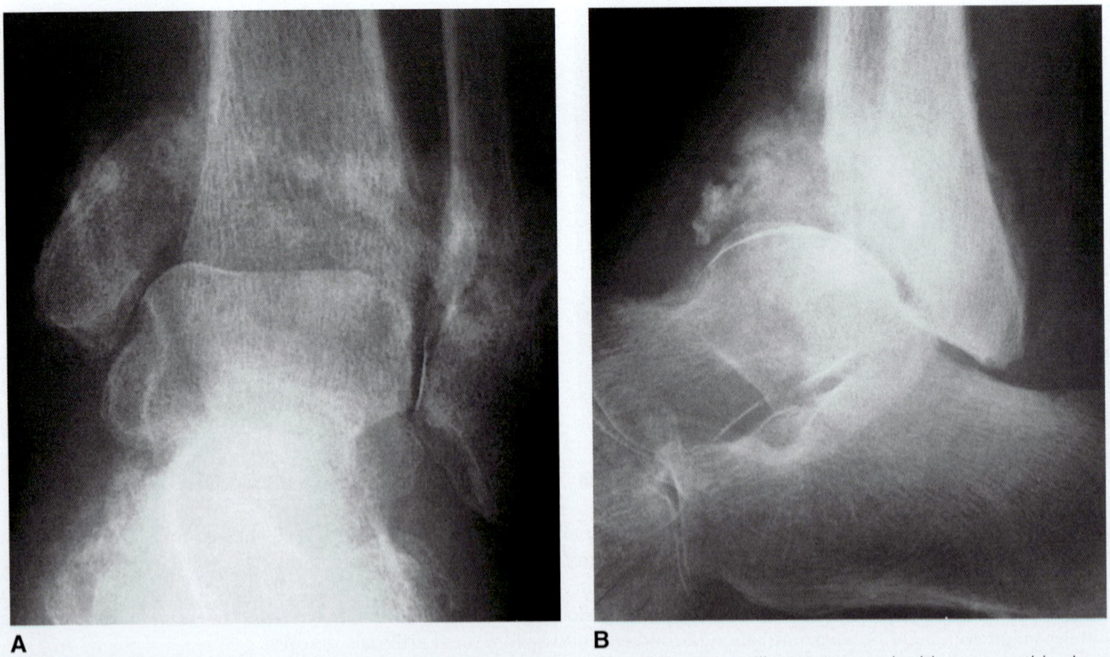

Figure 5.96 ■ **Neuropathic joint.** A 59-year-old woman with long-standing diabetes mellitus presented with neuropathic changes of left ankle joint, demonstrated here on the anteroposterior **(A)** and lateral **(B)** radiographs.

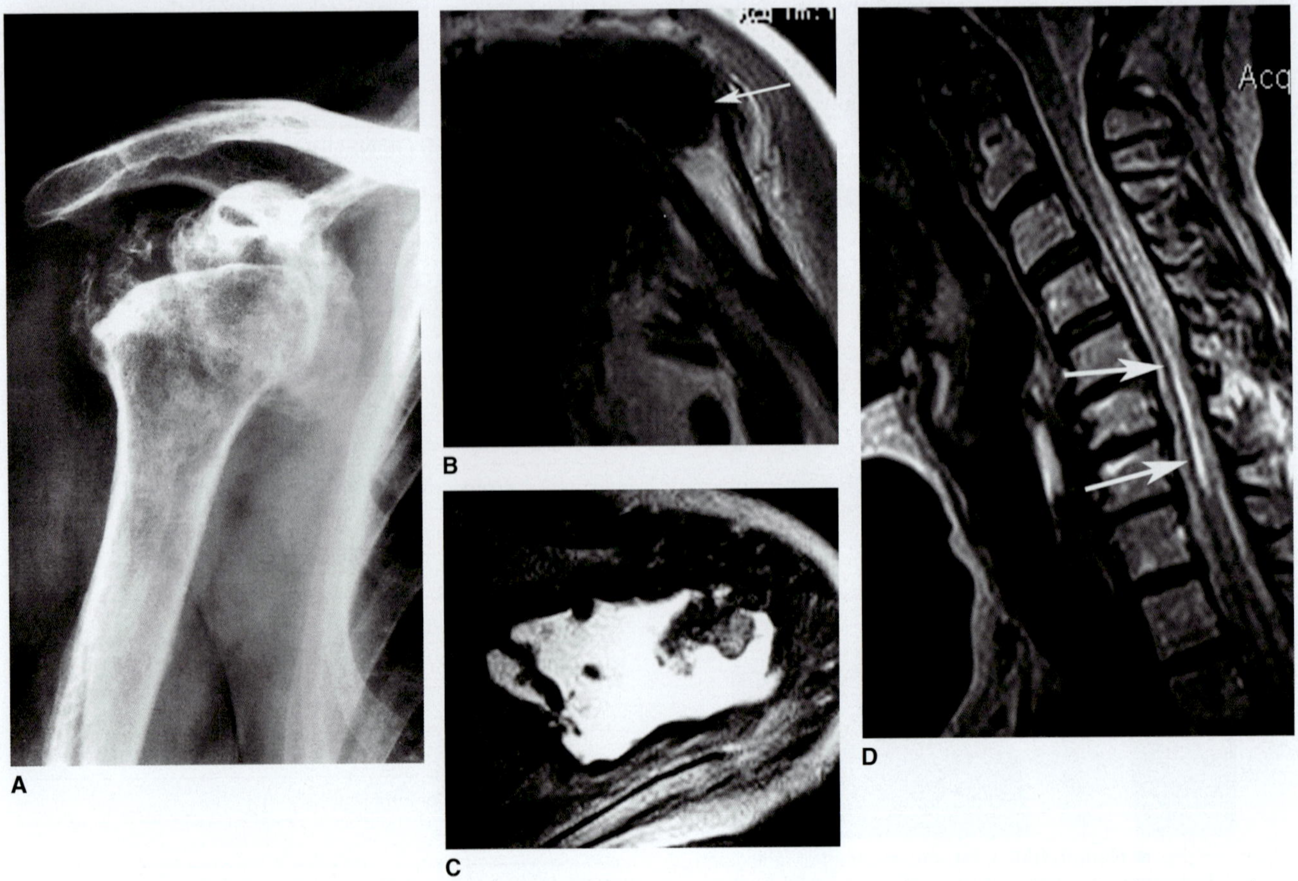

Figure 5.97 ■ **Neuropathic joint. A:** A 59-year-old woman with syringomyelia developed a neuropathic shoulder joint. Anteroposterior radiograph shows destruction of the joint, bony debris, and subluxation of the humeral head. **B:** Coronal T1-weighted MRI of the left shoulder in another patient demonstrates neuroarthropathy of the glenohumeral joint with complete destruction of the humeral head (*arrow*). **C:** Axial T2-weighted MRI demonstrates the fluid-filled space of the destroyed glenohumeral joint. **D:** Sagittal T2-weighted MRI demonstrates syringomyelia of the cervical cord (*arrows*).

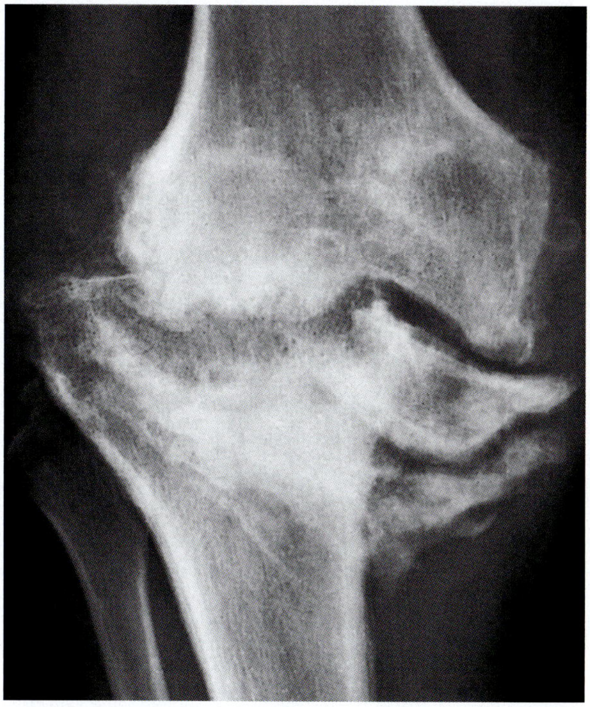

Figure 5.98 ■ Neuropathic joint. A 62-year-old man with syphilis presented with a typical neuropathic (Charcot) knee joint.

SUGGESTED READINGS

Abbott GT, Bucknall RC, Whitehouse GH. Osteoarthritis associated with distal interphalangeal joint involvement in rheumatoid arthritis. *Skeletal Radiol.* 1991;20:495–497.

Adamson TC III, Resnik CS, Guerra J Jr, et al. Hand and wrist arthropathies of hemochromatosis and calcium pyrophosphate deposition disease: distinct radiographic features. *Radiology.* 1983;147:377–381.

Agnesi F, Amrami KK, Frigo CA, Kaufman KR. Comparison of cartilage thickness with radiologic grade of knee osteoarthritis. *Skeletal Radiol.* 2008;37:639–643.

Ahlback S. Osteoarthritis of the knee: a radiographic investigation. *Acta Radiol Diagn (Stockh).* 1968;(suppl 277):7–72.

Alexander CJ. Osteoarthritis: a review of old myths and current concepts. *Skeletal Radiol.* 1990;19:327–333.

Alexander CJ. Idiopathic osteoarthritis: time to change paradigms? *Skeletal Radiol.* 2004;33:321–324.

Altman R, Asch E, Bloch D, et al. Development of criteria for the classification and reporting of osteoarthritis. Classification of osteoarthritis of the knee. Diagnostic and Therapeutic Criteria Committee of the American Rheumatism Association. *Arthritis Rheum.* 1986;29:1039–1049.

Audenaert EA, Baelde N, Huysse W, et al. Development of three-dimensional detection method of cam deformities in femoroacetabular impingement. *Skeletal Radiol.* 2011;40:921–927.

Bennett GL, Leeson MC, Michael A. Extensive hemosiderin deposition in the medial meniscus of a knee. Its possible relationship to degenerative joint disease. *Clin Orthop.* 1988;230:182–185.

Bennett GA, Waine H, Bauer W. Changes in the knee joint at various ages with particular reference to the nature and development of degenerative joint disease. In: The Commonwealth Fund. The New York Academy of Medicine; 1942:42–63.

Berenbaum F. Osteoarthritis. B. Pathology and pathogenesis. In: Klippel JH, Stone JH, Crofford LJ, White PH, eds. *Primer on the Rheumatic Diseases.* New York: Springer; 2008:229–234.

Bergman AG, Willen HK, Lindstand AL, Pettersson HTA. Osteoarthritis of the knee: correlation of subchondral MR signal abnormalities with histopathologic and radiographic features. *Skeletal Radiol.* 1994;23:445–448.

Bhalla S, Reinus WR. The linear intravertebral vacuum: a sign of benign vertebral collapse. *Am J Roentgenol.* 1998;170:1563–1569.

Bittersohl B, Hosalkar HS, Apprich S, et al. Comparison of pre-operative dGEMRIC imaging with intra-operative findings in femoroacetabular impingement: preliminary findings. *Skeletal Radiol.* 2011;40:553–561.

Blackburn WD Jr, Chivers S, Bernreuter W. Cartilage imaging in osteoarthritis. *Semin Arthritis Rheum.* 1996;25:273–281.

Bloem JL, Sartoris DJ, eds. *MRI and CT of the Musculoskeletal System. A Text-Atlas.* Baltimore, MD: Williams & Wilkins; 1992.

Bock GW, Garcia A, Weisman MH, et al. Rapidly destructive hip disease: clinical and imaging abnormalities. *Radiology.* 1993;186:461–466.

Boegard T, Jonsson K. Radiography in osteoarthritis of the knee. *Skeletal Radiol.* 1999;28:605–615.

Bora FW Jr, Miller G. Joint physiology, cartilage metabolism, and the etiology of osteoarthritis. *Hand Clin.* 1987;3:325–336.

Boutry N, Paul C, Leroy X, et al. Rapidly destructive osteoarthritis of the hip: MR imaging findings. *Am J Roentgenol.* 2002;179:657–663.

Braunstein EM, Brandt KD, Albrecht M. MRI demonstration of hypertrophic articular repair in osteoarthritis. *Skeletal Radiol.* 1990;19:335–339.

Broderick LS, Turner DA, Renfrew DL, et al. Severity of articular cartilage abnormality in patients with osteoarthritis: evaluation with fast spin-echo MR vs arthroscopy. *Am J Roentgenol.* 1994;162:99–103.

Brossmann J, Preidler K-W, Daenen B, et al. Imaging of osseous and cartilaginous intraarticular bodies in the knee: comparison of MR imaging and MR arthrography with CT and CT arthrography in cadavers. *Radiology.* 1996;200:509–517.

Brower AC, Downey EF. Kümmell disease: report of a case with serial radiographs. *Radiology.* 1981;141:363–364.

Buckwalter JA, Mankin HG. Articular cartilage. II. Degeneration and osteoarthritis, repair, regeneration, and transplantation. *J Bone Joint Surg Am.* 1997;79A:612–632.

Buckwalter JA, Mow VC. Cartilage repair in osteoarthritis. In: Moskowitz RW, Howell DS, Goldberg VM, Mankin HJ, eds. *Osteoarthritis.* 2nd ed. Philadelphia, PA: WB Saunders; 1992:71–107.

Bullough PG. *Atlas of Orthopedic Pathology with Clinical and Radiologic Correlation.* 2nd ed. New York, NY: Gower Medical Publishing; 1992:10.1–10.10.

Bullough PG. The pathology of osteoarthritis. In: Moskowitz RW, Howell DS, Goldberg VM, Mankin HJ, eds. *Osteoarthritis.* 2nd ed. Philadelphia, PA: WB Saunders; 1992:39–69.

Bullough PG, Bansal M. The differential diagnosis of geodes. *Radiol Clin North Am.* 1988;26:1165–1184.

Bullough PG, Boachie-Adjei O. *Atlas of Spinal Diseases.* Philadelphia, PA: JB Lippincott Company/Gower Medical Publishing; 1988:76–117.

Chan WP, Lang P, Stevens MP, et al. Osteoarthritis of the knee: comparison of radiography, CT, and MR imaging to assess extent and severity. *Am J Roentgenol.* 1991;157:799–806.

Charcot JM. Sur quelques arthropathies qui paraissent dépendre d'une lesion du cervean ou de la moëlle épindère. *Arch Physiol Norm Pathol.* 1868;1:161–178.

Charran AK, Tony G, Lalam R, et al. Destructive discovertebral degenerative disease of the lumbar spine. *Skeletal Radiol.* 2012;41:1213–1221.

Chen L, Boonthathip M, Cardoso F, et al. Acetabulum protrusio and center edge angle: new MR-imaging measurement criteria—a correlative study with measurement derived from conventional radiography. *Skeletal Radiol.* 2009;38:123–129.

Chou L, Knight R. Idiopathic avascular necrosis of a vertebral body: a case report and literature review. *Spine.* 1997;22:1928–1932.

Cicuttini FM, Spector TD. Genetics of osteoarthritis. *Ann Rheum Dis.* 1996;55:665–667.

Cohn EL, Maurer EJ, Keats TE, et al. Plain film evaluation of degenerative disk disease at the lumbosacral junction. *Skeletal Radiol.* 1997;26:161–166.

Crema MD, Roemer FW, Marra MD, et al. Articular cartilage in the knee: current MR imaging techniques and applications in clinical practice and research. *Radiographics.* 2011;31:37–62.

Dandachli W, Najefi A, Iranpour F, et al. Quantifying the contribution of pincer deformity to femoro-acetabular impingement using 3D computerized tomography. *Skeletal Radiol.* 2012;41:1295–1300.

Davis MA. Epidemiology of osteoarthritis. *Clin Geriatr Med.* 1988;4:241–255.

Della Torre P, Picuti G, Di Filippo P. Rapidly progressive osteoarthritis of the hip. *Ital J Orthop Traumatol.* 1987;13:187–200.

Dieppe P. Osteoarthritis. A.Clinical features. In: Klippel JH, Stone JH, Crofford LJ, White PH, eds. *Primer on the Rheumatic Diseases.* New York, NY: Springer; 2008:224–228.

Dieppe P, Cushnaghan J. The natural course and prognosis of osteoarthritis. In: Moskowitz RW, Howell DS, Goldberg VM, Mankin HJ, eds. *Osteoarthritis.* 2nd ed. Philadelphia, PA: WB Saunders; 1992:399–412.

Disler DG, Recht MP, McCauley TR. MR imaging of articular cartilage. *Skeletal Radiol.* 2000;29:367–377.

Emrani PS, Katz JN, Kessler CL, et al. Joint space narrowing and Kellgren-Lawrence progression in knee osteoarthritis: an analytic literature synthesis. *Osteoarthritis Cartilage.* 2008;16:873–882.

Epstein BS, Epstein JA, Jones MD. Lumbar spinal stenosis. *Radiol Clin North Am.* 1977;15:227–239.

Erkintalo MO, Salminen JJ, Alanen AM, et al. Development of degenerative changes in the lumbar intervertebral disk: results of a prospective MR imaging study in adolescents with and without low-back pain. *Radiology.* 1995;196:529–533.

Fairbank TJ. Knee joint changes after meniscectomy. *J Bone Joint Surg Br.* 1948;30B:664–670.

Felson DT. The course of osteoarthritis and factors that affect it. *Rheum Dis Clin North Am.* 1993;19:607–615.

Felson DT. Clinical practice. Osteoarthritis of the knee. *N Engl J Med.* 2006;354:841–848.

Forestier J, Rotes-Querol J. Senile ankylosing hyperostosis of the spine. *Ann Rheum Dis.* 1950;9:321–330.

Ganz R, Parvizi J, Beck M, et al. Femoroacetabular impingement: a cause for osteoarthritis of the hip. *Clin Orthop Relat Res.* 2003;417:112–120.

Giori NJ, Trousdale RT. Acetabular retroversion is associated with osteoarthritis of the hip. *Clin Orthop Relat Res.* 2003;417:263–269.

Golimbu C, Firooznia H, Rafii M. The intravertebral vacuum sign. *Spine.* 1986;11:1040–1043.

Grainger AJ, Farrant JM, O'Connor PJ, et al. MR imaging of erosions in interphalangeal joint osteoarthritis: is all osteoarthritis erosive? *Skeletal Radiol.* 2007;36:737–745.

Greenspan A, Beltran J. *Orthopedic Imaging—A Practical Approach.* 6th ed. Philadelphia, PA: Wolters Kluwer; 2015:550–581.

Greenspan A, Norman A, Tchang FKM. "Tooth" sign in patellar degenerative disease. *J Bone Joint Surg Am.* 1977;59A:483–485.

Gross A, Ma CB. Approach to the patient with knee pain. In: Imboden JB, Hellmann DB, Stone JH, eds. *Current Diagnosis and Treatment. Rheumatology.* 3rd ed. New York, NY: McGraw Hill; 2013:110–123.

Hardi CF, Sokoloff L. Secondary osteonecrosis in osteoarthritis of the femoral head. *Hum Pathol.* 1984;15:79–83.

Harris J, Carter AR, Glick EN, Storey GO. Ankylosing hyperostosis. Clinical and radiological features. *Ann Rheum Dis.* 1974;33:210–215.

Harrison MH, Schajowicz F, Trueta J. Osteoarthritis of the hip: a study of the nature and evolution of the disease. *J Bone Joint Surg Br.* 1953;35B:598–629.

Hart DJ, Spector TD. The classification and assessment of osteoarthritis. *Baillieres Clin Rheumatol.* 1995;9:407–432.

Hashemi SA, Dehghani J, Vosoughi AR. Can crossover sign be a reliable marker of global retroversion of the acetabulum? *Skeletal Radiol.* 2017;46:17–21.

Hayward I, Bjorkengren AG, Pathria MN, et al. Patterns of femoral head migration in osteoarthritis of the hip: a reappraisal with CT and pathologic correlation. *Radiology.* 1988;166:857–860.

Hill CL, Gale DG, Chaisson CE, et al. Knee effusions, popliteal cysts, and synovial thickening: association with knee pain in osteoarthritis. *J Rheumatol.* 2001;28:1330–1337.

Hodler J, Resnick D. Current status of imaging of articular cartilage. *Skeletal Radiol.* 1996;25:703–709.

Huetink K, van 't Klooster R, Kaptein BL, et al. Automatic radiographic quantification of hand osteoarthritis; accuracy and sensitivity to change in joint space width in a phantom and cadaveric study. *Skeletal Radiol.* 2012;41:41–49.

Jacobsen S, Romer L, Soballe K. Degeneration in dysplastic hips. A computer tomography study. *Skeletal Radiol.* 2005;34:778–784.

Jacobson JA, Girish G, Jiang Y, Sabb BJ. Radiographic evaluation of arthritis: degenerative joint disease and variations. *Radiology.* 2008;248:737–747.

Jeffcoate W. The causes of the Charcot syndrome. *Clin Podiatr Med Surg.* 2008;25:29–42.

Jones EA, Manaster BJ, May DA, Disler DG. Neuropathic osteoarthropathy: diagnostic dilemmas and differential diagnosis. *Radiographics.* 2000;20:S279–S293.

Jungmann PM, Liu F, Link TM. What has imaging contributed to the epidemiological understanding of osteoarthritis? *Skeletal Radiol.* 2014;43:271–275.

Kassarjian A, Yoon LS, Belzile E, et al. Triad of MR arthrographic findings in patients with cam-type femoroacetabular impingement. *Radiology.* 2005;236:588–592.

Kellgren JH, Lawrence JS. Radiological assessment of osteo-arthrosis. *Ann Rheum Dis.* 1957;16:494–502.

Kellgren JH, Moore R. Generalized osteoarthritis and Heberden's nodes. *Br Med J.* 1952;1:181–187.

Kerr R, Resnick D, Pineda C, Haghighi P. Osteoarthritis of the glenohumeral joint: a radiologic-pathologic study. *Am J Roentgenol.* 1985;144:967–972.

Kijowski R, Stanton P, Fine J, De Smet A. Subchondral bone marrow edema in patients with degeneration of the articular cartilage of the knee joint. *Radiology.* 2006;238:943–957.

Kim JA, Park JS, Jin W, et al. Herniation pits in the femoral neck: a radiographic indicator of femoroacetabular impingement? *Skeletal Radiol.* 2011;40:167–172.

Kirkaldy-Willis WH, Farfan HF. Instability of the lumbar spine. *Clin Orthop.* 1982;165:110–123.

Knutsson F. The vacuum phenomenon in the intervertebral discs. *Acta Radiol.* 1942;23:173–175.

Komiya S, Inoue A, Sasaguri Y, et al. Rapidly destructive arthropathy of the hip. Studies on bone resorptive factors in joint fluid with a theory of pathogenesis. *Clin Orthop.* 1992;284:273–282.

Kornaat PR, Ceulemans RYT, Kroon HM, et al. MRI assessment of knee osteoarthritis: Knee Osteoarthritis Scoring System (KOSS)—inter-observer and intra-observer reproducibility of a compartment-based scoring system. *Skeletal Radiol.* 2005;34:95–102.

Kumpan W, Salomonowitz E, Seidl G, Wittich GR. The intervertebral vacuum phenomenon. *Skeletal Radiol.* 1986;15:444–447.

Kuo A, Ezzet KA, Patti S, Colwell CW Jr. Total hip arthroplasty in rapidly destructive osteoarthritis of the hip: a case series. *HSS J.* 2009;5:117–119.

Laborie LB, Lehmann TG, Engesaeter IO, et al. Prevalence of radiographic findings thought to be associated with femoroacetabular impingement in a population-based cohort of 2081 healthy young adults. *Radiology.* 2011;260:494–502.

Lawrance JAL, Athanasou NA. Rapidly destructive hip disease. *Skeletal Radiol.* 1995;24:639–641.

Laxafoss E, Jacobsen S, Gosvig KK, Sonne-Holm S. Case definitions of knee osteoarthritis in 4,151 unselected subjects: relevance for epidemiologic studies. The Copenhagen Osteoarthritis Study. *Skeletal Radiol.* 2010;39:859–866.

Leach RE, Gregg T, Siber FJ. Weight-bearing radiography in osteoarthritis of the knee. *Radiology.* 1970;97:265–268.

Lefkowitz DM, Quencer RM. Vacuum facet phenomenon: a computed tomographic sign of degenerative spondylolisthesis. *Radiology.* 1982;144:562.

Leone A, Cassar-Pullicino VN, Guglielmi G, Bonomo L. Degenerative lumbar intervertebral instability: what is it and how does imaging contribute? *Skeletal Radiol.* 2009;38:529–533.

Leone A, Cassar-Pullicino VN, Semprini A, et al. Neuropathic osteoarthropathy with and without superimposed osteomyelitis in patients with a diabetic foot. *Skeletal Radiol.* 2016;45:735–754.

Lequesne M. La coxarthrose destructrice rapide. *Rhumatologie.* 1970;22:51–63.

Lequesne MG, Laredo J-D. The faux profil (oblique view) of the hip in the standing position. Contribution to the evaluation of osteoarthritis of the adult hip. *Ann Rheum Dis.* 1998;57:676–681.

Link TM. The Founder's Lecture 2009: advances in imaging of osteoporosis and osteoarthritis. *Skeletal Radiol.* 2010;39:943–955.

Maldague BE, Noel HM, Malghem JJ. The intravertebral vacuum cleft: a sign of ischemic vertebral collapse. *Radiology.* 1978;129:23–29.

Mankin HJ, Brandt KD. Biochemistry and metabolism of articular cartilage in osteoarthritis. In: Moskowitz RW, Howell DS, Goldberg VM, Mankin HJ, eds. *Osteoarthritis.* 2nd ed. Philadelphia, PA: WB Saunders; 1992:109–154.

Martel W, Snarr JW, Horn JR. The metacarpophalangeal joints in interphalangeal osteoarthritis. *Radiology.* 1973;108:1–7.

McAfee PC, Ullrich CG, Yuan HA, et al. Computed tomography in degenerative lumbar spinal stenosis: the value of multiplanar reconstruction. *Radiographics.* 1982;2:529–537.

McCauley TR, Disler DG. Magnetic resonance imaging of articular cartilage of the knee. *J Am Acad Orthop Surg.* 2001;9:2–8.

McCauley TR, Kornaat PR, Jee WH. Central osteophytes in the knee: prevalence and association with cartilage defects on MR imaging. *Am J Roentgenol.* 2001;176:359–364.

Melville DM, Taljanovic MS, Scalcione LR, et al. Imaging and management of thumb carpometacarpal joint osteoarthritis. *Skeletal Radiol.* 2015;44:165–177.

Milgram JE. Recurrent articular spondylolisthesis: common cause of vertebral instabilities, root pain, sciatica, and ultimately spinal stenosis. Early detection and blocking of specific dislocations. *Bull Hosp Jt Dis Orthop Inst.* 1986;46:47–51.

Mitchell NS, Cruess RL. Classification of degenerative arthritis. *Can Med Assoc J.* 1977;117:763–765.

Mitrovic DR, Riera H. Synovial, articular cartilage and bone changes in rapidly destructive arthropathy (osteoarthritis) of the hip. *Rheumatol Int.* 1992;12:17–23.

Modic MT, Masaryk TJ, Ross JS, Carter JR. Imaging of degenerative disk disease. *Radiology.* 1988;168:177–186.

Modic MT, Steinberg PM, Ross JS, et al. Degenerative disk disease: assessment of changes in vertebral body marrow with MR imaging. *Radiology.* 1988;166:193–199.

Norman A. Roentgenologic diagnosis. In: Moskowitz RW, et al., eds. *Osteoarthritis—Diagnosis and Management.* Philadelphia, PA: WB Saunders; 1984:155–184.

Norman A, Robbins H, Milgram JE. The acute neuropathic arthropathy—a rapid severely disorganizing form of arthritis. *Radiology.* 1968;90:1159–1164.

Notzli HP, Wyss TF, Stoecklin CH, et al. The contour of the femoral head-neck junction as a predictor for the risk of anterior impingement. *J Bone Joint Surg Br.* 2002;84B:556–560.

Oettmeier R, Abendroth K. Osteoarthritis and bone: osteologic types of osteoarthritis of the hip. *Skeletal Radiol.* 1989;18:165–174.

Pepper HW, Noonan CD. Radiographic evaluation of total hip arthroplasty. *Radiology.* 1973;108:23–29.

Peterfy CG, Genant HK. Emerging applications of magnetic resonance imaging in the evaluation of articular cartilage. *Radiol Clin North Am.* 1996;34:195–213.

Peyron JG. Epidemiologic and etiologic approach of osteoarthritis. *Semin Arthritis Rheum.* 1979;8:288–306.

Peyron JG, Altman RD. The epidemiology of osteoarthritis. In: Moskowitz RW, Howell DS, Goldberg VM, Mankin HJ, eds. *Osteoarthritis.* 2nd ed. Philadelphia, PA: WB Saunders; 1992:15–37.

Pfirrmann CWA, Mengiardi B, Dora C, et al. Cam and pincer femoroacetabular impingement: characteristic MR arthrographic findings in 50 patients. *Radiology.* 2006;240:778–785.

Pollard TCB. A perspective on femoroacetabular impingement. *Skeletal Radiol.* 2011;40:815–818.

Pope TL Jr, Keats TE, de Lange EE, Fechner RE. Case report 426. Unilateral, rapidly destructive arthropathy of the hip ("analgesic hip"). *Skeletal Radiol.* 1987;16:342–345.

Postel M, Kerboull M. Total prosthetic replacement in rapidly destructive arthrosis of the hip joint. *Clin Orthop.* 1970;72:138–144.

Ranawat AS, Schulz B, Baumbach SF, et al. Radiographic predictors of hip pain in femoroacetabular impingement. *HSS J.* 2011;7:115–119.

Recht M, Bobic V, Burstein D, et al. Magnetic resonance imaging of articular cartilage. *Clin Orthop.* 2001;391(suppl):S379–S396.

Reichenbach S, Juni P, Werlen S, et al. Prevalence of cam-type deformity on hip magnetic resonance imaging in young males: a cross-sectional study. *Arthritis Care Res.* 2010;62:1319–1327.

Resnick D. Degenerative diseases of the vertebral column. *Radiology.* 1985;156:3–14.

Resnick D. Patterns of migration of the femoral head in osteoarthritis of the hip. Roentgenographic-pathologic correlation and comparison with rheumatoid arthritis. *Am J Roentgenol.* 1975;124:62–74.

Resnick D, Niwayama G. Degenerative disease of extraspinal locations. In: Resnick D, ed. *Diagnosis of Bone and Joint Disorders.* 3rd ed. Philadelphia, PA: WB Saunders; 1995:1263–1371.

Resnick D, Niwayama G. Diffuse idiopathic skeletal hyperostosis (DISH): ankylosing hyperostosis of Forestier and Rotes-Querol. In: Resnick D, ed. *Diagnosis of Bone and Joint Disorders.* 3rd ed. Philadelphia, PA: WB Saunders; 1995:1463–1495.

Resnick D, Niwayama G. Entheses and enthesopathy. Anatomical, pathological and radiological correlation. *Radiology.* 1983;146:1–9.

Resnick D, Niwayama G, Coutts RD. Subchondral cysts (geodes) in arthritic disorders: pathologic and radiographic appearance of the hip joint. *Am J Roentgenol.* 1977;128:799–806.

Resnick D, Niwayama G, Goergen TG. Degenerative disease of the sacroiliac joint. *Invest Radiol.* 1975;10:608–621.

Resnick D, Shaul SR, Robins JM. Diffuse idiopathic skeletal hyperostosis (DISH). Forestier's disease with extraspinal manifestations. *Radiology.* 1975;115:513–524.

Rosenberg ZS, Shankman S, Steiner GC, et al. Rapid destructive osteoarthritis: clinical, radiographic, and pathologic features. *Radiology.* 1992;182:213–216.

Ross JS, Modic MT, Masaryk TJ, et al. Assessment of extradural degenerative disease with Gd DTPA-enhanced MR imaging: correlation with surgical and pathologic findings. *Am J Neuroradiol.* 1989;10:1243–1249.

Ryu KN, Kim EJ, Yoo MC, et al. Ischemic necrosis of the entire femoral head and rapidly destructive hip disease: potential causative relationship. *Skeletal Radiol.* 1997;26:143–149.

Sandell LJ. Etiology of osteoarthritis: genetics and synovial joint involvement. *Nat Rev Rheumatol.* 2012;8:77–89.

Schiebler ML, Grenier N, Fallon M, et al. Normal and degenerated intervertebral disk: in vivo and in vitro MR imaging with histopathologic correlation. *Am J Roentgenol.* 1991;157:93–97.

Schmorl G, Junghanns H. *The Human Spine in Health and Disease.* 2nd ed. New York, NY: Grune & Stratton; 1971.

Schumacher HR. Articular cartilage in the degenerative arthropathy of hemochromatosis. *Arthritis Rheum.* 1982;25:1460–1468.

Sharma L. Osteoarthritis. C. Treatment. In: Klippel JH, Stone JH, Crofford LJ, White PH, eds. *Primer on the Rheumatic Diseases.* New York, NY: Springer; 2008:235–240.

Sienbenrock KA, Schoeniger R, Ganz R. Anterior femoroacetabular impingement due to acetabular retroversion: treatment with periacetabular osteotomy. *J Bone Joint Surg Am.* 2003;85-A:278–286.

Sokoloff L. Pathology and pathogenesis of osteoarthritis. In: Hollander JL, McCarty DJ, eds. *Arthritis and Allied Conditions.* 8th ed. Philadelphia, PA: Lea & Febiger; 1972:1009–1031.

Spector TD, MacGregor AJ. Risk factors for osteoarthritis: genetics. *Osteoarthritis Cartilage.* 2004;12(suppl A):S39–S44.

Stecher RM. Heberden's nodes: the clinical characteristic of osteo-arthritis of the fingers. *Ann Rheum Dis.* 1948;7:1–8.

Stoller DW. *MRI in Orthopaedics and Sports Medicine.* Philadelphia, PA: JB Lippincott; 1993.

Stoller DW, Cannon WD Jr, Anderson LJ. The knee. In: *Magnetic Resonance Imaging in Orthopaedics and Sports Medicine.* Philadelphia, PA: JB Lippincott; 1993:139–372.

Taljanovic MS, Graham AR, Benjamin JB, et al. Bone marrow edema pattern in advanced hip osteoarthritis: quantitative assessment with magnetic resonance imaging and correlation with clinical examination, radiographic findings, and histopathology. *Skeletal Radiol.* 2008;37:423–431.

Tamai M, Sagawa K, Kawabata R, et al. Production of IL-6 by T cells from the femoral head of patients with rapidly destructive coxopathy (RDC). *Clin Exp Immunol.* 1996;103:506–513.

Theodorou DJ. The intravertebral vacuum cleft sign. *Radiology.* 2001;221: 787–788.

Trepman E, Nihal A, Pinzur MS. Current topics review: Charcot neuroarthropathy of the foot and ankle. *Foot Ankle Int.* 2005;26:46–63.

Utsinger PD, Resnick D, Shapiro R. Diffuse skeletal abnormalities in Forestier disease. *Arch Intern Med.* 1976;136:763–768.

Waldschmidt JG, Braunstein EM, Buckwalter KA. Magnetic resonance imaging of osteoarthritis. *Rheum Dis Clin North Am.* 1999;25:451–465.

Watt I. Arthritis or arthrosis—that is the question? An overview of concept in osteoarthritis. *Osteologiai Kozlem.* 2005;3:131–136.

Watt I. Osteoarthritis revisited–again! *Skeletal Radiol.* 2009;38:419–423.

Watt I, Dieppe P. Osteoarthritis revisited. *Skeletal Radiol.* 1990;19:1–3.

Weber BG. Total hip replacement: rotating versus fixed and metal versus ceramic heads. In: Salvati EA, ed. *The hip. Proceedings of the Ninth Open Scientific Meeting of the Hip Society, 1981.* St. Louis, MO: CV Mosby; 1981:264–275.

Werner CML, Copeland CE, Stromberg J, et al. Correlation of the cross-over ratio of the cross-over sign on conventional pelvic radiographs with computed tomography retroversion measurements. *Skeletal Radiol.* 2010;39:655–660.

Wukich DA, Sung W. Charcot arthropathy of the foot and ankle: modern concepts and management review. *J Diabetes Complications.* 2009;23:409–426.

Xu L, Hayashi D, Guermazi A, et al. The diagnostic performance of radiography for detection of osteoarthritis-associated features compared with MRI in hip joints with chronic pain. *Skeletal Radiol.* 2013;42:1421–1428.

Yamamoto T, Bullough PG. The role of subchondral insufficiency fracture in rapid destruction of the hip joint. *Arthritis Rheum.* 2000;43:2423–2427.

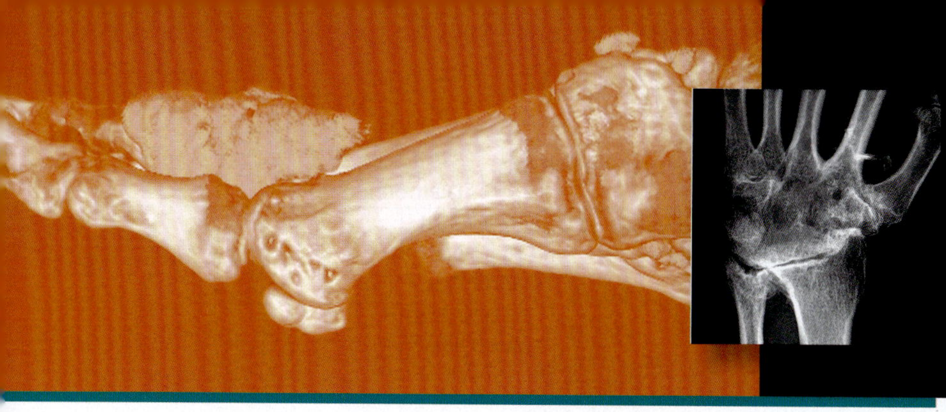

CHAPTER 6

Inflammatory Arthritides

The inflammatory arthritides constitute a group of diverse monoarticular and systemic disorders that have in common one important feature: inflammatory pannus eroding articular cartilage and bone (Fig. 6.1). An overview of the clinical and imaging hallmarks of the various inflammatory arthritides is shown in Table 6.1.

EROSIVE OSTEOARTHRITIS (EOA)

Erosive osteoarthritis was first described by Kellgren and Moore in 1952 and reintroduced in 1961 by Crain, who called it *interphalangeal osteoarthritis.* He defined this disorder as a localized variant of osteoarthritis involving the finger joints, characterized by degenerative changes with intermittent inflammatory episodes leading to deformities and ankylosis. In 1966, Peter and Pearson coined the term *erosive osteoarthritis*, and Ehrlich in 1972 described it as *inflammatory osteoarthritis*, based on the clinical symptoms of swelling, tenderness, erythema, warmth, and limitation of function. It can be defined as a progressive disorder of the interphalangeal joints with severe synovitis, superimposed on the changes of degenerative joint disease. Although the cause is still unclear, several investigators have suggested hormonal influences, metabolic background, autoimmunity, and heredity as being involved.

Clinical Features

EOA is a progressive inflammatory arthritis seen predominantly in middle-aged women. Only rarely are men affected, with an estimated female-to-male ratio of 12:1. Patients' ages range from 36 to 83 years, and mean age of onset is 50.5 years. This condition combines certain clinical manifestations of rheumatoid arthritis with certain imaging features of degenerative joint disease. Generally, involvement is limited to the hands, with the proximal and distal interphalangeal joints being the most commonly affected. Large joints, such as the hip or shoulder, are only rarely involved. The arthritis usually begins abruptly and is characterized by pain, swelling, and tenderness of the small joints of the hands. Also described are throbbing paresthesias of the fingertips and morning stiffness.

Pathology

Proliferative synovitis is the most common histopathologic feature of EOA and cannot be distinguished from that of seen in rheumatoid arthritis. Moreover, Peter et al. described findings in some patients consisting of degenerative cartilage with prominent subchondral granulation tissue, lymphocyte aggregates, plasma cell infiltration, and subsynovial fibrosis. Loose fibrin-like material was noted interstitially as well as villous hypertrophy, hyperemia and thickening of the blood vessel walls, and organizing amorphous exudates that overlaid the synovium. Generally speaking, the pathologic synovium of EOA exhibits features that are consistent with both RA and OA.

Imaging Features

In the early stage of the disease, the main feature is symmetric synovitis of the interphalangeal joints. Later, this is followed by articular erosions, which exhibit a characteristic radiographic feature named the "gull-wing" deformity by Martel. This configuration is seen as a result of central erosion and marginal proliferation of bone (Figs. 6.2 and 6.3); Heberden nodes may also be present. Periosteal reaction taking the form of linear or fluffy bone apposition over the cortex near the affected joints is occasionally

(Continued on page 203)

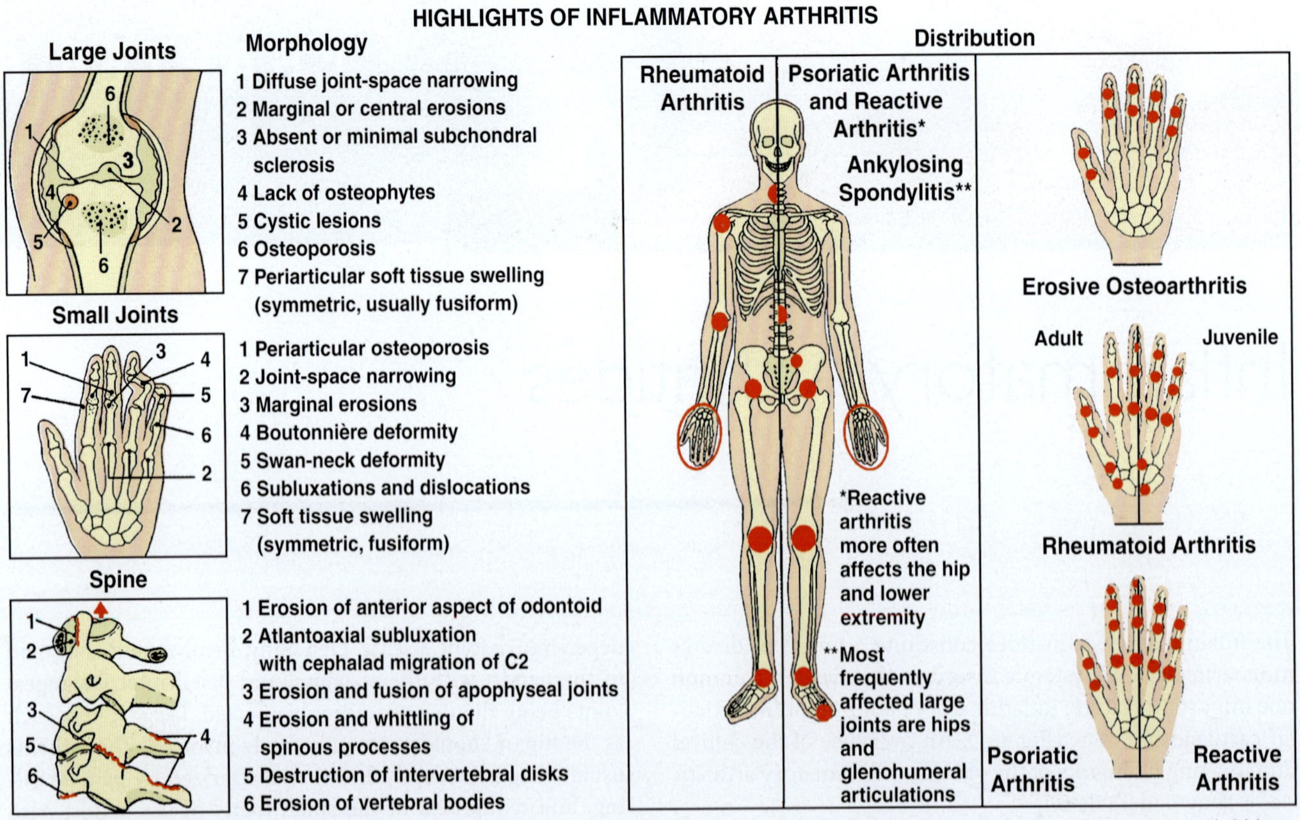

Figure 6.1 ■ Inflammatory arthritides. Highlights of the morphology and distribution of arthritic lesions in the inflammatory arthritides.

Table 6.1 CLINICAL AND IMAGING HALLMARKS OF INFLAMMATORY ARTHRITIDES

Type of Arthritis	Site	Crucial Abnormalities	Technique[a]/Projection
Erosive Osteoarthritis (F; middle age)	Hands	Involvement of Proximal interphalangeal joints Distal interphalangeal joints Gull-wing deformities associated with erosions Heberden nodes Joint ankylosis	Dorsovolar view
Rheumatoid Arthritis (F > M; presence of rheumatoid factor and DRW4)	Hands and wrists	Involvement of	Dorsovolar view
		Metacarpophalangeal joints	Dorsovolar and Norgaard views, MRI
		Proximal interphalangeal joints	
		Central and marginal erosions	
		Periarticular osteoporosis	Dorsovolar view
		Joint deformities: swan-neck, boutonnière, main-en-lorgnette, hitchhiker's thumb	Dorsovolar view
		Synovitis	Postcontrast MRI
		Pre-erosive edema	MRI
	Hip	Narrowing of joint space	Anteroposterior and lateral views
		Erosions	Anteroposterior and lateral views MRI
		Acetabular protrusion	Anteroposterior view
	Knee	Narrowing of joint space	Anteroposterior and lateral views
		Erosions	
		Synovial cysts	MRI
	Ankle and foot	Involvement of subtalar joint	Lateral view
		Erosions of calcaneus	Lateral and Broden views Lateral view (heel)
	Hands	Joint ankylosis	Dorsovolar view (wrist and hand)

Table 6.1 CLINICAL AND IMAGING HALLMARKS OF INFLAMMATORY ARTHRITIDES (*Continued*)

Type of Arthritis	Site	Crucial Abnormalities	Technique[a]/Projection
Juvenile Idiopathic Arthritis		Periosteal reaction Growth abnormalities	
	Knees	Growth abnormalities	Anteroposterior and lateral views
	Cervical spine	Fusion of apophyseal joints C1–C2 subluxation	Anteroposterior, lateral, and oblique views Lateral view in flexion
Ankylosing spondylitis (M > F; young adult; 95% positive for HLA-B27)	Spine	Squaring of vertebral bodies Syndesmophytes "Bamboo" spine Paravertebral ossifications "Shiny corners"	Anteroposterior and lateral views Lateral view
	Sacroiliac joints	Inflammatory changes Fusion	Posteroanterior and Ferguson views
	Pelvis	Whiskering of iliac crests and ischial tuberosity	Anteroposterior view
Reactive arthritis (M > F)	Foot	Involvement of great toe articulations Erosions of calcaneus	Anteroposterior and lateral views
	Spine	Single, coarse syndesmophyte	Anteroposterior and lateral views
	Sacroiliac joints	Unilateral or bilateral but asymmetric involvement	Posteroanterior and Ferguson views Computed tomography Postcontrast MRI
Psoriatic arthritis (M ≥ F; skin changes; HLA-B27 positive)	Hands	Involvement of distal interphalangeal joints Erosion of terminal tufts Mouse-ear erosions Pencil-in-cup deformities Sausage digit Joint ankylosis Fluffy periosteal reaction	Dorsovolar view
	Foot	Involvement of distal interphalangeal joints Erosions of terminal tufts and calcaneus	Anteroposterior and lateral views (ankle and foot)
	Spine	Single, coarse syndesmophyte	Anteroposterior and lateral views
	Sacroiliac joints	Unilateral or bilateral symmetric or asymmetric involvement	Posteroanterior and Ferguson views Postcontrast MRI
Enteropathic arthropathies	Sacroiliac joints	Symmetric involvement	Posteroanterior and Ferguson views Computed tomography Postcontrast MRI
SAPHO syndrome	Sternoclavicular, costosternal, and manubriosternal joints	Osteosclerosis, hyperostosis, cortical thickening	Computed tomography

[a]Radionuclide bone scan is used to determine the distribution of arthritic lesions in the skeleton.

observed. Swelling of soft tissue, usually fusiform, may be present around involved articulations (see Figs. 6.2A and 6.3E, F); however, periarticular osteoporosis is rarely present. Later in the disease process, bone ankylosis of the phalanges may develop (see Fig. 6.3G). Approximately 15% of patients with erosive osteoarthritis may have clinical, laboratory, and imaging manifestations of rheumatoid arthritis (Fig. 6.4). The exact relationship between these two conditions is still unclear. Some investigators believe that erosive osteoarthritis is actually rheumatoid arthritis originating in unusual sites but subsequently progressing to the articulations that are more typically involved. Others suggest that each is a distinct entity, citing as evidence the fact that the synovial fluid of patients with rheumatoid arthritis does not resemble that of patients with erosive osteoarthritis, that the immunologic abnormalities commonly seen in rheumatoid arthritis are absent in the latter condition, and that the serologic test for rheumatoid factor is negative.

Because imaging presentation of erosive and nonerosive osteoarthritis may be similar, the investigators were looking into the other means to distinguish these two conditions. The recent studies of serum biomarkers were very promising in this respect. They demonstrated elevation of myeloperoxidase,

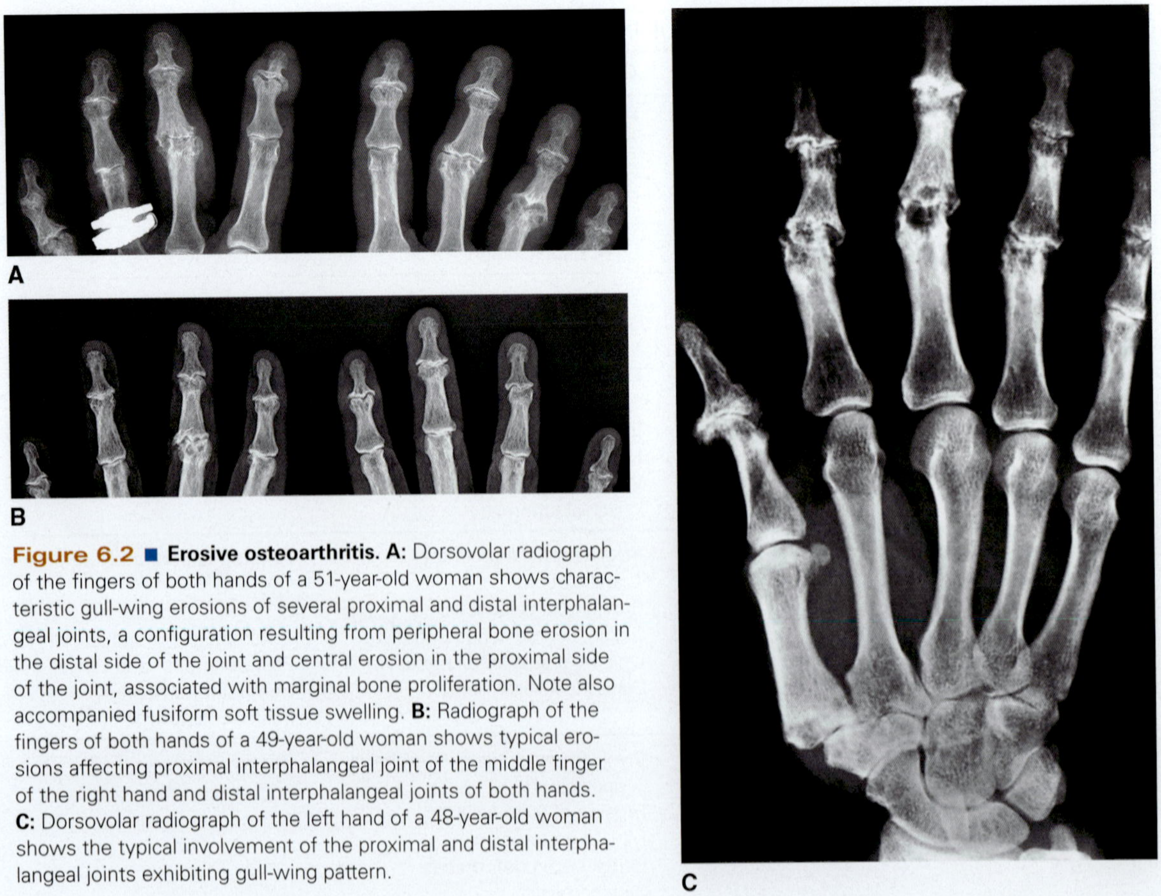

Figure 6.2 ■ **Erosive osteoarthritis. A:** Dorsovolar radiograph of the fingers of both hands of a 51-year-old woman shows characteristic gull-wing erosions of several proximal and distal interphalangeal joints, a configuration resulting from peripheral bone erosion in the distal side of the joint and central erosion in the proximal side of the joint, associated with marginal bone proliferation. Note also accompanied fusiform soft tissue swelling. **B:** Radiograph of the fingers of both hands of a 49-year-old woman shows typical erosions affecting proximal interphalangeal joint of the middle finger of the right hand and distal interphalangeal joints of both hands. **C:** Dorsovolar radiograph of the left hand of a 48-year-old woman shows the typical involvement of the proximal and distal interphalangeal joints exhibiting gull-wing pattern.

C-reactive protein, and serum levels of nitrated form of a marker of type II collagen denaturation (Coll2-1NO2) in patients with EOA.

Differential Diagnosis

The conditions to be considered in differential diagnosis of EOA include primarily classic interphalangeal osteoarthritis, rheumatoid arthritis, and psoriatic arthritis. In interphalangeal OA, certain features, including osteophytosis, subchondral sclerosis, narrowing of the joint spaces, and Heberden and Bouchard nodes, are similar to those of EOA. However, joint erosions and interphalangeal ankylosis are absent. The relationship of EOA to OA and RA still remains a matter of controversy. Some investigators regard EOA as an entirely separate entity, whereas others believe that it represents the end spectrum of OA or perhaps an interface between OA and RA. Ehrlich noted the superimposition of clinical, laboratory, and imaging features of RA in 62 of 170 patients (15%) whose initial diagnosis was EOA. He was first to suggest a relationship between EOA and RA. Conversely, Martel and associates hypothesize that erosions in EOA reflect the intensity and duration of inflammation, favoring the OA spectrum of the disease rather than separate disease entities. The distribution of affected joints in OA and EOA in the hand is identical, with a distinct propensity for DIP and PIP joints as well occasional involvement of the first carpometacarpal and metacarpophalangeal articulations. However, in classic OA affecting the hand, the articular erosions are absent. In addition, Smith and coworkers in their research study of OA and EOA observed that patients with EOA exhibited more severe imaging features of OA in those joints with erosive changes than in the joints without such changes. It is worthwhile to indicate that in adult onset of RA, unlike in EOA, the distal interphalangeal joints are commonly spared, and the erosions are marginal rather than central. In juvenile onset of RA (juvenile idiopathic arthritis), however, the DIP joints may also be affected. Both forms of RA are characterized by notable periarticular osteoporosis, which usually is absent in EOA. There are also differences in the clinical and laboratory findings. Latex agglutination tests for rheumatoid factor are typically negative, the ESR is normal or only minimally elevated, and the synovial fluid reveals no significant inflammatory changes. Moreover, patients do not experience prolonged morning stiffness. Subcutaneous nodules, a common clinical feature of RA, are absent, and no subluxation or dislocation is observed in the interphalangeal joints.

Another condition to be distinguished from EOA is psoriatic arthritis. Both arthritides preferentially affect the DIP joints, but the erosions of psoriatic arthritis are usually marginally located, similar to those of RA. Unlike EOA, which almost invariably has a symmetric distribution, most patients with psoriatic arthritis exhibit asymmetrical

(Continued on page 206)

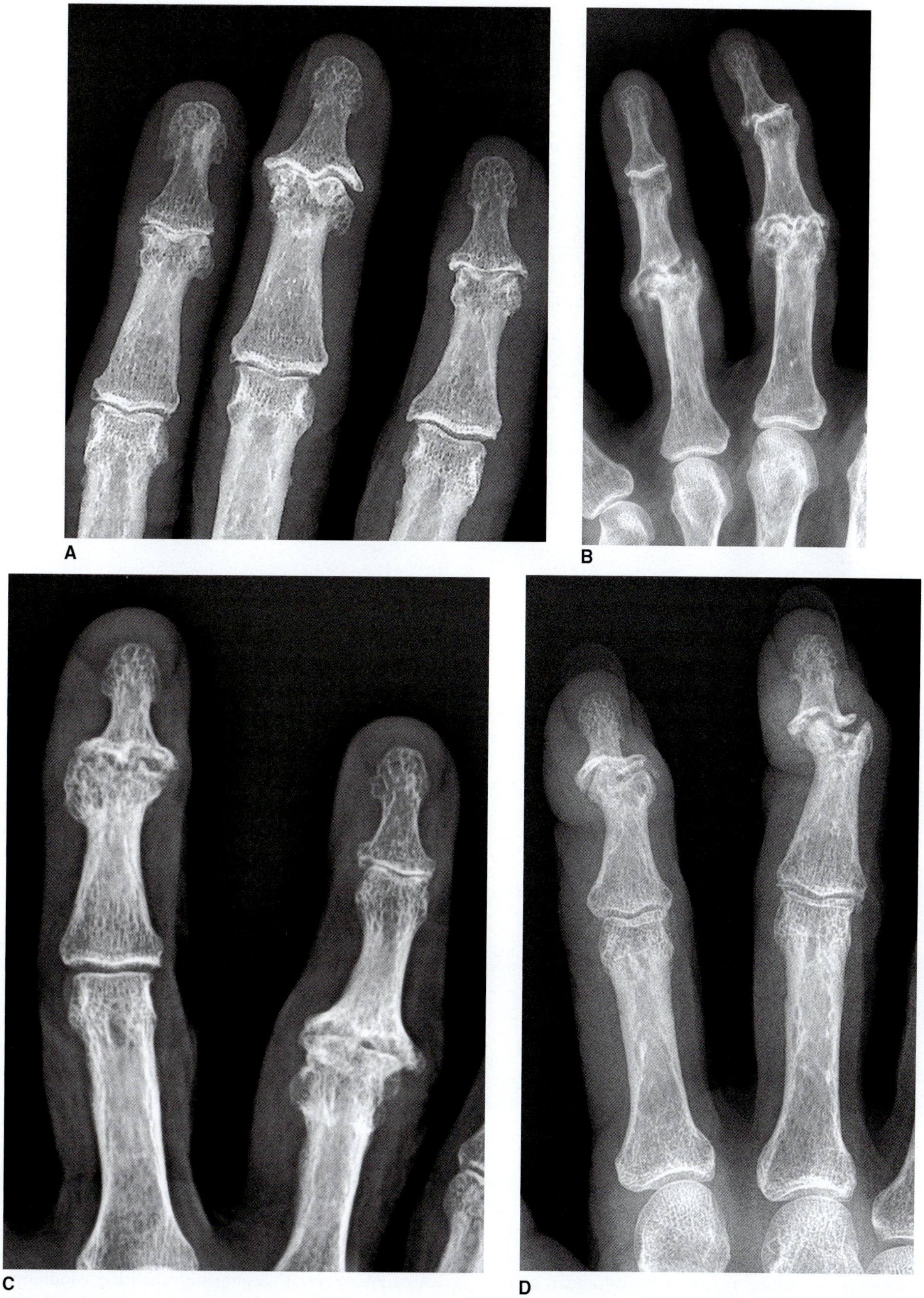

Figure 6.3 ■ **Erosive osteoarthritis. A:** Cone-down view of the index, middle, and ring fingers of a 70-year-old man shows gull-wing erosions of the distal interphalangeal joints. **B:** Cone-down view of the middle and ring fingers of a 66-year-old woman shows advanced erosions of the proximal interphalangeal joints and early erosions of the distal interphalangeal joints. **C:** Cone-down view shows characteristic erosion of the proximal interphalangeal joint of the ring finger and distal interphalangeal joint of the index finger of a 53-year-old woman. **D:** Radiograph of the index and middle fingers of a 50-year-old woman shows gull-wing erosions of the distal interphalangeal joints.

(Continued)

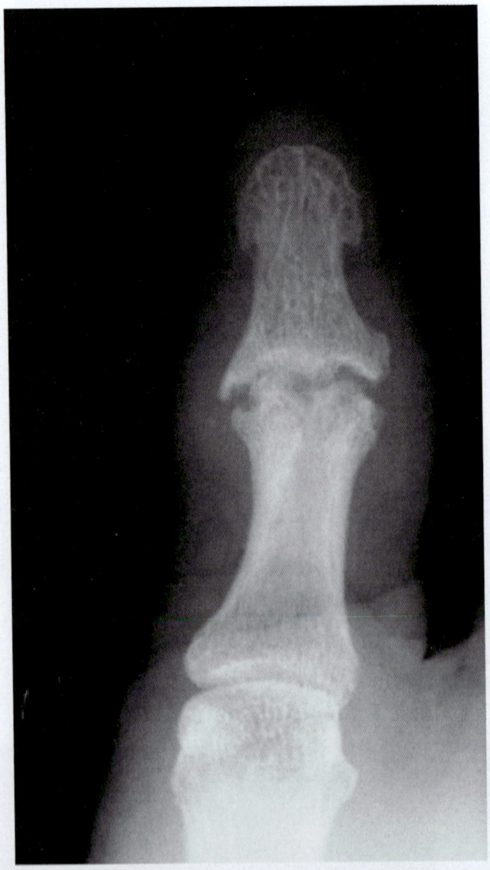

E

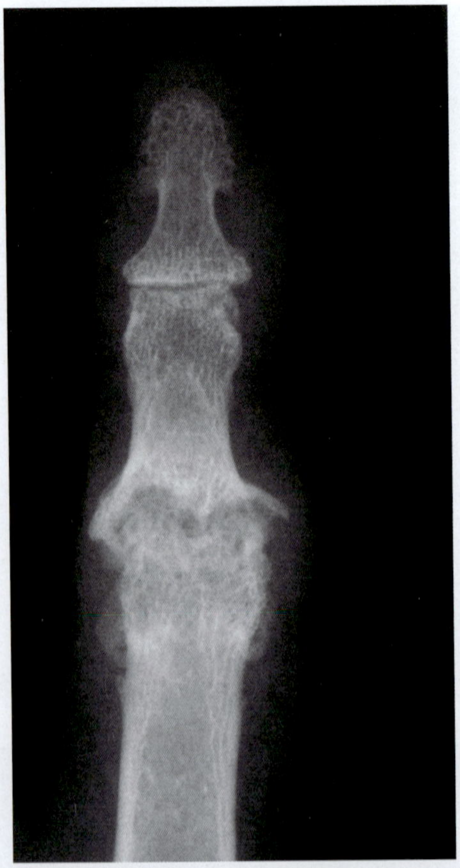

F

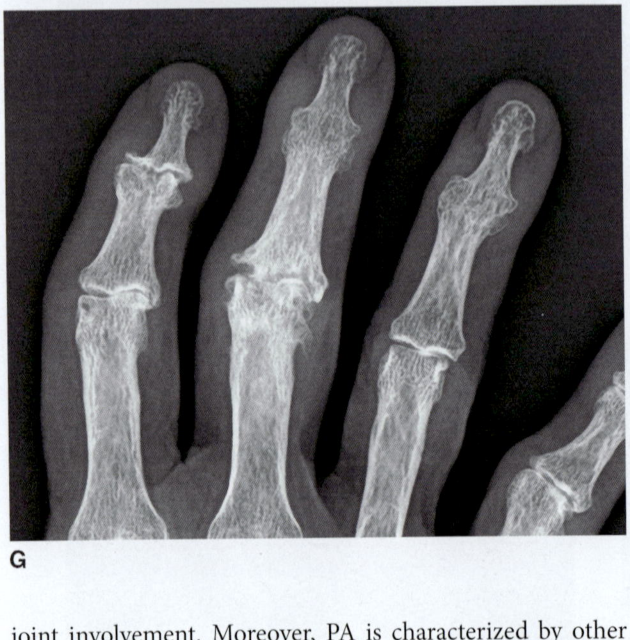

G

Figure 6.3 ■ (*Continued*) **E:** Dorsovolar radiograph of the left thumb of a 51-year-old woman shows characteristic gull-wing erosion of the interphalangeal joint. Note adjacent fusiform soft tissue swelling and lack of periarticular osteoporosis. **F:** In another patient, a 50-year-old woman, gull-wing erosion is accompanied by periosteal reaction and fusiform soft tissue swelling, very similar to psoriatic arthritis. **G:** In this patient, a 69-year-old woman, apart from the typical erosions of the proximal interphalangeal joint of the middle finger and distal interphalangeal joint of the index finger, observe also the fusion of the distal interphalangeal joints of the middle and ring fingers.

joint involvement. Moreover, PA is characterized by other abnormalities not seen in EOA, including skin lesions, nails abnormalities, involvement of sacroiliac joints (sacroiliitis), paraspinal ossifications, and formation of broad-based osteophytes at the plantar aspect of the calcaneus, accompanied by fluffy periostitis. Fluffy periostitis is also seen in the short tubular bones, unlike linear bone apposition observed in EOA. The articular erosions at the DIP joints are also different, with "mouse-ear" rather than "gull-wing" configuration. Lastly, acro-osteolysis and tapered erosions with pencil-like deformities, leading to the so-called arthritis mutilans, are absent in EOA. Although osteophytosis is a consistent phenomenon in EOA, it is almost never seen in RA or PA. When it accompanies the latter conditions, it is secondary because of superimposed degenerative changes rather than a primary feature.

Very rarely, erosive changes in the interphalangeal joints seen in hyperparathyroidism arthropathy can simulate

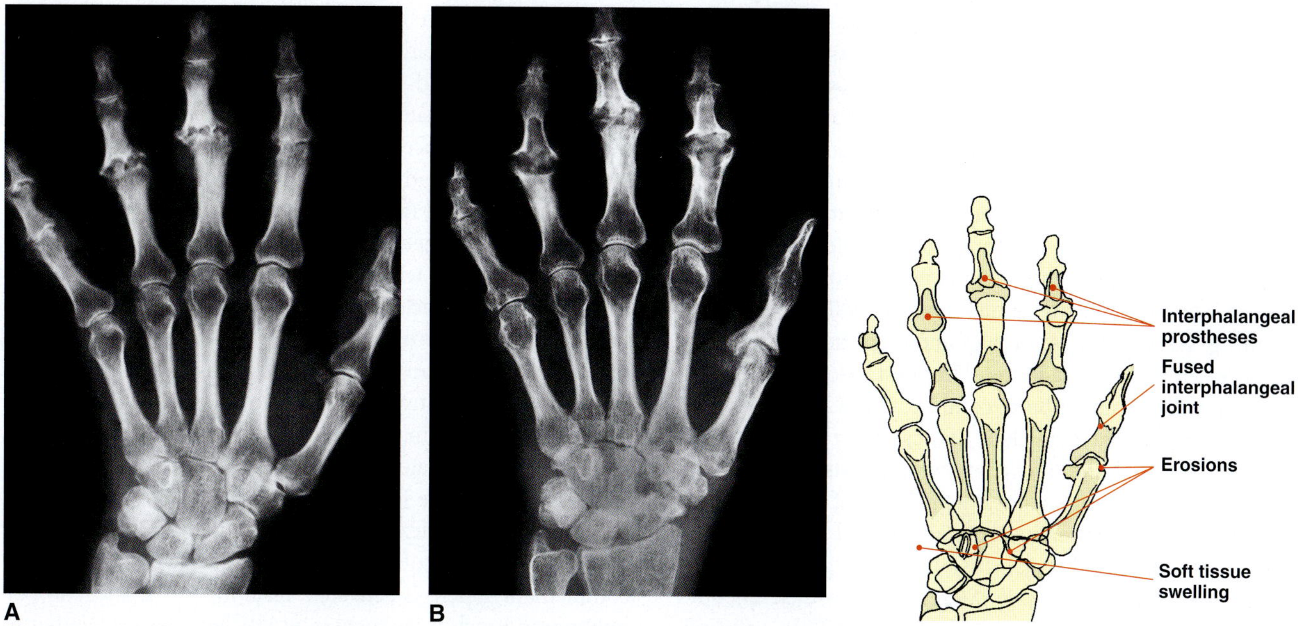

Figure 6.4 ■ Progression of erosive osteoarthritis into rheumatoid arthritis. A: Dorsovolar radiograph of the hand of a 58-year-old woman demonstrates the gull-wing configuration of erosive changes in the proximal interphalangeal joints and the distal interphalangeal joint of the small finger. Because of protracted pain and lack of response to conservative treatment, she underwent joint resection followed by implantation of silicone–rubber prostheses in the proximal interphalangeal joints of the index, middle, and ring fingers, together with fusion of the interphalangeal joint of the thumb and the distal interphalangeal joint of the small finger. Five years after surgery, the classic radiographic features of rheumatoid arthritis developed, involving the wrists **(B),** elbows, shoulders, hips, and cervical spine. Note the surgical fusion of interphalangeal joints of the thumb and fifth finger, as well as the spontaneous fusion of the distal interphalangeal joints of the index and ring fingers.

those present in EOA. However, differential features include osteopenia, invariably accompanying the changes of hyperparathyroidism, and frequent occurrence of acroosteolysis, a hallmark of former condition. Moreover, the erosions seen in hyperparathyroidism arthropathy are not as sharply demarcated as in EOA, being the result of periosteal, chondral, and subchondral resorption. Other features of hyperparathyroidism, including cortical "tunneling," "brown" tumors, soft tissue calcifications, and involvement of ligaments and tendons leading to joint laxity and instability, are additional differentiating features.

Occasionally, a variant of erosive osteoarthritis may be seen as one of the features of Cronkhite-Canada syndrome. This rare systemic disorder also manifests with generalized gastrointestinal polyposis, hyperpigmentation of the skin, and nail atrophy.

Treatment

The main objective of therapy in patients with inflammatory erosive osteoarthritis is relief of pain and restoration of joint function. Nonpharmacologic therapy includes physical and occupational therapy. Range-of-motion exercises and moist heat, in the form of a paraffin bath, are helpful. Pharmacologic methods include analgesics, nonsteroidal anti-inflammatory drugs (NSAIDs), and corticosteroids. Selected cases have also been treated in the past with methotrexate and oral gold salts. Recently, promising results have been achieved with administration of hydroxychloroquine in patients who did not respond to NSAIDs. Also good results have been reported after subcutaneous injections of adalimumab and intra-articular injections of infliximab. Surgical intervention is often necessary for the relief of persistent pain and the correction of severe deformities. One of the most effective procedures is joint replacement by means of silicone–rubber arthroplasties (see Fig. 6.4B). The indications for this type of surgery are loss of the joint space, synovial proliferation with joint destruction, loss of normal alignment, and uncontrollable pain.

RHEUMATOID ARTHRITIS (RA)

Rheumatoid arthritis is a progressive, chronic, systemic inflammatory disease affecting primarily the synovial joints, leading to synovial inflammation and proliferation, loss of articular cartilage, and erosions of subchondral bone. The pathophysiologic hallmark of this condition is formation of pannus, which refers to hypertrophied synovium that develops as inflammatory response. The destructive action of pannus is responsible for progressive erosions and joint surface damage and ligament and joint capsule tearing, all leading to joint deformities and instability. Women are affected three times more often than are men. The course of the disease varies from patient to patient, and there is a striking tendency toward spontaneous remissions and exacerbations.

Although it is much enigmatic, most rheumatologists also include under the rubric of "rheumatoid arthritis" a condition called *seronegative rheumatoid arthritis* (see text below), in which patients present without rheumatoid factor or antibodies to CCP but with the clinical and imaging picture of rheumatoid arthritis. Currently, rheumatoid arthritis is considered to be a heterogeneous autoimmune disorder, with genetic factors playing an important role in the disease expression. Multiple genome-wide association studies have been conducted, but the results have generally been disappointing. The genetics is complex and multifactorial and varies between ethnic populations. The best association is with the major histocompatibility complex (MHC), but the data have yielded no practical clues that can be translated to the bedside. Although the association with the susceptibility loci of *HLA-DRB1* (which encodes the β-chain of HLA-DR) and *PTPN22* genes is better understood, several non-HLA loci have been linked to this arthritis, including the 18q21 chromosome region of the *TNFRSR11A* gene, which encodes the receptor activator of nuclear factor kappaB. In addition, a common genetic variant at the *TRAF1-C5* locus on chromosome 9 is associated with an increased risk of anti-CCP-positive rheumatoid arthritis. Allelic variants of *HLA-DRB1* associated with risk for rheumatoid arthritis encode a similar sequence, namely, amino acids 70 to 74, known as the shared epitope (SE). The detection of antibodies to citrullinated proteins (CCP), representing specific autoantibodies in the patient's serum, is an important diagnostic finding.

In 2010, the American College of Rheumatology in collaboration with European League Against Rheumatism established new classification criteria for rheumatoid arthritis (RA). Their work "*focused on identifying, among patients newly presenting with undifferentiated inflammatory synovitis, factors that best discriminated between those who were and those who were not at high risk for persistent and/or erosive disease—this being the appropriate current paradigm underlying the disease construct 'rheumatoid arthritis.*'" The main advantage of this new classification is focusing on features at earlier stages of rheumatoid arthritis rather than defining the disease by its late-stage features, as it was practiced in the past. In the established new criteria, classification as "definite RA" was based on the presence of synovitis in at least one joint, absence of alternative diagnosis that better explains the synovitis, and achievement of a total score of 6 or greater (out of possible 10) from the individual scores in four categories: number and site of involved joints (score range from 0 to 5), serologic abnormality (score range from 0 to 3), elevated acute-phase response (score range from 0 to 1), and duration of symptoms (two levels; range from 0 to 1).

Serology of Rheumatoid Arthritis

Rheumatoid factors, so widely used by clinicians, are anti–gamma globulin antibodies that are generally IgM and combine with their antigens (immunoglobulin G [IgG]) to form immune complexes. These complexes activate the complement system, which releases mediators responsible for producing inflammation within the joint structures. Because rheumatoid factors can be found in the serum and in joint fluids of patients with nonrheumatoid disorders, their presence alone is not diagnostic of rheumatoid arthritis. They have been studied for decades and were once thought to be the only critical serologic marker of rheumatoid arthritis; this, however, is not the case, because rheumatoid factors can be found in the joint fluid of patients with nonrheumatoid disorders. Although the rheumatoid factor is still widely used, it has lost much of the luster of the past. Nevertheless, finding high titers of these factors in a joint effusion strongly suggests the diagnosis of rheumatoid arthritis. Early in the course of disease, rheumatoid factors may be demonstrated in the synovial fluid before they are positive in the serum, allowing early diagnosis. Rheumatoid factors do participate in the pathogenesis of rheumatoid arthritis through the formation of local and circulating antigen–antibody complexes. In synovial fluid, IgM and IgG rheumatoid factors can combine to form immune complexes. The complement system is activated, resulting in the attraction of polymorphonuclear leukocytes into the joint space. Discharge of their hydrolytic enzymes causes the destruction of joint tissues. The process initiating these events is as yet unknown. Patients with rheumatoid arthritis with subcutaneous nodules almost always will have positive rheumatoid factors, generally in high titer. Interesting, however, is the fact that frequency and severity of rheumatoid nodules has greatly deceased in population and the disease is strikingly different in this respect from two generations ago.

As already discussed in the text above, autoantibodies against the group of *citrullinated proteins (CCPs)* are more pathognomonic for rheumatoid arthritis than rheumatoid factors. The second-generation enzyme-linked immunosorbent assay (ELISA) tests for anti–cyclic citrullinated peptide 2 (anti-CCP2) antibodies have specificity for RA as high as 97%. These antibodies are directed at one or all of the following proteins: alpha enolase, fibrinogen, and vimentin. In all cases, the arginine in these proteins has been replaced by the plant amino acid citrulline. In people with a genetic predisposition to loss of tolerance, autoantibodies to these CCPs appear and may be detected many years before the clinical onset of rheumatoid arthritis. There are several factors known to accelerate this loss of tolerance, including smoking and infections, particularly *Proteus* infections of the gums.

Clinical Features

Articular and periarticular manifestations include joint swelling and tenderness to palpation, with morning stiffness and severe motion impairment in the affected joints. The clinical presentation varies between the patients, but an insidious onset of pain with symmetrical swelling of the joints of the hands is the most common finding. Some patients may present with palindromic onset, monoarticular presentation, extra-articular synovitis (such as tenosynovitis and bursitis), and general symptoms such as malaise, fatigue, anorexia, weight loss, and low-grade fever.

Imaging Features

Rheumatoid arthritis is characterized by a diffuse, usually multicompartmental, symmetric narrowing of the joint space associated with marginal or central erosions, periarticular osteoporosis, and periarticular soft tissue swelling; subchondral sclerosis is minimal or absent and formation of osteophytes is lacking.

Large Joint Involvement

Any of the large weight-bearing and non–weight-bearing joints can be affected by rheumatoid arthritis. Regardless of the size of the joint and the site of involvement, certain imaging features can be identified that are characteristic of this inflammatory process.

Osteoporosis

In rheumatoid arthritis, unlike osteoarthritis, osteoporosis is a striking feature. In the early stage of the disease, osteoporosis is localized to periarticular areas (juxta-articular osteoporosis), but with progression of the condition, a generalized osteoporosis can be observed.

Joint Space Narrowing

This is usually a symmetric process with concentric narrowing of the joint. Concentric narrowing in the hip joint leads to axial migration of the femoral head, which in more advanced stages may result in acetabular protrusio (Figs. 6.5 and 6.6). Similar concentric joint space narrowing is observed in the shoulder joint (Fig. 6.7). In

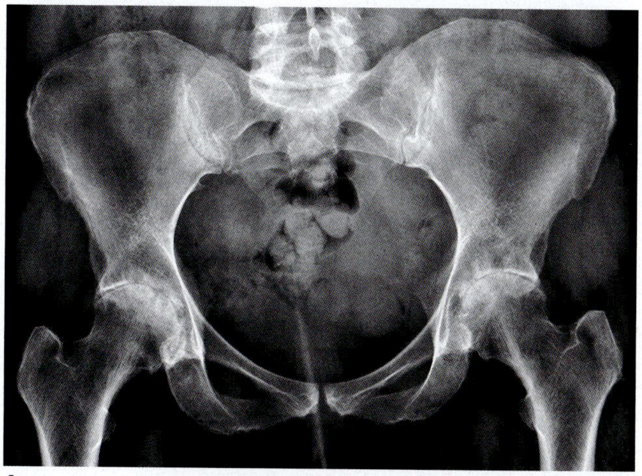

A

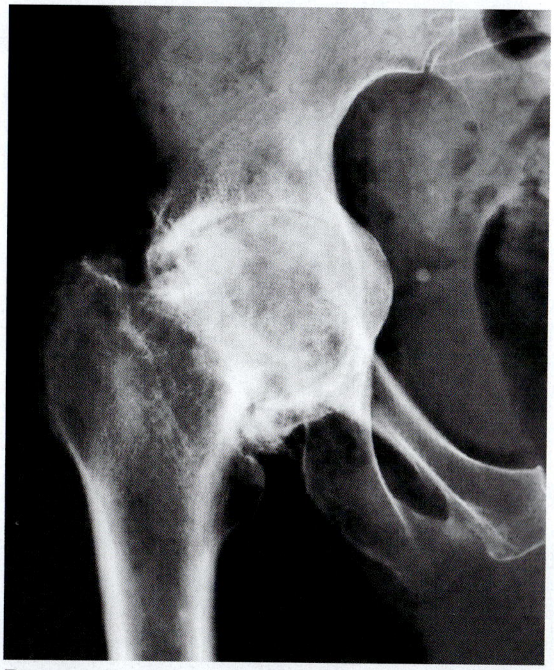

B

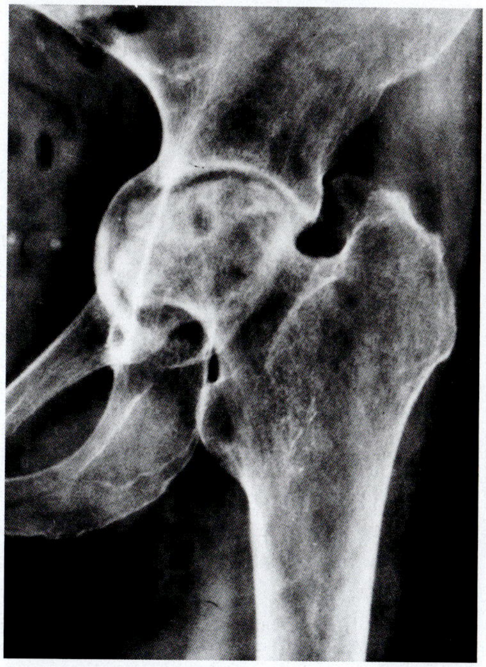

C

Figure 6.5 ■ Rheumatoid arthritis of the hip joints. **A:** Anteroposterior radiograph of the pelvis of a 47-year-old woman shows uniform narrowing of both hip joints accompanied by axial migration of the femoral heads. **B:** Anteroposterior radiograph of the right hip of a 60-year-old woman with advanced rheumatoid arthritis shows concentric joint space narrowing, with axial migration of the femoral head leading to acetabular protrusion. Some superimposed secondary osteoarthritic changes are also present. **C:** Anteroposterior radiograph of the left hip of a 64-year-old woman shows erosions of the femoral head and acetabulum, concentric narrowing of the hip joint, and acetabular protrusion.

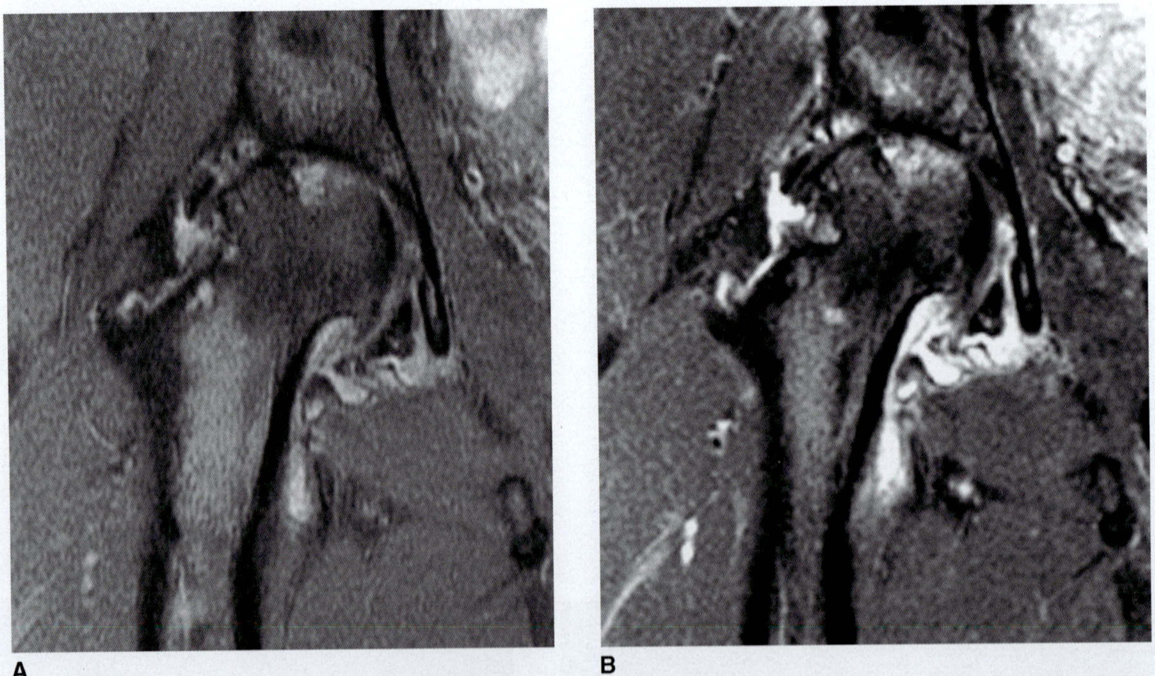

Figure 6.6 ■ **MRI of rheumatoid arthritis of the hip joint.** Coronal proton density-weighted fat-suppressed MRI **(A)** and coronal proton density-weighted fat-suppressed MR image **(B)** of the right hip joint of a 31-year-old woman obtained after intravenous administration of gadolinium show uniform narrowing of the joint space, joint effusion, synovitis, and erosions of the femoral head and acetabulum.

addition, cephalad migration of the humeral head may be seen secondary to destructive changes in the shoulder joint and rupture of the rotator cuff (Fig. 6.8A); resorption of the distal end of the clavicle, which assumes a pencil-like appearance, may also be observed. Tear of the rotator cuff in this condition (Fig. 6.8B, C) must be differentiated from the chronic traumatic form of this abnormality (Fig. 6.9). In the knee joint, all three compartments are commonly narrowed in a uniform manner (Fig. 6.10). The loss of the articular cartilage is caused by inflammation and pannus formation. There is little evidence of bone repair or osteophyte formation, and there is invariably associated joint effusion (Fig. 6.11). In the elbow and ankle, uniform joint space narrowing is observed (Figs. 6.12 to 6.14).

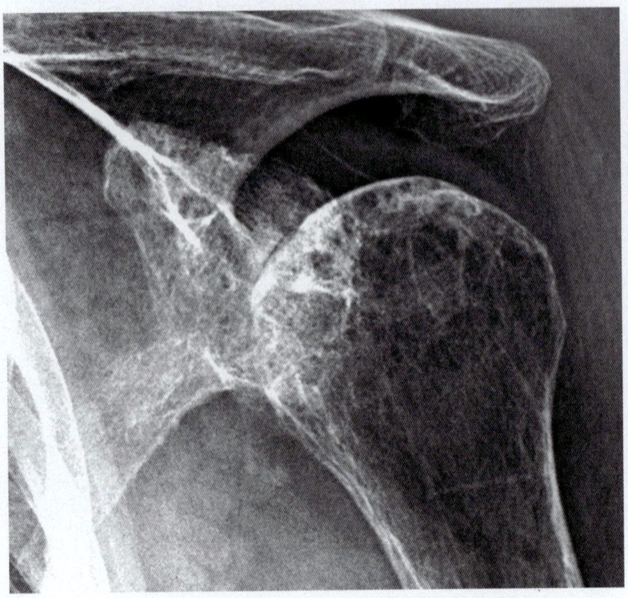

Figure 6.7 ■ **Rheumatoid arthritis of the shoulder joint.** Radiograph of the left shoulder of a 70-year-old woman shows periarticular osteoporosis and concentric narrowing of the glenohumeral joint.

Articular Erosions

Erosive destruction of a joint may be central or peripheral in location. As a rule, reparative processes are absent or very minimal; thus, there is no evidence of subchondral sclerosis or osteophytosis (Fig. 6.15), which may be present only if secondary degenerative changes are superimposed on the underlying inflammatory process (see Fig. 5.11).

Osseous Erosions

Loss of the normal radiolucent triangle between the posterosuperior margin of the calcaneus and the adjacent Achilles tendon is consistent with the presence of inflammatory fluid within the retrocalcaneal bursa (Fig. 6.16A), commonly associated with erosion of the calcaneus (Fig. 6.16B–D). In the hands, the carpal bones are commonly affected (Figs. 6.17 to 6.19).

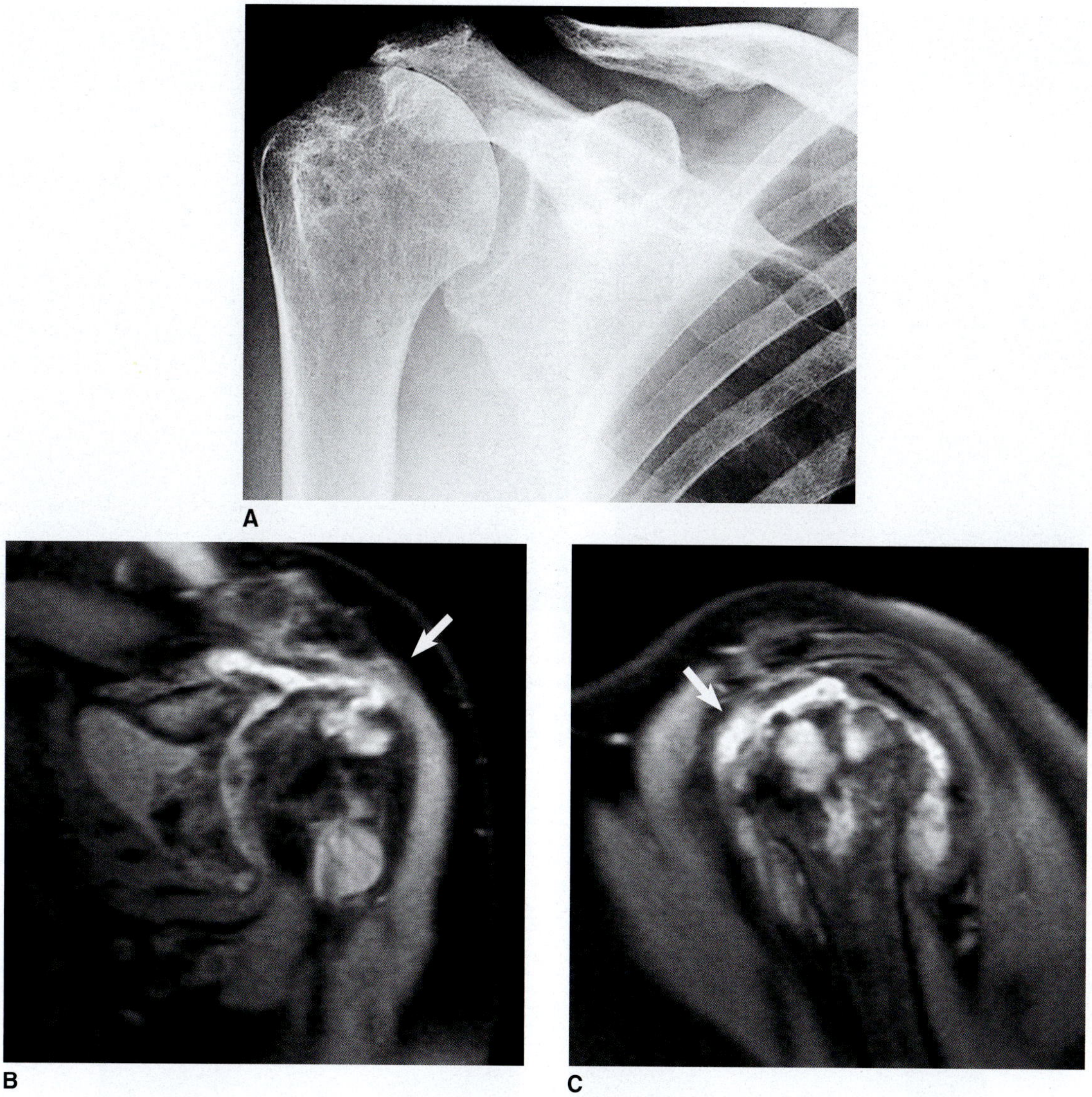

Figure 6.8 ■ **Rheumatoid arthritis, chronic rotator cuff tear. A:** Anteroposterior radiograph of the right shoulder of a 72-year-old man with advanced rheumatoid arthritis shows upward migration of the humeral head secondary to rotator cuff tear, a common complication of rheumatoid changes in the shoulder joint. Note the characteristic tapered erosion of the distal end of the clavicle, erosions of the humeral head, and the substantial degree of periarticular osteoporosis. Coronal oblique **(B)** and sagittal **(C)** proton density-weighted fat-suppressed MR images of the left shoulder of a 64-year-old woman show large articular and periarticular erosions, joint space narrowing, joint effusion, and a tear of the supraspinatus tendon (*arrows*), all the features of advanced rheumatoid arthritis.

Synovial Cysts and Pseudocysts

These radiolucent defects are usually seen in close proximity to the joint (Fig. 6.20). They may or may not communicate with the joint space.

Baker Cyst

Popliteal cyst is a common finding, seen in ~48% of patients with rheumatoid arthritis, and can be detected with ultrasound (Fig. 6.21, see also Fig. 2.76A) or with MRI (Fig. 6.22, see also Fig. 2.99). It extends posteriorly and may be directed inferiorly or superiorly in the soft tissues in the posterior aspect of the knee joint. Rupture of the Baker cyst leads to extravasation of the inflammatory content into the soft tissues of calf, producing pain and swelling that may be mistaken for thrombophlebitis (see Fig. 2.77).

Joint Effusion

Fluid can be best demonstrated in the knee joint on the lateral projection (see Fig. 6.10B). Fluid in the other large joints such as the shoulder, elbow, and hip can be best demonstrated by MRI (see Figs. 6.13 and 6.16).

Rice Bodies

Bearing macroscopic similarity to grains of polished white rice, these small, usually uniform in size intra-articular

(Continued on page 216)

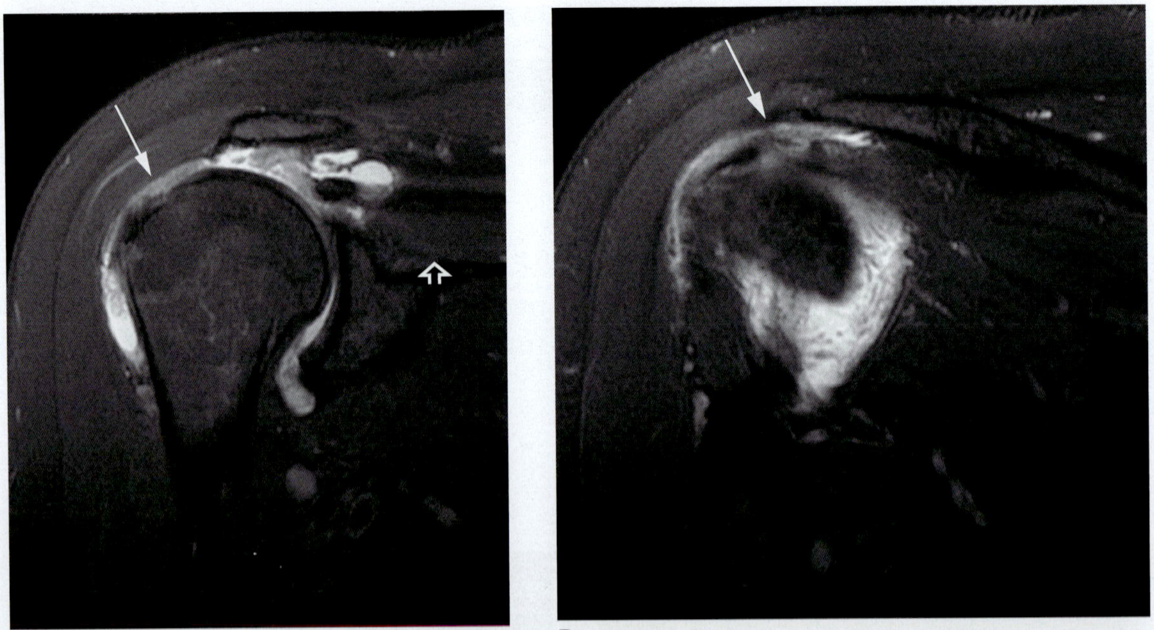

A B

Figure 6.9 ■ **Massive posttraumatic rotator cuff tear. A:** Coronal oblique proton density-weighted fat-suppressed MR arthrographic image of the right shoulder of a 32-year-old man, who sustained multiple injuries in a motorcycle accident, shows a full-thickness tear of the supraspinatus tendon (*arrow*). The supraspinatus muscle is medially retracted (*open arrow*). **B:** More posterior section shows also a tear of the infraspinatus tendon (*arrow*). Note lack of inflammatory features seen in rheumatoid arthritis.

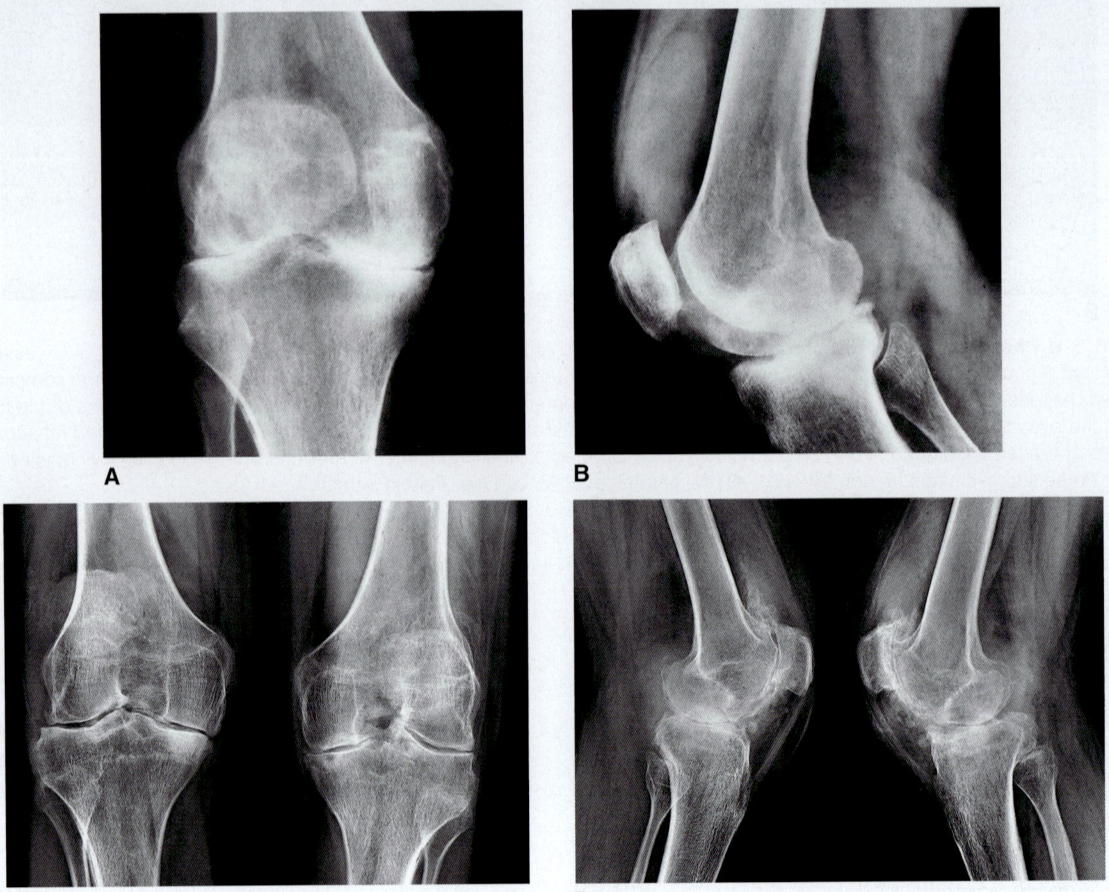

C D

Figure 6.10 ■ **Rheumatoid arthritis of the knee joints.** Anteroposterior **(A)** and lateral **(B)** radiographs of the right knee of a 52-year-old woman joints show tricompartmental involvement. Note the periarticular osteoporosis, joint effusion, and lack of osteophytosis. Anteroposterior **(C)** and lateral **(D)** radiographs of both knees of a 50-year-old man show uniform narrowing of the medial, lateral, and femoropatellar joint compartments associated with joint effusions.

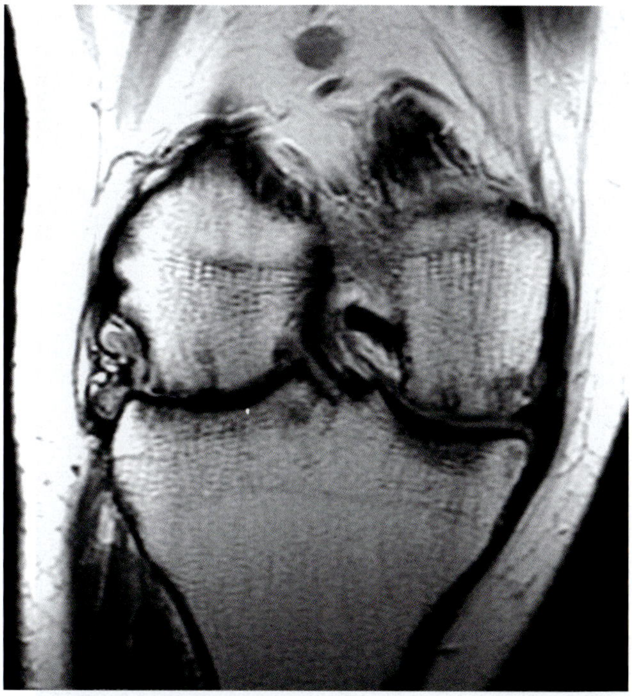

A

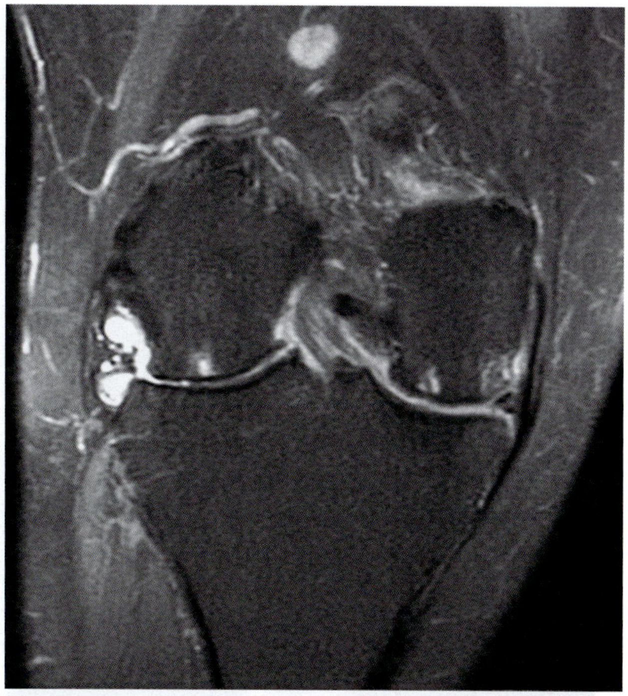

B

Figure 6.11 ■ **MRI of rheumatoid arthritis of the knee.** Coronal T1-weighted **(A)** and coronal proton density-weighted **(B)** fat-suppressed MR images of the left knee of a 50-year-old woman show uniform joint space narrowing of the lateral and medial compartments, destruction of the articular cartilage, subchondral bone erosions, and tear of the lateral and medial menisci. **C:** Coronal T1-weighted MRI of the right knee of another patient demonstrates a joint effusion with inflammatory pannus (*arrow*). Note the lower signal intensity of the fluid as compared to the slightly higher signal of the pannus.

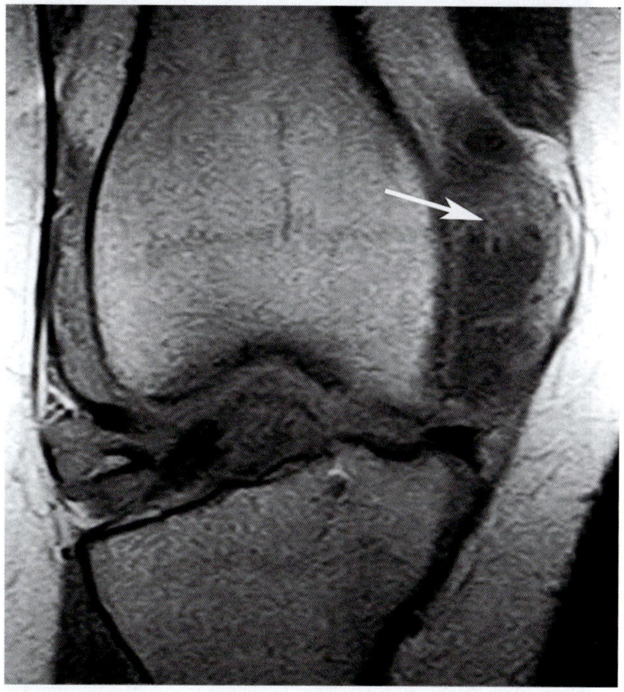

C

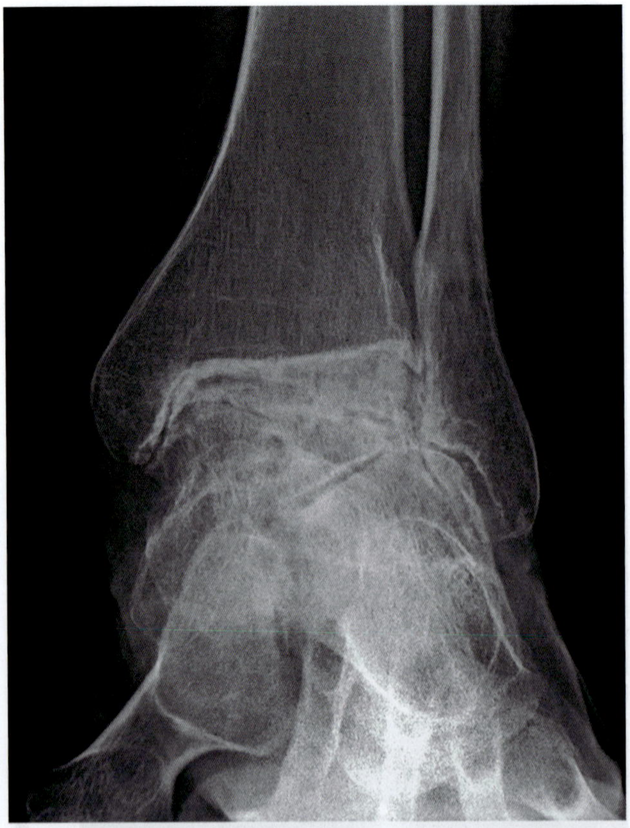

A

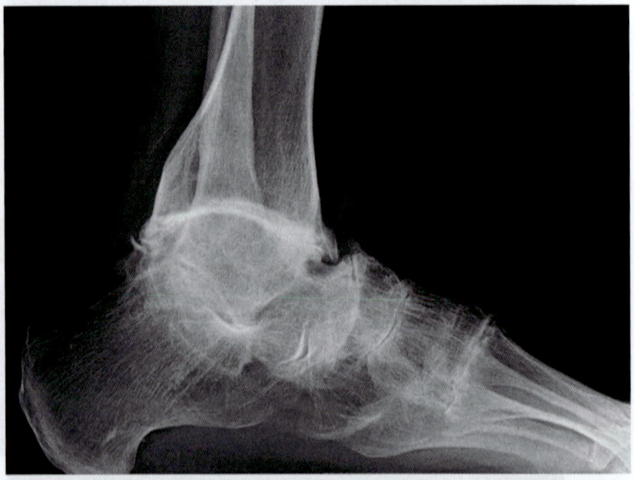

B

Figure 6.14 ■ Rheumatoid arthritis of the ankle joints. Anteroposterior **(A)** and lateral **(B)** radiographs of the ankle show uniform joint space narrowing of the tibiotalar, subtalar, Chopart, and Lisfranc joints.

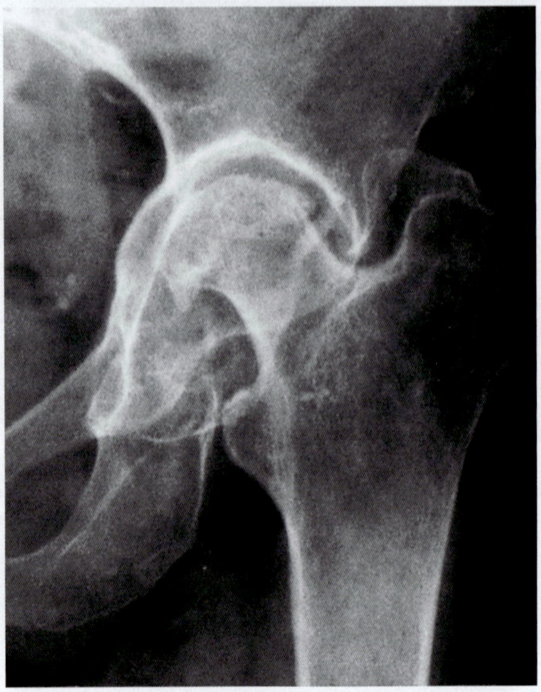

Figure 6.15 ■ Rheumatoid arthritis of the hip joint. Anteroposterior radiograph of the left hip of a 59-year-old woman with advanced rheumatoid polyarthritis demonstrates the typical erosions of the femoral head and acetabulum, and acetabular protrusio. Note the lack of osteophytosis and the only very minimal reactive sclerosis.

or intrabursal loose bodies are commonly associated with rheumatoid arthritis and are thought to represent a complication of chronic inflammatory process. Occasionally, they also may be seen in seronegative inflammatory arthritis and even in tuberculous arthritis. These particles contain collagen, fibrinogen, fibrin, reticulin, elastin, mononuclear cells, blood cells, and some amorphous material (Fig. 6.23). On radiography (Fig. 6.24), this condition occasionally can be mistaken for synovial chondromatosis (see Chapter 10). On MR T1-weighted images, rice bodies exhibit intermediate signal intensity, whereas on T2 weighting, they are only slightly hyperintense relative to muscle (Figs. 6.25 and 6.26).

Rheumatoid Nodules

They are relatively common, with a reported frequency of ~25%. They usually develop over pressure areas such as elbow (Fig. 6.27) or ischial tuberosities.

Small Joint Involvement

Rheumatoid arthritis characteristically affects the small joints of the wrist, as well as the metacarpophalangeal and proximal interphalangeal joints of the hands and feet. As a rule, the distal interphalangeal joints in the hand are spared, although in advanced stages of the disease even these may be

(Continued on page 222)

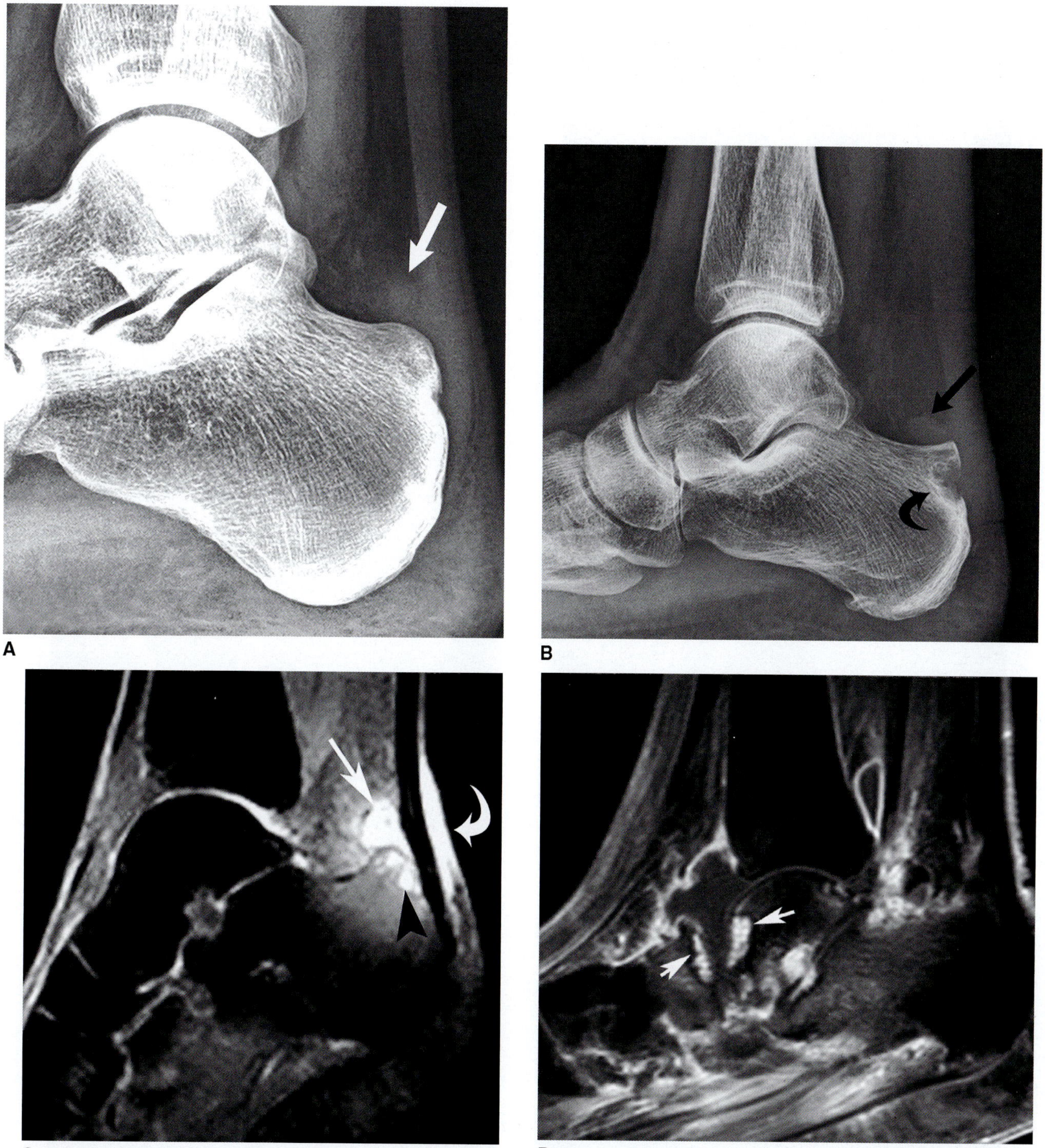

A B C D

Figure 6.16 ■ **Rheumatoid arthritis: osseous erosions. A:** Lateral radiograph of the heel of a 49-year-old woman shows retrocalcaneal bursitis (*arrow*) without osseous erosions. **B:** Lateral radiograph of the foot of a 55-year-old woman who presented with a heel pain shows fluid in the retrocalcaneal bursa (*arrow*) associated with erosion of the calcaneus (*curved arrow*). **C:** Sagittal STIR MR image in another patient demonstrates bone erosion in the posterior process of the calcaneus (*arrowhead*) associated with extensive surrounding bone marrow edema and retrocalcaneal and retro-Achilles bursitis (*arrows*). **D:** Sagittal T1-weighted fat-saturated postcontrast MRI of the ankle in another patient demonstrates a large tibiotalar joint effusion with enhancing synovium/pannus. Note the bone erosions in the talus and navicular bones containing enhancing inflammatory pannus (*arrows*).

Figure 6.17 ■ Rheumatoid arthritis: osseous erosions. Norgaard view of both hands of a 33-year-old woman shows early erosions of both pisiform bones (*arrows*).

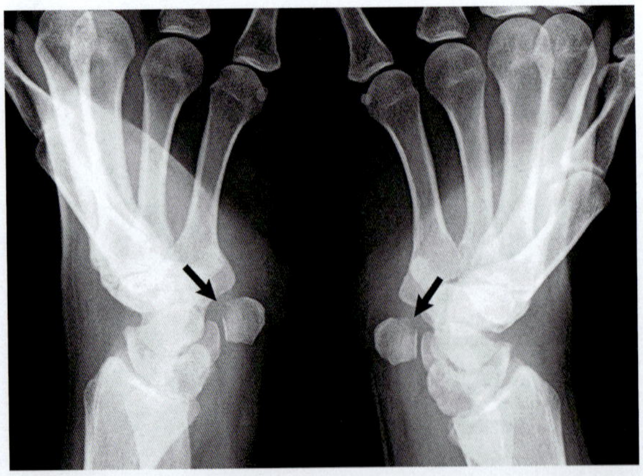

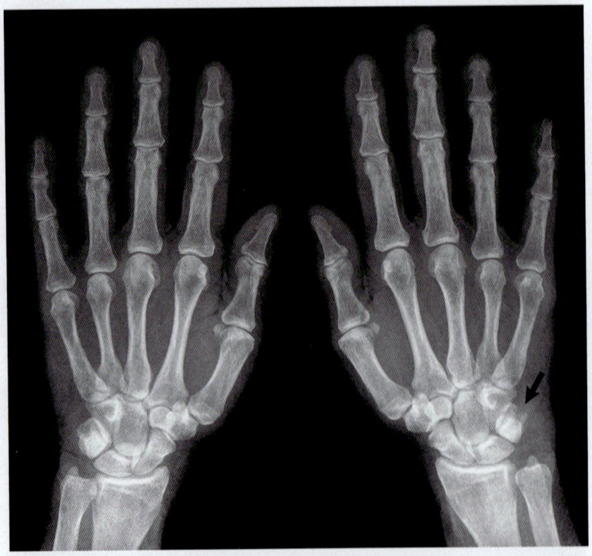

A

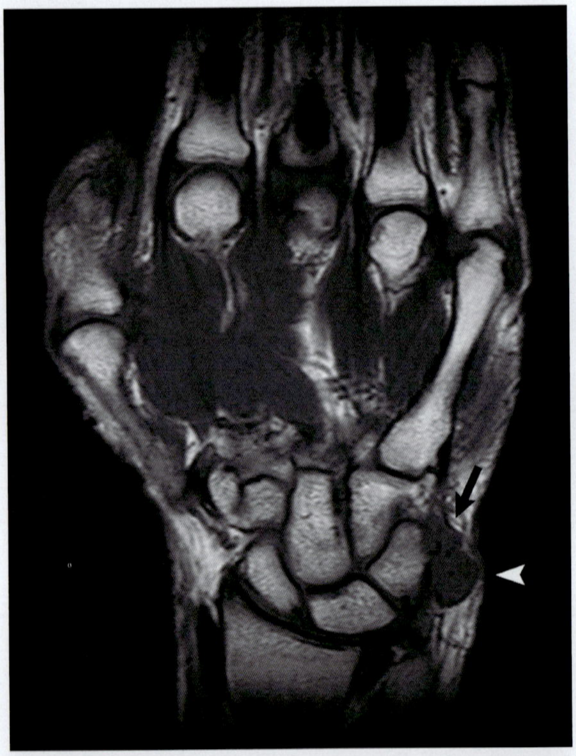

B

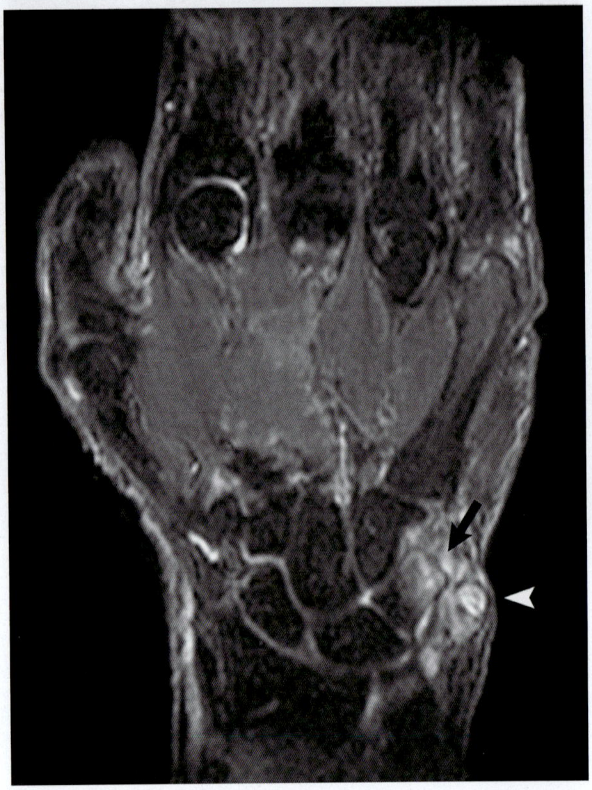

C

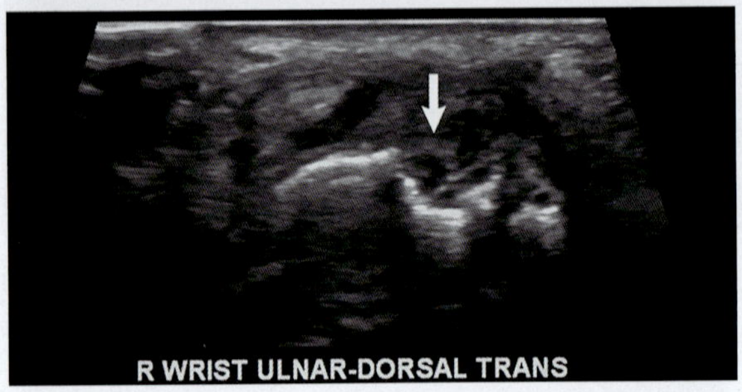

D

Figure 6.18 ■ Rheumatoid arthritis: osseous erosions. **A:** Dorsovolar radiograph of both hands of a 50-year-old woman shows erosion of the right triquetral bone (*arrow*). This was an isolated osseous abnormality in this patient. Coronal proton density-weighted **(B)** and coronal proton density-weighted **(C)** fat-suppressed MR images demonstrate erosion of the triquetrum associated with soft tissue edema (*arrows*). Note also edema in adjacent extensor carpi ulnaris tendon (*arrowheads*). **D:** Transverse US image of the same area also effectively depicts the triquetral erosion (*arrow*).

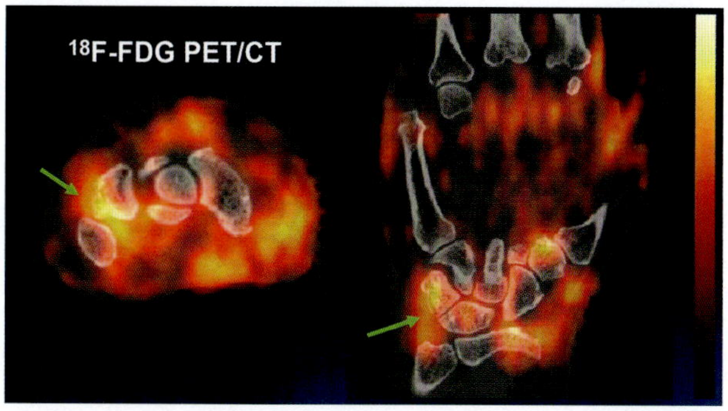

Figure 6.19 ■ PET/CT of osseous erosion. Axial and coronal reformatted fused 18F-FDG PET/CT images of the right wrist of a 59-year-old woman with rheumatoid arthritis show high glucose uptake in the pisiform–triquetral compartment and erosion of the triquetral bone (*arrows*).

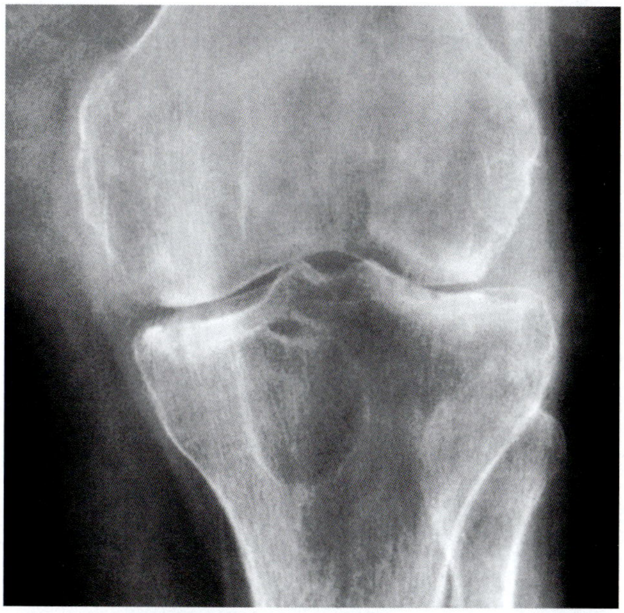

Figure 6.20 ■ Rheumatoid cyst. Anteroposterior radiograph of the left knee of a 35-year-old woman with rheumatoid arthritis shows a large synovial cyst in the proximal tibia. Note also articular erosions and periarticular osteoporosis.

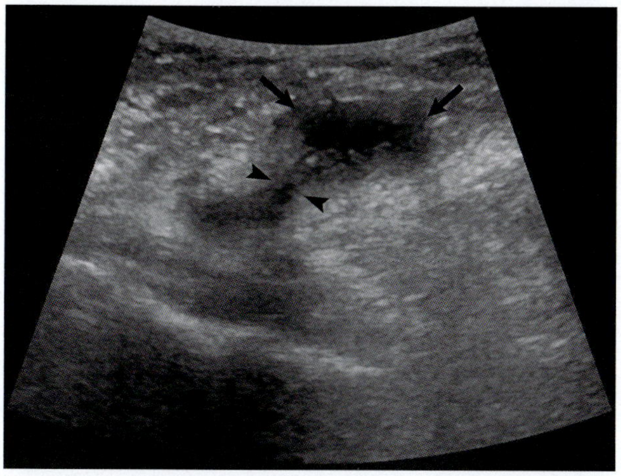

Figure 6.21 ■ US of the Baker cyst. Transverse US image of the knee of a 42-year-old woman with rheumatoid arthritis shows an oval in shape hypoechoic area (*arrows*) that communicates with the knee joint (*arrowheads*).

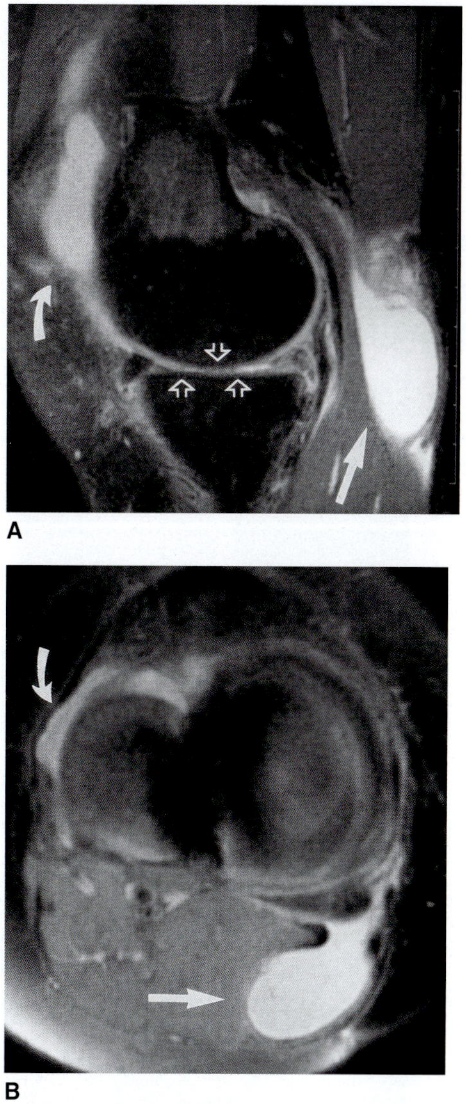

Figure 6.22 ■ MRI of the Baker cyst. Sagittal **(A)** and axial **(B)** T2-weighted fat-suppressed MR images of a 60-year-old woman with rheumatoid arthritis demonstrate a large popliteal cyst (*arrows*). *Open arrows* point to erosive changes of the articular cartilage; *curved arrows* indicate joint effusion.

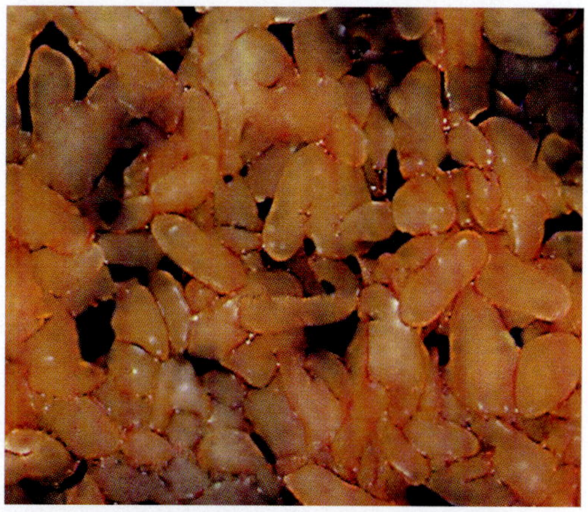

Figure 6.23 ■ Rice bodies. Photograph of fibrinous loose bodies recovered from the knee joint of the patient with rheumatoid arthritis. (From Bullough PG. *Atlas of Orthopedic Pathology with Clinical and Radiologic Correlation*. 2nd ed. New York, NY: Gower Medical Publishing; 1992, Fig. 11.18, p. 11.6.)

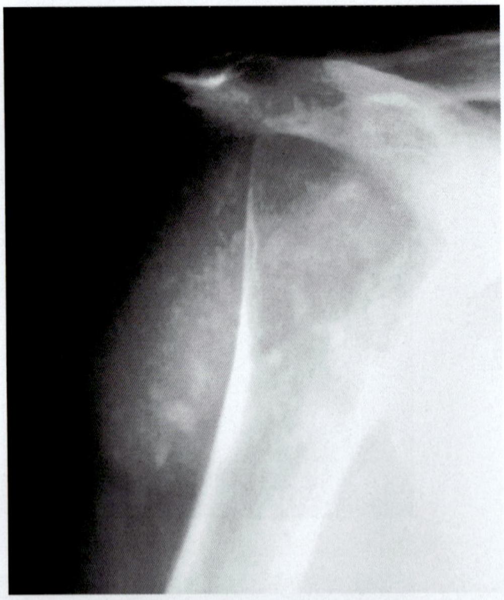

Figure 6.24 ■ **Rice bodies.** Anteroposterior radiograph of the right shoulder of a 60-year-old woman with advanced rheumatoid arthritis demonstrates multiple rice bodies within subacromial–subdeltoid bursae complex.

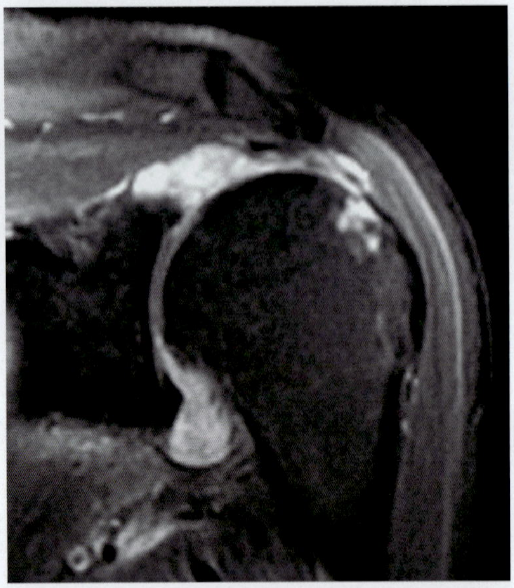

A

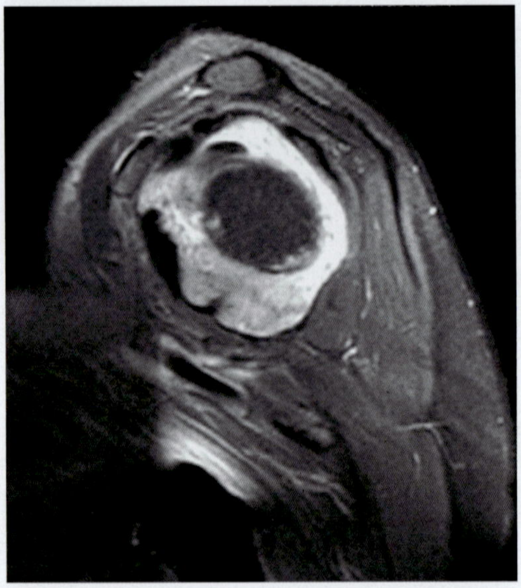

B

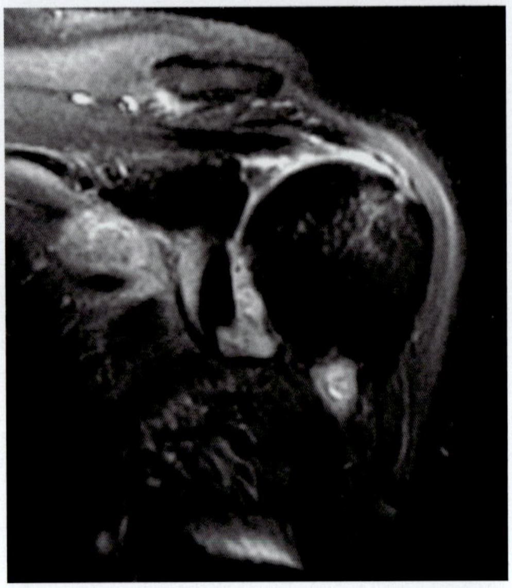

C

Figure 6.25 ■ **MRI of rice bodies.** Oblique coronal proton density-weighted **(A)**, sagittal proton density-weighted **(B)**, and oblique coronal T2-weighted **(C)** fat-suppressed MR images of the left shoulder of a 66-year-old woman with rheumatoid arthritis show numerous rice bodies within the shoulder joint.

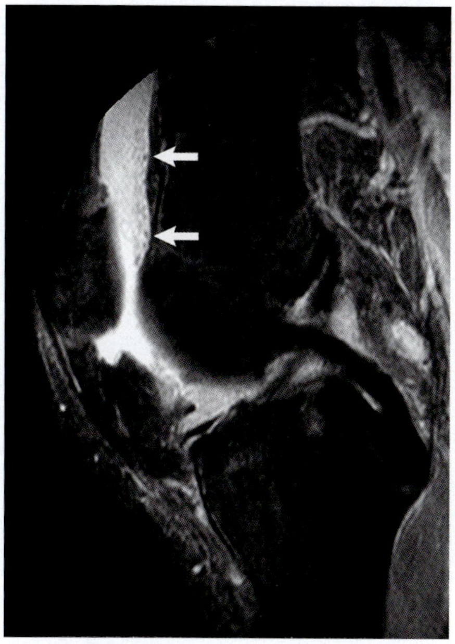

A

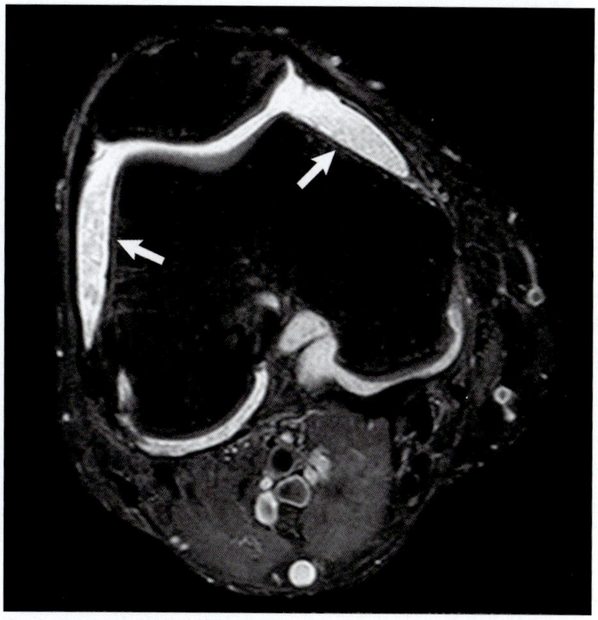

B

Figure 6.26 ■ **MRI of rice bodies.** Sagittal **(A)** and axial **(B)** fast spin-echo (FSE) proton density-weighted fat-suppressed MR images of the right knee of a 68-year-old woman with rheumatoid arthritis show numerous rice bodies within the joint fluid (*arrows*).

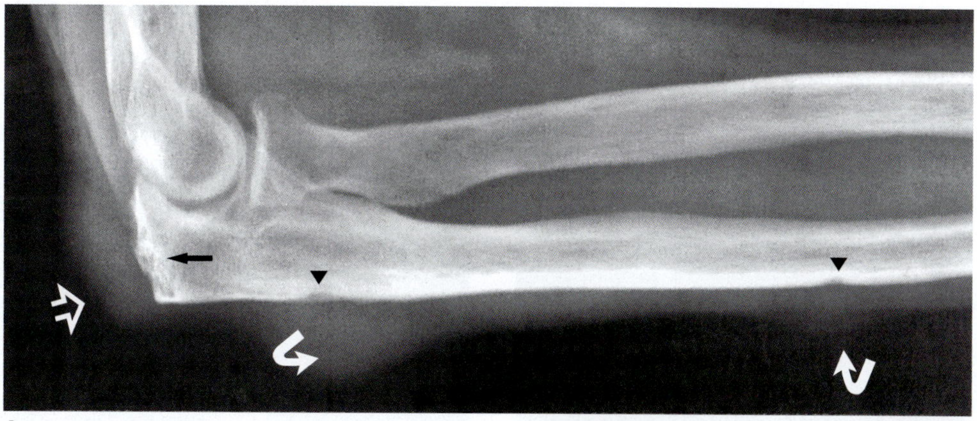

A

Figure 6.27 ■ **Rheumatoid nodules. A:** Lateral radiograph of the right elbow of a 39-year-old man demonstrates erosions of the olecranon process (*arrow*), olecranon bursitis (*open arrow*), and rheumatoid nodules on the dorsal aspect of the forearm (*curved arrows*). Note the characteristic pitlike cortical erosions at the site of the rheumatoid nodules (*arrowheads*). **B:** A 68-year-old woman with rheumatoid arthritis had a large rheumatoid nodule at the lateral side of the elbow joint. Note erosions at the radiocapitellar joint (*arrow*).

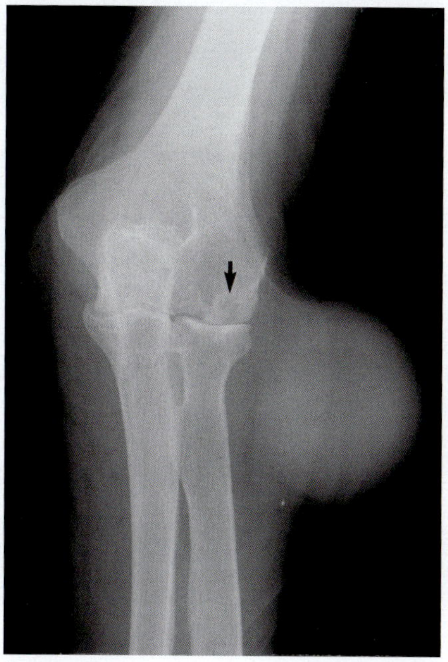

B

affected. This latter point, however, is controversial, because some investigators believe that if the distal interphalangeal joints are involved, the condition may represent juvenile idiopathic arthritis or another form of polyarthritis, not classic rheumatoid arthritis.

In addition to the characteristic changes exhibited in large joint involvement, the small joints may also show radiographic features specific for these sites.

Soft Tissue Swelling

This earliest sign of rheumatoid arthritis usually has a fusiform, symmetric shape. It is periarticular in location and represents a combination of joint effusion, edema, and tenosynovitis. Although it can be seen on the radiographs (see Fig. 6.34), the MRI provides a more effective way of demonstration of this critical feature of pre-erosive rheumatoid arthritis (Fig. 6.28). MRI also is a modality of choice to show early changes of tenosynovitis (Fig. 6.29), although ultrasound may effectively demonstrate soft tissue abnormalities at the joints (Fig. 6.30) as well as tenosynovitis in the hands and feet (Fig. 6.31, see also Figs. 2.80 and 2.81).

(Continued on page 224)

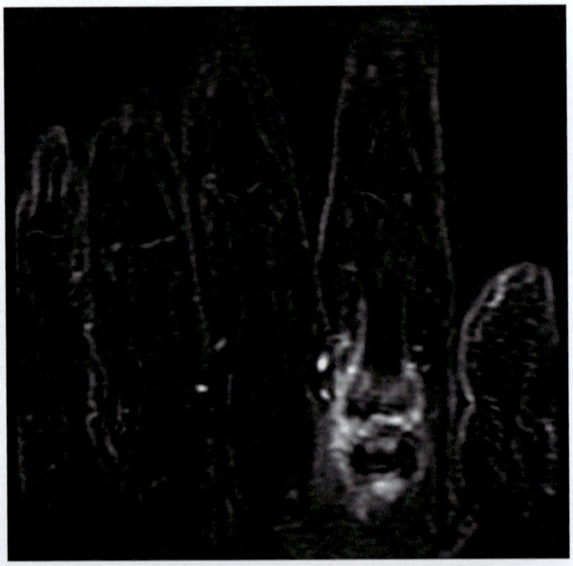

Figure 6.28 ■ MRI of very early changes of rheumatoid arthritis. Coronal STIR MR image of the hand demonstrates bone marrow edema involving the proximal phalanx and distal metacarpal of the second digit, with prominent periarticular soft tissue edema. Bone marrow edema may be seen on MRI before the bone erosions are seen on radiographs (pre-erosive edema). This feature makes MRI a good tool for establishing an early diagnosis thus leading to early therapy of rheumatoid arthritis.

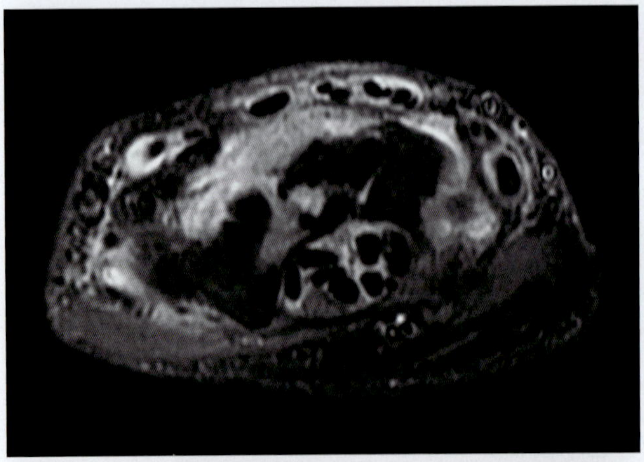

A

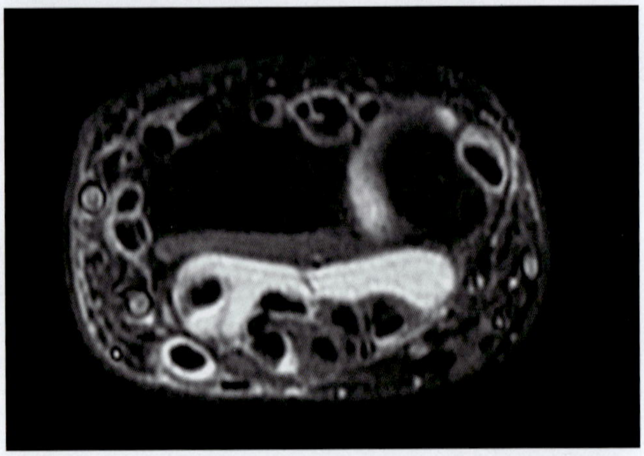

B

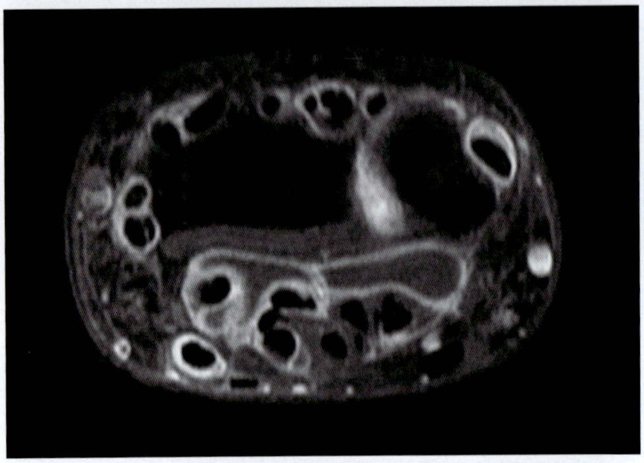

C

Figure 6.29 ■ MRI of tenosynovitis. Two axial STIR **(A, B)** and axial T1-weighted fat-suppressed **(C)** MR postcontrast images of the wrist of a 67-year-old woman with rheumatoid arthritis show synovial thickening and diffuse tenosynovitis of all flexor and extensor tendons.

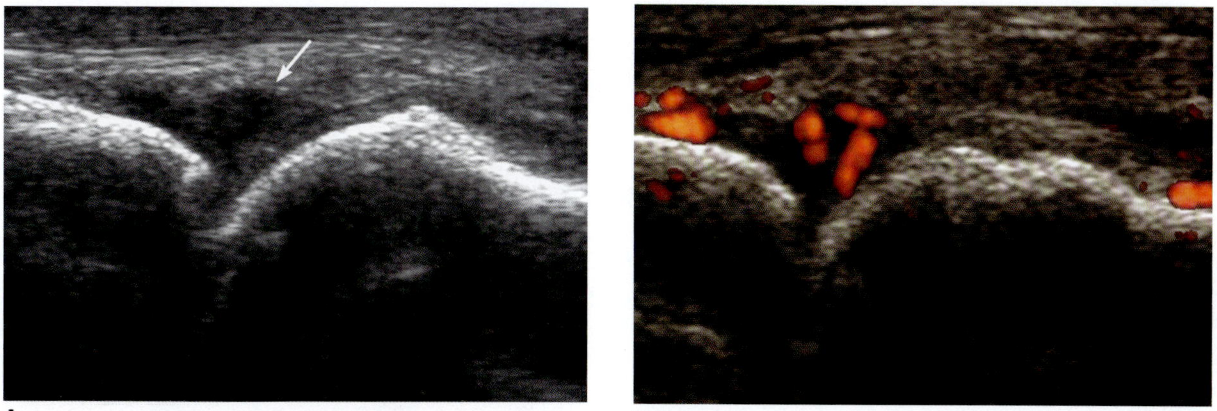

A B

Figure 6.30 ■ **US of small joint synovitis. A:** Longitudinal ultrasound image of the left second metacarpophalangeal joint of a 60-year-old man with rheumatoid arthritis shows hypoechoic triangular area at the site of distended joint capsule, representing joint effusion and synovial thickening. **B:** Power Doppler color scale of the same area shows increased vascularity consistent with synovial hyperemia from active inflammation. (Reprinted with permission from Klein MJ, Bonar SF, Freemont T, et al., eds. *Atlas of Nontumor Pathology. Non-neoplastic Diseases of Bones and Joints.* Washington DC: American Registry of Pathology and Armed Forces Institute of Pathology, 2011, Fig. 2-17, p. 68.)

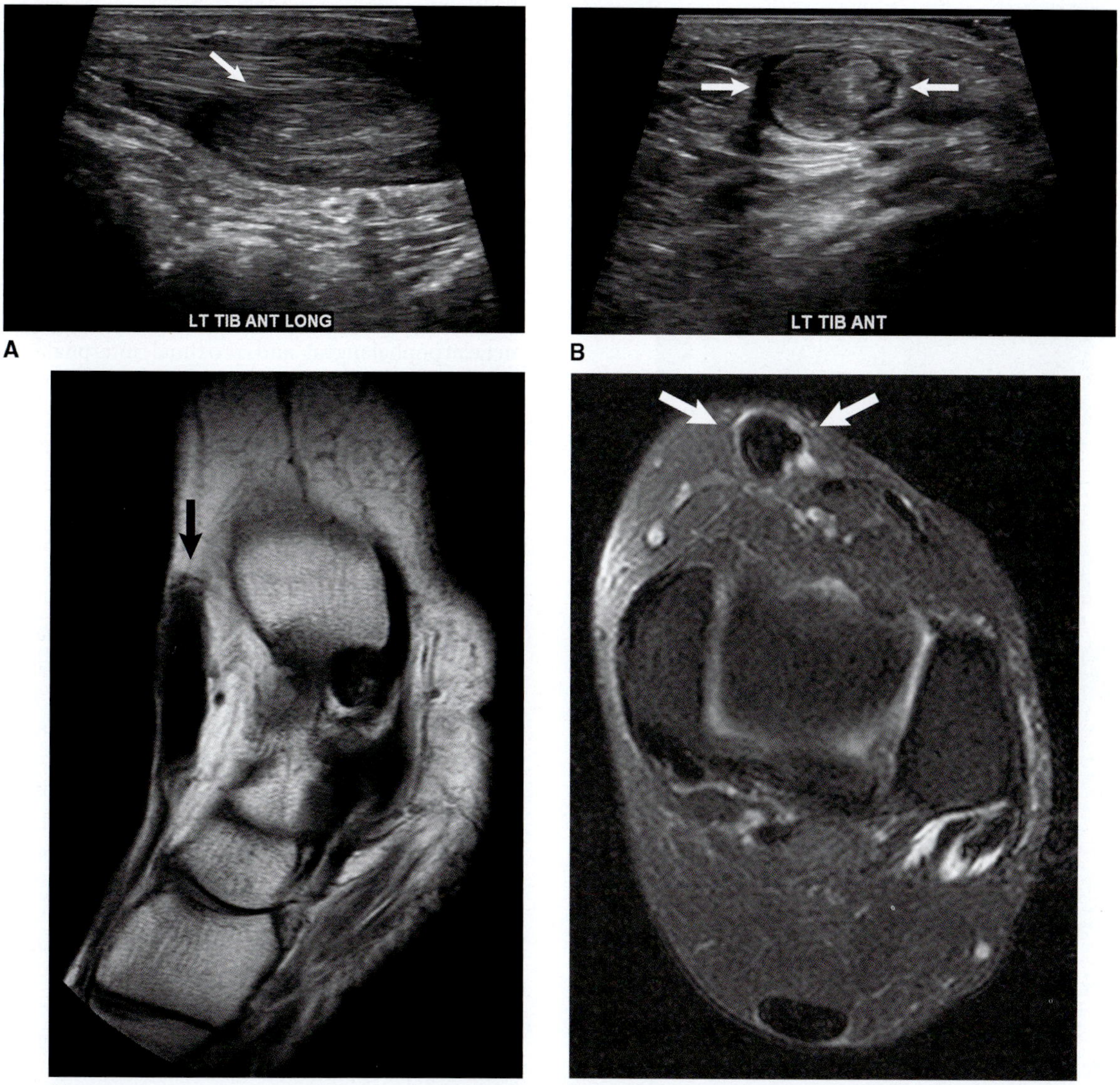

A B C D

Figure 6.31 ■ **US and MRI of tenosynovitis.** Longitudinal **(A)** and transverse **(B)** US images of the anterior aspect of the left ankle of a 65-year-old woman with rheumatoid arthritis show markedly thickened anterior tibialis tendon and fluid within the tendon sheath (*arrows*). **C:** Sagittal T1-weighted MR image confirms the thickening of the anterior tibialis tendon. **D:** Axial proton density-weighted fat-suppressed MR image shows in addition fluid within the anterior tibialis tendon sheath (*arrows*) and tenosynovitis of the peroneus longus and brevis tendons.

Loss of Articular Cortex

This is another early radiographic sign of inflammatory arthritis: the so-called articular (or subchondral) cortex becomes indistinct or completely lost (Fig. 6.32).

Marginal Erosions

Other early radiographic signs of articular abnormalities manifest as marginal erosions at so-called bare areas. These are the sites within the joint capsule that are not covered by articular cartilage (Fig. 6.33). The most common locations for these erosions are the radial aspects of the second and third metacarpal heads and the radial and ulnar aspects of the bases of the proximal phalanges (Fig. 6.34). Synovial inflammation in the prestyloid recess, a diverticulum of the radiocarpal joint that is intimate with the styloid process of ulna, as Resnick pointed out, produces marginal erosion of the styloid tip.

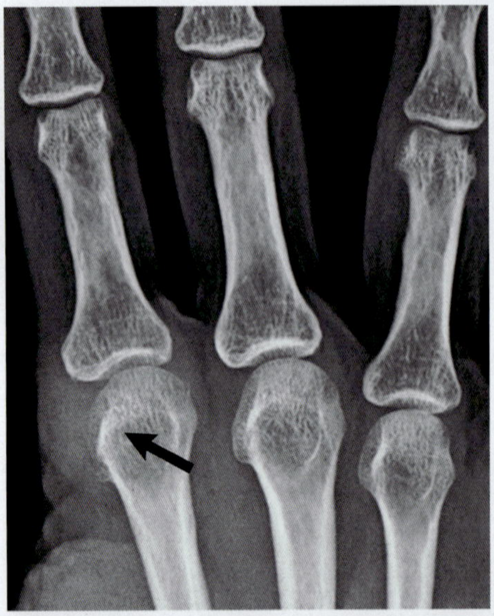

A

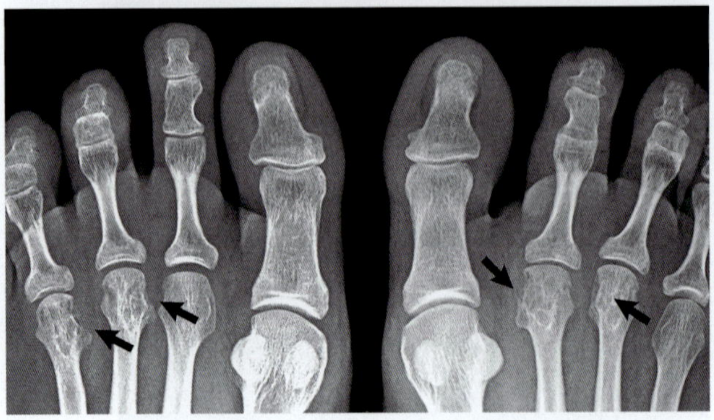

B

Figure 6.32 ■ Rheumatoid arthritis—loss of articular cortex. A: Very early radiographic feature is the loss of so-called articular cortex of the metacarpal head on the radial aspect (*arrow*). Compare with the intact outline of the normal third and fourth metacarpal heads. **B:** In another patient, the metatarsal heads are affected in similar manner (*arrows*), but to a slightly greater extent.

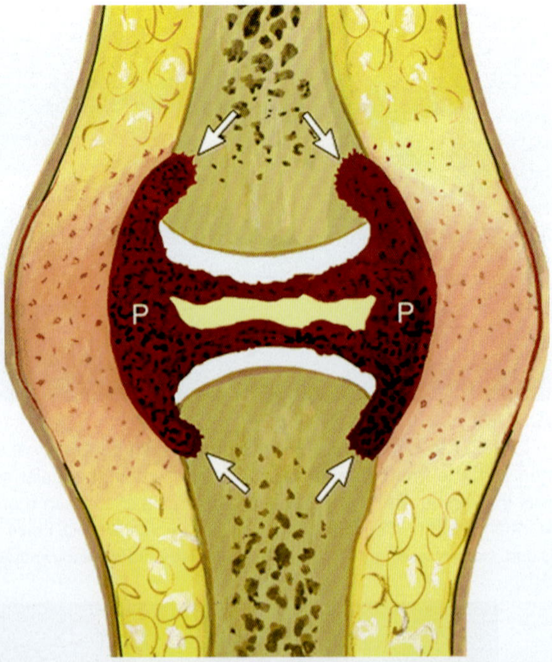

Figure 6.33 ■ Rheumatoid arthritis—erosions in bare areas. Invasion of inflammatory pannus (*P*) into the articular areas not covered by the articular cartilage (so-called bare areas) causes marginal erosions (*arrows*).

Articular Erosions

In more advanced stages of rheumatoid arthritis, articular erosions are commonly seen. In the hand, the metacarpophalangeal and proximal interphalangeal joints are usually affected (Fig. 6.35) as well as joints of the wrist (Figs. 6.36 and 6.37, see also Fig. 6.35A). In the foot, the metatarsophalangeal and proximal interphalangeal joints are commonly affected (Figs. 6.38 and 6.39). The subtalar joint may be affected as well (Fig. 6.40).

Joint Deformities

Although not pathognomonic for rheumatoid arthritis, certain deformations such as the *swan-neck deformity* and the *boutonniére deformity* are more often seen in this form of arthritis than in other inflammatory arthritides. The first of these represents hyperextension in the proximal interphalangeal joint and flexion in the distal interphalangeal joint, a configuration resembling a swan's neck (Fig. 6.41, see also Fig. 1.3C). In the boutonniére deformity, the configuration is just the opposite, with flexion in the proximal joint and extension in the distal interphalangeal joint (Fig. 6.42, see also Fig. 1.3A, B). The word *boutonniére* is French for "buttonhole," the term for this deformity deriving from the configuration of the finger while securing a flower to a lapel. A similar deformation of the thumb is called *hitchhiker's thumb* (see Fig. 1.2).

Moreover, subluxations and dislocations with malalignment of the fingers are common findings in advanced stages of rheumatoid arthritis. Particularly characteristic are ulnar deviation of the fingers in the metacarpophalangeal joints and

(Continued on page 227)

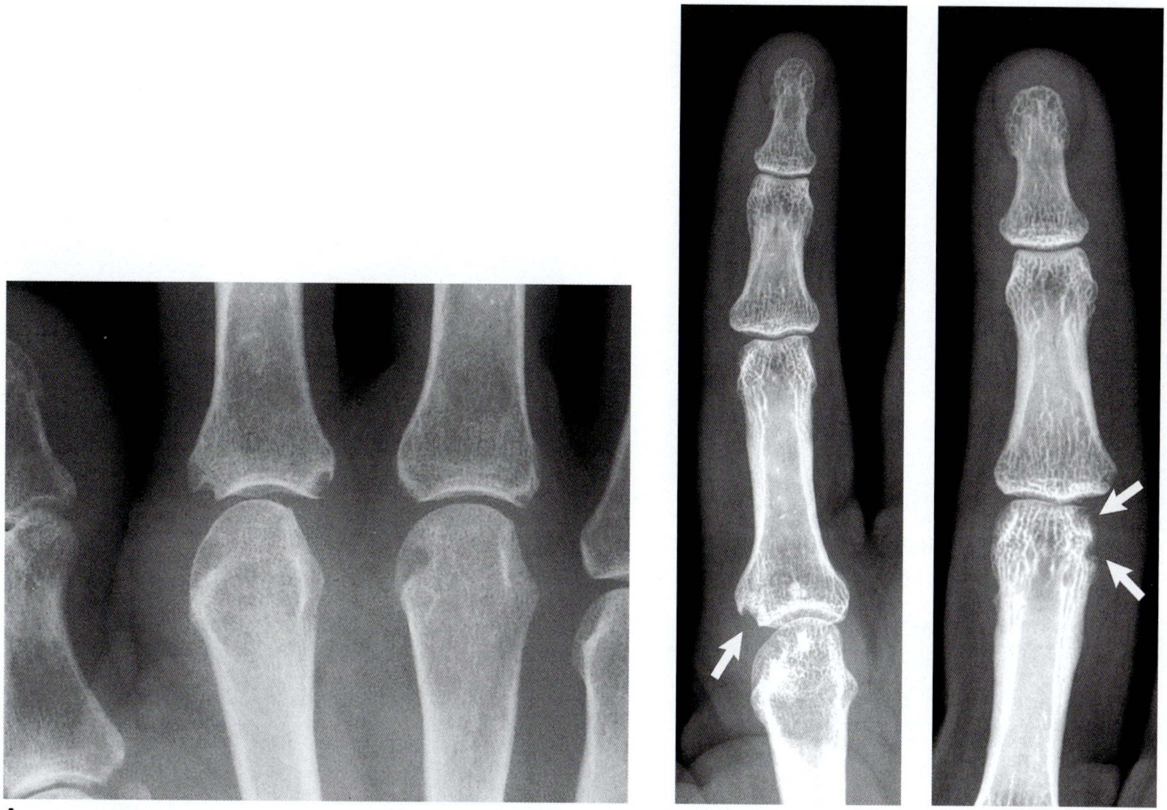

A B C

Figure 6.34 ■ Rheumatoid arthritis—erosions in bare areas. A: Typical erosions in the bare areas are seen in this 55-year-old woman with rheumatoid arthritis. Note also periarticular osteoporosis and soft tissue swelling. **B:** Radiograph of the index finger shows erosion in the bare area at the base of the proximal phalanx (*arrow*) associated with soft tissue swelling. **C:** Radiograph of the middle finger of another patient shows erosions in the bare areas at the distal end of the proximal phalanx (*arrows*).

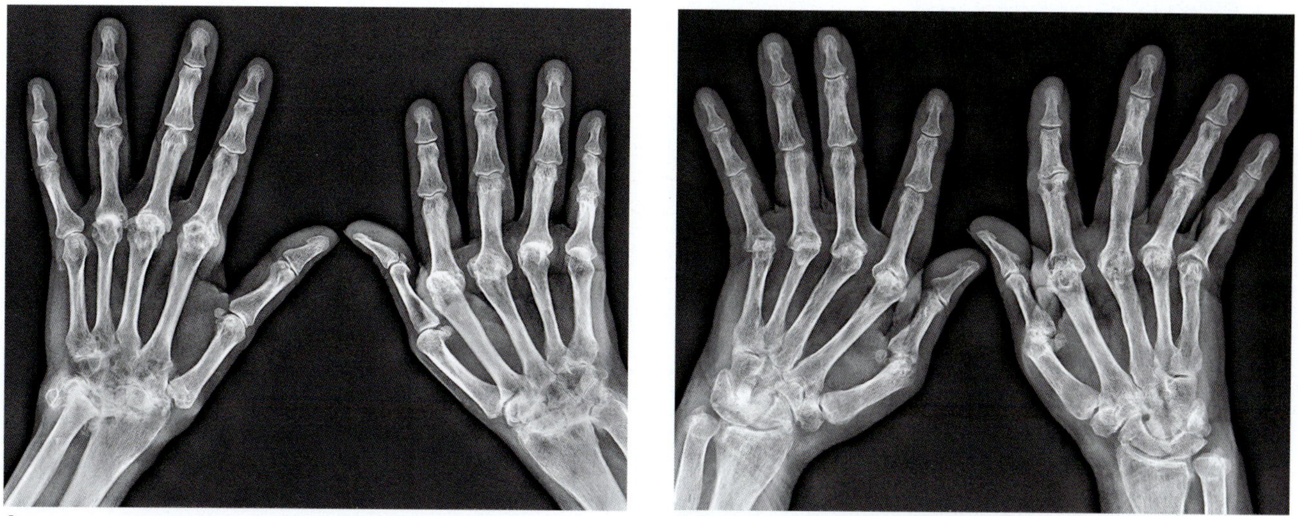

A B

Figure 6.35 ■ Rheumatoid arthritis of the hands. A: Dorsovolar radiograph of both hands of a 63-year-old woman shows typical for this disease loss of articular cartilage and subchondral erosions affecting predominantly metacarpophalangeal, radiocarpal, and intercarpal joints. Observe that the distal interphalangeal joints are spared. **B:** Dorsovolar radiograph of both hands of a 72-year-old woman shows articular erosions affecting metacarpophalangeal joints of both hands. The proximal interphalangeal joints of the left hand are also affected. The distal interphalangeal joints are normal.

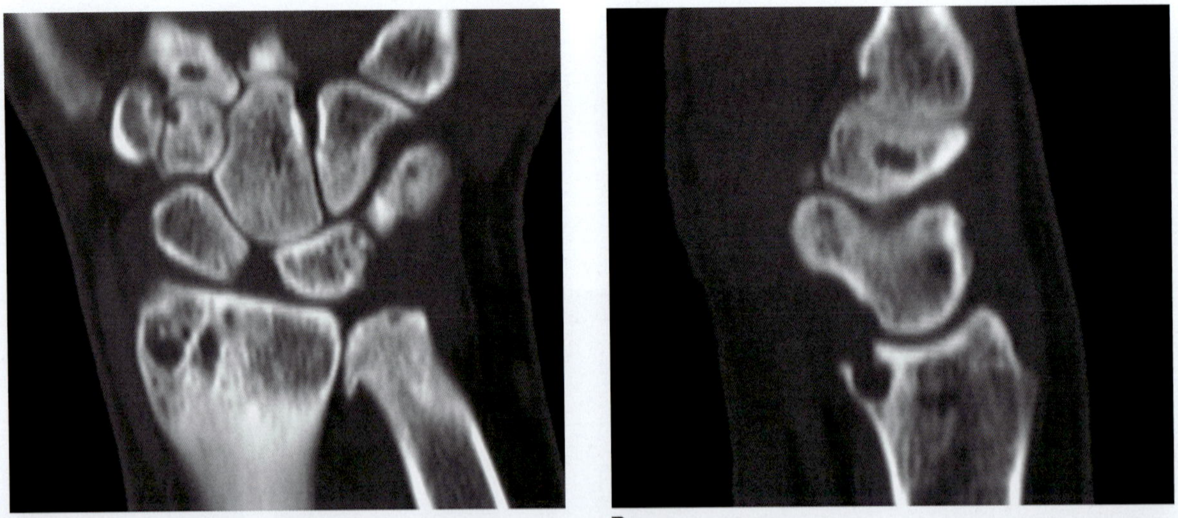

A B

Figure 6.36 ■ **CT of rheumatoid arthritis of the wrist.** Coronal **(A)** and sagittal **(B)** reformatted CT images of the left wrist of a 39-year-old woman show erosions of the radiocarpal joint and erosions of the several carpal bones.

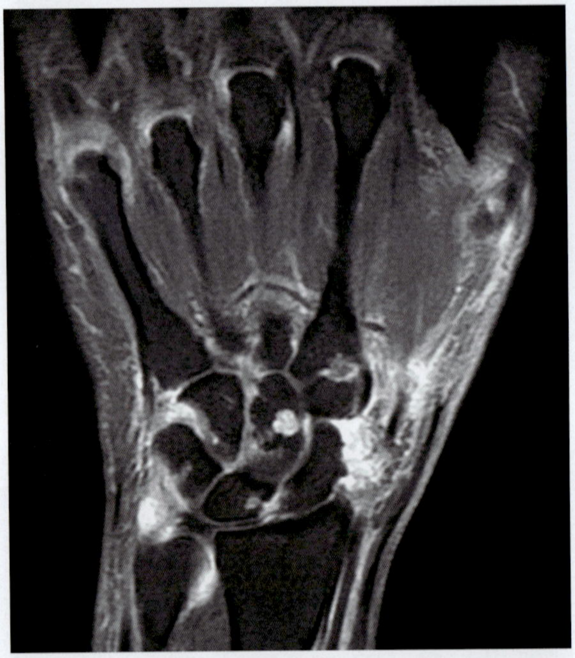

A

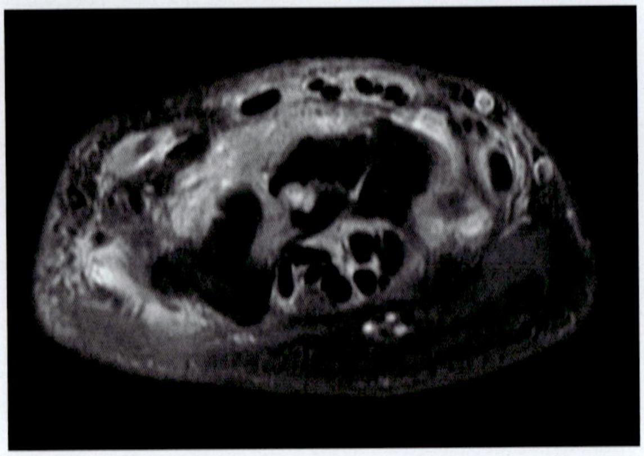

B

Figure 6.37 ■ **MRI of rheumatoid arthritis of the wrist.** Coronal **(A)** and axial **(B)** T1-weighted fat-suppressed MR images of the right wrist of a 60-year-old woman, obtained after intravenous administration of gadolinium, show erosions of the ulnar styloid and several carpal bones including the scaphoid, lunate, triquetrum, capitate, and hamate. There are also erosions of the second and third carpometacarpal joints. Note in addition extensive synovitis exhibiting high signal intensity.

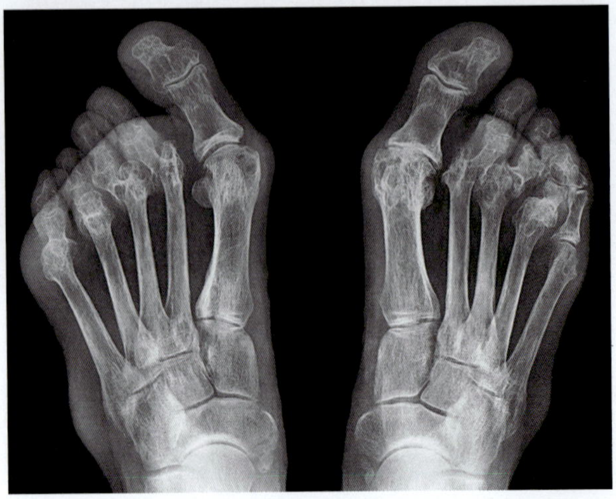

Figure 6.38 ■ **Rheumatoid arthritis of the feet.** Dorsoplantar radiograph of both feet of a 55-year-old woman shows erosions and subluxations of metatarsophalangeal joints.

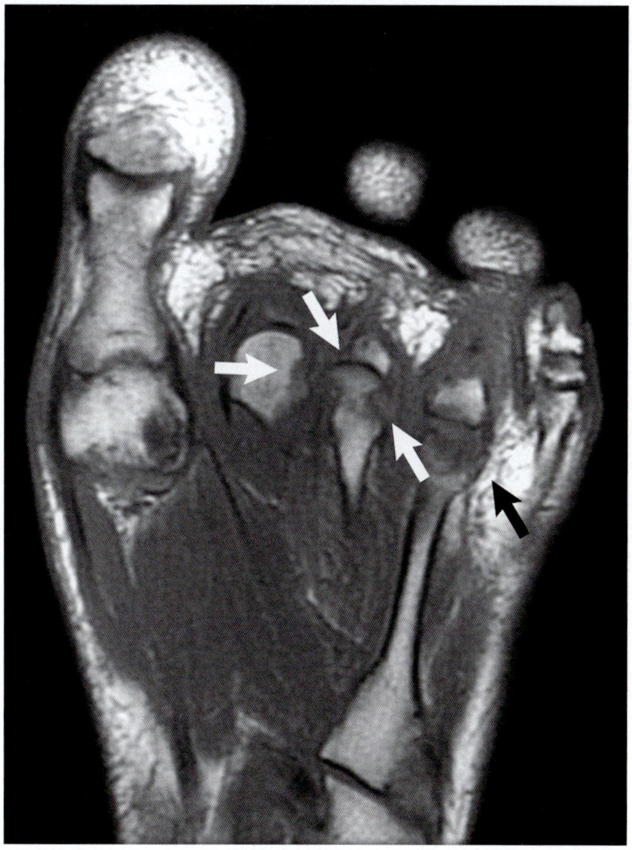

A

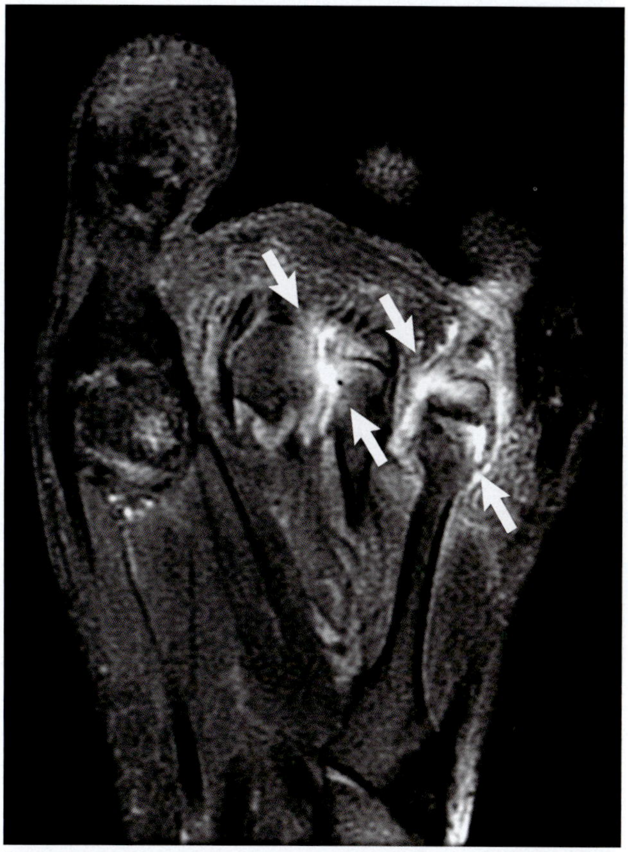

B

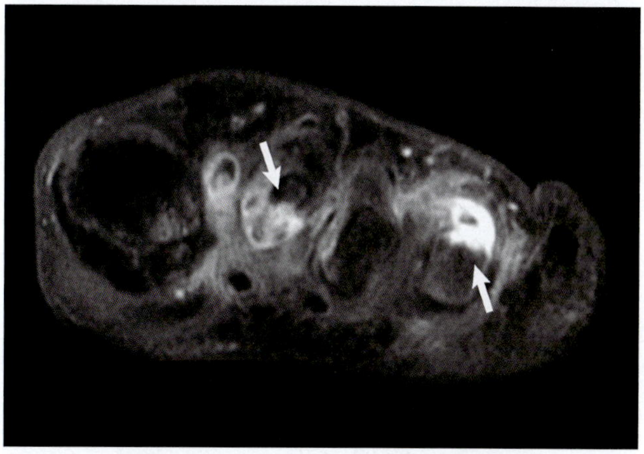

C

Figure 6.39 ■ MRI of rheumatoid arthritis of the foot. Long-axis T1-weighted **(A)**, long-axis proton density-weighted fat-suppressed **(B)**, and short-axis T1-weighted fat-suppressed **(C)** postcontrast MR images of the left foot of a 64-year-old woman show erosions of the second, third, and fourth metatarsophalangeal joints (*arrows*) accompanied by synovitis.

radial deviation of the wrist in the radiocarpal articulation (Fig. 6.43). In far-advanced stages of rheumatoid arthritis, shortening of several phalanges may be encountered secondary to destructive changes in the joints associated with dislocations in the metacarpophalangeal joints. This deformity appears as a "telescoping" of the fingers, hence its name, *main en lorgnette*, from the French name for the telescoping type of opera glass (Fig. 6.44). An abnormally wide space between the lunate and the scaphoid may also be encountered in advanced stages of the disease secondary to erosion and rupture of the scapholunate ligament (Fig. 6.45); this phenomenon is known in the literature as the Terry-Thomas sign. Joint deformities are also often seen in the foot, and subluxation in the metatarsophalangeal joints often leads to deformities such as hallux valgus and hammer toes (Fig. 6.46).

Joint Ankyloses

A rare finding that may be observed in advanced stages of rheumatoid arthritis is joint ankylosis, which is most commonly encountered in the midcarpal articulations (see Figs. 6.43 and 6.44). Ankylotic changes in the wrist are more common in patients with juvenile idiopathic arthritis and with so-called seronegative rheumatoid arthritis.

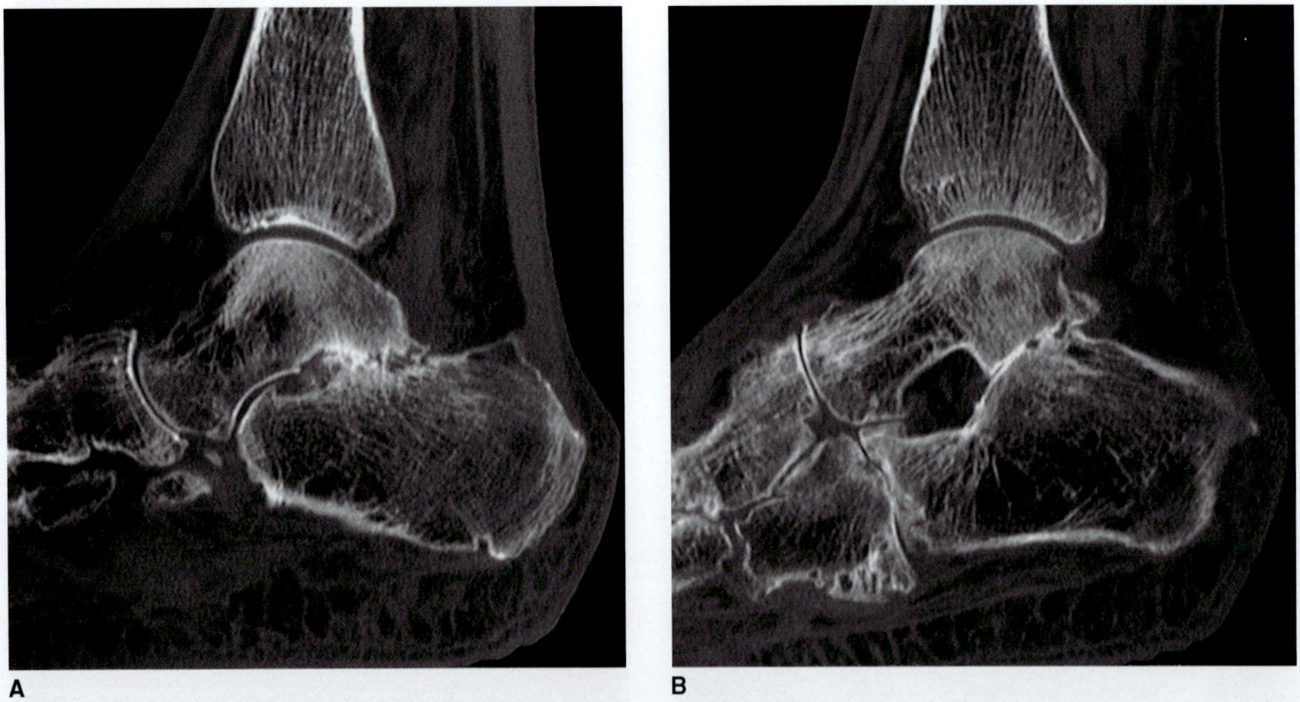

Figure 6.40 ■ CT of rheumatoid arthritis of the foot. A and B: Two sagittal reformatted CT images of the hindfoot of a 52-year-old man show erosions of the subtalar and calcaneocuboid joints.

Involvement of the Spine

The thoracic and lumbar segments are affected by rheumatoid arthritis only on rare occasions. The cervical spine, however, is involved in ~50% of individuals with this condition (Table 6.2). The most characteristic radiographic features of rheumatoid arthritis in the cervical spine can be observed in the odontoid process, the atlantoaxial joints, and the apophyseal joints. Erosive changes may be encountered in the odontoid process (Figs. 6.47 and 6.48) and in apophyseal joints (Fig. 6.49, see also Fig. 6.47), whereas subluxation is a common finding in the atlantoaxial joint secondary to erosion of the transverse ligament (connecting the odontoid process to the atlas) by inflammatory pannus. This laxity becomes apparent on the radiograph obtained in the lateral view of the flexed cervical spine (Fig. 6.50, see also Fig. 2.17) frequently accompanied by cephalad migration (so-called vertical translation) of the odontoid process, also known as cranial settling or atlantoaxial impaction (Fig. 6.51, see also Fig. 6.49). This complication often requires surgical intervention, and the most common procedure to correct this is posterior fusion.

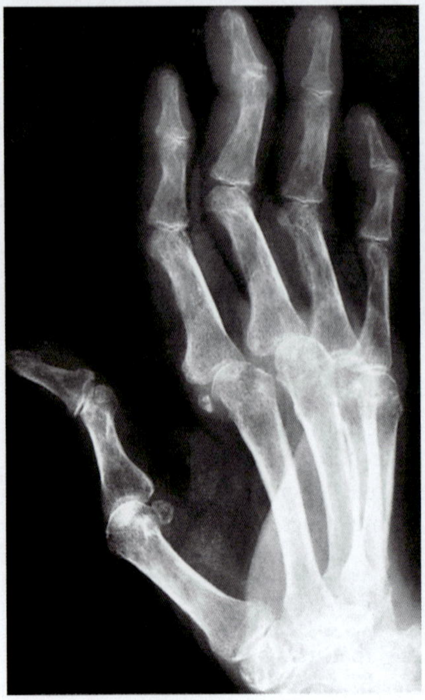

Figure 6.41 ■ Rheumatoid arthritis. Oblique radiograph of the hand of a 59-year-old woman shows the swan-neck deformity of the second through fifth fingers. Note the flexion in the distal interphalangeal joints and the extension in the proximal interphalangeal joints, the hallmarks of this abnormality.

Severe involvement of the apophyseal and uncovertebral joints (joints of Luschka) leads to subluxations. Multiple levels may be affected, resulting in a "stepladder" configuration of the spine. In extremely rare cases, in a manner similar to that in juvenile idiopathic arthritis, the apophyseal joints may ankylose. The other structures occasionally affected by rheumatoid process are the intervertebral disks and adjacent vertebral bodies, which become involved as a result of synovitis extending from the uncovertebral joints. Only a small percentage of patients with cervical disease may have cervical myelopathy. MRI is an ideal modality to evaluate spinal cord involvement in these patients (see Fig. 6.51).

(Continued on page 231)

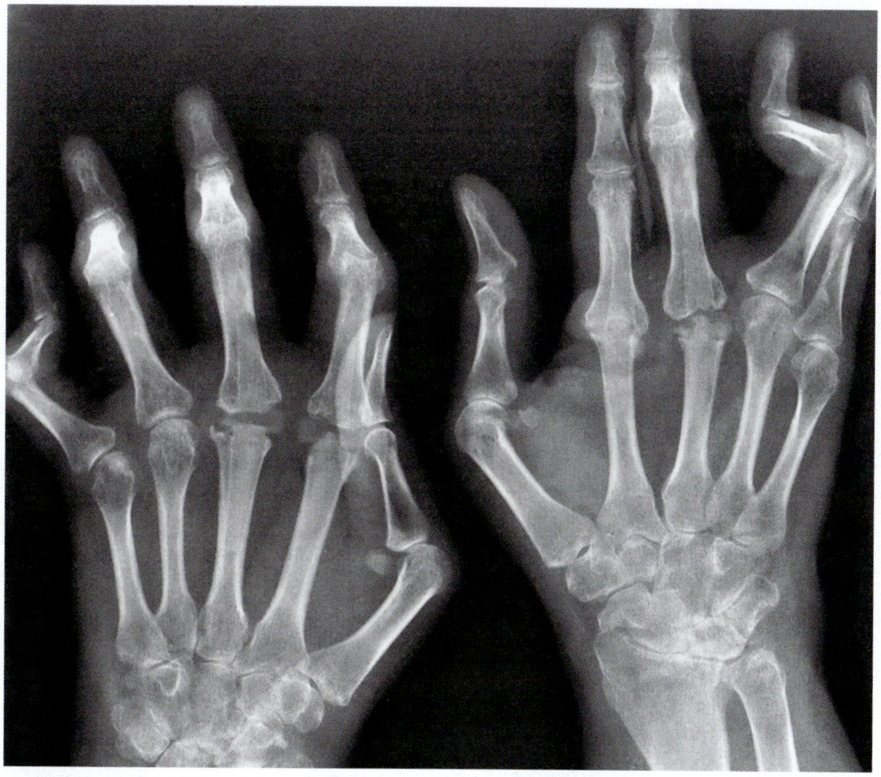

Figure 6.42 ■ **Rheumatoid arthritis.** Dorsovolar radiograph of the hands of a 48-year-old woman demonstrates the boutonniére deformity in the small and ring fingers of the right hand and in the ring finger of the left hand.

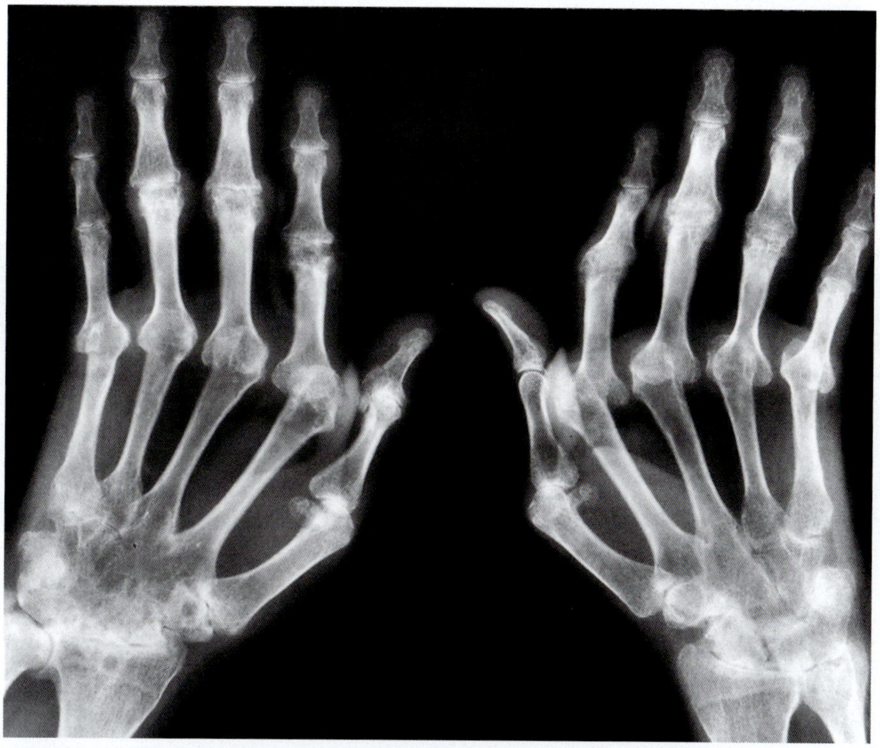

Figure 6.43 ■ **Rheumatoid arthritis.** Dorsovolar projection of both hands of a 51-year-old woman shows subluxation in the metacarpophalangeal joints resulting in ulnar deviation of the fingers and radial deviation in the radiocarpal articulations. Note also ankylosis of the midcarpal articulations of the right hand.

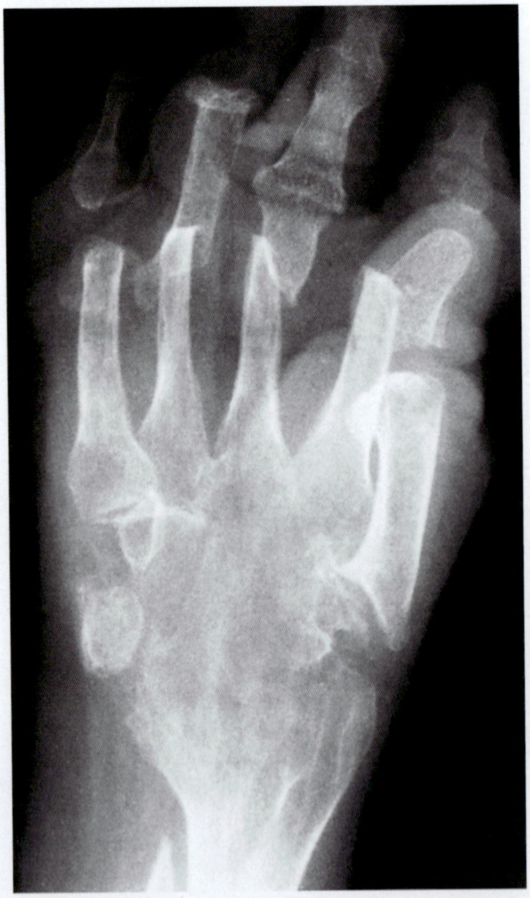

Figure 6.44 ■ Rheumatoid arthritis. Dorsovolar radiograph of the right hand of a 54-year-old woman with long-standing advanced rheumatoid arthritis demonstrates the *main-en-lorgnette* deformity. Note the telescoping of the fingers secondary to destructive joint changes and dislocations in the metacarpophalangeal joints. There is also ankylosis of the radiocarpal and intercarpal articulations and "penciling" of the distal ulna.

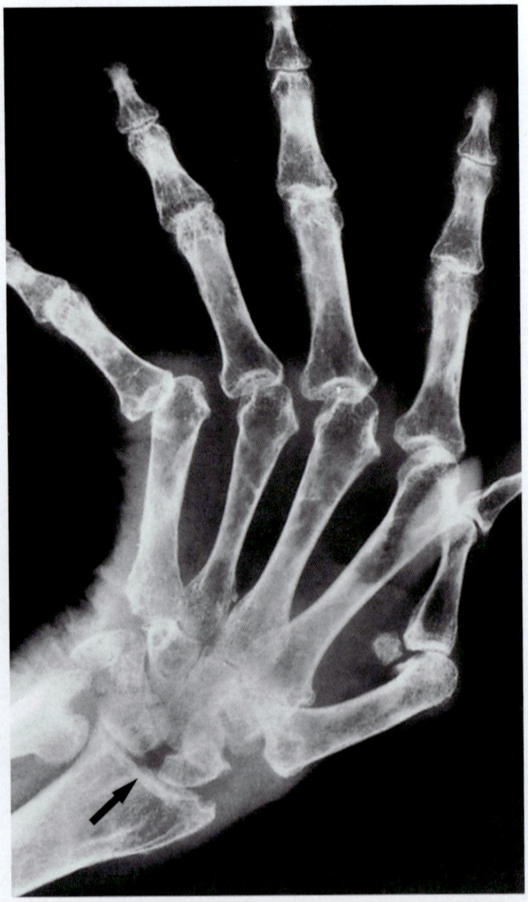

Figure 6.45 ■ Rheumatoid arthritis. Dorsovolar radiograph of the hand of a 60-year-old woman shows a gap between the scaphoid and lunate (*arrow*), known as a Terry-Thomas sign, indicating destruction of the scapholunate ligament. Note also the subluxation in the metacarpophalangeal joints resulting in ulnar deviation of the fingers.

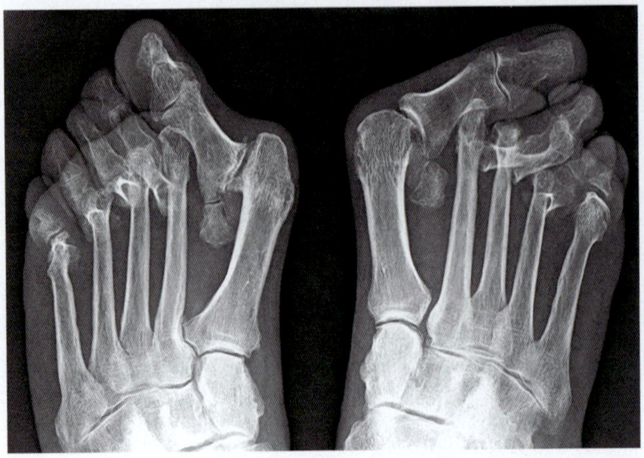

A

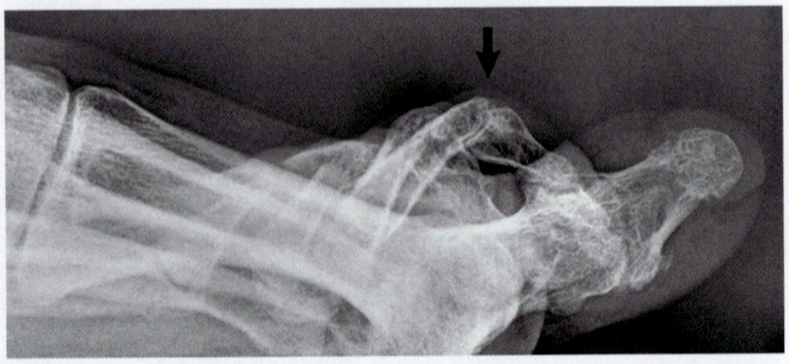

B

Figure 6.46 ■ Rheumatoid arthritis. Dorsoplantar radiograph of both feet **(A)** and lateral radiograph of the toes **(B)** of the left foot of a 71-year-old woman show erosions of the metatarsophalangeal joints associated with subluxations and dislocations, severe hallux valgus deformity, and hammer toes (*arrow*).

Table 6.2 ABNORMALITIES OF THE CERVICAL SPINE IN RHEUMATOID ARTHRITIS

Osteoporosis
Erosion of the odontoid process
Atlantoaxial (C1–C2) subluxation
Vertical translation of the odontoid (cranial settling)
Erosions of the apophyseal joints
Fusion of the apophyseal joints
Erosions of the uncovertebral (Luschka) joints
Disk space narrowing
Erosions and sclerosis of the vertebral body margins
Erosions (whittling) of the spinous processes
Subluxations of the vertebral bodies ("stepladder" or "doorstep" appearance on lateral radiographs)

Modified from Resnick D, Niwayama G. Rheumatoid arthritis and the seronegative spondyloarthropathies: radiographic and pathologic concepts. In: Resnick D, ed. *Diagnosis of Bone and Joint Disorders.* 3rd ed. Philadelphia, PA: WB Saunders; 1995:807–865, with permission.

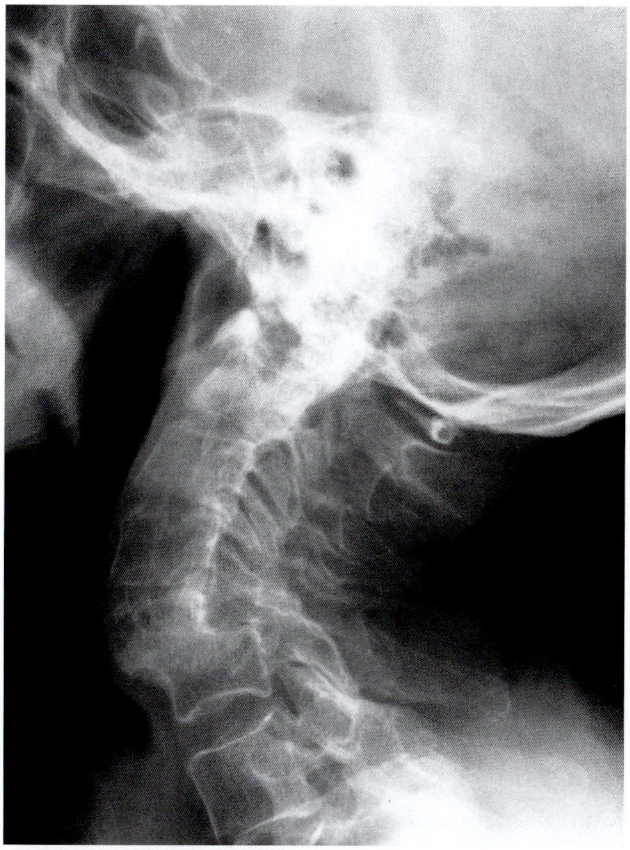

Figure 6.47 ■ Rheumatoid arthritis of the cervical spine. Lateral radiograph of the cervical spine of a 52-year-old woman with advanced rheumatoid arthritis shows erosive changes of the apophyseal joints. In addition, note osteoporosis, erosion of the odontoid, erosions at the diskovertebral junctions, and whittling of the spinous processes.

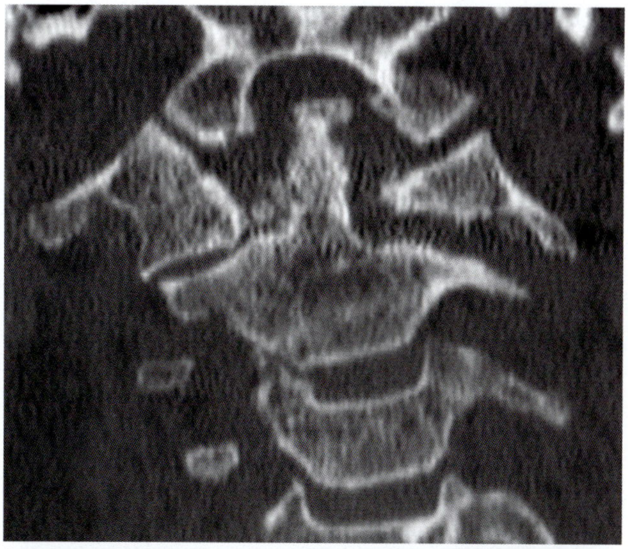

A

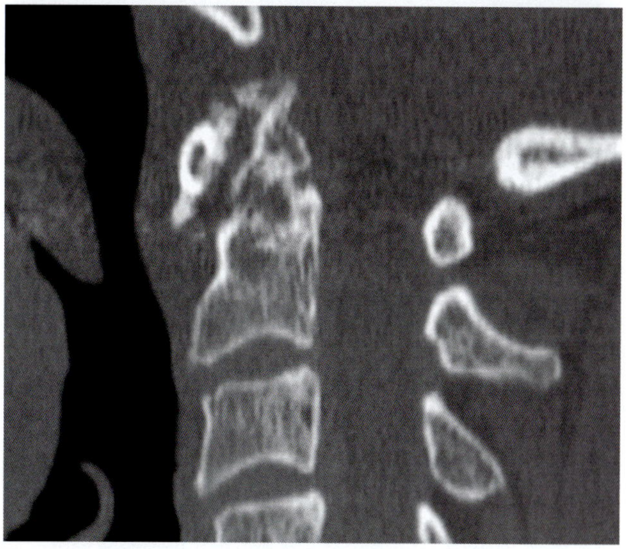

B

Figure 6.48 ■ CT of rheumatoid arthritis of the cervical spine. Coronal **(A)** and sagittal **(B)** reformatted CT images of the upper cervical spine of a 47-year-old woman show erosions of the odontoid process.

Differential Diagnosis of Rheumatoid Arthritis

The characteristic clinical and imaging features of rheumatoid arthritis have been extensively described in the literature. An accurate diagnosis is usually made without difficulty if the patient presents with symmetrical peripheral polyarthritis, synovial inflammatory changes, and subcutaneous nodules. Many conditions, however, can mimic RA. Clinically, acute viral syndromes such as hepatitis B, erythrovirus (Parvovirus B19), or Epstein-Barr virus can produce a polyarthritis with symptoms closely resembling those of RA, although those entities usually resolve over a 2- to 4-week period. From the radiologic point of view, the most important is to differentiate RA from psoriatic arthritis. Both diseases tend to involve multiple joints, and the articular erosions show similar morphologic features; however, the distribution of the lesions

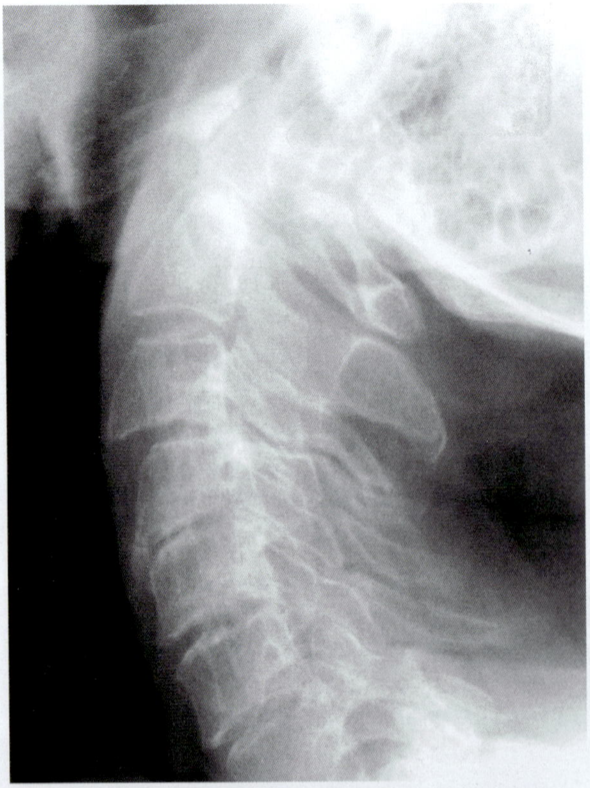

Figure 6.49 ■ Rheumatoid arthritis of the cervical spine. Lateral radiograph of the cervical spine of a 41-year-old woman shows a vertical translocation of the odontoid process (cranial settling). Note also erosive changes at the diskovertebral junctions, erosions of the apophyseal joints, and whittling of the spinous processes.

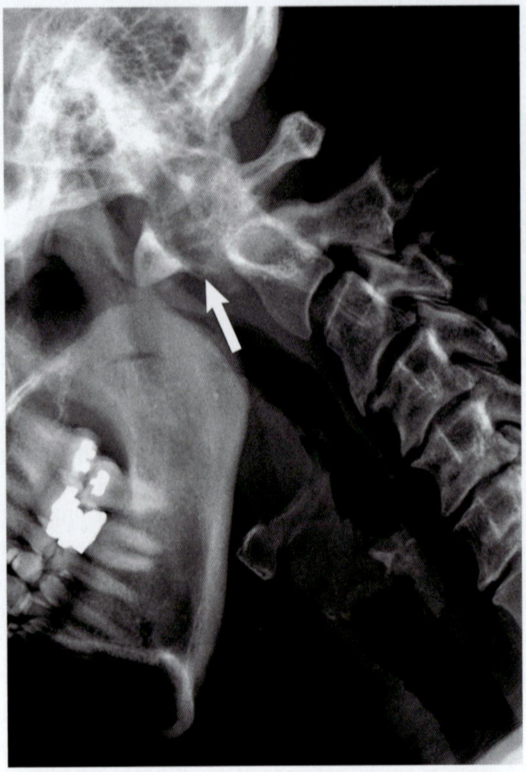

Figure 6.50 ■ Rheumatoid arthritis: C1–C2 instability. Flexion lateral radiograph of the cervical spine in a 51-year-old woman shows C1–C2 subluxation (*arrow*).

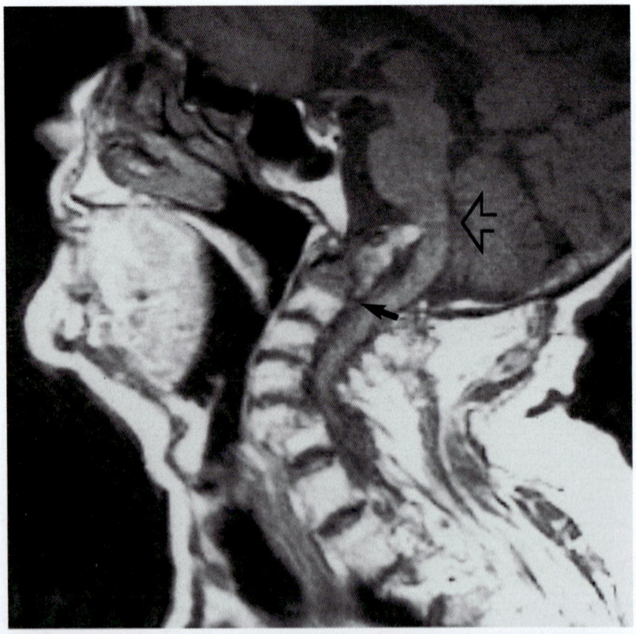

Figure 6.51 ■ MRI of rheumatoid arthritis of the cervical spine. A 52-year-old woman with advanced rheumatoid arthritis presented with chronic neck pain, weakness of the upper limbs, numbness in both hands, and occasional dyspnea and cardiac arrhythmia. A sagittal spin-echo T1-weighted MR image shows inflammatory pannus eroding odontoid (*arrow*) and cranial settling with cephalad migration of C2 impinging on the medulla oblongata (*open arrow*).

differs. Although the proximal interphalangeal joints of the hand and foot are affected in both conditions, the involvement of the distal interphalangeal joints should point to the latter diagnosis. Other connective tissue disorders that can cause polyarthritis with a rheumatoid-like distribution include systemic lupus erythematosus (SLE), scleroderma, and Sjögren syndrome. In most cases, the presence of extra-articular features in these conditions, such as Raynaud phenomenon, skin rash, the absence of anti-CCP reactivity, and the presence of antinuclear antibodies, is helpful in differential diagnosis. Furthermore, patients with SLE usually present with subluxations and dislocations of the small joints of the hand without articular erosions. Patients with rheumatoid nodules occasionally may be misdiagnosed as having gouty arthritis. The morphologic features of erosive changes of gout, however, particularly the characteristic overhanging edge and partial preservation of joint space, are not present in rheumatoid arthritis. Noninflammatory painful conditions affecting the joints, such as osteoarthritis, usually do not create serious diagnostic problems.

Complications of Rheumatoid Arthritis

The complications of rheumatoid arthritis are related not only to the inflammatory process itself but also to the sequelae of treatment (see the discussion on the complications of treatment in Chapter 4). The large doses of steroids that in the past have been commonly prescribed

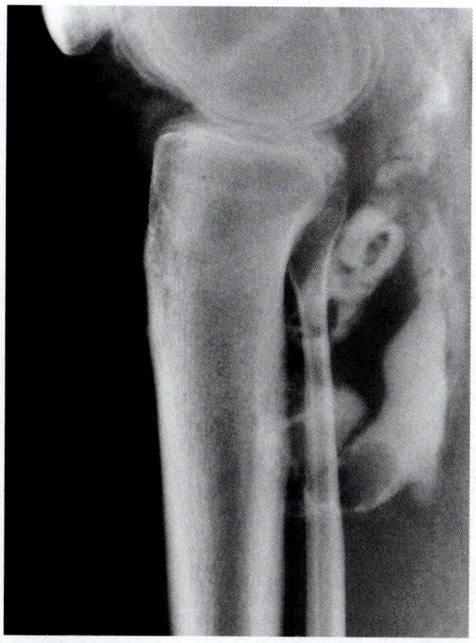

Figure 6.52 ■ Rheumatoid arthritis complicated by a Baker cyst. A 31-year-old woman with a 2-year history of seropositive rheumatoid arthritis developed swelling of the upper calf and tenderness in the popliteal fossa. A presumptive diagnosis of thrombophlebitis was made, but a venogram failed to corroborate this. This lateral view of a knee arthrogram shows a large popliteal (Baker) cyst dissecting into the medial aspect of the calf. This condition is a well-documented complication in patients with rheumatoid arthritis.

in therapy often led to the development of generalized osteoporosis and osteonecrosis (AVN). Severe osteoporosis and large bony erosions may in turn precipitate pathologic fracture, a frequent complication. Tear of the rotator cuff may also occur because of erosion by inflammatory pannus in the shoulder joint (see Fig. 6.8). In the knee, a large popliteal (Baker) cyst may complicate rheumatoid arthritic changes (Figs. 6.52 and 6.53, see also Figs. 6.21 and 6.22); this condition may be misdiagnosed as thrombophlebitis (see Fig. 2.76).

RHEUMATOID NODULOSIS

A variant of rheumatoid arthritis is rheumatoid nodulosis, which occurs predominantly in men. It is a nonsystemic disorder characterized by the presence of multiple subcutaneous nodules (Fig. 6.54) and a very high rheumatoid factor titer; as a rule, there are no joint abnormalities. Occasionally, small cystic lesions may be present in various bones. Nodules are usually different in size and consistency, and distribution is over the elbows, extensor surfaces of hands and feet, and other pressure points.

On histologic examination, the nodules show typical rheumatoid changes, including central necrosis surrounded by palisading histiocytes and fibroblasts, with an outer layer of connective tissue and chronic inflammatory cells. Only occasionally will the histologic appearance be atypical. In these cases, the nodule may contain abundant cholesterol clefts and lipid-loaded macrophages, suggestive of xanthoma or even multicentric reticulohistiocytosis.

In classic rheumatoid arthritis, small-vessel vasculitis is a primary factor in nodule development, and circulating immune complexes used by rheumatoid synovium are responsible for such extra-articular manifestations as vasculitis, polyserositis, and nodules. In rheumatoid nodulosis, however,

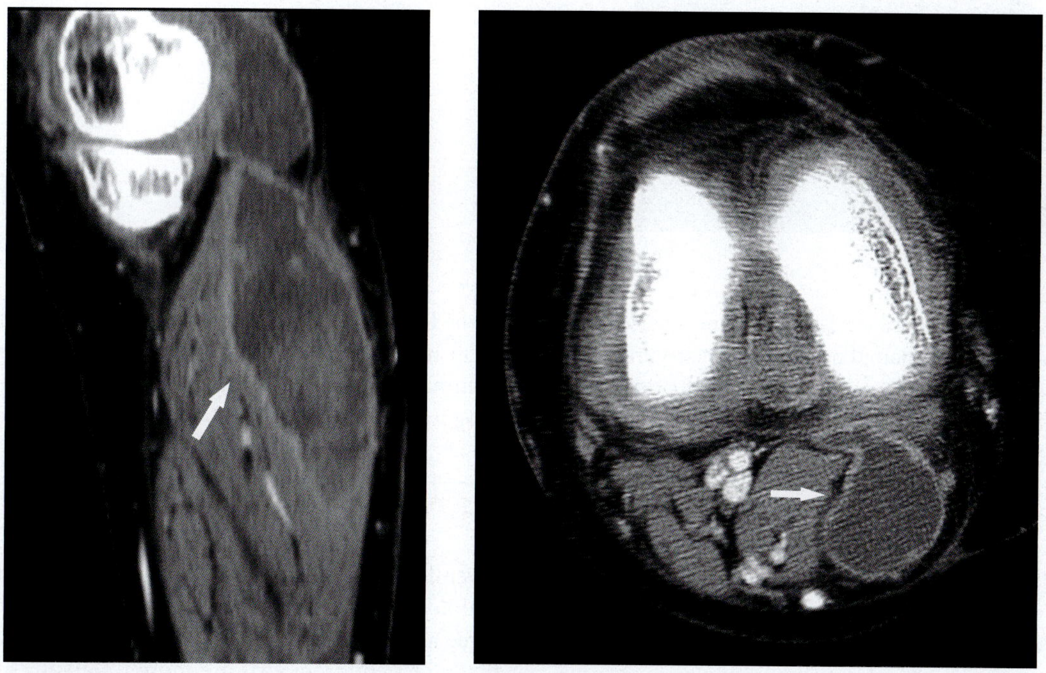

A B

Figure 6.53 ■ CT of a Baker cyst. Sagittal reformatted **(A)** and axial **(B)** CT images, obtained after intravenous administration of contrast agent, show a large Baker cyst (*arrows*) in a patient diagnosed with rheumatoid arthritis.

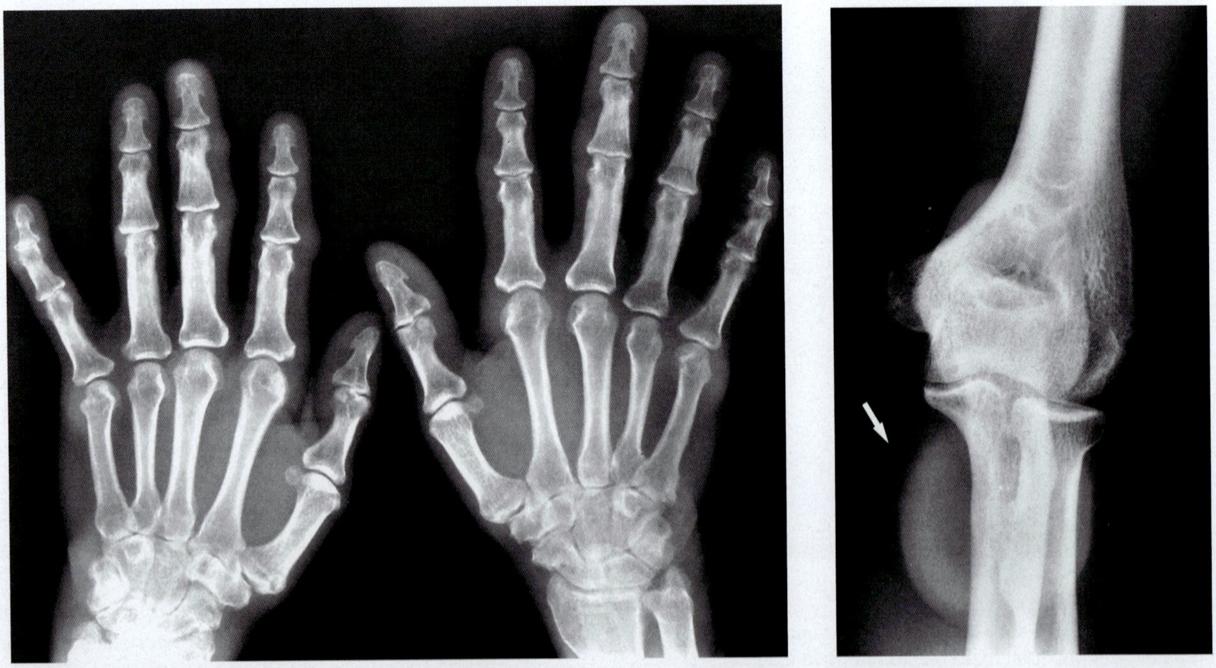

A B

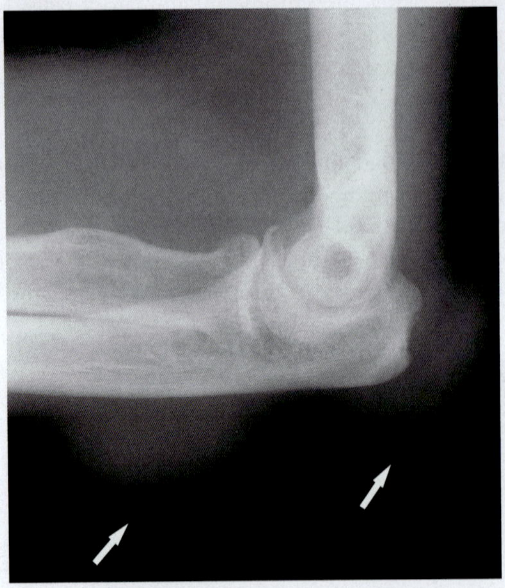

C

Figure 6.54 ■ Rheumatoid nodulosis. A 52-year-old man with a 15-year history of polyarthritis presented with large, fluctuant nodules on the dorsal aspect of the hands and elbows. A high titer of rheumatoid factor (1:1,280) was identified in his serum. **A:** Dorsovolar view of both hands shows several soft tissue nodules adjacent to joints (*arrows*). Note the lack of joint abnormalities. Anteroposterior **(B)** and lateral **(C)** radiographs of the left elbow demonstrate similar soft tissue masses at the dorsal aspect of the proximal forearm (*arrows*). The elbow joint is intact.

nodules develop in the absence of active joint disease. Thus, the pathogenesis of rheumatoid nodulosis remains unclear.

A positive family history of rheumatoid arthritis in some patients with rheumatoid nodulosis and the occurrence of familial nodulosis suggest the involvement of hereditary factors. The strong male preponderance suggests that androgens may modify disease expression in genetically predisposed individuals, but the most common feature in males with this disorder is a history of smoking. Rheumatoid nodulosis is often misdiagnosed as gout or xanthomatosis. Moreover, it should be kept in mind when evaluating this condition that ~20% of patients with classic rheumatoid arthritis have rheumatoid nodules, which are usually located at sites of pressure or stress such as the dorsal aspect of the hands and forearms (see Fig. 6.27). Articular involvement in nodular rheumatoid arthritis distinguishes it from rheumatoid nodulosis, which consequently has a better prognosis.

JUVENILE IDIOPATHIC ARTHRITIS (JIA)

Juvenile idiopathic arthritis, formerly termed juvenile rheumatoid arthritis (JRA), is a heterogeneous group of at least three autoimmune chronic inflammatory synovial diseases that affect children; girls are more frequently affected than are boys. The term JIA was introduced by the International League of Associations for Rheumatology (ILAR) to replace two other terms: juvenile rheumatoid arthritis and juvenile chronic arthritis. JIA is classified on the basis of the number of joints affected, variety of symptoms, family history, and serologic findings. The three defined subtypes are Still disease, polyarticular arthritis, and pauciarticular (oligoarticular) arthritis. Some investigators include under this rubric also enthesitis-related arthritis (ERA) and juvenile psoriatic arthritis. Each of these subgroups has distinct clinical and laboratory findings and different natural histories. There is no pathognomonic laboratory test for any of them, and the diagnosis is based on the clinical spectrum exhibited by a given patient. The etiology is unknown, and the genetic component is complex, making clear distinction between the various subtypes sometimes difficult. The involvement of tumor necrosis factor (TNF) protein and its receptors in the pathology of JIA has been suggested by multiple studies; however, in general, genome-wide association studies, much like in adult onset of RA, have been disappointing. Studies of non-HLA genes with the MHC, cytokine, and T-cell–related genes have been all positively associated with this arthritis, and most recently, link between MHC-encoded *LMP7* gene and early-onset pauciarticular JIA and between the gene-encoding Tapasin and systemic-onset JIA has been established. Nonetheless, these associations are weak and not much useful for genetic counseling or for diagnosis.

About 55% to 75% of patients with JIA present with monoarticular or pauciarticular disease. The most commonly affected joints include the knee, followed by the hand, wrist, hip, ankle, and tarsal joints. The cervical spine is also frequently affected. Patients with polyarticular involvement are at the greatest risk for disease progression and joint destruction.

Still Disease

Still disease, included by some authorities into the group of polyarticular juvenile idiopathic arthritis, is well known for sudden onset of spiking fever, lymphadenopathy, and an evanescent salmon-colored skin rash. Patients may exhibit hepatosplenomegaly, pleuritis, pericarditis, fatigue, anorexia, and weight loss. The majority of patients have chronic and recurrent arthralgias. A significant number of patients, depending on the series, may also subsequently have chronic polyarthritis. A poorly understood Still-like disease with fever and arthralgias may develop in some adult patients, recently designated as macrophage-activating syndrome (see text below). In all cases, etiology can be related to immunologic storm, namely, uncontrolled activation of macrophages and secretion of variety of proinflammatory cytokines.

Polyarticular Juvenile Idiopathic Arthritis

Polyarticular juvenile idiopathic arthritis accounts for only 2% to 7% of all cases of JIA and consists of inflammation of five or more joints within 6 months of onset, with associated findings of anorexia, weight loss, fatigue, and adenopathy. Growth retardation is common. This disorder also results in the following abnormalities: undergrowth of the mandible, early closure of the growth plates resulting in shortening of metacarpals and metatarsals, and overgrowths of the epiphyses at the knees, hips, and shoulders. Rheumatoid nodules are present in approximately one-third of the patients. Erosions are detected in nearly all children during the first 5 years from the onset of the disease. They are usually observed in the carpal, metacarpophalangeal, metatarsophalangeal, and interphalangeal joints. A worse prognosis occurs in patients with positive rheumatoid factors.

Juvenile Idiopathic Arthritis with Pauciarticular Onset (Oligoarthritis)

The third subtype of juvenile idiopathic arthritis has pauciarticular onset, with four or fewer joints involved within 6 months of onset in ~40% of patients. The girls are more commonly affected. The knee joint is usually affected first, followed by the ankle joint. Some of these patients may even present with negative rheumatoid factor, whereas others may have positive antigen HLA-B27. Pediatric rheumatologists have attempted to define other subgroups within this pauciarticular subgroup, but, with the exception of HLA-B27–positive children with sacroiliitis, such definitions are broad and clinically dependent on unique systemic features such as iridocyclitis. However, involvement of the sacroiliac joints is not a feature of juvenile idiopathic arthritis as was thought in the past; rather, it represents juvenile onset of ankylosing spondylitis. Similarly, some investigators believe that patients with pauciarticular arthritis, particularly those with positive histocompatibility antigen HLA-B27, may in fact have atypical ankylosing spondylitis syndrome or spondyloarthropathy; both these conditions are different from rheumatoid arthritis.

Arthritis with Enthesitis (ERA)

This type of arthritis constitutes about 5% to 10% of all JIA cases, predominantly affects boys over 6 years of age, and is typify by enthesopathy (enthesitis) at the site of attachment of Achilles tendon and fascia plantaris to the calcaneus, and quadriceps tendon into the patella, associated with asymmetric arthritis affecting articulations of the lower extremities and hip joint. Sacroiliac joints are usually affected. Most patients present with positive HLA-B27 antigen.

Juvenile Psoriatic Arthritis

This form of arthritis, first described by Ansell and Bywaters in 1962, is defined as a seronegative inflammatory arthritis presenting before the age of 16 years with either typical for

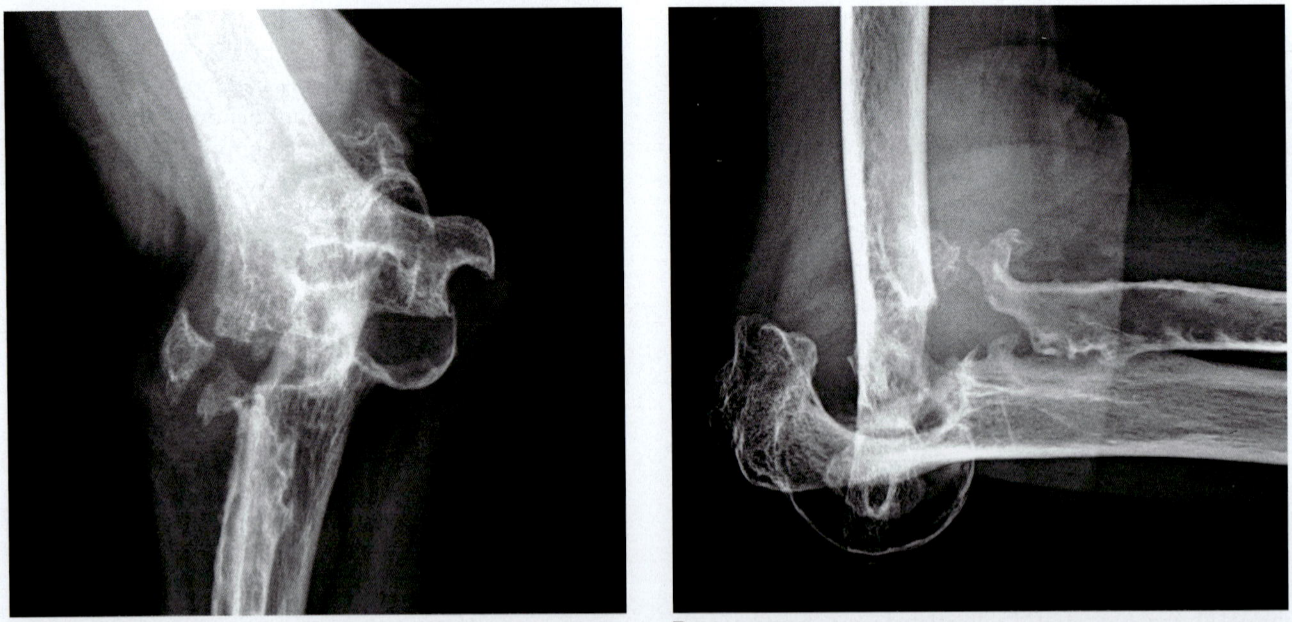

A B

Figure 6.55 ■ Juvenile idiopathic arthritis. Anteroposterior **(A)** and lateral **(B)** radiographs of the elbow of a 35-year-old woman show severe destruction and subluxation of the joint associated with joint effusion.

psoriasis features, or at least three of the four minor criteria: dactylitis, nail pitting, psoriasis-like skin changes, and family history of psoriasis. Girls are affected more commonly than boys. Clinically, the patients may present with joint pain and swelling, reddish scaly skin rash, nail changes, and ocular involvement. Early imaging findings can be demonstrated by MRI, including synovial abnormalities (thickening and enhancement), joint effusion, bone marrow edema, tendon abnormalities (thickening, edema, tenosynovitis), and joint abnormalities (joint space narrowing and articular erosions). Some patients may present with acro-osteolysis.

Imaging Features

Juvenile idiopathic arthritis exhibits many of the features of adult rheumatoid arthritis, although the destructive joint changes are much more striking (Fig. 6.55). However, some additional features that are almost pathognomonic for this condition have been identified.

Periosteal Reaction

This feature is usually seen along the shafts of the proximal phalanges and metacarpals (Fig. 6.56).

Joint Ankyloses

Ankylosis has been reported to occur within 3 to 5 years after onset of the disease. It may occur not only in the wrist (Figs. 6.57 and 6.58) but also in the interphalangeal articulations (Figs. 6.59 and 6.60), and in the tarsal bones. Intervertebral

(Continued on page 238)

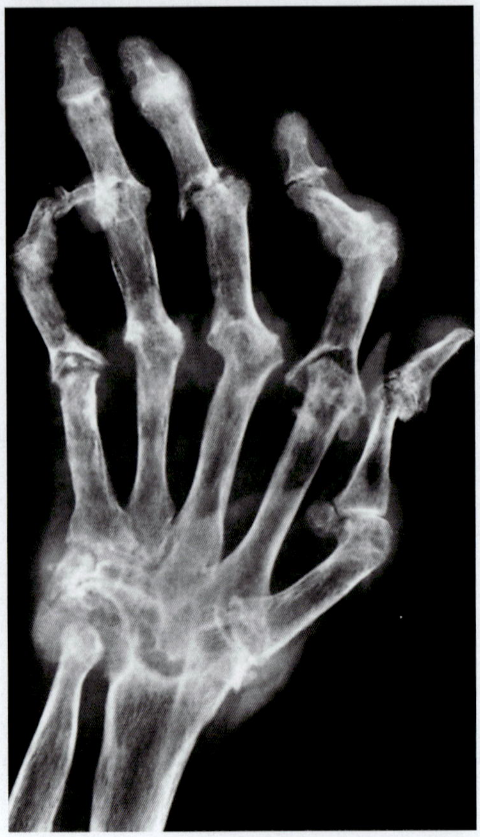

Figure 6.56 ■ Juvenile idiopathic arthritis. Dorsovolar radiograph of the wrist and hand of a 26-year-old woman with a 14-year history of arthritis shows severe destructive changes in the wrist and in the metacarpophalangeal and proximal interphalangeal articulations. Note the ankylosis of the third and fourth metacarpophalangeal joints and periostitis involving the proximal phalanges and metacarpals.

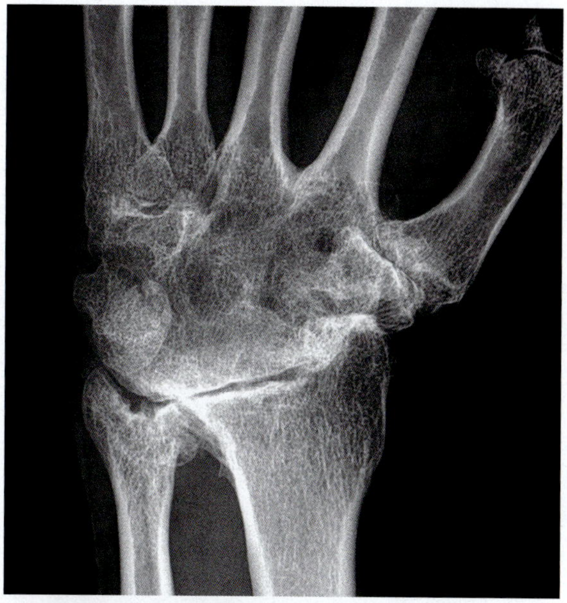

Figure 6.57 ■ Juvenile idiopathic arthritis. A dorsovolar radiograph of the right wrist of a 28-year-old man shows fusion of the several carpal and carpometacarpal joints.

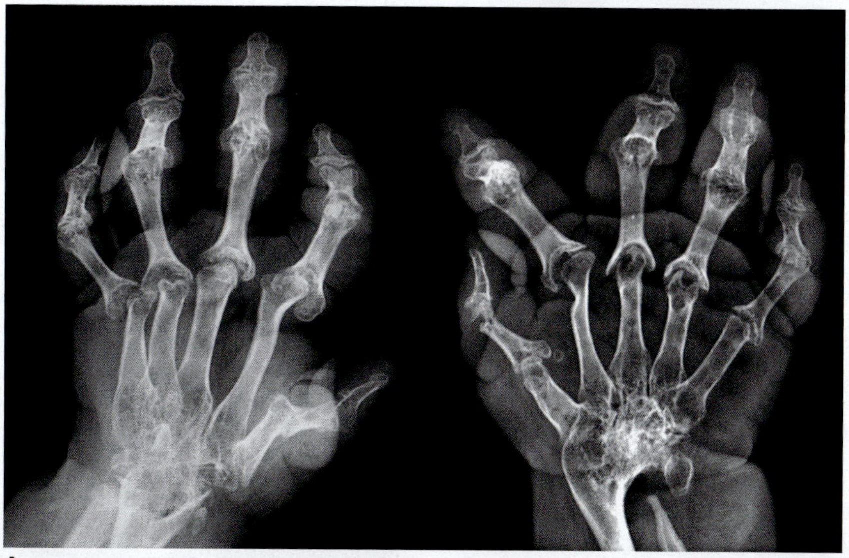

A

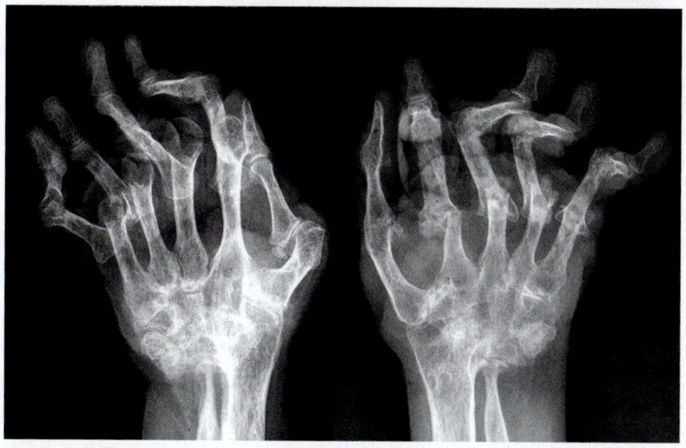

B

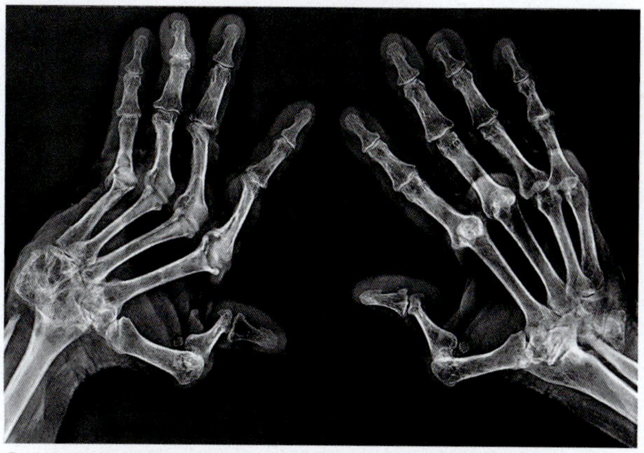

C

Figure 6.58 ■ Juvenile idiopathic arthritis. A: Dorsovolar radiograph of the hand of a 25-year-old woman with a 10-year history of juvenile idiopathic arthritis shows advanced destructive changes in multiple joints of the hand and wrist. Joint ankylosis is evident in several articulations. **B:** In another patient, a 51-year-old woman, observe erosions, subluxations, and dislocations in several metacarpophalangeal joints of both hands, and striking deformities of the fingers. In addition, there is fusion of the radiocarpal and midcarpal joints as well as of the first metacarpophalangeal and interphalangeal joints of the left thumb. **C:** Radiograph of both hands of a 62-year-old woman demonstrates erosions and subluxations of the radiocarpal, midcarpal, and metacarpophalangeal joints of the left hand. The radiocarpal and midcarpal joints of the right wrist are fused. The metacarpophalangeal joints of the right hand show status post Silastic arthroplasties.

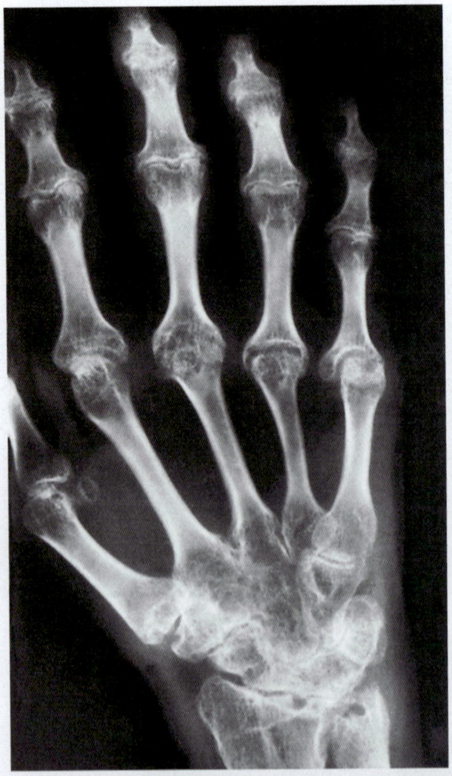

Figure 6.59 ■ Juvenile idiopathic arthritis. Dorsovolar radiograph of the hand of a 25-year-old woman with a 10-year history of JIA shows advanced destructive changes in multiple joints of the hand and wrist. Joint ankylosis is evident in several articulations.

fusion and ankylosis of the apophyseal joints of the cervical spine is also a characteristic finding (Figs. 6.61 and 6.62).

Growth Abnormalities

Because the onset of juvenile idiopathic arthritis frequently occurs before completion of skeletal maturation, alterations in growth of the bones is a common finding. The involvement of epiphyseal sites often leads to fusion of the growth plate, with resultant retardation of bone growth (Fig. 6.63); it may also precipitate acceleration of growth caused by stimulation of the growth plates by hyperemia. Enlargement of the epiphysis of the distal femur leads to characteristic overgrowth of the condyles in the knee associated with widening of the intercondylar notch and squaring of the patella (Fig. 6.64).

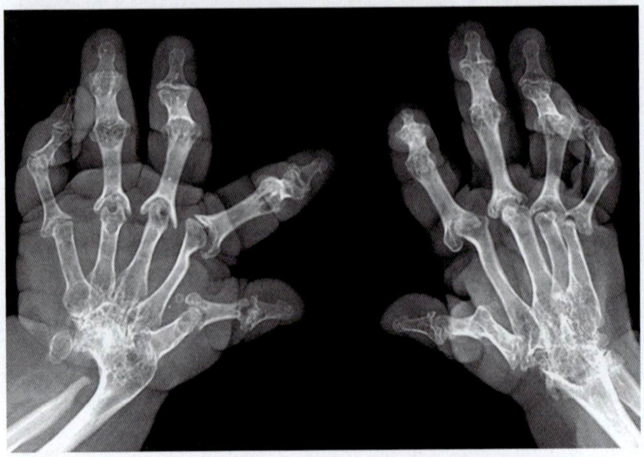

Figure 6.60 ■ Juvenile idiopathic arthritis. Dorsovolar radiograph of both hands of a 50-year-old woman shows erosions of the metacarpophalangeal and interphalangeal joints. Note also interphalangeal fusion of the index, middle, and ring fingers and fusion of the radiocarpal and midcarpal joints.

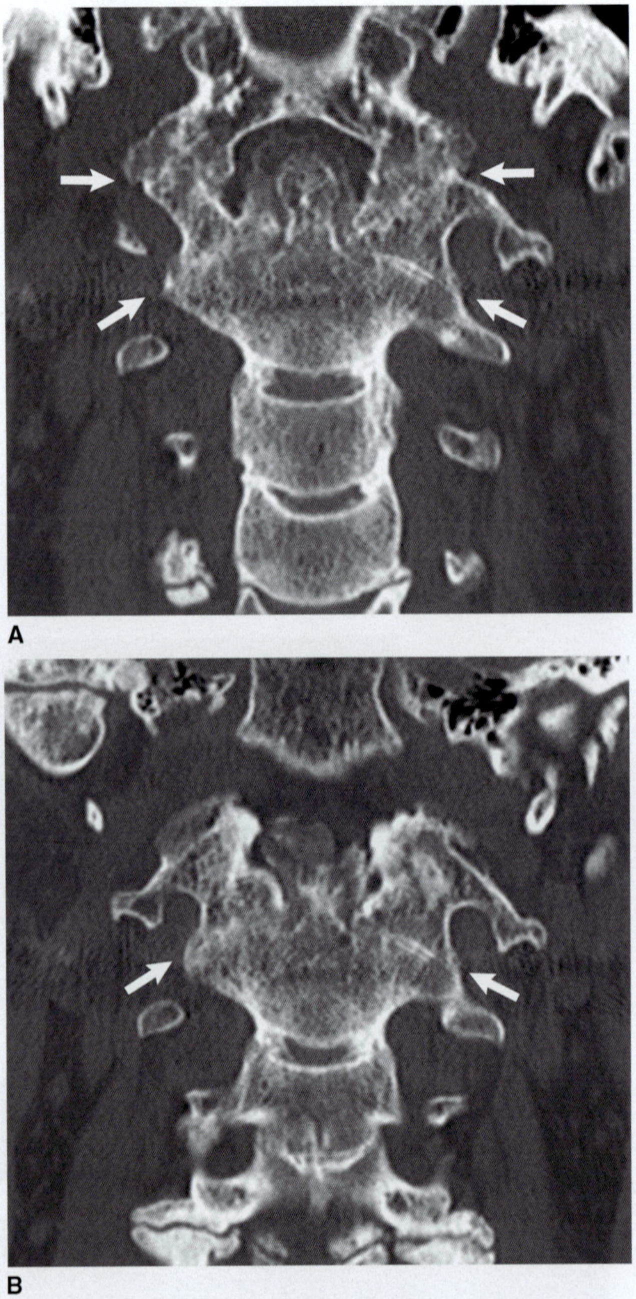

Figure 6.61 ■ Juvenile idiopathic arthritis. A and B: Two coronal reformatted CT sections of the upper cervical spine of a 56-year-old man show atlantoaxial fusion (*arrows*).

Acro-osteolysis

The resorption of the distal phalangeal tufts may be seen in juvenile psoriasis (Fig. 6.65).

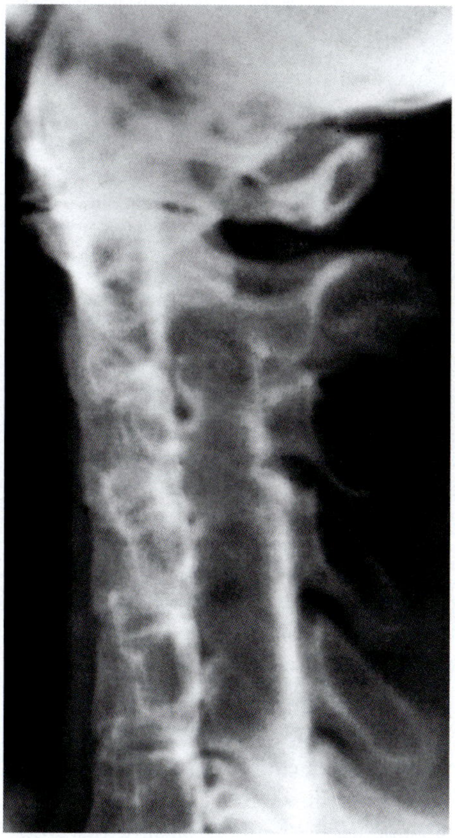

Figure 6.62 ■ **Juvenile idiopathic arthritis.** Lateral radiograph of the cervical spine in a 25-year-old woman with a 15-year history of polyarthritis shows fusion of the apophyseal joints, a common finding in this condition.

Sacroiliitis

This feature is seen in ~30% of patients with the ERA subtype of juvenile idiopathic arthritis. Imaging identification of this abnormality is crucial because, despite the inflammatory changes of sacroiliac joints, the clinical symptoms (pain) may be a relative late development in the pediatric population.

Although most of the features of JIA listed above can be effectively demonstrated on conventional radiography, MRI may provide additional information, particularly in early cases when osseous erosions are either absent or occult (Figs. 6.66 and 6.67). Among others, this technique is also effective in demonstration of synovial proliferation, pannus formation, and bone marrow edema. It also may uncover early abnormalities of the growth plates.

Macrophage Activation Syndrome (MAS)

MAS refers to a clinicopathologic entity caused by excessive uncontrolled activation and expansion of T lymphocytes and macrophagic histiocytes that exhibit hemophagocytic activity. The expansion of these cells leads to a massive systemic inflammatory response associated with pancytopenia, liver and spleen dysfunction, hypertriglyceridemia, hyperferritinemia, and coagulopathy resembling disseminated intravascular coagulation (DIC). Because expansion of tissue macrophages and histiocytes is often triggered by infections or modifications in the drug therapy, some investigators prefer the term reactive hemophagocytic lymphohistiocytosis

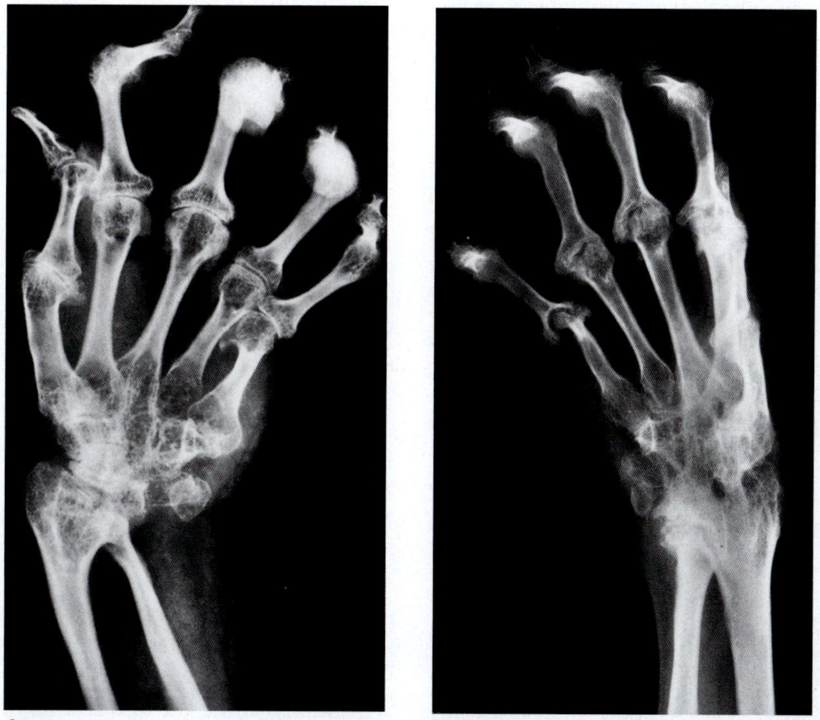

A B

Figure 6.63 ■ **Juvenile idiopathic arthritis. A and B:** Dorsovolar radiograph of the hands of a 24-year-old woman with advanced juvenile idiopathic arthritis, which was diagnosed when she was 7 years old, shows retarded growth of the bones caused by early fusion of the growth plates. Multiple deformities of the digits include hitchhiker's thumb and a boutonniére configuration of the fingers.

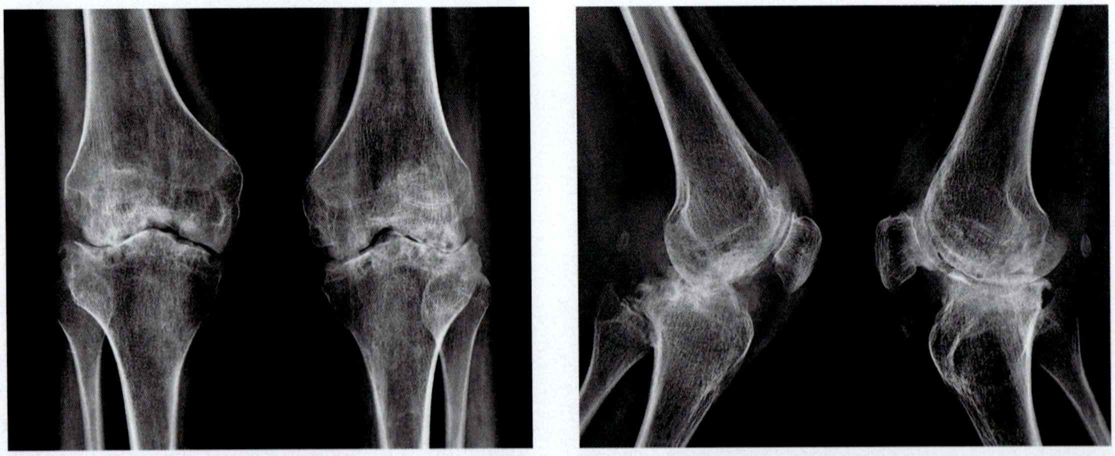

A B

Figure 6.64 ■ Juvenile idiopathic arthritis. Anteroposterior **(A)** and lateral **(B)** radiographs of both knees of a 20-year-old woman show uniform tricompartmental joint space narrowing, subchondral erosions, overgrowth of the femoral condyles, deep intercondylar notch, and "squaring" of the patellae, the characteristic features of this disorder.

for this condition. MAS is a severe and potentially life-threatening complication of several chronic rheumatologic disorders of childhood. It occurs most commonly with systemic juvenile idiopathic arthritis and adult-onset Still disease.

TREATMENT OF RHEUMATOID ARTHRITIS

Medical

Over the past several years, there has been significant change in treatment of rheumatoid arthritis that contributed to major improvement in clinical outcome of patients with this debilitating disease. These encouraging results were mainly achieved through the introduction of the newer biologic agents that have revolutionized the treatment of rheumatoid arthritis and should be offered and discussed with each and every patient with this disease. Historically, treatment included methotrexate, sulfasalazine, leflunomide, hydroxychloroquine, azathioprine, cyclosporine, etanercept, minocycline, and gold salts. However, now all patients receive methotrexate with or without biologic agents (see also text in Chapter 4). They comprise tumor necrosis factor (TNF)-blocking agents (so-called anti-TNF agents—infliximab, etanercept, and adalimumab), rituximab (monoclonal antibody against the protein CD20), abatacept (a fusion protein), and tocilizumab (interleukin-6 receptor–inhibiting monoclonal antibodies). In clinical trials, cyclosporine alone or in combination with methotrexate also has been shown to reduce the arthritic symptoms, and even to delay the development of articular erosions, but is rarely used. Similarly, low doses of glucocorticoids (such as prednisone) can provide rapid improvement of articular symptoms. If indicated, intra-articular injections of steroids can suppress joint inflammation. NSAIDs play only a minor role in the treatment, and their use is mainly reserve to symptomatic relief.

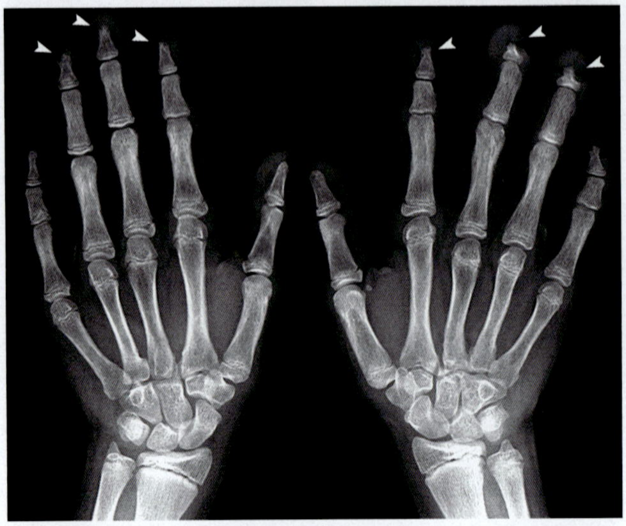

Figure 6.65 ■ Juvenile psoriasis. Dorsovolar radiographs of both hands of an 11-year-old girl with clinically documented psoriasis show acro-osteolysis of several fingers (*arrowheads*).

Surgical

Surgical treatment includes mainly total joint arthroplasties, performed not only on the large joints like hip, knee, shoulder, and elbow but also replacement of small joints of the hands and feet (see Chapter 4).

SERONEGATIVE SPONDYLOARTHROPATHIES (SPA)

Seronegative spondyloarthropathies constitute a heterogeneous group of inflammatory arthritides, predominantly involving axial and peripheral joints. In addition, the characteristic feature of these arthritides is inflammation of entheses (enthesitis) at the site of insertion of tendons and ligaments to bone. Diseases belonging to this group include ankylosing spondylitis, psoriatic arthritis, reactive arthritis, enteropathic arthritis, and undifferentiated spondyloarthritis.

(Continued on page 243)

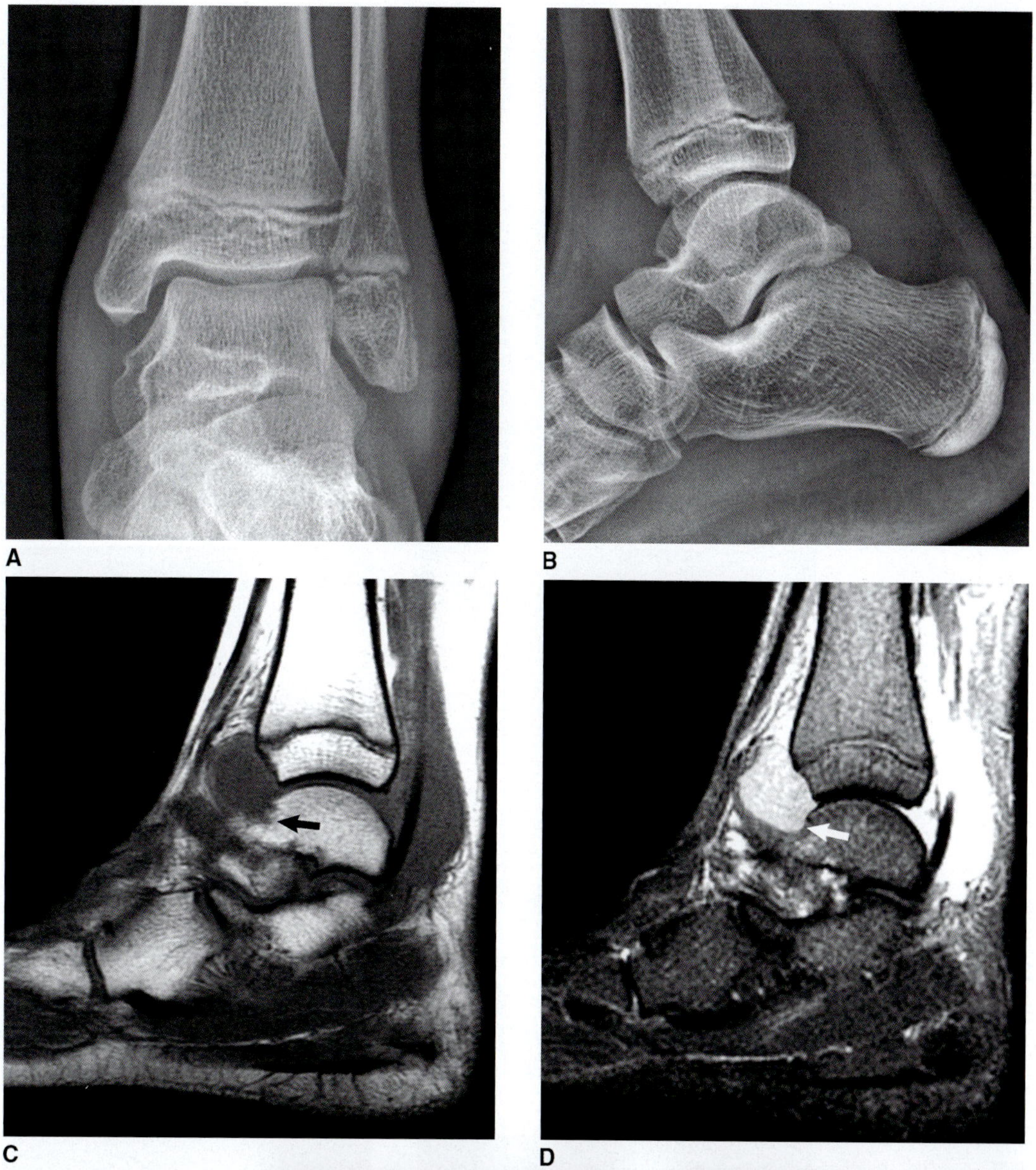

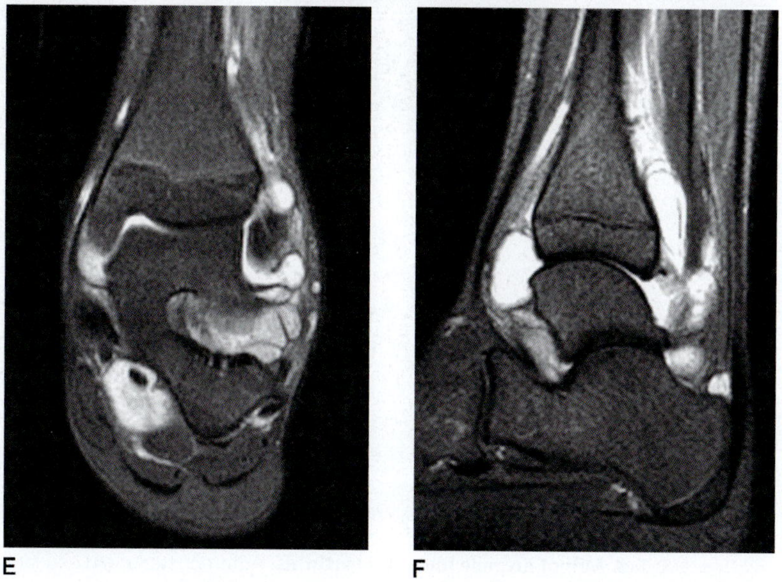

Figure 6.66 ■ MRI of juvenile idiopathic arthritis. Anteroposterior **(A)** and lateral **(B)** radiographs of the left ankle of a 10-year-old girl show soft tissue swelling and tibiotalar joint effusion. No obvious erosions are identified. Sagittal T1-weighted **(C)** and sagittal inversion recovery (IR) **(D)** MR images show inflammatory pannus eroding dorsal aspect of the talus (*arrows*). Coronal **(E)** and sagittal **(F)** T1-weighted fat-suppressed MR images obtained after intravenous administration of gadolinium show extensive synovitis and tenosynovitis.

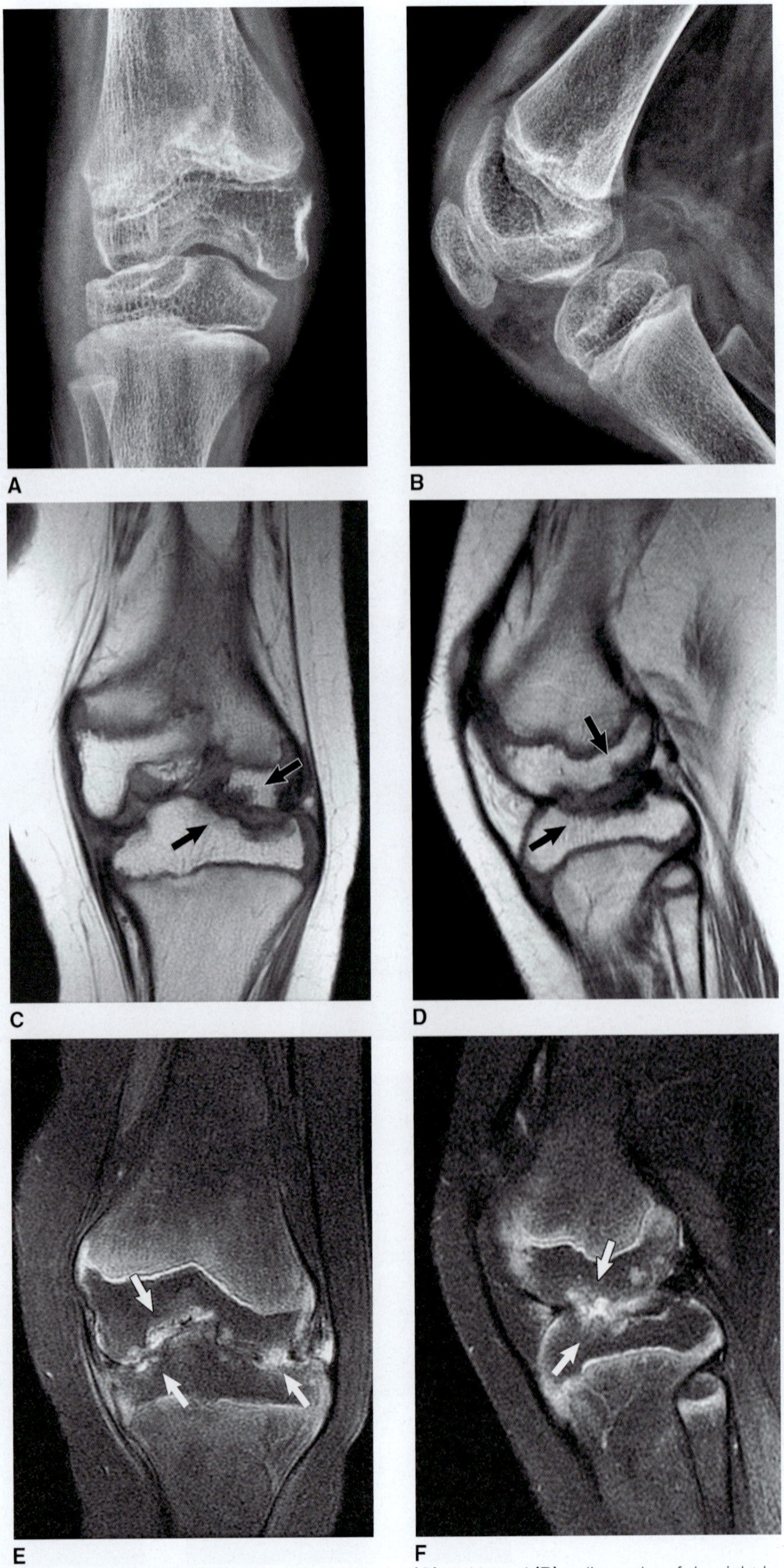

Figure 6.67 ■ **MRI of juvenile idiopathic arthritis.** Anteroposterior **(A)** and lateral **(B)** radiographs of the right knee of a 9-year-old girl show periarticular osteoporosis and joint effusion. Articular erosions are not well demonstrated. Coronal **(C)** and sagittal **(D)** proton density-weighted and coronal **(E)** and sagittal **(F)** proton density-weighted fat-suppressed MR images show significant loss of articular cartilage of distal femur and proximal tibia and subchondral bone erosions (*arrows*).

Ankylosing Spondylitis (AS)

Clinical and Pathologic Features

Ankylosing spondylitis, known in the European literature as *Bechterew disease* or *Marie-Strümpell disease*, is a chronic, progressive, inflammatory arthritis principally affecting the synovial joints of the spine and adjacent soft tissues as well as the sacroiliac joints. Sacroiliitis, which is the hallmark and usually the first manifestation of the disease, is typically bilateral and symmetric. Spinal involvement usually begins in the thoracolumbar or lumbosacral junction and extends symmetrically without skipping areas. The peripheral joints such as the hips, shoulders, and knees may also be involved. It is seen seven times more frequently in men than in women, and predominantly at a young age. Patients with ankylosing spondylitis commonly exhibit extra-articular features of disease including iritis, pulmonary fibrosis, cardiac conduction defects, aortic incompetence, spinal cord compression, and amyloidosis. Patients may also have low-grade fever, anorexia, fatigue, and weight loss. Early mortality has been reported, associated mainly with an increased risk of cardiovascular morbidity.

Rheumatoid factor is negative in patients with ankylosing spondylitis, which is the prototype of the seronegative spondyloarthropathies. A high percentage of patients (up to 95%), however, possess histocompatibility antigen HLA-B27. There is a strong familial association. Pathologically, ankylosing spondylitis is a diffuse proliferative synovitis of the diarthrodial joints exhibiting features similar to those seen in rheumatoid arthritis. In addition, there is inflammatory enthesopathy at the anterior and posterior aspects of the vertebral bodies, followed by a secondary process of progressive calcification and ossification, initially limited to the spinal ligaments and annulus fibrosus, and gradually spreading throughout the spine resulting in partial or total spine fusion (Fig. 6.68).

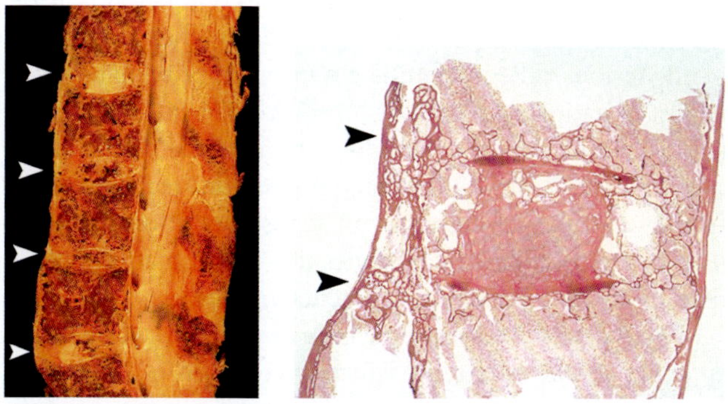

A B

Figure 6.68 ■ Pathology of ankylosing spondylitis. **A:** Photograph of the sagittal section of the lumbar spine shows anterior syndesmophytes (*arrowheads*) fusing the intervertebral disk spaces, which are not significantly narrowed. **B:** Photomicrograph shows marginal syndesmophytes (*arrowheads*) at the site of annulus fibrosus. (Modified from Bullough PG, Boachie-Adjei O. *Atlas of Spinal Diseases.* Philadelphia, JB Lippincott Company; New York, Gower Medical Publishing; 1988, Fig. 9.23, p. 109.)

Imaging Features

Squaring of the anterior border of the lower thoracic and lumbar vertebrae and so-called shiny corners or Romanus lesion, present at the anterosuperior and anteroinferior corners of the vertebral bodies, is one of the earliest radiographic features of ankylosing spondylitis, best demonstrated on the lateral radiograph of the spine (Fig. 6.69, see also Fig. 3.28A). As the condition progresses, syndesmophytes form, bridging the vertebral bodies (Fig. 6.70, see also Fig. 3.28B, C). The delicate appearance of these excrescences and their vertical rather than horizontal orientation distinguish them from the osteophytes of degenerative spine disease (Fig. 6.71). Paravertebral ossifications are common in ankylosing spondylitis. When the apophyseal joints and vertebral bodies fuse late in the course of the disease, a radiographic hallmark of this condition, the "bamboo" spine, can be observed (Fig. 6.72, see also Fig. 3.29). On the anteroposterior radiographs of the lumbar spine, a

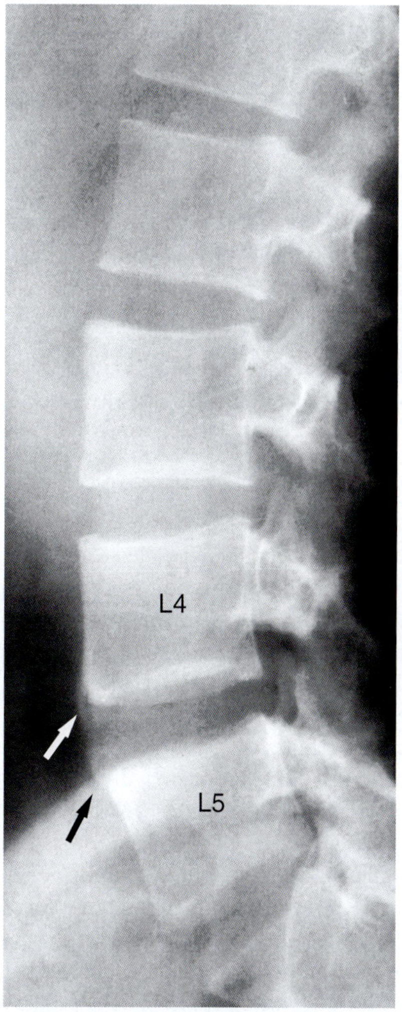

Figure 6.69 ■ Ankylosing spondylitis. Lateral radiograph of the lumbar spine in a 28-year-old man demonstrates squaring of the vertebral bodies secondary to small osseous erosions at the corners (osteitis) followed by repair/remodeling. The finding is an early radiographic feature of ankylosing spondylitis. Note also the formation of syndesmophytes at the L4–L5 disk space (*arrows*).

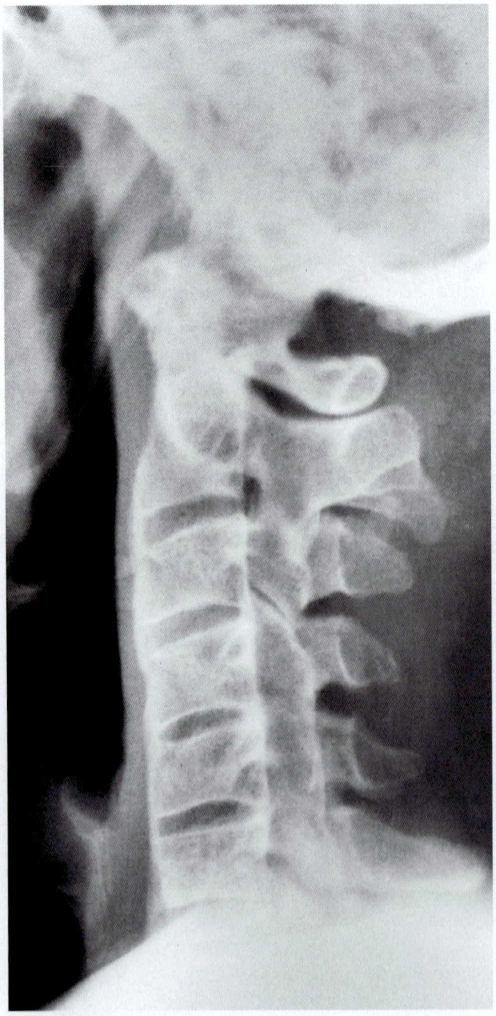

Figure 6.70 ■ Ankylosing spondylitis. Lateral radiograph of the cervical spine in a 31-year-old man demonstrates delicate syndesmophytes bridging the vertebral bodies, a common feature of ankylosing spondylitis. Note the fusion of several apophyseal joints.

single radiodense central line (so called a dagger sign) may be identified, representing ossification of the supraspinous and interspinous ligaments (Fig. 6.73). Sites of ankylosis are prone to "banana stick" fractures and subsequent pseudoarthrosis formation. The sacroiliac joints are also invariably affected in this process, exhibiting symmetric bilateral sacroiliitis (Fig. 6.74). In the initial stage of SI joints involvement, MRI detects subchondral marrow edema, ill-defined articular surfaces associated with bone erosions, and occasionally synovial enhancement. In the later stage of the disease, inflammation leads to complete fusion of sacroiliac joints (Fig. 6.75, see also Fig. 6.72B). MRI of the lumbar spine shows foci of end plate edema at the anterior corners, known as Romanus lesions. Among conditions affecting vertebral column that should not be mistaken for ankylosing spondylitis is progressive noninfectious anterior vertebral fusion, so-called *Copenhagen syndrome*. The disease usually presents in early childhood and adolescent age and is characterized by disk space obliteration and anterior osseous ankylosis with fusion of the vertebral bodies (Fig. 6.76).

In the peripheral joints, inflammatory changes may be indistinguishable from those seen in rheumatoid arthritis (see Fig. 6.72B). In the foot, erosions characteristically occur at certain tendinous insertions, particularly in the calcaneus (see Fig. 3.21). Involvement of the ischial tuberosities and iliac crests exhibits a lacelike formation of new bone called "whiskering."

Treatment

Physical therapy is important to prevent spinal deformity and loss of motion in the joints. Nonsteroidal anti-inflammatory drugs (NSAIDs) are used as first-line medical treatment to relieve the pain. Disease-modifying antirheumatic drugs (DMARDs) proved to be not very effective, although they can alleviate the symptoms from coexisting peripheral arthritis. Clinical trials showed that symptoms in some patients had improved after treatment with tumor necrosis factor (TNF) inhibitors. Surgery is usually limited to stabilization of spinal fractures, one of the complications of ankylosing spondylitis.

Reactive Arthritis (Reiter Syndrome)

Clinical Features

Reactive arthritis, an autoimmune condition that develops in response to an infection in another part of the body, usually gastrointestinal or genitourinary infection, affects five times more males than females and is characterized by arthritis, conjunctivitis, and urethritis. It was first reported in 1916 by the German military physician Hans Conrad Julius Reiter (who later was prosecuted in Nuremberg as a war criminal for his involvement in forced human experimentation in the Buchenwald concentration camp during the Second World War), and in the same year, it was described by the French physicians Fiessinger and LeRoy. Reactive arthritis is also well known for the presence of mucocutaneous rash, keratoderma blennorrhagica. Like in ankylosing spondylitis, eye involvement is common and can include conjunctivitis, iritis, uveitis, and episcleritis. About 20% to 40% of the men develop penile lesions called balanitis circinata. Approximately 60% to 80% of patients are positive for HLA-B27 gene on chromosome 6. This frequency varies according to the ethnic origin of the patient. Unlike ankylosing spondylitis, reactive arthritis may exhibit unilateral sacroiliac diseases. Prominent feature of reactive arthritis is enthesitis—inflammation of sites of tendon and ligament attachments to bone.

Two types of this syndrome have been identified. First, the sporadic or endemic type, which is common in the United States, is associated with nongonococcal urethritis, prostatitis, or hemorrhagic cystitis, although recently genital infections with *Chlamydia trachomatis* and *Neisseria gonorrhoeae* have been reported. It occurs almost exclusively in males, with male-to-female ratio ranging from 5:1 to 10:1, and the peak onset in the third decade. In Europe, a second type has been identified, which is an epidemic form associated with bacillary (*Shigella*) dysentery. This type may be seen in women as

(Continued on page 247)

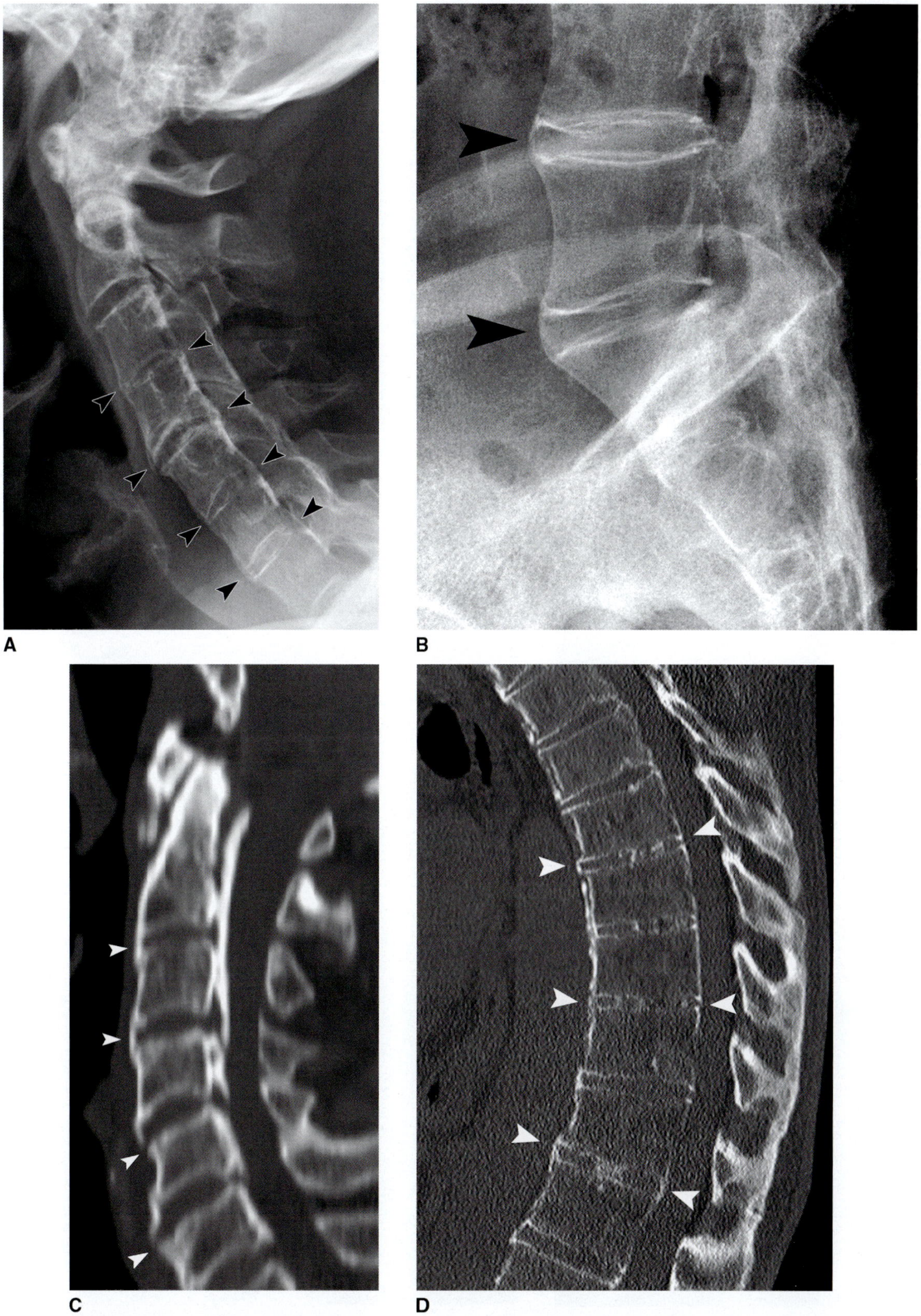

Figure 6.71 ■ **Ankylosing spondylitis. A:** Lateral radiograph of the cervical spine of a 32-year-old man shows delicate vertically oriented anterior and posterior syndesmophytes (*arrowheads*). **B:** Lateral cone-down radiograph of the lumbosacral segment of a 29-year-old man shows delicate vertically oriented anterior syndesmophytes (*arrowheads*). Sagittal reformatted CT image of the cervical spine **(C)** and sagittal reformatted image **(D)** of the thoracic spine of another patient demonstrate delicate vertically oriented anterior and posterior syndesmophytes (*arrowheads*).

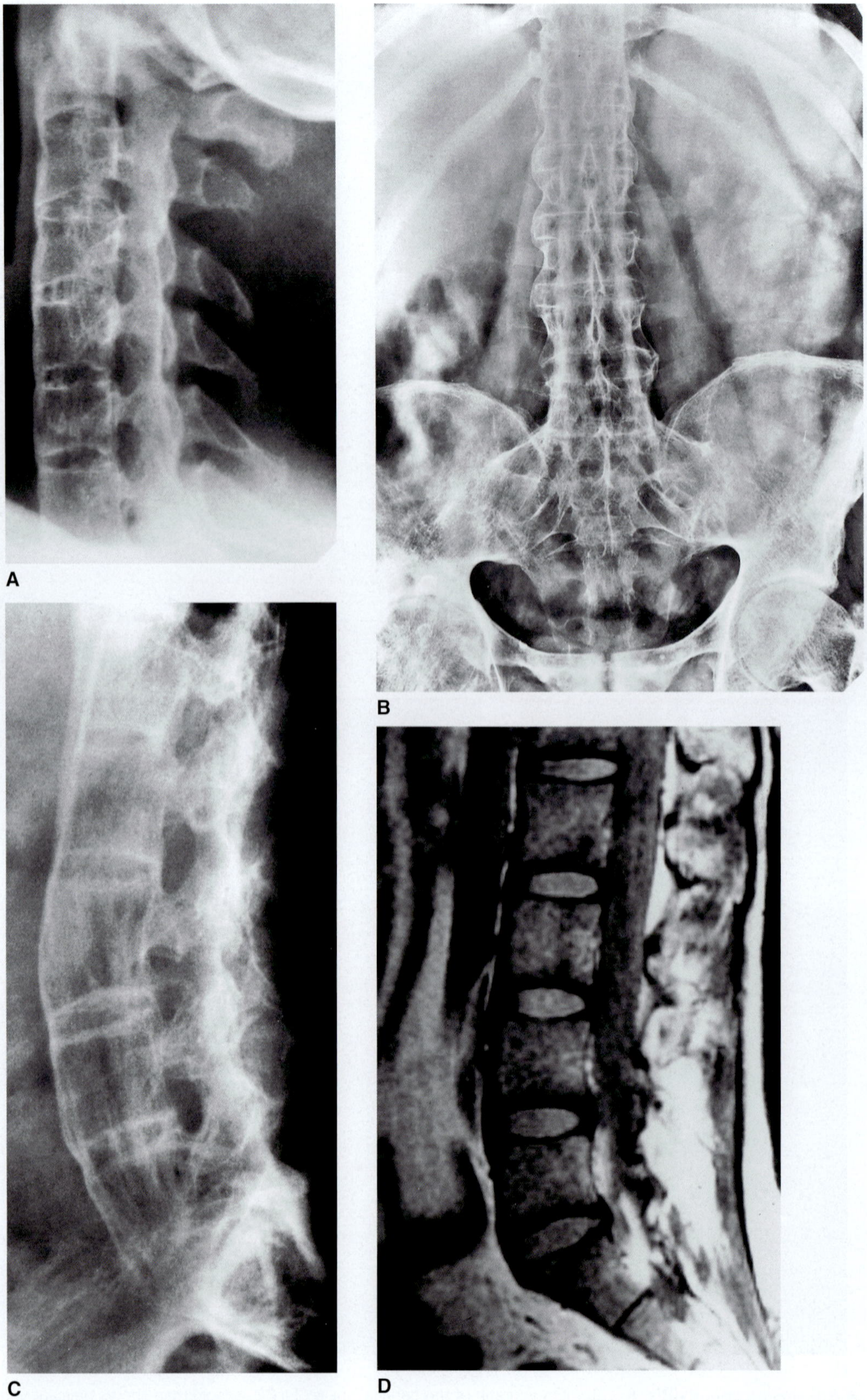

Figure 6.72 ■ **Ankylosing spondylitis. A:** Lateral radiograph of the cervical spine in a 53-year-old man with advanced ankylosing spondylitis shows anterior syndesmophytes bridging the vertebral bodies and posterior fusion of the apophyseal joints, together with paravertebral ossifications, producing a "bamboo-spine" appearance. The same phenomenon is seen on the anteroposterior **(B)** and lateral **(C)** radiographs of the lumbosacral spine. Note on the anteroposterior radiograph the fusion of the sacroiliac joints and the involvement of both hip joints, which show axial migration of the femoral heads similar to that seen in rheumatoid arthritis. **D:** Sagittal proton density-weighted MRI shows anterior syndesmophytes, calcification of the posterior longitudinal ligament, and preservation of the intervertebral disks.

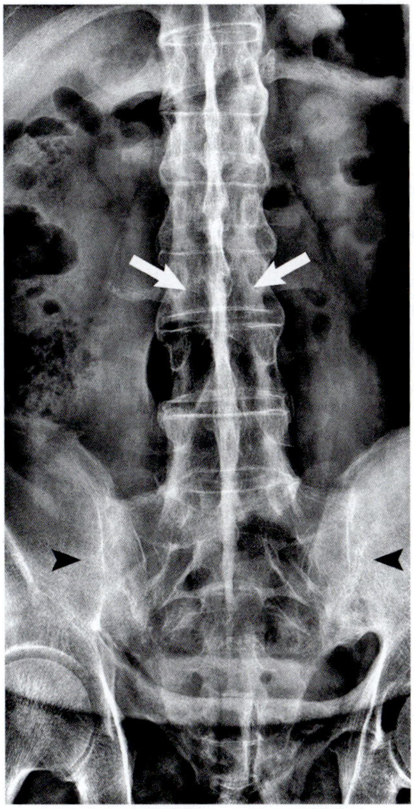

Figure 6.73 ■ Ankylosing spondylitis. Anteroposterior radiograph of the lumbar spine of a 42-year-old man shows ossifications of the supraspinous and interspinous ligaments, producing a "dagger sign" (*arrows*). Note symmetrical bilateral fusion of the sacroiliac joints (*arrowheads*).

well. There has been considerable research on the putative role of *Yersinia enterocolitica* in inducing disease, particularly in Scandinavia, where such infections are more prevalent than in North America. The frequency in the general population is estimated to be 3.5 to 5 cases per 100,000, but in the era before effective therapy for HIV, it was as high as 75% incidence in HIV-positive males expressing positive HLA-B27.

Imaging Features

Radiographically, reactive arthritis is marked by peripheral and usually asymmetric arthritis, with a predilection for the joints of the lower limb (Fig. 6.77). The foot is the most common site of involvement, particularly the metatarsophalangeal joints and the heels (Fig. 6.77B; see also Figs. 3.21 and 3.22D). Periosteal new bone formation is not uncommon. Involvement of the sacroiliac joints, which is frequently encountered, may be either asymmetric (unilateral [Fig. 6.78] or bilateral [Fig. 6.79]) or symmetric (bilateral [Figs. 6.80]). In the thoracic and lumbar spine, coarse syndesmophytes or paraspinal ossifications may be present, characteristically bridging adjacent vertebrae (Fig. 6.81, see also Fig. 3.30A). The symphysis pubis and manubriosternal joint may also be affected.

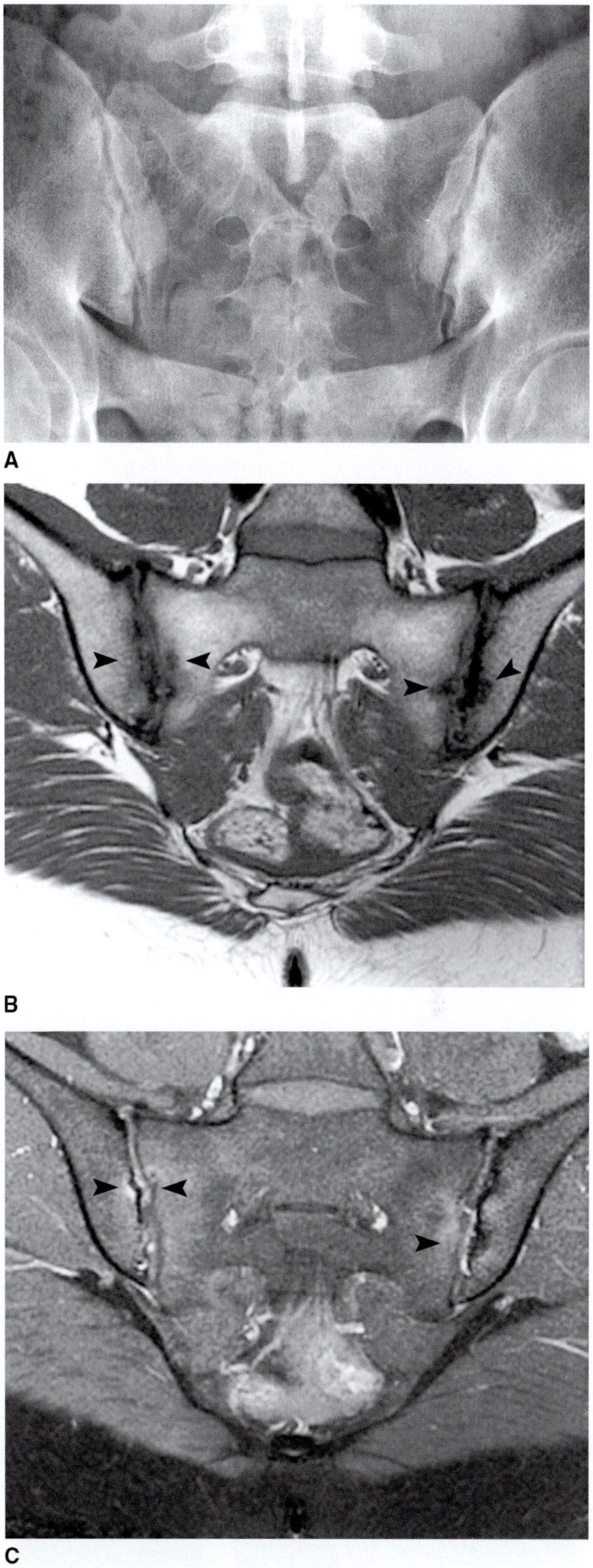

Figure 6.74 ■ Ankylosing spondylitis. Fergusson view of the pelvis of a 25-year-old man shows bilateral symmetric sacroiliitis **(A)**, confirmed on coronal T1-weighted **(B)** and coronal T1-weighted **(C)** fat-suppressed postcontrast MR images (*arrowheads*).

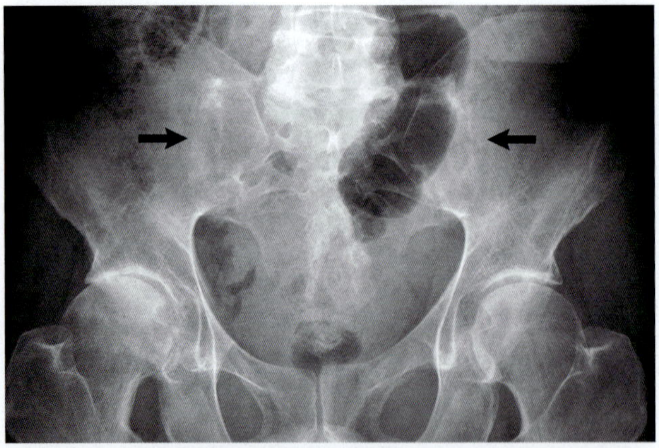

Figure 6.75 ■ **Ankylosing spondylitis.** Anteroposterior radiograph of the pelvis of a 49-year-old man shows fusion of both sacroiliac joints (*arrow*). Note also early inflammatory changes of both hip joints.

Differential Diagnosis

In the differential diagnosis, septic arthritis should always be considered. This diagnosis can be confirmed or excluded through the clinical presentation and synovial fluid analysis. Rheumatoid arthritis is usually distinguished by the pattern of joint involvement. Psoriatic arthritis and occasionally ankylosing spondylitis may exhibit some overlapping clinical features, but imaging findings in these conditions are extremely helpful in the differential diagnosis.

Treatment

NSAIDs remain the treatment of choice for the articular manifestations and in most cases provided adequate control of acute synovitis and enthesitis. DMARDs may be considered in patients not responding to treatment with NSAIDs and glucocorticoids. Appropriate short-term antibiotic therapy should be administered if the infection remains active.

Psoriatic Arthritis

Clinical Features

Psoriasis is a dermatologic disorder that affects ~1% to 2% of the population. The macular and papular skin lesions of psoriasis display characteristic focal plaques covered with silvery white scales and are commonly located over extensor surfaces of the extremities. Nail abnormalities, including

(Continued on page 250)

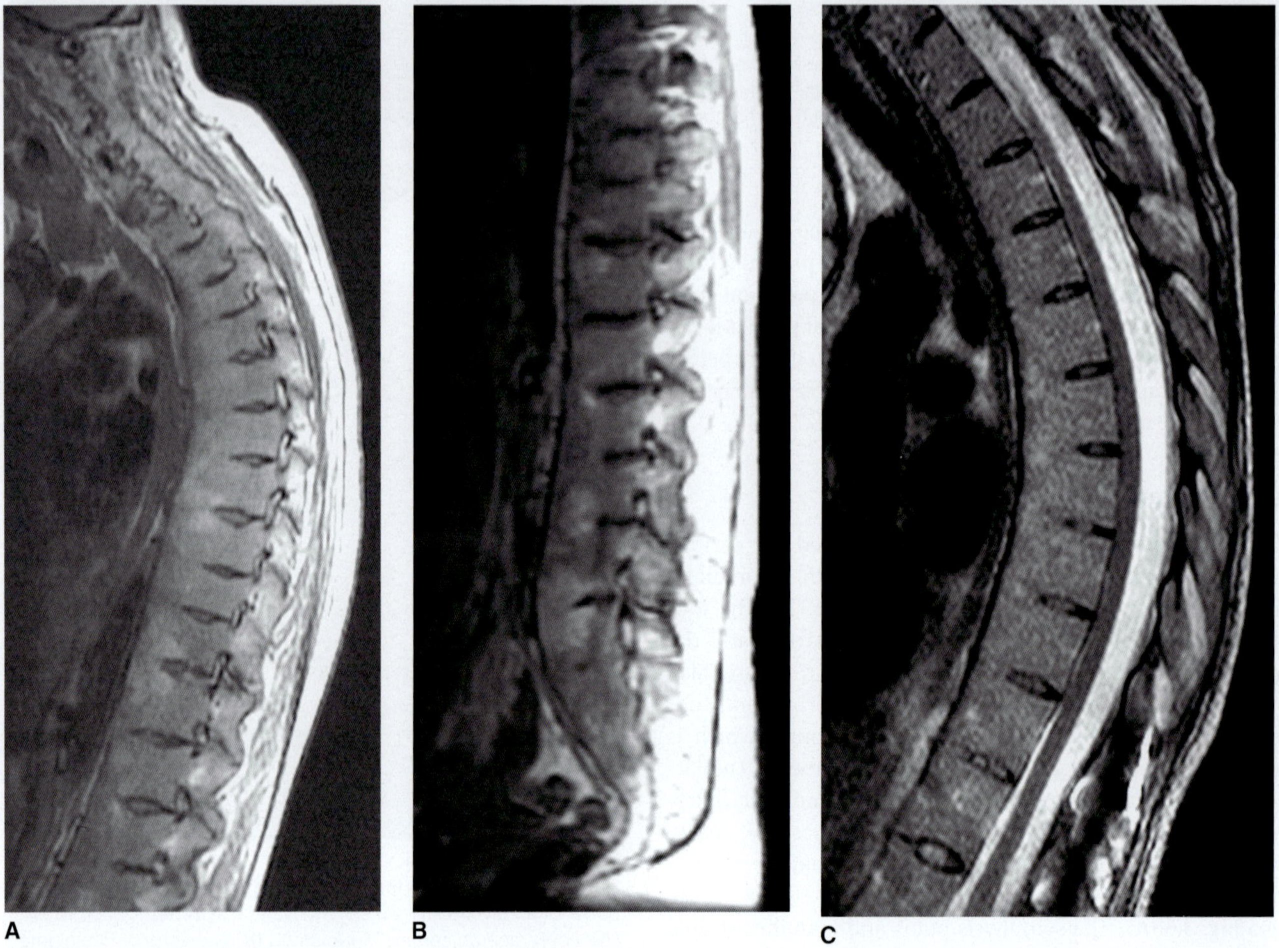

Figure 6.76 ■ **Copenhagen syndrome.** Sagittal T1-weighted MR images of the thoracic **(A)** and lumbar **(B)** spine and T2-weighted MRI of the thoracic spine **(C)** of a 16-year-old girl show fusion of the anterior aspects of the vertebral bodies. Unlike in ankylosing spondylitis, the apophyseal joints are normal.

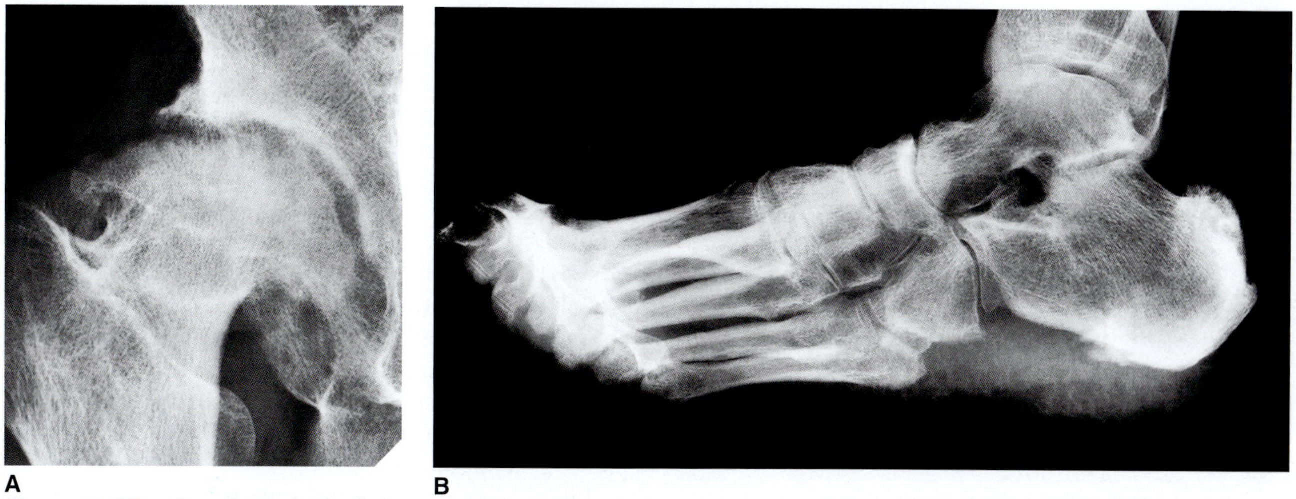

Figure 6.77 ■ **Reactive arthritis. A:** Anteroposterior radiograph of right hip joint of a 39-year-old man shows characteristic changes of inflammatory arthritis. **B:** Lateral radiograph of the foot of a 28-year-old man demonstrates the "fluffy" periostitis of the calcaneus and inflammatory changes of the metatarsophalangeal joints typical of this condition.

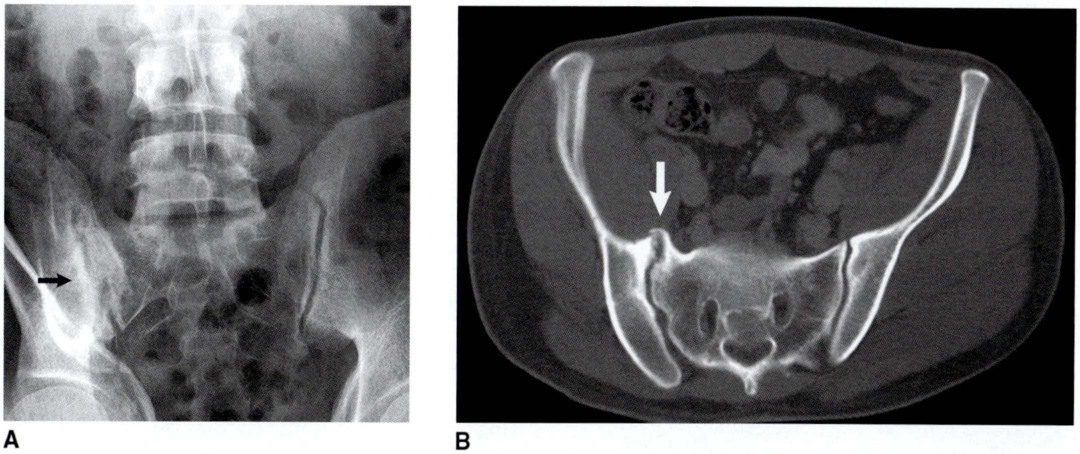

Figure 6.78 ■ **Reactive arthritis.** Fergusson view of the sacroiliac joints **(A)** and axial CT image of the pelvis **(B)** of a 38-year-old man show unilateral right-sided sacroiliitis (*arrows*).

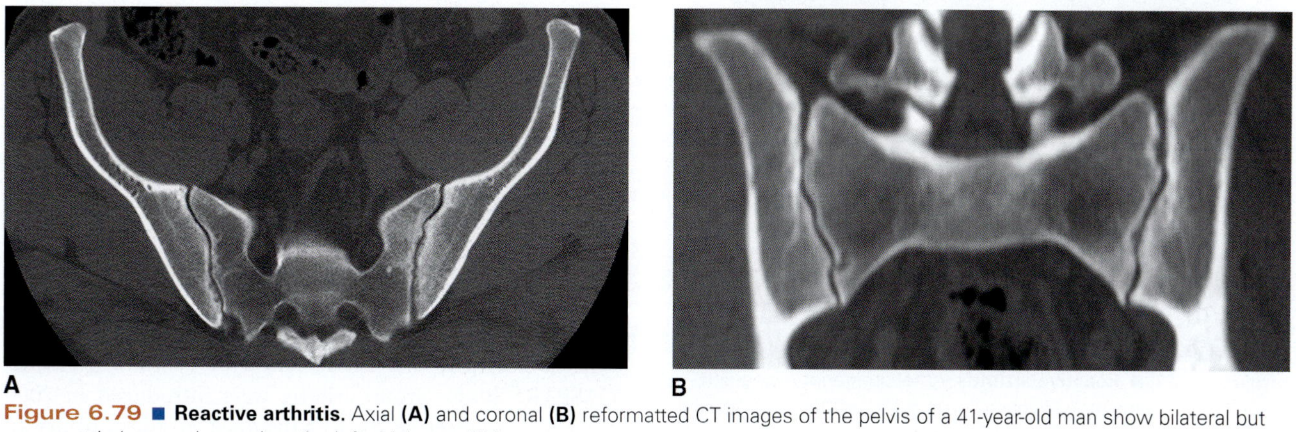

Figure 6.79 ■ **Reactive arthritis.** Axial **(A)** and coronal **(B)** reformatted CT images of the pelvis of a 41-year-old man show bilateral but asymmetric (more advanced on the left side) sacroiliitis.

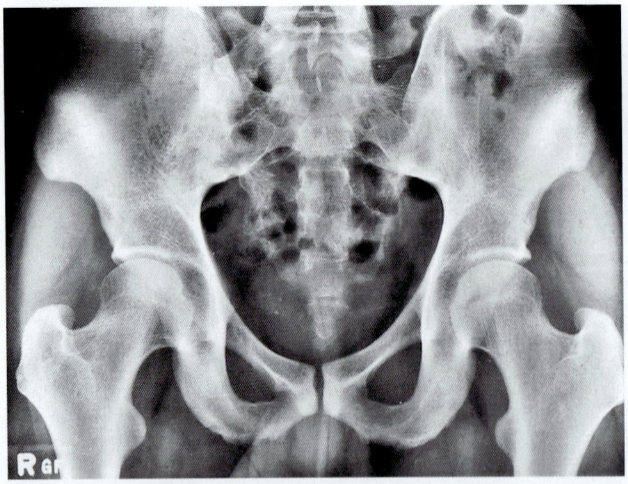

Figure 6.80 ■ **Reactive arthritis.** Anteroposterior radiograph of the pelvis of the patient shown in Figure 6.77B demonstrates symmetric bilateral involvement of the sacroiliac joints.

discoloration, fragmentation, pitting, and onycholysis, may provide an early diagnostic clue (see Figs. 1.4 and 3.2). Approximately 10% to 15% of patients with psoriasis develop inflammatory arthritis, which usually predates the onset of cutaneous abnormalities by about 10 years. Articular disease is more common in patients with moderate or severe skin abnormalities, and according to Wright, severe and mutilating arthropathy is often associated with extensive exfoliative skin abnormalities. The entheses are an important site of inflammation and subsequent pathology in this disorder. These are locations where tendons, ligaments, and fascia insert into bone. Histopathology is characterized by chronic inflammatory infiltrates similar to that present in rheumatoid arthritis.

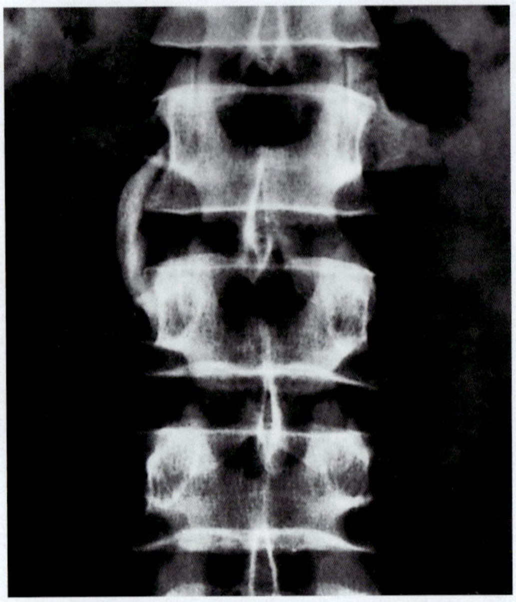

Figure 6.81 ■ **Reactive arthritis.** Anteroposterior radiograph of the lumbar spine of a 23-year-old man demonstrates a paraspinal ossification bridging the L2 and L3 vertebrae.

The cause of psoriatic arthritis is unknown, and its relationship to rheumatoid arthritis and spondyloarthropathies is still unsettled. It has been postulated that some mutations in the genes *CARD14*, *HLA-B*, *HLA-C*, *HLA-DRB1*, *IL12B*, *IL13*, *IL23R*, and *TRAF3IP2* are associated with this arthritis. Regarding HLA, a haplotype epidemiologic association involves the expression of both class I and class II HLA alleles, including HLA-B13, HLA-B17, HLA-B27, HLA-B38, HLA-B39, HLA-Cw6, HLA-DR4, and HLA-DR7. It is worthwhile to notice that HLA-B27 is present in 60% of patients with disease, as compared with 8% of the general population. Nonetheless, as noted, extensive genetic analysis has been disappointing in yielding any practical data that can be extrapolated for predictive therapies or genetic counseling.

The arthritis predominantly affects the distal interphalangeal joints of the hands and feet, although other sites of involvement—the proximal interphalangeal joints as well as the hips, knees, ankles, shoulders, and spine—may also be encountered.

According to the original classification of psoriatic arthritis by Moll and Wright, five specific subgroups of arthritic syndromes have been described in psoriatic arthritis.

Subgroup 1, or classic psoriatic arthritis, includes nail pathology with frequent erosion of the terminal tufts termed acro-osteolysis (Fig. 6.82). It is important, however, to remember that other conditions may also exhibit acro-osteolysis (Table 6.3). The involvement of the distal and occasionally proximal interphalangeal joints of the hand and foot is also a common finding (Figs. 6.83 and 6.84).

Subgroup 2, well known for the "opera-glass" deformity of the hand, is termed *arthritis mutilans* because of the extensive destruction of the phalanges and metatarsal and metacarpal joints, including the "pencil-in-cup" deformity (Fig. 6.85). Other joints such as hip or elbow (Fig. 6.86) are also frequently affected. Patients with arthritis mutilans often will have sacroiliitis.

Subgroup 3 is characterized by symmetric polyarthritis (Figs. 6.87 and 6.88) and may result in ankylosis of the proximal and distal interphalangeal joints. In this form, psoriatic arthritis is frequently indistinguishable from rheumatoid arthritis (Fig. 6.89).

Subgroup 4 is characterized by oligoarticular arthritis, and in contrast to subgroup 3, the joint involvement is asymmetric, generally including the proximal and distal interphalangeal and metacarpophalangeal articulations (Fig. 6.90). Patients with this oligoarticular arthritis form the most frequent subgroup of psoriatic arthritis and are known for the appearance of sausage-like swelling of digits (Fig. 6.91).

Subgroup 5 is axial spondyloarthropathy that has features similar to those of ankylosing spondylitis.

More recently, the Classification of Psoriatic Arthritis (CASPAR) Study Group criteria were introduced in 2006 as a new classification for this disorder. To the contrary to

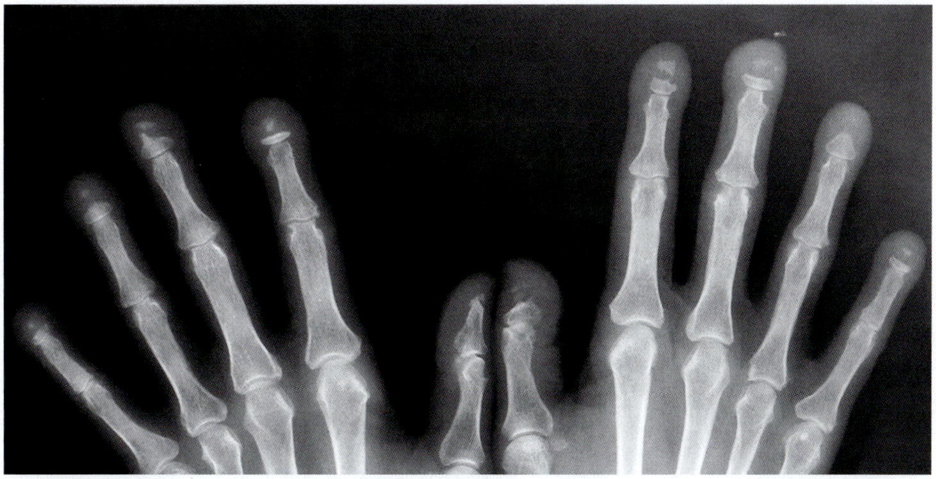

Figure 6.82 ■ **Psoriatic arthritis.** A 57-year-old woman with long-standing psoriasis developed resorption of the tufts of the distal phalanges (acro-osteolysis) of both hands, typical of this condition.

the original classification, CASPAR Study Group provided the diagnosis of psoriatic arthritis in patients without skin lesions. To increase the sensitivity, additional features were included, such as dactylitis ("sausage digit"), nail changes, and family history.

Table 6.3 MOST COMMON CAUSES OF ACRO-OSTEOLYSIS
Trauma
Diabetic gangrene
Psoriasis
Scleroderma
Dermatomyositis
Rheumatoid arthritis
Raynaud disease
Hyperparathyroidism (primary, secondary)
Frostbite
Burn (thermal, electrical)
Congenital (Hajdu-Cheney syndrome)
Leprosy
Gout
Pyknodysostosis
Sarcoidosis
Sjögren syndrome
Polyvinyl chloride
Pachydermoperiostosis
Thromboangiitis obliterans
Syringomyelia

Modified from Reeder MM. *Reeder and Felson's Gamuts in Radiology*. 4th ed. New York: Springer; 2003, with permission.

Imaging Features

In general, there are few characteristic radiographic features of psoriatic arthritis that help to make a correct diagnosis. In the phalanges of the hand or foot, a periosteal reaction in the form of a "fluffy" new bone apposition may often be noted (Fig. 6.92, see also Fig. 6.90). If this new bone is periarticular in location and associated with erosions of the interphalangeal joints, it exhibits a "mouse-ear" appearance (Fig. 6.93). Occasionally psoriatic hand arthropathy can cause significant enlargement of the thumb sesamoids, similar to one described in acromegaly (Fig. 6.94). In the advanced arthritis mutilans stage of psoriatic arthritis, severe deformities such as the "pencil-in-cup" configuration (see Fig. 6.85) and interphalangeal ankylosis may be observed. In the heel, late-stage changes may be seen in the formation of broad-based osteophytes and in the presence of erosions and a fluffy periostitis (see Figs. 3.21 and 3.22C). Very early inflammatory changes, not so obvious on other imaging modalities, can be demonstrated by 18F-FDG PET and PET/CT techniques (Fig. 6.95). Isolated tenosynovitis, especially of the flexor tendon sheaths, with additional synovitis and soft tissue edema results in dactylitis (sausage digit), which is a hallmark of psoriatic arthritis (see Figs. 6.90A and 6.91). Less commonly, the extensor tenosynovitis is observed (see Fig. 6.95A). Magnetic resonance imaging, in addition to articular erosions, may also detect proliferative synovitis, subarticular bone marrow edema, enthesitis, and tenosynovitis (Fig. 6.96).

Psoriatic arthritis of the spine is associated with a particularly high incidence of sacroiliitis, which may be bilateral and symmetric (Fig. 6.97), bilateral and asymmetric (Fig. 6.98B), or unilateral (Fig. 6.98A). Both synovial and syndesmotic parts of the joint may be affected. As in reactive arthritis, coarse asymmetric syndesmophytes and paraspinal ossifications may form (Figs. 6.99 and 6.100), and as Resnick pointed out, this may represent an early manifestation of the disease. In the axial skeleton, MRI is highly sensitive in detection of spondylitis and sacroiliitis (Fig. 6.101).

(Continued on page 255)

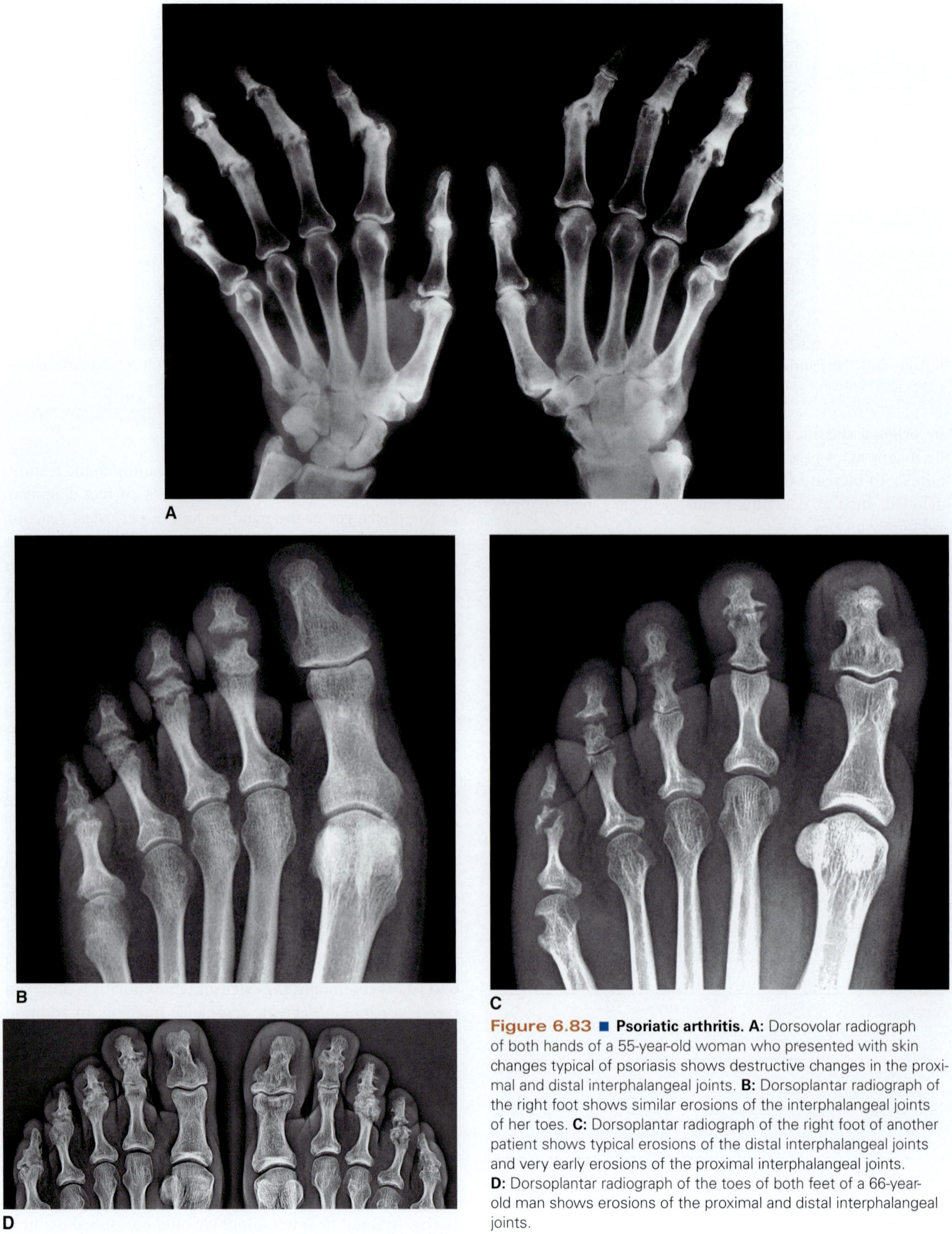

Figure 6.83 ■ **Psoriatic arthritis. A:** Dorsovolar radiograph of both hands of a 55-year-old woman who presented with skin changes typical of psoriasis shows destructive changes in the proximal and distal interphalangeal joints. **B:** Dorsoplantar radiograph of the right foot shows similar erosions of the interphalangeal joints of her toes. **C:** Dorsoplantar radiograph of the right foot of another patient shows typical erosions of the distal interphalangeal joints and very early erosions of the proximal interphalangeal joints. **D:** Dorsoplantar radiograph of the toes of both feet of a 66-year-old man shows erosions of the proximal and distal interphalangeal joints.

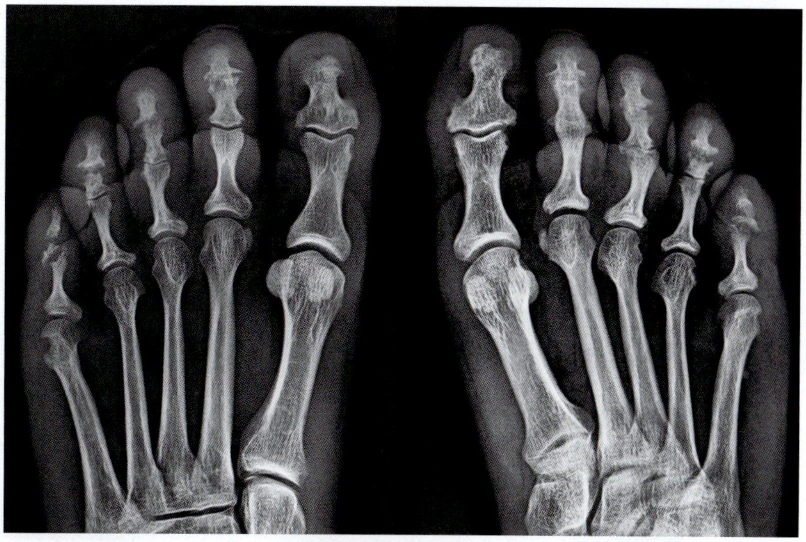

Figure 6.84 ■ Psoriatic arthritis. Anteroposterior radiograph of both feet of a 46-year-old woman shows characteristic erosions of several distal interphalangeal joints and erosion of the right fifth metatarsal head. Note also fusion of the proximal interphalangeal joint of the second left toe.

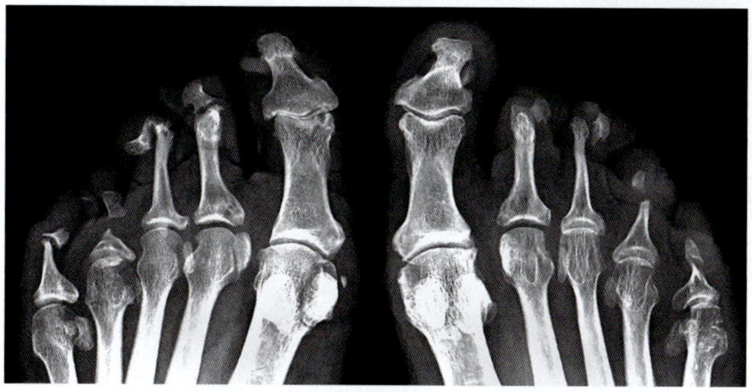

A

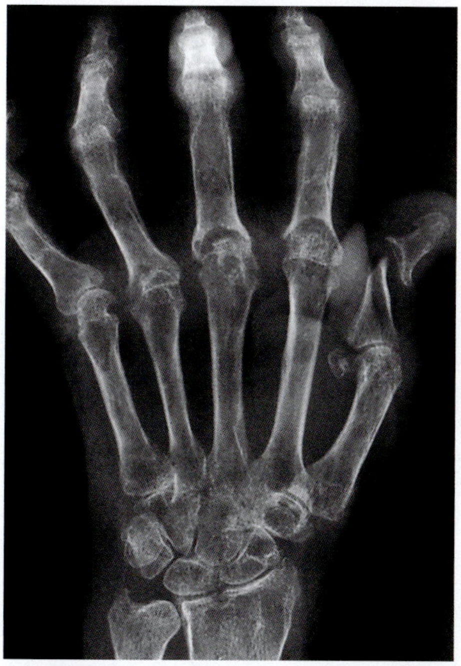

B

Figure 6.85 ■ Psoriatic arthritis mutilans. A: Radiograph of both feet of a 60-year-old man shows typical changes of arthritis mutilans affecting the toes. **B:** Dorsovolar radiograph of the hand of a 57-year-old woman shows the typical presentation of psoriatic polyarthritis. The "pencil-in-cup" deformity in the interphalangeal joint of the thumb is characteristic for this form of psoriasis.

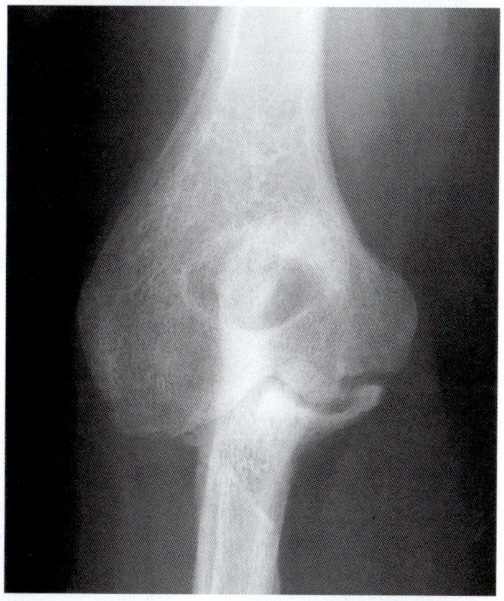

A

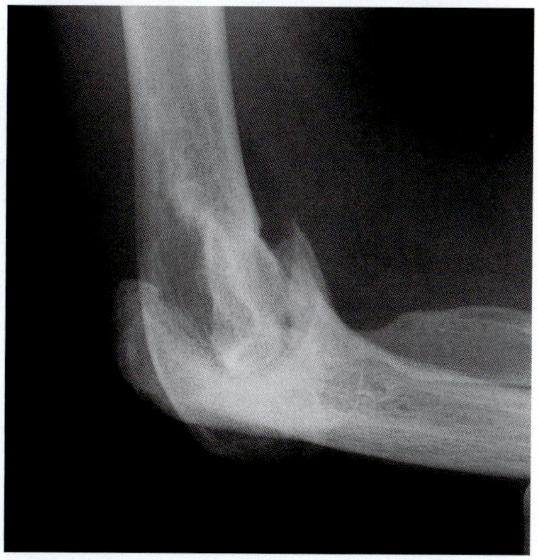

B

Figure 6.86 ■ Psoriatic arthritis. A 49-year-old man presented with psoriatic arthritis mutilans. Anteroposterior **(A)** and lateral **(B)** radiographs of the right elbow show extensive articular erosions. Elevated anterior fat-pad indicates a joint effusion.

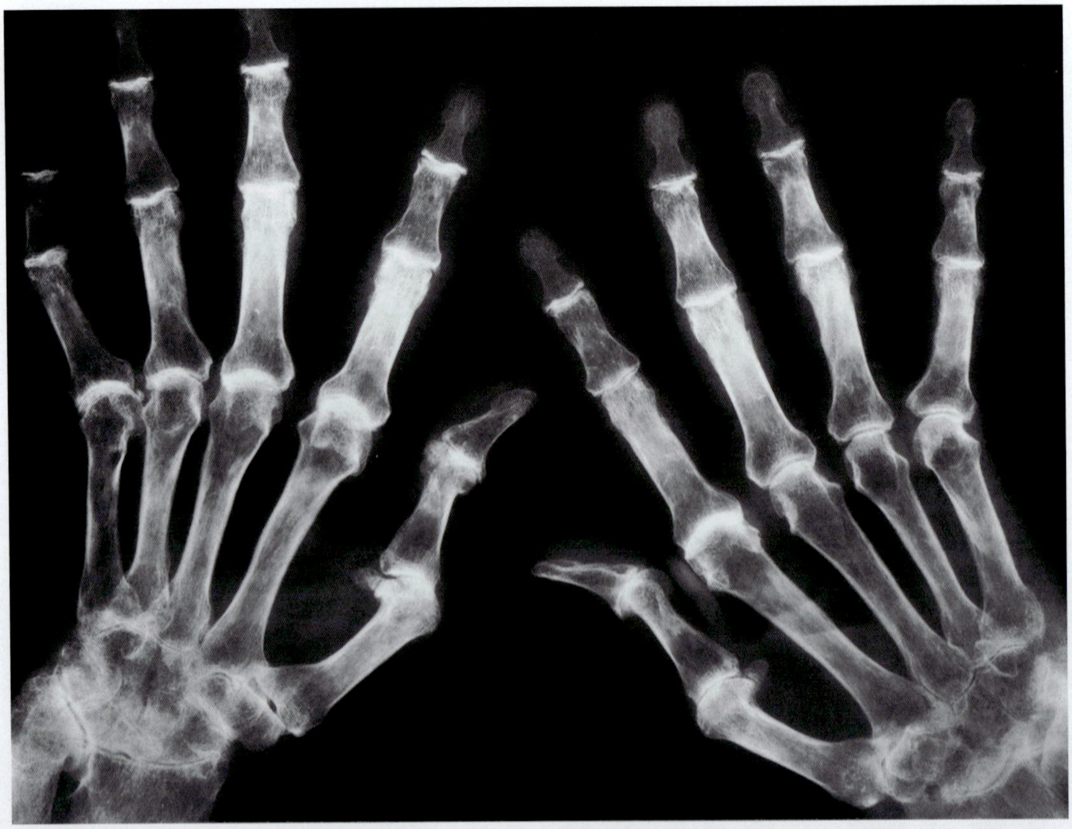

Figure 6.87 ■ **Psoriatic arthritis.** A 75-year-old woman presented with symmetric psoriatic polyarthritis affecting all joints of the hands and wrists. Unlike in adult-onset type of rheumatoid arthritis, the distal interphalangeal joints are also involved.

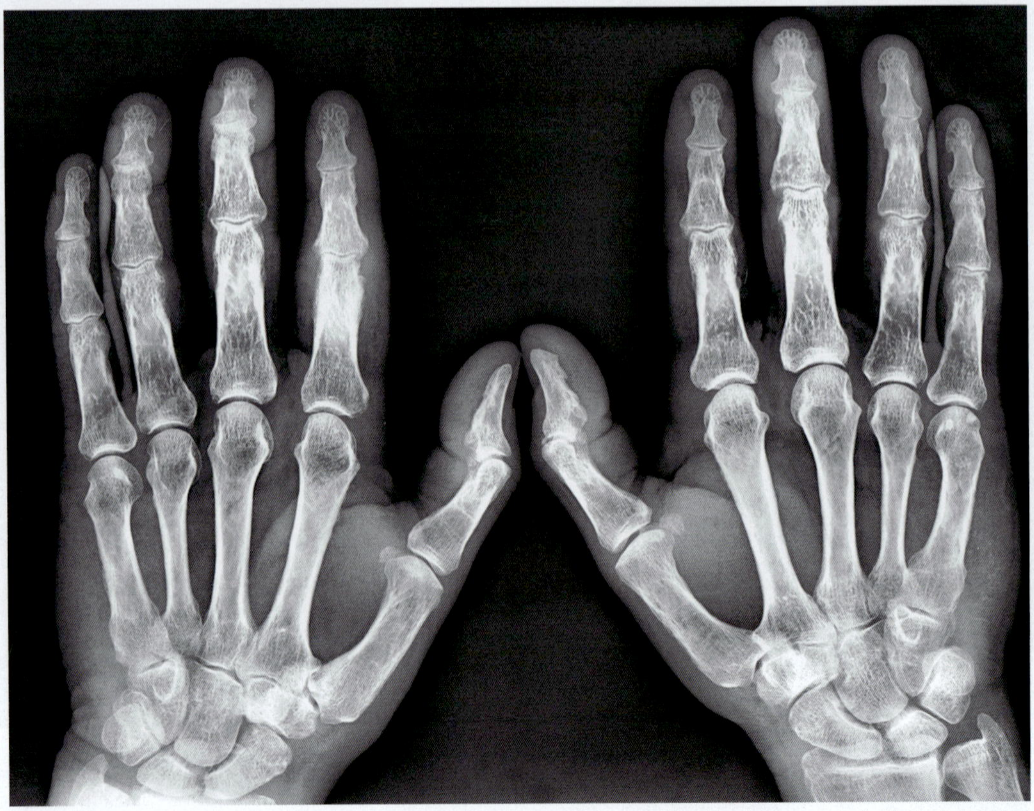

Figure 6.88 ■ **Psoriatic arthritis.** A 65-year-old man presented with psoriatic arthritis affecting symmetrically both hands. Note soft tissue swelling, articular erosions, and periostitis.

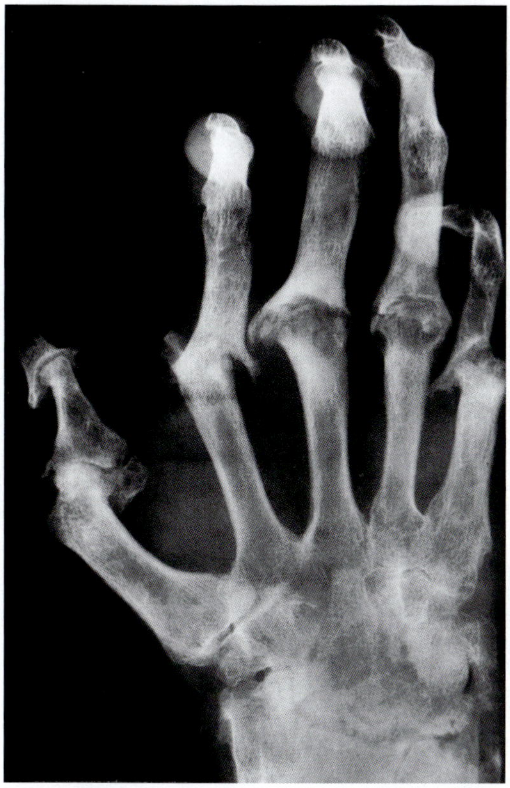

Figure 6.89 ■ **Psoriatic arthritis.** Dorsovolar radiograph of the left hand of a 67-year-old man with the polyarthritic form of psoriatic arthritis demonstrates erosions and fusion of multiple joints. The swan-neck deformity of the small finger is similar to that seen in patients with rheumatoid arthritis.

Differential Diagnosis

The diagnosis of psoriatic arthritis at times may be challenging, particularly when skin manifestations are subtle, or the arthritis antedates the skin lesions. The lack of clearly defined diagnostic criteria and the possibility of overlap syndromes of other rheumatologic disorders further add to the complexity of diagnosis. The differential diagnosis of psoriatic arthritis includes other forms of inflammatory arthritides, such as other seronegative spondyloarthropathies, in particular those associated with sacroiliitis and enthesitis, as well as rheumatoid arthritis. The appearance of periostitis and joint ankylosis in psoriatic arthritis usually leads to the correct diagnosis. Because on conventional radiography the appearance of articular erosions may be very similar in both diseases, some investigators suggested using dynamic contrast-enhanced MRI to discriminate these two entities. Schwenzer and collaborators found significant correlations between inflammatory parameters and dynamic contrast-enhanced findings in patients with rheumatoid arthritis but not in those with psoriatic arthritis. Specifically, they found a statistically significant difference in synovial enhancement 15 minutes after intravenous administration of gadolinium in patients with rheumatoid arthritis.

Treatment

Patients with psoriatic arthritis are also treated with biologic agents as first-line therapy, and this approach has

(Continued on page 259)

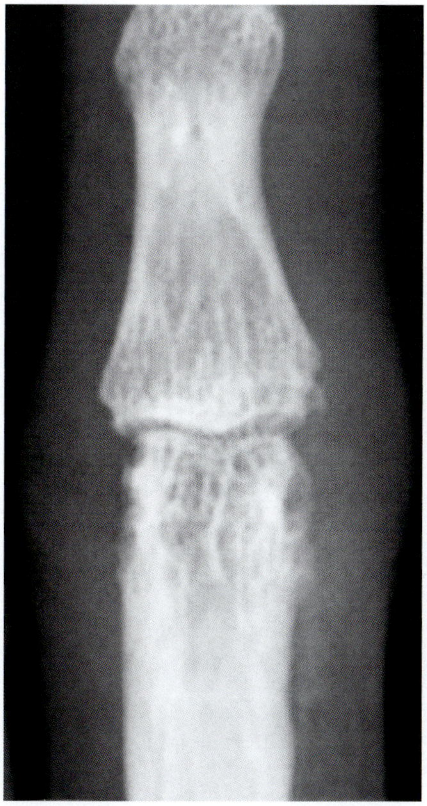

A

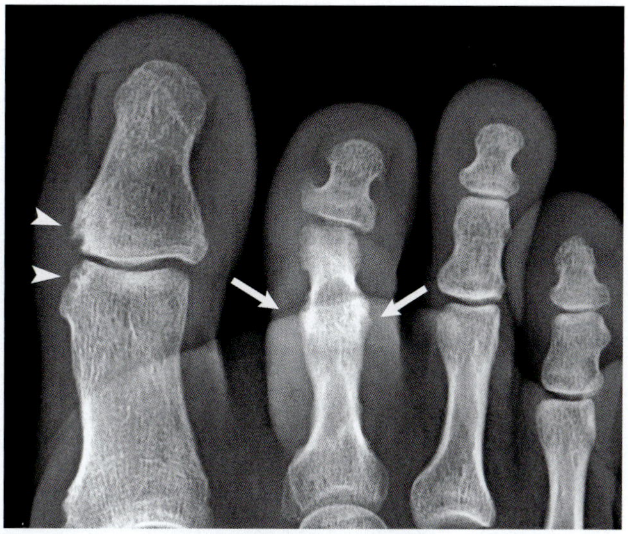

B

Figure 6.90 ■ **Psoriatic arthritis. A:** A 39-year-old man presented with a painful and swollen middle finger of his right hand (so-called sausage digit). Note subtle periarticular erosions, fluffy periosteal reaction, and soft tissue swelling, features characteristic of oligoarticular psoriatic arthritis. **B:** In another patient, a 32-year-old man, observe erosions at the interphalangeal joint of the left great toe (*arrowheads*) and fusion of the proximal interphalangeal joint of the second toe (*arrows*) associated with fusiform soft tissue swelling.

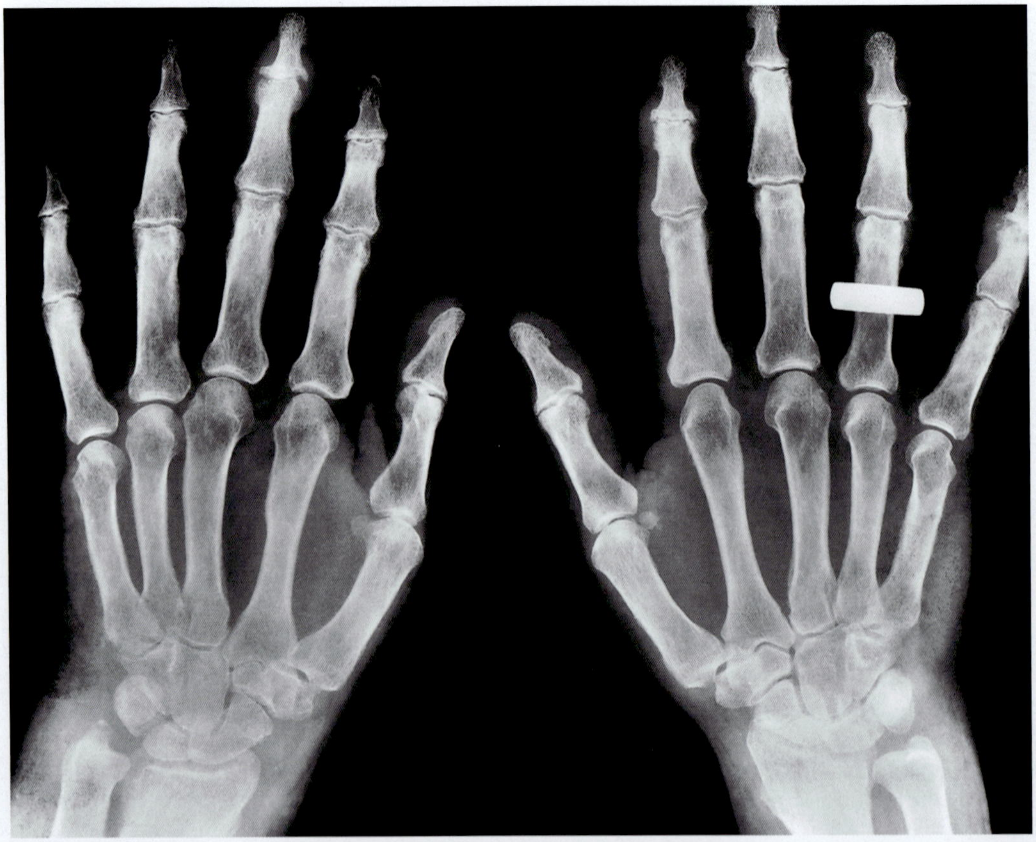

Figure 6.91 ■ **Psoriatic arthritis.** Dorsovolar radiograph of the hands of a 33-year-old man with psoriasis and oligoarticular involvement shows destructive changes in the distal interphalangeal joints of the right middle finger and the left index and small fingers. The right middle and left index fingers presented as "sausage digits."

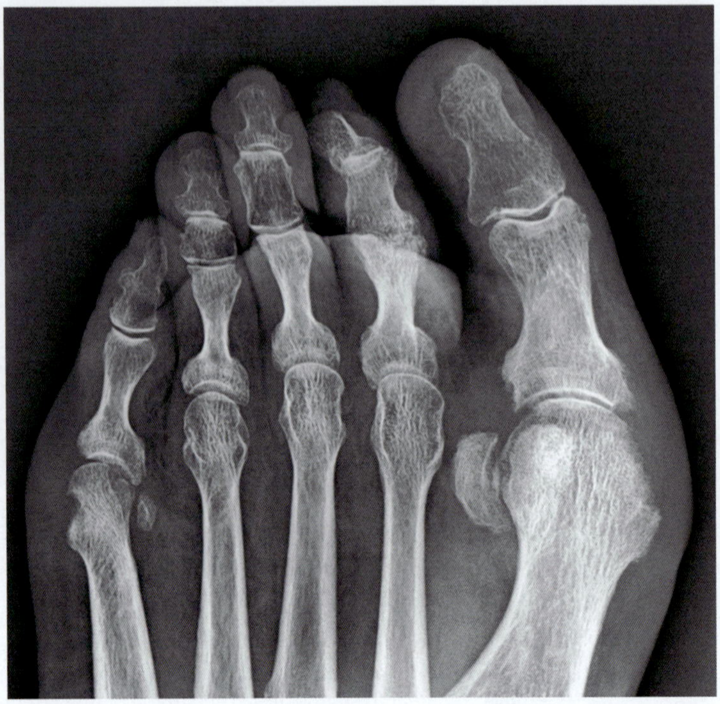

Figure 6.92 ■ **Psoriatic arthritis.** Periarticular erosions at the first metatarsophalangeal joint and proximal interphalangeal joint of the second toe are accompanied by fluffy periostitis.

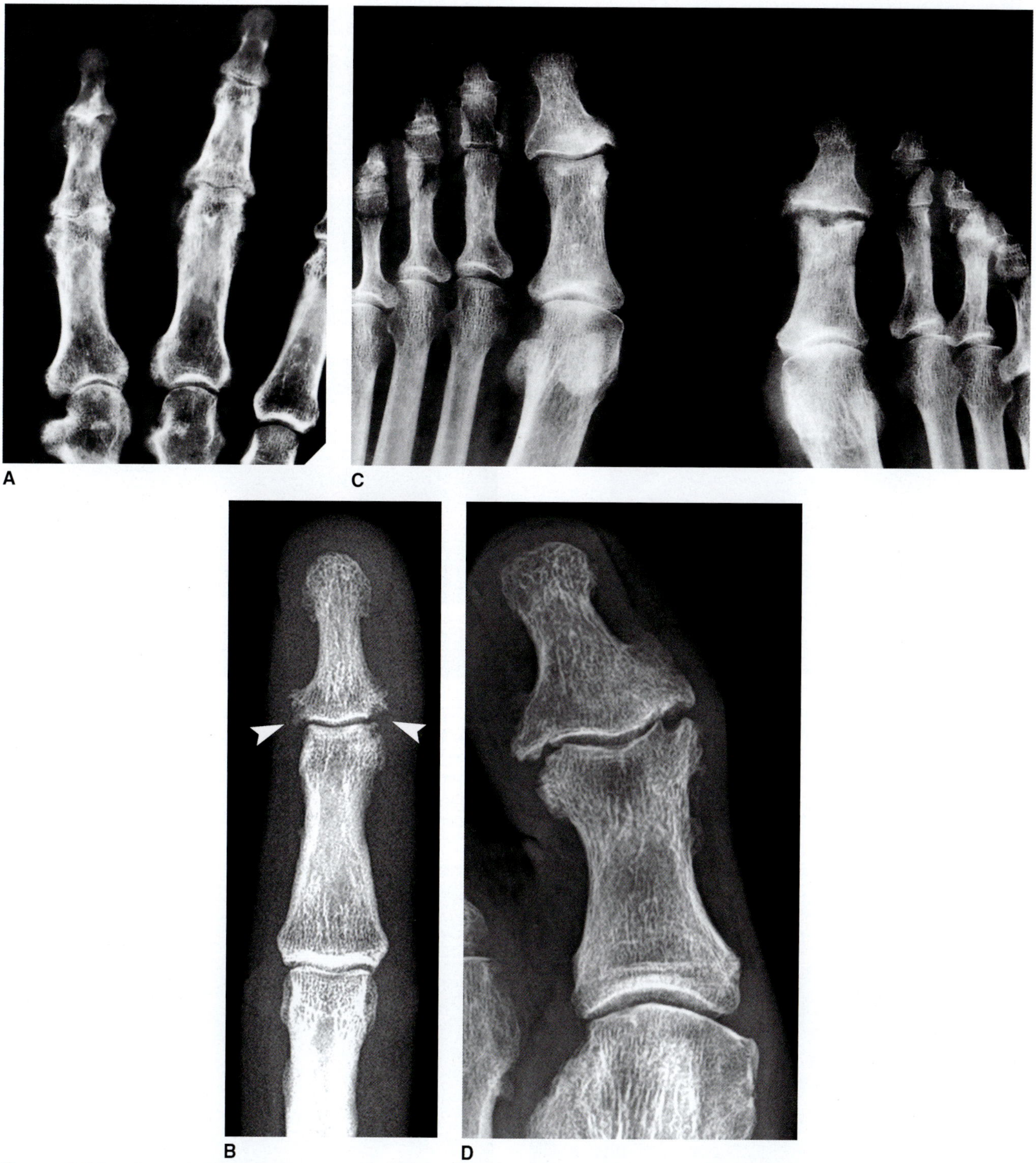

Figure 6.93 ■ **Psoriatic arthritis. A:** Dorsovolar radiograph of the ring and small fingers of a 48-year-old man who presented with clinically documented psoriasis shows marginal erosions and new bone apposition in the proximal and distal interphalangeal joints, resembling mouse ears. Note the fluffy periostitis in the juxta-articular areas of the phalanges and distal metacarpals. **B:** Mouse-ears appearance of erosion of the distal interphalangeal joint of the index finger (*arrowheads*) is seen in another patient. **C:** In the feet, the same process has led to a mouse-ear appearance at the interphalangeal joints of the great toes. **D:** In another patient, a 51-year-old man, observe the mouse-ear erosion of the interphalangeal joint of right great toe.

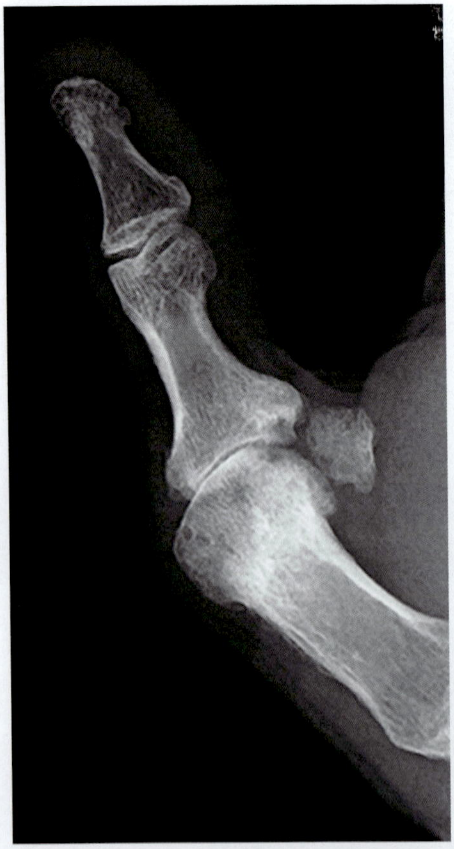

Figure 6.94 ■ **Psoriatic arthritis.** Radiograph of the left thumb of a 44-year-old man shows erosions at the first metacarpophalangeal joint and enlarged sesamoid bone.

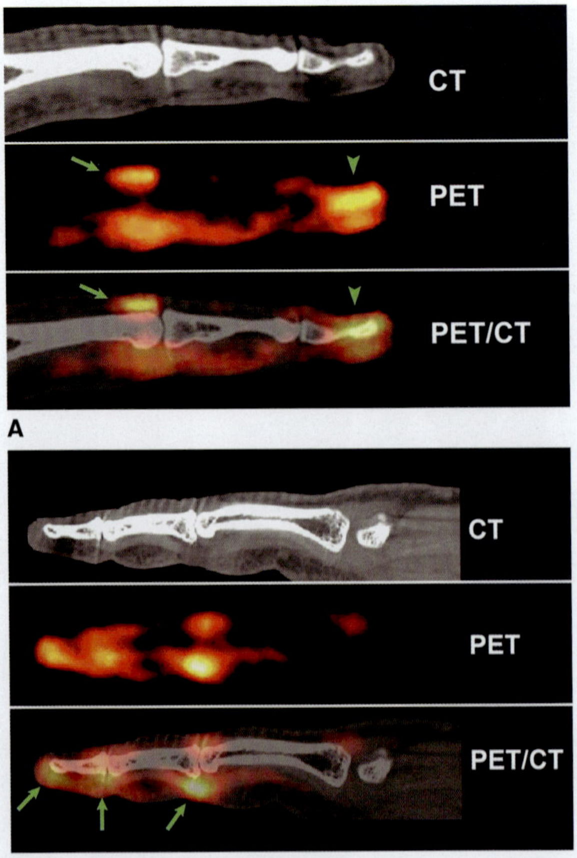

Figure 6.95 ■ **CT, 18F-FDG PET, and PET/CT of psoriatic arthritis. A:** Along the extensor tendon (*arrows*) and its insertion into the nail bed (*arrowheads*) of the middle finger of a 53-year-old man, the inflammatory changes are well demonstrated by increased metabolic activity. **B:** In another patient, a 50-year-old man, note the inflammatory changes at the flexor tendon of the index finger (*arrows*).

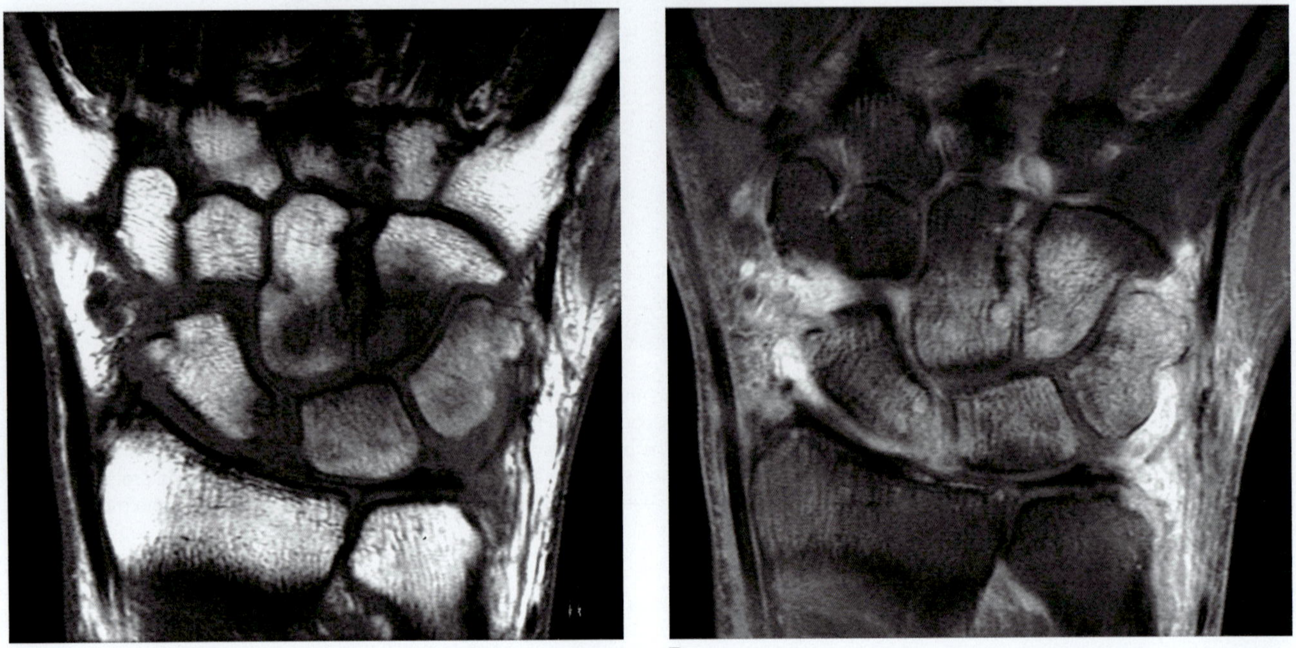

Figure 6.96 ■ **MRI of psoriatic arthritis.** Coronal T1-weighted **(A)** and coronal T1-weighted fat-suppressed **(B)** MR images of the left wrist obtained after intravenous administration of gadolinium show bone marrow edema, erosions of several carpal bones, and synovitis in a 50-year-old man.

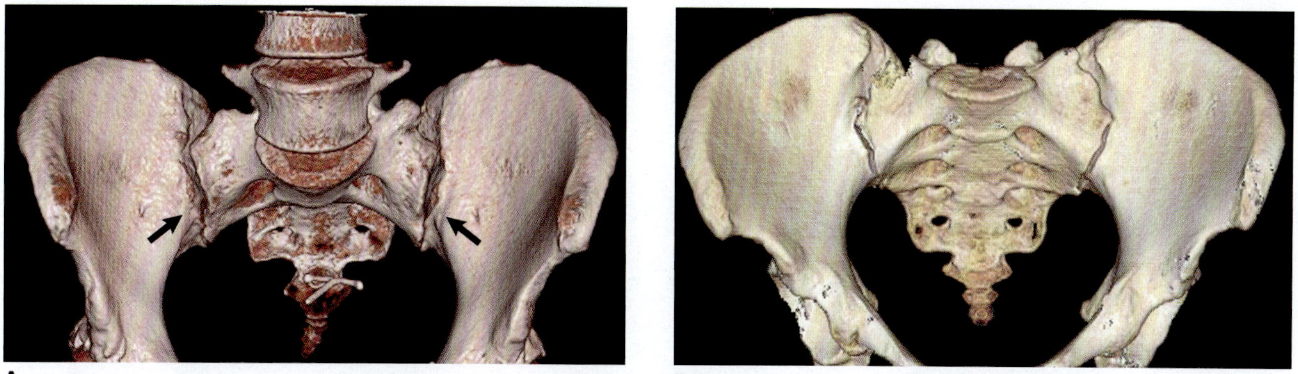

A B

Figure 6.97 ■ **3D CT of sacroiliitis in psoriatic arthritis. A:** Three-dimensional reconstructed CT image of the pelvis of a 38-year-old woman shows early subtle erosions of synovial portion of both sacroiliac joints (*arrows*). **B:** 3D CT of normal sacroiliac joints is shown for comparison.

dramatically improved the outcome of the disease. Biologic inhibitors of TNF including etanercept, adalimumab, certolizumab, infliximab, and golimumab decrease the symptoms of articular and skin manifestations of psoriasis. However, there are many other new drugs introduced to treat both psoriasis and psoriatic arthritis; therefore, the reader is referred to recent reviews in the literature on this important subject.

ENTEROPATHIC ARTHROPATHIES

This group, probably of autoimmune etiology, comprises arthritides associated with inflammatory intestinal diseases such as ulcerative colitis, regional enteritis (Crohn disease), and intestinal lipodystrophy (Whipple disease), the last of which predominantly affects men in their fourth and fifth

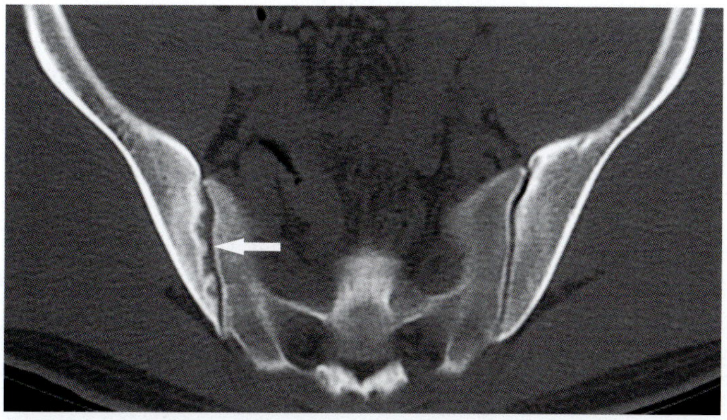

A

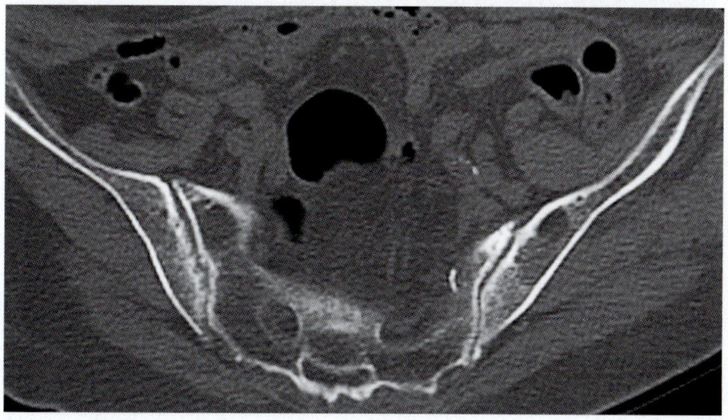

B

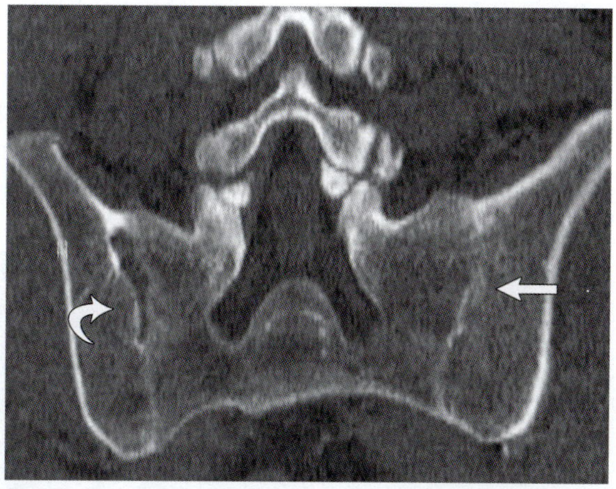

C

Figure 6.98 ■ **Sacroiliitis in psoriatic arthritis. A:** Axial CT section through the sacroiliac joints of a 28-year-old man with clinical diagnosis of psoriasis shows unilateral involvement of the right sacroiliac joint (*arrow*). **B:** Axial CT image of sacroiliac joints of a 61-year-old woman with psoriatic arthritis and bilateral sacroiliitis demonstrates asymmetric involvement. **C:** Coronal CT image of sacroiliac joints of a 70-year-old man shows complete fusion of the left (*arrow*) and incomplete fusion of the right (*curved arrow*) SI joint.

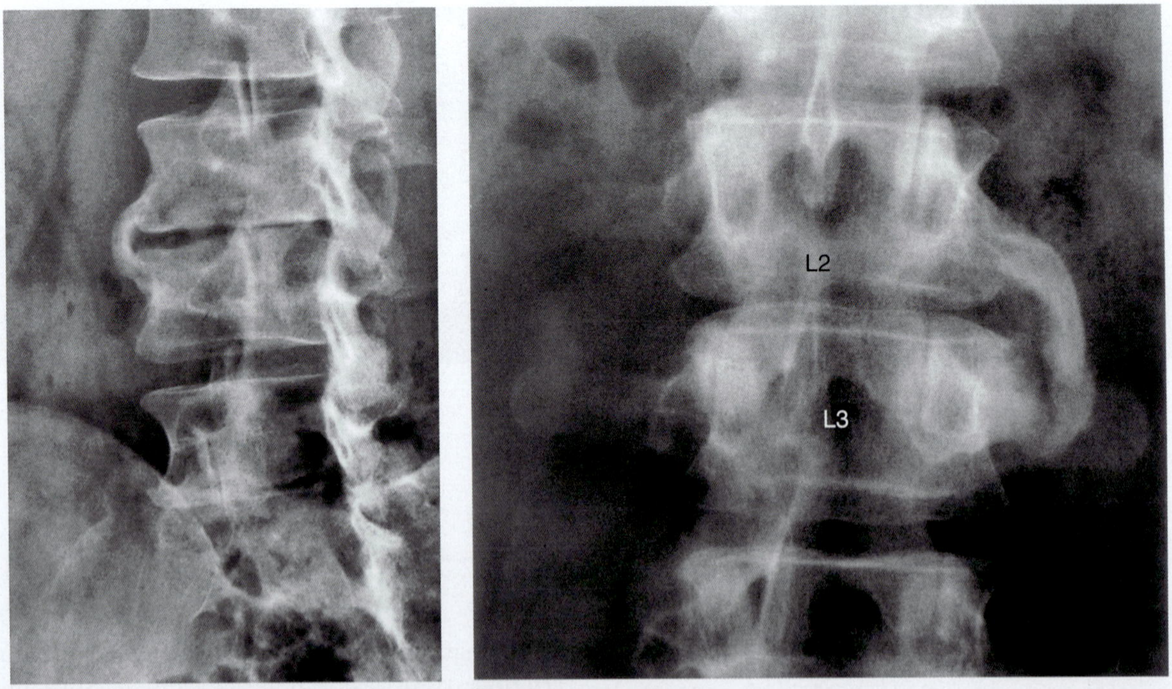

A B

Figure 6.99 ■ Spinal abnormalities in psoriatic arthritis. A: Oblique radiograph of the lumbar spine in a 30-year-old man with psoriasis shows a characteristic single coarse syndesmophyte bridging the bodies of L3 and L4. The right sacroiliac joint is also affected. **B:** Anteroposterior radiograph of the lumbar spine in a 45-year-old man with psoriasis reveals paraspinal ossification at the level of L2–L3.

decades. The histocompatibility antigen HLA-B27 is present in most patients with enteropathic abnormalities. In all three conditions, the spine, the sacroiliac joints, and peripheral joints may be affected. In the spine, squaring of the vertebral bodies and the formation of syndesmophytes, similar to the features of ankylosing spondylitis, are common imaging findings. Sacroiliitis, which is usually bilateral and symmetric, is radiographically indistinguishable from ankylosing spondylitis (Fig. 6.102). The severity of the spondylitis and sacroiliitis progresses independently of the course of the bowel disease or treatment of the primary intestinal problem. In addition, patients may also exhibit a peripheral arthritis, involving the knees, ankles, elbows, and wrists, usually in a bilateral and symmetric fashion, the activity of which generally approximates the activity of the bowel disease.

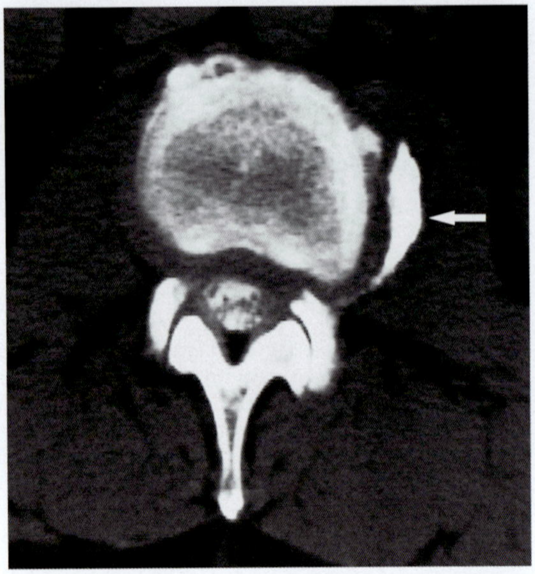

Figure 6.100 ■ Spinal abnormalities in psoriatic arthritis. A postmyelographic axial CT section of the lumbar spine shows a paraspinal ossification (*arrow*) in a 48-year-old man with psoriasis.

Finally, it should be noted that arthritis may follow intestinal bypass procedures. The synovitis is polyarticular and symmetric, but radiographically the lesions are nonerosive.

UNDIFFERENTIATED SPONDYLOARTHRITIS (USPA)

The term undifferentiated spondyloarthritis is applied to patients exhibiting increased HLA-B27 positivity, and who also have peripheral arthritis, sacroiliitis, and/or enthesitis, but who lack of clinical or imaging features allowing further subclassification. A subset of patients with this designation may progress to ankylosing spondylitis or psoriatic arthritis, but it is not clear which clinical or laboratory features may be predictive of such progression. According to Taurog et al., the concept of undifferentiated spondyloarthritis is becoming gradually subsumed under the general rubric of axial and peripheral spondyloarthropathy.

(Continued on page 263)

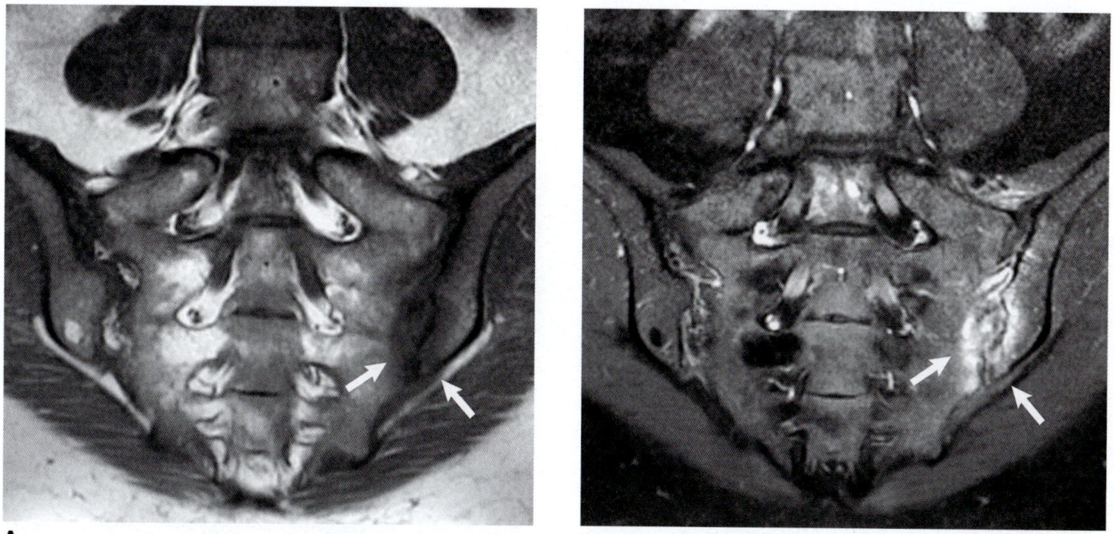

A B

Figure 6.101 ■ **MRI of sacroiliitis in psoriatic arthritis.** Coronal T1-weighted **(A)** and coronal T1-weighted fat-suppressed **(B)** MR image obtained after intravenous administration of gadolinium shows left sacroiliitis (*arrows*) in a 40-year-old woman.

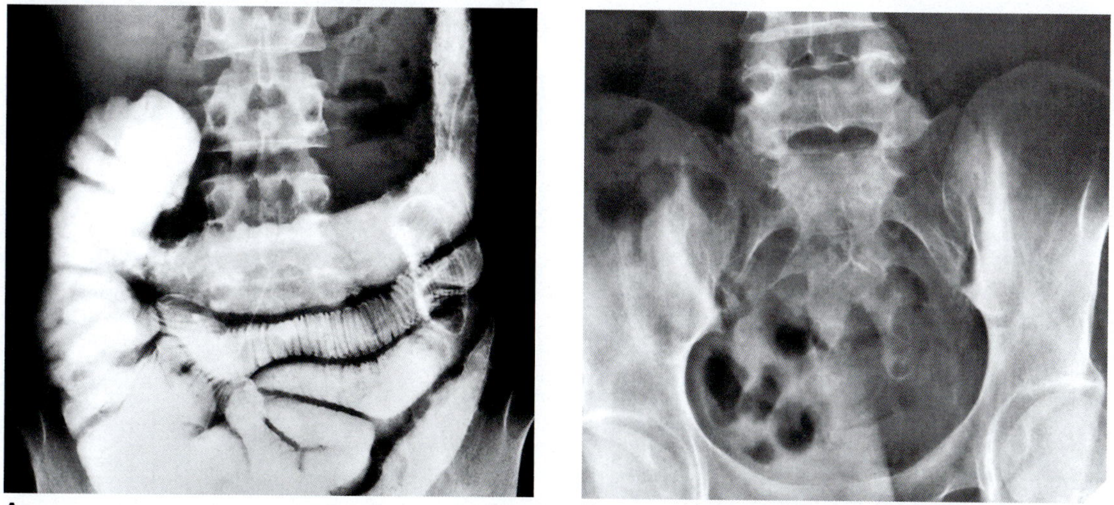

A B

Figure 6.102 ■ **Ulcerative colitis complicated by sacroiliitis.** A 20-year-old woman with known ulcerative colitis developed severe low back pain localized to the sacroiliac joints. **A:** Barium enema study shows extensive involvement of the transverse and descending colon, consistent with ulcerative colitis. **B:** Posteroanterior radiograph of the pelvis shows symmetric, bilateral sacroiliitis similar to that seen in ankylosing spondylitis.

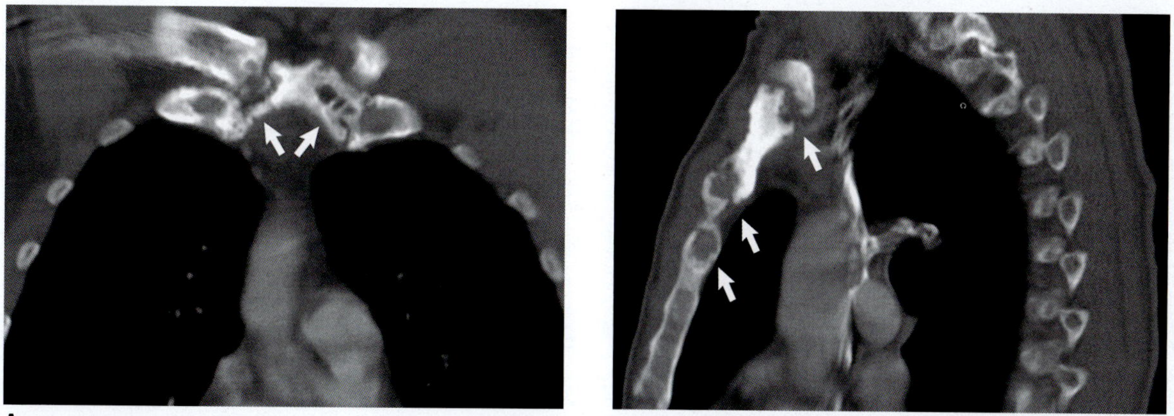

A B

Figure 6.103 ■ **SAPHO syndrome.** A 49-year-old man presented with pustulosis on his palms and soles and anterior chest wall pain. **A:** Coronal reformatted CT image of the sternum shows sclerotic changes and erosions of the sternoclavicular and costosternal joints (*arrows*). **B:** Sagittal reformatted CT image in addition shows osteolytic foci in the sternum (*arrows*).

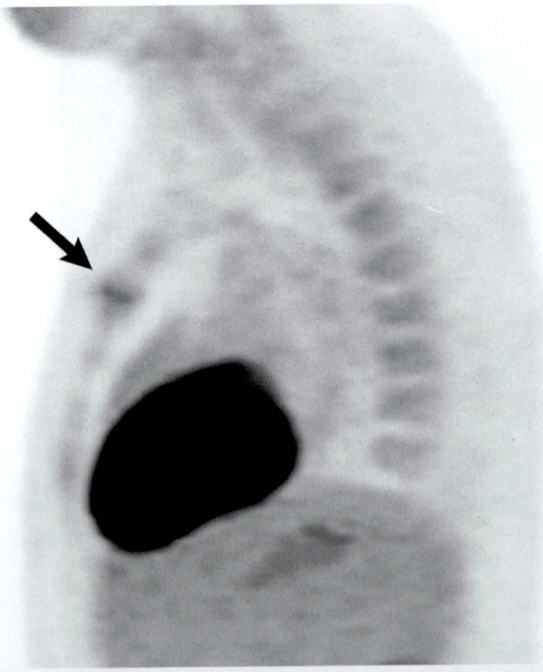

A

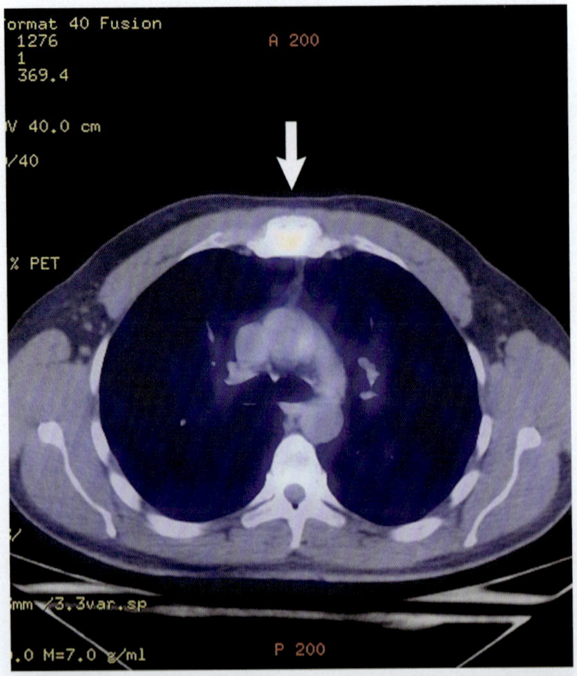

B

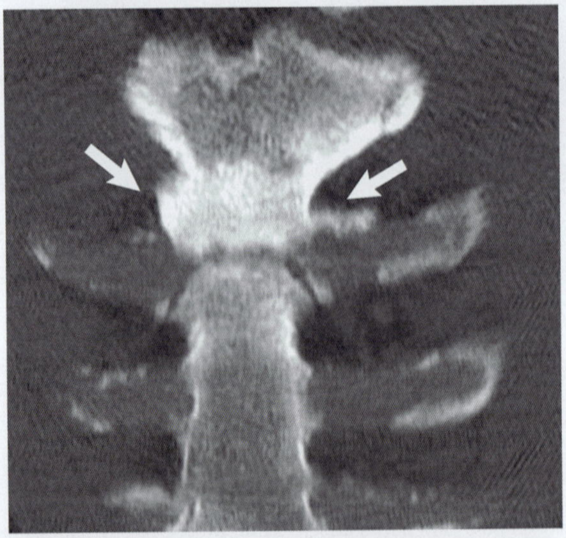

C

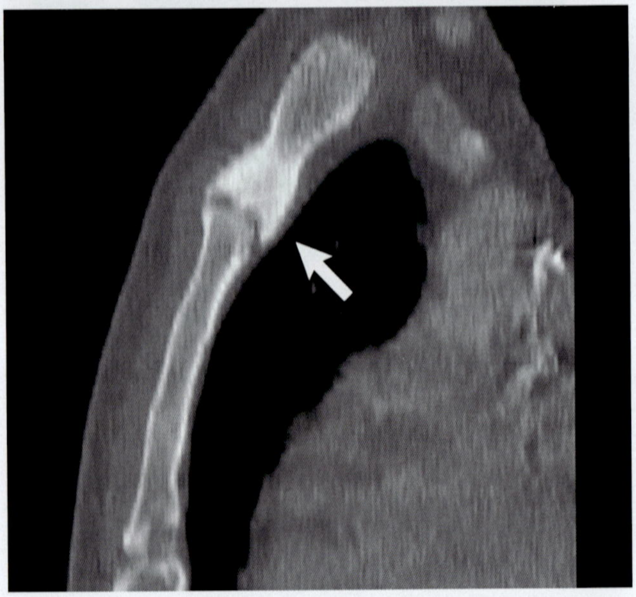

D

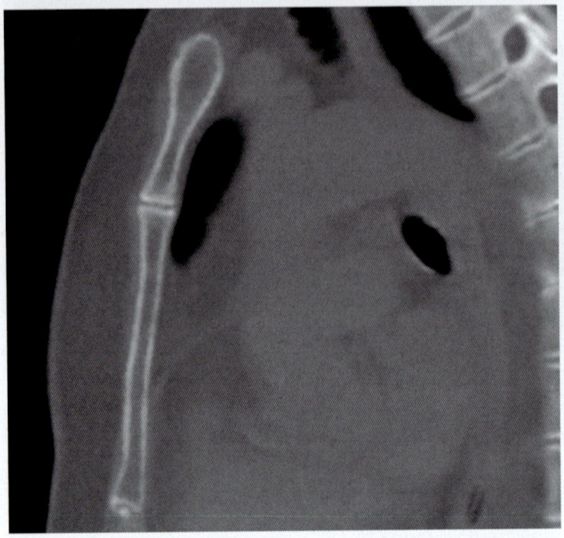

E

Figure 6.104 ■ **SAPHO syndrome.** 18F-FDG PET **(A)** and axial fused PET/CT **(B)** images of the upper thorax of a 52-year-old man show increased metabolic activity in the sternum (*arrows*). Coronal **(C)** and sagittal reformatted **(D)** CT images of the sternum show hyperostotic and sclerotic changes at the manubriosternal joint (*arrows*). **E:** Sagittal reformatted CT image of a normal manubriosternal joint is shown for comparison.

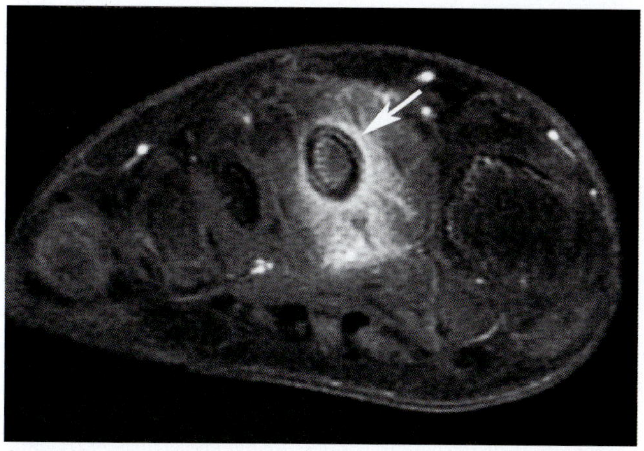

A

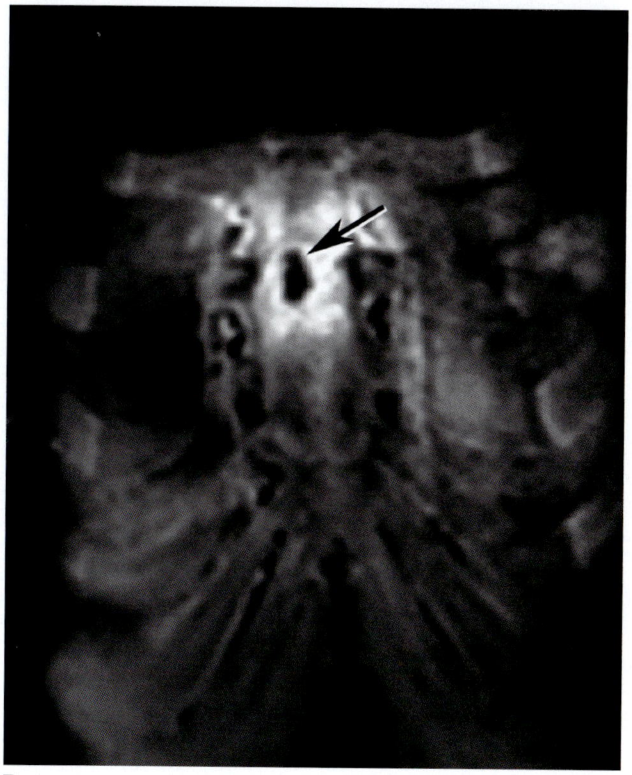

B

Figure 6.105 ■ MRI of chronic recurrent multifocal osteomyelitis. A 12-year-old girl presented with history of chronic foot pain and anterior chest wall pain. **A:** Short-axis T2-weighted fat-suppressed MR image of the forefoot shows signal alteration of the second metatarsal bone associated with periosteal reaction (*arrow*) and surrounding soft tissue edema. **B:** Coronal T1-weighted fat-suppressed MR image of the sternum obtained after intravenous administration of gadolinium shows a focal area of low signal intensity in the body of the sternum (*arrow*) surrounded by enhancing edema.

SAPHO SYNDROME

In 1987, Chomot and collaborators coined the acronym SAPHO (***s***ynovitis, ***a***cne, ***p***ustulosis, ***h***yperostosis, ***o***steitis) for a group of patients with pustular acne (palmoplantar pustulosis) and hyperostotic inflammation of bone. Some investigators link SAPHO syndrome with seronegative spondyloarthropathies, because significant number of patients with this condition fulfill the accepted criteria for spondyloarthropathy. However, not all of the individuals affected with this disorder have the genetic predisposition found in the patients with the other seronegative spondyloarthropathies discussed in the text above. Specifically, only some patients with this syndrome tested positive for human leukocyte antigen HLA-B27. SAPHO, whose etiology is still not known, affects patients in any age, more commonly women than men. The most common site of involvement is the sternoclavicular, manubriosternal, and costosternal joints. Imaging findings include osteosclerosis, hyperostosis, cortical thickening, and narrowing of the medullary canal, with external surface of bone appearing sometimes expanded, indistinct, or irregular (Figs. 6.103 and 6.104). Articular manifestations become apparent some time after the onset of skin lesions. Cutaneous manifestations include palmoplantar pustulosis, severe forms of acne (acne fulminans or conglobata, hidradenitis suppurativa), and various forms of psoriatic-like skin lesions. The treatment with antibiotics (clindamycin) and nonsteroidal anti-inflammatory drugs (lornoxicam) proved to be very effective in rapid symptoms resolution. Recent clinical trials suggested that pamidronate might be an effective drug for this condition.

Some researchers combine SAPHO together with chronic recurrent multifocal osteomyelitis (CRMO), an acute inflammatory multifocal process affecting more than one bone, occurring mostly in children and adolescents, with clinical and imaging manifestations similar to osteomyelitis (Fig. 6.105), but without infection and lack of known pathogen. Giedion et al. described this entity in 1972, and some authors contended that CRMO is in fact the pediatric presentation of SAPHO. Yet, there are also many investigators who believe that these are two separate entities with the different localization of inflammation: in pediatric CRMO, the extremities are more often affected, whereas in SAPHO, the axial skeleton, and particularly the costosternoclavicular region, is the focus of abnormalities. Moreover, CRMO is now considered to be an inherited autoinflammatory disease caused by immune dysregulation, without autoantibodies or antigen-specific T cells. Some investigators suggested a link between CRMO and a rare allele of marker D18S60, resulting in a haplotype relative risk (HRR) of chromosome 18 (18q21.3-18q22).

SUGGESTED READINGS

Adam G, Dammer M, Bohndorf K, et al. Rheumatoid arthritis of the knee: value of gadopentetate dimeglumine-enhanced MR imaging. *Am J Roentgenol.* 1991;156:125–129.

Agten CA, Zubler V, Rosskopf AB, et al. Enthesitis of lumbar spine ligaments in clinically suspected spondyloarthritis: value of gadolinium-enhanced MR images in comparison to STIR. *Skeletal Radiol.* 2016;45:187–195.

Aletaha D, Neogi T, Silman AJ, et al. 2010 Rheumatoid arthritis classification criteria. An American College of Rheumatology/European League Against Rheumatism Collaborative Initiative. *Arthritis Rheum.* 2010;62:2569–2581.

Algin O, Gokalp G, Baran B, et al. Evaluation of sacroiliitis: contrast-enhanced MRI with subtraction technique. *Skeletal Radiol.* 2009;38:983–988.

Amital H, Applbaum YH, Aamar S, et al. SAPHO syndrome treated with pamidronate: an open-label study of 10 patients. *Rheumatology (Oxford).* 2004;43:658–661.

Andonopoulos AP, Yarmentis S, Sfountouris H, et al. Baker's cyst in rheumatoid arthritis: an ultrasonographic study with a high resolution technique. *Clin Exp Rheumatol.* 1995;13:633–636.

Ansell BM, Wigley RA. Arthritic manifestations in regional enteritis. *Ann Rheum Dis.* 1964;23:64–72.

Arnett FC, Bias WB, Stevens MB. Juvenile-onset chronic arthritis. Clinical and roentgenographic features of a unique HLA-B27 subset. *Am J Med.* 1980;69:369–376.

Arnett FC, Edworthy SM, Bloch DA, et al. The American Rheumatism Association 1987 revised criteria for the classification of rheumatoid arthritis. *Arthritis Rheum.* 1988;31:315–324.

Ash Z, Marzo-Ortega H. Ankylosing spondylitis—the changing role of imaging. *Skeletal Radiol.* 2012;41:1031–1034.

Athreya BH. Is macrophage activation syndrome a new entity? *Clin Exp Rheumatol.* 2002;20:121–123.

Azouz EM, Duffy CM. Juvenile spondyloarthropathies: clinical manifestations and medical imaging. *Skeletal Radiol.* 1995;24:399–408.

Bakewell C, Dugowson C. Baker's cyst in a patient with rheumatoid arthritis. *N Engl J Med.* 2009;361:1098.

Bas S, Perneger TV, Seitz M, et al. Diagnostic tests for rheumatoid arthritis: comparison of anti-cyclic citrullinated peptide antibodies, anti-keratin antibodies and IgM rheumatoid factors. *Rheumatology.* 2002;41:809–814.

Behrens EM, Beukelman T, Paessler M, Cron RQ. Occult macrophage activation syndrome in patients with systemic juvenile idiopathic arthritis. *J Rheumatol.* 2007;34:1133–1138.

Belhorn LR, Hess EV. Erosive osteoarthritis. *Semin Arthritis Rheum.* 1993;22: 298–306.

Beresford MW. Juvenile idiopathic arthritis: new insights into classification, measures of outcome, and pharmacotherapy. *Paediatr Drugs.* 2011;13:161–173.

Björkengren AG, Geborek P, Rydholm U, et al. MR imaging of the knee in acute rheumatoid arthritis: synovial uptake of gadolinium-DOTA. *Am J Roentgenol.* 1990;155:329–332.

Björkengren AG, Pathria MN, Sartosis DJ, et al. Carpal alterations in adult-onset Still disease, juvenile chronic arthritis, and adult-onset rheumatoid arthritis: comparative study. *Radiology.* 1987;165:545–548.

Boden SD, Dodge LD, Bohlman HH, Rechtine GR. Rheumatoid arthritis of the cervical spine. *J Bone Joint Surg Am.* 1993;75A:1282–1297.

Bollow M, Braun J, Biedermann T, et al. Use of contrast-enhanced MR imaging to detect sacroiliitis in children. *Skeletal Radiol.* 1998;27:606–616.

Bonel HM, Schneider P, Seemann MD, et al. MR imaging of the wrist in rheumatoid arthritis using gadobenate dimeglumine. *Skeletal Radiol.* 2001;30:15–24.

Boutin RD, Resnick D. The SAPHO syndrome: an evolving concept for unifying several idiopathic disorders of bone and skin. *Am J Roentgenol.* 1998;170:585–591.

Boutry N, Morel M, Flipo R-M, et al. Early rheumatoid arthritis: a review of MRI and sonographic findings. *Am J Roentgenol.* 2007;189:1502–1509.

Bozgeyik Z, Ozgocmen S, Kocakoc E. Role of diffusion-weighted MRI in the detection of early active sacroiliitis. *AJR Am J Roentgenol.* 2008;191:980–986.

Breton S, Jousse-Joulin S, Cangemi C, et al. Comparison of clinical and ultrasonographic evaluation for peripheral synovitis in juvenile idiopathic arthritis. *Semin Arthritis Rheum.* 2011;41:272–278.

Brower AC, Allman RM. Pencil pointing: a vascular pattern of deossification. *Radiographics.* 1983;3:315–325.

Brower AC, Kransdorf MJ. Evaluation of disorders of the sacroiliac joint. *Appl Radiol.* 1992:31–43.

Burgos-Vargas R. Juvenile ankylosing spondylitis. *Rheum Dis Clin North Am.* 1992;18:123–142.

Burgos-Vargas R, Vazquez-Mellado J. The early clinical recognition of juvenile-onset ankylosing spondylitis and its differentiation from juvenile rheumatoid arthritis. *Arthritis Rheum.* 1995;38:835–844.

Calabro JJ, Gordon RD, Miller KI. Bechterew's syndrome in children: diagnostic criteria. *Scand J Rheumatol.* 1980;32(suppl):45–48.

Canella C, Schau B, Ribeiro E, et al. MRI in seronegative spondyloarthritis: imaging features and differential diagnosis in the spine and sacroiliac joints. *Am J Roentgenol.* 2013;200:149–157.

Carmona R, Harish S, Linda DD, et al. MR imaging of the spine and sacroiliac joints for spondyloarthritis: influence on clinical diagnostic confidence and patient management. *Radiology.* 2013;269:208–215.

Cassidy JT, Levinson JE, Bass JC, et al. A study of classification criteria for a diagnosis of juvenile rheumatoid arthritis. *Arthritis Rheum.* 1986;29:274–281.

Cassidy JT, Petty RE. Spondyloarthropathies. In: Cassidy JT, Petty RE, eds. *Text Book of Pediatric Rheumatology.* 2nd ed. New York, NY: Churchill Livingstone; 1990:221–259.

Chamot A, Benhamou CI, Kahn MF, et al. Le syndrome acne pustulose hyperostose osteitis (SAPHO). *Rev Rheumatol.* 1987;43:187–196.

Chen TS, Crues JV III, Ali M, Troum OM. Magnetic resonance imaging is more sensitive than radiographs in detecting change in size of erosions in rheumatoid arthritis. *J Rheumatol.* 2006;33:1957–1967.

Choy E, Aletaha D, Behrens F, et al. Monotherapy with biologic disease-modifying anti-rheumatic drugs in rheumatoid arthritis. *Rheumatology (Oxford).* 2016:pii:kew271.

Chung C, Coley BD, Martin LC. Rice bodies in juvenile rheumatoid arthritis. *Am J Roentgenol.* 1998;170:698–700.

Coates LC, Conaghan PG, Emery P, et al. Sensitivity and specificity of the classification of psoriatic arthritis criteria in early psoriatic arthritis. *Arthritis Rheum.* 2012;64:3150–3155.

Coates LC, Hodgson R, Conaghan PG, Freston JE. MRI and ultrasonography for diagnosis and monitoring of psoriatic arthritis. *Best Pract Res Clin Rheumatol.* 2012;26:805–822.

Cobby M, Cushnaghan J, Creamer P, Dieppe P, Watt I. Erosive osteoarthritis: is it a separate disease entity? *Clin Radiol.* 1990;42:258–263.

Cohen PA, Job-Deslandre CH, Lalande G, Adamsbaum C. Overview of the radiology of juvenile idiopathic arthritis (JIA). *Eur J Radiol.* 2000;33:94–101.

Colebatch-Bourn AN, Edwards CJ, Collado P, et al. EULAR—PreS points to consider for the use of imaging in the diagnosis and management of juvenile idiopathic arthritis in clinical practice. *Ann Rheum Dis.* 2015;74:1946–1957.

Crain DC. Interphalangeal osteoarthritis characterized by painful, inflammatory episodes, resulting in deformity of the proximal and distal articulations. *JAMA.* 1961;175:1949–1953.

Dale K, Paus AC, Laires K. A radiographic classification in juvenile rheumatoid arthritis applied to the knee. *Eur Radiol.* 1994;4:27–32.

Davidson J. Juvenile idiopathic arthritis: a clinical overview. *Eur J Radiol.* 2000;33:128–134.

Dihlmann W. Current radiodiagnostic concept of ankylosing spondylitis. *Skeletal Radiol.* 1979;4:179–188.

Earwaker JWS, Cotton A. SAPHO syndrome or concept? Imaging findings. *Skeletal Radiol.* 2003;32:311–327.

Ehrlich GE. Inflammatory osteoarthritis. I. The clinical syndrome. *J Chronic Dis.* 1972;25:317–328.

Ehrlich GE. Inflammatory osteoarthritis. II. The superimposition of rheumatoid arthritis. *J Chronic Dis.* 1972;25:635–643.

Ehrlich GE. Osteoarthritis beginning with inflammation. Definitions and correlations. *JAMA.* 1975;232:157–159.

Ehrlich GE. Erosive osteoarthritis: presentation, clinical pearls, and therapy. *Curr Rheumatol Rep.* 2001;3:484–488.

Einig M, Higer HP, Meairs S, et al. Magnetic resonance imaging of the craniocervical junction in rheumatoid arthritis: value, limitations, indications. *Skeletal Radiol.* 1990;19:341–346.

El-Khoury GY, Larson RK, Kathol MH, et al. Seronegative and seropositive rheumatoid arthritis: radiographic differences. *Radiology.* 1988;168:517–520.

el-Noueam KI, Giuliano V, Schweitzer ME, O'Hara BJ. Rheumatoid nodules: MR/pathological correlation. *J Comput Assist Tomogr.* 1997;21:796–799.

Eustace S, DiMasi M, Adams J, et al. In vitro and in vivo spin echo diffusion imaging characteristics of synovial fluid: potential non-invasive differentiation of inflammatory and degenerative arthritis. *Skeletal Radiol.* 2000;29:320–323.

Farrant JM, Grainger AJ, O'Connor PJ. Advanced imaging in rheumatoid arthritis. Part 2: erosions. *Skeletal Radiol.* 2007;36:381–389.

Farrant JM, O'Connor PJ, Grainger AJ. Advanced imaging in rheumatoid arthritis. Part 1: synovitis. *Skeletal Radiol.* 2007;36:269–279.

Fezoulidis I, Neuhold A, Wicke L, et al. Diagnostic imaging of the occipitocervical junction in patients with rheumatoid arthritis. *Eur J Radiol.* 1989;9:5–11.

Filipovich HA. Hemophagocytic lymphohistiocytosis. *Immunol Allergy Clin North Am.* 2002;22:281–300.

Flato B, Lien G, Smerdel A, et al. Prognostic factors in juvenile rheumatoid arthritis: a case-controlled study revealing early predictors and outcome after 14.9 years. *J Rheumatol.* 2003;30:386–393.

Forrester DM. Imaging of the sacroiliac joints. *Radiol Clin North Am.* 1990;28:1055–1072.

Galvez J, Sola J, Ortuno G, et al. Microscopic rice bodies in rheumatoid synovial fluid sediments. *J Rheumatol.* 1992;19:1851–1858.

Garg N, van den Bosch F, Deodhar F. The concept of spondyloarthritis: where are we now? *Best Pract Res Clin Rheumatol.* 2014;28:663–672.

Gaspersic N, Sersa I, Jevtic V, et al. Monitoring ankylosing spondylitis therapy by dynamic contrast-enhanced and diffusion-weighted magnetic resonance imaging. *Skeletal Radiol.* 2008;37:123–131.

Giedion A, Holthusen W, Masel LF, Vischer D. Subacute and chronic "symmetrical" osteomyelitis. *Ann Radiol (Paris).* 1972;15:330–342.

Ginsberg MH, Genant HK, Yü TF, McCarty D. Rheumatoid nodulosis: an unusual variant of rheumatoid disease. *Arthritis Rheum.* 1975;18:49–58.

Giovagnoni A, Grassi W, Terilli F, et al. MRI of the hand in psoriatic and rheumatical arthritis. *Eur Radiol.* 1995;5:590–595.

Gold RH, Bassett LW, Theros EG. Radiologic comparison of erosive polyarthritides with prominent interphalangeal involvement. *Skeletal Radiol.* 1982;8:89–97.

Golla A, Jansson A, Ramser J, et al. Chronic recurrent multifocal osteomyelitis (CRMO): evidence for a susceptibility gene located on chromosome 18q21.3-18q22. *Eur J Hum Genet.* 2002;10:217–221.

Gordon DA, Hastings DE. Rheumatoid arthritis: clinical features—early, progressive and late disease. In: Klippel JH, Dieppe PA, eds. *Rheumatology*. St. Louis, MO: CV Mosby; 1994:3.4.1–3.4.14.

Gran JT, Husby G. The epidemiology of ankylosing spondylitis. *Semin Arthritis Rheum.* 1993;22:319–334.

Grassi W, De Angelis R, Lamanna G, Cervini C. The clinical features of rheumatoid arthritis. *Eur J Radiol.* 1998;27(suppl 1):S18–S24.

Graudal NA, Jurik AG, de Carvalho A, Graudal HK. Radiographic progression in rheumatoid arthritis: a long-term prospective study of 109 patients. *Arthritis Rheum.* 1998;41:1470–1480.

Greenspan A. Erosive osteoarthritis. *Semin Musculoskelet Radiol.* 2003;7:155–159.

Greenspan A, Baker ND, Norman A. Rheumatoid arthritis simulating other lesions. *Bull Hosp Jt Dis Orthop Inst.* 1983;43:70–77.

Gregersen PK, Silver J, Winchester RJ. The shared epitope hypothesis: an approach to understanding the molecular genetics of susceptibility to rheumatoid arthritis. *Arthritis Rheum.* 1987;30:1205–1213.

Grom AA. NK dysfunctions: a common pathway in systemic onset juvenile rheumatoid arthritis, macrophage activation syndrome, and hemophagocytic lymphohistiocytosis. *Arthritis Rheum.* 2004;50:689–698.

Guillemin F, Billot L, Boini S, et al. Reproducibility and sensitivity to change of 5 methods for scoring hand radiographic damage in patients with rheumatoid arthritis. *J Rheumatol.* 2005;32:778–786.

Gylys-Morin VM, Graham TB, Blebea JS, et al. Knee in early juvenile rheumatoid arthritis. MR imaging findings. *Radiology.* 2001;220:696–706.

Hafner R, Michels H. Psoriatic arthritis in children. *Curr Opin Rheumatol.* 1996;23:166–170.

Handly B, Moore M, Creutzberg G, et al. Bisphosphonate therapy for chronic recurrent multifocal osteomyelitis. *Skeletal Radiol.* 2013;42:1777–1778.

Hazlewood GS, Barnabe C, Tomlison G, et al. Methotrexate monotherapy and methotrexate combination therapy with traditional and biologic disease modifying anti-rheumatic drugs for rheumatoid arthritis: a network meta-analysis. *Cochrane Database Syst Rev.* 2016;(8):CD010227. Doi: 10. 1002/14651858.

Helliwell PS, Porter G; CASPAR Study Group. Sensitivity and specificity of plain radiographic features of peripheral enthesopathy at major sites in psoriatic arthritis. *Skeletal Radiol.* 2007;36:1061–1066.

Helliwell PS, Wright V. Clinical features of psoriatic arthritis. In: Klippel JH, Dieppe PA, eds. *Practical Rheumatology*. London, UK: Mosby; 1995:235–242.

Hermann K-GA, Bollow M. Magnetic resonance imaging of sacroiliitis in patients with spondyloarthritis: correlation with anatomy and histology. *Rofo.* 2014;186:230–237.

Herregods N, Jaremko JL, Baraliakos X, et al. Limited role of gadolinium to detect active sacroiliitis on MRI in juvenile spondyloarthritis. *Skeletal Radiol.* 2015;44:1637–1646.

Herve-Somma CMP, Sebag GH, Prieur AM, et al. Juvenile rheumatoid arthritis of the knee: MR evaluation with Gd-DOTA. *Radiology.* 1992;182:93–98.

Hodgson RJ, Barnes T, Connolly S., et al. Changes undergoing the dynamic contrast-enhanced MRI response to treatment in rheumatoid arthritis. *Skeletal Radiol.* 2008;37:201–207.

Holoshitz J. The rheumatoid arthritis HLA-DRB1 shared epitope. *Curr Opin Rheumatol.* 2010;22:293–298.

Hughes RJ, Saifuddin A. Progressive non-infectious anterior vertebral fusion (Copenhagen Syndrome) in three children: features on radiographs and MR imaging. *Skeletal Radiol.* 2006;35:397–401.

Jamieson TW, De Smet AA, Stechschulte DJ. Erosive arthropathy associated with scleromyxedema. *Skeletal Radiol.* 1985;14:286–290.

Jevtic V, Kos-Golja M, Rozman B, McCall I. Marginal erosive discovertebral "Romanus" lesions in ankylosing spondylitis demonstrated by contrast enhanced Gd-DTPA magnetic resonance imaging. *Skeletal Radiol.* 2000;29:27–33.

Jevtic V, Watt I, Rozman B, et al. Distinctive radiological features of small hand joints in rheumatoid arthritis and seronegative spondyloarthritis demonstrated by contrast-enhanced (Gd-DTPA) magnetic resonance imaging. *Skeletal Radiol.* 1995;24:351–355.

Johnson K. Imaging of juvenile idiopathic arthritis. *Pediatr Radiol.* 2006;36:743–758.

Kahn MF. Why the "SAPHO" syndrome? *J Rheumatol.* 1995; 22: 2017–2019.

Kamishima T, Tanimura K, Aoki Y, et al. Simplified approach to MR image quantification of the rheumatoid wrist: a pilot study. *Skeletal Radiol.* 2011;40:65–74.

Kamishima T, Tanimura K, Shimizu M, et al. Monitoring anti-interleukin 6 receptor antibody treatment for rheumatoid arthritis by quantitative magnetic resonance imaging of the hand and power Doppler ultrasonography of the finger. *Skeletal Radiol.* 2011;40:745–755.

Kapasi OA, Ruby LK, Calney K. The psoriatic hand. *J Hand Surg [Am].* 1982;7A: 492–497.

Kaye BR, Kaye RL, Bobrove A. Rheumatoid nodules. *Am J Med.* 1984;76:279–292.

Keat A. Reiter's syndrome and reactive arthritis in perspective. *N Engl J Med.* 1983;309:1606–1615.

Keats TE, Johnstone WH, O'Brien WM. Large joint destruction in erosive osteoarthritis. *Skeletal Radiol.* 1981;6:267–269.

Kellgren JH, Moore R. Generalized osteoarthritis and Heberden's nodes. *Br Med J.* 1952;1:181–187.

Kelly JJ III, Weisiger BB. The arthritis of Whipple's disease. *Arthritis Rheum.* 1963;25:615–632.

Kettering JM, Towers JD, Rubin DA. The seronegative spondyloarthropathies. *Semin Roentgenol.* 1996;31:220–228.

Khalkhali I, Stadalnik RC, Wiesner KB, Shapiro RF. Bone imaging of the heel in Reiter's syndrome. *Am J Roentgenol.* 1979;132:110–112.

Khan MA, van der Linden SM. A wider spectrum of spondyloarthropathies. *Semin Arthritis Rheum.* 1990;20:107–113.

Kim NR, Choi J-Y, Hong SH, et al. "MR corner sign": value for predicting presence of ankylosing spondylitis. *Am J Roentgenol.* 2008;191:124–128.

Klecker R, Weissman BN. Imaging features of psoriatic arthritis and Reiter's syndrome. *Semin Musculoskelet Radiol.* 2003;7:115–126.

Klenerman L. The foot and ankle in rheumatoid arthritis. *Br J Rheumatol.* 1995;34:443–448.

König H, Sieper J, Wolf K-J. Rheumatoid arthritis: evaluation of hypervascular and fibrous pannus with dynamic MR imaging enhanced with Gd-DTPA. *Radiology.* 1990;176:473–477.

Kredich D, Patrone NA. Pediatric spondyloarthropathies. *Clin Orthop Relat Res.* 1990;259:18–22.

Küster W, Lenz W. Morbus Crohn und Colitis ulcerosa. Häufigkeit, familiäres Vorkommen und Schwangerschaftsverlauf. *Ergeb Inn Med Kinderheilkd.* 1984;53: 103–132.

Lacout A, Rousselin B, Pelage J-P. CT and MRI of spine and sacroiliac involvement in spondyloarthropathy. *Am J Roentgenol.* 2008;191:1016–1023.

Larbi A, Viala P, Molinari N, et al. Assessment of MRI abnormalities of the sacroiliac joints and their ability to predict axial spondyloarthritis: a retrospective pilot study on 110 patients. *Skeletal Radiol.* 2014;43:351–358.

Laxer RM, Babyn P, Liu P, Silverman ED, Shore A. Magnetic resonance studies of the sacroiliac joints in children with HLA-B27 associated seronegative arthropathies. *J Rheumatol.* 1992;19(suppl 33):123.

Lee EY, Sundel RP, Kim S, et al. MRI findings of juvenile psoriatic arthritis. *Skeletal Radiol.* 2008;37:987–996.

Lopez-Ben R, Bernreuter WK, Moreland LW, Alarcon GS. Ultrasound detection of bone erosions in rheumatoid arthritis: a comparison to routine radiographs of the hands and feet. *Skeletal Radiol.* 2004;33:80–84.

Louie GH, Bingham III CO. Reactive arthritis. In: Imboden JB, Hellmann DB, Stone JH, eds. *Current Diagnosis & Treatment—Rheumatology.* 3rd ed. New York, NY: McGraw Hill; 2007:167–170.

Louie GH, Bingham CO III. Psoriatic arthritis. In: Imboden JB, Hellmann DB, Stone JH, eds. *Current Diagnosis & Treatment—Rheumatology.* 3rd ed. New York, NY: McGraw Hill; 2007:171–176.

Louvel JP, Duvey A, Da Silva F, et al. Computed tomography of sternoclavicular joint lesions in spondyloarthropathies. *Skeletal Radiol.* 1997;26:419–423.

Lund PJ, Heikal A, Maricic MJ, Krupinski EA, Williams CS. Ultrasonographic imaging of the hand and wrist in rheumatoid arthritis. *Skeletal Radiol.* 1995;24:591–596.

Magni-Manzoni S, Epis O, Ravelli A, et al. Comparison of clinical versus ultrasound-determined synovitis in juvenile idiopathic arthritis. *Arthritis Rheum.* 2009;61:1497–1504.

Maksymowych WP, Crowther SM, Dhillon SS, et al. Systemic assessment of inflammation by magnetic resonance imaging in the posterior elements of the spine in ankylosing spondylitis. *Arthritis Care Res.* 2010;62:4–10.

Mak W, Hunter JC. MRI of early diagnosis of inflammatory arthritis. *J Musculoskelet Med.* 2009;26:478–486.

Maksymowych WP, Crowther SM, Dhillon S, et al. Systematic assessment of inflammation by magnetic resonance imaging in the posterior elements of the spine in ankylosing spondylitis. *Arthritis Care Res.* 2010;62:4–10.

Malattia C, Damasio MB, Basso C, et al. Dynamic contrast-enhanced magnetic resonance imaging in the assessment of disease activity in patients with juvenile idiopathic arthritis. *Rheumatology (Oxford).* 2010;49:178–185.

Malattia C, Damasio MB, Magnaguagno F, et al. Magnetic resonance imaging, ultrasonography, and conventional radiography in assessment of bone erosions in juvenile idiopathic arthritis. *Arthritis Rheum.* 2008;59:1764–1772.

Manaster BJ. Arthritis. In: Manaster BJ, Dister DG, May DA, eds. *Musculoskeletal Imaging. The Requisites.* 2nd ed. St Louis, MO: Mosby; 2002:105–187.

Marshall H, Bromilow J, Thomas AL, Arden NK. Pamidronate: a novel treatment for SAPHO. *Rheumatology (Oxford).* 2002;41:231–233.

Martel W, Braunstein EM, Borlaza G, et al. Radiologic features of Reiter disease. *Radiology.* 1979;132:1–10.

Martel W, Snarr JW, Horn JR. Metacarpophalangeal joints in interphalangeal osteoarthritis. *Radiology.* 1973;108:1–7.

Martel W, Stuck KJ, Dworin AM, Hylland RG. Erosive osteoarthritis and psoriatic arthritis: a radiologic comparison in the hand, wrist, and foot. *Am J Roentgenol.* 1980;134:125–135.

Martini A. It is time to rethink juvenile idiopathic arthritis classification and nomenclature. *Ann Rheum Dis.* 2012;71:1437–1439.

Martini A, Lovell DJ. Juvenile idiopathic arthritis: state of the art and future perspectives. *Ann Rheum Dis.* 2010;69:1260–1263.

Matzaroglou C, Velissaris D, Karageorgos A, et al. SAPHO syndrome diagnosis and treatment: report of five cases and review of the literature. *Open Orthop J.* 2009;3:100–106.

McEwen C. Osteoarthritis of the fingers with ankylosis. *Arthritis Rheum.* 1968;11:734–744.

McGonagle D. The history of erosions in rheumatoid arthritis: are erosions history? *Arthritis Rheum.* 2010;62:312–315.

McQueen FM, Ostergaard M. Established rheumatoid arthritis—new imaging modalities. *Best Pract Res Clin Rheumatol.* 2007;21:841–856.

Moldofsky PJ, Dalinka MK. Multiple loose bodies in rheumatoid arthritis. *Skeletal Radiol.* 1979;4:219–222.

Moll JHM, Wright V. Psoriatic arthritis. *Semin Arthritis Rheum.* 1973;3: 55–78.

Mutlu H, Silit E, Pekkafali Z, et al. Multiple rice body formation in the subacromial-subdeltoid bursa and knee joint. *Skeletal Radiol.* 2004;33:531–533.

Nakahara N, Uetani M, Hayashi K, et al. Gadolinium-enhanced MR imaging of the wrist in rheumatoid arthritis: value of the fat suppression pulse sequences. *Skeletal Radiol.* 1996;25:639–647.

Nakayamada S, Kubo S, Iwata S, Tanaka Y. Recent progress in JAK inhibitors for the treatment of rheumatoid arthritis. *BioDrugs.* 2016;30: 407–419.

Navalho M, Resende C, Rodrigues AM, et al. Bilateral MR imaging of the hand and wrist in early and very early inflammatory arthritis: tenosynovitis is associated with progression to rheumatoid arthritis. *Radiology.* 2012;264:823–833.

Navallas M, Ares J, Beltran B, et al. Sacroiliitis associated with axial spondyloarthropathy: new concepts and latest trends. *Radiographics.* 2013;33: 933–956.

Navallas M, Inarejos EJ, Iglesias E, et al. MR imaging of the temporomandibular joint in juvenile idiopathic arthritis: technique and findings. *Radiographics.* 2017;37:595–612.

Niewold TB, Harrison MJ, Paget SA. Anti-CCP antibody testing as a diagnostic and prognostic tool in rheumatoid arthritis. *QJM.* 2007;100: 193–201.

Nikpoor N, Aliabadi P, Poss R, et al. Case report 504. Unusual bilateral calcified giant cysts (geodes) in rheumatoid arthritis. *Skeletal Radiol.* 1988;17:515–517.

Olejarova M, Kupka K, Pavelka K, et al. Comparison of clinical, laboratory, radiographic, and scintigraphic findings in erosive and nonerosive hand osteoarthritis. *Joint Bone Spine.* 2000;67:107–112.

Oloff-Solomon J, Oloff LM, Jacobs AM. Rheumatoid nodulosis in the foot: a variant of rheumatoid disease. *J Foot Surg.* 1984;23:382–385.

Oppenheimer DA, Jones HH. Hypertrophic osteoarthropathy of chronic inflammatory bowel disease. *Skeletal Radiol.* 1982;9:109–113.

Ostendorf B, Mattes-Gyorgy K, Reichelt DC, et al. Early detection of bony alterations in rheumatoid and erosive arthritis of finger joints with high-resolution single photon emission computed tomography, and differentiation between them. *Skeletal Radiol.* 2010;39:55–61.

Ostensen H, Pettersson H, Davies AM, eds. *The WHO Manual of Diagnostic Imaging.* Geneva, Switzerland: World Health Organization; 2002: 129–142.

Paimela L. The radiographic criterion in the 1987 revised criteria for rheumatoid arthritis. *Arthritis Rheum.* 1992;35:255–258.

Paparo F, Ravelli M, Semprini A, et al. Seronegative spondyloarthropathies: what radiologists should know. *Radiol Med.* 2014;119:156–163.

Patton JT. Differential diagnosis of inflammatory spondylitis. *Skeletal Radiol.* 1976;1:77–85.

Pattrick M, Manhire A, Ward AM, Doherty M. HLA-A, B antigens and α_1-antitrypsin phenotypes in nodal generalized osteoarthritis and erosive osteoarthritis. *Ann Rheum Dis.* 1989;48:470–475.

Peter JB, Pearson CM, Marmor L. Erosive osteoarthritis of the hands. *Arthritis Rheum.* 1966;9:365–388.

Petty RE, Southwood TR, Baum J, et al. Revision of the proposed classification criteria for juvenile idiopathic arthritis: Durban, 1997. *J Rheumatol.* 1998;25:1991–1994.

Petty RE, Southwood TR, Manners P, et al. International League of Associations for Rheumatology classification of juvenile idiopathic arthritis: second revision, Edmonton, 2001. *J Rheumatol.* 2004;31: 390–392.

Plaza M, Nowakowska-Plaza A, Pracon G, Sudol-Szopinska I. Role of ultrasonography in the diagnosis of rheumatic diseases in light of ACR/ EULAR guidelines. *J Ultrason.* 2016;16:55–64.

Plenge RM, Seielstad M, Padyukov L, et al. TRAF1-C5 as a risk locus for rheumatoid arthritis—a genomewide study. *N Engl J Med.* 2007;357: 1199–1209.

Poleksic L, Zdravkovic D, Jablanovic D, et al. Magnetic resonance imaging of bone destruction in rheumatoid arthritis: comparison with radiography. *Skeletal Radiol.* 1993:22:577–580.

Polster JM, Winalski CS, Sundaram M, et al. Rheumatoid arthritis: evaluation with contrast-enhanced CT with digital bone masking. *Radiology.* 2009;252:225–231.

Punzi L, Ramonda R, Deberg M, et al. Coll2-1, Coll2-1NO2, and myeloperoxidase serum levels in erosive and non-erosive osteoarthritis of the hands. *Osteoarthritis Cartilage.* 2012;20:557–561.

Qubti MA, Flynn JA. Ankylosing spondylitis & the arthritis of inflammatory bowel disease. In: Imboden JB, Hellmann DB, Stone JH, eds. *Current Diagnosis & Treatment—Rheumatology.* 3rd ed. New York, NY: McGrawHill; 2007:159–166.

Ravelli A, Martini A. Juvenile idiopathic arthritis. *LaEncet.* 2007;369:767–778.

Raychaudhuri SB, Deodhar A. The classification and diagnostic criteria of ankylosing spondylitis. *J Autoimmunity* 2014;48–49:128–133.

Reeder MM. *Reeder and Felson's Gamuts in Radiology.* 4th ed. New York: Springer; 2003.

Reijnierse M, Bloem JL, Dijkmans BAC, et al. The cervical spine in rheumatoid arthritis: relationship between neurologic signs and morphology on MR imaging and radiographs. *Skeletal Radiol.* 1996;25:113–118.

Reiter H. Ueber eine bisher unerkannte spirochaeteninfektion (spirochaetosis arthritica). *Dtsch Med Wochenschr.* 1916;42:1535–1536.

Resnick D. Erosive arthritis of the hand and wrist in hyperparathyroidism. *Radiology.* 1974;110:263–269.

Resnick D. Rheumatoid arthritis of the wrist: why the ulnar styloid? *Radiology.* 1974;112:29–35.

Resnick D. Common disorders of synovium-lined joints: pathogenesis, imaging abnormalities, and complications. *Am J Roentgenol.* 1988;151:1079–1093.

Resnick D, Niwayama G. Rheumatoid arthritis and the seronegative spondyloarthropathies: radiographic and pathologic concepts. In: Resnick D, ed. *Diagnosis of Bone and Joint Disorders.* 3rd ed. Philadelphia, PA: WB Saunders; 1995:807–865.

Reynolds H, Carter SW, Murtagh FR, et al. Cervical rheumatoid arthritis: value of flexion and extension views in imaging. *Radiology.* 1987;164:215–218.

Roberton DM, Cabral DA, Malleson PN, Petty RE. Juvenile psoriatic arthritis: follow up and evaluation of diagnostic criteria. *J Rheumatol.* 1996;23:166–170.

Roderick MR, Ramanan AV. Chronic recurrent multifocal osteomyelitis. *Adv Exp Med Biol.* 2013;764:99–107.

Rominger MB, Bernreuter WK, Kenney PJ, et al. MR imaging of the hands in early rheumatoid arthritis: preliminary results. *Radiographics.* 1993;13:37–46.

Rossi F, Di Dia F, Galipo O, et al. Use of the Sharp and Larsen scoring methods in the assessment of radiographic progression in juvenile idiopathic arthritis. *Arthritis Rheum.* 2006;55:717–723.

Rovetta G, Bianchi G, Monteforte P. Joint failure in erosive osteoarthritis of the hands. *Int J Tissue React.* 1995;17:33–42.

Rudwaleit M, Taylor WJ. Classification criteria for psoriatic arthritis and ankylosing spondylitis/axial spondyloarthritis. *Best Pract Res Clin Rheumatol.* 2010;24:589–604.

Rukavina I. SAPHO syndrome: a review. *J Child Orthop.* 2015;9:19–27.

Rundback JH, Rosenberg ZS, Solomon G. The radiographic features of rheumatoid arthritis in HLA-B27-positive patients. *Skeletal Radiol.* 1993;263–267.

Sanders KM, Resnik CS, Owen DS. Erosive arthritis in Cronkhite-Canada syndrome. *Radiology.* 1985;156:309–310.

Sankowski AJ, Lebkowska UM, Cwikla J, et al. Psoriatic arthritis. *Pol J Radiol.* 2013;78:1–17.

Sawhney S, Woo P, Murray KJ. Macrophage activation syndrome: a potentially fatal complication of rheumatic disorders. *Arch Dis Child.* 2001;85:421–426.

Scarpa R, Mathieu A. Psoriatic arthritis: evolving concepts. *Curr Opin Rheumatol.* 2000;12:274–280.

Schellekens G, Visser H, de Jong B, et al. The diagnostic properties of rheumatoid arthritis antibodies recognizing a cyclic citrullinated peptide. *Arthritis Rheum.* 2000;43:155–163.

Schoellnast H, Deutschmann HA, Hermann J, et al. Psoriatic arthritis and rheumatoid arthritis: findings in contrast-enhanced MRI. *AJR Am J Roentgenol.* 2006;187:351–357.

Schueller-Weidekamm C, Lodemann K-P, Grisar J, et al. Contrast-enhanced MR imaging of hand and finger joints in patients with early rheumatoid arthritis: do we really need a full dose of gadobenate dimeglumine for assessing synovial enhancement at 3T? *Radiology.* 2013;268: 161–169.

Schwenzer NF, Kotter I, Henes JC, et al. The role of dynamic contrast-enhanced MRI in the differential diagnosis of psoriatic and rheumatoid arthritis. *AJR Am J Roentgenol.* 2010;194:715–720.

Scott WW, Fishman EK, Kuhlman JE, et al. Computed tomography evaluation of the sacroiliac joints in Crohn disease. *Skeletal Radiol.* 1990;19:207–210.

Scott C, Meiorin S, Filocamo G, et al. A reappraisal of intra-articular corticosteroid therapy in juvenile idiopathic arthritis. *Clin Exp Rheumatol.* 2010;28:774–781.

Sheybani EF, Khanna G, White AJ, Demertzis JL. Imaging of juvenile idiopathic arthritis: a multimodality approach. *Radiographics.* 2013;33:1253–1273.

Smith D, Braunstein EM, Brandt KD, Katz BP. A radiographic comparison of erosive osteoarthritis and idiopathic nodal osteoarthritis. *J Rheumatol.* 1992;19:896–904.

Smukler NM, Edeiken J, Giuliano VJ. Ankylosis in osteoarthritis of the finger joints. *Radiology.* 1971;100:523–530.

Soldatos T, Pezeshk P, Ezzani F, et al. Cross-sectional imaging of adult crystal and inflammatory arthropathies. *Skeletal Radiol.* 2016;45: 1173–1191.

Sommer OJ, Kladosek A, Weiler V, et al. Rheumatoid arthritis: a practical guide to state-of-the-art imaging, image interpretation, and clinical implications. *Radiographics.* 2005;25:381–398.

Spira D, Kottar I, Henes J, et al. MRI findings in psoriatic arthritis of the hands. *Am J Roentgenol.* 2010;195:1187–1193.

Stadalnik RC, Dublin AB. Sesamoid periostitis in the thumb in Reiter's syndrome. *Am J Roentgenol.* 1961;86:344–350.

Stecher RM. Heberden's nodes. A clinical description of osteoarthritis in the finger joint. *Ann Rheum Dis.* 1955;14:1–10.

Stephan JL, Kone-Paut I, Galambrun C, et al. Reactive haemophagocytic syndrome in children with inflammatory disorders: a retrospective study of 24 patients. *Rheumatology (Oxford).* 2001;40:1285–1292.

Stewart NR, Crabbe JP, McQueen FM. Magnetic resonance imaging of the wrist in rheumatoid arthritis: demonstration of progression between 1 and 6 years. *Skeletal Radiol.* 2004;33:704–711.

Stiskal MA, Neuhold A, Szolar DH, et al. Rheumatoid arthritis of the craniocervical region by MR imaging: detection and characterization. *Am J Roentgenol.* 1995;165:585–592.

Sudol-Szopinska I, Grochowska E, Gietka P, et al. Imaging of juvenile idiopathic arthritis. Part II: ultrasonography and MRI. *J Ultrasound.* 2016;16:237–251.

Sudol-Szopinska I, Jans L, Teh J. Rheumathoid arthritis: what do MRI and ultrasound show. *J Ultrason.* 2017;17:5–16.

Sudol-Szopionska I, Jurik AG, Eshed I, et al. Recommendations of the ESSR Arthritis Subcommittee for the use of magnetic resonance imaging in musculoskeletal rheumatic diseases. *Semin Musculoskelet Radiol.* 2015;19:396–411.

Sudol-Szopinska I, Kwiatkowska B, Prochorec-Sobieszek M, et al. Enthesopathies and enthesitis. Part 2: imaging studies. *J Ultrasound.* 2015;15:196–207.

Sudol-Szopinska I, Matuszewska G, Gietka P, et al. Imaging of juvenile idiopathic arthritis. Part I: clinical classifications and radiographs. *J Ultrasound.* 2016;16:225–236.

Sudol-Szopinska I, Matuszewska G, Kwiatkowska B, Pracon G. Diagnostic imaging of psoriatic arthritis. Part I: etiopathogenesis, classification and radiographic features. *J Ultrasound.* 2016;16:65–77.

Sudol-Szopinska I, Pracon G. Diagnostic imaging of psoriatic arthritis. Part II: magnetic resonance imaging and ultrasonography. *J Ultrasound.* 2016;16:163–174.

Sundaram M, Patton JT. Paravertebral ossification in psoriasis and Reiter's disease. *Br J Radiol.* 1975;48:628–633.

Swett HA, Jaffe RB, McIff EB. Popliteal cysts: presentation as thrombophlebitis. *Radiology.* 1975;115:613–615.

Taurog JD, Chhabra A, Colbert RA. Ankylosing spondylitis and axial spondyloarthritis. *N Engl J Med.* 2016;374:2563–2574.

Taouli B, Zaim S, Peterfy CG, et al. Rheumatoid arthritis of the hand and wrist: comparison of three imaging techniques. *Am J Roentgenol.* 2004;182:937–943.

Tehranzadeh J, Ashikyan O, Anavim A, Shin J. Detailed analysis of contrast-enhanced MRI of hands and wrists in patients with psoriatic arthritis. *Skeletal Radiol.* 2008;37:433–442.

Tehranzadeh J, Ashikyan O, Dascalos J. Magnetic resonance imaging in early detection of rheumatoid arthritis. *Semin Musculoskelet Radiol.* 2003;7:79–94.

Tehranzadeh J, Ashikyan O, Dascalos J, Dennehey C. MRI of large intraosseous lesions in patients with inflammatory arthritis. *Am J Roentgenol.* 2004;183:1453–1463.

Thompson W, Donn R. Juvenile idiopathic arthritis genetics—What's new? What's next? *Arthritis Res.* 2002;4:302–306.

Turesson C, Matteson EL. Genetics of rheumatoid arthritis. *Mayo Clin Proc.* 2006;81:94–101.

Turesson C, O'Fallon W, Crowson C, et al. Extra-articular disease manifestations in rheumatoid arthritis: incidence, trends and risk factors over 46 years. *Ann Rheum Dis.* 2003;62:722–727.

Uhl M, Allmann KH, Ihling C, et al. Cartilage destruction in small joints by rheumatoid arthritis: assessment of fat-suppressed three-dimensional gradient-echo MR pulse sequences in vitro. *Skeletal Radiol.* 1998;27: 677–682.

Ustinger PD, Resnick D, Shapiro RF, et al. Roentgenologic, immunologic and therapeutic study of erosive (inflammatory) osteoarthritis. *Arch Intern Med.* 1978;138:693–697.

Valeri G, Ferrara C, Ercolani P, et al. Tendon involvement in rheumatoid arthritis of the wrist: MRI findings. *Skeletal Radiol.* 2001;30:138–143.

Van der Kooij SM, Allaart CF, Dijkmans BA, Breedveld FC. Innovative treatment strategies for patients with rheumatoid arthritis. *Curr Opin Rheumatol.* 2008;20: 287–294.

Van der Woude D, Rantapaa-Dahlqvist S, Ioan-Fascinay A, et al. Epitope spreading of the anti-citrullinated protein antibody response occurs before disease onset and is associated with the disease course of early arthritis. *Ann Rheum Dis.* 2010;69:54–60.

Villeneuve E, Emery P. Rheumatoid arthritis: what has changed? *Skeletal Radiol.* 2009;38:109–112.

Vinson EN, Major NM. MR imaging of ankylosing spondylitis. *Semin Musculoskelat Radiol.* 2003;7:103–113.

Yang H, Rivoire J, Hoppe M, et al. Computer-added and manual quantification of MRI synovitis, bone marrow edema-like lesions, erosion and cartilage loss in rheumatoid arthritis of the wrist. *Skeletal Radiol.* 2015;44:539–547.

Yu W, Feng F, Dion E, et al. Comparison of radiography, computed tomography and magnetic resonance imaging in the detection of sacroiliitis accompanying ankylosing spondylitis. *Skeletal Radiol.* 1998;27: 311–320.

Wamser G, Bohndorf K, Vollert K, et al. Power Doppler sonography with and without echo-enhancing contrast agent and contrast-enhanced MRI for evaluation of rheumatoid arthritis of the shoulder joint: differentiation between synovitis and joint effusion. *Skeletal Radiol.* 2003;32:351–359.

Weber U, Ostergaard M, Lambert RGW, Maksymowych WP. The impact of MRI on the clinical management of inflammatory arthritides. *Skeletal Radiol.* 2011;40:1153–1173.

Weishoupt D, Schweitzer ME, Alam F, et al. MR imaging of inflammatory joint diseases of the foot and ankle. *Skeletal Radiol.* 1999;28:663–669.

Weissman BN. Imaging techniques in rheumatoid arthritis. *J Rheumatol Suppl.* 1994;42:14–19.

Whitehouse RW, Aslam R, Bukhari M, et al. The sesamoid index in psoriatic arthropathy. *Skeletal Radiol.* 2005;34:217–220.

Wisnieski JJ, Askari AD. Rheumatoid nodulosis. A relatively benign rheumatoid variant. *Arch Intern Med.* 1981;141:615–619.

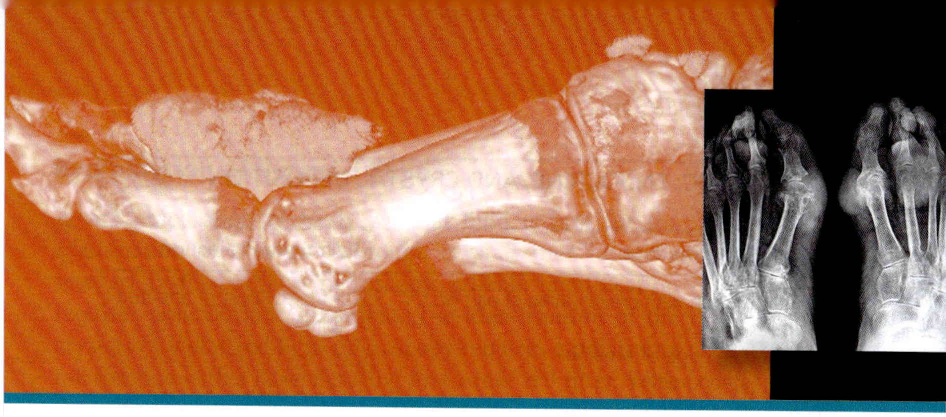

CHAPTER 7

Metabolic, Endocrine, and Crystal Deposition Arthropathies

An overview of the clinical and imaging hallmarks of the arthropathies associated with metabolic, endocrine, and crystal deposition abnormalities is shown in Table 7.1.

GOUT

Clinical Features

Gout is a metabolic disorder of purine metabolism characterized by recurrent episodes of acute arthritis associated with the presence of monosodium urate monohydrate crystals in the synovial fluid leukocytes and, in many cases, gross deposits of sodium urate (tophi) in periarticular soft tissues. Tophi, a pathognomonic feature of gout, typically form on pressure points in and around the inflamed joints. Serum uric acid concentrations are elevated; however, hyperuricemia does not necessarily lead to gout, and patients with gout may occasionally present with normal serum uric acid levels. Crystal deposits cause acute inflammation of the articular and paraarticular soft tissues, whereas recurrent acute intermittent flares can result in chronic gouty arthritis leading to cartilage and bone destruction.

Gouty arthritis accounts for ~5% of all arthritides. Four stages of the disease have been recognized: asymptomatic hyperuricemia, acute gouty arthritis, intercritical gout, and chronic tophaceous gout. Articular manifestations occur in the different stages of the disease. Ninety percent of the first gout attacks are monoarticular. The great toe is the most common site of involvement in gouty arthritis; the condition known as *podagra*, which involves the first metatarsophalangeal joint, occurs in ~75% of patients. Other frequently affected sites include the ankles, knees, hands, wrists, and elbows. Most patients are men, showing the higher prevalence after the age of 65 years, but gouty arthritis is seen in postmenopausal women as well (men-to-women ratio being 20:1). Recent data from genome-wide association studies (GWAS) show that genetic variants of SLC2A9/GLUT9 were associated with lower serum uric acid levels, and the values were higher among women, and, conversely, genetic variants of protein ABCG2 were associated with higher serum uric acid levels, and the values were higher among men. These studies point to GLUT9 and ABCG2 as being important modulators of uric acid levels and playing important role in the risk of gout.

Hyperuricemia

Uric acid is the end product of catabolism of purine, a component of nucleic acid (DNA and RNA), and because humans lack the enzyme uricase, increased synthesis of uric acid or decreased secretion of uric acid by the kidneys leads to hyperuricemia. In another way, an increased miscible pool of uric acid with resulting hyperuricemia can occur only in two principal ways: first, urate is produced in such large quantities that, even though excretion routes are of normal capacity, they are inadequate to handle the excessive load; second, the capacity for uric acid excretion is critically reduced so that even a normal quantity of uric acid cannot be eliminated.

In 25% to 30% of gouty patients, a primary defect in the rate of purine synthesis causes excessive uric acid

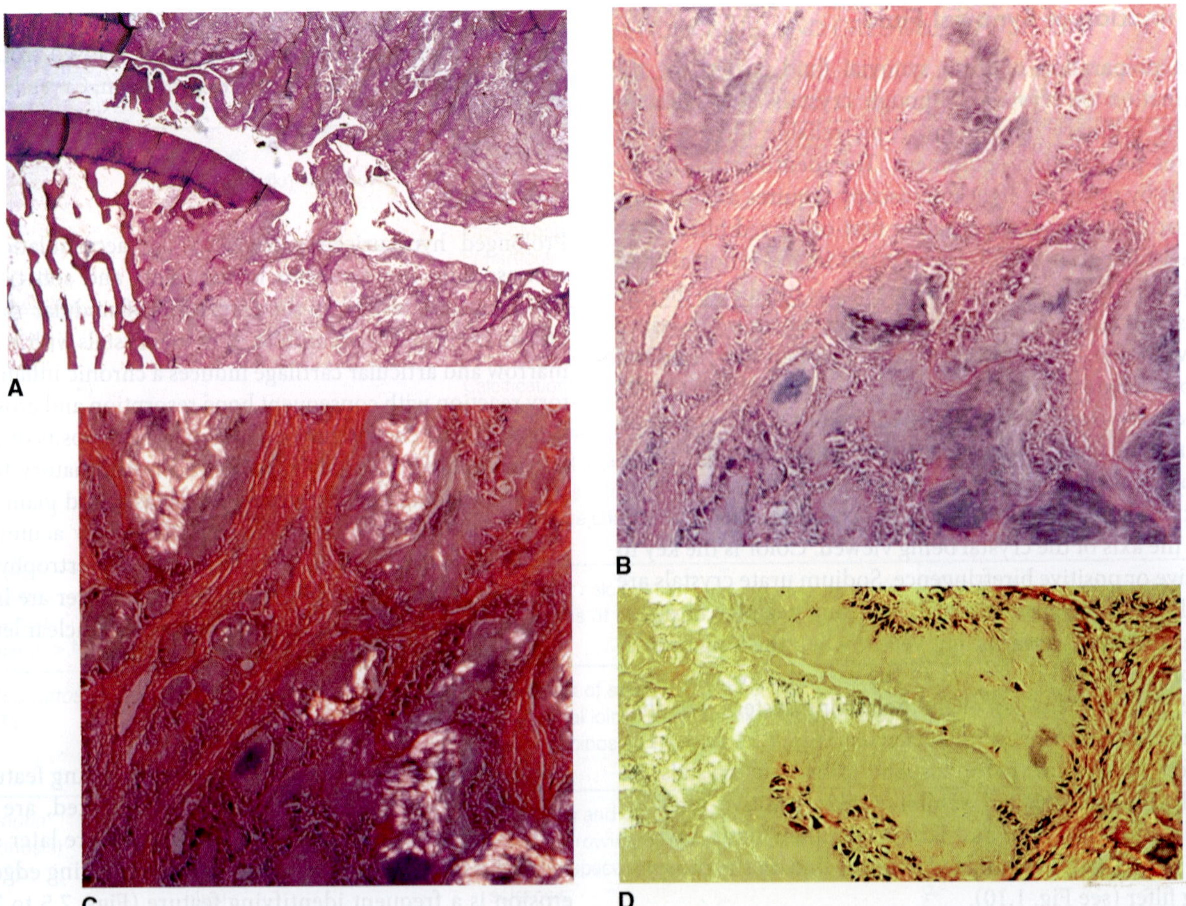

Figure 7.2 ■ **Histopathology of gouty arthritis. A:** Low-power photomicrograph of a portion of the joint shown in Figure 7.1 depicts the erosion of the bone and articular cartilage by an amorphous material (H&E, original magnification ×2.5). **B:** On slightly higher magnification observe bluish amorphous material surrounded by bundles of dense collagenized tissue and inflammatory cells (H&E, original magnification ×4). **C:** Same field examined by polarized light demonstrates the birefringence of the crystalline material (H&E, polarize light, original magnification ×4). **D:** On the higher magnification, note a thin layer of mononuclear and giant cells surrounding the amorphous crystalline deposit, with an occasional sprinkling of chronic inflammatory cells (H&E, polarized light, original magnification ×25). (From Bullough PG. *Atlas of Orthopedic Pathology with Clinical and Radiologic Correlation*. 2nd ed. New York, NY: Gower Medical Publishing; 1992, Figs. 11.37, 11.38, and 11.39.)

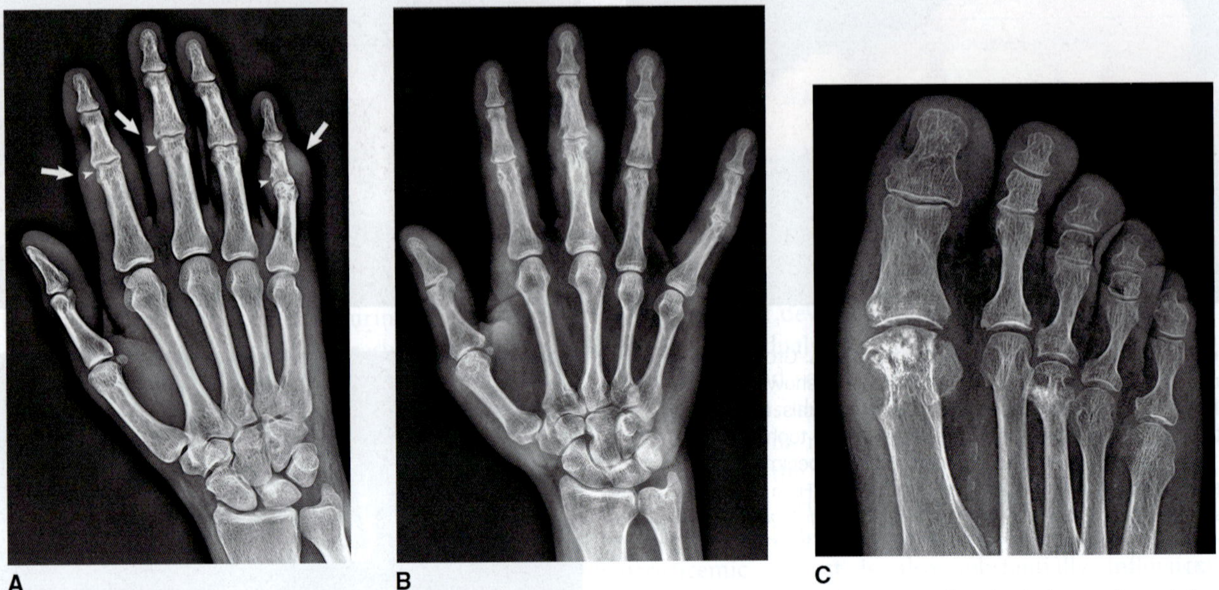

Figure 7.3 ■ **Gouty arthritis. A:** Dorsovolar radiograph of the left hand of a 55-year-old man shows small periarticular erosions at the proximal interphalangeal joints of the index, middle, and small fingers (*arrowheads*) with associated soft tissue tophi (*arrows*). **B:** Dorsovolar radiograph of the left hand of a 51-year-old man shows small periarticular erosions at the proximal interphalangeal joints of the index, middle, and small fingers and at the first metacarpophalangeal joint with associated soft tissue tophi. **C:** Dorsoplantar radiograph of the left forefoot of a 68-year-old man shows periarticular erosions of the first, second, and third metatarsal heads, as well as at the bases of the proximal phalanges of the great, second, and third toes. Note preservation of the joint spaces.

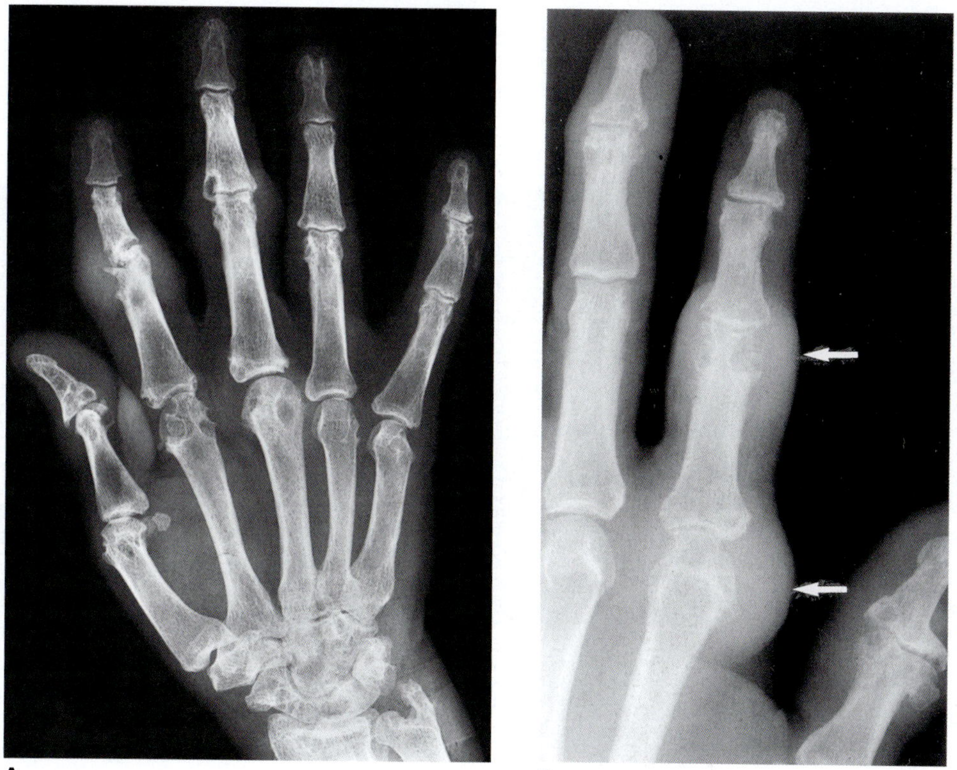

A B

Figure 7.4 ■ **Gouty arthritis. A:** Dorsovolar radiograph of the left hand of a 43-year-old man with tophaceous gout shows multiple sharply marginated articular and periarticular erosions and soft tissue masses at the proximal interphalangeal joints of the index and middle fingers, representing tophi. **B:** Dorsovolar radiograph of the fingers of a 70-year-old man with gouty arthritis shows multiple articular and periarticular erosions associated with large tophi (*arrows*).

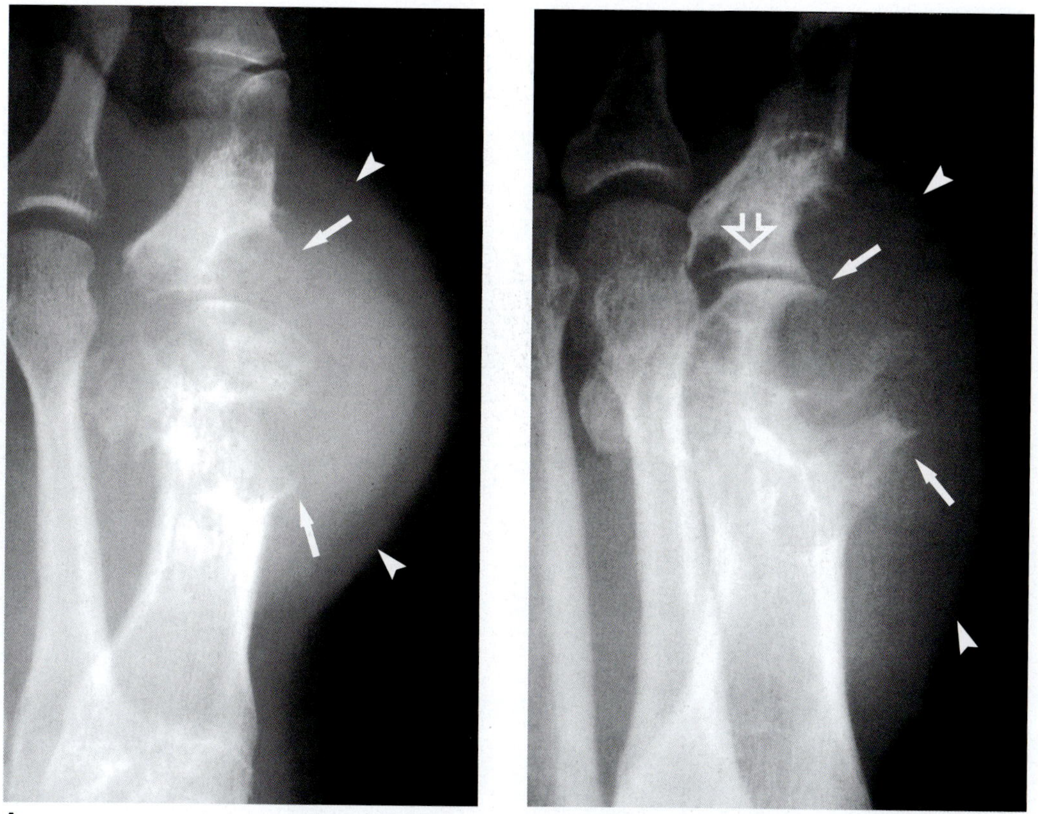

A B

Figure 7.5 ■ **Gouty arthritis.** Anteroposterior **(A)** and oblique **(B)** radiographs of the right great toe of a 58-year-old man with a 3-month history of gout shows the typical involvement of the first metatarsophalangeal joint. Note the characteristic "overhanging edge" of the erosive changes (*arrows*), preservation of the lateral portion of the joint (*open arrow*), and a large tophus (*arrowheads*).

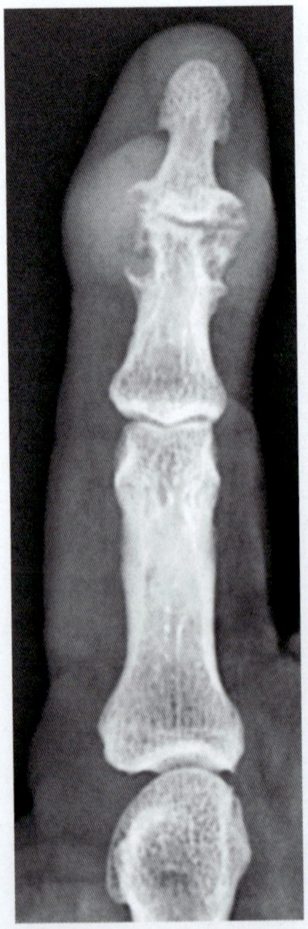

Figure 7.6 ■ Gouty arthritis. Typical para-articular erosions in the distal interphalangeal joint of the index finger exhibiting an "overhanging edge" are associated with a large tophus.

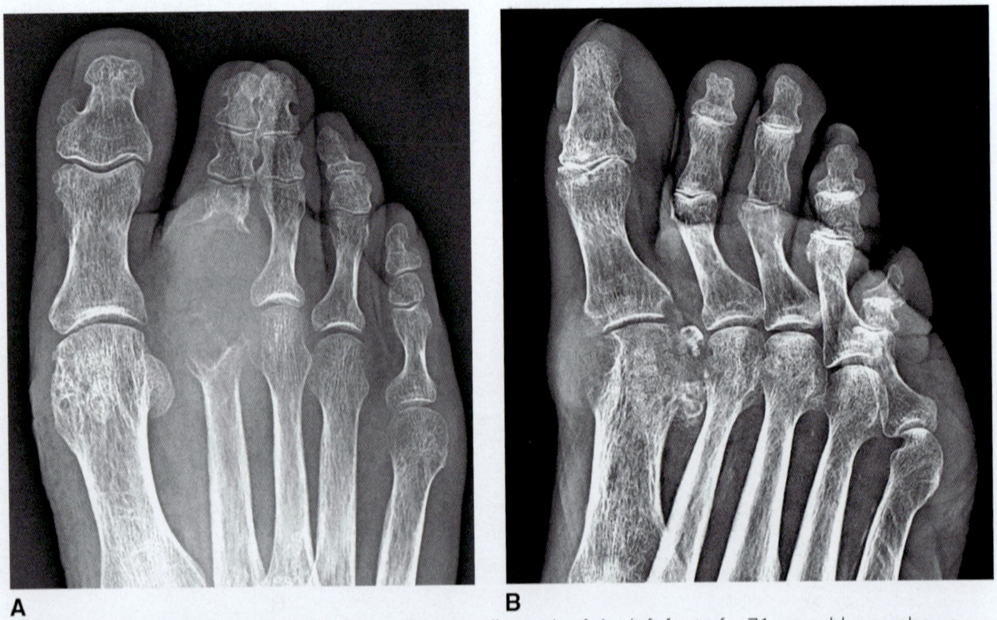

Figure 7.7 ■ Gouty arthritis. A: Dorsoplantar radiograph of the left foot of a 71-year-old man shows destruction of the second metatarsophalangeal joint exhibiting overhanging edges. **B:** Oblique radiograph of the left foot of an 80-year-old man shows erosions at the first metatarsophalangeal joint. Observe overhanging edge and preservation of part of the joint.

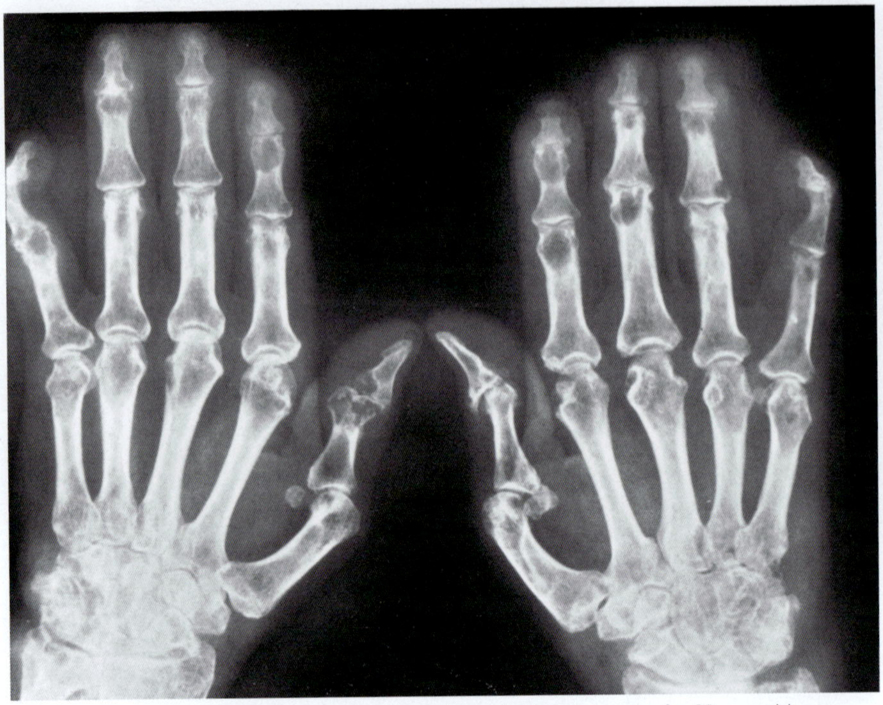

Figure 7.8 ■ Gouty arthritis. Dorsovolar radiograph of both hands of a 60-year-old man shows articular and periarticular erosions. In addition, note the presence of intraosseous defects in the phalanges consistent with intraosseous tophi.

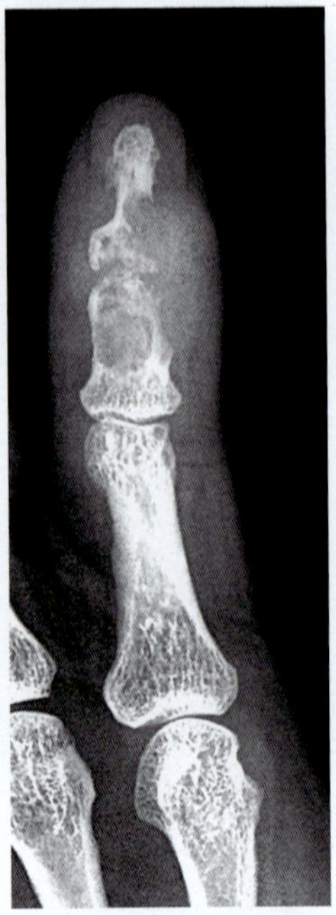

Figure 7.9 ■ Gouty arthritis. Radiograph of the index finger of a 65-year-old man shows the intraosseous tophi within the middle and distal phalanges.

helps differentiate this condition from rheumatoid arthritis. The reason for the absence of osteoporosis is that the duration of an acute gouty attack is too short to allow the development of the disuse osteoporosis so often seen in patients with rheumatoid arthritis. If erosion involves the articular end of the bone and extends into the joint, part of the joint is usually preserved (Fig. 7.10A, see also Fig. 7.5). Unlike rheumatoid arthritis, periarticular and articular erosions are asymmetric in distribution (Fig. 7.11). In chronic tophaceous gout, monosodium urate crystal deposit in and around the joint is seen, creating dense masses in the soft tissues called tophi, which frequently exhibit calcifications (Figs. 7.12 to 7.15, see also Figs. 7.1 and 7.2). Characteristically, tophi are randomly distributed

(Continued on page 279)

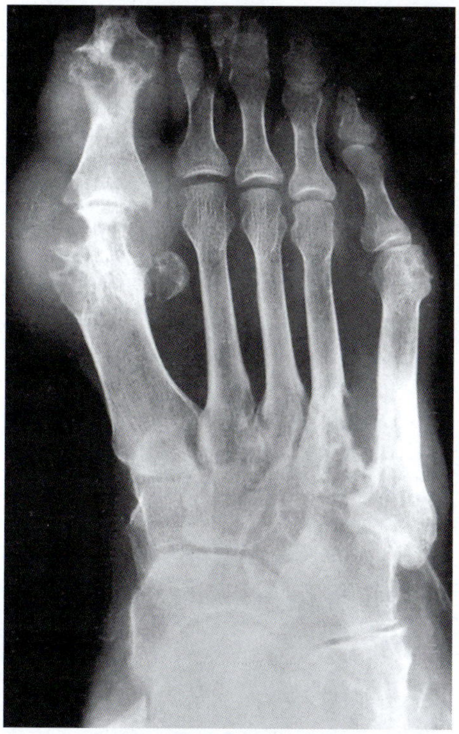

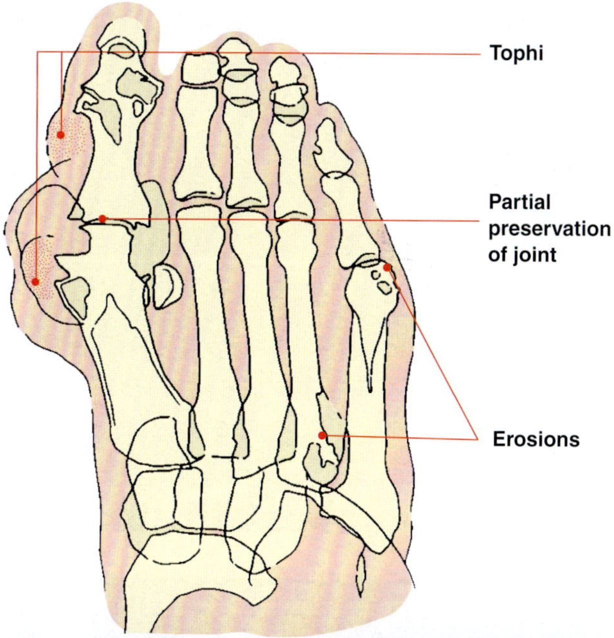

A

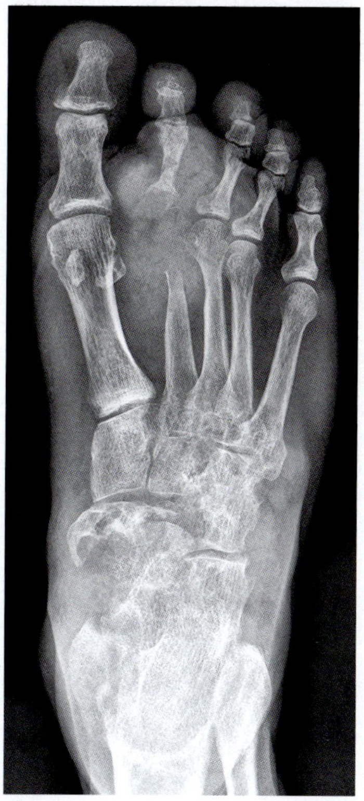

B

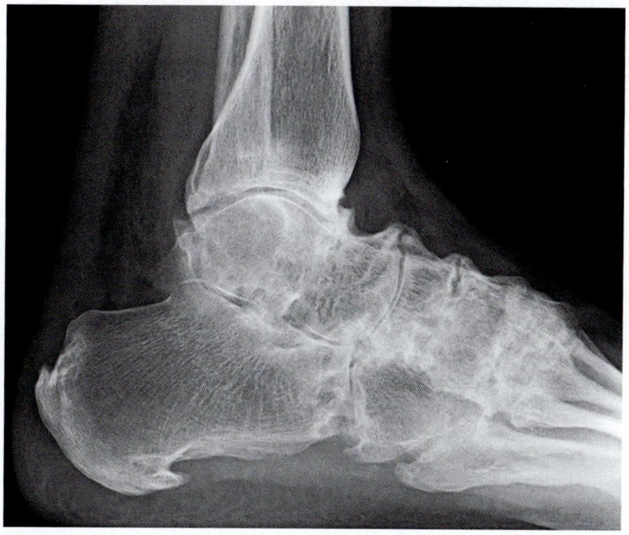

C

Figure 7.10 ■ **Gouty arthritis. A:** Dorsoplantar radiograph of the left foot of a 62-year-old man with a long history of tophaceous gout shows multiple erosions involving the joints of the great and small toes and the base of the fourth and fifth metatarsals. The first metatarsophalangeal joint is partially preserved, a characteristic feature of gouty arthritis. A large soft tissue mass of the great toe represents a tophus. Dorsoplantar radiograph of the left foot **(B)** and lateral radiograph of the left ankle **(C)** of a 49-year-old man show numerous articular and periarticular erosions of the midfoot and Lisfranc joint and destruction of the second metatarsophalangeal joint associated with several soft tissue tophi.

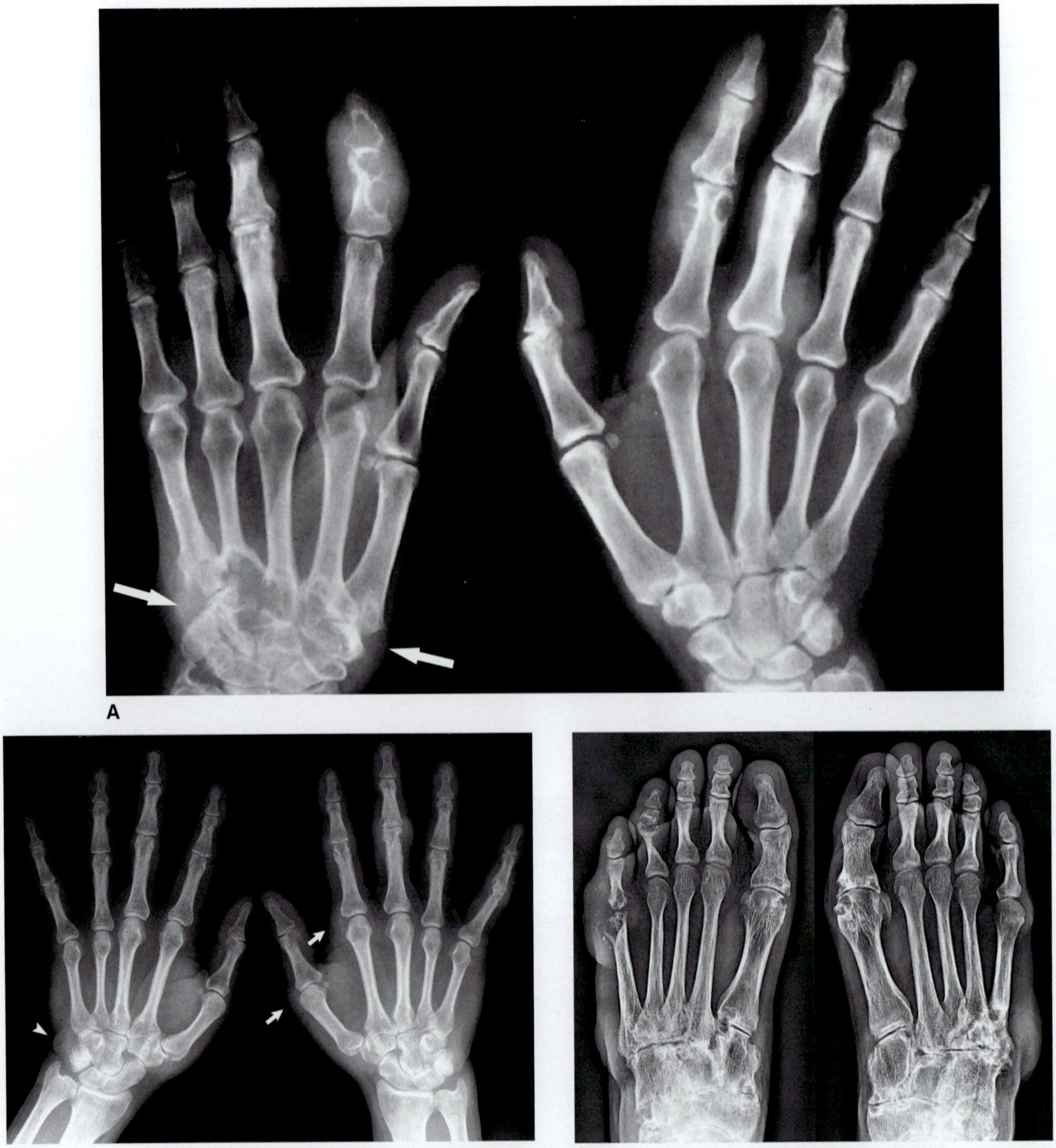

Figure 7.11 ■ **Gouty arthritis. A:** Dorsovolar radiograph of the hands of a 64-year-old woman shows the typical asymmetric distribution of periarticular and articular erosions. Note involvement of the carpometacarpal joints of the right hand (*arrows*), a typical site for gout. **B:** Dorsovolar radiograph of the hands of a 58-year-old man shows periarticular erosions and soft tissue tophi of the proximal interphalangeal joints of the index, middle, and small fingers of the left hand. There are also tophi at the first and second metacarpophalangeal joints (*arrows*), but no erosions are present. In the right hand, a soft tissue tophus is seen adjacent to the hamate bone (*arrowhead*). **C:** Dorsoplantar radiograph of the feet of a 46-year-old man shows asymmetric distribution of the articular and periarticular erosions, some of them associated with soft tissue tophi.

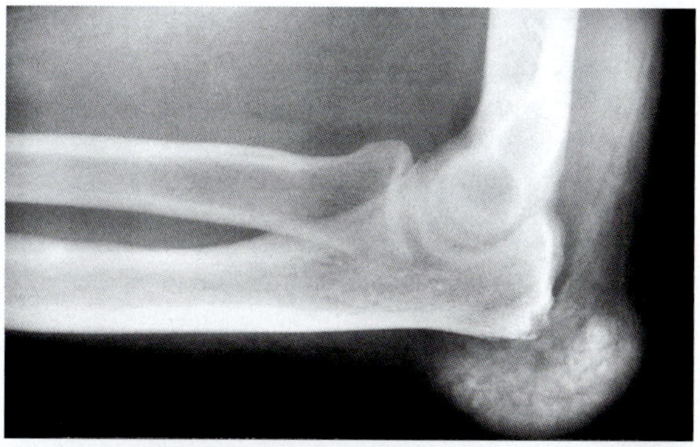

A

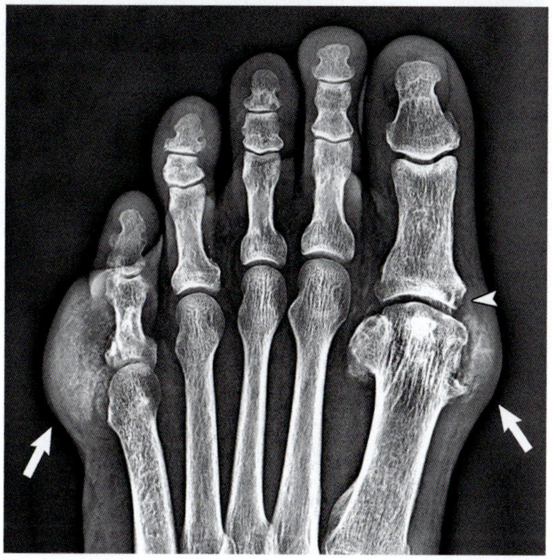

B

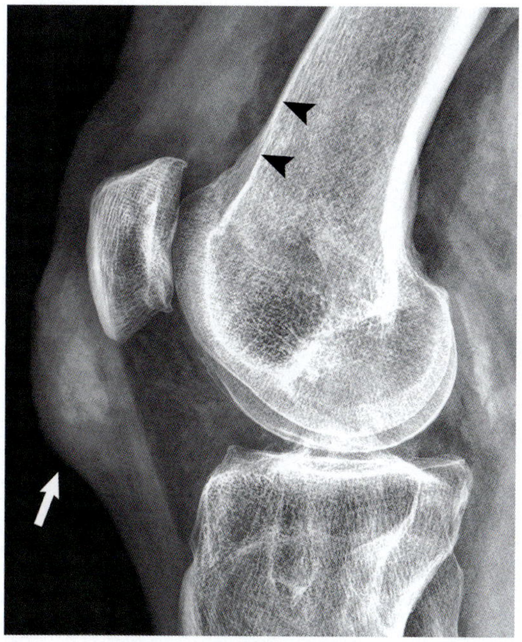

C

Figure 7.12 ■ Gouty tophi. A: Lateral radiograph of the elbow of a 73-year-old man with a 30-year history of gout shows a tophus with dense calcifications adjacent to the olecranon process, which exhibits small erosion. **B:** Dorsoplantar radiograph of the right forefoot of a 69-year-old man shows densely calcified prominent tophi at the fifth and first metatarsophalangeal joints (*arrows*). Note small periarticular erosion at the base of the proximal phalanx of the great toe (*arrowhead*). **C:** Lateral radiograph of the right knee of a 60-year-old man shows a large infrapatellar tophus (*arrow*). There are no articular erosions present, but there is a small suprapatellar joint effusion (*arrowheads*).

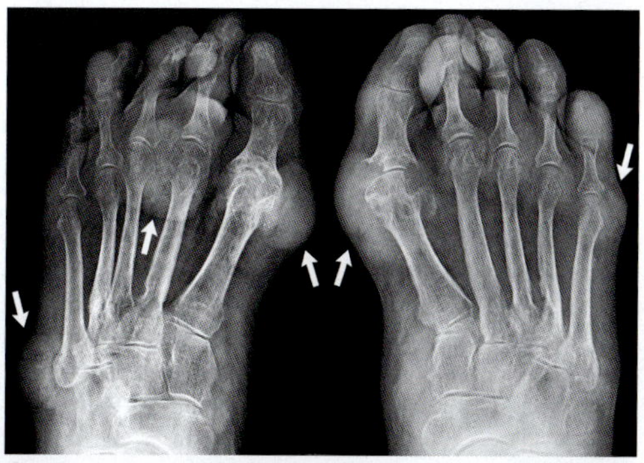

A

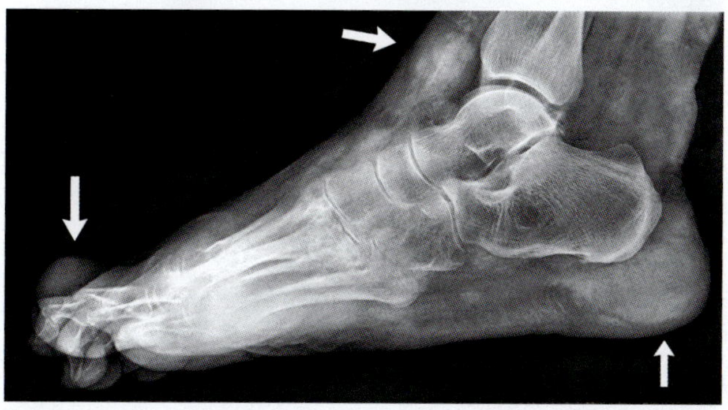

B

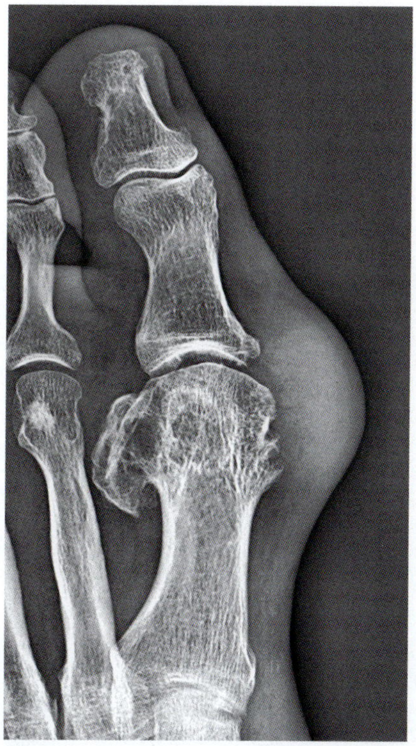

C

Figure 7.13 ■ Gouty tophi. Anteroposterior radiograph of both feet **(A)** and lateral radiograph of the left foot **(B)** of a 69-year-old man show numerous gouty tophi (*arrows*). Note also a characteristic for this arthritis erosion of the first metatarsophalangeal joint of the left foot. **C:** Radiograph of the great toe of a 54-year-old man shows a large tophus adjacent to the first metatarsophalangeal joint. Note also small erosions at the base of the proximal phalanx and at the medial aspect of the first metatarsal head.

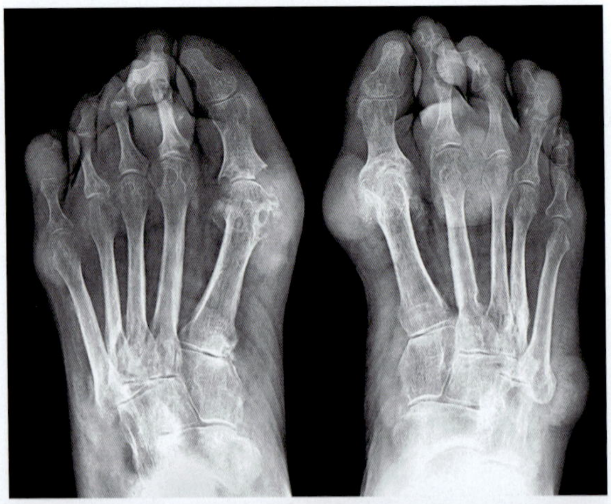

A

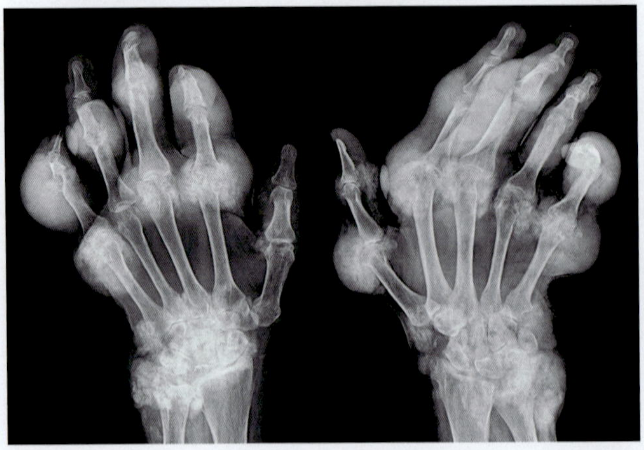

B

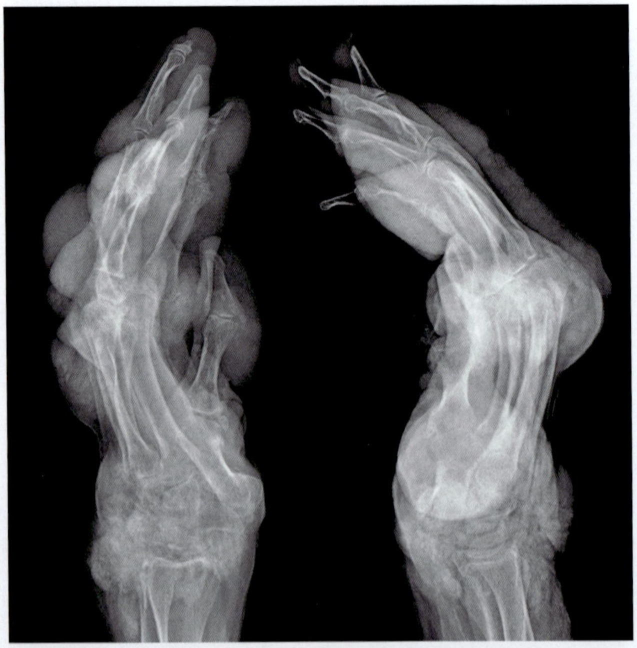

C

Figure 7.14 ■ Gouty tophi. Dorsoplantar radiograph of both feet **(A)** and dorsovolar **(B)** and lateral **(C)** radiographs of both hands of an 81-year-old man show numerous calcified tophi associated with periarticular and articular erosions.

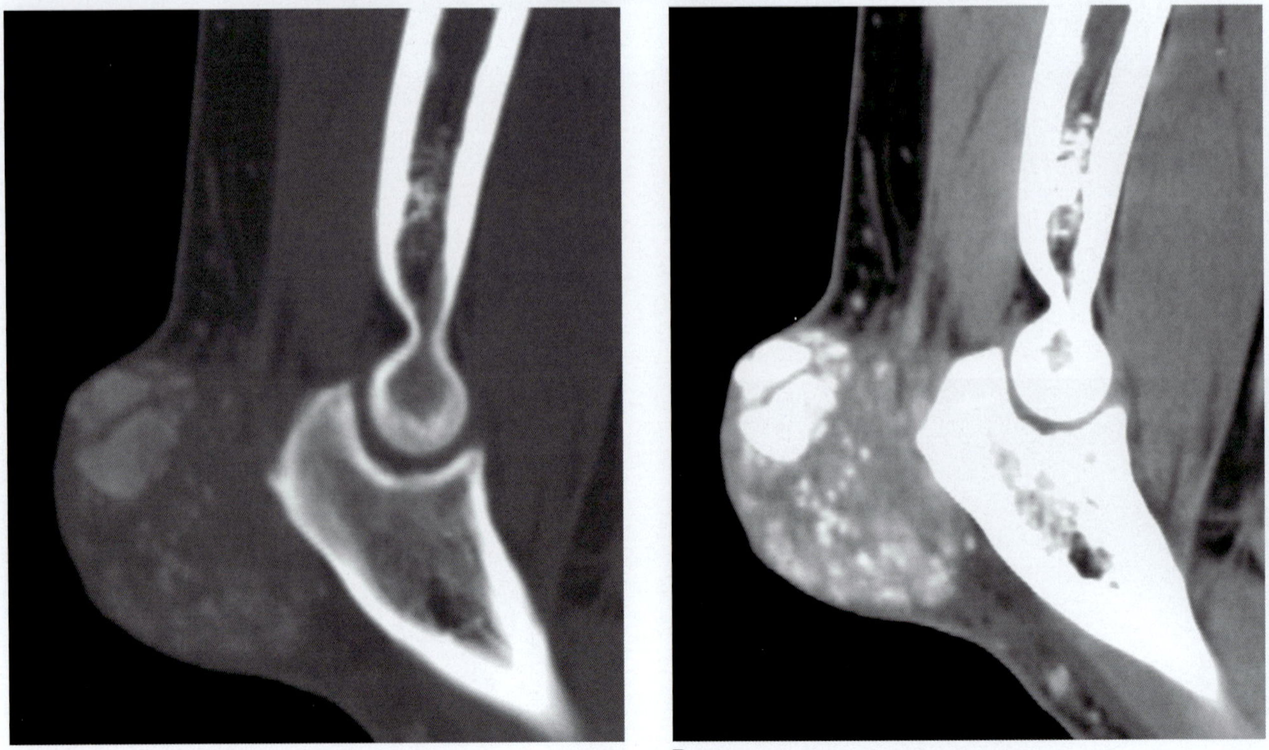

A B

Figure 7.15 ■ CT of gouty tophus. Sagittal reformatted CT images of the elbow viewed in bone **(A)** and soft tissue **(B)** window show a large soft tissue mass with numerous calcifications adjacent to the olecranon process of ulna.

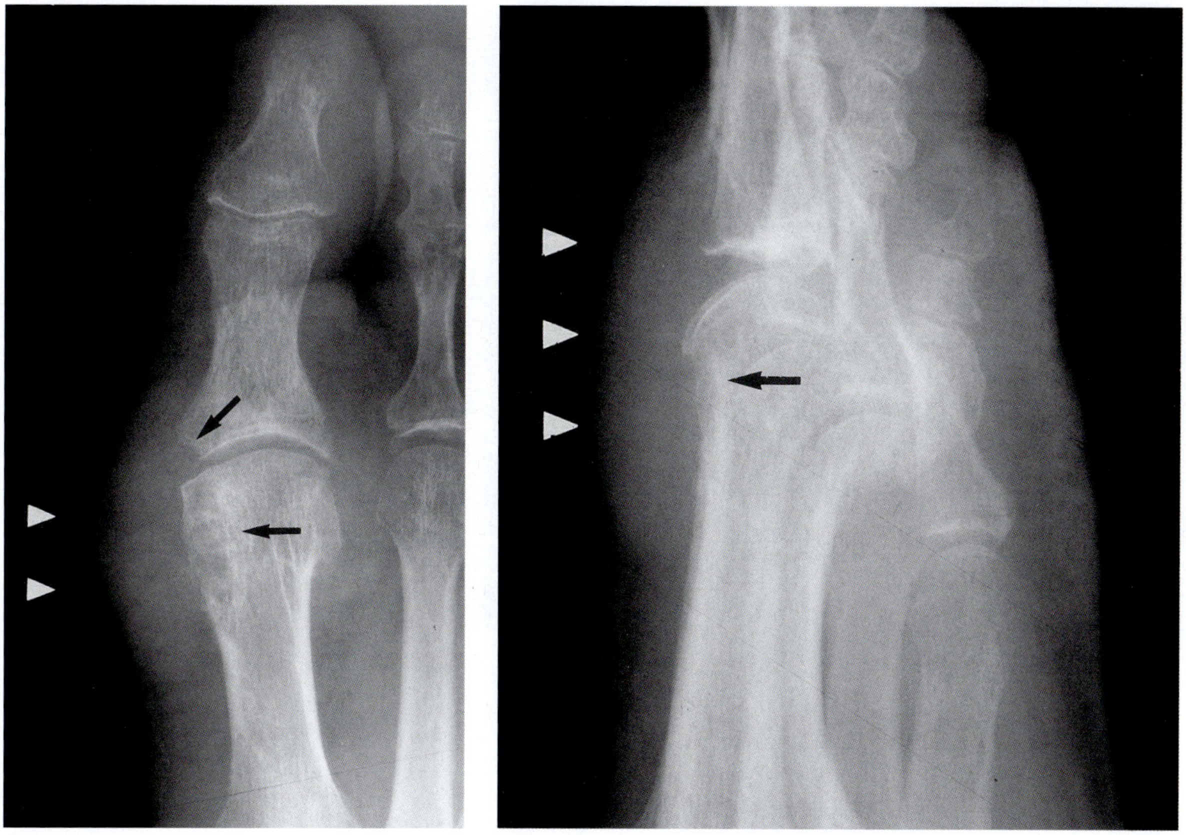

A B

Figure 7.16 ■ **Gouty tophus.** Dorsoplantar **(A)** and lateral **(B)** radiographs of the great toe show articular and periarticular erosions (*arrows*) associated with a large tophus on the dorsal aspect of the first metatarsophalangeal joint (*arrowheads*).

and are usually asymmetric; if they occur in the hands or feet, they are more often seen on the dorsal aspect (Fig. 7.16). Currently, dual-energy CT (DECT) color-coded images can accurately depict gouty tophi (Figs. 7.17 to 7.20, see also Figs. 2.27 and 2.28). DECT has ability to extract information and characterize the chemical composition of material according to the differential x-ray photon energy–dependent attenuation of compounds being examined at two different energy levels. Reported sensitivity of this technique varies between 78% and 100% and specificity between 89% and 100%. Magnetic resonance imaging is also an effective way to detect articular and soft tissue abnormalities of gouty arthritis. Tophaceous gouty deposits exhibit a wide spectrum of signal intensities characteristics, which reflects their variable composition and relative proportion of protein, fibrous tissue, crystals,

(Continued on page 282)

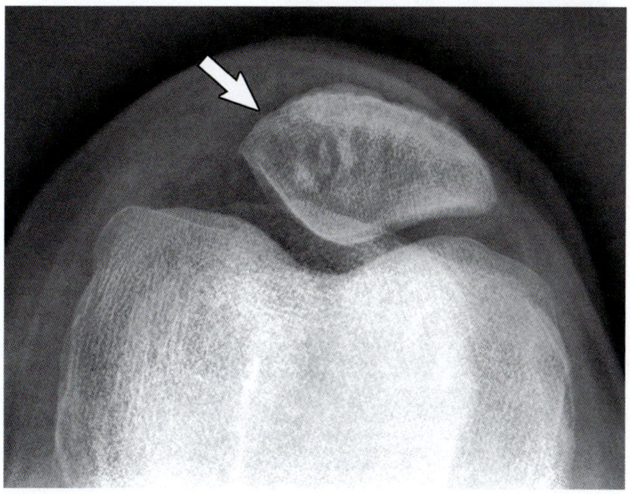

A

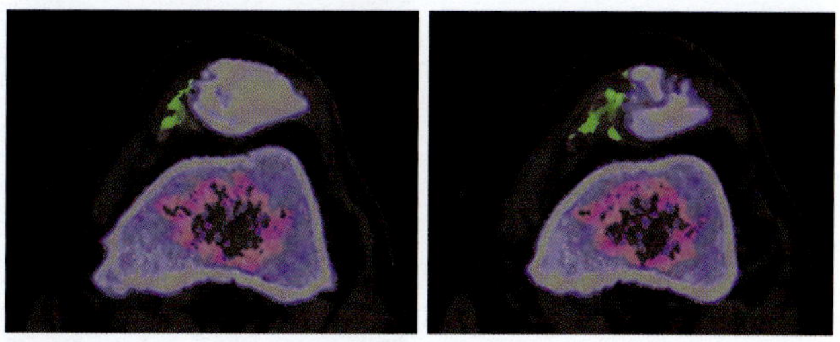

B

Figure 7.17 ■ **Dual-energy CT of tophaceous gout.**
A: Merchant view of the left knee of a 68-year-old man shows a radiolucent defect in the medial aspect of the patella (*arrow*).
B: Two dual-energy color-coded axial CT images show a soft tissue, monosodium urate crystal–containing tophus (*green foci*) eroding medial aspect of the patella.

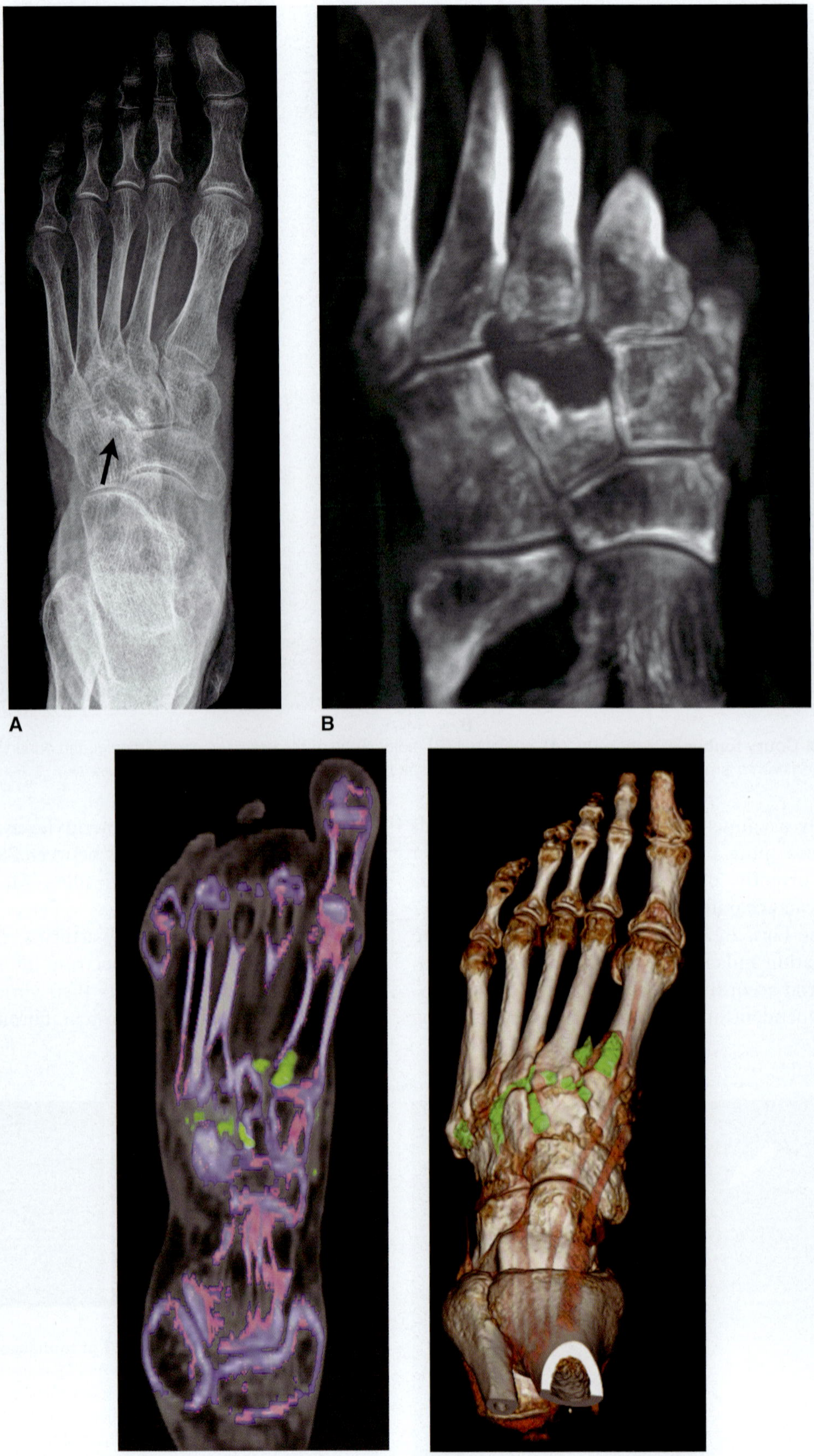

A B C D

Figure 7.18 ■ Dual-energy CT of tophaceous gout. Anteroposterior radiograph of the right foot **(A)** of a 48-year-old man shows nonspecific erosion at the third tarsometatarsal joint (*arrow*), confirmed on the coronal reformatted CT image **(B)**. Dual-energy coronal **(C)** and 3D reconstructed **(D)** color-coded CT images show in addition several masses (*green areas*) representing uric acid crystals within the gouty tophi.

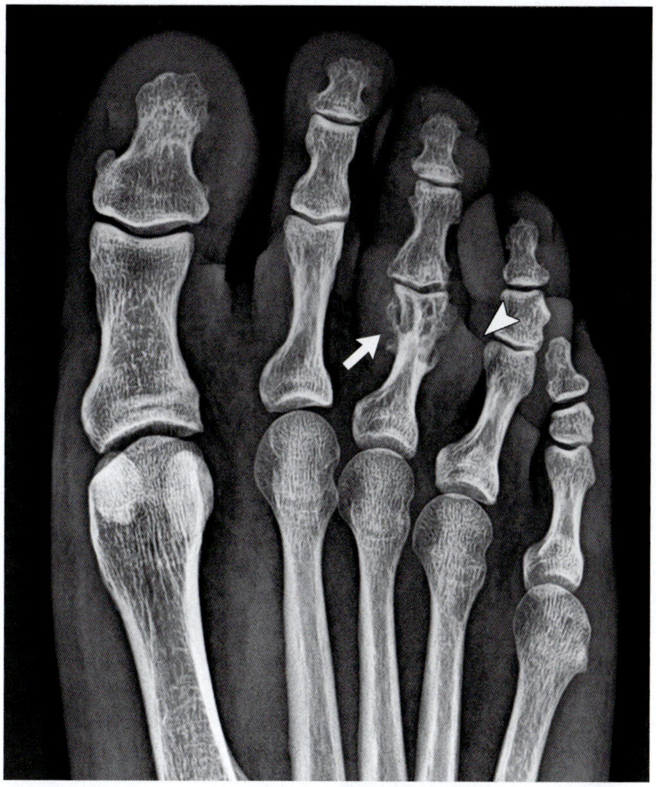

A

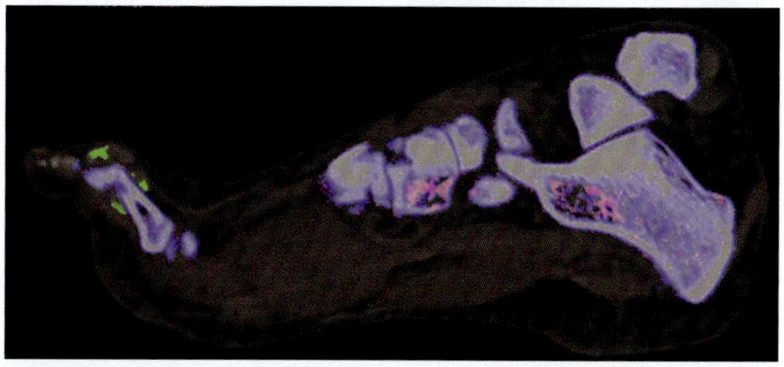

B

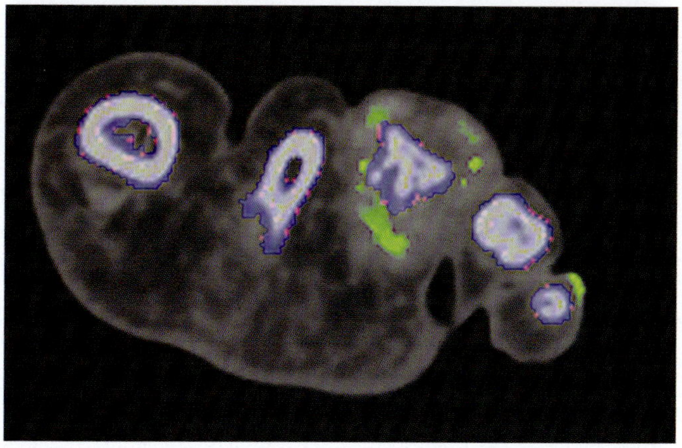

C

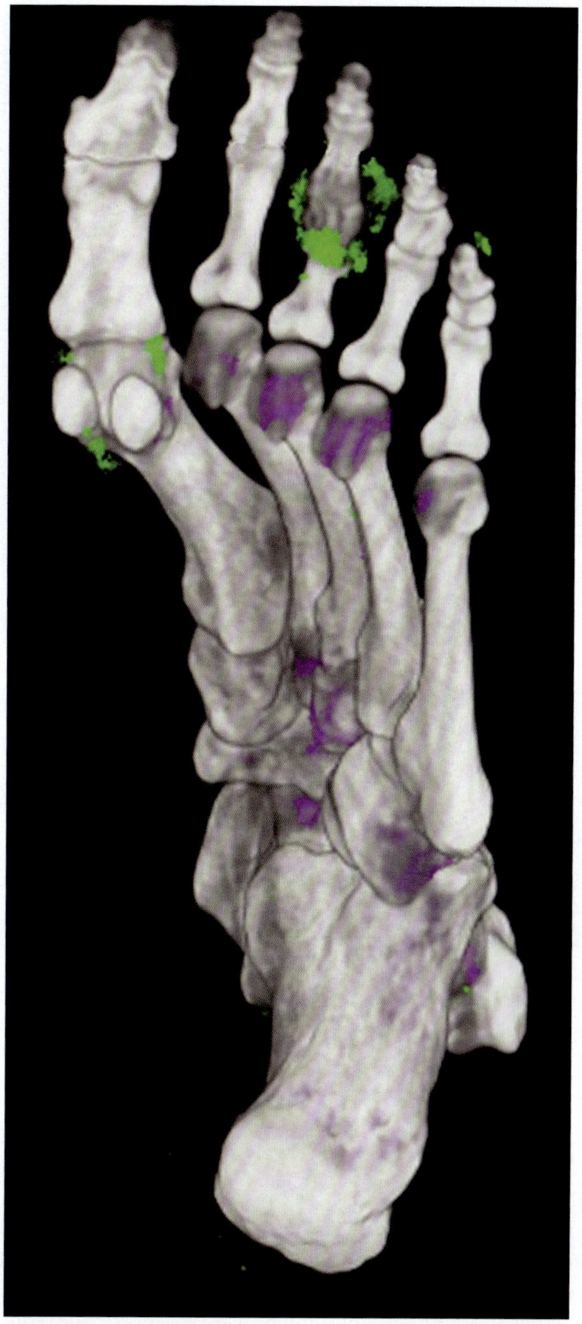

D

Figure 7.19 ■ **Dual-energy CT of tophaceous gout.** A 50-year-old man presented with painful swollen third toe of the left foot. **A:** Anteroposterior radiograph shows a para-articular erosion of the proximal phalanx of the third toe (*arrow*), associated with a fusiform mass (*arrowhead*). Dual-energy sagittal reformatted **(B)** and axial color-coded **(C)** CT images supplemented with 3D reconstructed CT color-coded image **(D)** viewed from the plantar aspect of the foot were diagnostic of gouty tophi in several locations (*green areas*).

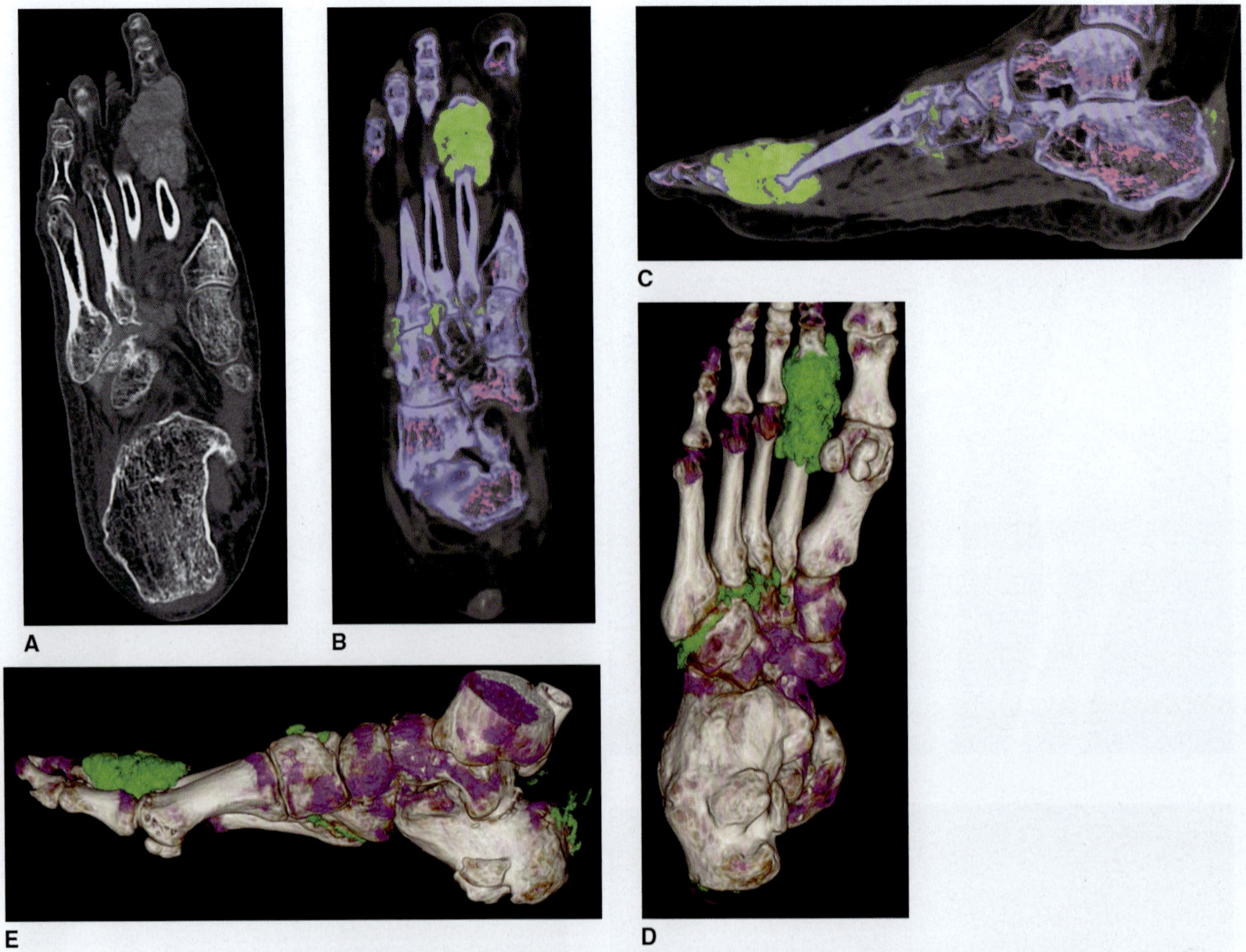

Figure 7.20 ■ **Dual-energy CT of tophaceous gout. A:** Long-axis CT image of the right foot of a 71-year-old man (same patient as shown in Fig. 7.7A) shows a nonspecific low-attenuation mass in the region of the second toe. Long-axis **(B)** and sagittal **(C)** reformatted dual-energy color-coded CT images identify the mass as being a large tophus containing monosodium urate crystals (*green area*). In addition, several smaller tophi are identified at the site of Lisfranc joint and at the site of Achilles tendon attachment to the calcaneus. Three-dimensional reconstructed dual-energy CT color-coded images viewed from the plantar **(D)** and medial **(E)** aspects of the foot better demonstrate the spatial distribution of the urate tophi.

and hemosiderin. Most lesions are isointense relative to muscle on T1-weighted images, and low-to-intermediate heterogeneous signal intensity on proton density–weighted and water-sensitive (IR, T2) sequences (Fig. 7.21). There is strong enhancement following intravenous injection of gadolinium, although contrast enhancement of the tophus is variable and depends on the vascularity of the affected synovium and surrounding granulation tissue (Fig. 7.22). Concomitant enhancement of adjacent tendon sheaths, ligaments, muscles, and bone marrow may also be present, reflecting intense inflammatory reaction.

Although imaging findings of gouty arthritis are generally very characteristic and most of the time even pathognomonic, clinical presentation of acute gouty arthritis may be sometimes mistaken for septic arthritis. The two conditions may present with similar symptoms including joint pain, swelling, tenderness, and occasionally similar laboratory findings such as elevated white blood cell count and sedimentation rate. Soft tissue tophi may at times mimic rheumatoid nodules. Intraosseous tophi may have aggressive appearance and thus may simulate malignant bone tumor. On radiography, articular gouty erosions, particularly affecting the proximal and distal interphalangeal joints, may sometimes mimic erosive osteoarthritis. Amyloid infiltrate of the articular structures may cause soft tissue masses accompanied by cystic and erosive lesions indistinguishable from those of gout. Finally, it has to be pointed out that gout may coexist with other arthropathic conditions such as rheumatoid arthritis, osteoarthritis, and infectious arthritis.

Treatment

The treatment of gout depends upon the stages of the disease. Recently, The American College of Physicians (ACP) developed guidelines and clinical recommendations on the management of gout. The acute gouty attacks respond well to colchicine, as well as to nonsteroidal anti-inflammatory drugs (NSAIDs) such as ibuprofen, naproxen, or indomethacin. In chronic stages, corticosteroids control inflammation and pain. In addition, the drugs that block uric acid

(Continued on page 285)

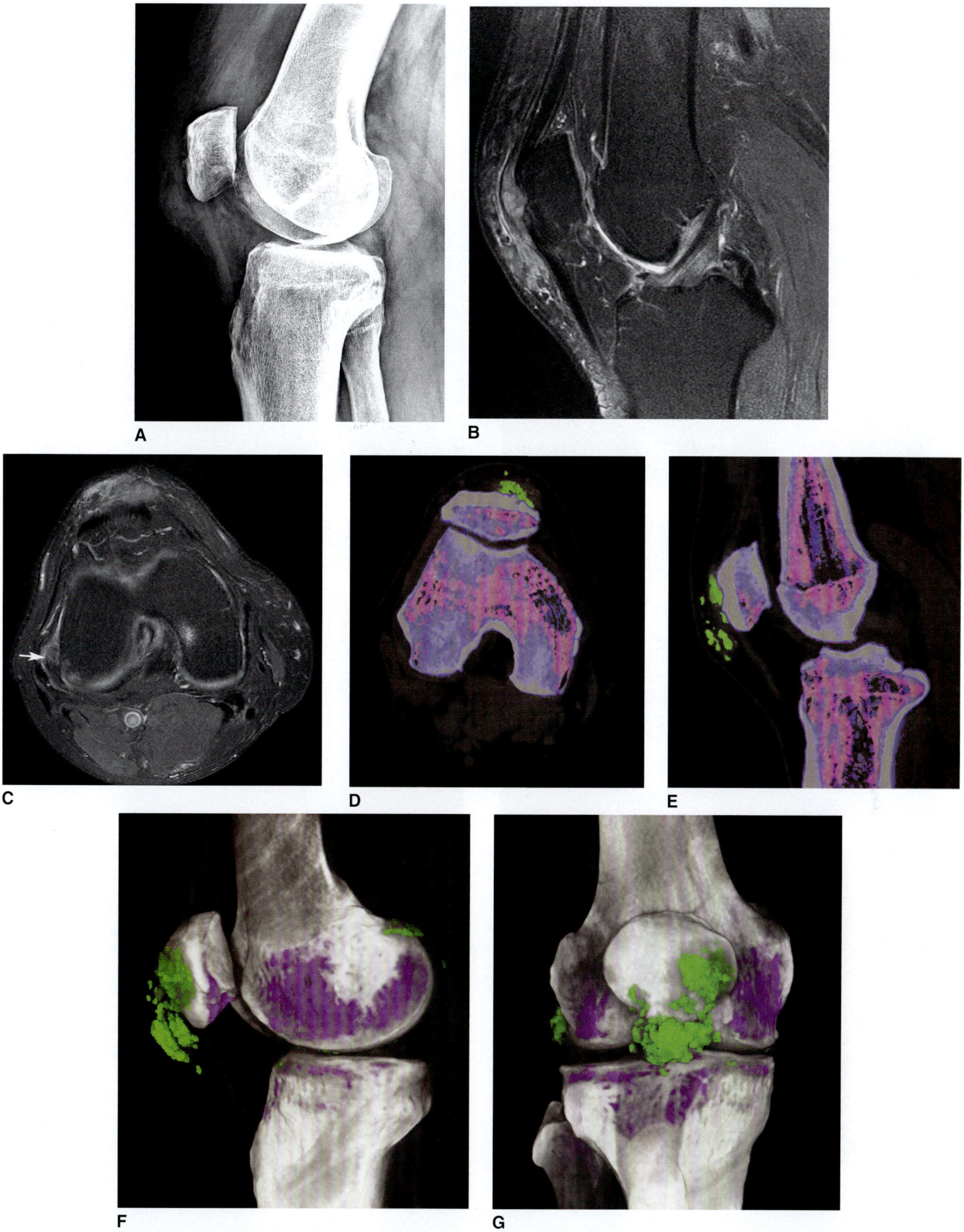

Figure 7.21 ■ **MRI and dual-energy CT of tophaceous gout. A:** Lateral radiograph of the knee of a 65-year-old man, who presented with right knee pain, shows prepatellar soft tissue mass eroding the anterior cortex of the patella. Sagittal **(B)** and axial **(C)** proton density–weighted fat-suppressed MR images demonstrate heterogeneous mass adjacent to the patella and smaller mass eroding the lateral femoral condyle (*arrow*). Axial **(D)** and sagittal **(E)** dual-energy color-coded CT images are diagnostic for the presence of gouty tophi containing monosodium urate crystals (*green areas*). Three-dimensional reconstructed color-coded CT images viewed from the lateral **(F)** and frontal **(G)** aspects of the knee more accurately depict the gouty tophi.

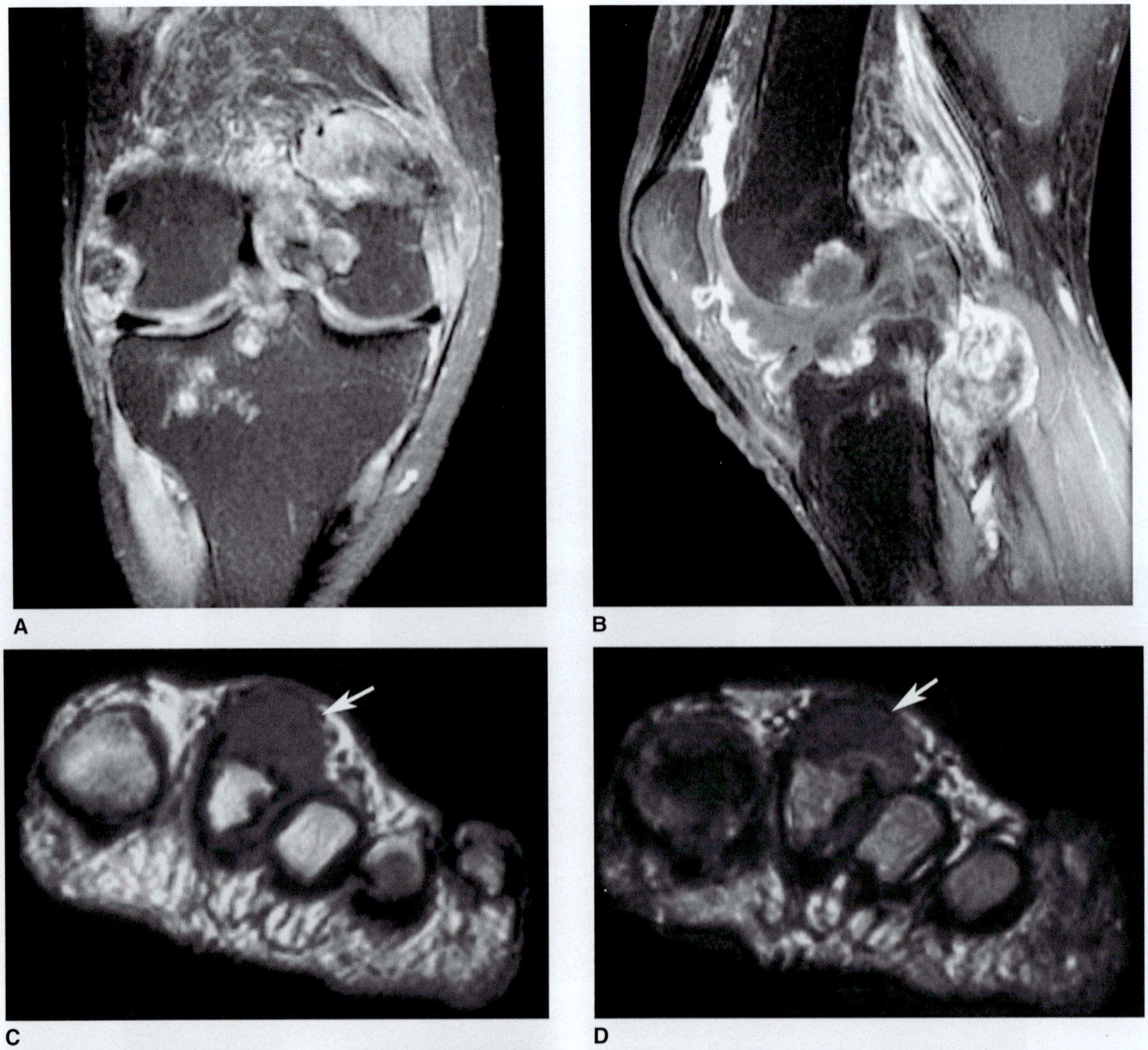

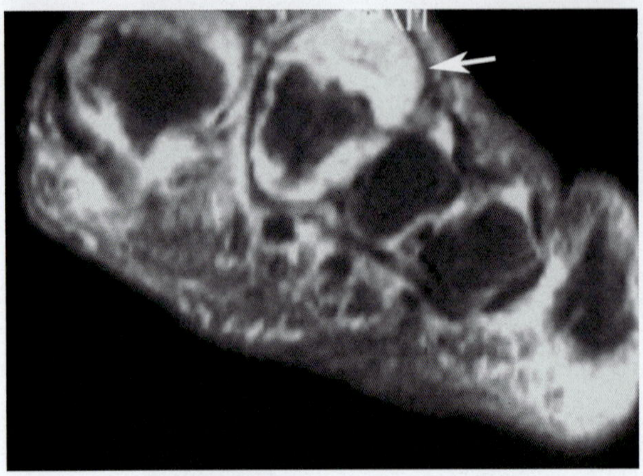

Figure 7.22 ■ **MRI of gouty arthritis.** Coronal proton density–weighted fat-suppressed **(A)** and sagittal T1-weighted fat-suppressed contrast-enhanced **(B)** MR images of the right knee of a 53-year-old man show multiple articular and para-articular erosions associated with intraosseous as well as soft tissue tophi. **C:** Short-axis T1-weighted MRI of the foot in another patient with gouty arthritis demonstrates a low signal intensity tophaceous deposit in the dorsal aspect of the second metatarsal (*arrow*). **D:** Short axis T2-weighted MRI of the same patient shows the low signal intensity tophaceous deposit (*arrow*). **E:** Short axis postcontrast T1-weighted fat-saturated MRI demonstrates strong enhancement of the tophaceous deposit (*arrow*).

production, such as xanthine oxidase inhibitors (allopurinol or febuxostat), and medications that improve removal of uric acid from the body (probenecid), are used to prevent complications of gout. Most recently, rheumatologists reported that urate-lowering therapy using pegloticase, a pegylated mammalian (porcine-like) recombinant uricase, resulted in reduction of the gouty tophus size both at subcutaneous sites and within the joints. However, ACP recommends that clinicians should discuss benefits, harms, costs, and individual preferences with patients before initiating urate-lowering therapy in patients with recurrent gout attacks. This includes the risk of Stevens-Johnson syndrome in patients receiving allopurinol.

CALCIUM PYROPHOSPHATE DIHYDRATE (CPPD) CRYSTAL DEPOSITION DISEASE

Clinical and Pathologic Features

CPPD crystal deposition disease is a metabolic disorder, which is characterized by the accumulation of calcium pyrophosphate dihydrate crystals in intra-articular and periarticular tissues, most commonly within fibrocartilage and hyaline cartilage. In addition, synovial, bursal, ligamentous, and tendinous calcifications are encountered. It rarely presents as a soft tissue mass in extra-articular location, which is known as tumoral or tophaceous pseudogout. The condition may occur as a hereditary or sporadic disorder. Some investigators suggested that a putative pyrophosphate transporter, the progressive ankylosis protein homolog, a protein encoded by *ANKH* gene, might be responsible for this disease. *ANKH* may also play a role in modulating the enzymes involved in mineralization, such as alkaline phosphatase, thus potentially contributing to the disease process. The men and women are equally affected; most commonly, patients are middle aged and older. The disease may be asymptomatic, in which case the only imaging finding may be *chondrocalcinosis* (see text below). When symptomatic, it is called *pseudogout*. There is, however, a great deal of confusion about these terms, and they are often misused.

In an effort to explain the relationship between chondrocalcinosis, calcium pyrophosphate arthropathy, and the pseudogout syndrome, Resnick has proposed an integration of these terms under the rubric CPPD crystal deposition disease. *Chondrocalcinosis*, a condition in which calcification of the hyaline (articular) cartilage or fibrocartilage (menisci) occurs, may be seen in other disorders as well, such as gout, hyperparathyroidism, hemochromatosis, hepatolenticular degeneration (Wilson disease), and degenerative joint disease (Table 7.2). *Calcium pyrophosphate arthropathy* refers to CPPD crystal deposition disease affecting the joints and producing structural damage to the articular cartilage. It displays distinctive imaging abnormalities such as narrowing of the joint space, subchondral sclerosis, and osteophytosis, similar to osteoarthritis. The *pseudogout syndrome* represents a condition in which symptoms such as acute pain are similar to those seen in gouty arthritis; however, it does not respond to the usual treatment (colchicine) for the latter disease.

Table 7.2 MOST COMMON CAUSES OF CHONDROCALCINOSIS

Senescent (aging process)
Osteoarthritis
Posttraumatic
Calcium pyrophosphate arthropathy (CPPD crystal deposition disease)
Gout
Hemochromatosis
Hyperparathyroidism
Hypophosphatasia
Ochronosis
Oxalosis
Wilson disease
Acromegaly
Idiopathic

Modified from Reeder MM, Felson B, 1975, with permission.

Calcium pyrophosphate crystals, the pathogens in pseudogout, range up to 10 µm in length. As in gout, many intracellular crystals are seen during an acute episode. The colors are usually but not always much less intense than urates, that is, they are weakly birefringent. Pyrophosphate crystals are generally chunkier and often show a line down the middle. The most common form of calcium pyrophosphate crystal is a rhomboid. Pyrophosphate crystals are positively birefringent in that they are blue when the longitudinal axis of the crystal is parallel to the slow vibrations axis of the red compensator and yellow when it is perpendicular (see previous text and Figs. 1.9 and 1.10). Pathologic findings consist of punctate or linear calcium deposits, usually in the hyaline cartilage paralleling the subchondral bone end plate, also referred to as a "subchondral" or "articular" cortex (Fig. 7.23). Punctate calcifications may also be seen in synovial tissue (Fig. 7.24). On microscopic examination, the chalky white deposits appear either crystalline or amorphous. In the vascularized tissue, there is associated inflammatory infiltrate that includes monophages and phagocytic polykaryons. In nonvascularized tissue, no inflammatory reaction is present. The pyrophosphate crystals are distinguished from urate crystals by their rhomboid shape (Fig. 7.25) and by their weakly positive birefringence (see prior text).

(Continued on page 287)

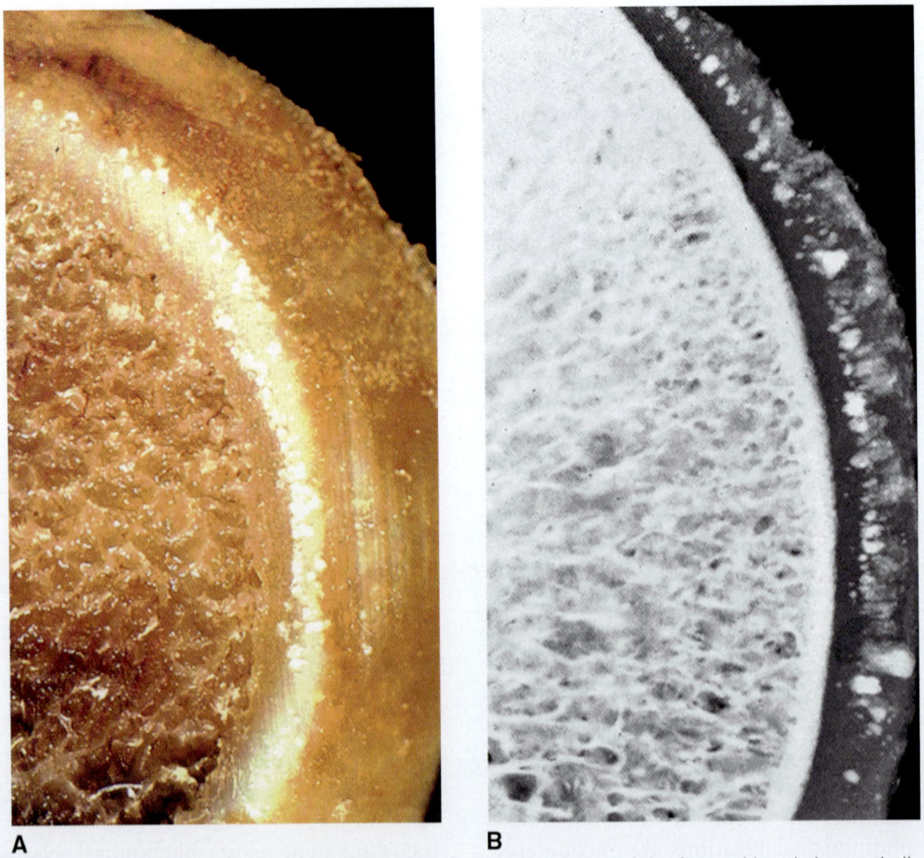

Figure 7.23 ■ **Pathology of CPPD crystal deposition disease. A:** Sagittal section of the femoral head shows chalky white deposits of calcium pyrophosphate dihydrate within the articular cartilage. **B:** Radiograph of the specimen clearly demonstrates the calcific nature of the deposit. (Reprinted from Bullough PG. *Atlas of Orthopedic Pathology with Clinical and Radiologic Correlation.* 2nd ed. New York, NY: Gower Medical Publishing; 1992, Fig. 11.46, p. 11.15.)

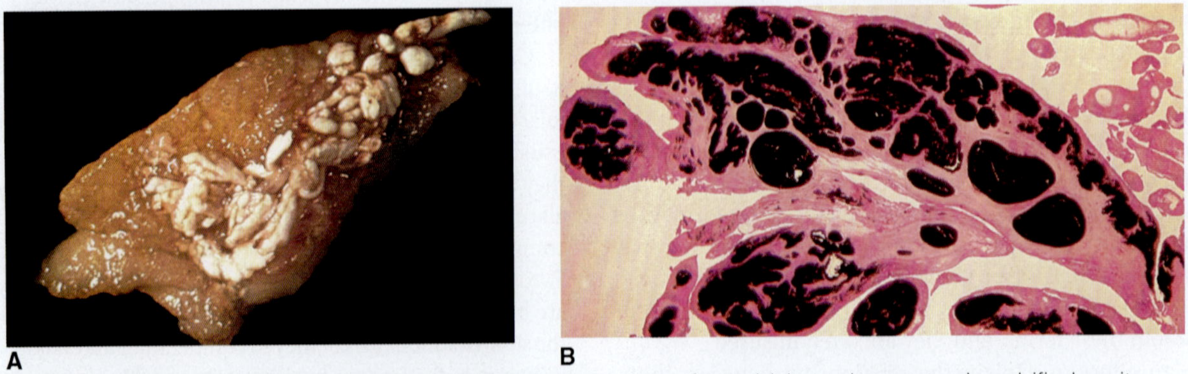

Figure 7.24 ■ **Pathology of CPPD crystal deposition disease. A:** Fragment of synovial tissue shows extensive calcific deposit. **B:** Histopathologic section of the specimen stained with von Kossa stain demonstrates the calcium deposits (*black*) (original magnification ×1). (Reprinted from Bullough PG. *Atlas of Orthopedic Pathology with Clinical and Radiologic Correlation.* 2nd ed. New York, NY: Gower Medical Publishing; 1992, Figs. 11.47 and 11.48, p. 11.16.)

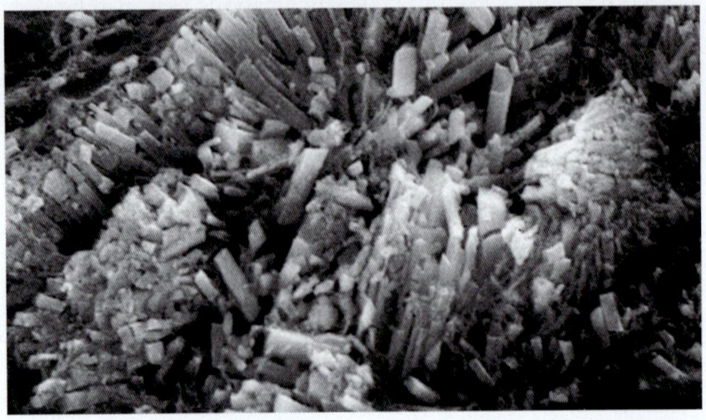

Figure 7.25 ■ **Electron microscopy of CPPD crystal deposition disease.** Scanning electron photomicrograph of calcium pyrophosphate dihydrate deposits shows characteristic rhomboidal crystals (original magnification ×2400). (Reprinted from Bullough PG. *Atlas of Orthopedic Pathology with Clinical and Radiologic Correlation.* 2nd ed. New York, NY: Gower Medical Publishing; 1992, Fig. 11.51, p. 11.16.)

Imaging Features

The radiographic appearance of asymptomatic CPPD crystal deposition disease is merely marked by chondrocalcinosis (Fig. 7.26). The arthritic changes encountered in this condition are similar to those seen in osteoarthritis. Any joint in the body may be affected, including the spine. The most common sites, however, are the knee (Fig. 7.27) and the wrist/hand (particularly the second and third metacarpophalangeal joints) (Figs. 7.28 and 7.29). Other joints affected in descending frequency include elbow (Fig. 7.30), shoulder (see Fig. 7.26A), ankle, and hip (Fig. 7.31). One of the complications of the wrist involvement is development of scapholunate advanced collapse (SLAC) deformity. In the knee joint, typically, the femoropatellar joint compartment is affected to significantly greater degree then medial or lateral joint compartments (Figs. 7.32 and 7.33). As mentioned, CPPD crystal deposition disease is characterized by calcification of the articular cartilage and fibrocartilage; the tendons, ligaments, and joint capsule may exhibit calcifications as well (see Figs. 7.27B and 7.33D).

Differential diagnosis of CPPD crystal deposition disease arthropathy should include osteoarthritis and neuropathic arthropathy, and if the second ant third metacarpophalangeal joints are affected, hemochromatosis and acromegalic arthropathy should be additional considerations.

Rarely, CPPD deposits can assume the form of bulky tumor-like masses located in the joint and paraarticular soft tissues. In these instances, it may mimic a malignant tumor; hence, this form of CPPD deposition was termed by Sissons and associates, "tumoral calcium pyrophosphate deposition disease." The mineral deposits are associated with a tissue reaction characterized by the presence of histiocytes and multinucleated giant cells, sometimes with bone and cartilage formation. The differential diagnosis should include tumoral calcinosis, a disorder characterized by the presence of single or multiple lobulated cystic masses in the soft tissues, usually near the major joints, containing chalky material consisting of calcium phosphate, calcium carbonate, or hydroxyapatite. The calcified deposits fail to show a crystalline appearance when examined by polarization microscopy. In this condition, the masses are painless and usually occur in children and adolescents, a majority of whom are black.

(Continued on page 292)

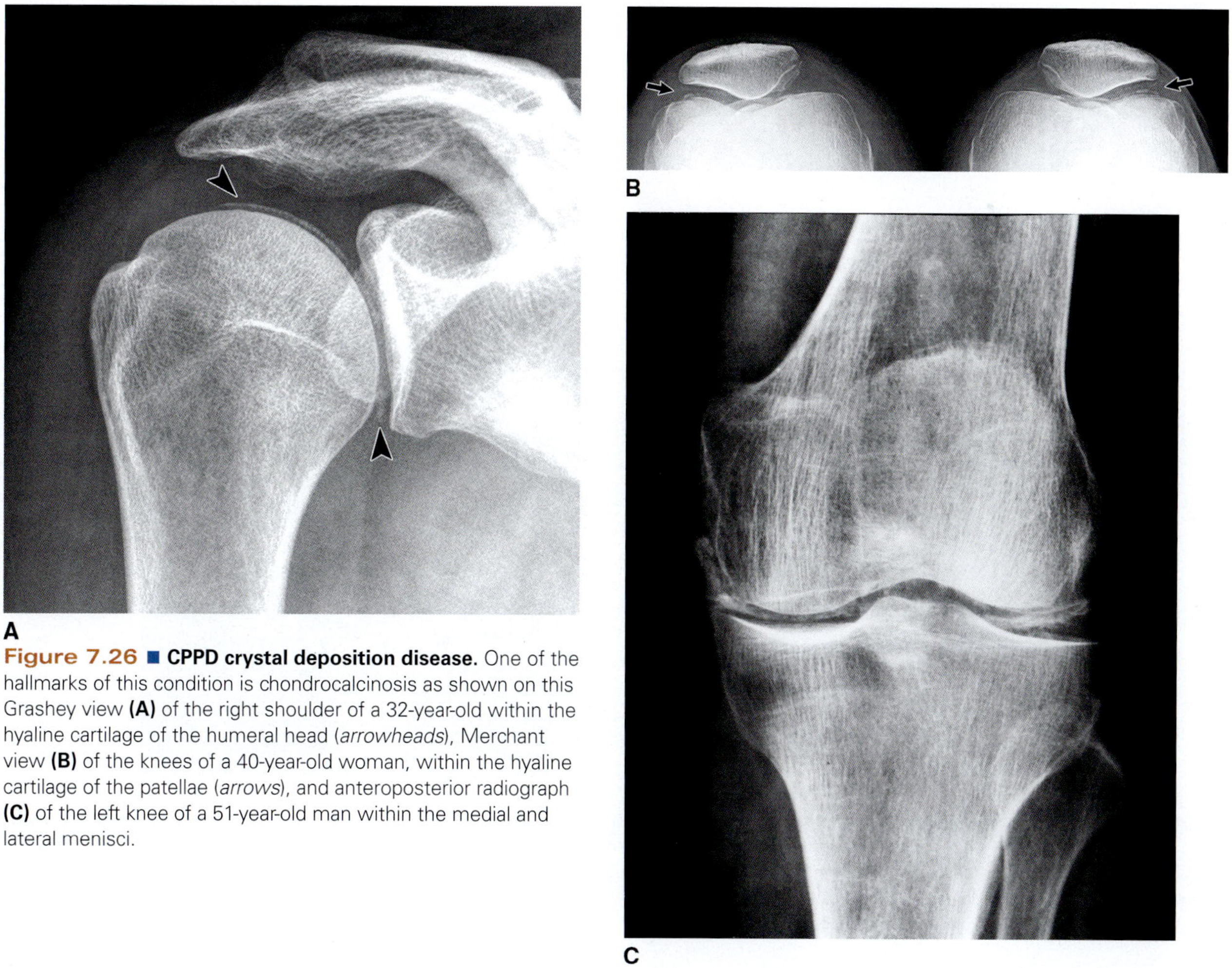

Figure 7.26 ■ CPPD crystal deposition disease. One of the hallmarks of this condition is chondrocalcinosis as shown on this Grashey view **(A)** of the right shoulder of a 32-year-old within the hyaline cartilage of the humeral head (*arrowheads*), Merchant view **(B)** of the knees of a 40-year-old woman, within the hyaline cartilage of the patellae (*arrows*), and anteroposterior radiograph **(C)** of the left knee of a 51-year-old man within the medial and lateral menisci.

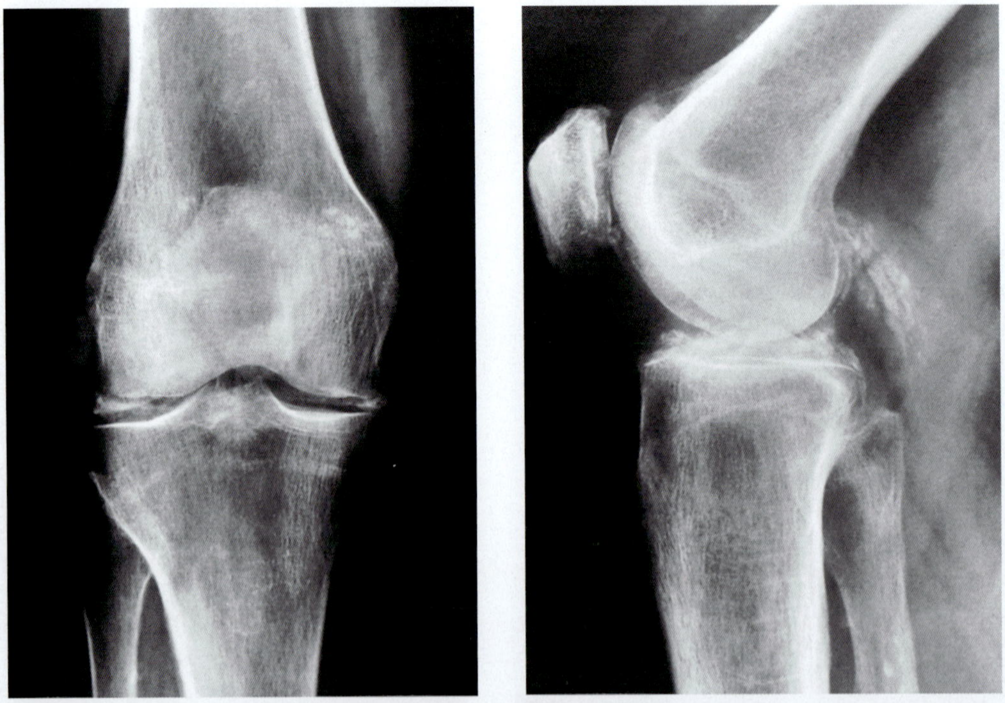

A B

Figure 7.27 ■ **CPPD crystal deposition disease.** A 70-year-old woman presented with acute onset of pain in her right knee and was treated with colchicine for acute gouty arthritis without relief of her pain. Synovial fluid yielded calcium pyrophosphate crystals. Anteroposterior **(A)** and lateral **(B)** radiographs of the knee demonstrate calcification of the hyaline and fibrocartilage. Capsular and tendinous calcifications are also apparent, as well as narrowing of the femoropatellar joint compartment, a characteristic feature of this disorder.

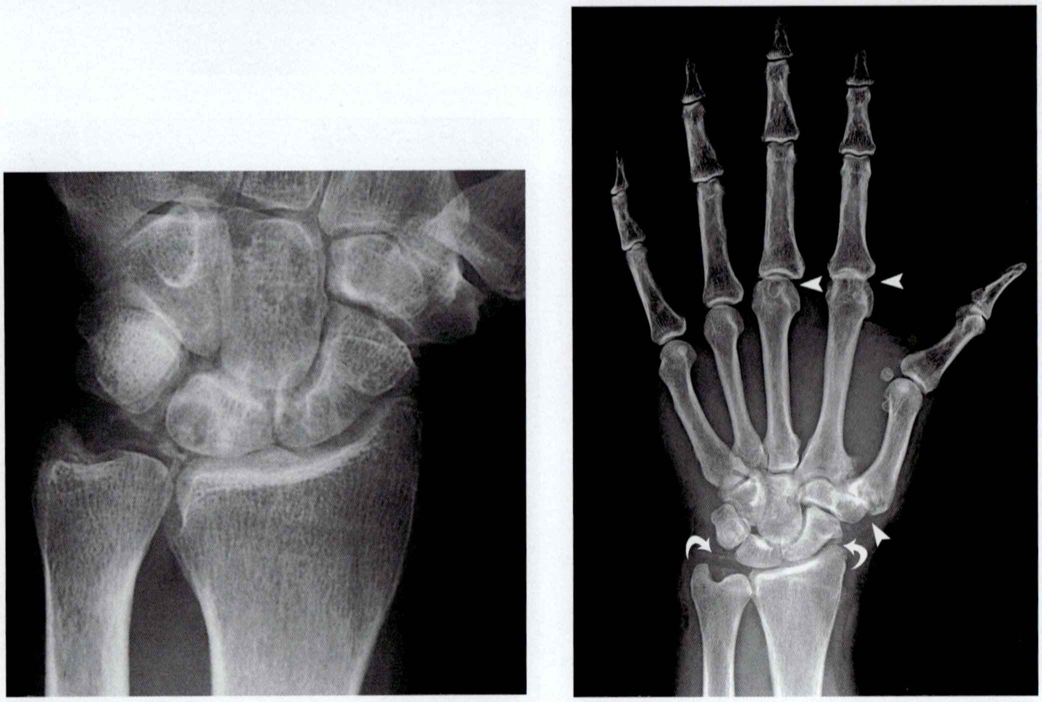

A B

Figure 7.28 ■ **CPPD crystal deposition disease. A:** Dorsovolar radiograph of the right wrist of a 63-year-old man who presented with an acute onset of pain shows chondrocalcinosis of the triangular fibrocartilage, cystic changes in the scaphoid and lunate, and narrowing of the radiocarpal joint. **B:** Dorsovolar radiograph of the right hand of a 55-year-old woman shows chondrocalcinosis within the triangular fibrocartilage complex and radiocarpal joint (*curved arrows*), in addition to typical arthritic changes affecting second and third metacarpophalangeal and first carpometacarpal joints (*arrowheads*).

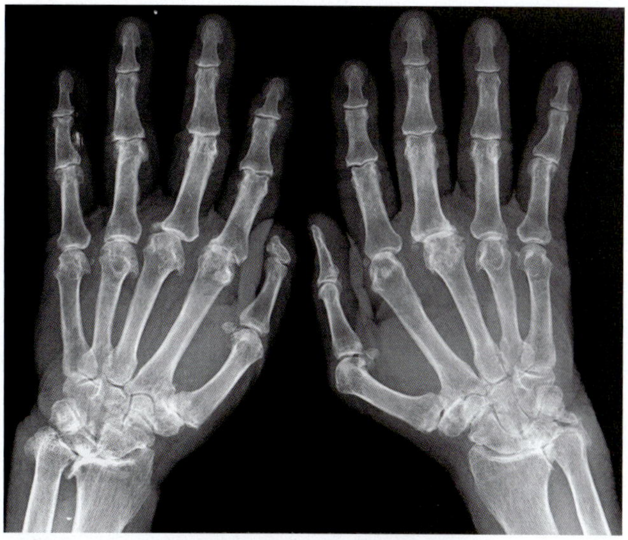

Figure 7.29 ■ CPPD crystal deposition disease. Dorsovolar radiograph of both hands of a 60-year-old man shows typical for this condition arthropathy of the radiocarpal, metacarpophalangeal, and proximal interphalangeal joints.

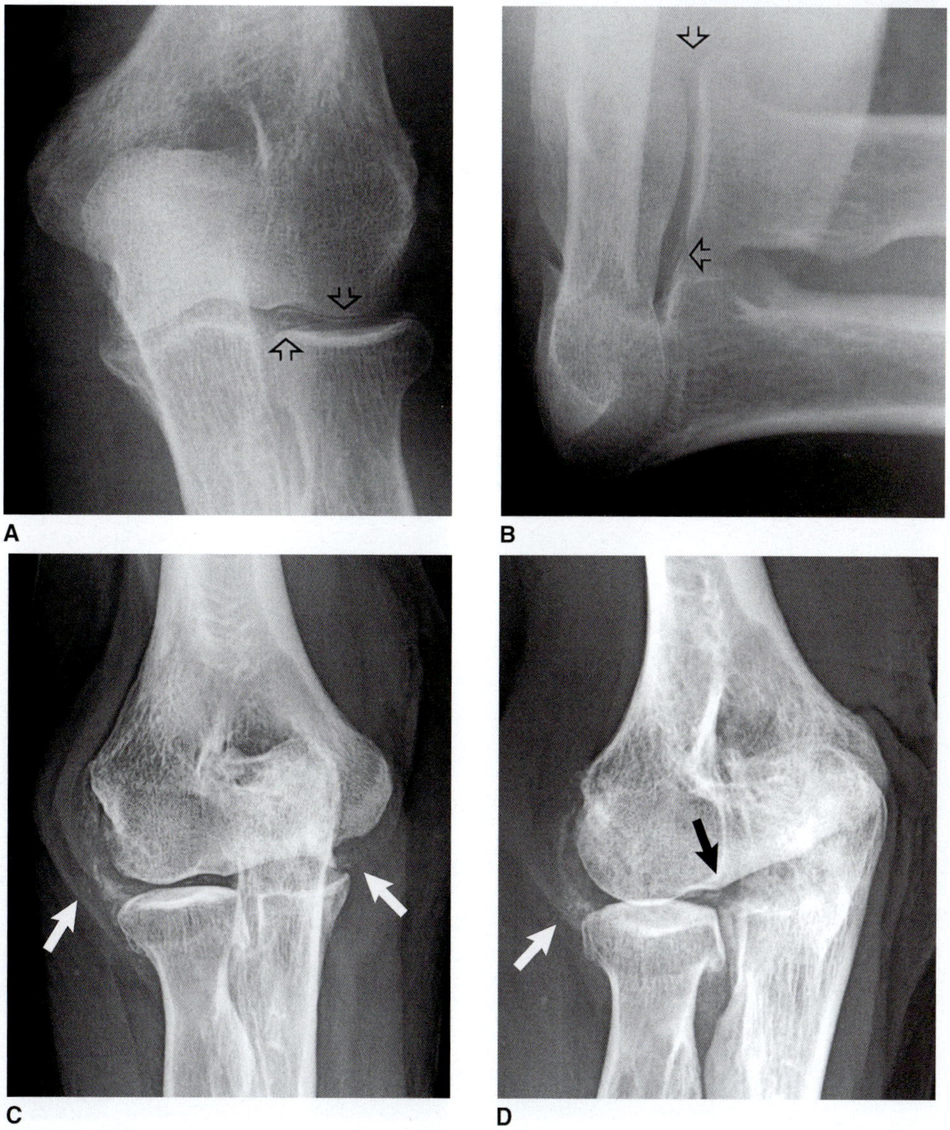

Figure 7.30 ■ CPPD crystal deposition disease. Anteroposterior **(A)** and radial head–capitellum **(B)** views of the right elbow of a 52-year-old woman with pseudogout syndrome demonstrate chondrocalcinosis (*open arrows*) but no other alterations of the joint space. Anteroposterior **(C)** and external oblique **(D)** radiographs of the right elbow of a 57-year-old man, in addition to extensive chondrocalcinosis (*arrows*) demonstrate also early osteoarthritic-like changes of the radiocapitellar joint.

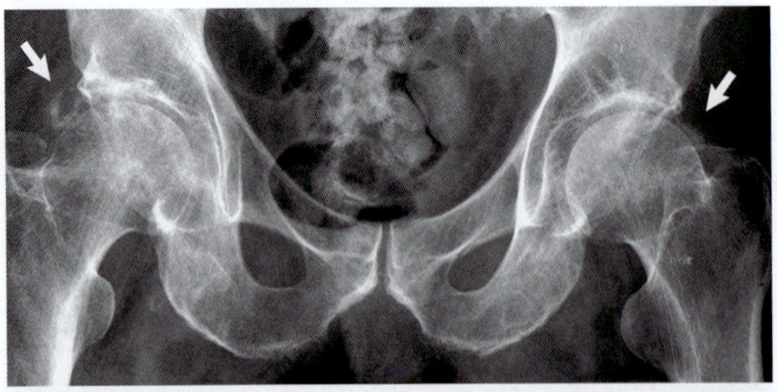

A

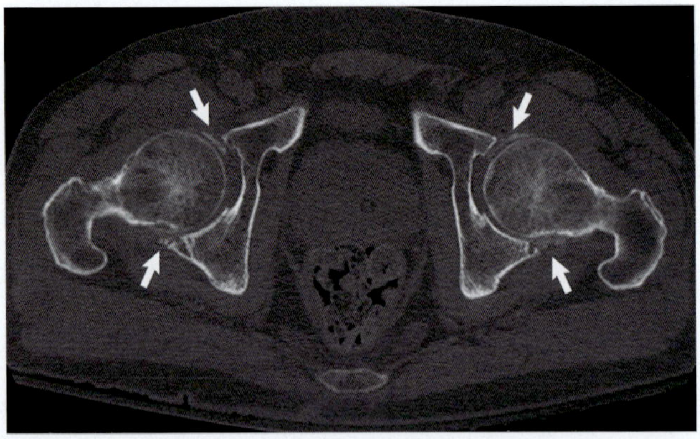

B

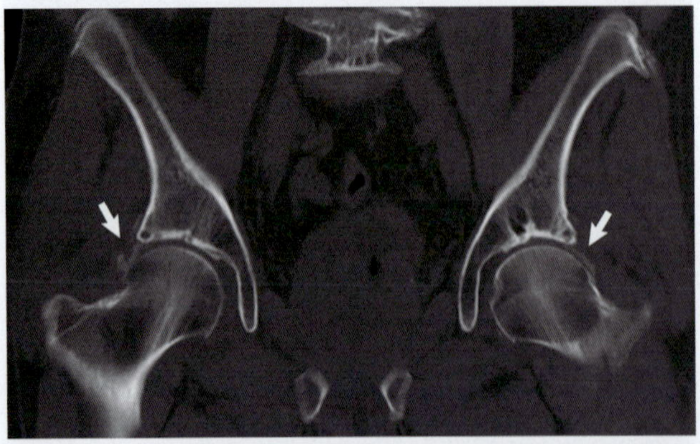

C

Figure 7.31 ■ **CPPD crystal deposition disease.** **A:** Anteroposterior radiograph of the pelvis of a 61-year-old man shows chondrocalcinosis within the hyaline cartilage of the femoral heads and in the fibrocartilaginous acetabular labra (*arrows*). Axial **(B)** and coronal reformatted **(C)** CT images demonstrate more accurately the calcific deposits within the hip joints (*arrows*). Note also subchondral cystlike lesions of both acetabula.

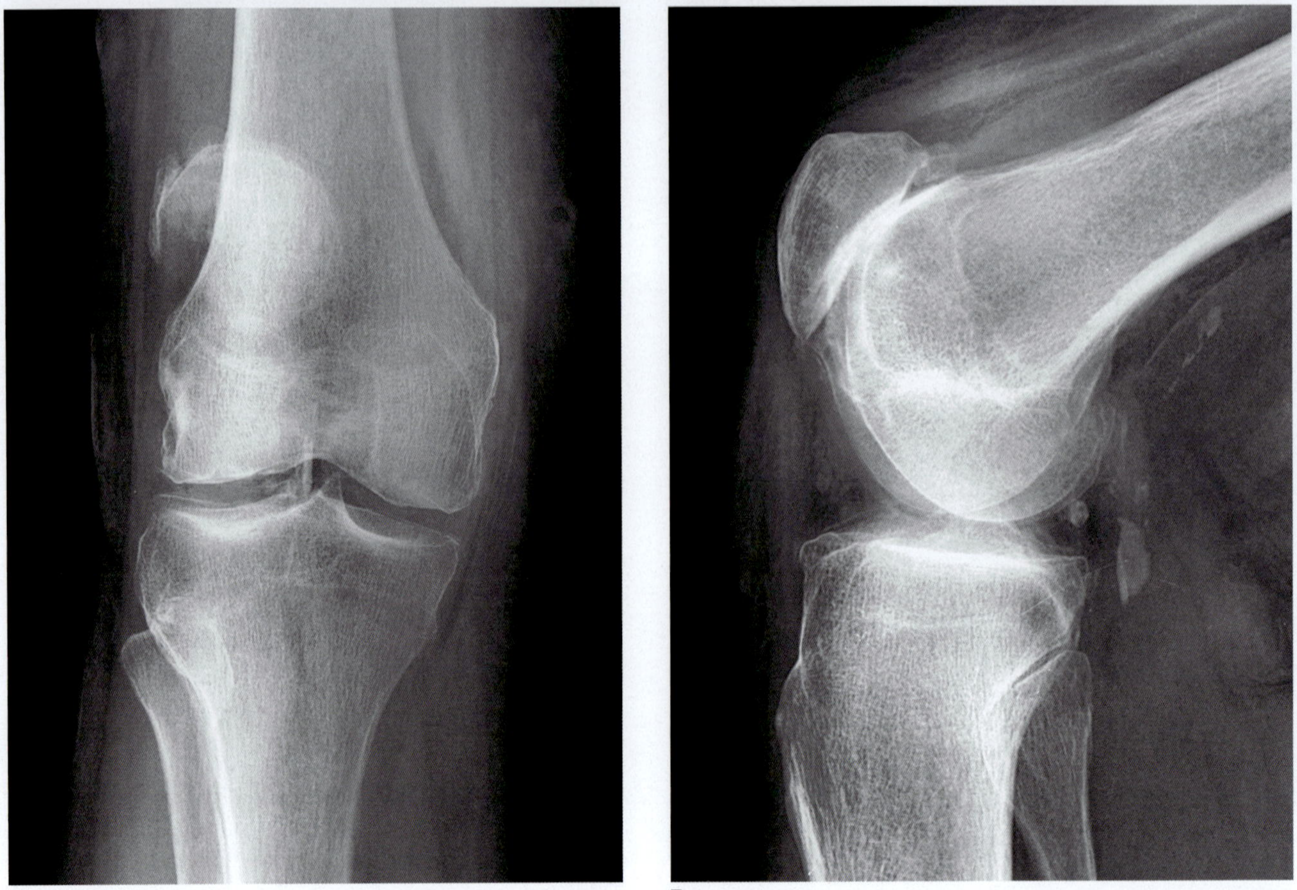

A B

Figure 7.32 ■ **CPPD crystal deposition disease.** Anteroposterior **(A)** and lateral **(B)** radiographs of the right knee of a 58-year-old woman, whose knee joint aspiration revealed calcium pyrophosphate crystals, show chondrocalcinosis and marked narrowing of the femoropatellar joint.

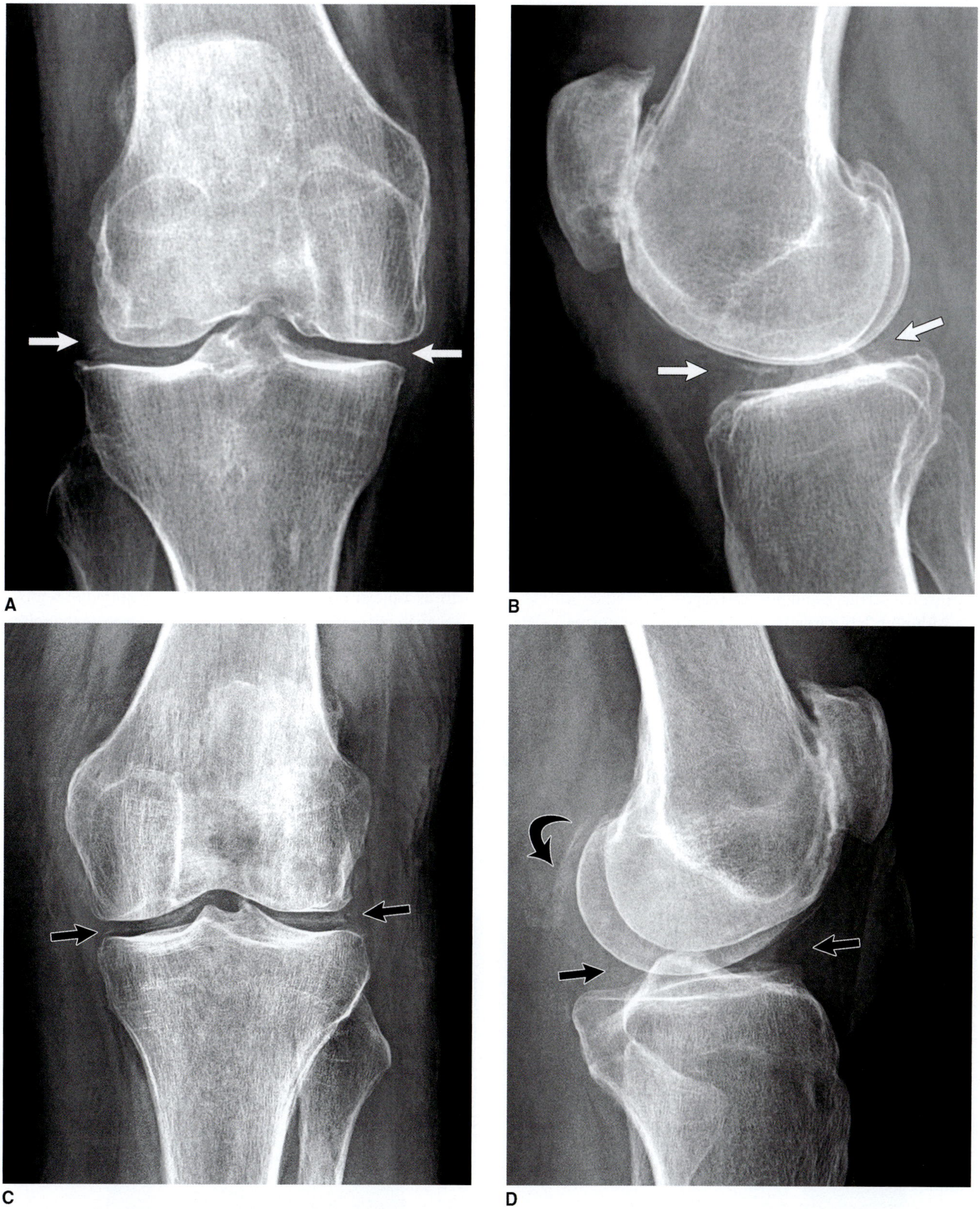

Figure 7.33 ■ **CPPD crystal deposition disease.** Anteroposterior **(A)** and lateral **(B)** radiographs of the right knee of a 67-year-old woman show extensive chondrocalcinosis of the fibrocartilaginous menisci (*arrows*) and advanced arthrosis of the femoropatellar joint compartment. Note that the medial and lateral joint compartments are only slightly narrowed. Anteroposterior **(C)** and lateral **(D)** radiographs of the left knee of a 75-year-old woman demonstrate very similar findings: there is severe narrowing and subchondral sclerosis of the femoropatellar joint compartment, but the medial and lateral compartments are essentially within normal range. The *arrows* are pointing to chondrocalcinosis, and the *curved arrow* to calcification within gastrocnemius tendon.

CALCIUM HYDROXYAPATITE (CHA) CRYSTAL DEPOSITION DISEASE

Clinical Features

Resulting from abnormal deposition of calcium hydroxyapatite crystals in and around the joints, CHA crystal deposition disease is more common in women and may at times simulate gout or pseudogout syndrome. Acute symptoms include pain, tenderness on palpation, and local swelling and edema. The syndrome may be associated with other disorders, such as scleroderma, dermatomyositis, MCTD, and chronic renal disease, particularly one treated by hemodialysis. Recent investigations suggested a genetic predisposition for this condition. Amor and associates raised the possibility of an inherited defect that might be responsible for the development of CHA crystal deposition disease by demonstrating an increased prevalence of the histocompatibility antigen of HLA-A2 and HLA-BW35 in patients affected by this disorder.

CHA crystals are most frequently deposited in periarticular locations, usually in and around tendons, joint capsule, or bursae. This is the feature that distinguishes the syndrome from CPPD crystal deposition disease, which affects primarily hyaline cartilage and fibrocartilage.

Although laboratory findings are usually normal, CHA crystal deposition disease may occasionally cause fever, elevated concentration of C-reactive protein, and elevated ESR.

Imaging Features

Radiographic features depend on the site of involvement, but usually cloudlike or dense homogeneous calcific deposits are seen around the joint and tendons. The most common location is around the shoulder joint at the site of the supraspinatus tendon (Figs. 7.34 and 7.35A). At this location, it is commonly referred to as calcific peritendinitis or tendinitis (tendinosis or tendinopathy), calcific periarthritis, or periarthritis calcarea. The MRI manifestations of calcific peritendinitis include low signal intensity deposits adjacent to the tendon with marked inflammatory reaction (Fig. 7.35B, C). Calcific deposits can migrate into the adjacent bone, into the adjacent bursa, or into the tendon extending along the myotendinous plane (Fig. 7.35D, E).

Treatment

Treatment of this condition includes application of shockwave therapy (using sound waves), acetic acid iontophoresis, and drugs such as corticosteroids and cimetidine. Occasionally, arthroscopic or open shoulder surgery is required to remove the calcific deposits. However, it has to be stressed that often the results of the treatment are disappointing.

(Continued on page 294)

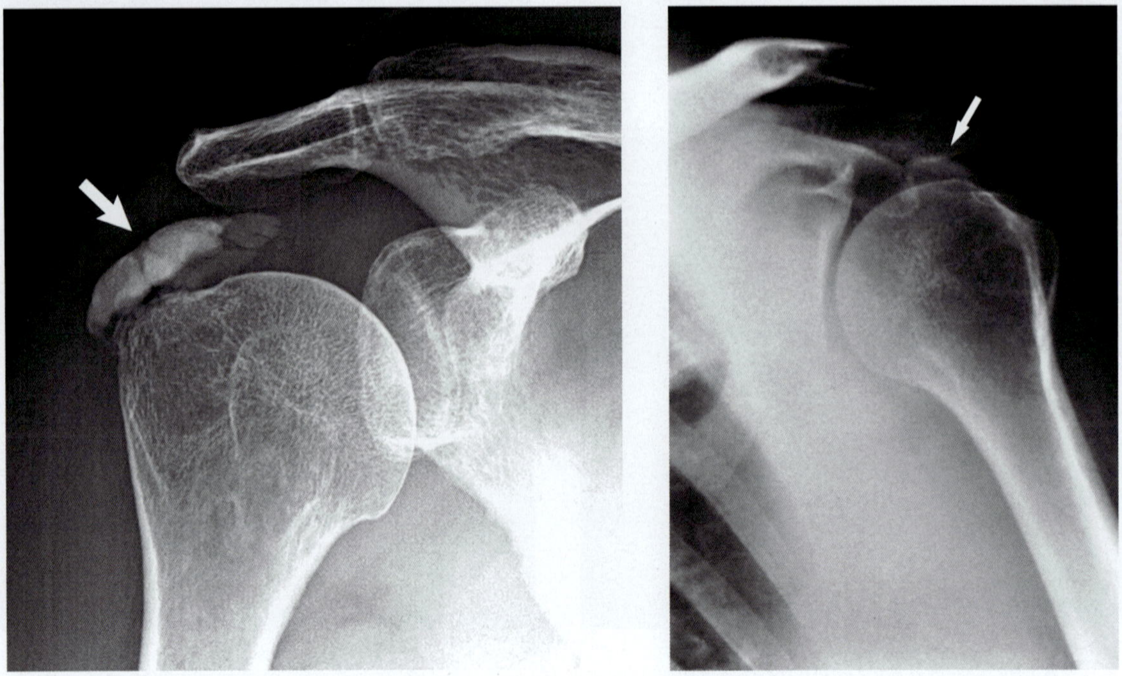

A B

Figure 7.34 ■ CHA crystal deposition disease. A: Anteroposterior radiograph of the right shoulder of a 41-year-old man shows calcific deposit within the attachment of the supraspinatus tendon to the greater tuberosity of the humerus (*arrow*). **B:** Anteroposterior radiograph of the left shoulder (Grashey view) of a 50-year-old woman who had been experiencing pain in this region for several months demonstrates an amorphous, homogenous calcific deposit in the soft tissues at the site of supraspinatus tendon (*arrow*).

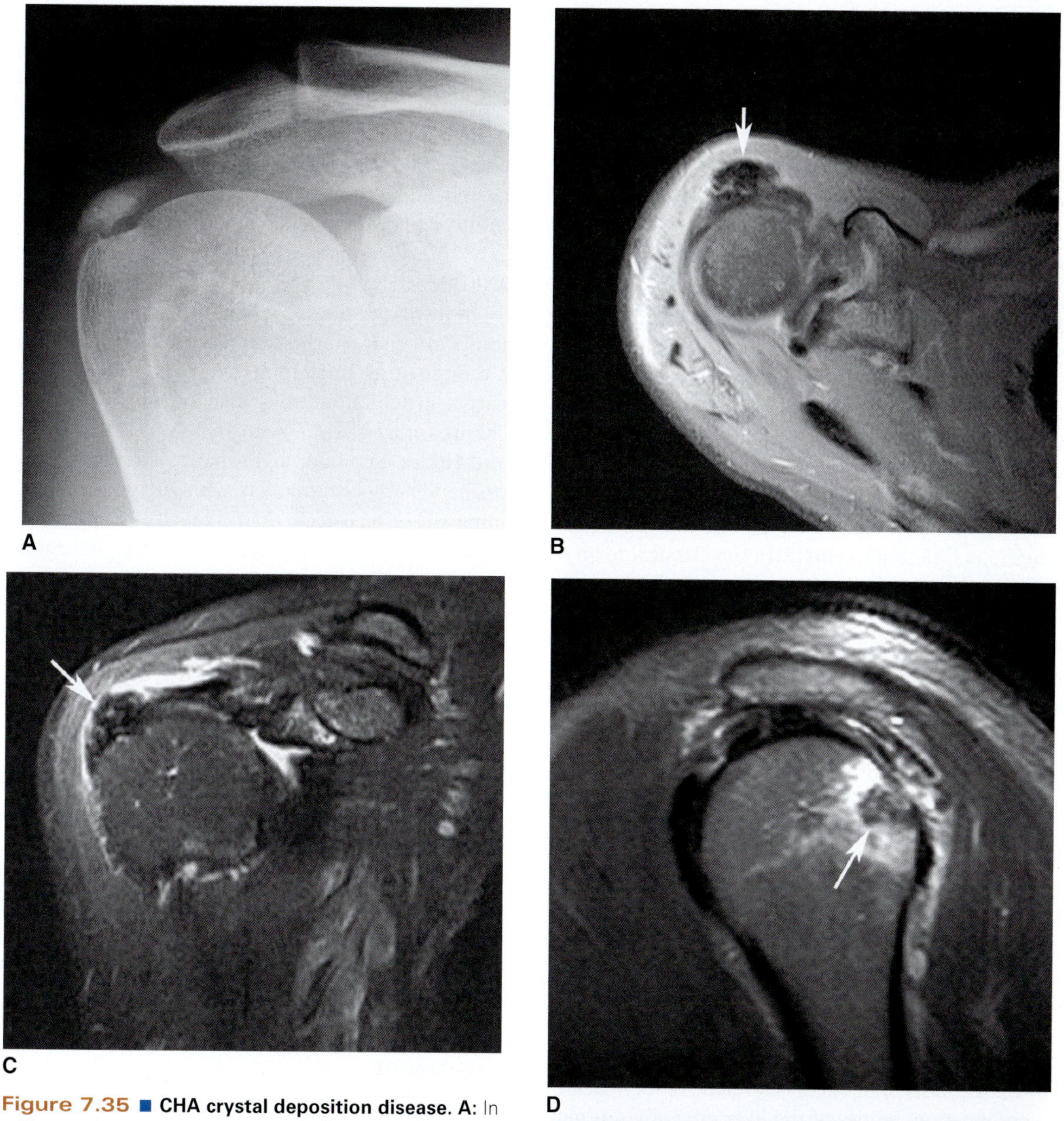

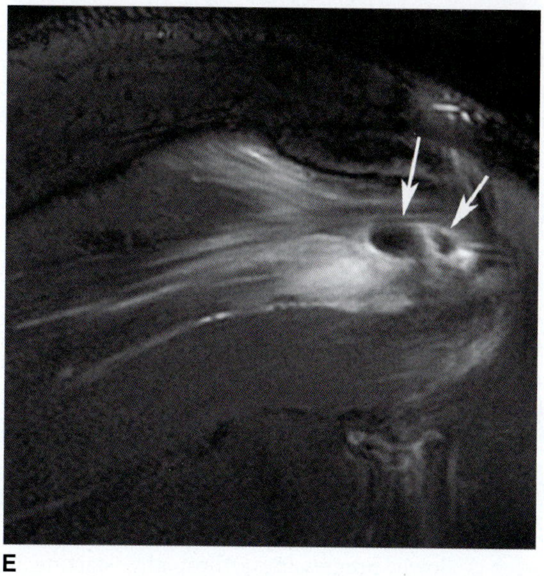

Figure 7.35 ■ **CHA crystal deposition disease. A:** In a 38-year-old woman who presented with left shoulder pain, a calcific deposit is seen at the site of insertion of the supraspinatus tendon to the greater tuberosity of the humerus. **B:** Axial proton density fat-saturated MRI of the shoulder in another patient demonstrates low signal intensity calcium deposit adjacent to the supraspinatus tendon (*arrow*). **C:** Coronal oblique T2-weighted MRI of the same patient shows the hypointense calcific deposit (*arrow*) with surrounding inflammatory changes and subacromial–subdeltoid bursitis. **D:** Sagittal oblique T2-weighted MRI of the shoulder in another patient demonstrates intraosseous migration of the calcific deposits (*arrow*). **E:** Oblique coronal T2-weighted MRI of the shoulder in the same patient shows intramuscular migration of the calcific deposits (*arrows*). Note the severe muscular inflammatory reaction.

HEMOCHROMATOSIS

Clinical and Pathologic Features

Hemochromatosis is a rare autosomal recessive disorder of iron metabolism, characterized by increased intestinal absorption of iron from a normal diet and presenting with iron deposition in various organs, particularly the liver, skin, and pancreas. It may be primary (endogenous or idiopathic), caused by an error in metabolizing iron, or secondary, caused by iron overload. Idiopathic hemochromatosis, with a prevalence of about 4 cases per 1,000 in Europe and North America, may be familial and has been linked with histocompatibility antigens HLA-A3 (placing the gene on the short arm of chromosome 6), HLA-B7, and HLA-B14. The newest studies using a positional cloning technique discovered a novel MHC class 1–type gene, originally called HLA-H, and now termed HFE, containing two missense mutations C282Y and H63D. In the classical form of the disease, cysteine is substituted by tyrosine at amino acid 282 in both alleles. The so-called compound heterozygote is less common (representing about 10% of cases) but is also compatible with hereditary hemochromatosis. In this form, histidine is substituted by aspartic acid at amino acid 63 in one allele and cysteine by tyrosine at amino acid 282 in the other (C282Y/H63D). More recently, additional mutations in other molecules involved in iron metabolism, including hepcidin, hemojuvelin, and ferroportin, have been identified.

The secondary form of hemochromatosis is related to increased intake and accumulation of iron (iron overload) such as occurs in patients with alcoholic liver cirrhosis, multiple blood transfusions, refractory anemia, and in those with chronic excessive oral iron ingestion. Hemochromatosis affects men ten times more frequently than women. It is generally diagnosed between the ages of 40 and 60 on the basis of markedly elevated serum iron levels. For confirmation, biopsy of the liver or synovium may be performed.

Pathologic findings include hemosiderin granules accumulation either in the synovioblasts or in the perivascular histiocytes. Occasionally, synovial villous hypertrophy may be present. Calcification may be seen within the fibrocartilage and hyaline cartilage (chondrocalcinosis). The explanation of the mechanism of this abnormality is based on the fact that ferric salts promote the formation and deposition of intraarticular calcium pyrophosphate crystals by inhibiting the activity of synovial pyrophosphates and decreasing the clearance of intraarticular immune complexes by inhibiting the activity of synovial reticuloendothelial cells.

Imaging Features

Fifty to eighty percent of patients with hemochromatosis will develop a slowly progressing arthropathy, starting in the small joints of the hands, but eventually, the large joints such as hips, knees, and shoulders may become affected (Fig. 7.36). The development of arthropathy appears to be intimately related to the deposition of small amounts of iron or hemosiderin within the affected joints. The intervertebral disks in the cervical and lumbar region may become affected as well. Some investigators believe that the arthropathy seen in this condition differs from typical degenerative joint disease and warrants classification in the group of metabolic arthritides.

In the hand, the second and third metacarpophalangeal joints are characteristically affected (Figs. 7.37 and 7.38), although other small joints such as the interphalangeal and carpal articulations may also be involved. Degenerative changes may also be seen in the shoulders, knees, hips, and ankles. Shoulder arthropathy is relatively common in primary hemochromatosis with imaging findings resembling those of osteoarthritis or CPPD crystal deposition disease. Loss of the articular space, eburnation, subchondral cyst formation, and osteophytosis are the most prominent radiographic features. The morphologic abnormalities may occasionally mimic those seen in rheumatoid arthritis.

MRI has been used for detection and quantification of iron overload in the liver, spleen, and pancreas, as the strong paramagnetic properties of the stored iron cause a significant decrease in T2 relaxation times of the affected tissues. However, accumulation of iron in the synovium or in articular cartilage is less pronounced, unless gradient echo sequences, which are more susceptible to the paramagnetic properties of iron, are used (Fig. 7.39). Nevertheless, MR imaging may demonstrate abnormalities of the menisci and articular cartilage including erosive changes and cyst formation.

Treatment

The treatment of hemochromatosis consists of phlebotomy on a regular basis. Early diagnosis is essential to positive results. Unfortunately, one survey of 2,851 patients with hemochromatosis showed that patients had consulted a physician after an average 2 years of symptoms, and on average, it took additional 10 years before the diagnosis was made.

WILSON DISEASE

Clinical and Pathologic Features

Known also as hepatolenticular degeneration, Wilson disease is a rare autosomal recessive inherited genetic disorder of copper metabolism. A defective *ATP7B* gene and related mutations have been mapped to chromosome 13 (13q14.3). The gene encodes intracellular copper-transporting P-type ATPase that transports copper into bile and incorporates

(Continued on page 297)

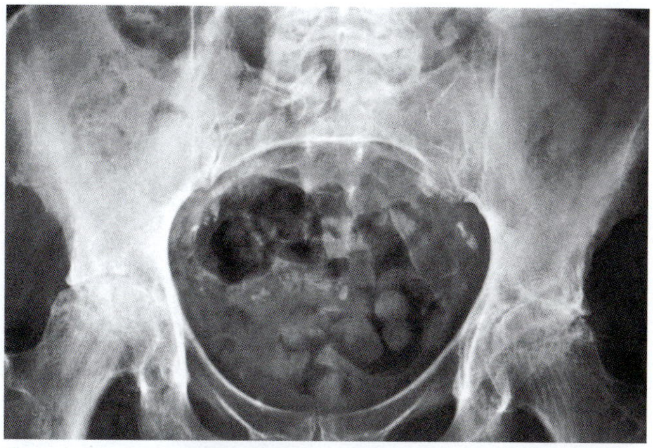

A

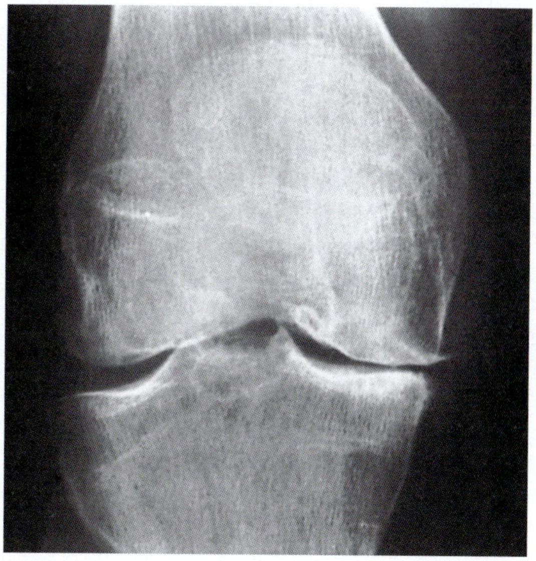

B

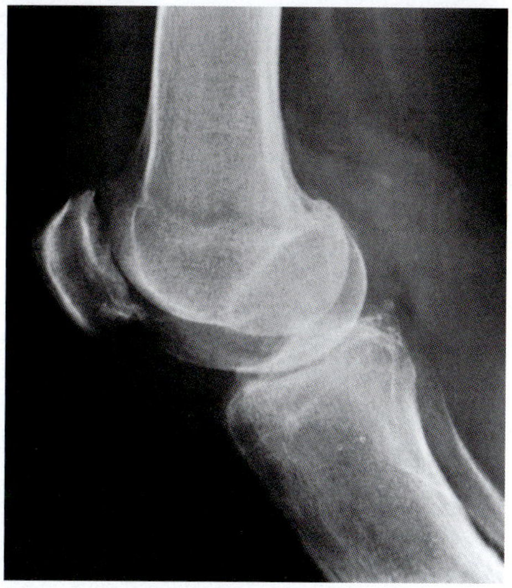

C

Figure 7.36 ■ **Hemochromatosis.** A 67-year-old woman was diagnosed with hemochromatosis arthropathy. **A:** Anteroposterior radiograph of the pelvis shows advanced arthritis of both hip joints. Severe concentric narrowing of joint space, subchondral sclerosis, and periarticular cysts are typical of hemochromatosis. Anteroposterior **(B)** and lateral **(C)** radiographs of the right knee demonstrate predilection for medial and femoropatellar compartments. Joint space narrowing and marked subarticular sclerosis with small osteophyte formation are characteristic.

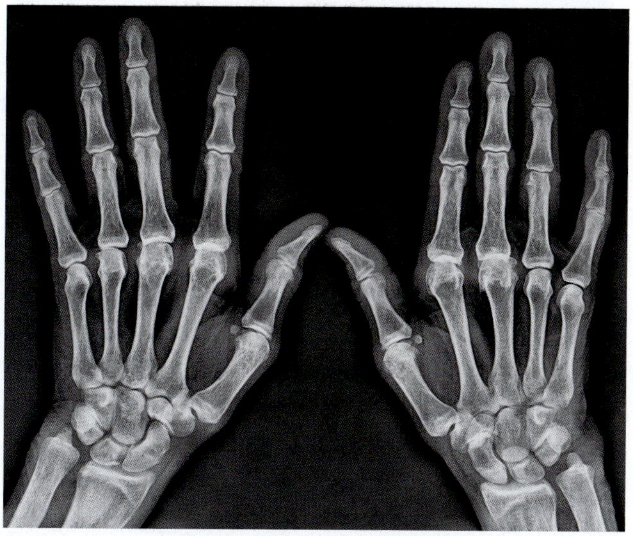

A

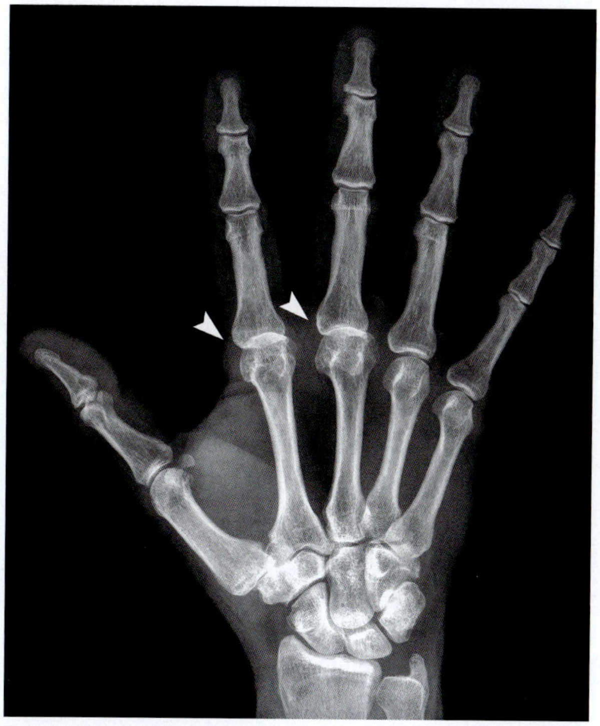

B

Figure 7.37 ■ **Hemochromatosis. A:** Dorsovolar radiograph of the hands of a 50-year-old man shows characteristic involvement of the second and third matacarpophalangeal joints. **B:** In another patient, a 41-year-old man, observe arthropathy of the second and third matacarpophalangeal joints of the left hand (*arrowheads*).

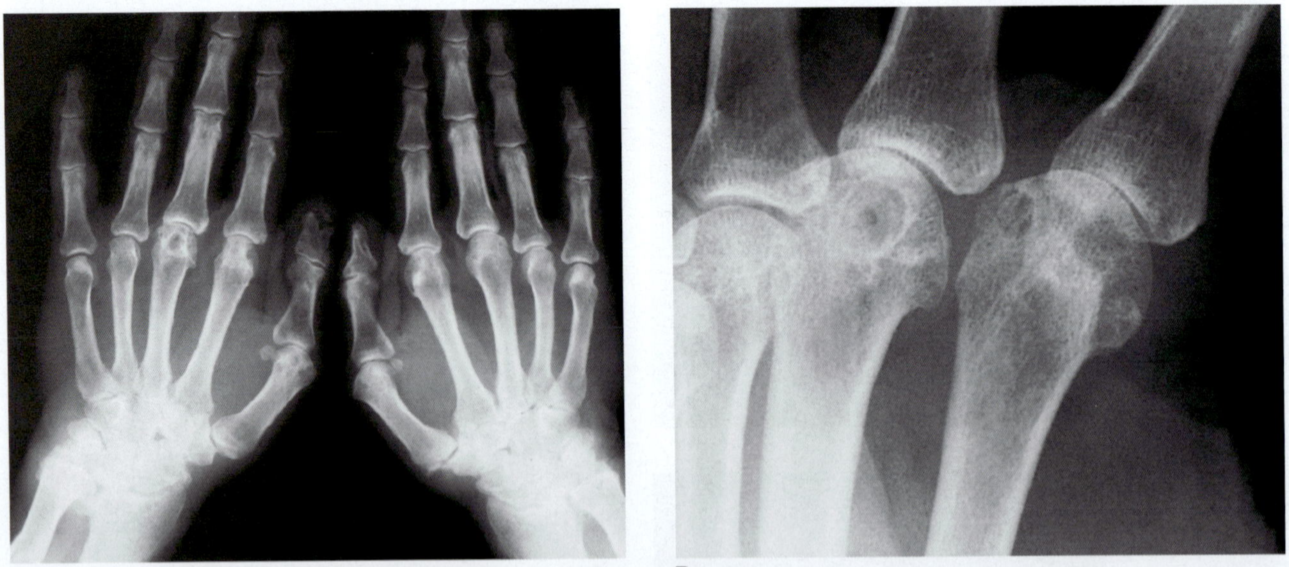

A B

Figure 7.38 ■ Hemochromatosis. A: Dorsovolar radiograph of both hands of a 45-year-old man shows typical abnormalities of hemochromatosis predominantly affecting wrists and metacarpophalangeal joints. **B:** A coned-down magnified radiograph of the second and third metacarpophalangeal joints of the right hand demonstrates characteristic involvement of the metacarpal heads.

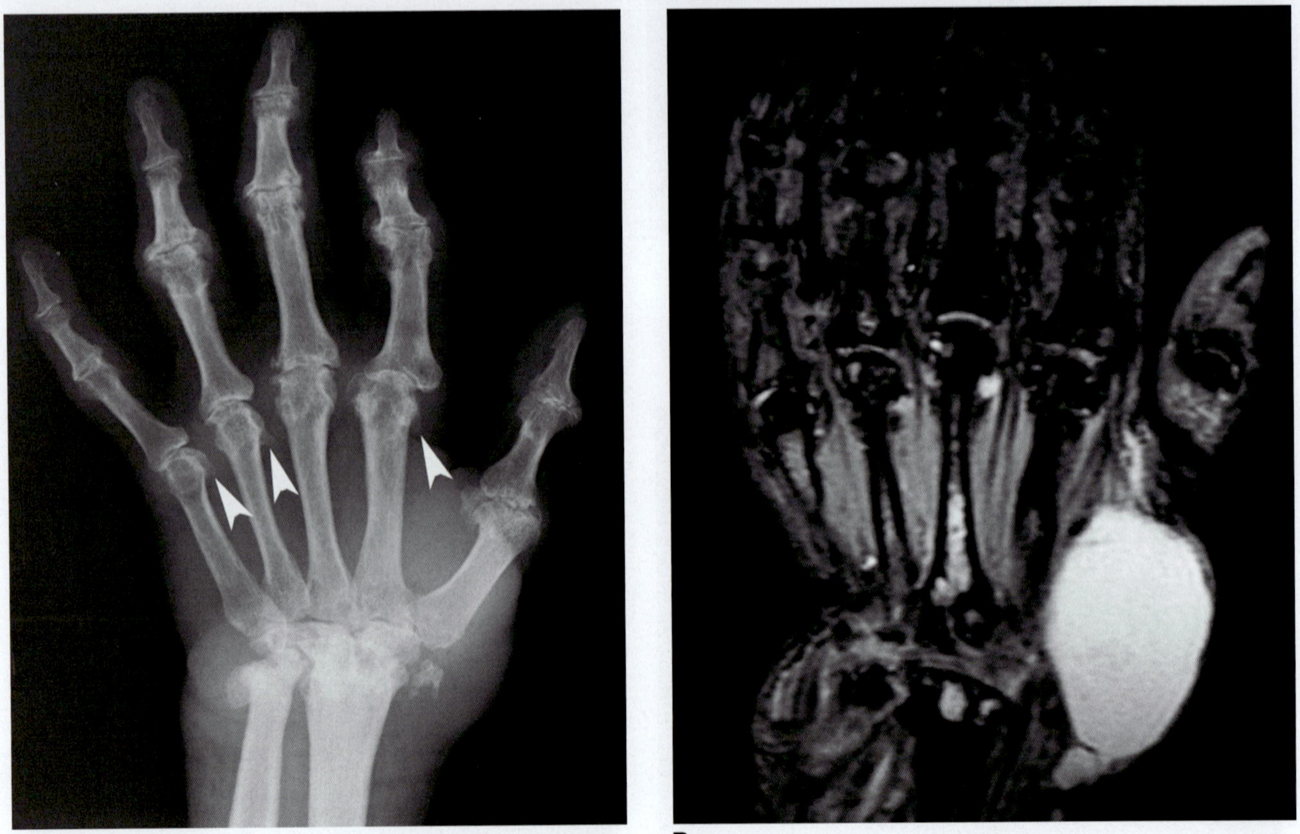

A B

Figure 7.39 ■ Hemochromatosis. A: Dorsovolar radiograph of the right hand of the patient with advanced arthropathy because of hemochromatosis shows the characteristic "hooks" of the heads of the metacarpals (*arrowheads*). **B:** Coronal gradient echo (GRE) MR image demonstrates the multiple erosions of the distal radius, metacarpals, and phalanges, and the secondary severe degenerative arthropathy. The incidental finding, not related to hemochromatosis, is a high signal intensity large ganglionic cyst in the radial aspect of the wrist.

it into ceruloplasmin, a 132 kDa protein produced by the liver. The condition is more common in men than in women. It is characterized by degenerative changes in the brain (basal ganglia), cirrhosis of the liver, and pathognomonic Kayser-Fleischer rings of greenish-brown pigment deposited in the Descemet membrane in the limbus of the cornea. The clinical symptoms result from accumulation of copper in the body, particularly in the liver and brain. Increased amount of copper within the liver overwhelms the proteins that normally bind it, causing oxidative damage through the process known as Fenton chemistry (or Fenton reaction). This damage eventually leads to chronic hepatitis, fibrosis, and liver cirrhosis. Lenticular degeneration leads to neurologic symptoms, including tremor, rigidity, dysarthria, and dyscoordination. Articular abnormalities may be present in about 50% of affected adults. The affected joints include those of the hand, wrist, elbow, shoulder, hip, and knee. Light and electron microscopy failed to detect crystal-containing calcium neither in synovial fluid nor in synovial biopsies. Synovial biopsies showed hyperplasia of synovial lining cells with mild inflammatory response. In the serum, levels of copper and copper-binding protein ceruloplasmin are decreased, and urinary copper excretion is increased. Electron microscopic detection of copper-containing hepatocytic lysosomes, in addition to the quantification of hepatic copper by atomic absorption spectrophotometry, is helpful in the diagnosis of the early stages of Wilson disease.

Imaging Features

Subchondral bone fragmentation, cyst formation, cortical irregularities and sclerosis, and joint narrowing have been described in the literature. The imaging findings resemble those present in CPPD crystal deposition disease and hemochromatosis. Articular cartilage calcification may occur but generally are rare.

Treatment

Copper chelating agents such as trientine, zinc salt, and D-penicillamine along with dietary copper restriction is the treatment of choice. A diet low in copper-containing foods is recommended with avoidance of mushrooms, nuts, chocolate, dried fruit, liver, and shellfish.

ALKAPTONURIA (OCHRONOSIS)

Clinical and Pathologic Features

Alkaptonuria is a rare autosomal-recessive inherited disease characterized by the presence of homogentisic acid in the urine that turns black when oxidized (Fig. 7.40). This metabolic abnormality results from the absence of the enzyme homogentisic acid oxidase, which plays a part in the normal degradation process of the aromatic amino acids tyrosine and phenylalanine. As a consequence, there is significant accumulation of homogentisic acid in various organs, with predilection for connective tissues. The genetic defect is caused by mutations within the homogentisate 1,2-dioxygenase (*HGD*) mapping to the chromosome 3q13.33. The deposition of an abnormal brown–black pigment, a polymer of homogentisic acid, within the intervertebral disks and in the articular cartilage is termed ochronosis (Fig. 7.41). This deposition leads to spondylosis and peripheral arthropathy. As a rule, ochronotic arthropathy is a manifestation of long-standing alkaptonuria. The condition affects men and women equally and is more common in certain areas in Slovakia, Dominican Republic, Jordan, and India. In general, the affected individuals are asymptomatic until adult life, at which time ochronotic arthropathy may develop in the joints of the axial and appendicular skeleton. The clinical signs consist of mild pain and a decreased range of motion in various joints. When the spine is involved, back pain and stiffness are the usual symptoms. Nonarticular features of ochronosis include bluish discoloration and calcification of the ear pinnae, triangular pigmentation of the sclera, and pigmentation over the nose, axillae, and groins.

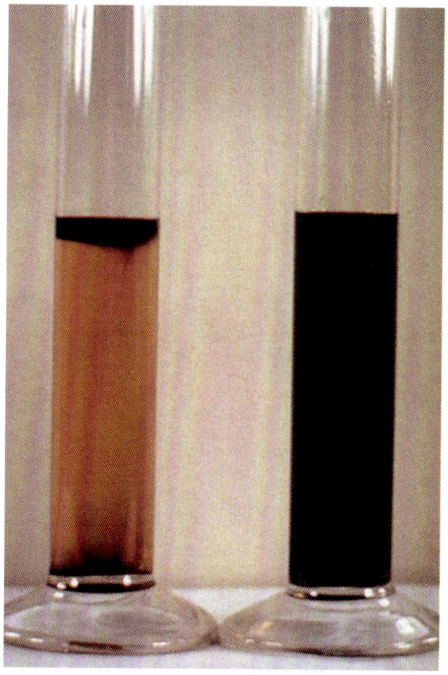

Figure 7.40 ■ Alkaptonuria. Two flasks contain urine from a patient with ochronosis. In the flask, on the left-hand side, the urine has been left to stand for 15 minutes. Some darkening is apparent on the surface because of oxidation of homogentisic acid. In the flask on the right, after 2 hours the urine has become entirely black. (From Bullough PG, Boachie-Adjei O. *Atlas of Spinal Diseases.* New York, NY: Gower Medical Publishing; 1988, Fig. 6.13, p. 75.)

Imaging Features

The radiographic presentation includes dystrophic calcifications, most commonly in the intervertebral disks and the articular cartilage, tendons, and ligaments (Fig. 7.42). Osteoporosis is usually present. Disk spaces are narrowed,

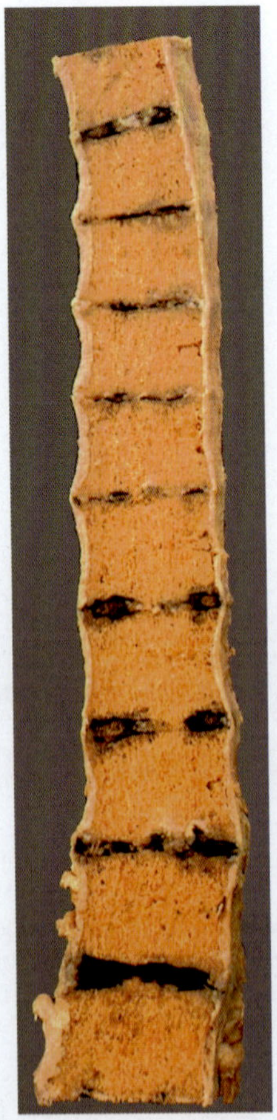

Figure 7.41 ■ Pathology of ochronosis. Sagitally sectioned spine specimen shows black pigmentation within the narrowed intervertebral disks. (From Bullough PG, Boachie-Adjei O. *Atlas of Spinal Diseases*. New York, NY: Gower Medical Publishing; 1988, Fig. 6.15, p. 75.)

with occasional vacuum phenomena. The extraspinal abnormalities are limited to involvement of the sacroiliac joints, the symphysis pubis, and the large peripheral joints, which are likewise narrowed and show periarticular sclerosis with occasional small osteophytes. Tendinous calcifications and ossifications may occur, at times leading to tendon rupture. The radiographic appearance may mimic that of degenerative joint disease or CPPD.

Treatment

The medical treatment includes the high doses of ascorbic acid (vitamin C), and herbicide drug nitisinone, that blocks the synthesis of homogentisic acid. The latter medication acts as an inhibitor of the enzyme 4-hydroxyphenylpyruvate dioxygenase, which mediates formation of homogentisic acid from 4-hydroxyphenulpyruvic acid. The surgical intervention includes diskectomy and spinal fusion, and arthroplasties of the affected joints.

HYPERPARATHYROIDISM

Clinical and Pathologic Features

Hyperparathyroidism, also known as *generalized osteitis fibrosa cystica* or *Recklinghausen disease of bone*, is the result of overactivity of the parathyroid glands, which produce parathormone (PTH). Increased production of this hormone is secondary to either adenoma (90% of cases) or hyperplasia of glands (9% of cases); only in very rare instances (1%) does hyperparathyroidism occur secondary to parathyroid

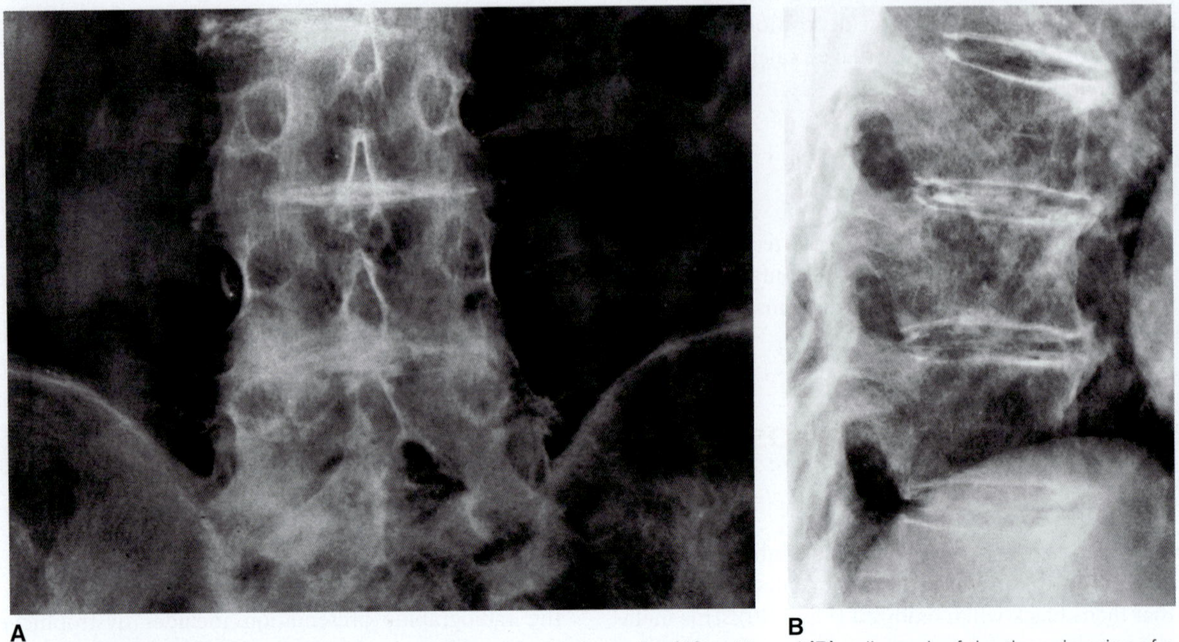

Figure 7.42 ■ Ochronosis. Anteroposterior radiograph of the lumbar spine **(A)** and lateral **(B)** radiograph of the thoracic spine of a 64-year-old woman with a clinical diagnosis of alkaptonuria demonstrate narrowing of several intervertebral disk spaces associated with marginal anterior osteophytes and moderate osteoporosis. Characteristic calcifications of multiple intervertebral disks are a hallmark of ochronosis.

carcinoma. Excessive secretion of PTH, which acts on the kidneys and on bones, leads to disturbances in calcium and phosphorus metabolism, resulting in hypercalcemia, hyperphosphaturia, and hypophosphatemia. Renal excretion of calcium and phosphate is increased, and serum levels of calcium are elevated, whereas those of phosphorous are reduced; serum levels of alkaline phosphatase are also elevated.

Hyperparathyroidism can be divided into primary, secondary, and tertiary forms. The classic form of the disorder, *primary hyperparathyroidism*, is marked by increased secretion of parathormone by the parathyroid glands. PTH secretion is mediated by an increase in serum ionized calcium levels, which affects the calcium-sensing receptors on the plasma membranes of parathyroid cells. If parathyroid glands do not respond to this feedback loop, PTH secretion remains elevated because of hypercalcemia, and the result is primary hyperparathyroidism. Women are affected about three times as often as men, and the condition is most commonly seen in the patient's third to fifth decade. Primary hyperparathyroidism is generally a heterogeneous disorder caused by mutations in the *MEN1*, *CDC73*, or *CASR* genes. The *MEN1* gene regulates production of a protein menin, which is a tumor suppressor. The *CDC73* gene provides instructions for making the parafibromin protein, another tumor suppressor. The loss of parafibromin's tumor suppressor function leads to the development of parathyroid adenoma or parathyroid carcinoma. The *CASR* gene provides instructions for production protein called the calcium-sensing receptor (CaSR) responsible for regulating the amount of calcium in the body, in part by controlling the production of parathormone.

An increased secretion of PTH in response to a sustained hypocalcemic state causes *secondary hyperparathyroidism*. Usually, the fundamental cause of parathyroid gland hyperfunction is impaired renal function. Hyperphosphatemia because of renal failure results in chronic hypocalcemia, which in turn promotes increased parathyroid secretion. Although secondary hyperparathyroidism is usually hypocalcemic, it may be normocalcemic as an adaptive response to the hypocalcemic state. *Tertiary hyperparathyroidism* represents a transformation from a hypocalcemic to a hypercalcemic state. The parathyroid glands "escape" from the regulatory effect of serum calcium levels. Patients in whom this escape occurs are usually receiving kidney hemodialysis; they are considered to have autonomous hyperparathyroidism.

Although primary hyperparathyroidism is traditionally synonymous with the hypercalcemic form of the disorder, some patients nonetheless may have normal or even reduced serum calcium levels. For this reason, Reiss and Canterbury proposed an alternative method of classifying hyperparathyroidism based on serum calcium levels. In this system, hyperparathyroidism is considered *hypercalcemic*, *normocalcemic*, or *hypocalcemic*.

Clinical features of hyperparathyroidism are usually fairly characteristic. Classic medical textbooks have described hyperparathyroidism as a disease of "stones and bones," in reference to nephrolithiasis and bone abnormalities encountered in this condition. Patient may present with kidney stones and bone pain and occasionally with a pathologic fracture because of osteopenia.

Pathologic findings consist of ragging and scalloping of bone trabeculae and increased number of osteoclasts on the bone surfaces resulting in characteristic "tunneling" or "dissecting resorption" of trabeculae (Figs. 7.43 and 7.44). In addition noted is fibrovascular proliferation that displaces the bone marrow in a paratrabecular distribution. Other findings include increased amounts of woven bone and marrow fibrosis, particularly abutting trabecular surfaces (Fig. 7.45).

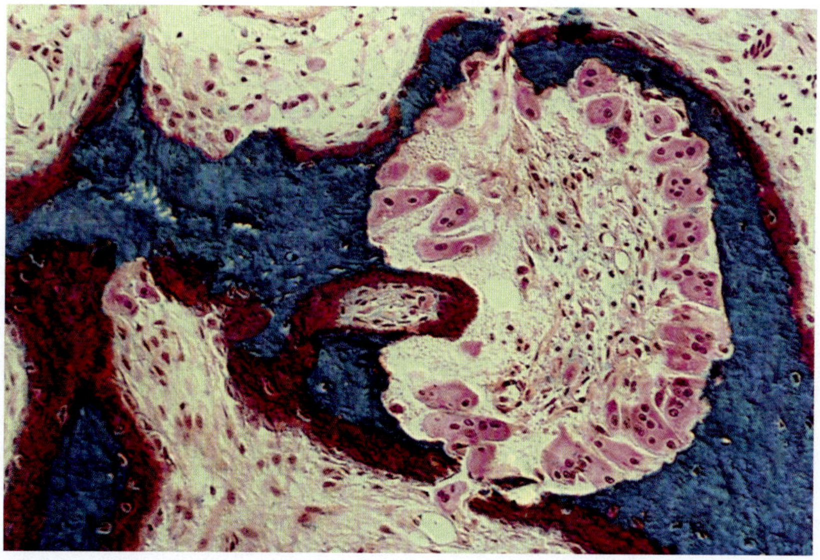

Figure 7.43 ■ Histopathology of hyperparathyroidism. Photomicrograph shows the osteoclastic cancellous bone tunneling, known as "tunneling resorption"' (Goldener stain, original magnification ×10). (From Bullough PG. *Atlas of Orthopedic Pathology with Clinical and Radiologic Correlation.* 2nd ed. New York, NY: Gower Medical Publishing; 1992, Fig. 7.1.)

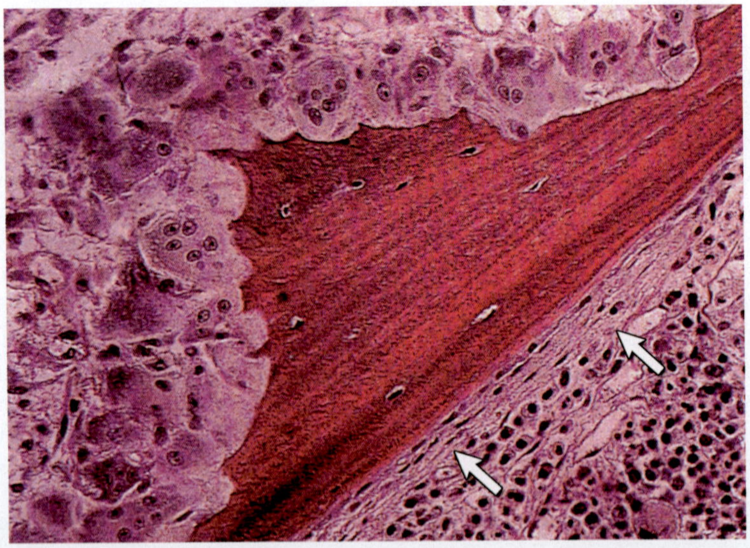

Figure 7.44 ■ Histopathology of hyperparathyroidism. Photomicrograph shows severe osteoclastic resorption of the bone trabecula. Note also peritrabecular fibrosis (*arrows*). (H&E, original magnification ×25). (Modified from Bullough PG. *Atlas of Orthopedic Pathology with Clinical and Radiologic Correlation*. 2nd ed. New York, NY: Gower Medical Publishing; 1992, Fig. 7.17.)

Imaging Features

Application of radiologic techniques in this condition is directed toward detection of parathyroid adenoma, particularly if the tumor is ectopic in location, and imaging the typical features of hyperparathyroidism. Recently, technetium 99m sestamibi (^{99m}Tc-MIBI) single-photon emission CT (SPECT) combined with image-fused CT gained wide acceptance in localizing of ectopic parathyroid adenomas causing primary hyperparathyroidism. Using a hybrid SPECT/CT instrument that couples a SPECT camera with CT camera in a single integrated unit affords the advantage of obtaining the three-dimensional (3D) functional information offered by SPECT with precise anatomic location provided by CT, thus improving the preoperative localization of parathyroid adenoma (Fig. 7.46). Trials using C-11 methionine positron emission tomography also confirmed the effectiveness of this technique to correctly localize abnormal parathyroid glands in patients with hyperparathyroidism.

One of the most characteristic imaging features of hyperparathyroidism is subperiosteal and subchondral bone resorption (Fig. 7.47). Trabecular, intracortical, endosteal, subligamentous, and subtendinous bone resorption can also occur. In the skull, bone resorption is described as a salt-and-pepper appearance and can lead to deceased differentiation between the inner and outer tables. The other imaging feature, although seen not only in this condition but also in other diseases associated with osteopenia,

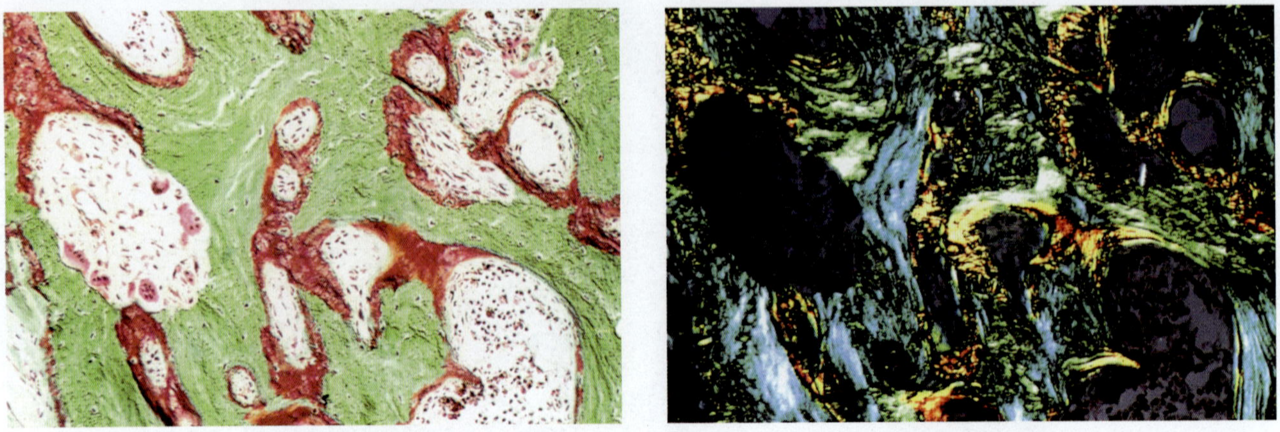

A B

Figure 7.45 ■ Histopathology of hyperparathyroidism. A: Photomicrograph shows bone marrow fibrosis, dissecting trabecular resorption, and increased amount of unmineralized bone (*staining red*) (Goldener stain, original magnification ×5). **B:** In polarized light the increased amount of osteoid and extensive amount of woven bone is more clearly depicted (Goldener stain, original magnification ×5). (From Bullough PG. *Atlas of Orthopedic Pathology with Clinical and Radiologic Correlation*. 2nd ed. New York, NY: Gower Medical Publishing; 1992, Fig. 7.20.)

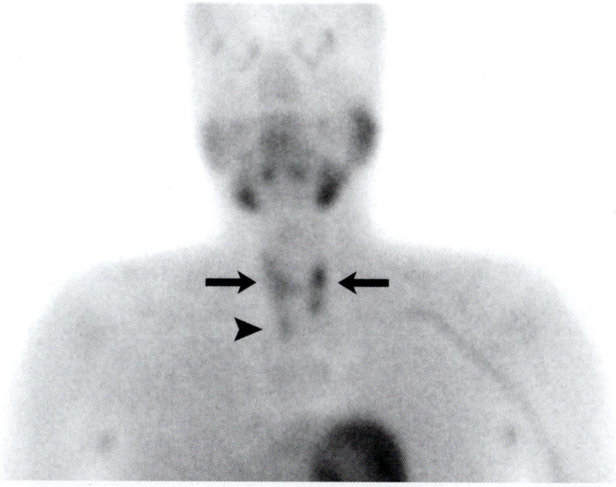
A

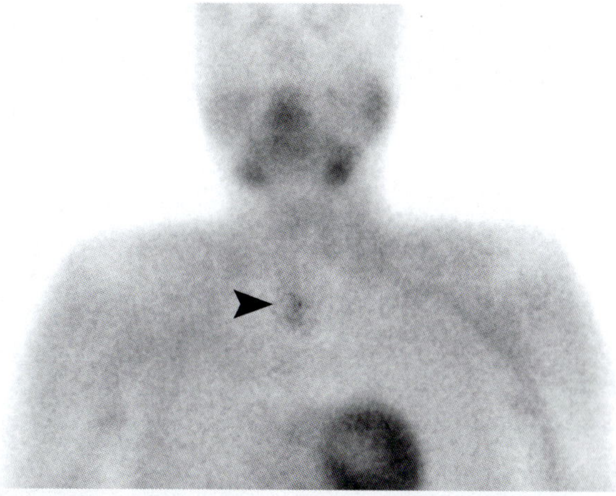
B

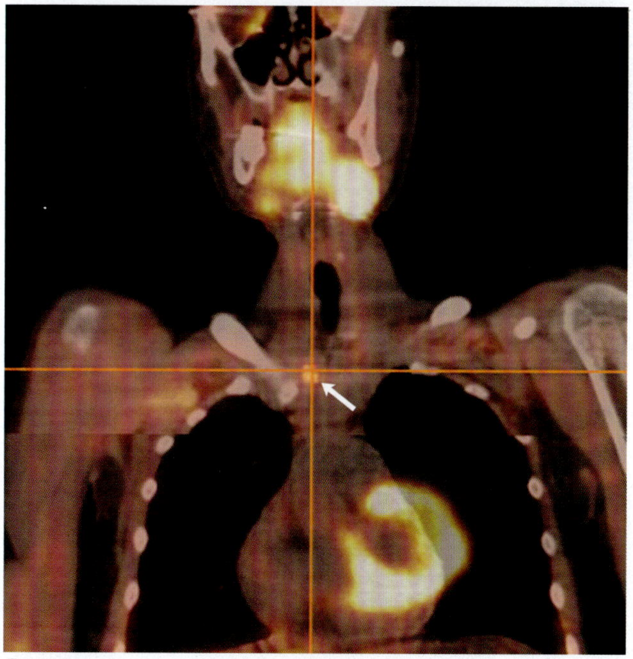
C

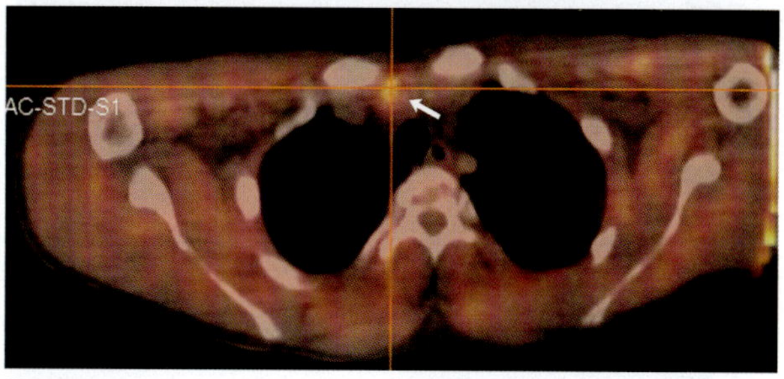

D

Figure 7.46 ■ **SPECT/CT of ectopic parathyroid adenoma.** A 26-year-old man with a clinical and laboratory signs and imaging features of primary hyperparathyroidism was investigated for the presence of parathyroid glands abnormalities. After intravenous injection of 23.8 mCi of ^{99m}Tc-MIBI, the static planar early **(A)** and delayed **(B)** frontal images of the neck and chest were obtained. The early image shows increased uptake of technetium sestamibi in the thyroid gland (*arrows*) and in the parathyroid adenoma, located inferiorly to the thyroid (*arrowhead*). The delayed image shows normal washout from the thyroid gland but persistent activity within the parathyroid adenoma, which is in ectopic location (*arrowhead*). SPECT/CT color-fusion coronal **(C)** and axial (transverse) **(D)** images demonstrate at the crosshairs focus of increased activity consistent with ectopic location of the parathyroid adenoma in the upper right mediastinum (*arrows*).

is cortical tunneling (Fig. 7.48). It occurs very early in a pathologic process and may be found even in the absence of other radiographic abnormalities of hyperparathyroidism. When subchondral bone resorption appears at the margins of certain articulations, it leads to the widening and irregular appearance of the joints, which accounts for articular manifestation or "arthropathy" of hyperparathyroidism. This is frequently noted at the acromioclavicular joint, more pronounced along the clavicular side (Fig. 7.49); at the sternoclavicular joint, sacroiliac articulations, more pronounced at the iliac side (Fig. 7.50); at the symphysis pubis, and sometimes at the metacarpophalangeal and interphalangeal joints (Fig. 7.51). The erosions can mimic rheumatoid arthritis, although they are usually asymptomatic, involve more commonly distal interphalangeal joints (Fig. 7.52), and almost invariably are associated with subperiosteal bone resorption, typical for hyperparathyroidism. Brown tumors, also known as osteoclastomas, are lytic lesions that result from the parathyroid hormone-driven activation of osteoclasts. Although generally solitary, they may be multifocal, commonly involving the facial bones, ribs, pelvic bones, and long and short tubular bones, and can have associated soft tissue component.

The other feature of hyperparathyroidism arthropathy is chondrocalcinosis, which involves calcium deposition in the articular cartilage and fibrocartilage. This finding may mimic degenerative joint disease and CPPD crystal deposition arthropathy. It may be distinguished from the calcification of degenerative joint disease by the absence of arthritic changes in the joint and from CPPD crystal deposition by the presence of osteopenia and other typical features of hyperparathyroidism.

(Continued on page 304)

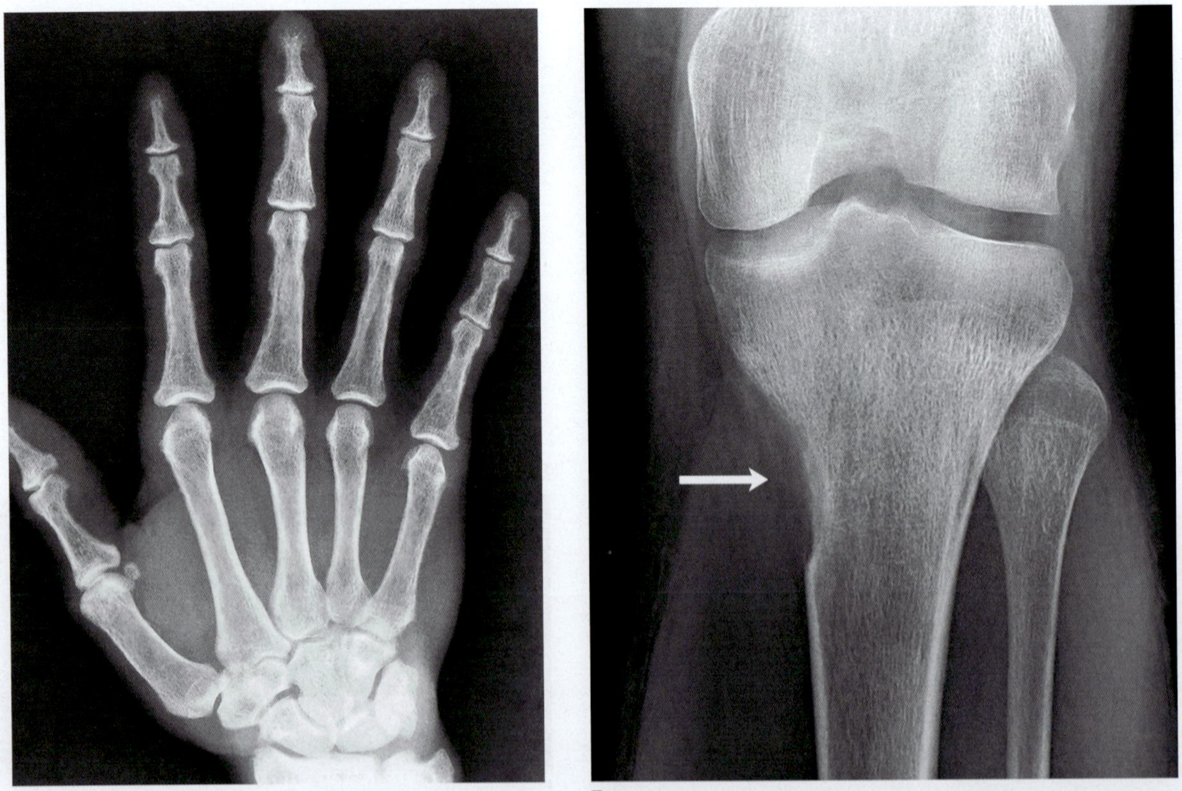

A B

Figure 7.47 ■ Primary hyperparathyroidism. A: Dorsovolar radiograph of the left hand of a 42-year-old man diagnosed with hyperplasia of the parathyroid glands shows typical subperiosteal resorption affecting primarily the radial aspects of the middle phalanges of the middle and index fingers. **B:** Anteroposterior radiograph of the left knee of a 32-year-old man shows a subperiosteal and cortical resorption of the medial aspect of the tibia (*arrow*).

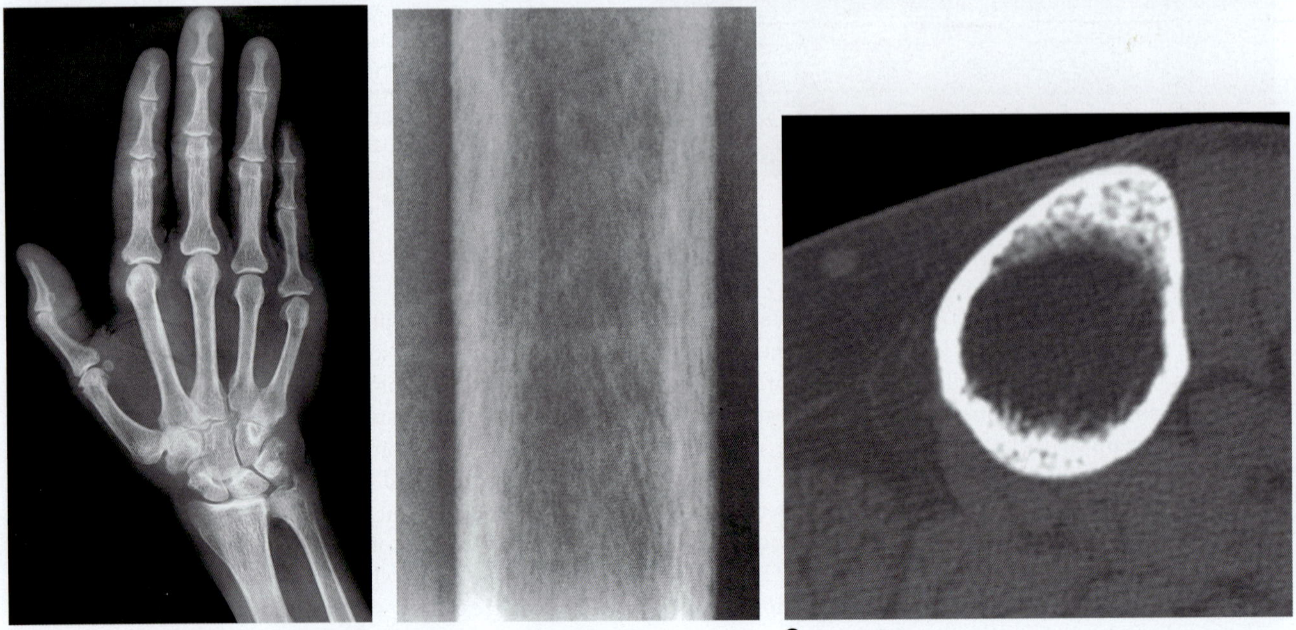

A B C

Figure 7.48 ■ Primary hyperparathyroidism. A: Dorsovolar radiograph of the left hand of a 52-year-old woman demonstrates the typical features of this condition. Note increased bone radiolucency (osteopenia), subperiosteal resorption at the radial aspects of the middle phalanges of the index, middle, and ring fingers, acroosteolysis of the terminal tufts of the index and middle fingers, and loss of osseous trabeculae resulting in cortical tunneling. This latter abnormality is better demonstrated on the magnified radiograph of the femur **(B)**, and on axial CT image **(C)**.

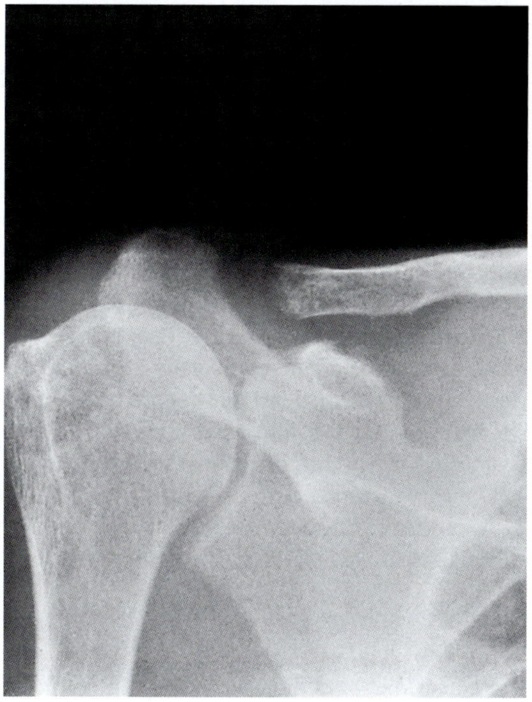

Figure 7.49 ■ **Primary hyperparathyroidism arthropathy.** Anteroposterior radiograph of the right shoulder of a 36-year-old woman shows resorption of the acromial end of the clavicle.

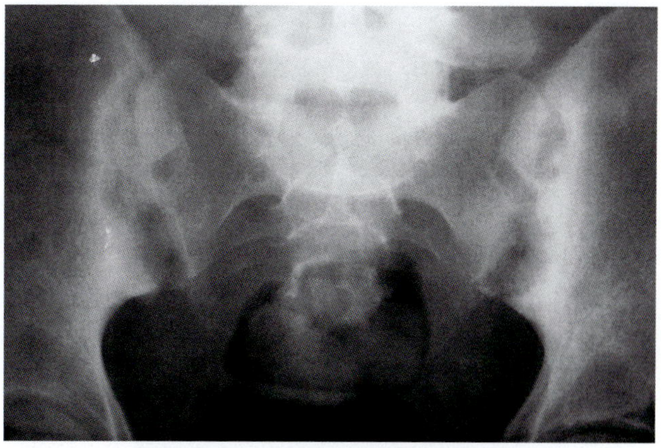

Figure 7.50 ■ **Primary hyperparathyroidism arthropathy.** Subchondral resorption resulted in widening of the sacroiliac joints in this 39-year-old man.

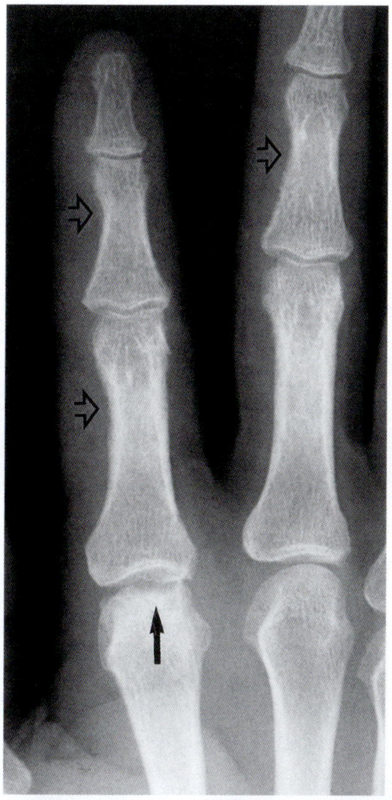

Figure 7.51 ■ **Primary hyperparathyroidism arthropathy.** Subchondral resorption is present at the head of the second metacarpal (*arrow*). Note also subperiosteal resorption at the proximal and distal phalanges (*open arrows*).

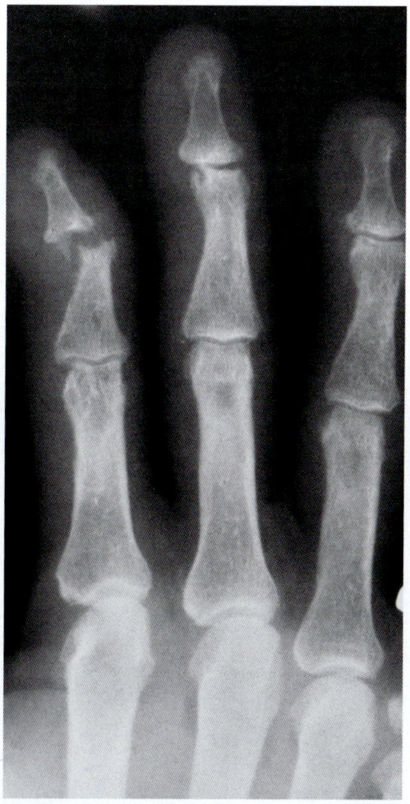

Figure 7.52 ■ **Primary hyperparathyroidism arthropathy.** Typical abnormalities of this condition are manifested in this patient at the distal interphalangeal joints of the index and middle fingers. Note also beginning of the resorption of the distal tufts (acroosteolysis).

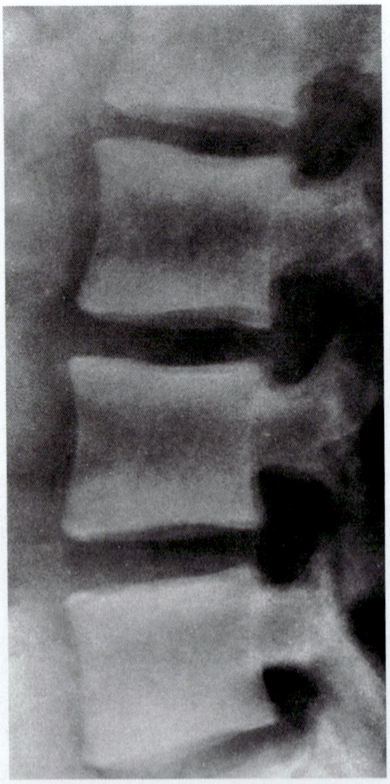

Figure 7.53 ■ **Secondary hyperparathyroidism.** A 17-year-old boy with chronic renal failure developed secondary hyperparathyroidism. Lateral radiograph of the lumbar spine demonstrates sclerotic bands adjacent to the vertebral end plates—the so-called *rugger jersey spine*.

In the secondary hyperparathyroidism, other characteristic features may be present in addition to the imaging findings discussed in the prior text. A generalized increased in bone density occurs, particularly in younger patients. In the spine, this change is reflected in dense sclerotic bands seen adjacent to the vertebral end plates, giving the vertebrae a sandwich-like appearance. This phenomenon is termed *rugger jersey spine* because the sclerotic bands form horizontal stripes resembling those of rugby shirts (Fig. 7.53). Deposition of calcium in fibrocartilage, articular cartilage, and soft tissue is common (Fig. 7.54). Localized destructive changes in bones, similar to those seen in the patients with primary hyperparathyroidism, take the form of cystic lesions of various sizes, commonly referred to as brown tumors (Fig. 7.55). Likewise, subchondral resorption at the site of sacroiliac joints leads to similar widening of these structures as sees in the primary form of this disease (Fig. 7.56).

Treatment

Surgery, consisting of removal of the parathyroid gland/glands, is the most common treatment for primary hyperparathyroidism and provides a cure in about 95% of all cases. Medical treatment includes calcimimetic drugs and hormone replacement therapy.

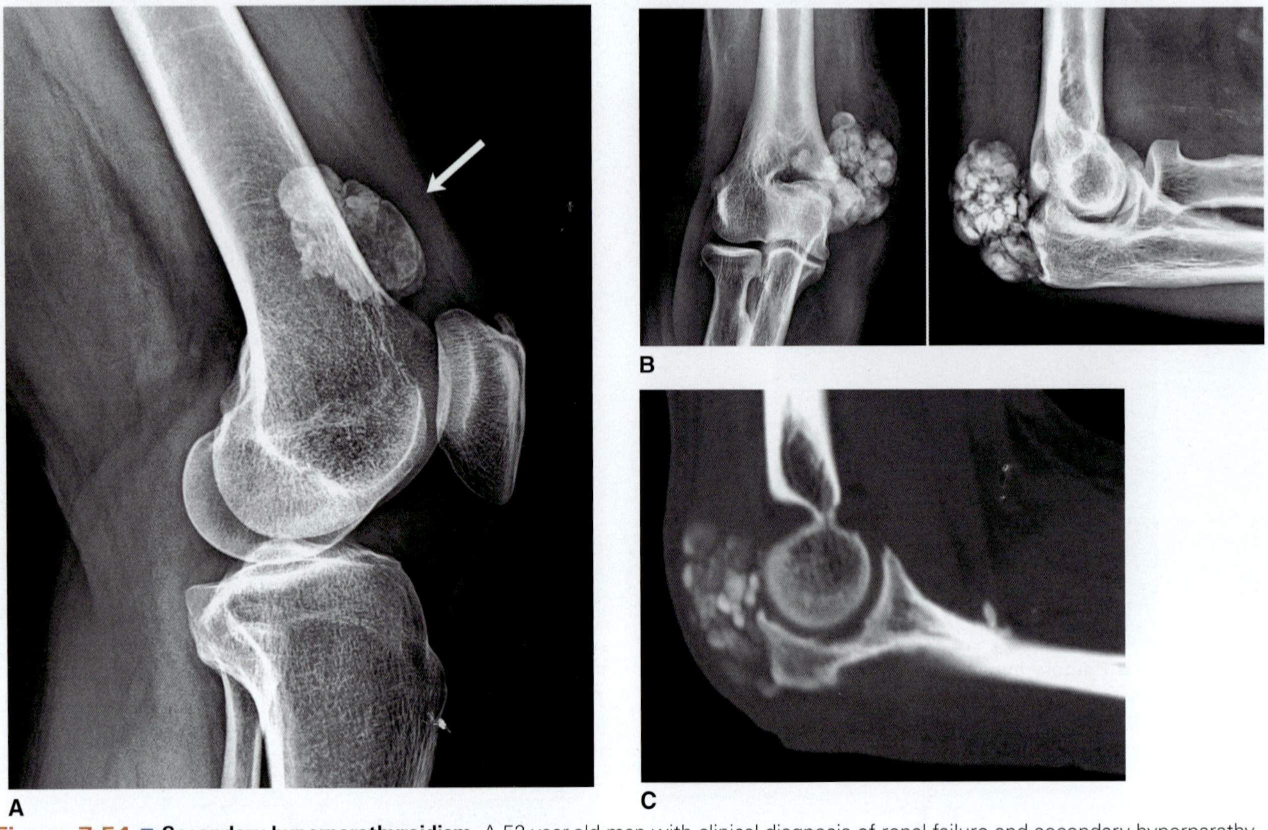

Figure 7.54 ■ **Secondary hyperparathyroidism.** A 52-year-old man with clinical diagnosis of renal failure and secondary hyperparathyroidism presented with soft tissue calcifications at several sites including the knee (*arrow*) **(A)** and elbow **(B, C)**.

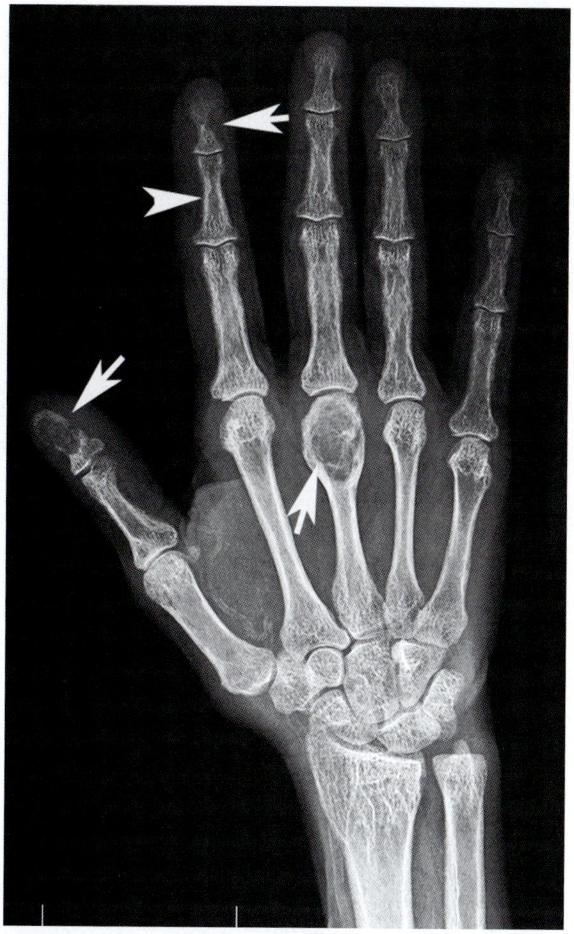

A

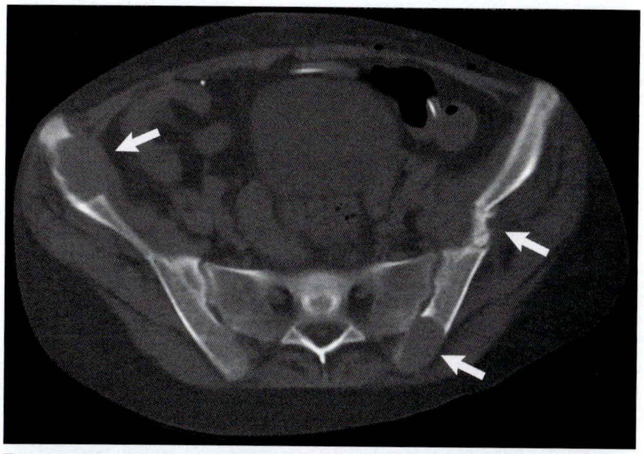

B

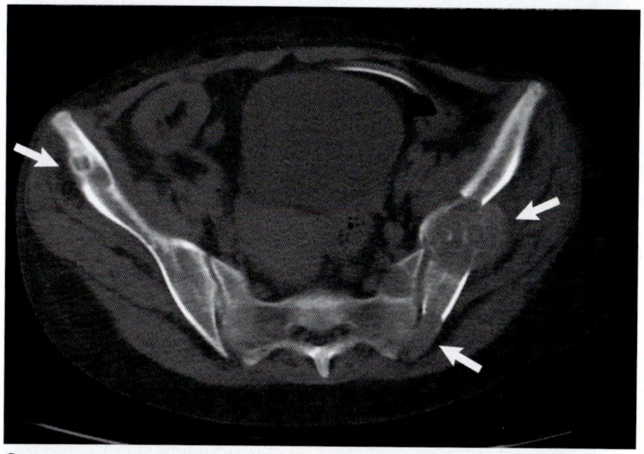

C

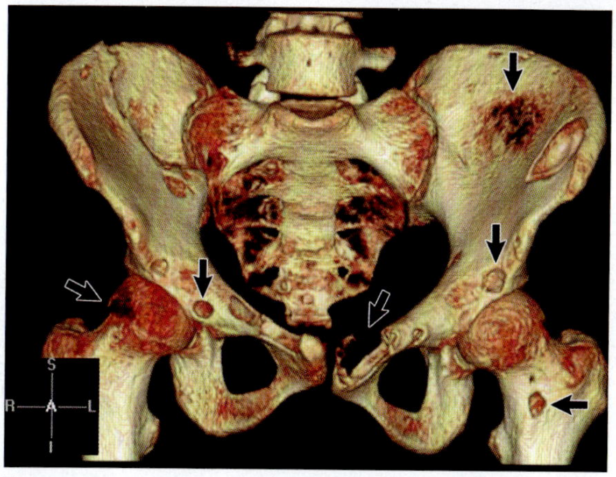

D

Figure 7.55 ■ Secondary hyperparathyroidism. A: Dorsovolar radiograph of the left hand of a 40-year-old woman with chronic renal failure demonstrates several lytic lesions in the third metacarpal head, distal phalanx of the thumb, and distal phalanx of the index finger (*arrows*), representing brown tumors. In addition note subperiosteal bone resorption of the middle phalanx of the index finger (*arrowhead*). Two axial **(B, C)** and 3D reconstructed **(D)** CT images of the pelvis of a 37-year-old man with chronic renal failure show multiple brown tumors exhibiting soft tissue component (*arrows*).

ACROMEGALY

Clinical Features

Acromegaly (from Greek *akros* [extreme or extremities] and *megalos* [large]) is a syndrome resulting from the overproduction of growth hormone (somatotropin or HGH—human growth hormone) by the eosinophilic cells of the anterior lobe of the pituitary gland, as a result of either hyperplasia of the gland or a tumor, after the closure of the growth plates. The onset of clinical symptoms is usually insidious. Gradual enlargement of the hands and feet and exaggeration of the facial features are the earliest manifestations. The characteristic facial changes result from overgrowth of the frontal sinuses, protrusion of the jaw (prognathism), accentuation of the orbital ridges, enlargement of the nose and lips, and thickening and coarsening of the soft tissues of the face. Degenerative joint changes in this condition are the result of hypertrophy of articular cartilage, which is not adequately nourished by synovial fluid because of its abnormal thickness. Arthritis-like symptoms including pain and stiffness are common, and limitation of joint motion becomes apparent.

Imaging Features

The hands exhibit revealing radiographic features. The heads of the metacarpals are enlarged, and irregular bone thickening along the margins results in formation of beaklike osteophytes. Characteristic changes are also seen in the distal phalanges; their bases enlarge and the terminal tufts form spurlike projections (Fig. 7.57). Hypertrophy of the

(Continued on page 307)

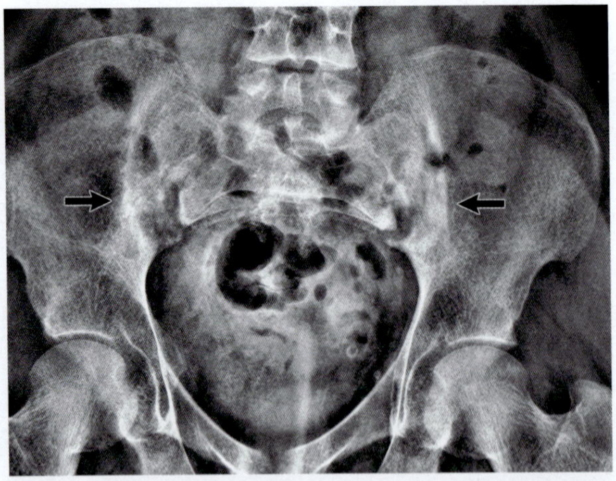

A

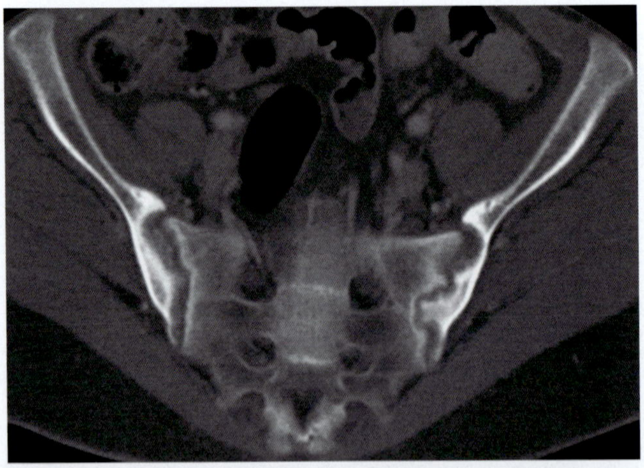

B

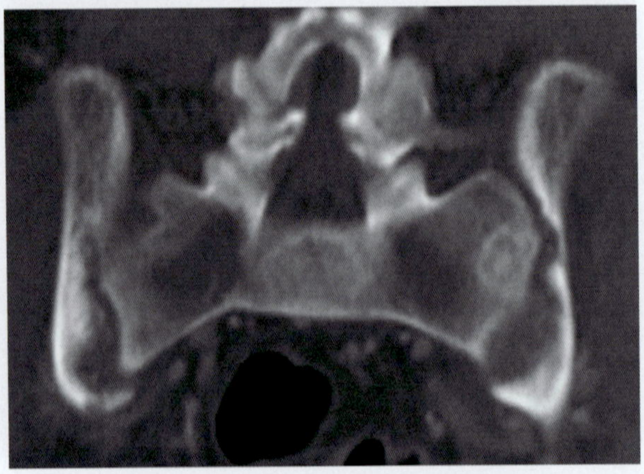

C

Figure 7.56 ■ Secondary hyperparathyroidism arthropathy. Anteroposterior radiograph **(A)** of the pelvis of a 27-year-old woman with chronic renal failure shows widening and peripheral sclerosis of both sacroiliac joints (*arrows*), better demonstrated on axial **(B)** and coronal reformatted **(C)** CT images.

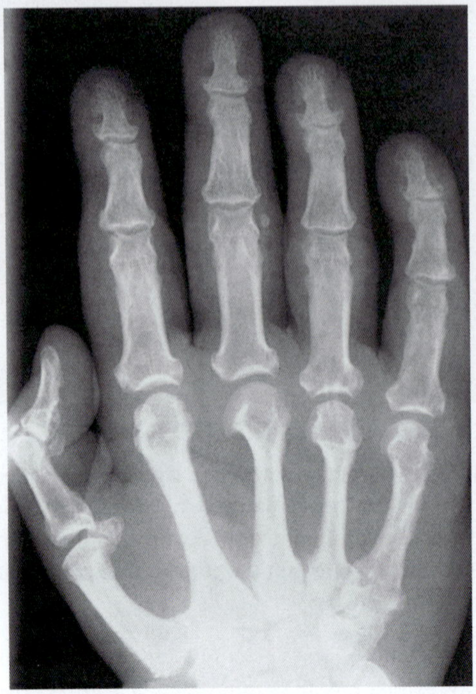

Figure 7.57 ■ Acromegalic arthropathy. Characteristic abnormalities in acromegalic hand include prominence of the soft tissue, enlargement of the tufts and bases of the distal phalanges, widening of the metacarpophalangeal joints, and beaklike osteophytes at the radial aspect of the metacarpal heads. Note also markedly enlarged sesamoid bone at the first metacarpophalangeal joint.

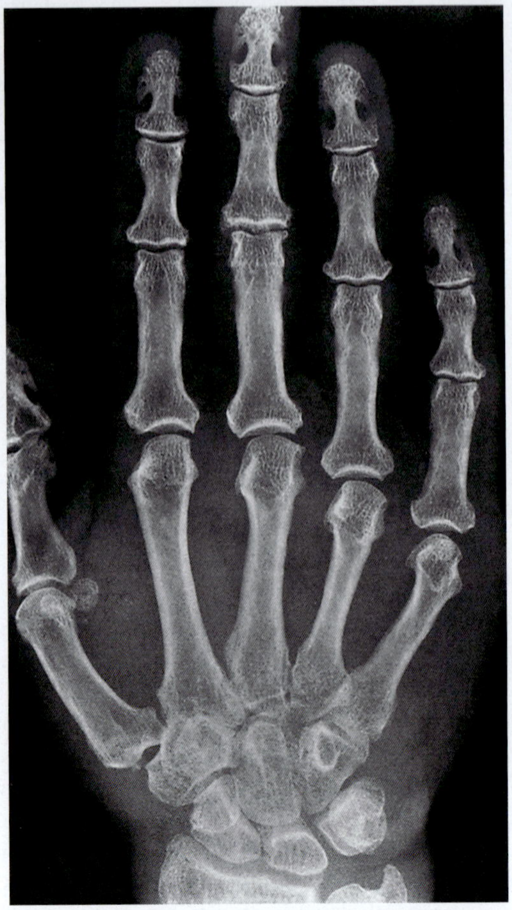

Figure 7.58 ■ Acromegalic arthropathy. Dorsovolar radiograph of the hand of a 38-year-old woman shows characteristic overgrowth of the terminal tufts and spurlike projections. The bases of the terminal phalanges are also enlarged, and the radiographic joint spaces are widened.

soft tissues may occur, leading to the development of square, spadeshaped fingers. After initial overgrowth of cartilage, as reflected by widening of the radiographic joint spaces in the hand, particularly at the metacarpophalangeal joints (Fig. 7.58), a later manifestation of this disorder is thinning of the joint cartilages with osteophyte formation caused by secondary osteoarthritis.

Besides articulations of the hands, large joints such as the hip, knee, and even shoulder or elbow may be affected. In particular, beaklike osteophytes on the inferior aspect of the humeral head, the lateral aspect of the acetabulum, the superior margin of the symphysis pubis, and radial aspects of the heads of metacarpals are characteristic.

Treatment

Surgical treatment of acromegaly consists of transsphenoidal removal of the pituitary tumor. Radiation is used as adjuvant therapy following surgery in those cases where some tumor still remains viable, and medications are not controlling the progression of acromegaly. Radiation treatment may be instituted in one of three ways: conventional radiation therapy, proton beam therapy, and stereotactic radiosurgery, also known as Gamma Knife radiosurgery.

SUGGESTED READINGS

Abreu M, Johnson K, Chung CB, et al. Calcification in calcium pyrophosphate dihydrate (CPPD) crystalline deposits in the knee: anatomic, radiographic, MR imaging, and histologic study in cadavers. *Skeletal Radiol.* 2004;33:392–398.

Adamson TC III, Resnik CS, Guerra J Jr, et al. Hand and wrist arthropathies of hemochromatosis and calcium pyrophosphate deposition disease: distinct radiographic features. *Radiology.* 1983;147:377–381.

Ala A, Walker AP, Ashkan K. Wilson's disease. *Lancet.* 2007;369:397–408.

Alustiza JM, Artetxe J, Castiella A, et al. MR quantification of hepatic iron concentration. *Radiology.* 2004;230:479–484.

Amor B, Cherot A, Delbarre F, et al. Hydroxyapatite rheumatism and HLA markers. *J Rheumatol.* 1977;4(Suppl 3):101–104.

Axford JS, Bomford A, Revell P, et al. Hip arthropathy in genetic hemochromatosis. *Arthritis Rheum.* 1991;34:357–361.

Baker ND, Jahss MH, Leventhal GH. Unusual involvement of the feet in hemochromatosis. *Foot Ankle.* 1984;4:212–215.

Barthelemy CR, Nakayama DA, Carrera GF, et al. Gouty arthritis: a prospective radiographic evaluation of sixty patients. *Skeletal Radiol.* 1984;11:1–8.

Beltran J, Marty-Delfaut E, Bencardino J, et al. Chondrocalcinosis of the hyaline cartilage of the knee: MRI manifestations. *Skeletal Radiol.* 1998;27:369–374.

Beutler E, Felitti VJ, Koziol JA, et al. Penetrance of 845G-A (C282Y) *HFE* hereditary haemochromatosis mutations in the USA. *Lancet.* 2002;359:211–218.

Bloch C, Hermann G, Yu TF. A radiologic reevaluation of gout: a study of 2,000 patients. *Am J Roentgenol.* 1980;134:781–787.

Boskey AL, Vigorita VJ, Sencer O, et al. Chemical, microscopic, and ultrastructural characterization of the mineral deposits in tumoral calcinosis. *Clin Orthop.* 1983;178:258–269.

Brandi ML, Falchetti A. Genetics of primary hyperparathyroidism. *Urol Int.* 2004;72(Suppl 1):11–16.

Braunstein EM, Menerey K, Martel W, et al. Radiologic features of pyrophosphate-like arthropathy associated with long-term dialysis. *Skeletal Radiol.* 1987;16:437–411.

Brown EM, MacLeod RJ. Extracellular calcium sensing and extracellular calcium signaling. *Physiol Rev.* 2001;81:239–297.

Brown EM, Juppner H. Parathyroid hormone synthesis, secretion, and action. In: Favus MJ, ed. *Primer on the metabolic bone diseases and disorders of mineral metabolism.* Washington, DC: The American Society for Bone & Mineral Research, 2006:90–99.

Brown TW, Genant HK, Hattner RS, et al. Multiple brown tumors in a patient with chronic renal failure and secondary hyperparathyroidism. *Am J Roentgenol.* 1977;128:131–134.

Bull PC, Thomas GR, Rommens JM. The Wilson disease gene is a putative copper transporting P-type ATPase similar to the Menkes gene. *Nat Genet.* 1993;5:327–337.

Burke BJ, Escobedo EM, Wilson AJ, et al. Chondrocalcinosis mimicking a meniscal tear on MR imaging. *Am J Roentgenol.* 1998;170:69–70.

Bywaters EGL, Dixon ASJ, Scott JT. Joint lesions of hyperparathyroidism. *Ann Rheum Dis.* 1963;22:171–187.

Carlsson A. Hereditary hemochromatosis: a neglected diagnosis in orthopedics. *Acta Orthop.* 2009;80:371–374.

Chang CY, Rosenthal DI, Mitchell DM, et al. Imaging findings of metabolic bone disease. *Radiographics.* 2016;36:1871–1887.

Chen C, Chandnani VP, Kang HS, et al. Scapholunate advanced collapse: a common wrist abnormality in calcium pyrophosphate dihydrate crystal deposition disease. *Radiology.* 1990;177:459–461.

Chen CKH, Chung CB, Yeh LR, et al. Carpal tunnel syndrome caused by tophaceous gout: CT and MR imaging features in 20 patients. *Am J Roentgenol.* 2000;175:655–659.

Chen CKH, Yeh LR, Pan H-B, et al. Intra-articular gouty tophi of the knee: CT and MR imaging in 12 patients. *Skeletal Radiol.* 1999;28:75–80.

Choi HK, Burns LC, Shojania K, et al. Dual energy CT in gout: a prospective validation study. *Ann Rheum Dis.* 2012;71:1466–1471.

Choi HK, Zhu Y, Mount DB. Genetics of gout. *Curr Opin Rheumatol.* 2010;22:144–151.

Choi HK, Curhan G. Soft drinks, fructose consumption, and the risk of gout in men: prospective cohort study. *BMJ.* 2008;336:309–312.

Choi HK, Mount DB, Reginato AM. Pathogenesis of gout. *Ann Intern Med.* 2005;143:499–516.

Choi HK, Al-Arfaj A, Nicolaou S, et al. Dual energy computed tomography in tophaceous gout. *Ann Rheum Dis.* 2008;19:13–23.

Choi HK, Al-Arfaj AM, Eftekhari A, et al. Dual-energy computed tomography in tophaceous gout. *Ann Rheum Dis.* 2009;68:1609–1612.

Chung CB, Mohana-Borges A, Pathria M. Tophaceous gout in an amputation stump in a patient with chronic myelogenous leukemia. *Skeletal Radiol.* 2003;32:429–431.

Coombs RJ, Padanilam TG, Phillips E. Tumoral pseudogout of the metatarsal. *Skeletal Radiol.* 2002;31:39–42.

Dabbagh AJ, Trenam CW, Morris CJ, et al. Iron in joint inflammation. *Ann Rheum Dis.* 1993;51:67–73.

Dalbeth N, Doyle AJ, McQueen FM, et al. Exploratory study of radiographic change in patients with tophaceous gout treated with intensive urate-lowering therapy. *Arthritis Care Res.* 2014;66:82–85.

Dalinka MK, Reginato AJ, Golden DA. Calcium deposition diseases. *Semin Roentgenol.* 1982;17:39–48.

Demertzis JL, Rubin DA. MR imaging assessment of inflammatory, crystalline-induced, and infectious arthritides. *Magn Reson Imaging Clin N Am.* 2011;19:339–363.

Desai MA, Peterson JJ, Garner HW, et al. Clinical utility of dual-energy CT for evaluation of tophaceous gout. *Radiographics.* 2011;31:1365–1375.

Dhanda S, Jagmohan P, Quek ST. A re-look at an old disease: a multimodality review on gout. *Clin Radiol.* 2011;66:984–992.

Diekhoff T, Sheel M, Hermann S, et al. Osteitis: a retrospective feasibility study comparing single-source dual-energy CT to MRI in selected patients with suspected acute gout. *Skeletal Radiol.* 2017;46:185–190.

Diekhoff T, Kiefer T, Stroux A, et al. Detection and characterization of crystal suspensions using single-source dual-energy computed tomography: a phantom model of crystal arthropathies. *Invest Radiol.* 2015;50:255–260.

Dymock IW, Hamilton EB, Laws JW, et al. Arthropathy of haemochromatosis: clinical and radiologic analysis of 63 patients with iron overload. *Ann Rheum Dis.* 1970;29:469–476.

Ebenbichler GR, Erdogmus CB, Resch KL, et al. Ultrasound therapy for calcific tendinitis of the shoulder. *N Engl J Med.* 1999;340:1533–1538.

El-Khoury GY, Foucar E, Blair WF, et al. Case report 364. Massive calcium pyrophosphate dihydrate crystal deposition disorder (MCPDD) involving thumb. *Skeletal Radiol.* 1986;15:313–315.

Eustace S, Buff B, McCarthy C, et al. Magnetic resonance imaging of hemochromatosis arthropathy. *Skeletal Radiol.* 1994;23:547–549.

Eustace S, Baker N, Lan HC, et al. Vignettes in arthritis: hemochromatosis arthropathy. *Radiol Clin North Am.* 1996;34:441–445.

Fam AG, Topp JR, Stein HB, et al. Clinical and roentgenographic aspects of pseudogout: a study of 50 cases and a review. *Can Med Assoc J.* 1981;124:545–551.

Farpour F, Phan SJ, Burns J, et al. Enhanced MR imaging of the shoulder, and sternoclavicular and acromioclavicular joint arthritis in primary hemochromatosis. *Rheumatol Int.* 2011;31:395–398.

Feder JN, Gnirke A, Thomas W, et al. A novel MHC class I-like gene is mutated in patients with hereditary haemochromatosis. *Nat Genet.* 1966;13:399–408.

Felitti VJ. Hemochromatosis: a common, rarely diagnosed disease. *Permanent J.* 1999;3:10–22.

Fenton HJH. Oxidation of tartaric acid in presence of iron. *J Chem Soc Trans.* 1894;65:399–911.

Feydy A, Liote F, Carlier R, et al. Cervical spine and crystal-associated diseases: imaging findings. *Eur Radiol.* 2006;16:459–468.

Fletcher LM, Powell LW. Hemochromatosis and alcoholic liver disease. *Alcohol.* 2003;30:131–136.

Garcia GM, McCord GC, Kumar R. Hydroxyapatite crystal deposition disease. *Semin Musculoskelet Radiol.* 2003;7:187–193.

Glazebrook KN, Guimaraes LS, Murthy NS, et al. Identification of intraarticular and periarticular uric acid crystals with dual-energy CT: initial evaluation. *Radiology.* 2011;261:516–524.

Gochee PA, Powell LW, Cullen DJ, et al. A population-based study of the biochemical and clinical expression of the H63D hemochromatosis mutation. *Gastroenterology.* 2002;122:646–651.

Goldstein S, Meyerstein D, Czapski G. The Fenton reagents. *Free Rad Biol Med.* 1993;15:435–445.

Guglielmi G, Muscarella S, Leone A, et al. Imaging of metabolic bone diseases. *Radiol Clin North Am.* 2008;46:734–754.

Hammoudeh M, Siam AR. Pseudogout in a young patient. *Clin Rheumatol.* 1998;17:242–245.

Hayashi M, Matsunaga T, Tanikawa H. Idiopathic widespread calcium pyrophosphate dihydrate crystal deposition disease in a young patient. *Skeletal Radiol.* 2002;31:246–250.

Hayes CW, Conway WF. Calcium hydroxyapatite deposition disease. *Radiographics.* 1990;10:1031–1048.

Hirsch JH, Killien FC, Troupin RH. The arthropathy of hemochromatosis. *Radiology.* 1976;118:591–596.

Hughes AE, McGibbon D, Woodward E, et al. Localization of a gene for chondrocalcinosis to chromosome 5q. *Hum Mol Genet.* 1995;4:1225–1228.

Ishida T, Dorfman HD, Bullough PG. Tophaceous pseudogout (tumoral calcium pyrophosphate dihydrate crystal deposition disease). *Hum Pathol.* 1995;26:587–593.

Jensen PS. Chondrocalcinosis and other calcifications. *Radiol Clin North Am.* 1988;26:1315–1325.

Janssens HJ, Janssen M, van de Lisdonk EH, et al. Limited validity of the American College of Rheumatology criteria for classifying patients with gout in primary care. *Ann Rheum Dis.* 2010;69:1255–1256.

Justesen P, Andersen PE Jr. Radiologic manifestations in alkaptonuria. *Skeletal Radiol.* 1984;11:204–208.

Janssens HJ, Janssen M, van de Lisdonk EH, et al. Use of oral prednisolone or naproxen for the treatment of gout arthritis: a double-blind, randomized equivalence trial. *Lancet.* 2008;371:1854–1860.

Johnson TR, Krauss B, Sedlmair M, et al. Material differentiation by dual-energy CT: initial experience. *Eur Radiol.* 2007;17:1510–1517.

Kim KY, Ralph SH, Hunsche E, et al. A literature review of the epidemiology and treatment of acute gout. *Clin Ther.* 2003;25:1593–1617.

Khanna D, Fitzgerald JD, Khanna PP, et al. American College of Rheumatology guidelines for management of gout. Part 1: systematic nonpharmacologic and pharmacologic therapeutic approaches to hyperuricemia. *Arthritis Care Res (Hoboken).* 2012;64:1431–1446.

Klontzas ME, Vassalou EE, Karantanas AH. Calcific tendinopathy of the shoulder with intraosseous extension: outcomes of ultrasound-guided percutaneous irrigation. *Skeletal Radiol.* 2017;46:201–208.

Klontzas ME, Vassalou EE, Zibis AH, et al. Hydroxyapatite deposition disease around the hip: outcomes of CT-guided treatment. *Diagn Interv Radiol.* 2016;22:466–470.

Kobylecka M, Plazinska MT, Chudzinski W, et al. Comparison of scintigraphy and ultrasound imaging in patients with primary, secondary and tertiary hyperparathyroidism-own experience. *J Ultrason.* 2017;17:17–22.

Laborde JM, Green DL, Ascari AD, et al. Arthritis in hemochromatosis. *J Bone Joint Surg [Am].* 1977;59A:1103–1107.

Lansa E, Banfi G, Serafini G, et al. Ultrasound-guided percutaneous irrigation in rotator cuff calcific tendinopathy: what is the evidence? A systematic review with proposals for future reporting. *Eur Radiol.* 2015;25:2176–2183.

Lemire JA, Harrison JJ, Turner RJ. Box 3: the Fenton reaction, free radical chemistry and metal poisoning. *Nature Rev Microbiol.* 2013;11:371–384.

Liote F, Ea HK. Recent developments in crystal-induced inflammation, pathogenesis and management. *Curr Rheumatol Rep.* 2007;9:243–250.

Llauger J, Palmer J, Roson N, et al. Nonseptic monoarthritis: imaging features with clinical and histopathologic correlation. *Radiographics.* 2000;20:S263–S278.

Mallinson PI, Reagan AC, Coupal T, et al. The distribution of urate deposition within the extremities in gout: a review of 148 dual-energy CT cases. *Skeletal Radiol.* 2014;43:277–281.

Mannoni A, Selvi E, Lorenzini S, et al. Alkaptonuria, ochronosis, and ochronotic arthropathy. *Sem Arthritis Rheum.* 2004;33:239–248.

Martel W. The overhanging margin of bone: a roentgenologic manifestation of gout. *Radiology.* 1968;91:755–756.

Martel W, McCarter DK, Solsky MA, et al. Further observation of the arthropathy of calcium pyrophosphate dihydrate crystal deposition disease. *Radiology.* 1981;141:1–15.

McCarty DJ. Calcium pyrophosphate dihydrate crystal deposition disease: pseudogout—articular chondrocalcinosis. In: McCarty DJ, ed. *Arthritis and Allied Conditions: A Textbook of Rheumatology.* 11th ed. Philadelphia: Lea & Febiger; 1989:1714–1720.

McCarthy DJ. Crystal and arthritis. *Dis Mon.* 1994;40:253–299.

McCarty DJ Jr, Haskin ME. The roentgenographic aspects of pseudogout (articular chondrocalcinosis). An analysis of 20 cases. *Am J Roentgenol.* 1963;90:1248–1257.

McDonell S, Preston B, Jewell S, et al. A survey of 2,851 patients with hemochromatosis: symptoms and response to treatment. *Am J Med.* 1999;106:619–625.

McQueen FM, Reeves Q, Dalbeth N. New insights into an old disease: advanced imaging in the diagnosis and management of gout. *Postgrad Med J.* 2013;89:87–93.

McQueen FM, Doyle A, Dalbeth N. Imaging in gout: what can we learn from MRI, CT, DECT and US? *Arthritis Res Ther.* 2011;13:246.

Merolla G, Bhat MG, Paladini P, Porcellini G. Complications of calcific tendinitis of the shoulder: a concise review. *J Orthop Traumatol.* 2015;16:175–183.

Milman N, Pedersen O, Ovesen L, et al. Frequency of the C282Y and H63D mutations of the hemochromatosis gene (HFE) in 2501 ethnic Danes. *Ann Hematol.* 2004;83:654–657.

Mitchell DM, Regan S, Cooley MR, et al. Long-term follow-up of patients with hyperparathyroidism. *J Clin Endocrinol Metab.* 2012;97:4507–4514.

Montgomery KD, Williams JR, Sculco TP, DiCarlo E. Clinical and pathologic findings in hemochromatosis hip arthropathy. *Clin Orthop.* 1998;347:179–187.

Monu JU, Pope TL Jr. Gout: a clinical and radiologic review. *Radiol Clin Noorth Am.* 2004;42:169–184.

Moore EA, Vennart W, Jacoby RK, et al. Magnetic resonance manifestations of idiopathic hemochromatosis in the wrist. *Br J Rheumatol.* 1993;32:917–922.

Netter P, Bardin T, Bianchi A, et al. The ANKH gene and familial calcium pyrophosphate dihydrate deposition disease. *J Bone Spine.* 2005;71:365–368.

Newberry SJ, FitzGerald JD, Motala A, et al. Diagnosis of gout: a systemic review in support of an American College of Physicians Clinical Practice Guideline. *Ann Intern Med.* 2017;166:27–36.

Nichols GM, Bacon BR. Hereditary hemochromatosis: pathogenesis and clinical features of a common disease. *Am J Gastroenterol.* 1989;84:851–854.

Nicolaou S, Liang T, Murphy DT, et al. Dual-energy CT: a promising new technique for assessment of the musculoskeletal system. *Am J Roentgenol.* 2012;199:S78–S86.

Nicolaou S, Yong-Hing CJ, Galea-Soler S, et al. Dual-energy CT as a potential new diagnostic tool in the management of gout in the acute setting. *Am J Roentgenol.* 2010;66:984–992.

Nussbaum AJ, Doppman JL. Shoulder arthropathy in primary hyperparathyroidism. *Skeletal Radiol.* 1982;9:98–102.

Olsen KM, Chew FS. Tumoral calcinosis: pearls, polemics, and alternative possibilities. *Radiographics.* 2006;26:871–885.

O'Neil J, Powell L. Clinical aspects of hemochromatosis. *Semin Liver Dis.* 2005;25:381–391.

Papakonstantinou O, Mohana-Borges AVR, Campell L, et al. Hip arthropathy in a patient with primary hemochromatosis: MR imaging findings with pathologic correlation. *Skeletal Radiol.* 2005;34:180–184.

Park HJ, Chung HW, Oh TS, et al. Tumoral pseudogout of the proximal interphalangeal joint of a finger: a case report and literature review. *Skeletal Radiol.* 2016;45:1007–1012.

Patil M, Sheth KA, Krishnamurthy AC, et al. A review and current perspective on Wilson disease. *J Clin Exp Hepatol.* 2013;3:321–336.

Pattamapaspong N, Vuthiwong W, Kanthawang T, et al. Value of ultrasonography in the diagnosis of gout in patients presenting with acute arthritis. *Skeletal Radiol.* 2017;46:759–767.

Phornphutkul C, Introne WJ, Perry MB, et al. Natural history of alkaptonuria. *N Engl J Med.* 2002;347:2111–2121.

Pietrangelo A. Hereditary hemochromatosis – a new look at an old disease. *N Engl J Med.* 2004;350:2383–2397.

Qaseem A, McLean RM, Starkey M, et al. Diagnosis of acute gout: a clinical practice guideline from the American College of Physicians. *Ann Intern Med.* 2017;166:52–57.

Qaseem A, Harris RP, Forciea MA, et al. Management of acute and recurrent gout: a clinical practice guideline from the American College of Physicians. *Ann Intern Med.* 2017;166:58–68.

Recht MP, Seragini F, Kramer J, et al. Isolated or dominant lesions of the patella in gout: a report of seven patients. *Skeletal Radiol.* 1994;23:113–116.

Reginato AM, Olsen BR. Genetics and experimental models of crystal-induced arthritis. Lessons learned from mice and men: is it crystal clear? *Curr Opin Rheumatol.* 2007;19:134–145.

Reiss E, Canterbury JM. Spectrum of hyperparathyroidism. *Am J Med.* 1974;56:794–799.

Resnick D, Niwayama G. Subchondral resorption of bone in renal osteodystrophy. *Radiology.* 1976;118:315–321.

Resnick CS, Resnick D. Crystal deposition disease. *Semin Arthritis Rheum.* 1983;12:390–403.

Resnick D. Calcium hydroxyapatite crystal deposition disease. In: Resnick D, ed. *Diagnosis of Bone and Joint Disorders.* 3rd ed. Philadelphia: WB Saunders; 1995:1615–1648.

Resnick D. Hemochromatosis and Wilson's disease. In: Resnick D, ed. *Diagnosis of Bone and Joint Disorders.* 3rd ed. Philadelphia, PA: WB Saunders; 1995:1649–1669.

Resnick D. Alkaptonuria. In: Resnick D, ed. *Diagnosis of Bone and Joint Disorders.* 3rd ed. Philadelphia, PA: WB Saunders; 1995:1670–1685.

Resnick D, Niwayama G. Gouty arthritis. In: Resnick D, ed. *Diagnosis of Bone and Joint Disorders.* 3rd ed. Philadelphia, PA: WB Saunders; 1995:1511–1555.

Resnick D, Niwayama G. Calcium pyrophosphate dihydrate (CPPD) crystal deposition disease. In: Resnick D, ed. *Diagnosis of Bone and Joint Disorders.* 3rd ed. Philadelphia, PA: WB Saunders; 1995:1556–1614.

Resnick D, Niwayama G, Goergen TC, et al. Clinical, radiographic and pathologic abnormalities in calcium pyrophosphate dihydrate crystal deposition disease (CPPD): pseudogout. *Radiology.* 1977;122:1–15.

Rivera-Sanfeliz G, Resnick D, Haghighi P, et al. Tophaceous pseudogout. *Skeletal Radiol.* 1996;25:699–701.

Rogachefsky RA, Carneiro R, Altman RD, et al. Gout presenting as infectious arthritis. *J Bone Joint Surg [Am].* 1994;76A:269–273.

Rosencrantz R, Schilsky M. Wilson disease: pathogenesis and clinical considerations in diagnosis and treatment. *Semin Liver Dis.* 2011;31:245–259.

Rousseau I, Cardinal E, Raymond-Tremblay D, et al. Gout: radiographic findings mimicking infection. *Skeletal Radiol.* 2001;30:565–569.

Ryan LM, McCarthy DJ. Understanding inorganic pyrophosphate metabolism: toward prevention of calcium pyrophosphate dihydrate crystal deposition. *Ann Rheum.* 1995;54:939–941.

Schmid H, Struppler C, Braun GS, et al. Ankle and hindfoot arthropathy in hereditary hemochromatosis. *J Rheumatol.* 2003;30:196–199.

Schumacher HR Jr, Becker MA, Edwards NL, et al. Magnetic resonance imaging in the quantitative assessment of gouty tophi. *Int J Clin Pract.* 2006;60:408–414.

Shekelle PG, Newberry SJ, FitzGerald JD, et al. Management of gout: a systematic review in support of an American College of Physicians Clinical Practice Guideline. *Ann Intern Med.* 2017;166:37–51.

Seil R, Litzenburger H, Kohn D, et al. Arthroscopic treatment of chronically painful calcifying tendinitis of the supraspinatus tendon. *Arthroscopy.* 2006;22:521–527.

Simon M. Genetics of hemochromatosis. *N Engl J Med.* 1979;301:1291–1292.

Sissons HA, Steiner GC, Bonar F, et al. Tumoral calcium pyrophosphate deposition disease. *Skeletal Radiol* 1989;18:79–87.

Smith HS, Bracken D, Smith JM. Gout: current insights and future perspectives. *J Pain.* 2011;12:1113–1129.

Soldatos T, Pezeshk P, Ezzati F, et al. Cross-sectional imaging of adult crystal and inflammatory arthropathies. *Skeletal Radiol.* 2016;45:1173–1191.

Stapelbroek JM, Bollen CW, Amstel JK. The H1069Q mutation in ATP7B is associated with late and neurologic presentation in Wilson disease: results of meta-analysis. *J Hepatol.* 2004;41:758–763.

Steinbach LS, Resnick D. Calcium pyrophosphate dihydrate crystal deposition disease revisited. *Radiology.* 1996;200:1–9.

Steinbach LS, Resnick D. Calcium pyrophosphate dihydrate crystal deposition disease: imaging perspectives. *Curr Probl Diagn Radiol.* 2000;11:209–228.

Stremmel W, Meyerrose KW, Niederau C. Wilson's disease: clinical presentation, treatment, and survival. *Ann Intern Med.* 1991;115:720–726.

Sussmann AR, Cohen J, Nomikos GC, et al. Magnetic resonance imaging of shoulder arthropathies. *Magn Reson Imaging Clin N Am.* 2012;20:349–371.

Suwannarat P, O'Brien K, Perry MB, et al. Use of nitisinone in patients with alkaptonuria. *Metabolism.* 2005;54:719–728.

Thiele RG, Schlesinger N. Diagnosis of gout by ultrasound. *Rheumatology.* 2007;46:1116–1121.

Valenti L, Rametta R, Dongiovanni P, et al. The hand arthropathy of hereditary hemochromatosis is strongly associated with iron overload. *J Rheumatol.* 2008;35:153–158.

Yang BY, Sartoris DJ, Djukic S, et al. Distribution of calcification in the triangular fibrocartilage region in 181 patients with calcium pyrophosphate dihydrate crystal deposition disease. *Radiology.* 1995;196:547–550.

Yokoyama M, Aono H, Takeda A, et al. Cimetidine for chronic calcifying tendinitis of the shoulder. *Reg Anesth Pain Med.* 2003;28:248–252.

Yu JS, Chung CB, Recht M, et al. MR imaging of tophaceous gout. *Am J Roentgenol.* 1997;168:523–527.

Williams CJ. Familial calcium pyrophosphate dihydrate deposition disease and the ANKH gene. *Curr Opin Rheumatol.* 2003;15:326–331.

Wilson SAK. Progressive lenticular degeneration: a familial nervous disease associated with cirrhosis of the liver. *Brain.* 1912;34:295–507.

Winterbourn CC. Toxicity of iron and hydrogen peroxide: the Fenton reaction. *Toxical Lett.* 1995;82:969–974.

Zhang Y, Brown MA. Genetic studies of chondrocalcinosis. *Curr Opin Rheumatol.* 2005;17:330–335.

Zhang W, Doherty M, Bardin T, et al. European league against rheumatism recommendations for calcium pyrophosphate deposition. Part I: terminology and diagnosis. *Ann Rheum Dis.* 2011;70:563–570.

Zhang W, Doherty M, Pascual E, et al. EULAR evidence based recommendations for gout. Part I: Diagnosis. Report of a task force of the Standing Committee for International Clinical Studies Including Therapeutics (ESCISIT). *Ann Rheum Dis.* 2006;65:1301–1311.

CHAPTER 8

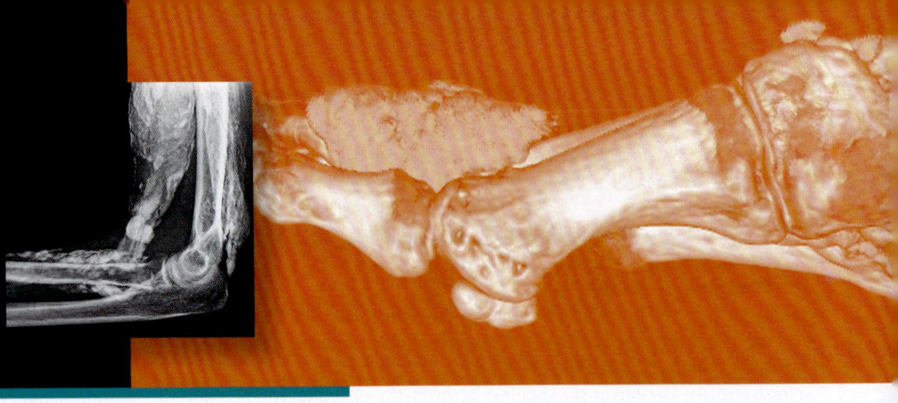

Connective Tissue Arthropathies

An overview of the clinical and imaging hallmarks of the forms of arthropathies associated with connective tissue disorders is presented in Table 8.1.

SYSTEMIC LUPUS ERYTHEMATOSUS (SLE)

Clinical Features

Systemic lupus erythematosus (SLE) is a chronic, inflammatory, connective tissue disorder of unknown cause characterized by significant immunologic abnormalities and involvement of multiple organs. Although the etiology of this disorder still remains unsettled, genetic, hormonal, and environmental influence play a role in disease pathogenesis. SLE is characterized by activation of polyclonal B cells to a variety of antigens and may be associated with hypergammaglobulinemia. Abnormalities of cytokines have been also reported including IL-1, IL-2, IL-6, and IL-10. There is increasing evidence that interferon-α (IFN-α) plays an important role in the pathogenesis of SLE. Various investigations have shown that plasmacytoid dendritic cells are responsible for release of IFN-α factor stimulation with immune complexes containing nucleic acid. The risk of acquiring SLE is in part genetic, but it is a complex genetic disorder with no clear mendelian pattern of inheritance, although it occurs in families. Genome-wide association studies have been disappointing and have implicated both genetic and epigenetic influences, but importantly, there are no clear applicable genetic tools. The first described genetic link to SLE was the major histocompatibility complex (MHC) on chromosome 6, which contains the human lymphocyte antigens (HLA)-DR. The other genes implicated included those that encode components of the complement pathway, Fc γ receptors, protein tyrosine phosphatase nonreceptor type 22 (PTPN22), and cytotoxic T lymphocyte–associated antigen 4 (CTLA4). Eight of the best-supported SLE susceptibility loci are 1q23, 1q25-31, 1q41-42, 2q35-37, 4p16-15.2, 6p11-21, 12p24, and 16q12. More recent investigations concluded that *PDCD1* (programmed cell death 1) gene is responsible for the linkage at chromosome 2q34 or 2q37 and is associated with lupus nephritis. Women, particularly adolescents and young adults, are affected nine times as frequently as men, and this prevalence may be linked to *TLR7* gene. In men with Klinefelter syndrome (47, XXY), the risk of SLE is 14-fold higher than in healthy male controls. Smoking is a risk factor as well and has been associated with anti-dsDNA production. SLE is more common in blacks in the United States, but it is rare among blacks in Africa. Cumulative results have shown that hereditary deficiencies of complement component C4A (a MHC class III gene) confer risk for SLE in almost all ethnic groups studied.

The clinical manifestations of SLE vary according to the distribution and extent of systemic alterations. The most common symptoms are malaise, weakness, fever, anorexia, and weight loss. Arthropathy and skin rashes are common findings. Cerebral infarction and renal disease are life-threatening complications. Consistent and characteristic features of this disease are serologic abnormalities, including a variety of serum autoantibodies including those directed against the nuclear antigens (antinuclear antibodies ANA). In addition, SLE is characterized by the production of cytoplasmic antigens, cell surface antigens, and soluble antigens in the circulation, such as IgG and phospholipids. Antinuclear antibodies are useful in the differential diagnosis of SLE, and changes in the titer of antibodies to DNA are useful in following disease activity. Antinuclear antibodies are a heterogeneous group of antibodies directed against a number of discrete nuclear macromolecular proteins. They represent what has classically been referred to as "autoantibodies" because they are directed against components normally present in all nucleated cells. They generally lack tissue or species

Table 8.1 CLINICAL AND IMAGING HALLMARKS OF CONNECTIVE TISSUE ARTHRITIDES (ARTHROPATHIES)

Type of Arthritis	Site	Crucial Abnormalities	Technique/Projection
Systemic Lupus Erythematosus (F > M; young adults; blacks > whites; skin changes: rash)	Hands Hips, ankles, shoulders	Flexible joint contractures Osteonecrosis	Lateral view Standard views of affected joints Scintigraphy Magnetic resonance imaging
Scleroderma (F > M; skin changes: edema, thickening)	Hands	Soft tissue calcifications Acroosteolysis Tapering of distal phalanges Interphalangeal destructive changes	Dorsovolar and lateral views
	Gastrointestinal tract	Dilatation of esophagus Decreased peristalsis Dilatation of duodenum and small bowel	Esophagram Esophagram (cine or video study) Upper gastrointestinal and small bowel series
Polymyositis/ Dermatomyositis		Pseudodiverticulosis of colon	Barium enema
	Upper and lower extremities (proximal parts)	Soft tissue calcifications	Xeroradiography; digital radiography
	Hands	Periarticular osteoporosis Erosions and destructive changes in distal interphalangeal articulations	Dorsovolar and lateral views
Mixed Connective Tissue Disease (overlap of clinical features of SLE, scleroderma, dermatomyositis, and rheumatoid arthritis)	Hands, wrists	Erosions and destructive changes in proximal interphalangeal, metacarpophalangeal, radiocarpal and midcarpal articulations, associated with joint space narrowing Symmetric soft tissue swelling Soft tissue atrophy and calcifications	Dorsovolar and lateral views Magnetic resonance imaging Magnetic resonance imaging Posteroanterior and lateral views
	Chest	Pleural and pericardial effusions	Ultrasound

specificity; therefore, they will cross-react with nuclei from different sources. The primary sources for study of these antibodies are patients with SLE and related systemic rheumatic diseases. Many studies have centered on defining the specificity of these antibodies and have contributed extensively to our understanding of their immunopathologic role in connective tissue disorders. It is worthwhile to state that 100% of patients with SLE are ANA positive; the concept of ANA-negative lupus is no longer valid. Furthermore, autoantibodies against small nuclear ribonucleoprotein (snRNP), also known as anti-Smith antibodies, were found to be highly specific for SLE, although they are present in only 15% to 30% of SLE patients. They are present more frequently (about 60%) in young black women with SLE. The immunobiology of lupus is well beyond the scope of this text, but we have to emphasize that despite exhaustive studies of tolerance and the existence of mouse model of lupus, there have not been any clinically significant advances in the specific treatment of SLE in nearly two decades.

Pathology reveals widespread vasculitis affecting capillaries, arterioles, and venules. There is villous hypertrophy of the synovium covered by fibrin. In addition, a low-grade lymphoplasmacytic inflammatory cell infiltrate in the subintima may be encountered. The synovial fluid is characterized by an inflammatory pattern in which lymphocytes often predominate, and LE cells are commonly seen.

Imaging Features

The musculoskeletal system is a common site of involvement in SLE, and joint abnormalities, exhibited by 90% of patients during the course of the disease, represent a significant part of the clinical and radiologic picture. Arthritic involvement is symmetric, and articular deformities without fixed contractures are a hallmark of this disorder. The hands are the predominant sites of involvement. Typically, the conventional radiography discloses malalignments, most commonly at the metacarpophalangeal and proximal interphalangeal joints of the fingers and the first carpometacarpal, metacarpophalangeal, and the interphalangeal joints of the thumb (Fig. 8.1). These abnormalities may not be apparent on a dorsovolar radiograph because the malalignments are flexible and are corrected by the pressure of the hand against the radiographic cassette (Fig. 8.2). These pathognomonic deformities usually occur secondary to a loss of support from the ligamentous and capsular structures about the joint and, at least in the early stage of disease, are completely reducible. Only very seldom are these abnormalities fixed

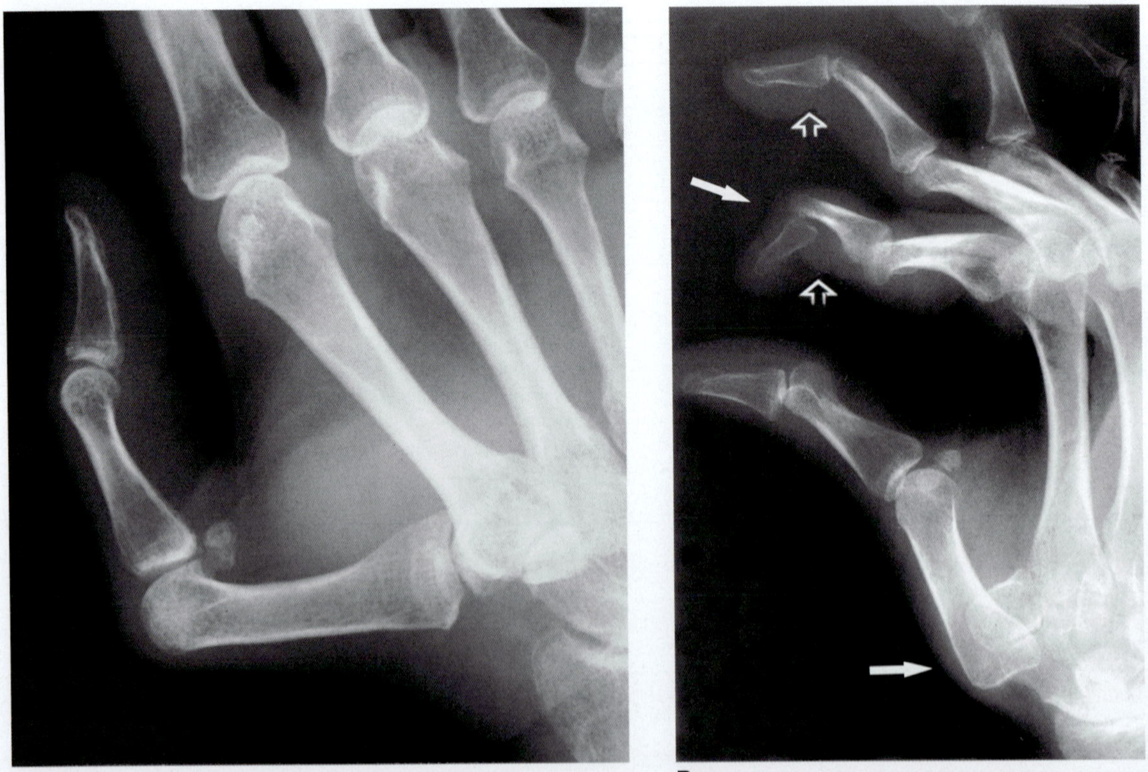

A B

Figure 8.1 ■ **Systemic lupus erythematosus. A:** Typical appearance of the thumb in a 43-year-old woman with SLE. Note subluxations in the first carpometacarpal and metacarpophalangeal joints without articular erosions. **B:** In another patient, a 32-year-old woman, the oblique radiograph of her left hand shows dislocations at the first carpometacarpal joint and distal interphalangeal joint of the index finger (*arrows*) and subluxations in the metacarpophalangeal joints of the index and middle fingers associated with swan neck deformities (*open arrows*).

and/or accompanied by articular erosions (Fig. 8.3). Some patients present with sclerosis of the distal phalanges (acral sclerosis) (Fig. 8.4) or with resorption of the terminal tufts (acroosteolysis). Osteonecrosis, which is frequently seen, has been attributed to complications of treatment with corticosteroids (Fig. 8.5). However, current investigations suggest the vital role of the inflammatory process (vasculitis) in the development of this complication.

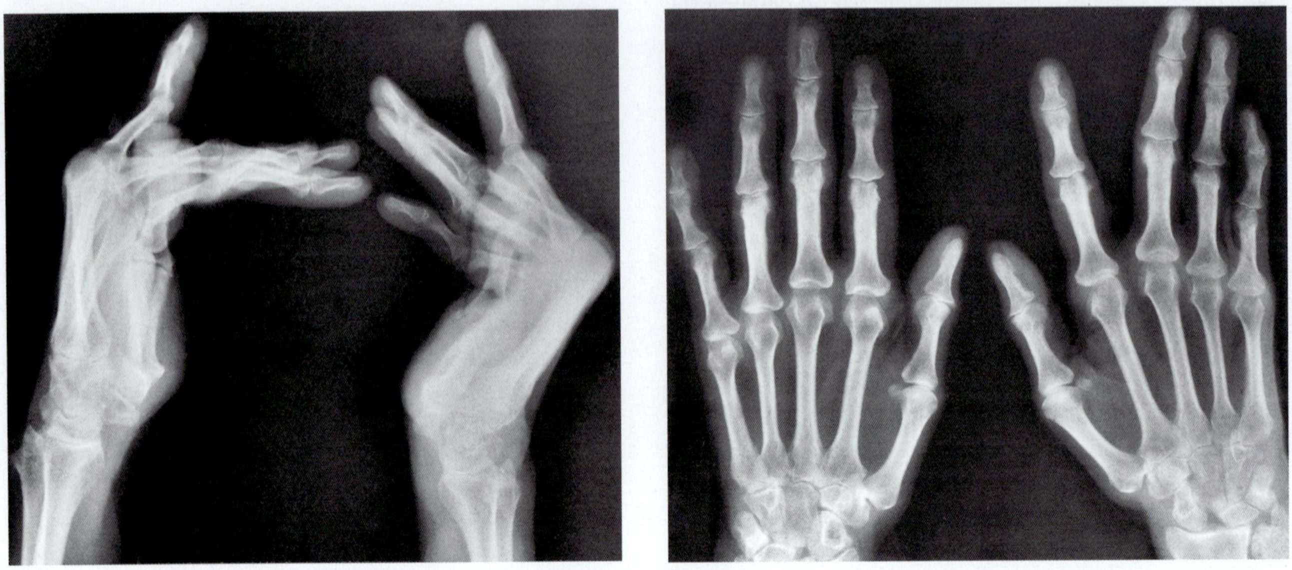

A B

Figure 8.2 ■ **Systemic lupus erythematosus. A:** Lateral radiograph of both hands of a 42-year-old woman with documented SLE for the past 4 years demonstrates flexion deformities in the metacarpophalangeal joints. **B:** On the dorsovolar projection, the flexion deformities have been corrected by the pressure of the hands against the radiographic cassette.

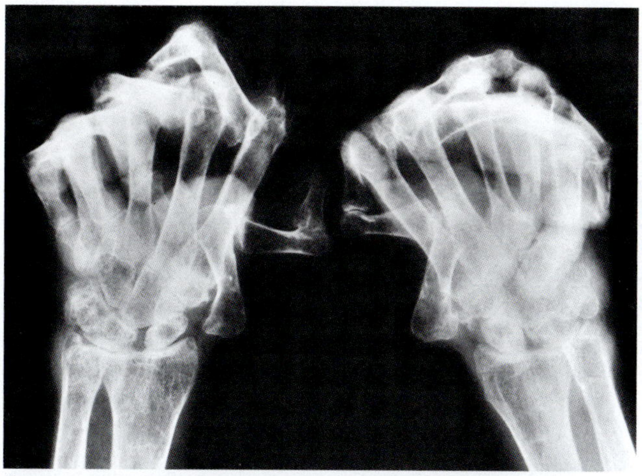

A

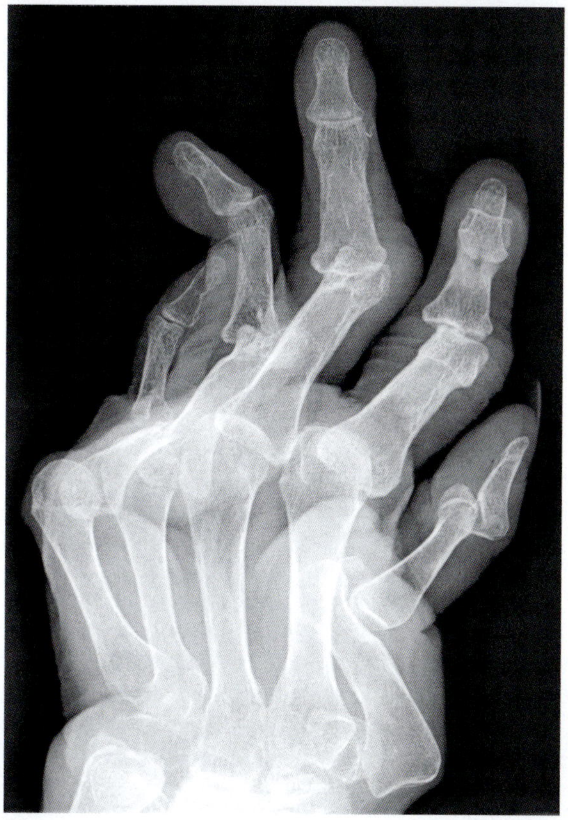

B

Figure 8.3 ■ Systemic lupus erythematosus. A: A 62-year-old woman presented with a 15-year history of SLE. Dorsovolar radiograph of both hands shows severe deformities, subluxations, and articular erosions. Note the advanced osteoporosis secondary to disuse of the extremities and treatment with corticosteroids. **B:** In another patient, a 51-year-old woman, note flexion contractions, subluxations, and dislocations in the several joints of the right hand.

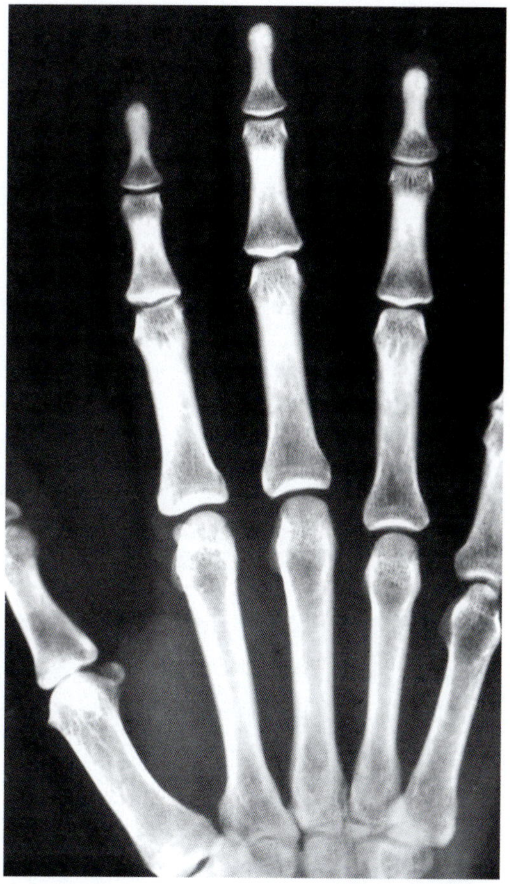

Figure 8.4 ■ Systemic lupus erythematosus. Dorsovolar radiograph of the hand of a 29-year-old woman demonstrates sclerosis of the distal phalanges (acral sclerosis). Similar sclerotic changes are also occasionally seen in rheumatoid arthritis and scleroderma.

Treatment

The treatment of SLE consists of using antimalarial drugs (such as hydroxychloroquine), corticosteroids (such as prednisone), and especially immunosuppressants (such as cyclophosphamide, azathioprine, mycophenolate, and methotrexate). Rituximab, a humanized monoclonal antibody against B cells, plasmaphoresis, and intravenous administration of immunoglobulin (IVIG) are also used under special circumstances. The details of the therapy, which is frequently individualized, are beyond the scope of this chapter; however, it is worthwhile to mention that SLE may become one of the first rheumatic diseases with a personalized therapeutic approach.

SCLERODERMA

Clinical Features

Scleroderma (progressive systemic sclerosis) is a generalized disorder of unknown cause. It is seen predominantly in young women, usually becoming apparent in their third and fourth decades. Primarily a connective tissue disorder characterized by deposition of collagen and other components of extracellular matrix in the skin and internal organs, it is distinguished by thickening and fibrosis of the skin and subcutaneous tissues, with frequent involvement of the musculoskeletal system. Scleroderma has an autoimmune basis with disease-specific ANAs, most commonly antitopoisomerase-1 and

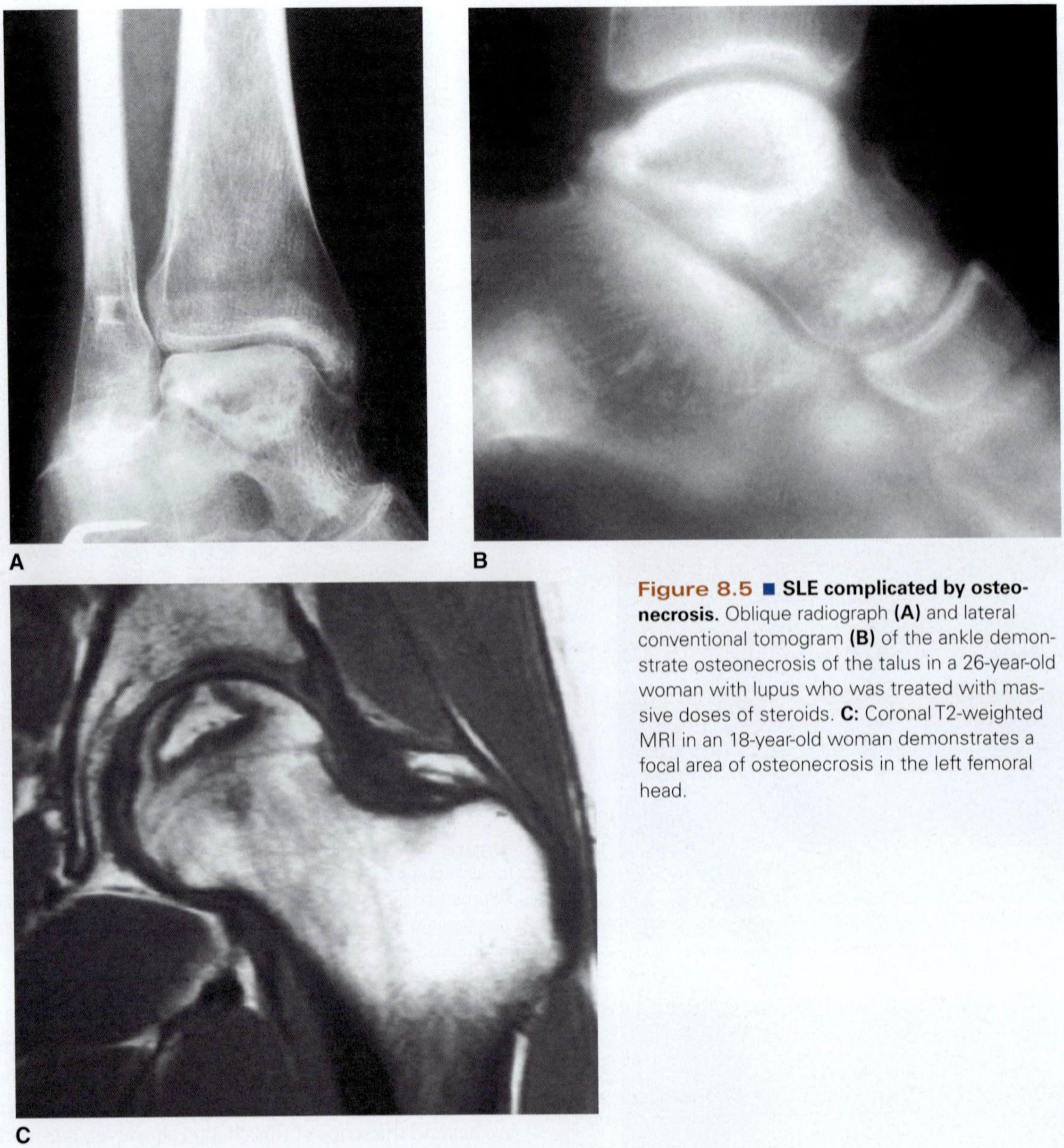

Figure 8.5 ■ SLE complicated by osteonecrosis. Oblique radiograph **(A)** and lateral conventional tomogram **(B)** of the ankle demonstrate osteonecrosis of the talus in a 26-year-old woman with lupus who was treated with massive doses of steroids. **C:** Coronal T2-weighted MRI in an 18-year-old woman demonstrates a focal area of osteonecrosis in the left femoral head.

anticentromere. Recently, researchers have identified a new genetic link to systemic form of scleroderma, a susceptibility locus involving the genome *CD247* (that encodes the T-cell receptor zeta subunit modulating T-cell activation), in addition to previously known genes *MHC*, *IRF5*, and *STAT4* (that encodes a regulatory protein important to immune system). However, these linkages are weak and do not provide a clear-cut genetic tool that is useful for patients. Clinically, many patients develop joint involvement, which is manifesting as arthralgia and arthropathy leading to flexion contractions of the fingers. Most patients have the so-called CREST syndrome, which refers to the coexistence of calcinosis, Raynaud phenomenon (episodes of intermittent pallor of the fingers and toes on exposure to cold, secondary to vasoconstriction of the small blood vessels), esophageal abnormalities (dilatation and hypoperistalsis), sclerodactyly, and telangiectasia; 30% to 40% of patients have a positive serologic test for rheumatoid factor and a positive antinuclear antibody (ANA) test.

Pathology shows symmetrical intimal thickening of affected arteries associated with endothelial necrosis and telangiectasia of capillaries. In the dermis, there is excessive deposition of fibrous tissue.

Imaging Features

Radiographically, scleroderma presents with characteristic abnormalities of the bone and soft tissues. The hands usually exhibit atrophy of the soft tissues at the tips of the fingers (Fig. 8.6), resorption of the distal phalanges (acroosteolysis), osteopenia, subcutaneous and periarticular calcifications (Figs. 8.7 to 8.9), and destructive changes of the small articulations, usually the interphalangeal joints (Figs. 8.9A and 8.10). Soft tissue

(Continued on page 316)

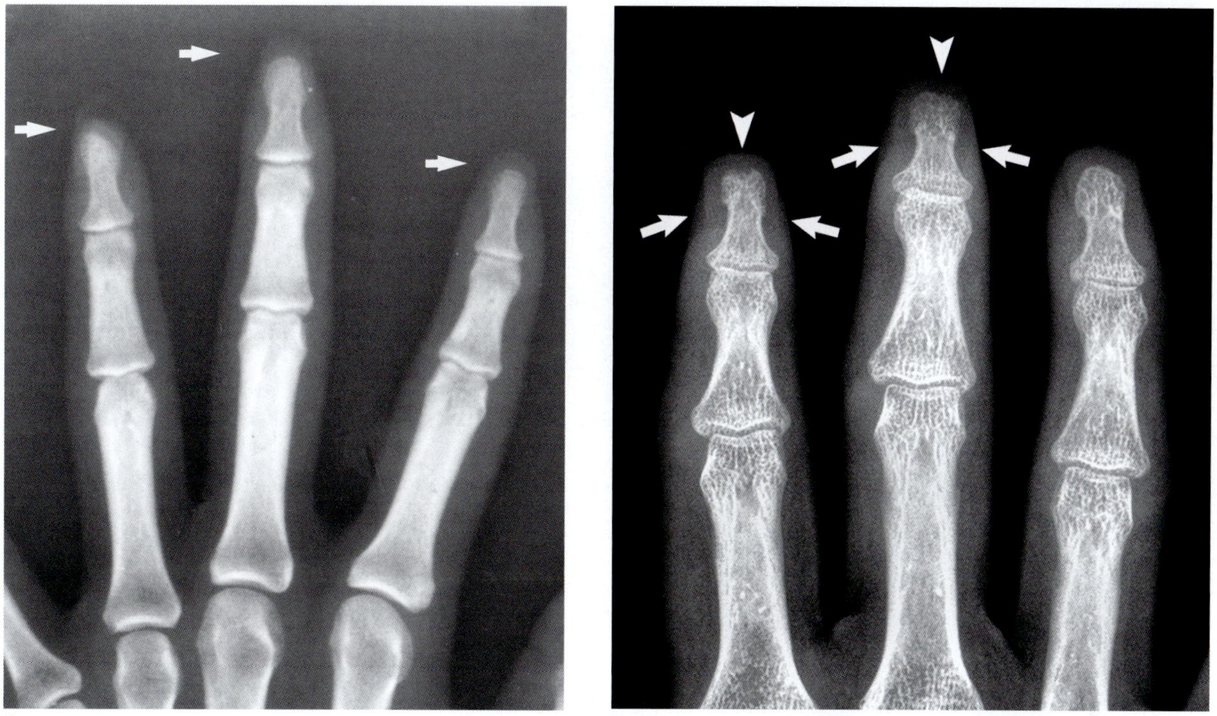

A B

Figure 8.6 ■ **Scleroderma. A:** A 24-year-old woman presented with atrophy of the soft tissues at the distal phalanges of the index, middle, and ring fingers (*arrows*). **B:** A radiograph of the fingers of the left hand of a 36-year-old woman shows atrophy of the soft tissue at the tip of the index and middle fingers (*arrows*) and early resorption of the terminal tufts (*arrowheads*). Compare with normal ring finger.

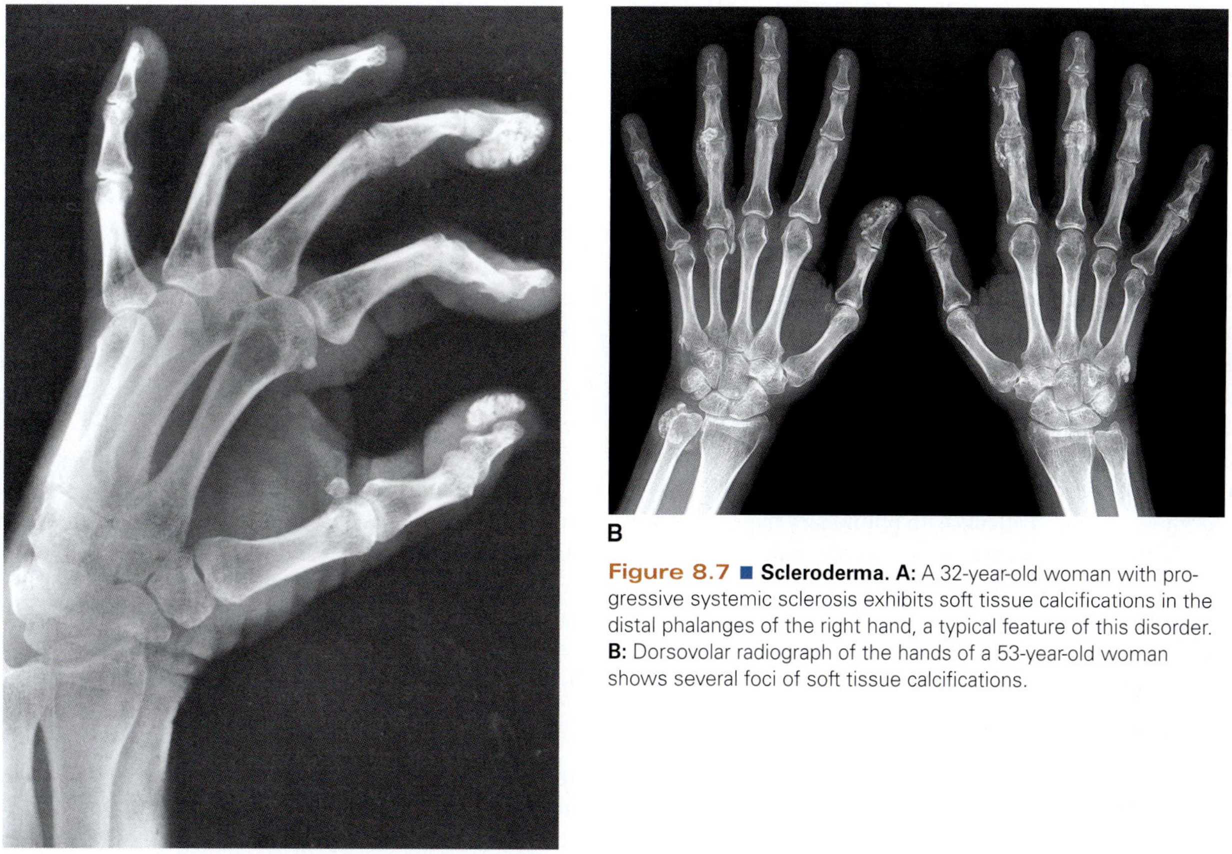

A B

Figure 8.7 ■ **Scleroderma. A:** A 32-year-old woman with progressive systemic sclerosis exhibits soft tissue calcifications in the distal phalanges of the right hand, a typical feature of this disorder. **B:** Dorsovolar radiograph of the hands of a 53-year-old woman shows several foci of soft tissue calcifications.

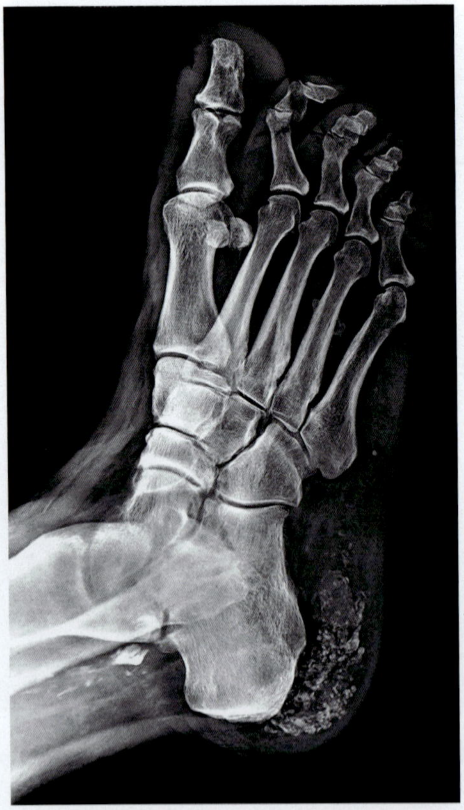

A

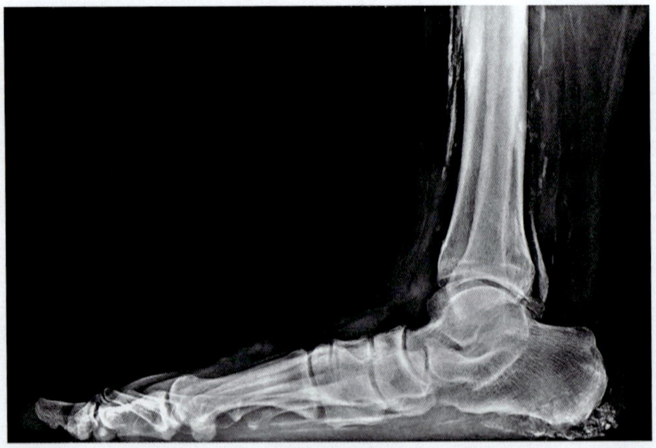

B

Figure 8.8 ■ **Scleroderma.** Oblique **(A)** and lateral **(B)** radiographs of the left foot of a 35-year-old man show calcifications of the soft tissues of the distal leg and adjacent to the calcaneus.

calcifications within the upper and lower limbs can occasionally be quite prominent (see Figs. 8.8 and 8.9B, C). Corroborative findings are seen in the gastrointestinal tract, where dilatation of the esophagus and small bowel, together with a pseudo-obstruction pattern, is characteristic (Fig. 8.11). Pseudodiverticula in the colon are also commonly seen.

Treatment

The treatment of scleroderma is elusive and there are no specific guidelines. Therapy includes the use of anti-inflammatory drugs such as NSAIDs, corticosteroids such as prednisone, immunosuppressive therapy, that is, cyclophosphamide, anti-interferon agents such as sifalimumab, anti-B-cell agents such as rituximab, and anticytokine therapy (anti-IL6R). Recent trials using autologous bone marrow transplantation yielded promising results but are not practical for most patients. Patients with pulmonary hypertension, a complication of scleroderma, are treated with prostaglandin inhibitors to reduce wedge pressure.

POLYMYOSITIS AND DERMATOMYOSITIS

Clinical Features

Polymyositis and dermatomyositis belong to the rare heterogeneous group of autoimmune myopathies. They represent disorders of striated muscle and skin and are characterized by diffuse, nonsuppurative inflammation, as well as degeneration. In adults, they can occur at any age, but the peak is seen between 45 and 60 years of age. Most patients have both skin and muscle involvement. Early diagnosis and subsequent management of patients with any type of myopathy, including polymyositis and dermatomyositis, can be facilitated by the use of appropriate laboratory tests. The four tests most helpful in evaluating muscle disorders include (1) serum enzymes, (2) urinary creatine and creatinine excretion, (3) electromyogram, and (4) muscle biopsy.

Different serum muscle enzyme determinations have been advocated, but the most valuable tests include serum creatine phosphokinase (CPK), aldolase (ALD), aspartate aminotransferase (AST), alamine aminotransferase (ALT), lactate dehydrogenase (LDH), glutamic oxaloacetic transaminase (SGOT), and serum glutamic pyruvic transaminase (SGPT). Further, the determination of serum enzyme levels and urinary creatine excretion is helpful for the clinical management of polymyositis and dermatomyositis, because the two tests provide a broader perspective than either test alone.

Polymyositis is characterized by a cytotoxic T-cell response targeting as yet unidentified muscle antigens presented by MHC class I molecules and can occur in isolation or more often as a part of multisystem overlap syndrome. Over the past decade, myositis-specific autoantibodies (MSAs) have been better characterized, including those directed against

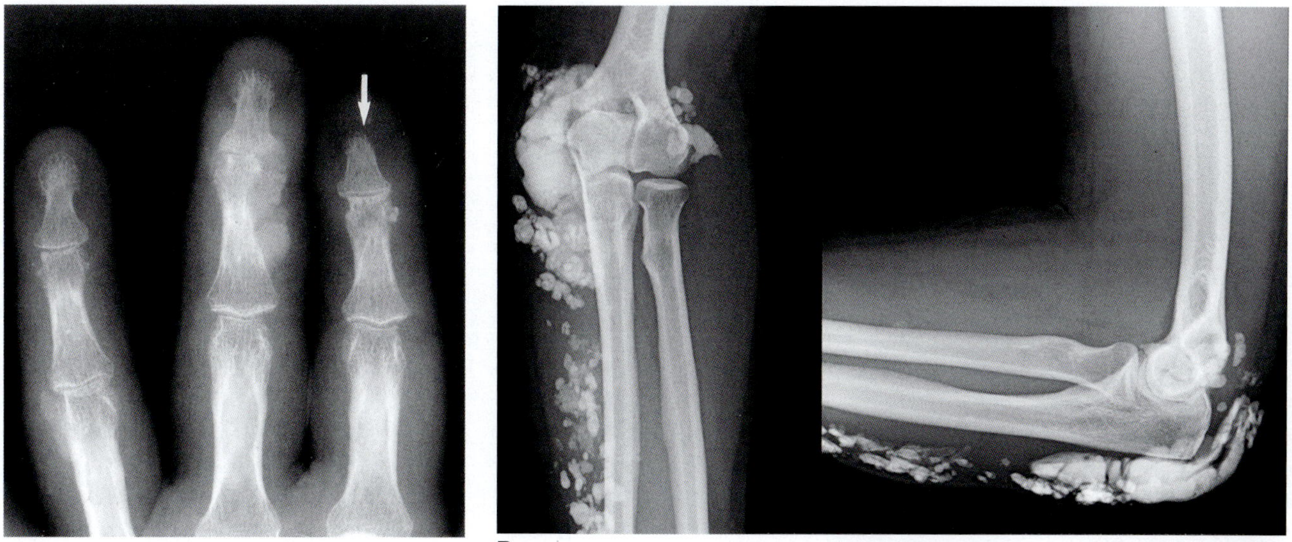

A B

Figure 8.9 ■ **Scleroderma. A:** Dorsovolar radiograph of the fingers of a 44-year-old woman reveals acroosteolysis (*arrow*), soft tissue calcifications, and destructive changes of the distal interphalangeal joint of the middle finger. **B:** In another patient, a 46-year-old woman, extensive soft tissue calcifications are present around the elbow and the forearm. **C:** Calcifications are present in the soft tissues of the posterior aspect of distal arm and proximal forearm in this 37-year-old woman.

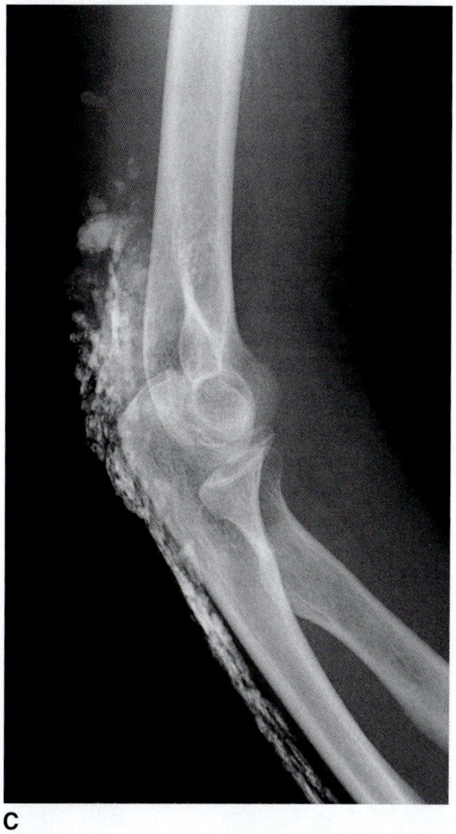

C

the aminoacyl-tRNA synthetase enzymes, the signal recognition particle and the Mi-2 protein. In addition, clinically significant novel autoantibodies—anti-CADM-140, anti-SAE (small ubiquitin-like modifier activating enzyme), anti-p155/140, and anti-p140—have been described. MSAs are directed against cytoplasmic or nuclear components involved in key regulatory intracellular processes including protein synthesis, translocations, and gene transcriptions. A number of different autoantibodies are found exclusively in dermatomyositis. Antibodies directed against the chromatin-remodeling enzyme Mi-2 are found in about 20% of patients. The anti-MDA5 antibodies have been reported in patients with amyopathic dermatomyositis, particularly in those with interstitial lung disease. In some patients, anti-small ubiquitin-like modifier 1 (SUMO-1) antibodies have been identified. Antinuclear antibodies were found in about 50% of patients with polymyositis and dermatomyositis and were found to be associated with the presence of antibodies directed against a nuclear protein Mi-2.

A positive biopsy may not only demonstrate that the disease process is myopathy, thus enabling the physician to rule out a neurogenic lower motor neuron lesion, but may also

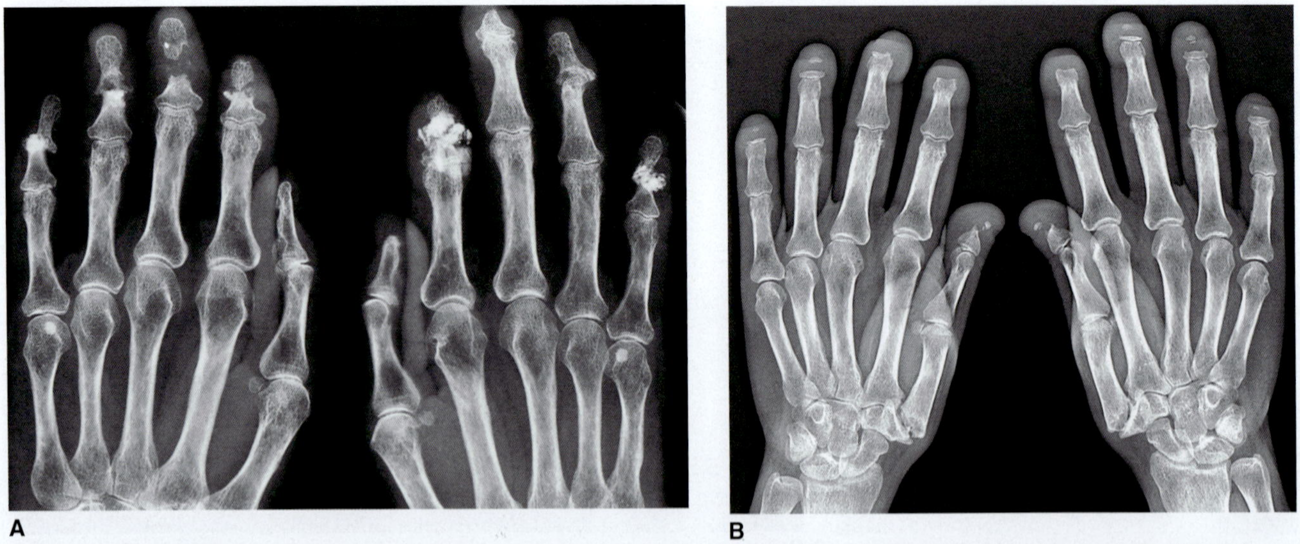

Figure 8.10 ■ Scleroderma. A: Dorsovolar radiograph of the hands of a 50-year-old man shows destructive changes in the distal interphalangeal joints, as well as soft tissue calcifications and resorption of the tip of the distal phalanx of the left middle finger. **B:** Dorsovolar radiograph of the hands of a 53-year-old woman with long-standing systemic sclerosis shows acroosteolysis of all distal phalanges. Note also erosions of the first carpometacarpal joints.

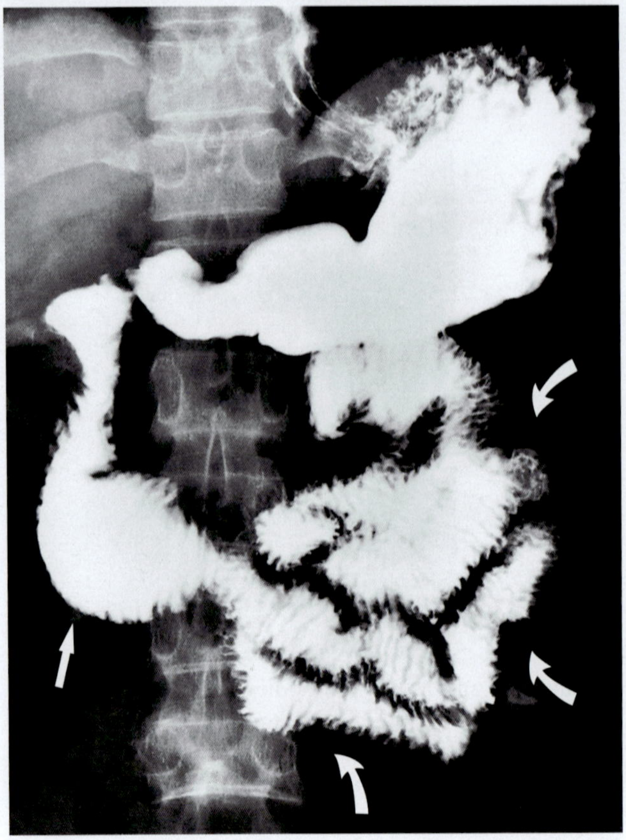

Figure 8.11 ■ Scleroderma. Upper gastrointestinal series and small bowel study in the patient shown in Figure 8.10A demonstrate dilatation of the second and third portions of the duodenum (*arrow*) and jejunum (*curved arrows*), with a pseudoobstruction pattern.

identify those patients whose muscle disease is more severe pathologically than was suspected on clinical grounds. This is important with respect to prognosis. With the aid of histochemical and electron microscopic techniques, muscle biopsy will occasionally enable the pathologist to diagnose one of the rare forms of myopathy that can clinically mimic polymyositis. Such diseases include sarcoid myopathy, central core disease, and muscle diseases associated with abnormal mitochondria.

The pathologic changes found on muscle biopsy in polymyositis have been well described. The degree of pathologic change may vary widely; one patient may show only negligible pathologic changes in muscle fibers on biopsy results, whereas another patient presenting similar clinical features may show extensive necrosis and fiber replacement. This variability in histologic findings is probably responsible for the frequent normal muscle biopsy results from patients with otherwise classic polymyositis. The overall rate of positive findings from muscle biopsy in several studies of polymyositis was in the range of 55% to 80%. The most common finding is lymphocytic infiltration. Areas of myonecrosis may be encountered.

Clinical symptoms consist of symmetric muscle weakness, especially in the proximal parts of the extremities. Additional symptoms include arthralgias, myalgias, and severe fatigue; Raynaud phenomenon may also be encountered. Dyspnea may reflect diaphragmatic weakness. Patients with dermatomyositis may present with cutaneous manifestations, including Gottron papules (raised violaceous lesions on the extensor surfaces of the elbows, knees, and the hands—particularly at the site of metacarpophalangeal and

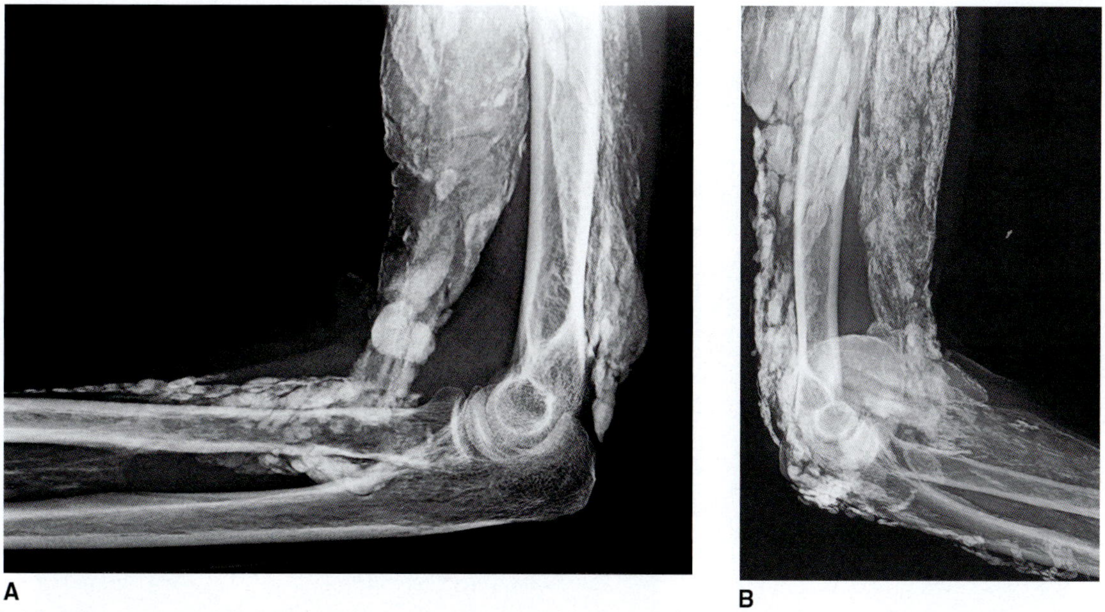

Figure 8.12 ■ **Dermatomyositis.** Lateral radiographs of the left **(A)** and right **(B)** elbow of a 50-year-old-woman show extensive calcifications of the muscles of the arm and forearm.

interphalangeal joints) and heliotrope rash (red or purple discoloration of the eyelids). Less common, erythematous or poikilodermatous rash across the posterior neck and shoulders (the shawl sign) and on the anterior neck and chest (the V-sign) may be observed. Some patients exhibit hyperkeratotic skin thickening, often associated with painful crackings either on the radial surfaces of the fingers (so-called mechanic's hands) or toes (mechanic's feet). Periungual telangiectasias and nail fold capillary changes identical to those seen in scleroderma also have been reported.

Imaging Features

Imaging abnormalities in polymyositis and dermatomyositis are divided into two types: those involving soft tissues and those involving joints. The most characteristic soft tissue abnormality in both conditions is soft tissue calcifications. The favorite sites of intramuscular calcification are the large muscles in the proximal parts of upper and lower extremities (Figs. 8.12 and 8.13). In addition, subcutaneous calcifications similar to those of scleroderma are seen

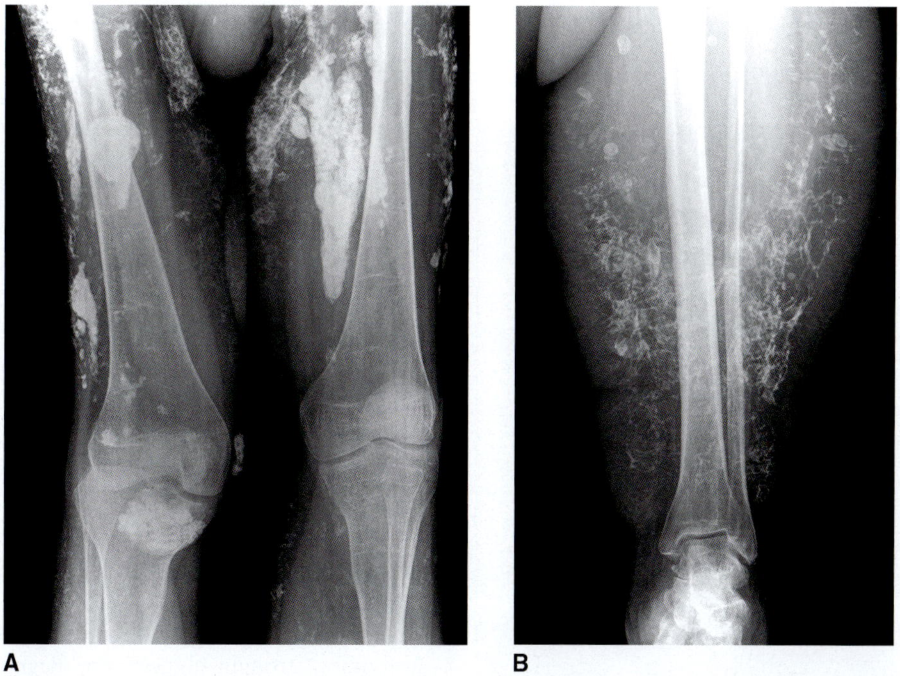

Figure 8.13 ■ **Dermatomyositis. A:** Anteroposterior radiograph of both knees shows extensive calcifications within the muscles. Observe also subcutaneous calcifications. The bones are markedly osteoporotic. **B:** Anteroposterior radiograph of the left leg of a 66-year-old woman shows subcutaneous and muscle calcifications.

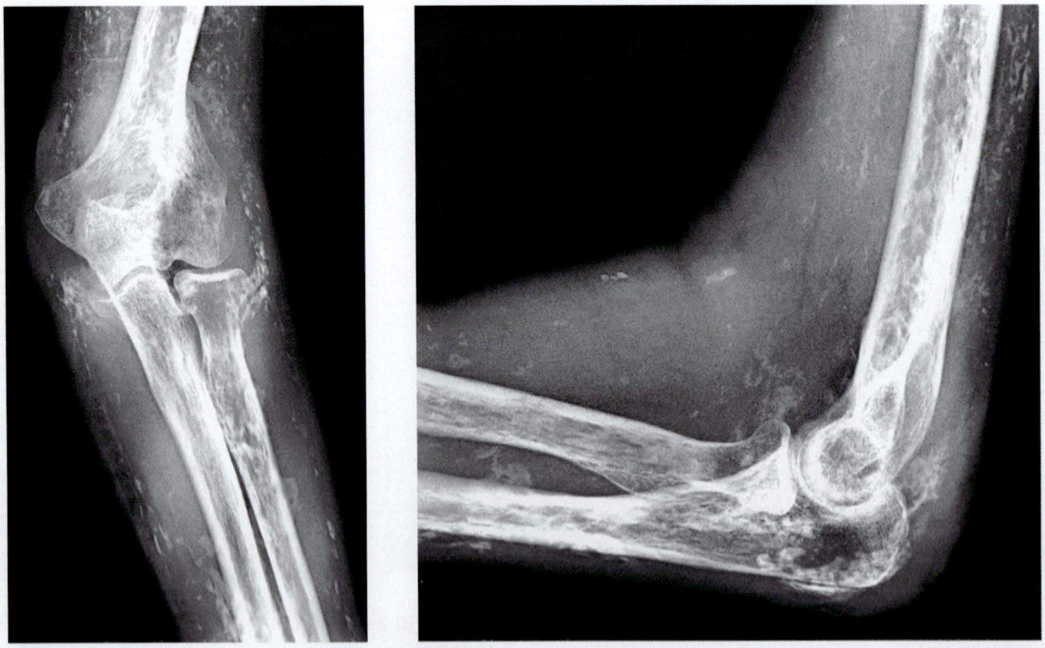

A B

Figure 8.14 ■ **Dermatomyositis.** External oblique **(A)** and lateral **(B)** radiographs of the left elbow of a 64-year-old woman show extensive soft tissue calcifications, characteristic for this disorder. Note also prominent periarticular osteoporosis.

(Figs. 8.14 and 8.15). MRI offers the best evaluation of abnormalities of the soft tissues including muscles. Muscle edema is an indicator of active inflammation (Figs. 8.16 and 8.17), and fatty infiltration is an indicator of chronic process (Fig. 8.18). MRI is also an effective modality to determine the site for muscle biopsy. It is also an important technique in monitoring the disease progression and response to therapy.

Articular abnormalities are rare. The most frequently reported, however, is periarticular osteoporosis. Destructive joint changes have been reported only occasionally and primarily in the distal interphalangeal articulations of the hands.

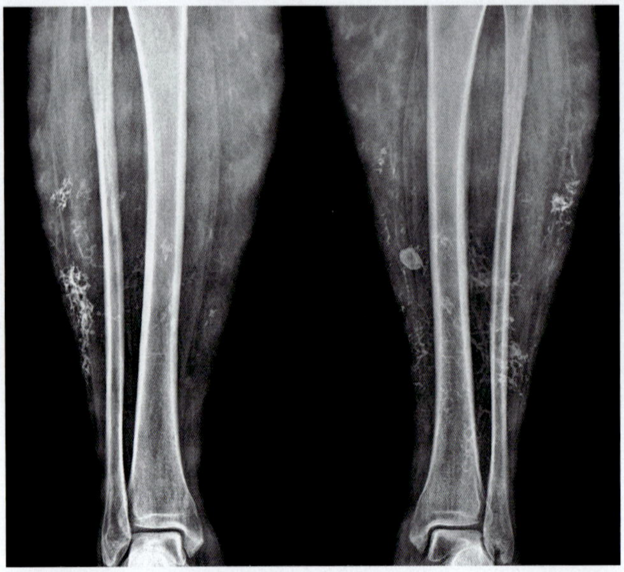

Figure 8.15 ■ **Dermatomyositis.** Anteroposterior radiograph of both legs of a 55-year-old woman shows predominantly cutaneous and subcutaneous calcifications.

Treatment

The therapy is directed to control inflammation through corticosteroids drugs. Immunosuppressive agents, including methotrexate, azathioprine, cyclophosphamide, cyclosporine A, and chlorambucil may be used for patients who do not respond to corticosteroids. Rituximab and mycophenolate mofetil have shown some benefit in patients who have been resistant to other therapies. Combination therapy such as azathioprine plus methotrexate and methotrexate plus cyclosporine A also has been tried. Intravenous administration of gamma globulins has been tried with mixed results.

MIXED CONNECTIVE TISSUE DISEASE (MCTD)

Mixed connective tissue disease (MCTD) was first reported as a distinctive syndrome by Sharp and associates in 1972. This syndrome is characterized by clinical abnormalities that combine the features of SLE, scleroderma, dermatomyositis, and rheumatoid arthritis. The one feature that distinguishes MCTD as a separate entity is a positive serologic test for antibody to the ribonucleoprotein (RNP) component of extractable nuclear antigen (ENA). Furthermore, anti-RNP antibodies, particularly those directed against ribonuclear protein U1-RNP, were found to be associated with MCTD. Detection of anti-RNP antibodies, in the absence of other antibodies, strongly suggests the diagnosis of MCTD. The typical clinical pattern of this condition consists of Raynaud phenomenon, polyarthralgia, swelling of the hands and

(Continued on page 322)

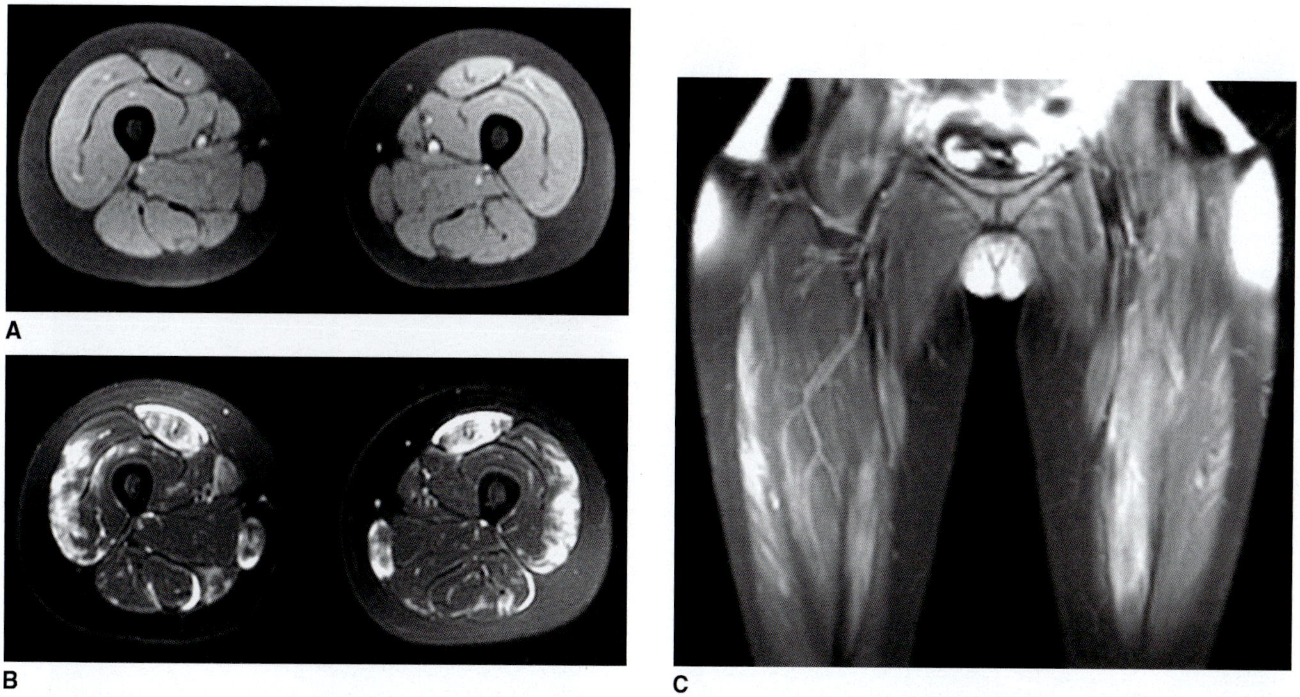

Figure 8.16 ■ MRI of polymyositis. Axial T1-weighted **(A)**, and axial **(B)** and coronal **(C)** T1-weighted fat-suppressed MR images obtained after intravenous administration of gadolinium, show enhancement of several group of muscles of the thighs of a 23-year-old woman, including abductors, rectus femoris, vastus lateralis, vastus intermedius, sartorius, gracilis, semimembranosus, and semitendinosus.

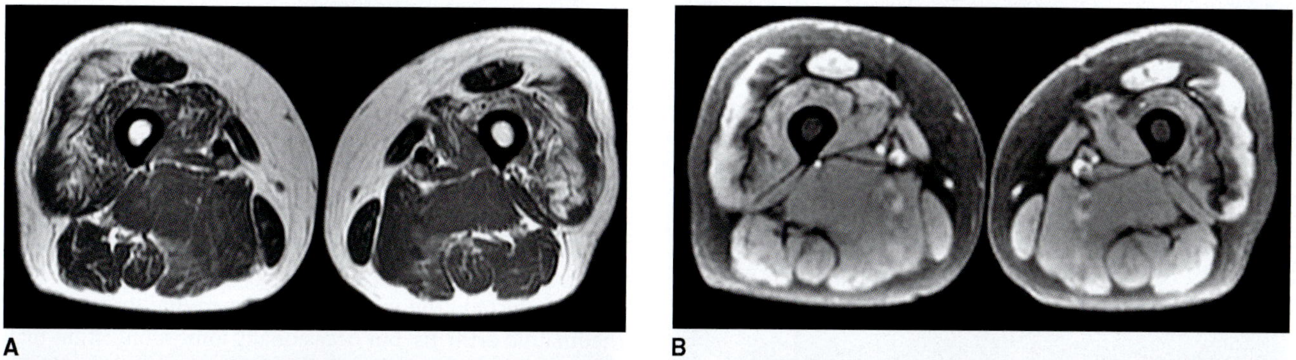

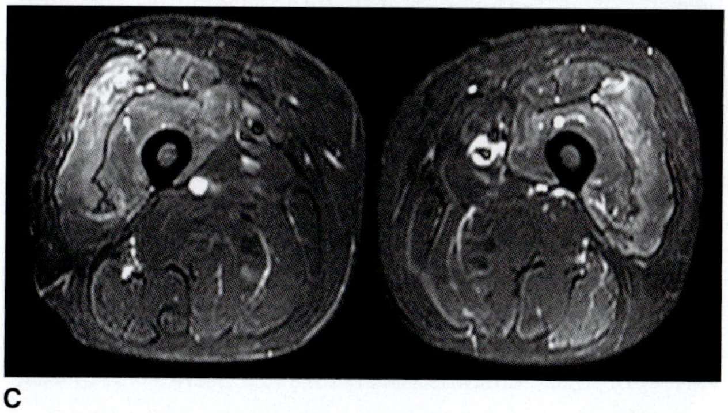

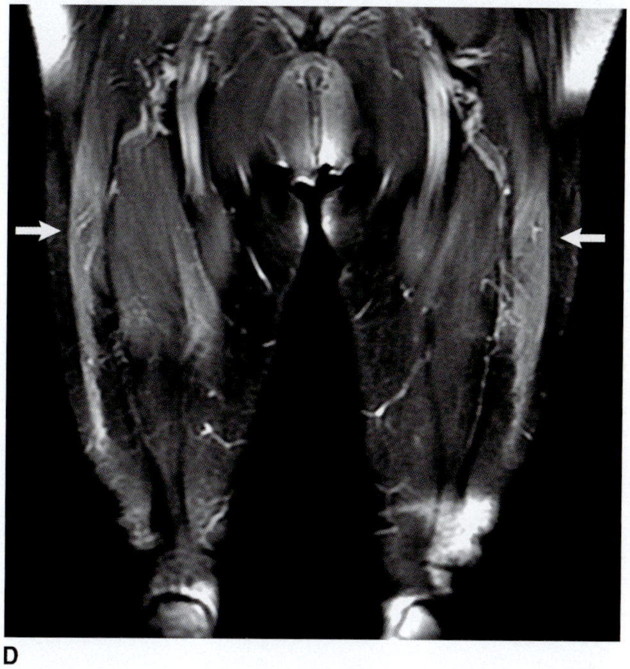

Figure 8.17 ■ MRI of polymyositis. A: Axial T1-weighted MR image of both thighs of a 65-year-old woman shows fatty atrophy predominantly affecting vastus lateralis and rectus femoris muscles. **B:** Axial T1-weighted fat-suppressed image shows areas of high signal intensities within the muscle structures. **C:** Axial STIR image shows high signal within the vastus lateralis muscles representing edema. **D:** Coronal T1-weighted fat-suppressed image obtained after intravenous administration of gadolinium shows subtle symmetrical enhancement of vastus lateralis (*arrows*).

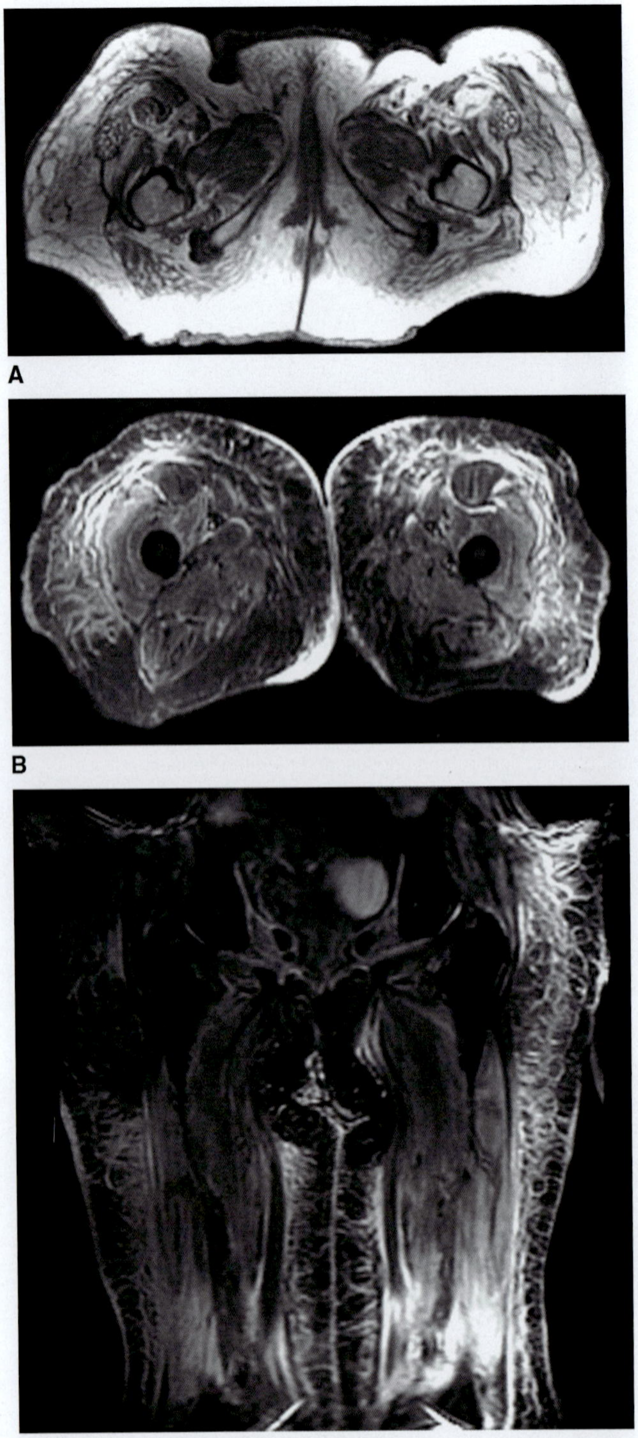

Figure 8.18 ■ MRI of polymyositis. A: Axial T1-weighted MR image of the proximal thighs of a 57-year-old woman shows fatty atrophies of all groups of muscles. Axial **(B)** and coronal **(C)** inversion recovery (IR) MR images demonstrate extensive subcutaneous fat and muscle edema.

fingers, esophageal hypomotility, inflammatory myopathy, lymphadenopathy, and pulmonary disease. Women constitute approximately 80% of affected patients. Patients with MCTD have prominent joint abnormalities, with typical involvement of the small articulations of the hand, wrist, and foot; large joints such as the knee, elbow, and shoulder may also be affected. The joint deformities mimic those seen in rheumatoid arthritis, but occasionally joint subluxation may be nonerosive, as in SLE. Soft tissue abnormalities are identical to those encountered in scleroderma (Figs. 8.19 to 8.23).

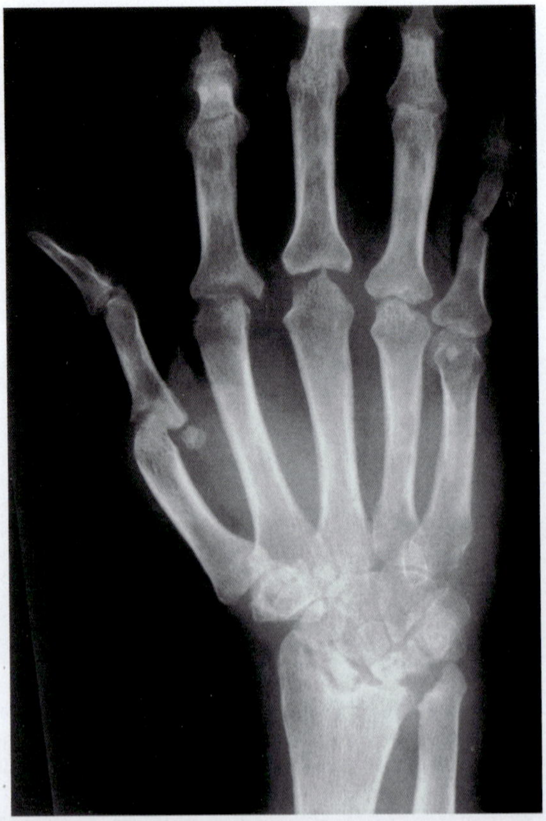

Figure 8.19 ■ Mixed connective tissue disease. A 44-year-old woman presented with clinical and imaging features of rheumatoid arthritis. In addition, she had clinically documented dermatomyositis. A dorsovolar radiograph of her left hand shows extensive articular erosions at radiocarpal, metacarpophalangeal, and proximal interphalangeal joints, typical for rheumatoid arthritis. The muscle biopsy result was consistent with polymyositis.

VASCULITIS

There is a diverse clinical spectrum of the vasculitides that includes systemic necrotizing vasculitis, hypersensitivity vasculitis, Wegener granulomatosis, lymphomatoid granulomatosis, giant cell arteritis (Takayasu arteritis), and a variety of miscellaneous syndromes (e.g., Kawasaki disease, Behçet disease, Churg-Strauss syndrome, and others). A discussion of these diverse but often overlapping diseases is far beyond the scope of this volume, and the reader is referred to several key references at the end of this chapter. The demonstration of vasculitis by angiograms can often be documented by the presence of aneurysmal dilatation in affected vessels. Generally, an angiogram is performed when the diagnosis cannot be established by tissue biopsy. Most recently, more advanced imaging modalities are

(Continued on page 324)

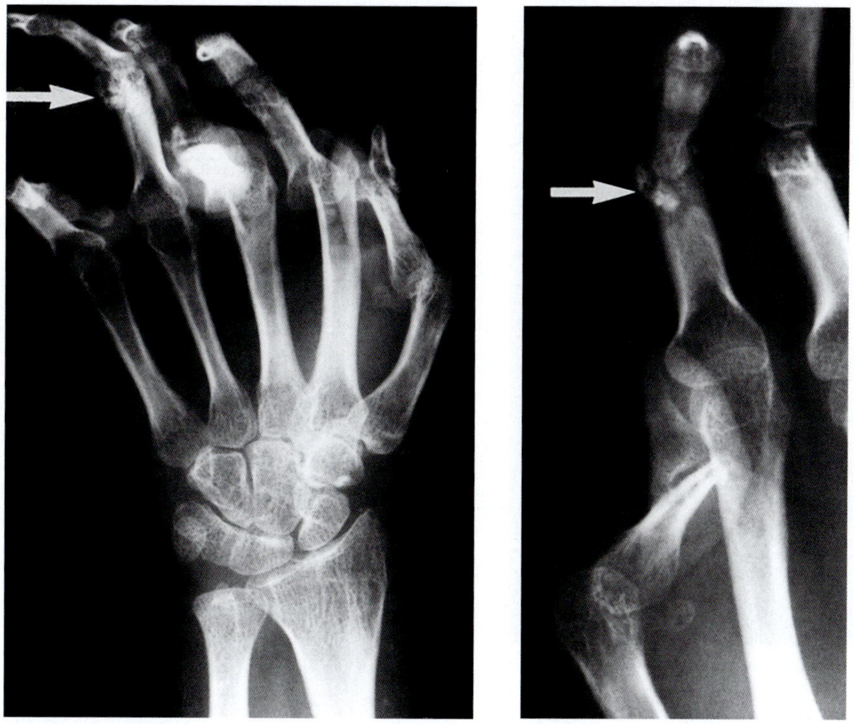

A B

Figure 8.20 ■ **Mixed connective tissue disease.** A 26-year-old woman presented with swelling of hands, polyarthralgia, and Raynaud phenomenon. She tested positively for the rheumatoid factors and antinuclear antibodies, and her clinical findings were characteristic for SLE and scleroderma. Oblique radiograph **(A)** of the right hand and coned-down view **(B)** of the thumb and index finger of the left hand show flexion deformities and subluxations in the multiple joints. Deformities of both thumbs are characteristic for SLE, whereas soft tissue calcifications (*arrows*) are typical for scleroderma.

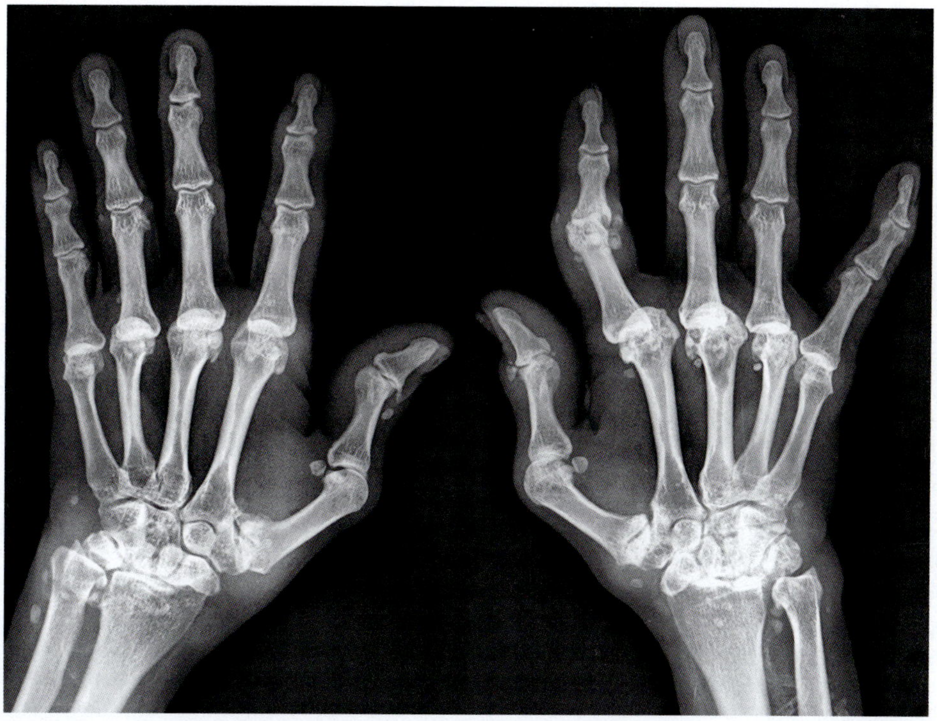

Figure 8.21 ■ **Mixed connective tissue disease.** Dorsovolar radiograph of the hands of a 55-year-old woman with documented long-standing rheumatoid arthritis, lupus erythematosus, and scleroderma shows erosive changes in both wrists, subluxations in the metacarpophalangeal joints, and soft tissue calcifications.

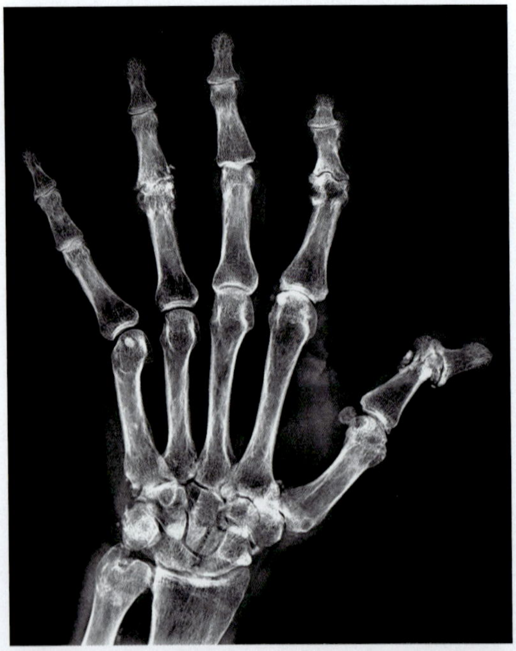

Figure 8.22 ■ Mixed connective tissue disease. Dorsovolar radiograph of the right hand of a 60-year-old man with a positive rheumatoid factor and skin changes typical for scleroderma shows erosions of the proximal interphalangeal joints of the index and ring fingers, second metacarpophalangeal joint, and the interphalangeal joint of the thumb. Note also soft tissue calcifications.

applied for diagnosis of the above-referenced condition, including CT angiography (see Figs. 2.32 and 2.33), MR angiography (see Fig. 2.36), and ^{18}F-FDG PET and PET/CT (see Fig. 2.72).

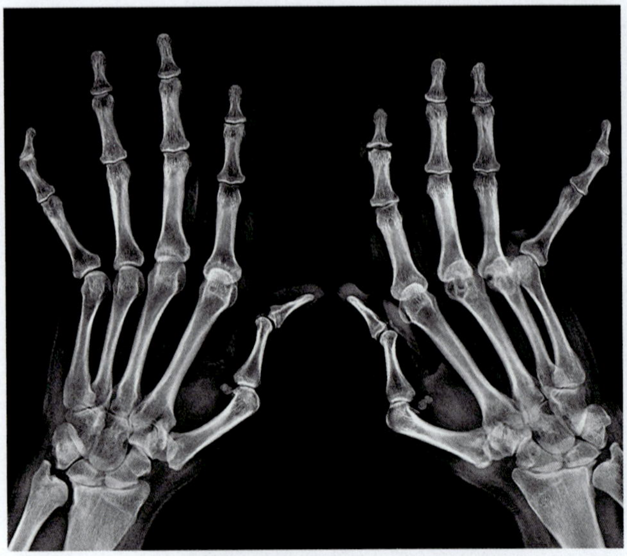

Figure 8.23 ■ Mixed connective tissue disease. Dorsovolar radiograph of the hands of a 52-year-old woman with clinically documented long-standing lupus erythematosus and rheumatoid arthritis shows features of both conditions, including erosions of the metacarpophalangeal joints, and subluxations in the first carpometacarpal joints and in the left fifth metacarpophalangeal joint.

SUGGESTED READINGS

Alexoudi I, Kapsimali V, Vaiopoulos A, et al. Evaluation of current therapeutic strategies in Behçet's disease. *Clin Rheumatol.* 2011;30:157–163.

Appel GB, Contreras G, Dooley MA, et al. Mycophenolate mofetil versus cyclophosphamide as lupus nephritis induction treatment. *J Am Soc Nephrol.* 2009;20:1103.

Arbuckie MR, McClain MT, Rubertone MV, et al. Development of antibodies before the clinical onset of systemic lupus erythematosus. *N Engl J Med.* 2003;349:1526–1533.

Assassi S, Radstake T, Mayes MD, et al. Genetics of scleroderma: implications for personalized medicine? *BMC Med.* 2013;11:9–16.

Barron KS, Shulman ST, Rowley A, et al. Report of the National Institute of Health workshop on Kawasaki disease. *J Rheumatol.* 1999;26:170–190.

Betteridge Z, Gunawardena H, North J, et al. Identification of a novel autoantibody directed against small ubiquitin-like modifier activating enzyme in dermatomyositis. *Arthritis Rheum.* 2007;56:3132–3137.

Borchers AT, Leibushor N, Naguwa SM, et al. Lupus nephritis: a critical review. *Autoimmun Rev.* 2012;12:174–194.

Borchers AT, Naguwa SM, Shoenfeld Y, et al. The geoepidemiology of systemic lupus erythematosus. *Autoimmun Rev.* 2010;9:277–287.

Brower AC, Resnick D, Karlin C, et al. Unusual articular changes of the hand in scleroderma. *Skeletal Radiol.* 1979;4:119–123.

Bunch TW. Prednisone and azathioprine for polymyositis: long-term follow-up. *Arthritis Rheum.* 1981;24:45–48.

Churg A. Recent advances in the diagnosis of Churg-Strauss syndrome. *Mod Pathol.* 2001;14:1284–1293.

Dajani AS, Taubert KA, Takahashi M, et al. Guidelines for long-term management of patients with Kawasaki disease. *Circulation.* 1994;89:916–922.

Dalakas MC. Calcifications in dermatomyositis. *N Engl J Med.* 1995;333:978–979.

Dalakas MC. Clinical, immunologic and therapeutic considerations of inflammatory myopathies. *Clin Neuropharmacol.* 1992;15:327–351.

Dalakas MC. Current treatment of the inflammatory myopathies. *Curr Opin Rheumatol.* 1994;6:595–601.

Dalakas M, Hohlfeld R. Polymyositis and dermatomyositis. *Lancet.* 2003;362:971–982.

Dell'Era M, Wofay D. Lupus clinical trials – an interim analysis. *Nat Rev Rheumatol.* 2009;5:348–351.

Denslow SA, Wade PA. The human Mi-2/NuRD complex and gene regulation. *Oncogene.* 2007;26:5433–5438.

Doria A, Gershwin ME, Selmi C. From old concerns to new advances and personalized medicine in lupus: the end of the tunnel is approaching. *J Autoimmun.* 2016;74:1–5.

Endo M, Tomizawa Y, Nishida H, et al. Angiographic findings and surgical treatment of coronary artery involvement in Takayasu arteritis. *J Thorac Cardiovasc Surg.* 2003;125:570–577.

Ferri C, Mascia MT. Cryoglobulinemic vasculitis. *Curr Opin Rheumatol.* 2006;18:54–63.

Fox R, Robinson C, Curd J, et al. Sjögren's syndrome. Proposed criteria for classification. *Arthritis Rheumatol.* 1986;29:577–585.

Garcia-Carrasco M, Ramos-Casals M, Rosas J, et al. Primary Sjögren's syndrome. Clinical and immunologic disease patterns in a cohort of 400 patients. *Medicine.* 2002;81:270–280.

Godman G, Churg J. Wegener's granulomatosis: pathology and review of the literature. *Arch Pathol Lab Med.* 1954;58:533–553.

Godman G. Wegener's granulomatosis. *Am J Med.* 1954;17:168–179.

Gottenberg J, Busson M, Loiseau P, et al. In primary Sjögren's syndrome, HLA class II is associated exclusively with autoantibody production and spreading of the autoimmune response. *Arthritis Rheumatol.* 2003;48:2240–2245.

Grundtman C, Lundberg IE. Pathogenesis of idiopathic inflammatory myopathies. *Curr Opin Rheumatol.* 2006;8:188–195.

Guerra SG, Vyse TJ, Cunninghame Graham DS. The genetics of lupus: a functional prospective. *Arthritis Res Ther.* 2012;14:211.

Gunawardena H, Belteridge ZE, McHugh NJ. Myositis-specific autoantibodies: their clinical and pathogenic significance in disease expression. *Rheumatology (Oxford).* 2009;48:607–612.

Hall JC, Casciola-Rosen L, Samedy L-A, et al. Anti-MDA5-associated dermatomyositis: expanding the clinical spectrum. *Arthritis Care Res.* 2013;65:1307–1315.

Helmick C, Felson DT, Lawrence R, et al. Estimates of the prevalence of arthritis and other rheumatic conditions in the United States. Part I. *Arthritis Rheum.* 2008;58:15–25.

Helmick C, Felson DT, Lawrence R, et al. Estimates of the prevalence of arthritis and other rheumatic conditions in the United States. Part II. *Arthritis Rheum.* 2008;58:26–35.

Hochberg MC. Updating the American College of Rheumatology revised criteria for 463 the classification of systemic lupus erythematosus. *Arthritis Rheum.* 1997;40:1725.

Hunder GG, Bloch DA, Mitchel BA, et al. The American College of Rheumathology 1990 criteria for the classification of giant cell arteritis. *Arthritis Rheum.* 1990;33:1122–1128.

International Study Group for Behçet's Disease. Criteria for diagnosis of Behçet's disease. *Lancet.* 1990;335:1078–1080.

Jennette JC, Falk RJ, Andrassy K, et al. Nomenclature of systemic vasculitides. Proposal of an international consensus conference. *Arthritis Rheum.* 1994;37:187–192.

Johansson M, Arlestig L, Moller B, et al. Association of a PDCD1 polymorphism with renal manifestations in systemic lupus erythematosus. *Arthritis Rheum.* 2005;52:1665–1669.

Kaklamani VG, Vaiopoulos G, Kaklamanis PG. Behçet's disease. *Semin Arthritis Rheum.* 1998;27:197–217.

La Montagna G, Sodano A, Capurro V, et al. The arthropathy of systemic sclerosis: a 12 month prospective clinical and imaging study. *Skeletal Radiol.* 2005;34:35–41.

Lang BA, Laxer RM, Morphy G, et al. Treatment of dermatomyositis with intravenous gammaglobulin. *Am J Med.* 1991;91:169–172.

Leavitt RY, Fauci AS, Bloch DA, et al. The American College of Rheumathology 1990 criteria for classification of Wegener's granulomatosis. *Arthritis Rheum.* 1990;33:1101–1107.

Long H, Yin H, Wang L, et al. The critical role of epigenetics in systemic lupus erythematosus and autoimmunity. *J Autoimmun.* 2016;74:118–138.

Luo Y-B, Mastaglia FL. Dermatomyositis, polymyositis and immune-mediated necrotizing myopathies. *Biochemica Biophys Acta.* 2015;1852: 622–632.

Malcus Johnsson P, Sandquist G, Bengtsson A, et al. Hand function and performance of daily activities in systemic lupus erythematosus. *Arthritis Rheum.* 2008;59:1432–1438.

Mammen AL, Truong A, Christopher-Stine L. Dermatomyositis, polymyositis, & immune-mediated necrotizing myopathy. In: Imboden JB, Hellmann DB, Stone JH, eds. *Current diagnosis & treatment: rheumatology*. 3rd ed. New York, NY: McGraw Hill Medical; 2013:232–241.

Martin J, Fonseca C. The genetics of scleroderma. *Curr Rheumatol Rep.* 2011;13:13–20.

Martin JE, Bossini-Castillo L, Martin J. Unraveling the genetic component of systemic sclerosis. *Hum Genet.* 2012;131:1023–1037.

Mastaglia FL, Phillips BA, Zilko P. Treatment of inflammatory myopathies. *Muscle Nerve.* 1997;20:651–664.

Mattaj IW, Habets WJ, van Venrooij WJ. Monospecific antibodies reveal details of U2 snRNP structure and interaction between U1 and U2 snRNPs. *EMBO J.* 1986;5:997–1002.

Migliorini P, Baldini C, Rocchi V, et al. Anti-Sm and anti-RNP antibodies. *Autoimmunity.* 2005;38:47–54.

Misra R, Darton K, Jewkes RF, et al. Arthritis in scleroderma. *Br J Rheumatol.* 1995;34:831–837.

Matsunga N, Hayahi K, Sahamoto I, et al. Takayasu arteritis: protean radiologic manifestations and diagnosis. *Radiographics.* 1997;17:579–594.

Mosca M, Boumpas DT, Bruce IN, et al. Treat-to-target in systemic lupus erythematosus: where are we today? *Clin Exp Rheumatol.* 2012;30: S112–S115.

Mosca M, Tani C, Filice ME, et al. TNF-alpha inhibitors in systemic lupus erythematosus. A case report and systematic literature review. *Mod Rheumatol.* 2015;25:642–645.

Pipitone N, Versari A, Salvarani C. Role of imaging studies in the diagnosis and follow-up of large-vessel vasculitis: an update. *Rheumatology.* 2008;47:403–408.

Presley BC, Bush JS, Watson S. Dermatomyositis with extensive calcifications in an adult. *West J Emerg Med.* 2012;13:136–138.

Sarova-Pinhas I, Siegal T, Turgman J, et al. Methotrexate treatment in dermatomyositis. *Eur Neurol.* 1977;16:149–154.

Schanz S, Fierlbeck G, Ulmer A, et al. Localized scleroderma: MR findings and clinical features. *Radiology.* 2011;260:817–824.

Scofield RH, Bruner GR, Namjou B, et al. Klinefelter's syndrome (47,XXY) in male systemic lupus erythematosus patients: support for the notion of a gene-dose effect from the X chromosome. *Arthritis Rheum.* 2008;58: 2511–2517.

Sestak AL, Nath SK, Sawalha AH, et al. Current status of lupus genetics. *Arthritis Res Ther.* 2007;9:210–224.

Sharp GC, Irvin WS, Tan EM, et al. Mixed connective tissue disease—an apparently distinct rheumatic disease syndrome associated with a specific antibody to an extractable nuclear antigen (ENA). *Am J Med.* 1972;52:148–159.

Sultan SM. Clinical assessment in adult onset idiopathic inflammatory myopathy. *Curr Opin Rheumatol.* 2004;16:668–672.

Tani C, D'Aniello D, Possemato N, et al. MRI pattern of arthritis in systemic lupus erythematosus: a comparative study with rheumatoid arthritis and healthy subjects. *Skeletal Radiol.* 2015;44:261–266.

Targoff I. Laboratory testing in the diagnosis and management of idiopathic inflammatory myopathies. *Rheum Dis Clin North Am.* 2002;28: 859–890.

Taroff IN, Reichlin M. The association between Mi-2 antibodies and dermatomyositis. *Arthritis Rheum.* 1985;28:796–803.

Taubert KA. Epidemiology of Kawasaki disease in the United States and worldwide. *Prog Pediatr Cardiol.* 1997;6:181–185.

Tsao BP. Update on human systemic lupus erythematosus genetics. *Curr Opin Rheumatol.* 2004;16:513–521.

Udoff EJ, Genant HK, Kozin F, et al. Mixed connective tissue disease: the spectrum of radiographic manifestations. *Radiology.* 1977;124: 613–618.

Vencovsky J, Jarosova K, Machacek S, et al. Cyclosporine A versus methotrexate in the treatment of polymyositis and dermatomyositis. *Scand J Rheumatol.* 2000;29:95–102.

Villalba L, Adams EM. Update on therapy for refractory dermatomyositis and polymyositis. *Curr Opin Rheumatol.* 1996;8:544–551.

Wang Y, Ladunga I, Miller AR, et al. The small ubiquitin-like modifier (SUMO) and SUMO-conjugating system of Chlamydomonas reinhardtii. *Genetics.* 2008;179:177–192.

Weinel S, Callen J. Calcinosis cutis complicating adult-onset dermatomyositis. *Arch Dermat.* 2004;140:365–366.

Weiss JE, Eberhard BA, Chowdury D, et al. Infliximab as a novel therapy for refractory Kawasaki disease. *J Rheumatol.* 2004;3:808–810.

Wung PK, Stone JH. Therapeutics for Wegener's granulomatosis. *Nat Clin Pract Rheumatol.* 2006;2:192–200.

Zhang Y, LeRoy G, Seelig H-S, et al. The dermatomyositis-specific autoantigen Mi2 is a component of a complex containing histone deacetylase and nucleosome remodeling activities. *Cell.* 1998;95:279–289.

Zieglschmid-Adams ME, Pandya AG, Cohen SB, et al. Treatment of dermatomyositis with methotrexate. *J Am Acad Dermatol.* 1995;32:754–757.

CHAPTER 9

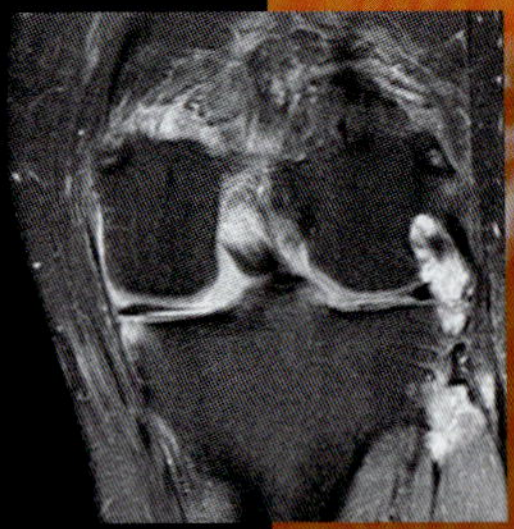

Musculoskeletal Infections

Infections of the musculoskeletal system can be subdivided into three categories: (a) those involving bones (osteomyelitis), (b) those involving joints (infectious arthritis), and (c) those involving soft tissues (cellulitis). Because of the complexity of the vertebrae and their soft tissue structures, infectious processes of the spine are considered under a separate heading.

INFECTIOUS ARTHRITIS

Three basic mechanisms allow an infectious organism—whether bacterium, virus, mycoplasma, rickettsia, or fungus—to reach the bone: (a) *hematogenous spread* via the bloodstream from a remote site of infection, such as the skin, tonsils, gallbladder, or urinary tract; (b) spread from a *contiguous source* of infection, such as from the soft tissues, teeth, or sinuses; and (c) *direct implantation*, such as through a puncture or missile wound or an operative procedure (Fig. 9.1). Hematogenous spread is common in children, and the usual focus of infection develops in the metaphysis. The metaphyseal location of infection in children is related to an osseous–vascular anatomy that differs in the infant, child, and adult. In the child (ages 1 to 16 years), there is separation of the blood supply to the metaphysis and epiphysis, each having its own source. Moreover, the arteries and capillaries of the metaphysis turn sharply without penetrating the open growth plate; in the region where capillaries become venules, the rate of blood flow is sluggish. Also contributing to the greater incidence of metaphyseal osteomyelitis in children is secondary thrombosis of end arteries with bacteria during transient bacteremia. In the infant (up to 1 year), however, osteomyelitis may sometimes have its focus in the epiphysis because some metaphyseal vessels may penetrate the growth plate and reach the epiphysis. With obliteration of the growth plate in the adult, there is vascular continuity between the shaft and the articular ends of the bone; hence, the focus of osteomyelitis can develop in any part of a bone. Contiguous spread and direct implantation are more common in adults. The sites of bone infection via either of these routes are directly related to the focus of soft tissue infection or the location of the wound.

An infectious agent (Table 9.1) may enter the joint by the same basic routes as in osteomyelitis: by direct invasion of the synovial membrane, either secondary to a penetrating wound or after a joint-replacement procedure, from an infection of the adjacent soft tissues, or indirectly via a blood-borne infection. Infectious arthritis may also occur secondary to a focus of osteomyelitis in the adjacent bone (Fig. 9.2).

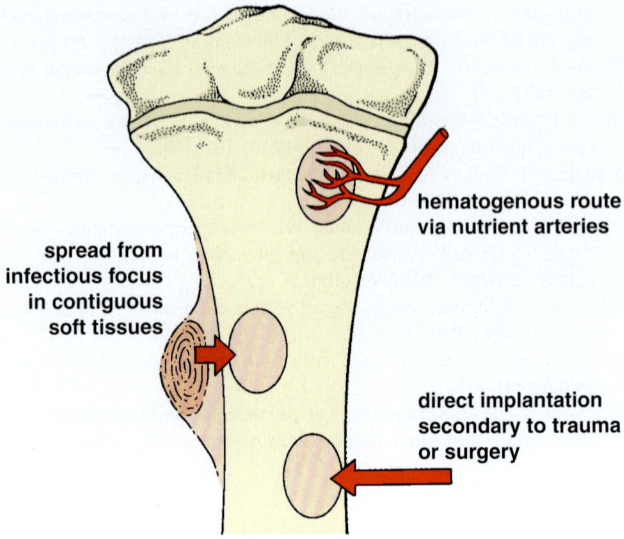

Figure 9.1 ■ Entry routes of an infectious organism into a bone. Infectious agents may gain entry to a bone through hematogenous spread, a source of infection in the contiguous soft tissues, or through direct implantation secondary to trauma or surgery.

Table 9.1 COMMON ETIOLOGIC AGENTS IN SEPTIC ARTHRITIS

Bacteria	Mycobacteria	Fungi	Spirochetes
Staphylococcus	*Mycobacterium tuberculosis*	*Actinomyces*	*Treponema pallidum*
Diplococcus	*Mycobacterium bovis*	*Coccidioides*	*Treponema pertenue*
Enterococcus	*Mycobacterium leprae*	*Cryptococcus*	*Borrelia burgdorferi*
Serratia	*Mycobacterium avium*	*Histoplasma*	
Pseudomonas	*Mycobacterium ulcerans*	*Blastomyces*	
Proteus		*Aspergillus*	
Clostridium		*Sporothrix*	
Bacteroides		*Candida*	
Escherichia		*Madurella*	
Klebsiella		*Nocardia*	
Neisseria			
Brucella			

PYOGENIC JOINT INFECTIONS

Clinical and Pathologic Features

Pyogenic (septic) arthritis is usually (80% to 90%) monoarticular with predilection for large weight-bearing joints, such as the knee or hip. The clinical signs and symptoms depend on the site and extent of involvement as well as the specific infectious organism. Although most cases of septic arthritis are caused by *Staphylococcus aureus*, *Escherichia coli*, and *Neisseria gonorrhoeae*, other pathogens—including *Pseudomonas aeruginosa*, *Enterobacter cloacae*, *Klebsiella pneumoniae*, *Candida albicans*, and *Serratia marcescens*—are being encountered with increasing frequency in joint infections in drug users caused by the contamination of injected drugs or needles. New strains of *Staphylococcus aureus* may be methicillin (MRSA) or vancomycin resistant. MRSA's secretion of the necrotizing toxin Panton-Valentine leukocidin results in more invasive infection and higher complication rates. Any large or small joint can be affected by septic arthritis, and hematogenous spread in drug addicts is characterized by unusual locations of the lesion, such as the spine (vertebrae and intervertebral disks), sacroiliac joints, sternoclavicular and acromioclavicular articulations, and pubic symphysis. Furthermore, with the increased usage of biologics and immunosuppressive drugs, clinicians should always keep in mind the possibility that an autoimmune disease has become complicated by an infection. This statement is particularly valid for the patients with rheumatoid arthritis who underwent surgery.

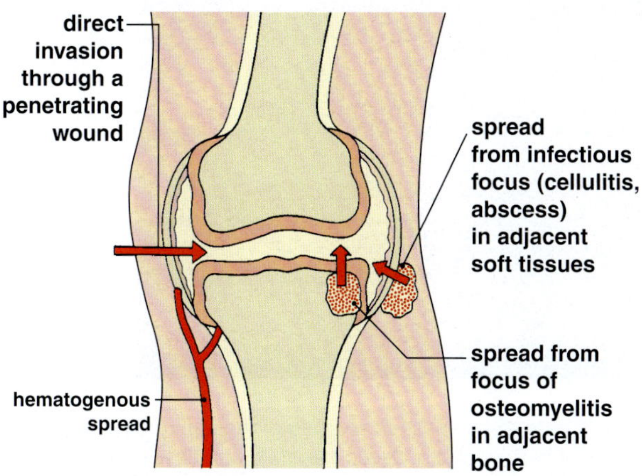

Figure 9.2 ■ Entry routes of an infectious organism into a joint. The routes of infection in infectious arthritis are similar to those of osteomyelitis, which itself may be a source of spread.

The classic clinical presentation of septic arthritis is an abrupt, acute onset of joint pain accompanied by swelling and warm sensation. The joint becomes tender to palpation, and there is marked restriction of both active and passive motion. Fever is encountered in about 60% to 80% of cases. Some patients may experience chills. Laboratory findings include elevation of white blood cell (WBC) count, elevation of erythrocyte sedimentation rate, and positive blood cultures. Pathologic findings include progressive and increasing neutrophilic infiltrate of the synovium, associated with vascular dilatation and congestion, and increased number of type A and B synoviocytes. This is followed by cartilage necrosis and subchondral bone erosion. Infiltrates of polymorphonuclear leukocytes on the articular cartilage surface are a common finding (Fig. 9.3). Synovial fluid appears opaque or frankly purulent. The nucleated cell count is very high, up to 50,000 cells per mm^3 (see also discussion in Chapter 1). Percutaneous aspiration and US-guided, CT-guided, or fluoroscopy-guided biopsy of a suspected focus of infection may be performed in the radiology suite. It can rapidly confirm a suspected diagnosis of infection and reveal the causative organism. For bacteriologic examination, synovial fluid should be placed into an empty sterile container (not carrying any media) and taken immediately to the laboratory for gram staining

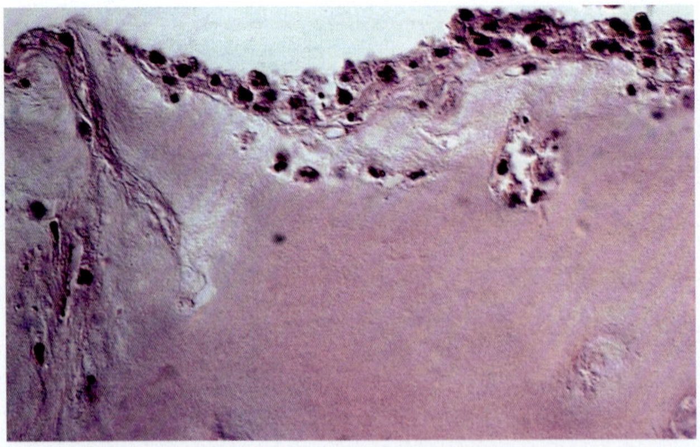

Figure 9.3 ■ Pathology of infectious arthritis. Photomicrograph of a portion of articular cartilage obtained from an acutely inflamed joint shows polymorphonuclear leukocytes on the cartilage surface and underlying erosion of the cartilage (H&E, original magnification ×25). (From Bullough PG. *Atlas of Orthopedic Pathology with Clinical and Radiologic Correlation*. 2nd ed. New York, NY: Gower Medical Publishing; 1992. Fig. 4.20, p. 4.11.)

and plating on appropriate media. Chocolate agar (CHOC), Thayer-Martin, or Transgrow media should be used when gonococcal arthritis is considered; Löwenstein-Jensen media, when tuberculous arthritis is suspected; Mannitol salt agar, for staphylococcus infection; and potato dextrose agar or Sabouraud agar for fungi infection.

Imaging Features

In most instances, conventional radiography is sufficient to demonstrate the pertinent features of a bone or joint infection, particularly with the advantage of digital radiography and newest technology of PACS (Picture Archive and Communication System) allowing filmless high-resolution image-display format. Most infectious arthritides demonstrate a very similar radiographic picture, including joint effusion and destruction of cartilage and subchondral bone with consequent joint space narrowing (Fig. 9.4, see also Fig. 3.19). However, certain radiographic features are characteristic of individual infectious processes as demonstrated at various target sites (Table 9.2) and may be helpful in arriving at the correct diagnosis. Generally, a single joint is affected, most commonly a weight-bearing joint like the knee or hip. The early stage of joint infection may be seen simply as joint effusion, soft tissue swelling, and periarticular osteoporosis, but "radiographic" joint space is usually preserved (Fig. 9.5). In the later phase of pyogenic arthritis, articular cartilage is destroyed; characteristically, both subarticular plates are involved and the joint space narrows (Figs. 9.6 to 9.9).

Scintigraphy has a very prominent role in diagnosing musculoskeletal infections, including infectious arthritis. In cases of suspected infection, radionuclide bone scan using

(Continued on page 331)

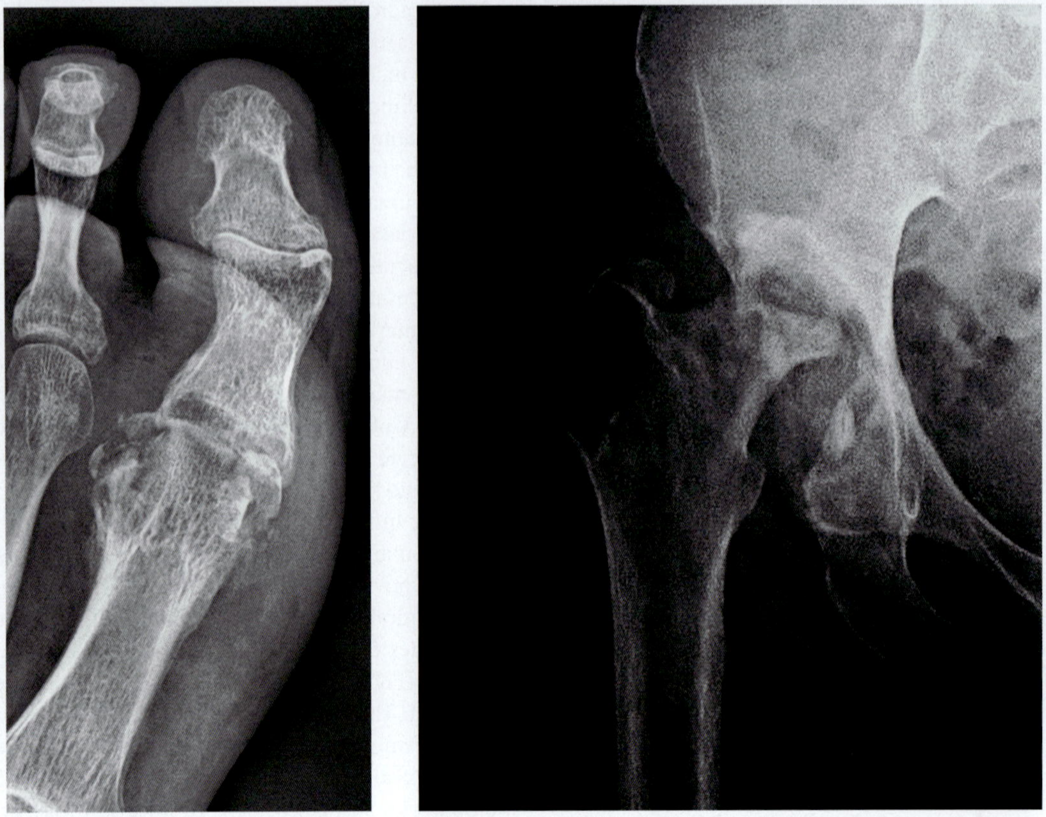

A B

Figure 9.4 ■ Infectious arthritis. A: A 48-year-old diabetic man presented with pain and soft tissue swelling of the right great toe for the past 3 months. Anteroposterior radiograph shows destruction of the first metatarsophalangeal joint associated with soft tissue swelling and edema typical for septic joint. **B:** In another patient, a 45-year-old HIV-positive man, who presented with a history of right hip pain for several months, anteroposterior radiograph shows extensive destruction of the right femoral head and right acetabulum. Hip joint aspiration and culture revealed methicillin-resistant *Staphylococcus aureus* (MARSA) infection.

Table 9.2 CLINICAL AND IMAGING HALLMARKS OF INFECTIOUS ARTHRITIS AT VARIOUS TARGET SITES

Type	Site	Crucial Abnormalities	Techniques/Projections
*Pyogenic Infections**	Peripheral joints	Periarticular osteoporosis	Radionuclide bone scan (early)
		Joint effusion	Standard views specific for site of involvement
		Destruction of subchondral bone (on both sides of joint)	Aspiration and arthrography
			MRI
	Spine	Narrowing of disk space	Anteroposterior and lateral views
		Loss of definition of vertebral end plate	
		Paraspinal mass	CT, MRI
		Partial or complete obstruction of intrathecal contrast flow	Myelogram
		Destruction of disk	Diskogram and aspiration
Nonpyogenic Infections			
Tuberculosis	Large joints	Monoarticular involvement (similar to rheumatoid arthritis)	Radionuclide bone scan
		"Kissing" sequestra (knee)	Standard views
		Sclerotic changes in subchondral bone	CT
	Spine	Gibbous formation	Anteroposterior and lateral views
		Lytic lesion in vertebral body	
		Destruction of disk	Diskogram and aspiration
		Paraspinal mass	CT, MRI
		Soft tissue abscess ("cold" abscess)	
		Obstruction of intrathecal contrast flow	Myelogram
Lyme disease	Knee	Narrowing of femoropatellar compartment	Lateral view
		Edematous changes in infrapatellar fat pad	CT, MRI

*In IV drug users, unusual sites of infection are encountered, including the vertebra; the sacroiliac, sternoclavicular, and acromioclavicular joints; and the pubic symphysis. The radiologic techniques used to evaluate infections at these sites, as well as the crucial radiographic abnormalities, are the same as those for the more common sites.

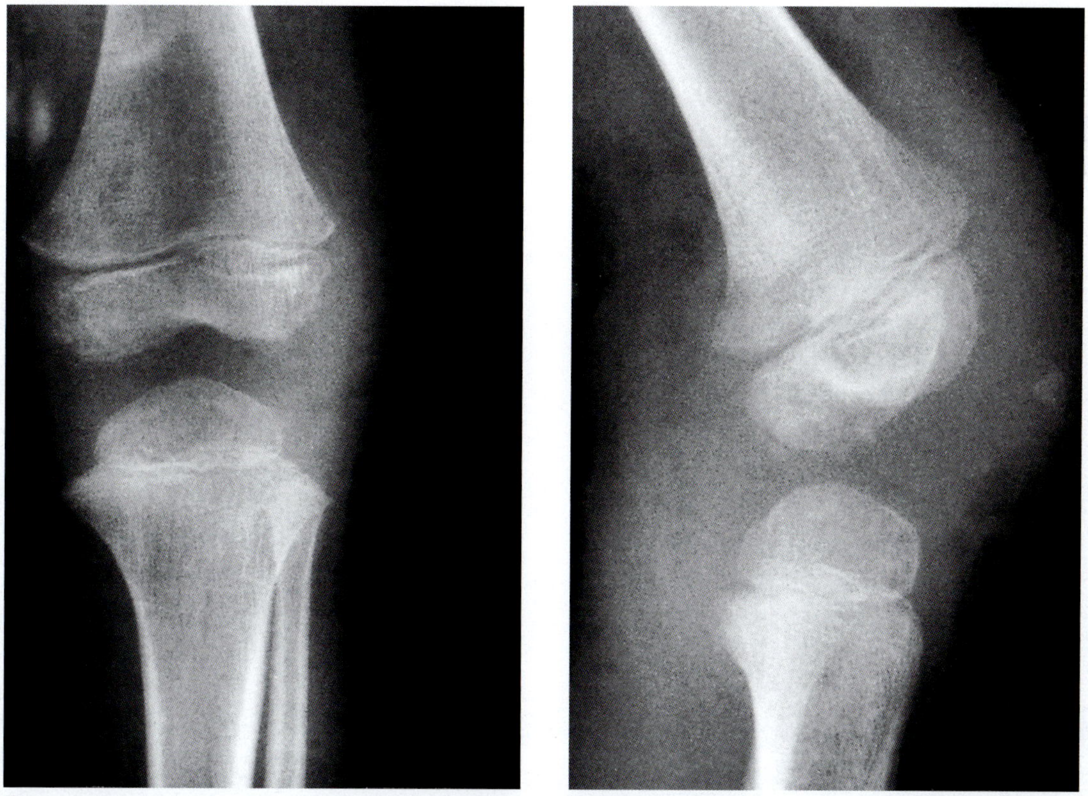

A B

Figure 9.5 ■ **Infectious arthritis.** Anteroposterior **(A)** and lateral **(B)** radiographs of the left knee of a 4-year-old child demonstrate a significant degree of periarticular osteoporosis and a large joint effusion. Note the small erosions of the distal epiphysis of the femur and the preservation of the joint space. Aspiration revealed hematogenous spread of a staphylococcal urinary tract infection.

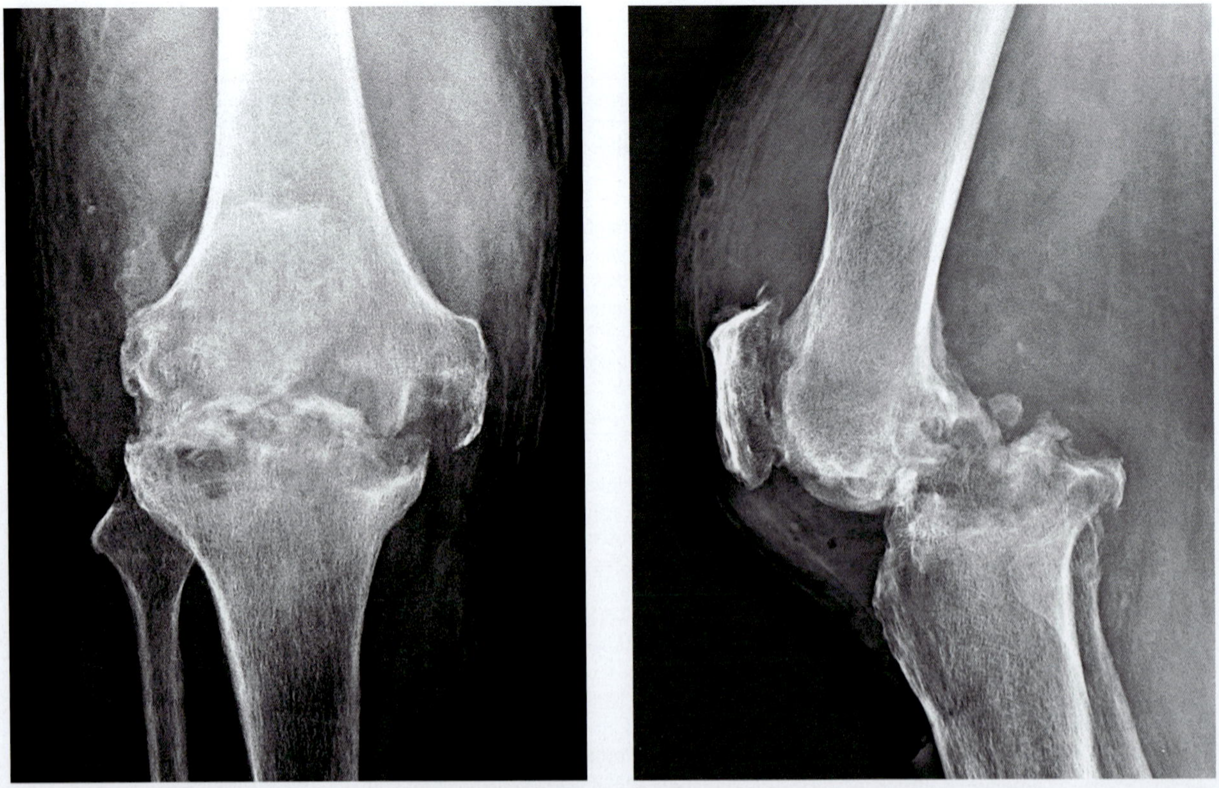

A B

Figure 9.6 ■ **Infectious arthritis.** Anteroposterior **(A)** and lateral **(B)** radiographs of the right knee of an 80-year-old man show destruction of articular cartilage of all three joint compartments, erosions of the subchondral bone, posterolateral subluxation, and a large joint effusion.

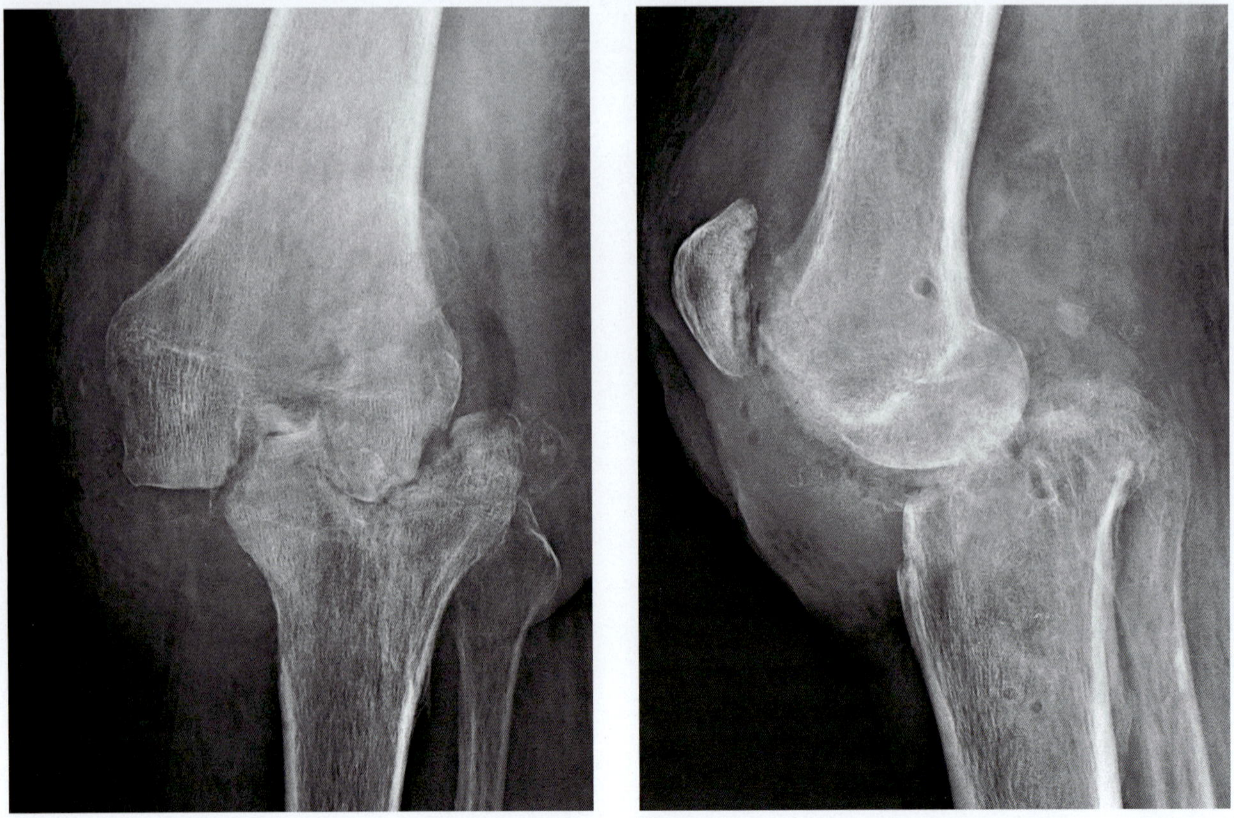

A B

Figure 9.7 ■ **Infectious arthritis.** Anteroposterior **(A)** and lateral **(B)** radiographs of the left knee of a 66-year-old man show destruction of the articular cartilage of all three joint compartments, large erosions of the subchondral bone, posterolateral subluxation, large joint effusion, and soft tissue swelling.

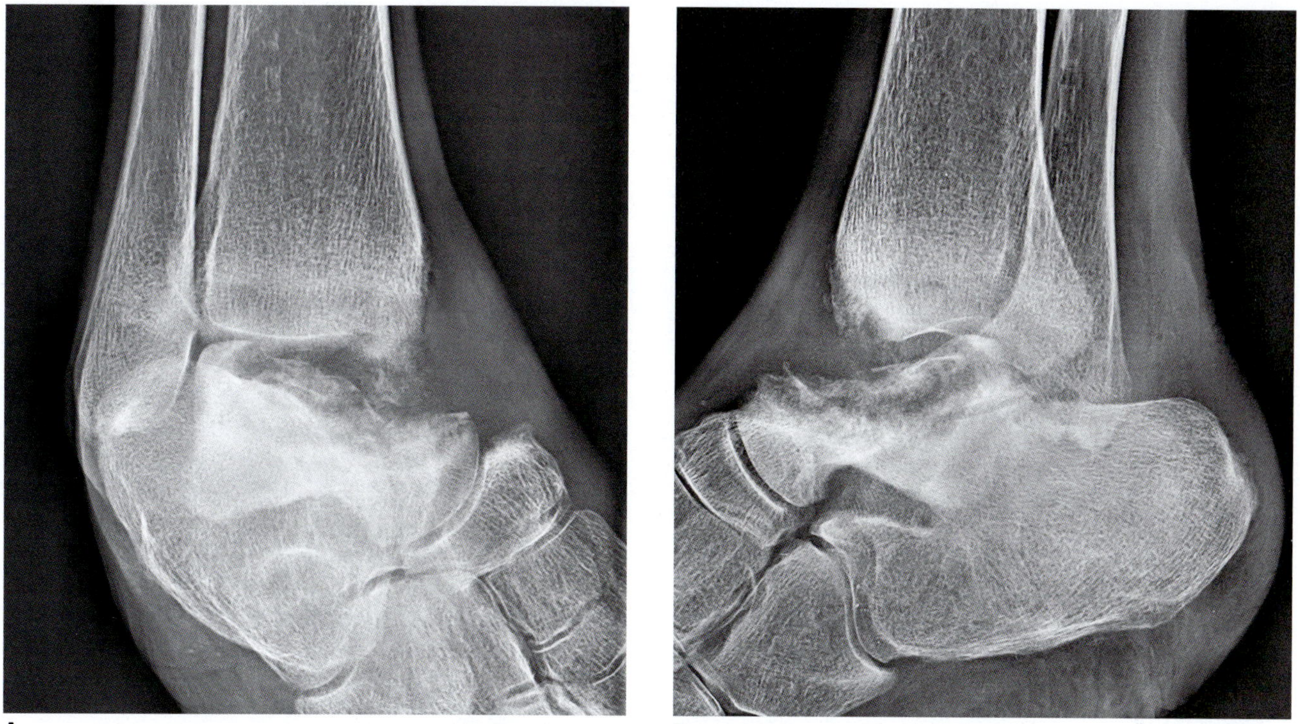

A B

Figure 9.8 ■ Infectious arthritis. Oblique **(A)** and lateral **(B)** radiographs of the right ankle of a 31-year-old man show destruction of the articular cartilage of the medial malleolus, anterior tibia, and dorsal aspect of the talus, associated with ankle joint effusion.

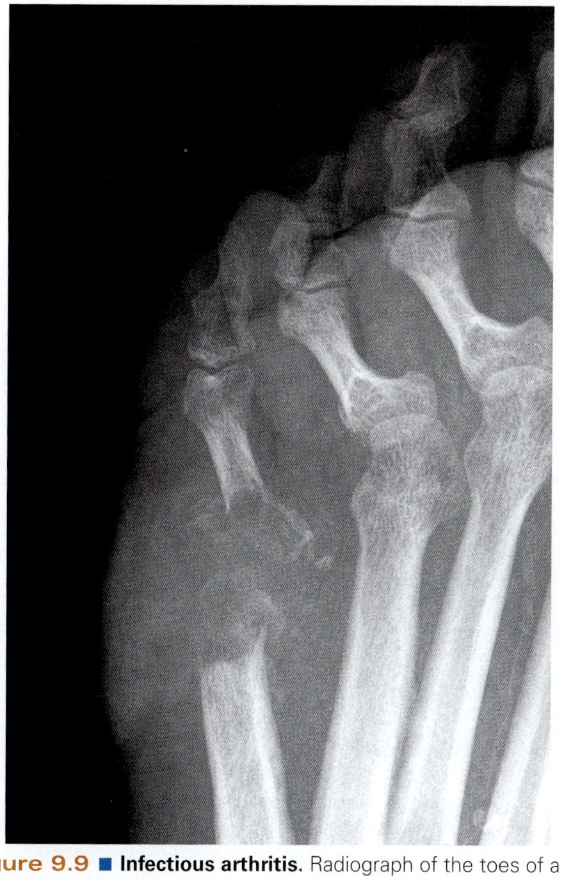

Figure 9.9 ■ Infectious arthritis. Radiograph of the toes of a 53-year-old woman shows destruction of the fifth metatarsophalangeal joint associated with a soft tissue swelling and edema.

technetium-99m-labeled (^{99m}Tc) phosphonates is routinely used, because there is an accumulation of tracer in the infected areas (see Fig. 2.54). A three- or four-phase technique is particularly useful for distinguishing infected joint from infected periarticular soft tissues if radiography is not diagnostic. With cellulitis, diffuse increased uptake is present in the first two phases, but there is no significant increase in uptake in the bone in the third and fourth delayed phases (see Fig. 2.53). Conversely, osteomyelitis causes focally increased uptake in all four phases. The four-phase bone scan can also be useful in diagnosing septic arthritis in situ or with extension into the adjacent bone.

Once the bone sustains an injury, such as surgery, fracture, or neuropathic osteoarthropathy, that causes increased bone turnover, routine scintigraphy with technetium-labeled phosphonate becomes less specific for infection. However, radionuclide studies using gallium (a ferric analog) and indium are more specific in these instances. There is still no general agreement on the exact mechanism of gallium localization in infected tissues. After intravenous injections of gallium, more than 99% is bound to various plasma proteins, including transferrin, haptoglobin, lactoferrin, albumin, and ferritin. At least five mechanisms of gallium transfer from the plasma into inflammatory exudates and cells have been suggested. These include direct leukocyte uptake, direct bacteria uptake, the protein-bound tissue uptake, increased vascularity, and increased bone turnover. Because gallium binds to the iron-binding molecule transferrin, the mechanism of gallium uptake in infectious processes is best explained by hyperemia and elevated permeability that increase delivery of the protein-bound tracer transferrin into the area of inflammation. Cells associated with the inflammatory response, particularly polymorphonuclear white cells in which lactoferrin is carried within intracytoplasmic granules, deposit iron-binding proteins extracellularly at the site of inflammation, serving to combat the infection by sequestering needed iron from bacteria. Lactoferrin, which has a high binding affinity for iron, takes the gallium away from the transferrin.

The other tracer used in infections is indium. Because indium-labeled white blood cells are usually not incorporated into areas of increased bone turnover, scintigraphy with indium-111 (^{111}In) oxine-labeled leukocytes is used as a sensitive and specific test in the general diagnosis of infection of the musculoskeletal system and in specific instances when infection complicates previous fracture or surgery. Like other imaging procedures in nuclear medicine, this test monitors the internal distribution of a tracer agent to provide diagnostic information. The inherent ability of white blood cells to accumulate at sites of inflammation makes their use in this test particularly effective in the diagnosis of infections (Fig. 9.10, see also Fig. 2.62). Merkel reported the sensitivity of indium scintigraphy in detecting infections to be 83%,

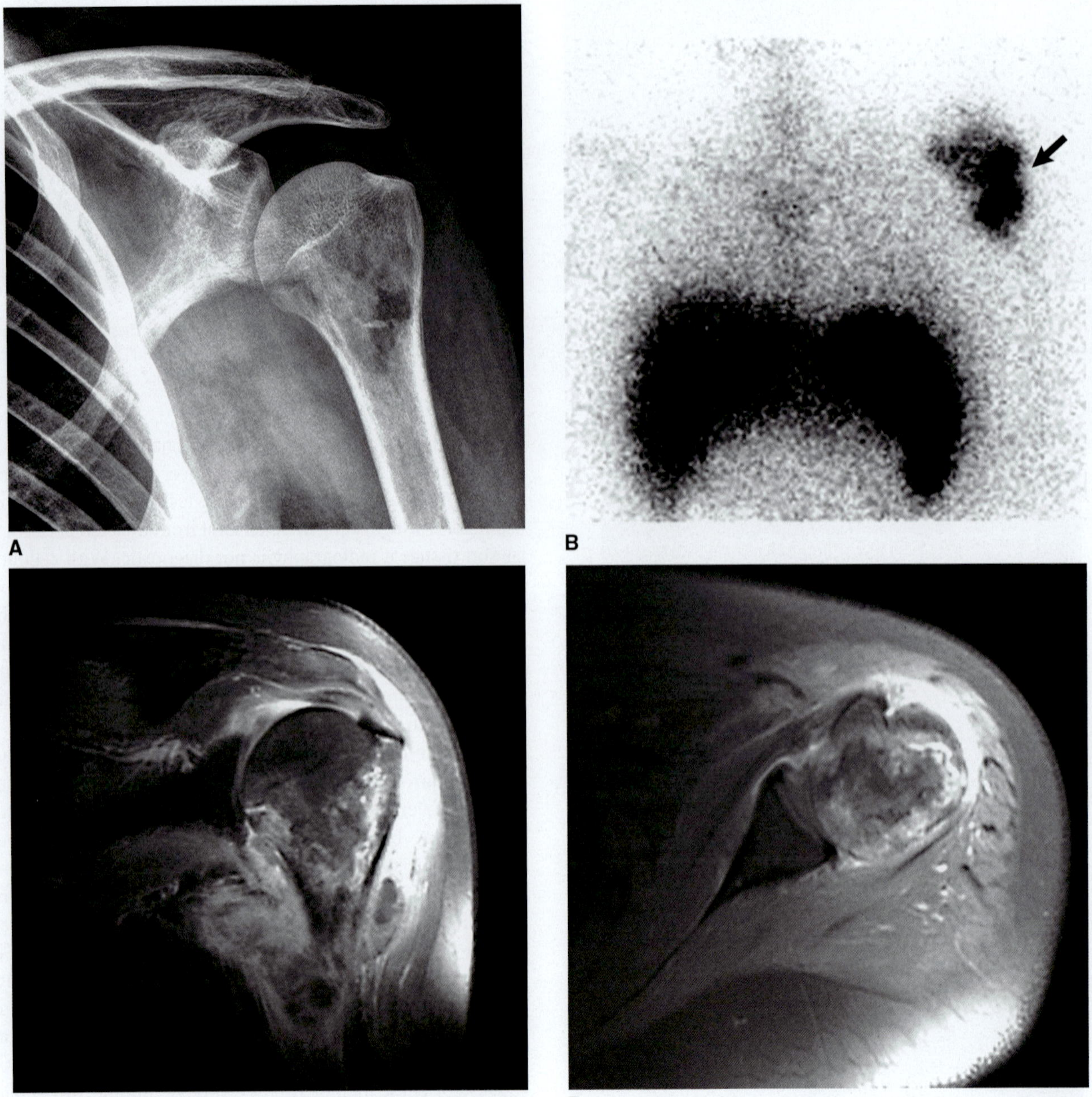

A B C D

Figure 9.10 ■ Scintigraphy and MRI of infectious arthritis. A: Anteroposterior radiograph of the left shoulder of a 20-year-old woman shows moderate periarticular osteoporosis, osteolytic ill-defined lesions in the glenoid and proximal humerus, and periosteal reaction at the lateral aspect of the humeral shaft. **B:** ^{111}In oxine-labeled white blood cell scintigraphy shows increased uptake of the radiopharmaceutical agent in the right shoulder (*arrow*). Coronal **(C)** and axial **(D)** T1-weighted fat-suppressed MR images obtained after administration of gadolinium show significant enhancement of the bones and surrounding soft tissues. The aspiration/biopsy followed by bacteriologic examination revealed *Bacteroides fragilis*.

with a specificity of 94% and an accuracy of 88%. It must be stressed, however, that because the ^{111}In-labeled leukocytes also accumulate in active bone marrow, the sensitivity for the detection of chronic osteomyelitis is reduced. To improve the diagnostic ability of this technique, a combined ^{99m}Tc-sulfur colloid bone marrow/^{111}In-labeled leukocyte study is advocated. A particularly difficult problem is the patient with diabetic foot neuropathy in whom superimposed infection is suspected. In this circumstance, radiography and even MRI are not very specific. Although soft tissue infection can be detected by the latter technique, early changes of osteomyelitis and septic arthritis may be missed. Often, no single imaging method can provide the correct diagnosis, and a combination of several imaging techniques should be used. The traditional sequential use of ^{67}Ga citrate in conjunction with the ^{99m}Tc-methylene diphosphonate (MDP) bone scan as an aid to diagnose osteomyelitis and infectious arthritis in the diabetic foot has been supplanted in recent years by the use of ^{111}In-labeled leukocytes. The drawback of this technique is that there remain difficulties in differentiating infection in the bone (osteomyelitis) from that in the adjacent tissue (cellulitis). A more recent attempt to improve this situation is the use of a combined ^{99m}Tc-bone scan/^{111}In-labeled leukocyte study to determine whether the leukocyte collection is in the bone or in the soft tissue. A new challenger to ^{111}In leukocyte scanning is the ^{99m}Tc-hexamethylpropylene amino oxine (HMPAO)–labeled leukocyte scan. At the time of this writing, other methods are being tested, namely, isotope-labeled (^{99m}Tc, ^{111}In, or ^{123}I) monoclonal antigranulocyte antibodies, isotope-labeled polyclonal IgG, isotope-labeled monocytes, isotope-labeled chemotactic polypeptide analogs, and isotope-labeled specific antibodies against bacteria.

Over the past decade, FDG-PET/CT has emerged as a rapidly evolving diagnostic tool for evaluation of infections. In particular, recent studies by Diaz and collaborators using a combination of [^{124}I] FIAU-positron emission tomography and CT demonstrated positive signals at the site of infection at two hours after administration of 2mCi (74 MBq) of radiopharmaceutical agent. FIAU [1-(2′-deoxy-2″fluoro-beta-D-arabinofuranosyl)-5-iodouracil], a nucleoside analog that freely enters and exits cells, is a substrate for the native thymidine kinase (TK) from a wide variety of bacteria. Once phosphorylated by TK, [^{124} I] FIAU becomes trapped within bacteria and can be detected with PET/CT.

Arthrography has rather limited application in the diagnosis of joint infections. This radiologic technique, which is often performed after aspiration of the joint to obtain a fluid specimen for bacteriologic examination, helps determine the extent of joint destruction and demonstrate the presence of synovitis (see Fig. 2.30). CT plays a determining role in demonstrating the extent of infection in bones and joints (Figs. 9.11 and 9.12). Ultrasound (US) can occasionally be used in diagnosing soft tissue and joint infections, as well as osteomyelitis. This modality has the advantage of being easily accessible and available at relatively reasonable cost. In addition, this technique does not expose the patient to ionizing radiation. Real-time capability of US is unique in providing a means to evaluate structures under dynamic conditions. Furthermore, US plays an important role in the guidance of percutaneous biopsy and aspiration of infectious lesions, as well as the therapeutic drainage of abscesses.

At the present time, MRI established its place in the evaluation of musculoskeletal infections. As several studies have indicated, osteomyelitis, soft tissue abscesses, joint and tendon sheath effusions, and various forms of cellulitis are well depicted by this modality. MRI is as sensitive as ^{99m}Tc-MDP in demonstrating osteomyelitis and infectious arthritis and more sensitive and more specific than other scintigraphic

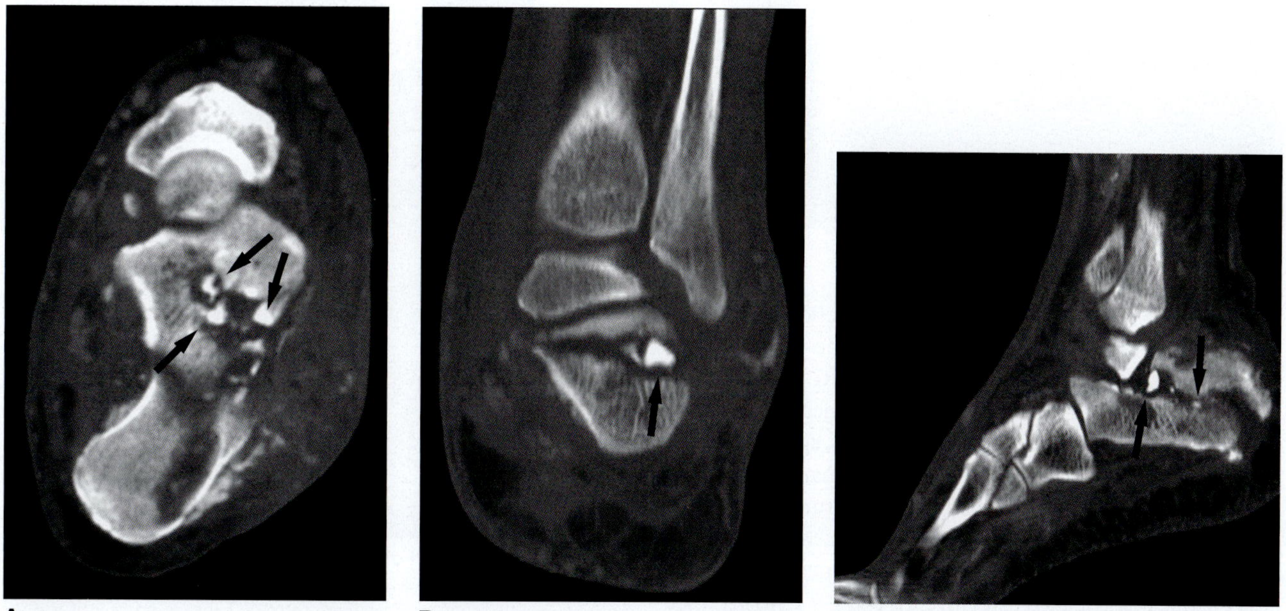

A B C

Figure 9.11 ■ **CT of osteomyelitis and infectious arthritis.** Axial **(A)**, coronal reformatted **(B)**, and sagittal reformatted **(C)** CT images of the left foot of a 72-year-old diabetic man demonstrate an active osteomyelitis of calcaneus and infection of the subtalar joint. Note several sclerotic osseous fragments representing sequestra (*arrows*).

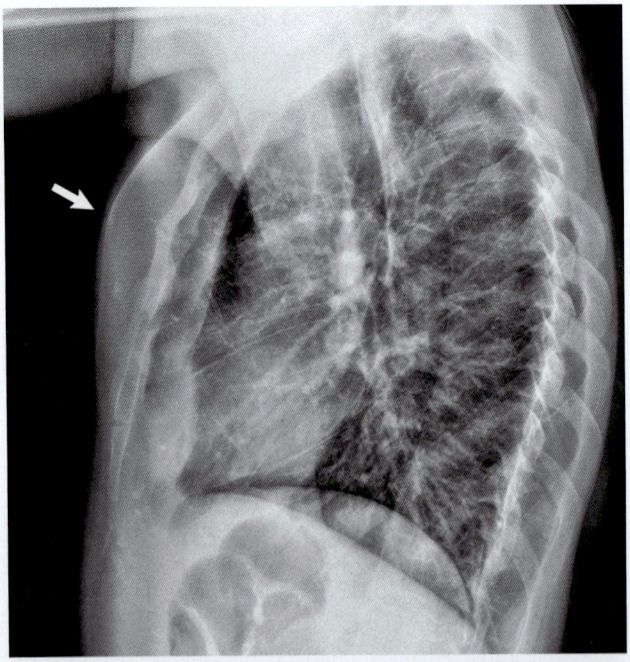

A

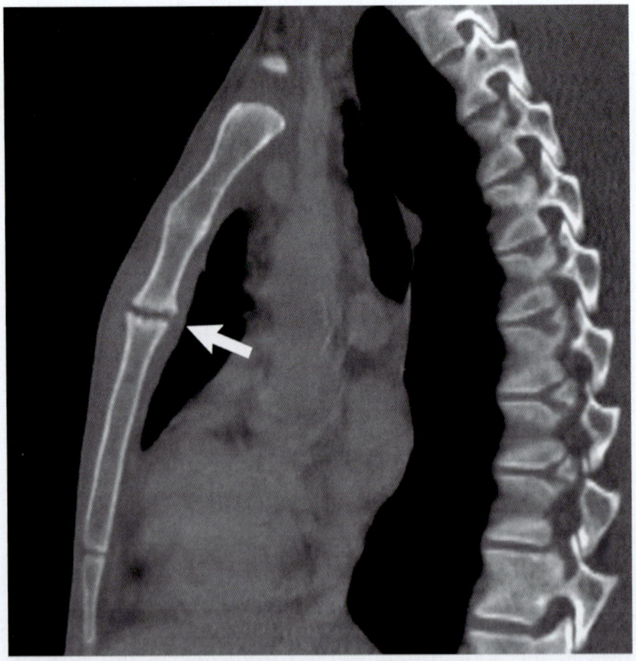

B

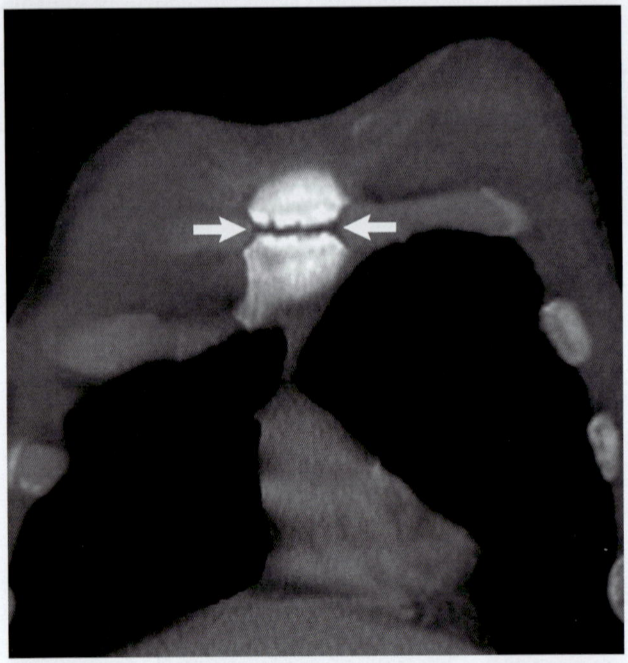

C

Figure 9.12 ■ CT of infectious arthritis. A 31-year-old IV drug abuser presented with anterior chest pain and fever. **A:** Lateral radiograph of the chest shows a large soft tissue swelling anteriorly to the upper sternum (*arrow*). **B:** Sagittal CT image of the chest demonstrates erosive changes of the manubriosternal joint (*arrow*). **C:** Coronal reformatted CT image shows more clearly the joint erosions (*arrows*).

techniques in demonstrating soft tissue infections, primarily because of its superior spatial resolution. The proper evaluation of musculoskeletal infections with MRI requires both T1- and T2-weighted images in at least two imaging planes. In anatomically complex areas such as the pelvis, spine, foot, and hand, three planes may be necessary. MRI manifestations of pyogenic arthritis include joint effusion with surrounding soft tissue edema and bone marrow edema (Figs. 9.13 and 9.14). In more advanced stages, cartilage and bone destruction may be seen, due to associated osteomyelitis (Figs. 9.15 to 9.17, see also Fig. 9.4). "Lamellated" joint effusion demonstrated with MRI has been described as a reliable sign of septic arthritis.

(Continued on page 336)

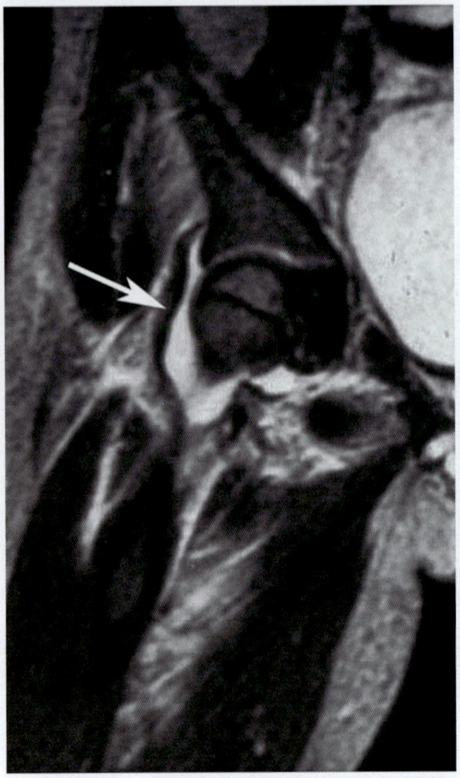

Figure 9.13 ■ MRI of septic arthritis. Coronal T2-weighted MRI of the right hip in a 12-year-old boy demonstrates a joint effusion with capsular distension (*arrow*). There is edema of the surrounding muscles. There are no signs of osteomyelitis. The arthrocentesis and bacteriologic studies of the obtained fluid confirmed the presence of joint infection.

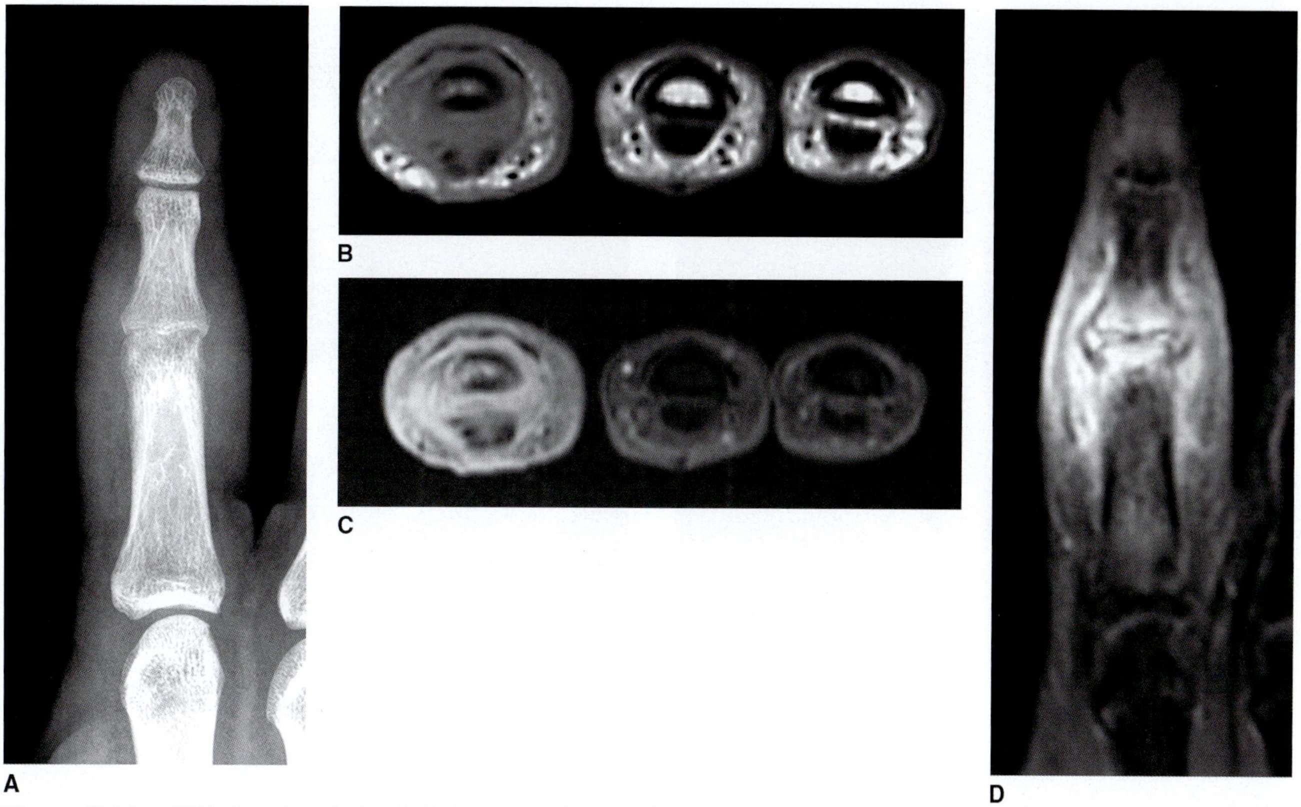

Figure 9.14 ■ MRI of septic arthritis. A: Radiograph of the index finger of a 22-year-old man shows narrowing of the proximal interphalangeal joint, periarticular osteoporosis, and soft tissue swelling. **B:** Axial T1-weighted MR image shows low-intensity signal of the bone marrow and surrounding soft tissues of the index finger (compare with normal middle and ring fingers). Axial **(C)** and coronal **(D)** T1-weighted fat-suppressed MR images obtained after intravenous administration of gadolinium show significant enhancement consistent with infectious synovitis, cellulitis, and osteomyelitis.

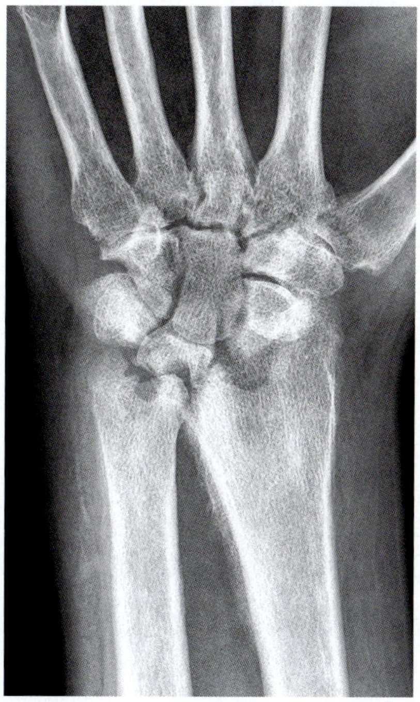

A

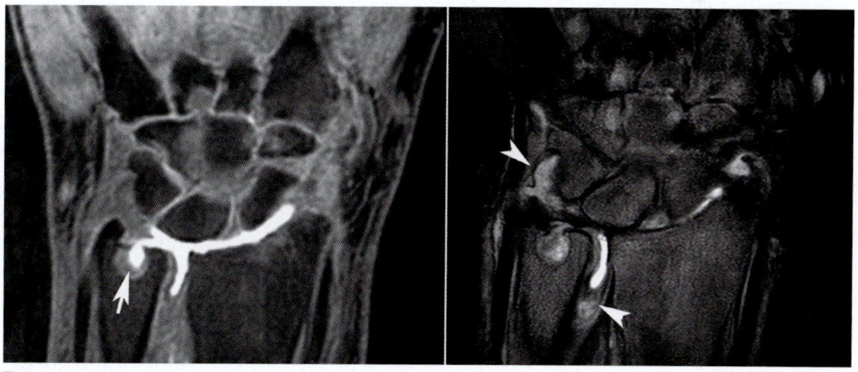

B

Figure 9.15 ■ MRI of septic arthritis. A: Dorsovolar radiograph of the right wrist of a 43-year-old man shows destruction of the radiocarpal joint and erosive changes of the distal radius, distal ulna, lunate, and scaphoid bones. Note also involvement of the carpometacarpal articulation. There is periosteal reaction of the distal radius and ulna and soft tissue swelling. **B:** Coronal 3D GRE fat-suppressed and coronal proton density-weighted fat-suppressed MR images demonstrate an erosion of the distal ulna (*arrow*) with a radiocarpal joint effusion extending to the distal radioulnar joint through a complete tear of the triangular fibrocartilage complex. Note the intermediate-to-low signal intensity of most of the effusion and mild surrounding soft tissue edema (*arrowheads*) consistent with synovitis due to septic arthritis.

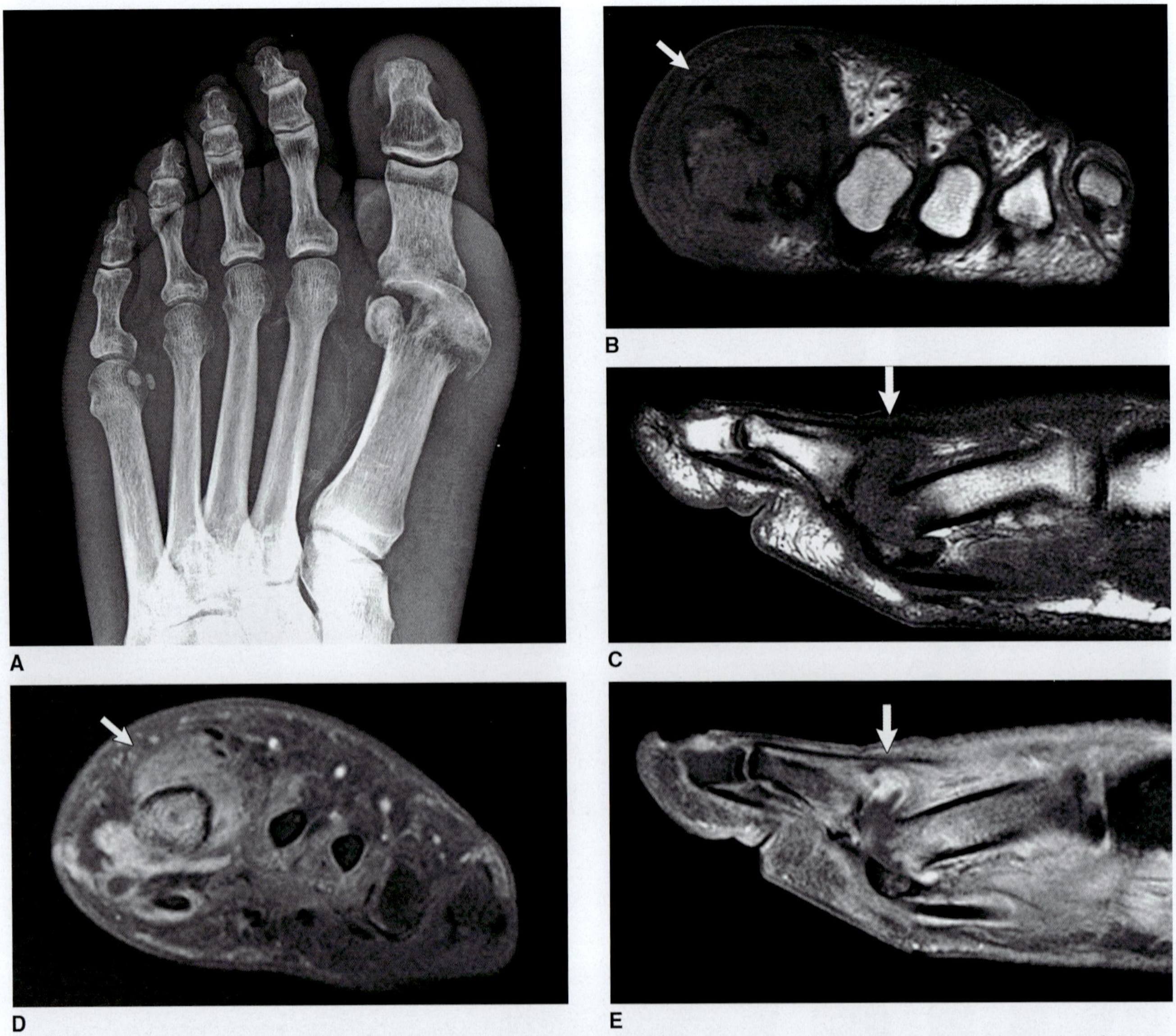

Figure 9.16 ■ MRI of septic arthritis. A: Dorsoplantar radiograph of the right forefoot of a 52-year-old man shows destruction of the first metatarsophalangeal joint, erosions of the head of the first metatarsal bone, and a large soft tissue swelling. Short-axis **(B)** and sagittal **(C)** T1-weighted MR images show low-intensity signal of partially destroyed head of the first metatarsal bone and surrounding soft tissues (*arrows*). Short-axis **(D)** and sagittal **(E)** T1-weighted fat-suppressed MR images obtained after administration of gadolinium show enhancement within the joint and bone marrow (*arrows*) indicative of joint infection and osteomyelitis.

Complications

Infectious arthritis of peripheral joints in children may lead to the destruction of the growth plate, with resulting growth arrest (Fig. 9.18). The infection may also spread to an adjacent bone, causing osteomyelitis. Secondary osteoarthritis and intra-articular bone ankylosis (Fig. 9.19) may also occur.

Treatment

Treatment of septic arthritis is based on clinical, laboratory, and microbiologic findings. Arthrocentesis and synovial fluid analysis are the cornerstone procedures leading to the adequate treatment of the septic joint. After confirmation of susceptibility of recovered organism, specific antibiotics are administered. Drainage of the infected joint must also be performed in order to relieve pain and eradicate the infection. Physical therapy is usually instituted as soon as the patient can tolerate mobilization of the inflamed joint.

NONPYOGENIC JOINT INFECTIONS

Tuberculous Arthritis

Musculoskeletal tuberculosis accounts for 1% to 3% of tuberculous infections, and most commonly results from

(Continued on page 338)

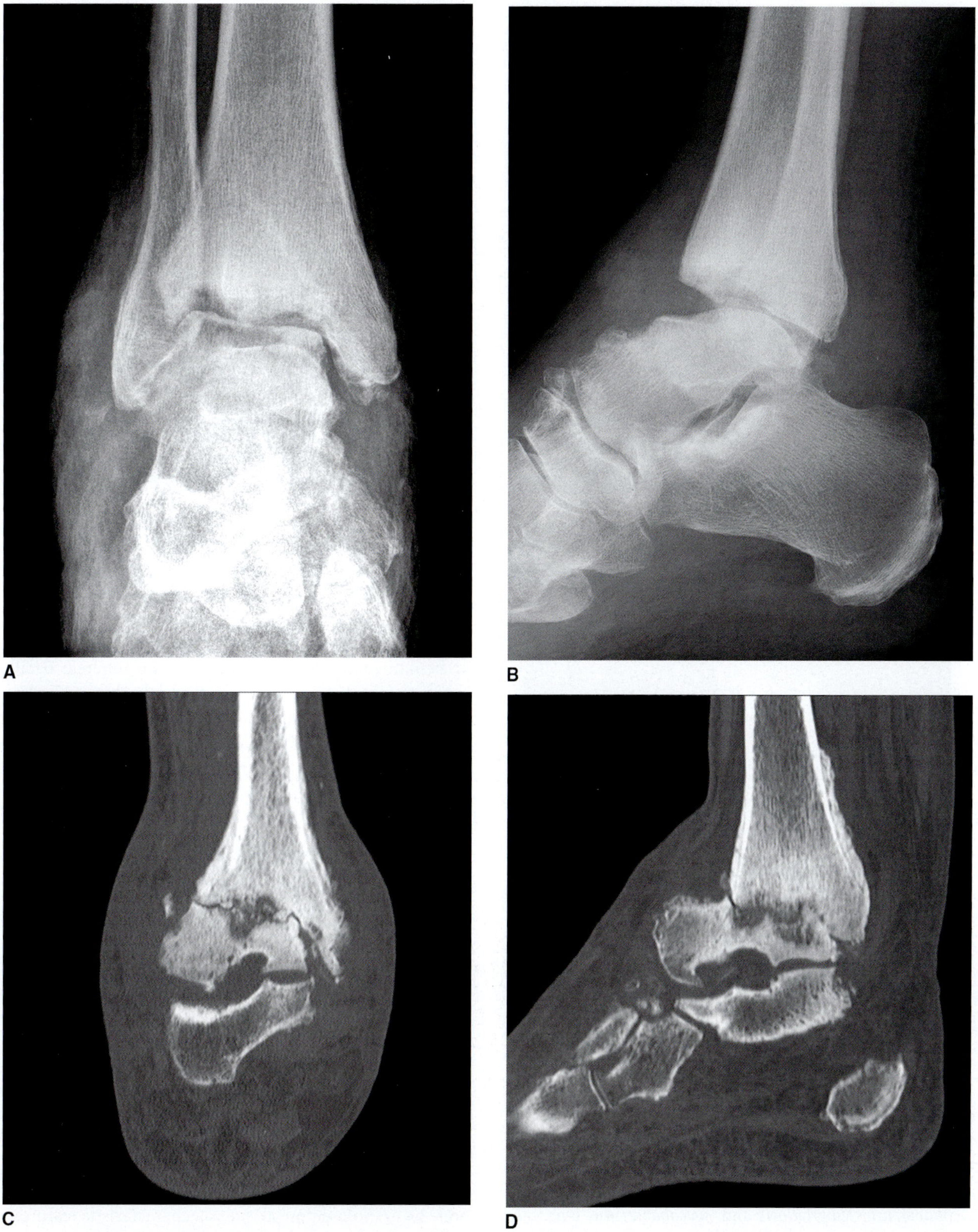

Figure 9.17 ■ **CT and MRI of septic arthritis.** Anteroposterior **(A)** and lateral **(B)** radiographs of the right ankle of a 65-year-old man show narrowing of the ankle joint, erosions of the distal tibia and talus, ankle joint effusion, and soft tissue swelling. Coronal **(C)** and sagittal reformatted **(D)** CT images show destructive joint changes more effectively. In addition, there are several small bone fragments within the joint space representing sequestra. Observe also periosteal reaction.

(Continued)

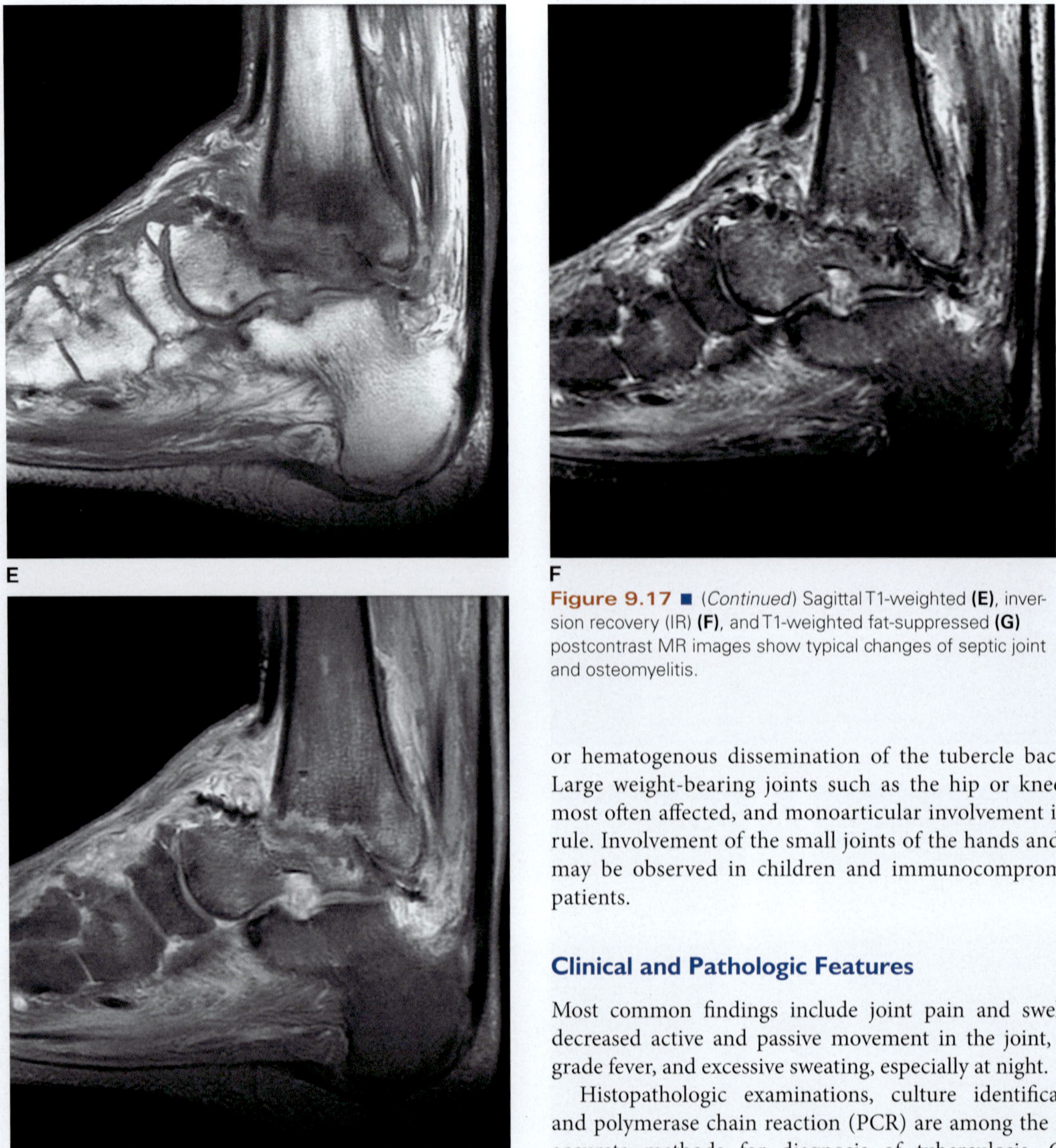

E

F

G

Figure 9.17 ■ (*Continued*) Sagittal T1-weighted **(E)**, inversion recovery (IR) **(F)**, and T1-weighted fat-suppressed **(G)** postcontrast MR images show typical changes of septic joint and osteomyelitis.

hematogenous or lymphatic dissemination of mycobacterium. Tuberculous arthritis represents 1% of all forms of extrapulmonary tuberculosis, although the number of cases has recently been on the rise. The acid-fast tubercle bacilli *Mycobacterium tuberculosis* and *Mycobacterium bovis* are the causative organisms. The infection may be found in all groups, but more commonly in children and young adults. Predisposing factors such as trauma, alcoholism, drug abuse, intra-articular injection of steroids, or prolonged systemic illness are found in most patients with tuberculous arthritis. The joint infection usually is caused by either direct invasion from an adjacent focus of osteomyelitis or hematogenous dissemination of the tubercle bacillus. Large weight-bearing joints such as the hip or knee are most often affected, and monoarticular involvement is the rule. Involvement of the small joints of the hands and feet may be observed in children and immunocompromised patients.

Clinical and Pathologic Features

Most common findings include joint pain and swelling, decreased active and passive movement in the joint, low-grade fever, and excessive sweating, especially at night.

Histopathologic examinations, culture identification, and polymerase chain reaction (PCR) are among the most accurate methods for diagnosis of tuberculosis. Gross pathologic examination of the areas affected by tuberculosis shows thickened edematous tissue, commonly studded with small grayish nodules, exhibiting white opaque center (granulomas). They may become confluent and produce larger areas of white necrotic material representing caseation (cheesy) necrosis. In the joint, separation of the articular cartilage dissected from underlying subchondral bone by granulomatous tissue is a characteristic feature. On microscopic examination, the typical tubercle consists of a central necrotic area surrounded by pale epithelioid histiocytes. Among these cells noted are scattered giant cells with nuclei typically arranged at the periphery of the cell, known as Langhans giant cells (Fig. 9.20). At the periphery of the tubercle, there is a rim of mixed chronic inflammatory cells present.

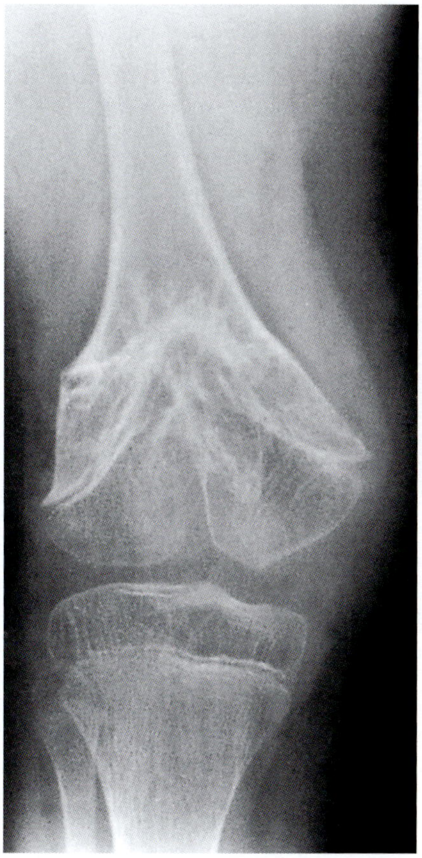

Figure 9.18 ■ Complication of joint infection. Anteroposterior radiograph of the right knee of an 8-year-old girl shows growth disturbance as a sequela of joint infection. Note the hypoplasia of the femur secondary to disuse of the limb, and deformity of the distal femoral epiphysis. The cone-shaped growth plate shows almost complete fusion.

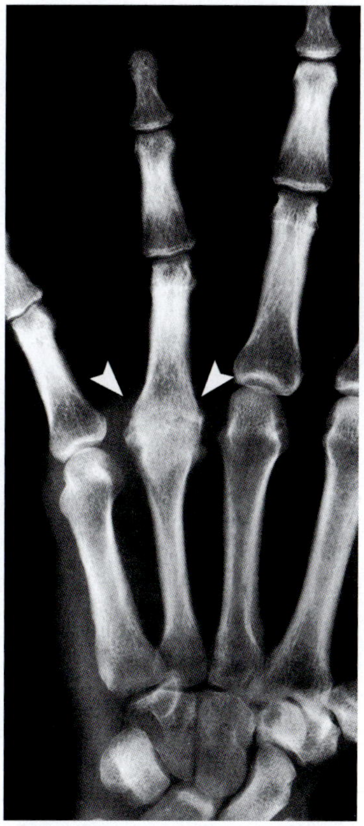

Figure 9.19 ■ Complication of joint infection. A 27-year-old man with septic arthritis of the fourth metacarpophalangeal joint of the left hand developed ankylosis of this articulation (*arrowheads*).

Imaging Features

Conventional radiography is usually sufficient to demonstrate the identifying features of tuberculous arthritis, although its early radiographic appearance is often indistinguishable from that of monoarticular rheumatoid arthritis. However, the involvement of only one joint, as demonstrated by scintigraphy, favors an infectious process (Fig. 9.21). A triad of radiographic abnormalities (Phemister triad), composed of periarticular osteoporosis, peripherally located osseous erosions, and gradual diminution of the joint space, should suggest the correct diagnosis;

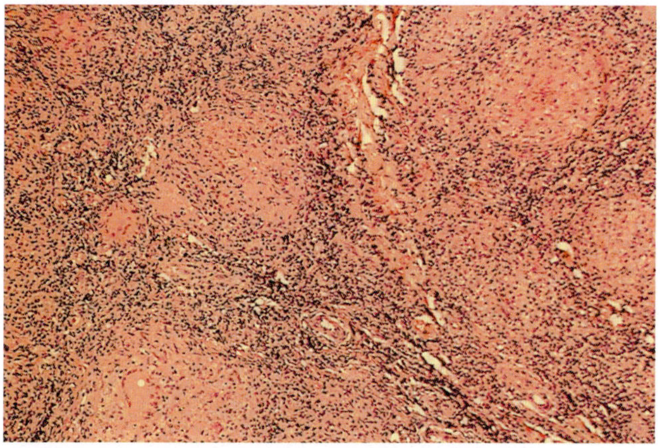

A

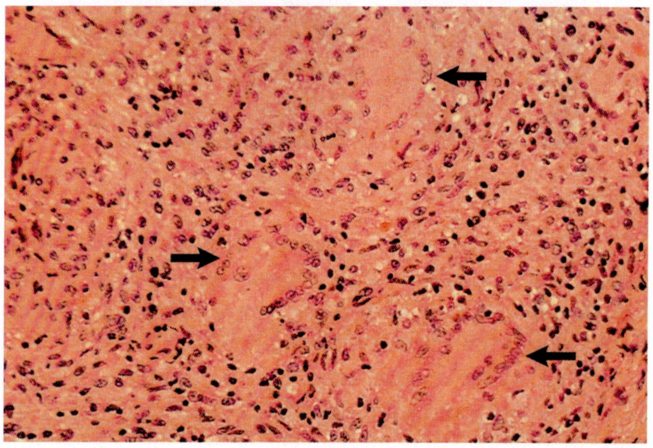

B

Figure 9.20 ■ Histopathology of tuberculous arthritis. A: Photomicrograph of granulomatous tissue obtained from the synovium of a knee joint shows focal giant cells, nodular collections of histiocytes, and an infiltration of chronic inflammatory cells (H&E, original magnification ×4). **B:** Higher magnification shows typical for tuberculosis Langhans giant cells (*arrows*) with peripherally arranged nuclei (H&E, original magnification ×10). (From Bullough PG. *Atlas of Orthopedic Pathology with Clinical and Radiologic Correlation.* 2nd ed. New York, NY: Gower Medical Publishing; 1992, Figs. 4.45 and 4.46, p. 4.23.)

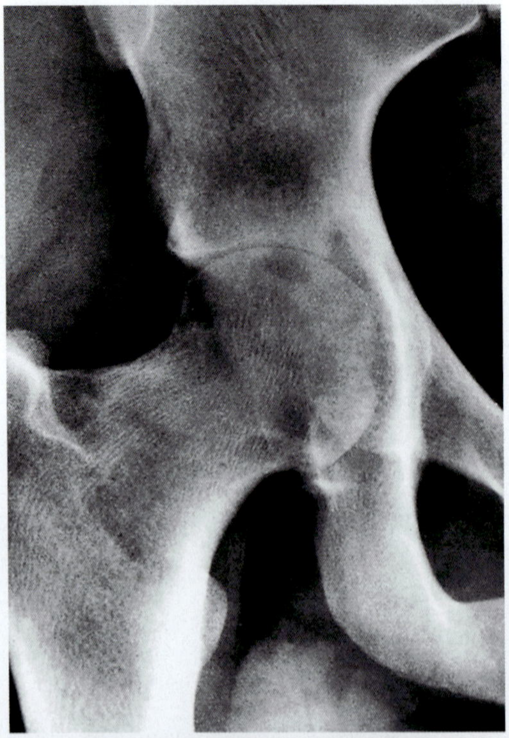

A

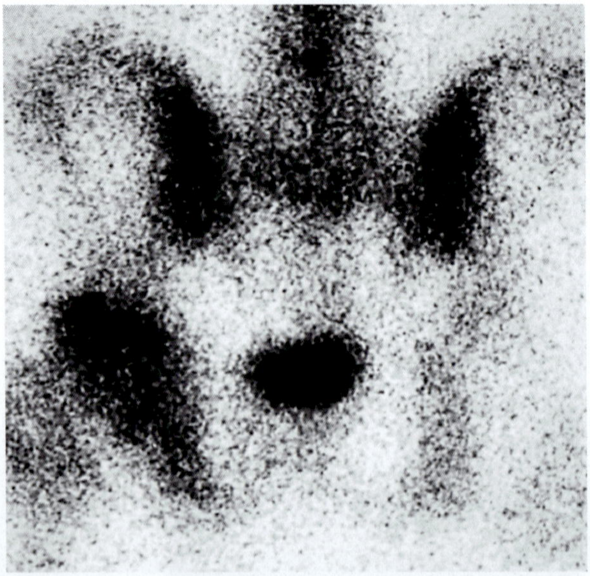

B

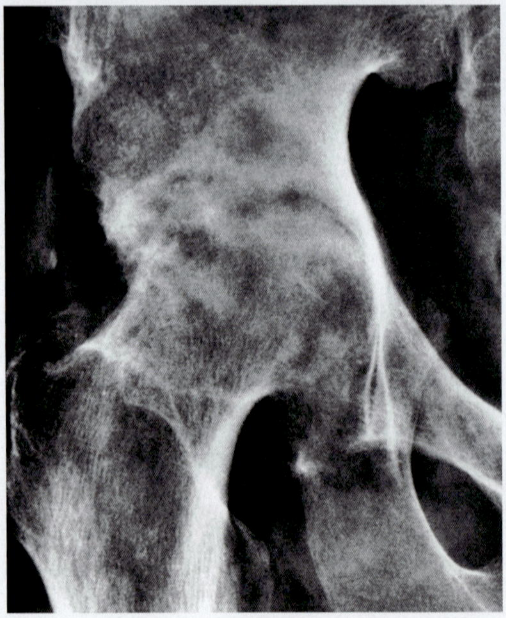

C

Figure 9.21 ■ **Tuberculous arthritis.** A 29-year-old woman with history of chronic alcoholism presented with right hip pain. **A:** Anteroposterior radiograph demonstrates diminution of the joint space, particularly in the weight-bearing region, as well as periarticular osteoporosis. **B:** Radionuclide bone scan using ^{99m}Tc-labeled diphosphonate demonstrates increased uptake of the radiopharmaceutical agent in the right hip. The increased activity at both sacroiliac joints is a normal finding. The diagnosis of tuberculous arthritis was confirmed by joint aspiration, which yielded *Mycobacterium tuberculosis*. **C:** In another patient, a 40-year-old man, anteroposterior radiograph of the right hip shows significant periarticular osteoporosis, concentric narrowing of the joint space, and small erosions of the femoral head and acetabulum.

CT examination, however, can be helpful in delineating subtle features (Fig. 9.22). Occasionally, wedge-shaped necrotic foci, so-called kissing sequestra, may be present on both sides of the affected joint, especially in the knee. At a later stage of the disease, there may be complete destruction of the joint, and sclerotic changes in adjacent bones are more frequently encountered (Fig. 9.23). The MRI manifestations of tuberculous arthritis parallel the radiographic changes, with bone marrow edema, joint effusion, marginal erosions, and progressive cartilage loss. The presence of multiple intra-articular bodies ("rice" bodies) is characteristic of tuberculous arthritis, although they may be seen also in rheumatoid arthritis and synovial chondromatosis. Tuberculous bursitis is rare but should be considered in the differential diagnosis of bursitis, especially if the infected bursa is grossly distended (Fig. 9.24).

Treatment

The treatment of tuberculosis consists of combination of rifampicin, isoniazid, ethambutol, and pyrazinamide. Occasionally, other drugs, such as amikacin, ethionamide, moxifloxacin, and streptomycin, are used. As of this writing, there are increasing reports of new antibiotic-resistant organisms.

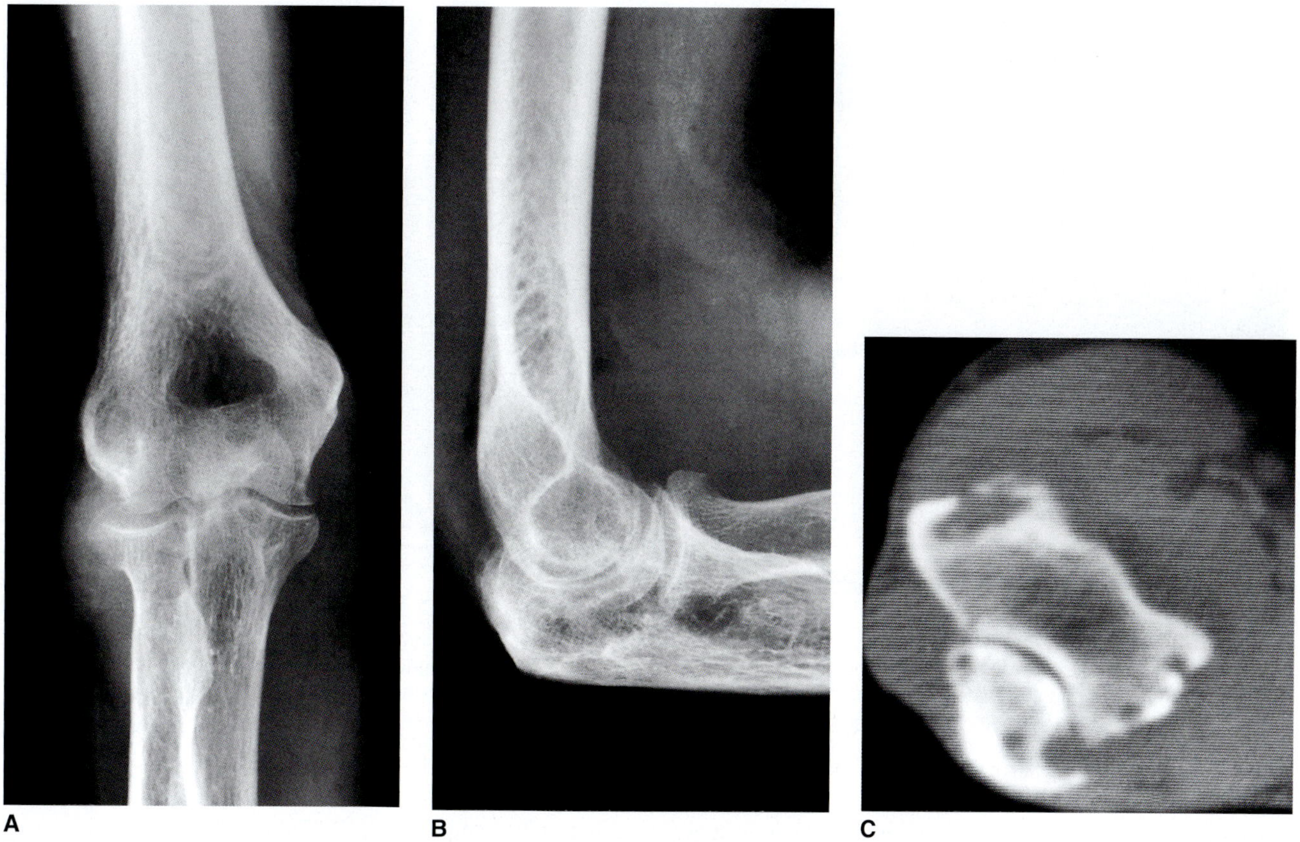

Figure 9.22 ■ **Tuberculous arthritis.** A 70-year-old man from India presented with pain in the left elbow for 4 months. According to his daughter, he had been treated for chronic lung disease. Anteroposterior **(A)** and lateral **(B)** radiographs of the elbow demonstrate a large joint effusion, as indicated by positive anterior and posterior fat pad signs on the lateral projection. Small periarticular erosions are not clear on these views. **C:** CT section shows narrowing of the joint and peripheral erosions typical of tuberculous infection.

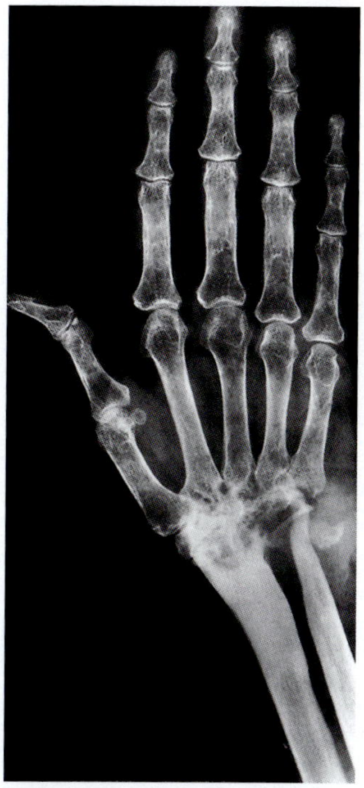

Figure 9.23 ■ **Tuberculous arthritis.** Posteroanterior radiograph of the left wrist and hand of a 52-year-old woman with pulmonary tuberculosis shows advanced arthritis involving the left carpus. There is complete destruction of the radiocarpal, midcarpal, and carpometacarpal articulations, as well as whittling and sclerotic changes in the distal radius and ulna. Note the osteoporosis distal to the affected joints and the soft tissue swelling.

SYPHILITIC INFECTION

Syphilis is a chronic systemic infectious disease caused by a spirochete, *Treponema pallidum.*

Primary form is typically acquired by direct sexual contact with infected person. *Secondary syphilis* occurs ~6 to 8 weeks after the primary infection. *Tertiary syphilis* may occur ~3 to 15 years after the initial infection. *Congenital syphilis,* which is transmitted from mother to fetus, may manifest as a chronic osteochondritis, periostitis, or osteitis.

Clinical presentation of syphilis varies considerably. It is worthwhile to remember that syphilis is one of the great masqueraders in medicine. Secondary syphilis, the result of hematogenous dissemination of *Treponema pallidum,* can mimic many other diseases, but cutaneous manifestations, such a generalized rash, are common. Fever, malaise, myalgias, and generalized lymphadenopathy are usually present. Patchy alopecia with a moth-eaten appearance is a classic finding. Joint pains may suggest syphilitic arthropathy.

The lesions of congenital syphilis, which most frequently involve the tibia, are characteristically widespread and symmetric in appearance; destructive changes are usually seen in the metaphysis at the junction with the growth plate, producing what is called the Wimberger sign. Joint involvement in syphilis may occur in either acquired (in the tertiary and less commonly in the secondary) or in congenital forms. In the latter, articular changes predominate in the late phases

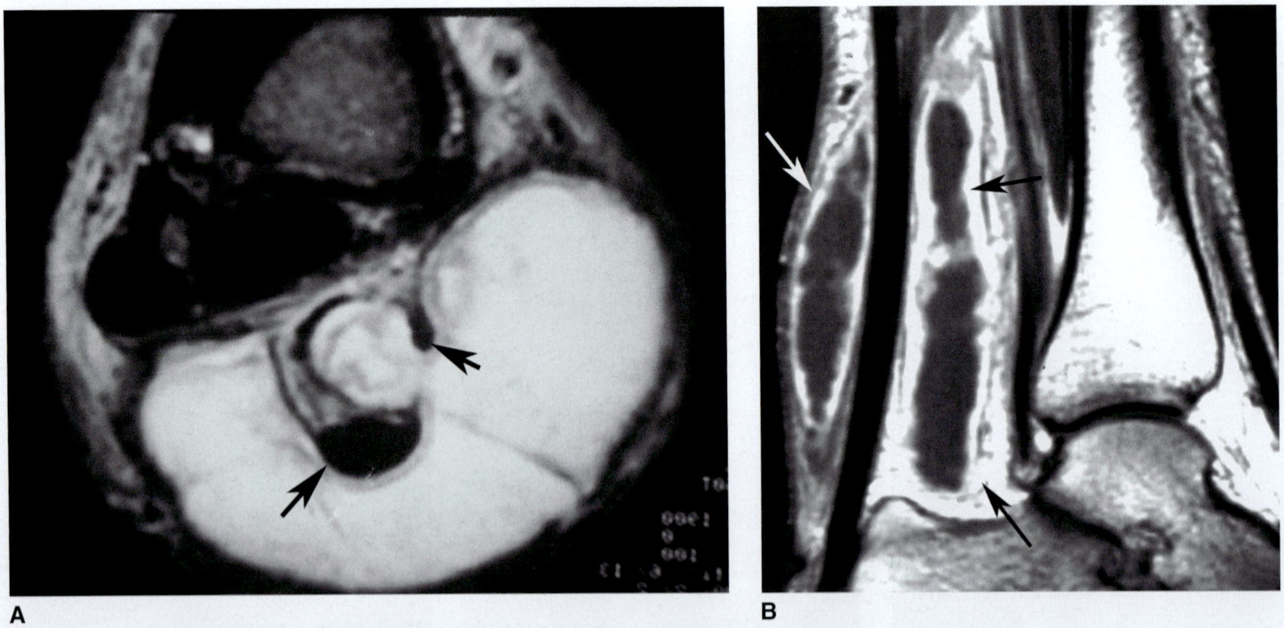

Figure 9.24 ■ **MRI of tuberculous bursitis. A:** Axial T2-weighted MRI of the ankle demonstrates a markedly distended retro-Achilles bursa surrounding posteriorly the Achilles and the plantaris tendons (*arrows*). **B:** Sagittal T1-weighted fat-saturated MRI obtained after intravenous administration of gadolinium demonstrates the enhancement of the wall of the bursa (*arrows*).

of the disease. Syphilitic arthritis presents nonspecific findings similar to those occurring in other infectious arthritides, including periarticular osteoporosis, joint effusion, joint space narrowing, subchondral bone destruction, and occasionally joint ankylosis. In congenital form, it usually causes symmetrical joint swelling due to synovitis and joint effusion (so-called Clutton joints).

Treatment of syphilis should follow current Center for Disease Control and Prevention (CDC) recommendations and should include consultation with the infection disease specialist. Intramuscular injections of benzathine penicillin G are the treatment of choice. The preparation used, dosage, and length of treatment depend on the stage and clinical manifestations of the disease.

OTHER INFECTIOUS ARTHRITIDES

Less frequently encountered than pyogenic or tuberculous arthritis are joint infections caused by fungi (actinomycosis, cryptococcosis, coccidioidomycosis, histoplasmosis, sporotrichosis, and candidiasis), viruses (smallpox), and spirochetes (syphilis, yaws).

Coccidioidomycosis

Among the fungal infections, coccidioidomycosis is of particular importance, not only because of an increase in the number of these infections in recent years but also because it may closely resemble skeletal tuberculosis. Also known as a San Joaquin Valley fever, it is a systemic disease caused by the soil dimorphic fungus *Coccidioides immitis*. This infection is endemic throughout the southwestern United States and the bordering regions of northern Mexico. Infection occurs through inhalation of dust containing the organism. The primary site of infection is the lung, and disease is commonly asymptomatic. When symptoms exist, they usually consist of mild flulike manifestations or mild lung disease. Dissemination of coccidioidomycosis is rare, but the incidence is increased in patients with specific risk factors. Those at increased risk include African Americans, Filipinos, Mexicans, males, pregnant women, children younger than 5 years, adults older than 50 years, and immunosuppressed patients. Patients with disseminated coccidioidomycosis usually present during the course of primary pulmonary infection. However, some patients with disseminated disease may have no clinical history or radiographic evidence of pulmonary disease. The skin and subcutaneous tissues are the most common sites of disseminated coccidioidal infection, followed by mediastinal involvement. The skeletal system is the third most common site of dissemination, and osseous manifestations occur in 10% to 50% of patients with disseminated disease.

Imaging presentation of the lesion of coccidioidomycosis is variable, but it is usually characterized by well-marginated, punched-out osteolytic lesions, commonly involving long and flat bones. The lesions are typically unilocular but occasionally may be multiloculated. The other pattern frequently observed is a permeative type of bone destruction, only occasionally accompanied by periosteal reaction. Soft tissue swelling and osteoporosis are much more common with the permeative pattern than with the punched-out lesions. The third most common pattern is joint involvement (septic arthritis), usually monoarticular (mostly of the ankle and knee joints), and is almost invariably associated with osseous involvement. Changes typically seen in joints include periarticular osteoporosis, a permeative/destructive pattern involving both articular surfaces, soft tissue swelling, and occasional periostitis. (Fig. 9.25). Joint involvement

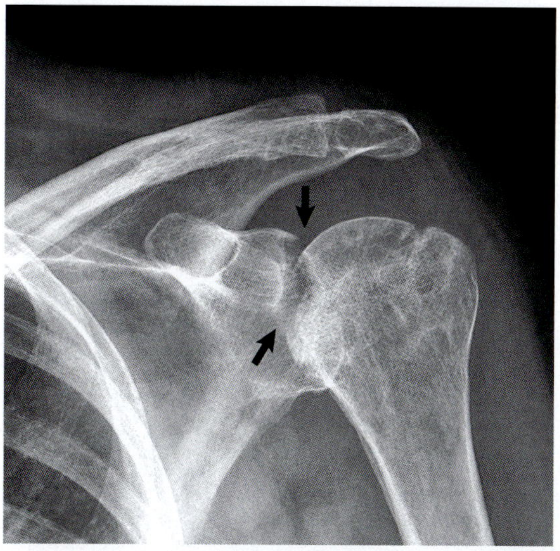

Figure 9.25 ■ Coccidioidomycosis of joint. Anteroposterior radiograph of the left shoulder of a 63-year-old woman diagnosed with pulmonary coccidioidomycosis shows erosions of the glenohumeral joint (*arrows*) and osteolytic lesions within the humeral head and greater tuberosity.

in coccidioidomycosis is indistinguishable from that seen with tuberculosis; however, the identification of *Coccidioides immitis* spherules in joint fluid is diagnostic.

Scintigraphy is valuable in the evaluation of patients with disseminated coccidioidomycosis. Radionuclide scans using gallium-67 (^{67}Ga) citrate and technetium-99m (^{99m}Tc) methylene diphosphonate (MDP) have been used to localize disease and can identify disseminated lesions that are clinically unsuspected (see Fig. 9.45). No false-negative bone scans have been reported. CT and magnetic resonance imaging (MRI) are helpful in defining osseous involvement and in determining the extent of joint and soft tissue disease (Figs. 9.26 to 9.28, see also Fig. 9.46). On CT, the lesions exhibit low-attenuation characteristics, often appearing bubbly and expansive. On MRI, the lesions show decreased signal intensity on T1-weighted images, with a corresponding increase on T2-weighted and gradient-echo sequences.

The infection can be difficult to eradicate, and treatment strategies vary widely from patient to patient, based on the patient's immune status and the severity of infection. The

(Continued on page 346)

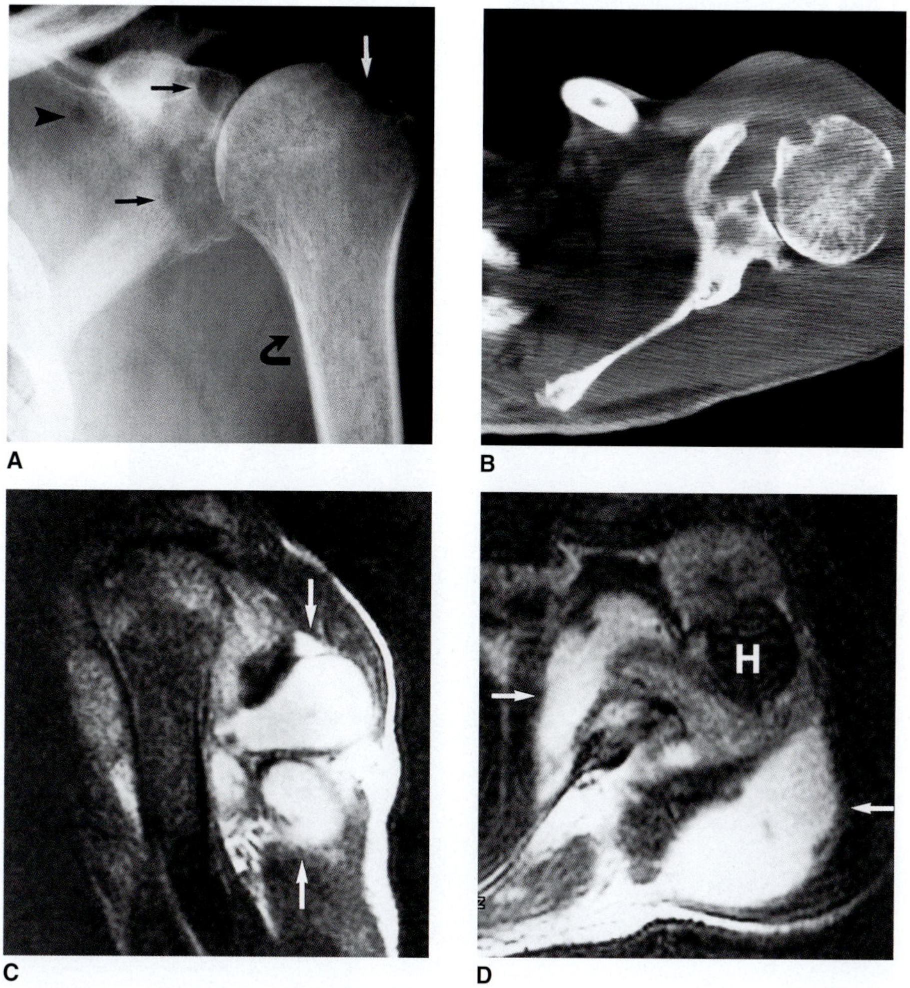

Figure 9.26 ■ CT and MRI of coccidioidomycosis infection of bone and joint. A 42-year-old man presented with a 4-week history of pain and decreased range of motion in the left shoulder. He had been previously hospitalized for pulmonary coccidioidomycosis. **A:** Anteroposterior radiograph shows several osteolytic lesions affecting the superolateral aspect of the humeral head and glenoid (*arrows*). Small punched-out lesion is noted in the body of the scapula (*arrowhead*). The *curved arrow* points to periosteal reaction along the medial humeral shaft. **B:** CT section reveals erosions of the anterior and posterolateral aspects of the humeral head. Also apparent are destruction of the articular surfaces of the humeral head and glenoid and narrowing of the glenohumeral joint. Sagittal **(C)** and axial **(D)** fast-spin echo (TR 4000/TE 102 ms) MR images show multiple, well-defined soft tissue abscesses displaying high signal intensity (*arrows*). *H*, humeral head.

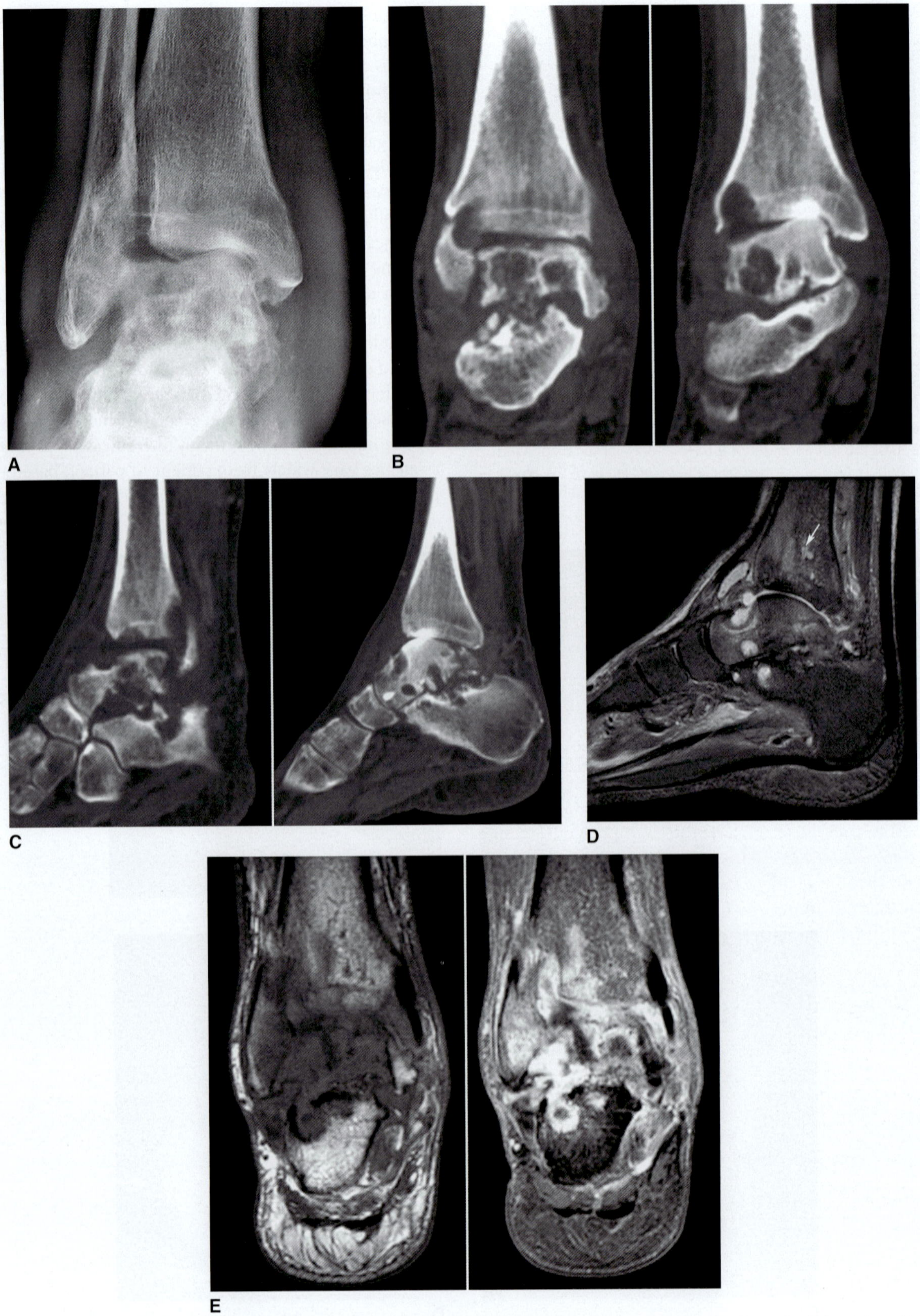

Figure 9.27 ■ **CT and MRI of coccidioidomycosis infection of bone and joints. A:** Anteroposterior radiograph of the right ankle of a 69-year-old man shows destruction of the tibiotalar joint, several radiolucent lesions in the talus, deformity of the ankle mortise, and large soft tissue swelling and edema. Two coronal **(B)** and two sagittal **(C)** CT sections demonstrate articular erosions of the ankle and subtalar joints, and several osteolytic lesions within the talus and calcaneus. **D:** Sagittal IR MR image shows multiple erosions of the talus and calcaneus with extensive bone marrow edema. Note also the tibial involvement (*arrow*). **E:** Coronal T1-weighted fat-suppressed MR images obtained before and after intravenous administration of gadolinium demonstrate diffuse signal abnormality of the talus, distal tibia, and fibula, with erosions in the calcaneus and inferior aspect of the talus. The bone marrow and the erosions show prominent enhancement.

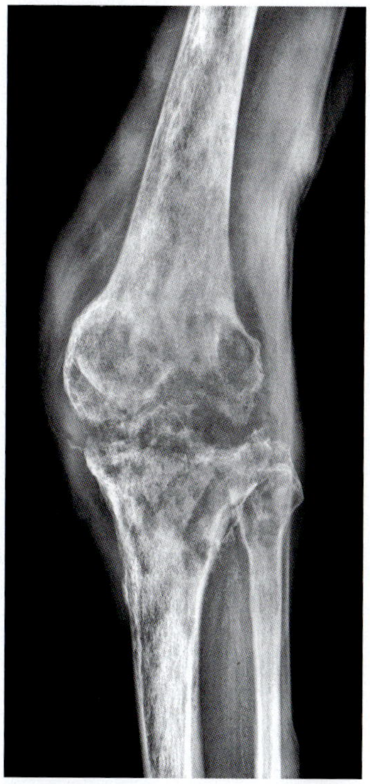

A

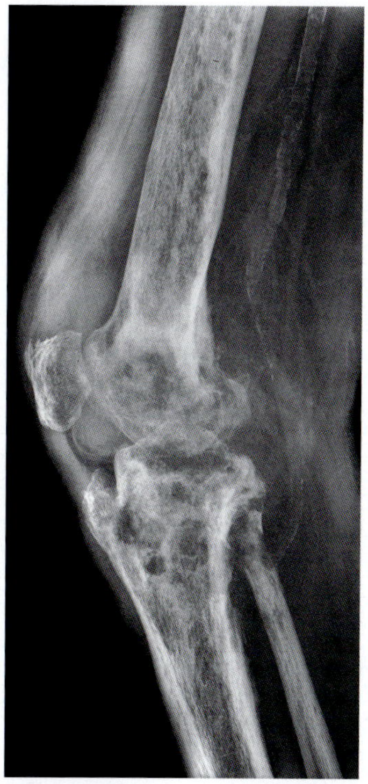

B

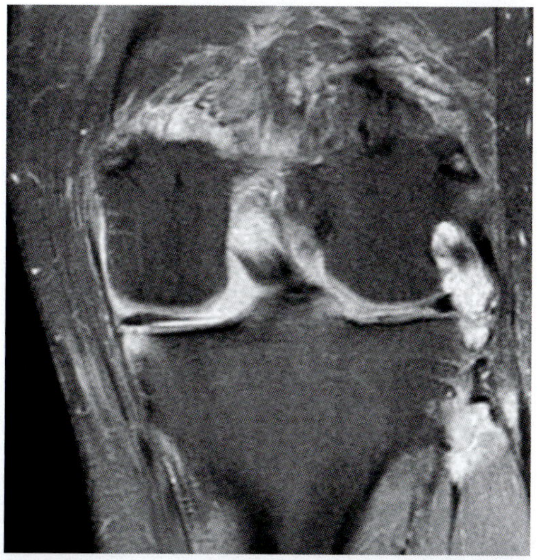

C

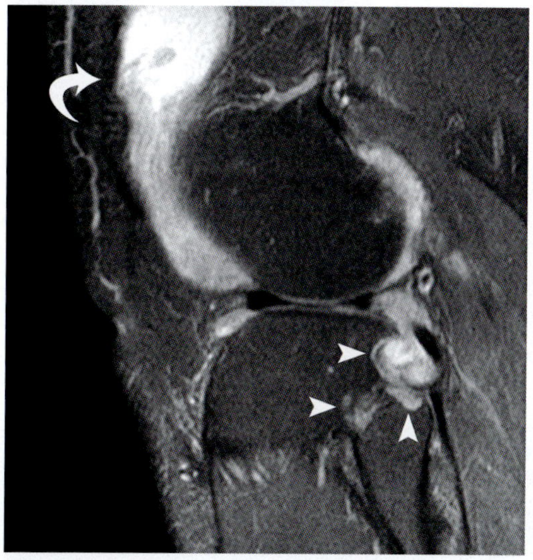

D

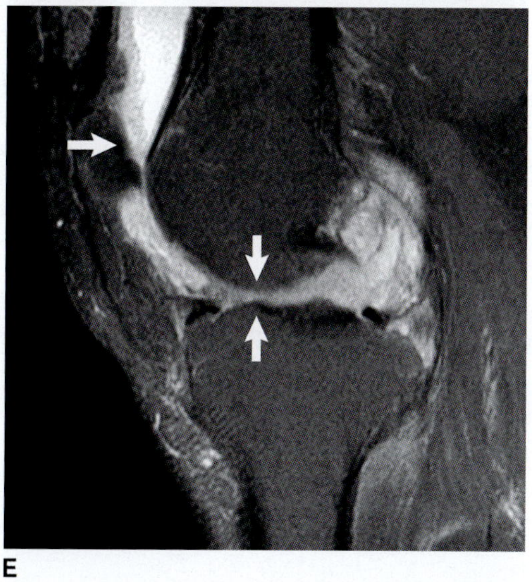

E

Figure 9.28 ■ **MRI of coccidioidomycosis infection of bone and joint.** Anteroposterior **(A)** and lateral **(B)** radiographs of the left knee of a 59-year-old woman show destruction of the articular cartilage and subchondral bone erosions, as well as several osteolytic lesions within the distal femur and proximal tibia and fibula. There is also a large joint effusion. Coronal **(C)** and two sagittal T2-weighted **(D, E)** MR images show articular cartilage destruction of the femorotibial and femoropatellar joints (*arrows*), erosions at the tibiofibular joint (*arrowheads*), and joint effusion (*curved arrow*).

antifungal drugs commonly used include amphotericin B, ketoconazole, fluconazole, and itraconazole.

Lyme Arthritis

Of interest is Lyme arthritis, an infectious articular condition caused by the spirochete *Borrelia burgdorferi*, which is transmitted to human by the deer tick *Ixodes dammini*, also known as *Ixodes scapularis*, or related ticks such as *Ixodes pacificus* and *Ixodes ricinus*. The illness, which was first described in patients from Lyme, Connecticut, usually begins in the summer with a characteristic skin lesion (erythema chronicum migrans) at the site of a tick bite and flulike symptoms; within weeks to months, a chronic arthritis develops that is characterized by erosions of cartilage and bone. The joint involvement has some similarities to juvenile idiopathic arthritis, reactive arthritis, and tuberculous arthritis. A joint effusion may be present in the early stages of the disease, and characteristic edematous changes of the infrapatellar fat pad may be noted in the knee (Fig. 9.29). MRI may show ribbon-like folds of hypertrophied synovium and frondlike extensions of synovium and synovial fluid into infrapatellar fat pad (Fig. 9.30). Generally, Lyme arthritis is frequently overdiagnosed by family physicians, and when suspected, consultation with rheumatologist is essential. The Infectious Disease Society of America has established guidelines for treatment of Lyme arthritis; therefore, an urgent consultation with an infectious disease specialist is indicated to determine the stage of disease and the most effective treatment protocol including monitoring. In early infection, the usual treatment consists of oral administration of antibiotics such as doxycycline, amoxicillin, azithromycin, and cefuroxime axetil. For late infection, intravenous administration of ceftriaxone is the treatment of choice. For chronic Lyme arthritis, synovectomy may be curative.

Parasitic Infections

Parasitic disease of the musculoskeletal system due to infestation by roundworms, flatworms, or tapeworms, such as hookworm disease, loiasis, filariasis, cysticercosis, or echinococcosis, is relatively uncommon in the western hemisphere, but in some endemic areas, parasitic infection needs to be considered in the differential diagnosis of bone and soft tissue lesions, especially when there are unusual imaging findings. The joints are affected exceptionally rarely, and there are only a few reports in the literature of articular infection caused by *Strongyloides stercoralis*.

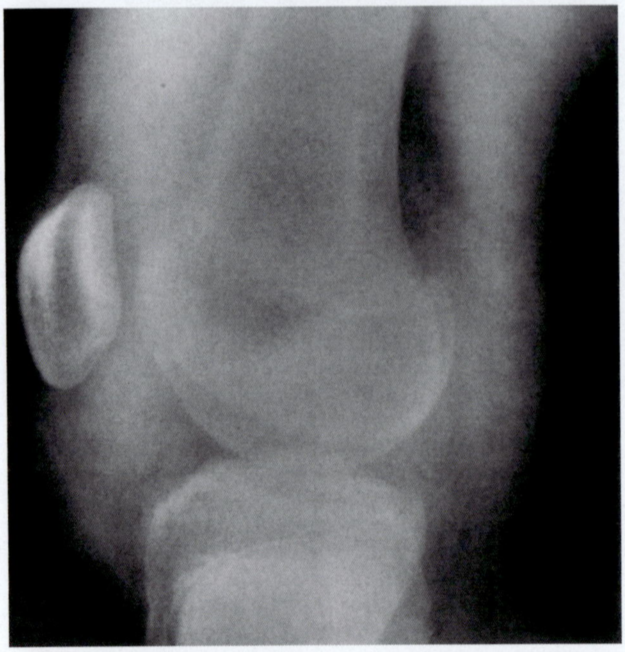

Figure 9.29 ■ **Lyme arthritis.** Lateral radiograph of the right knee of a 13-year-old boy, who presented with intermittent soft tissue swelling and knee effusion for several months, shows periarticular osteoporosis, joint effusion, soft tissue swelling, and areas of mottled density at the site of infrapatellar fat pad. (Reprinted from Lawson JP, Rahn DW. Lyme disease and radiologic findings in Lyme arthritis. *AJR Am J Roentgenol* 1992;158:1065–1069, with permission.)

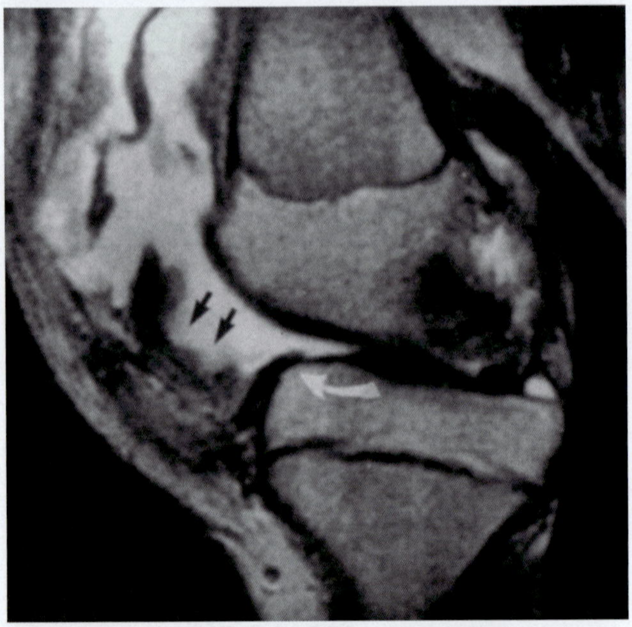

Figure 9.30 ■ **MRI of Lyme arthritis.** Sagittal T2-weighted MRI of the left knee of a 17-year-old boy, who presented with knee swelling for 7 months, reveals joint effusion that displaced medial meniscus anteriorly (*curved white arrow*). Note ribbon-like folds of hypertrophied synovium and frondlike extensions of synovium and synovial fluid into infrapatellar fat pad (*black arrows*). (Reprinted from Lawson JP, Rahn DW. Lyme disease and radiologic findings in Lyme arthritis. *AJR Am J Roentgenol* 1992;158:1065–1069, with permission.)

INFECTIONS OF THE SPINE

Infections in the spine may be located in a vertebral body, an intervertebral disk, the paravertebral soft tissues, or the epidural compartment; very rarely, an infection may involve the contents of the spinal canal or the spinal cord. The mechanisms of infection are the same as those of osteomyelitis and infectious arthritis (Fig. 9.31). An intervertebral disk infection, for example, may result from a puncture of the canal or of the disk itself during a procedure, as well as from a penetrating injury. It can also spread from a contiguous source of infection such as a paraspinal abscess. Most common, however, is hematogenous spread after surgical procedures such as laminectomy or spinal fusion, or during generalized bacteremia or sepsis. Regardless of the primary location of the infectious process, *Staphylococcus aureus* is responsible for more than 90% of all infections of the spine.

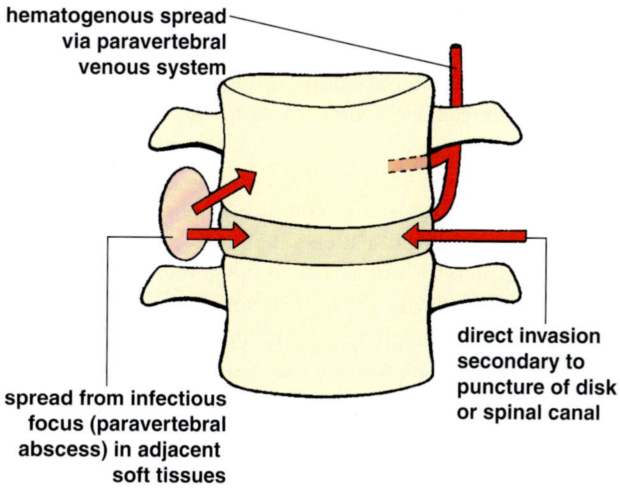

Figure 9.31 ■ Entry routes of an infectious organism into a vertebra. The potential routes of infection of a vertebra or an intervertebral disk are direct invasion, hematogenous spread, and extension from a focus of infection in the adjacent soft tissues.

Pyogenic Infections

Infectious organisms may reach the spine by several routes. Hematogenous spread occurs by way of arterial and venous routes (the Batson paravertebral venous system), and the organism lodges in the vertebral body, commonly in the anterior subchondral region. This osteomyelitic focus can spread to the intervertebral disk through perforation of the vertebral end plate, causing disk space infection (diskitis) (Fig. 9.32). Disk space infection can also be induced directly by the implantation of an organism through puncture of the spinal canal, either during spinal surgery or, rarely, by spread from a contiguous site of infection such as a paravertebral

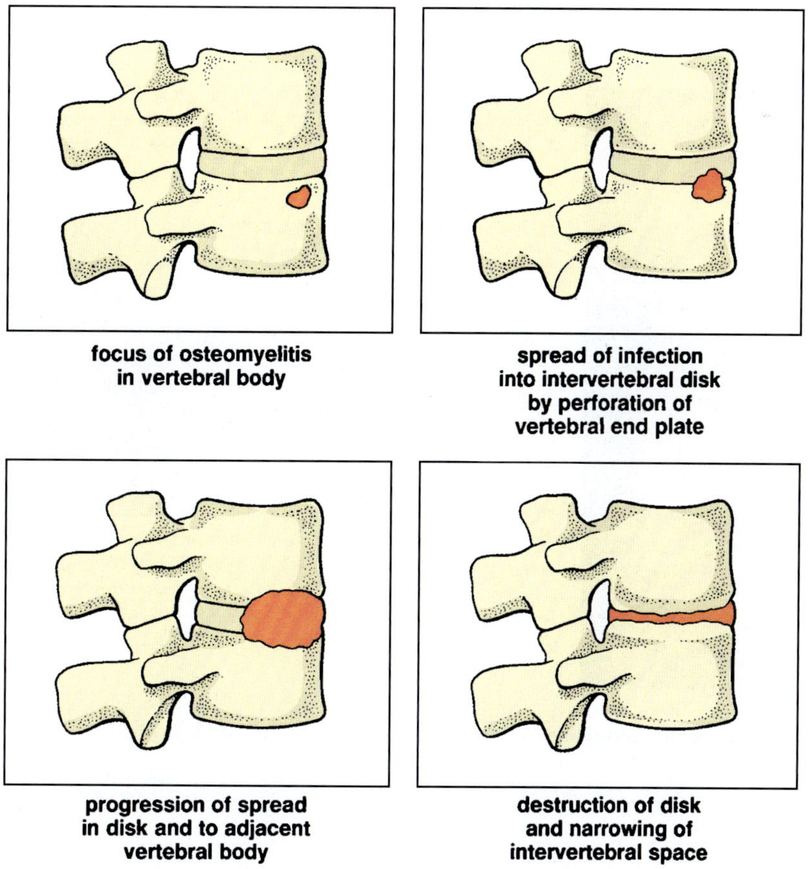

Figure 9.32 ■ Sequential stages of involvement of a vertebral body and disk by an infectious process.

abscess (see Fig. 9.31). The common organisms include *Staphylococcus aureus* and *Streptococcus pyogenes* and in intravenous drug abusers also Gram-negative bacilli, such as *Escherichia coli, Pseudomonas aeruginosa*, and *Klebsiella pneumoniae*. Predisposing factors include systemic urinary tract infection, diabetes mellitus, chronic hepatitis, sickle cell anemia, cardiovascular conditions, obesity, and intravenous drug addiction. Patients that have been treated with immunosuppressive drugs, including steroids and biologic agents, are also at risk. The lumbar spine is affected twice as common as the thoracic spine, and the cervical spine is only rarely involved. Disk infection may also occur in children via a hematogenous route because there is still a blood supply to the disk.

Clinical and Pathologic Features

Patients may range from being asymptomatic to having severe neurologic complications. The average period between the first symptoms and diagnosis has been reported to be between 2 and 6 months, the delay being the result of often nonspecific symptoms. Pain, which is the predominant symptom, is generally localized to the spine, exacerbated by movement, and occasionally radiating to the abdomen, hip, or groin. Radicular symptoms may also be present. Some patients have reported paravertebral muscle tenderness and spasm, and limitation of spine movement.

Because the segmental arteries supply blood to two consecutive vertebrae, vertebral osteomyelitis commonly involves two adjacent vertebral bodies. By extension, the infectious process is propagated from the vertebral body into the intervertebral disk. The vascular supply to intervertebral disk becomes compromised, leading to disk fragmentation, tissue necrosis, and total destruction. Microscopic changes depend upon the duration of the disease and reflect the stages of the infection: acute, subacute, or chronic. Early in the infectious process, an acute inflammatory reaction consists of leukocytic infiltration, edema, and necrosis of trabecular bone and bone marrow adjacent to the vertebral end plates (Fig. 9.33). In subacute and chronic phase of the disease, acute inflammation is gradually replaced by a lymphocytic and plasma cell infiltrate. Healing of infectious spondylitis and diskitis can lead to complete ankylosis of the adjacent vertebrae.

Imaging Features

Radiographically, disk infection is characterized by narrowing of the disk space, destruction of the adjacent vertebral end plates, and a paraspinal mass. Although most cases are obvious on standard anteroposterior and lateral radiographs of the spine (Fig. 9.34), CT (Fig. 9.35) may yield additional information. Radionuclide bone scan can detect early infection before any changes are noticed radiographically (Fig. 9.36). Occasionally, diskography is performed, but, as in the use of arthrography in joint infections, the primary objective is obtaining a specimen for bacteriologic examination. A contrast study, however, may outline the extent of a disk infection (Fig. 9.37). Myelography is still

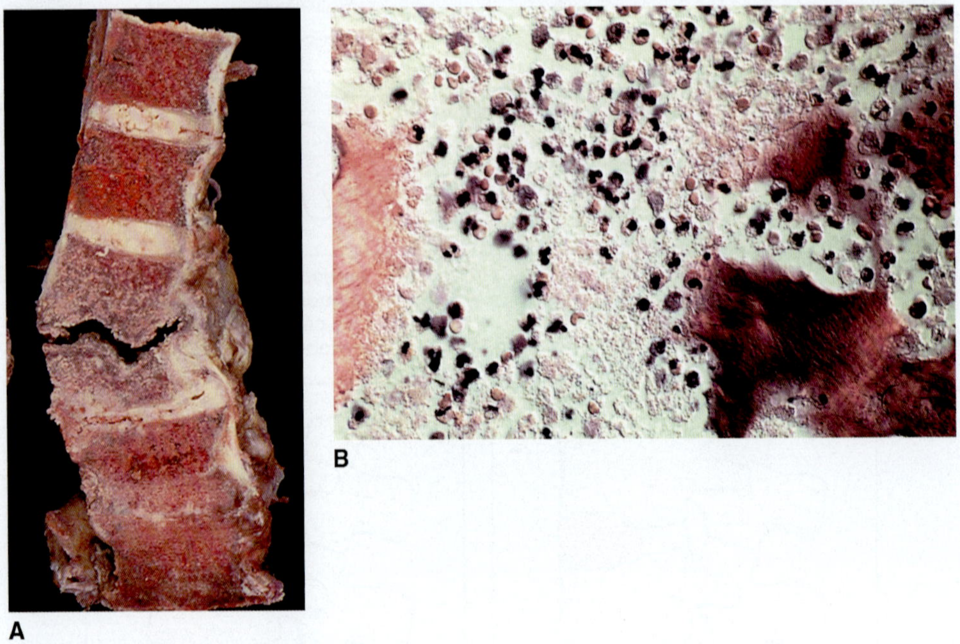

Figure 9.33 ■ **Pathology of pyogenic spondylitis. A:** Photograph of a sagittal section through the thoracolumbar spine shows involvement of the intervertebral disk and adjacent two vertebrae. **B:** Photomicrograph shows acute infection of the bone marrow spaces (H&E, original magnification ×25). (From Bullough PG, Boachie-Adjei O. *Atlas of Spinal Diseases*. New York, NY: JB Lippincott Company/Gower Medical Publishing; 1988, Figs. 12.8 and 12.9, pp. 161–162.)

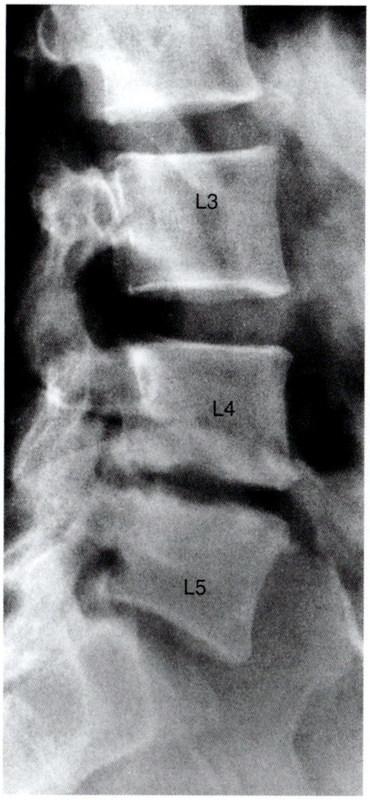

Figure 9.34 ■ **Intervertebral disk infection.** Lateral radiograph of the lumbar spine in a 32-year-old man demonstrates the typical radiographic changes of disk infection. There is narrowing of the disk space at L4–L5, and the inferior end plate of L4 and superior end plate of L5 are indistinctly outlined. Note the normal end plates at the L3–L4 disk space.

useful in evaluating infections within the spinal canal, as well as in vertebral osteomyelitis and disk infection (see Fig. 9.44B).

MRI has become the modality of choice in diagnosing and evaluating infections of the spine. Characteristic findings of disk space narrowing, disk destruction, paraspinal soft tissue thickening, and edematous changes in the paraspinal musculature are well demonstrated by this technique (Figs. 9.38 and 9.39).

More recently, positron emission tomography with 18 fluorine-labeled fluorodeoxyglucose (18F FDG PET) studies proved to be very effective in demonstrating spondylodiskitis.

Treatment

The reader is directed to The Infectious Diseases Society of America (IDSA) clinical practice guidelines for the diagnosis and treatment of native vertebral osteomyelitis (NVO) in adults. Generally, it involves the combination of antimicrobial therapy and surgical intervention with or without stabilization.

Nonpyogenic Infections

Tuberculosis

Infection of the spine by the tubercle bacillus is known as *tuberculous spondylitis* or *Pott disease*. The vertebral body or intervertebral disk may be involved, with the lower thoracic

(Continued on page 351)

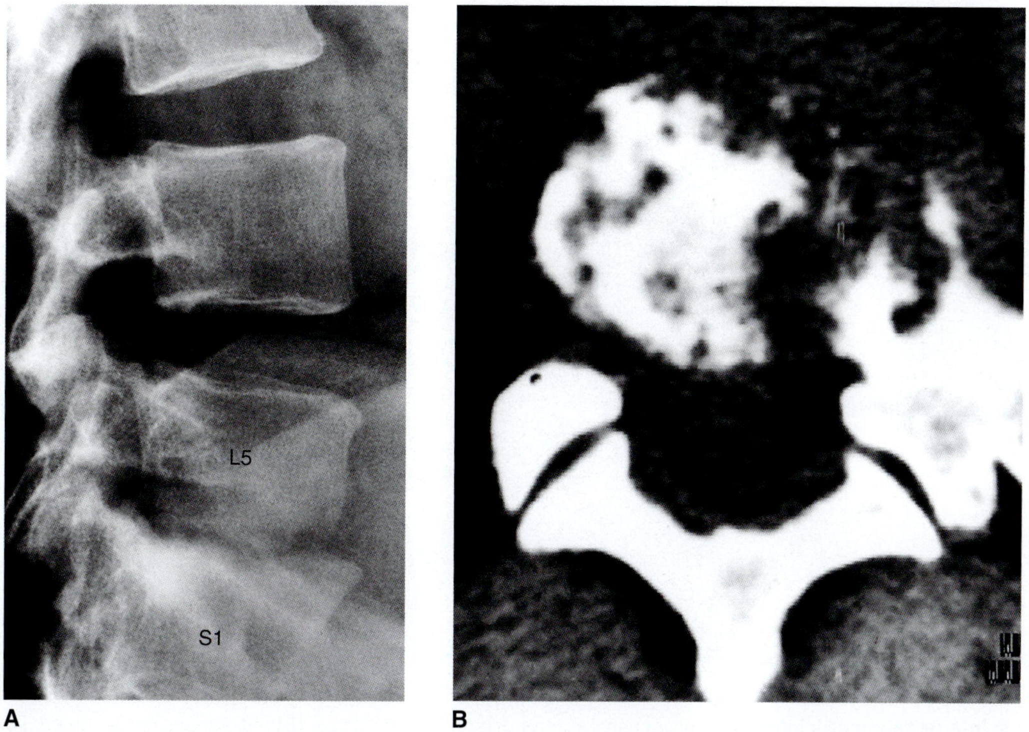

Figure 9.35 ■ **CT of intervertebral disk infection.** A 40-year-old man presented with lower back pain for 8 weeks, which he attributed to lifting a heavy object. **A:** Lateral radiograph of the lumbosacral spine shows narrowing of the L5–S1 disk space and suggests some fuzziness of the adjacent vertebral end plates. **B:** CT section through the disk space clearly shows destructive changes of the disk and vertebral end plate characteristic of infection.

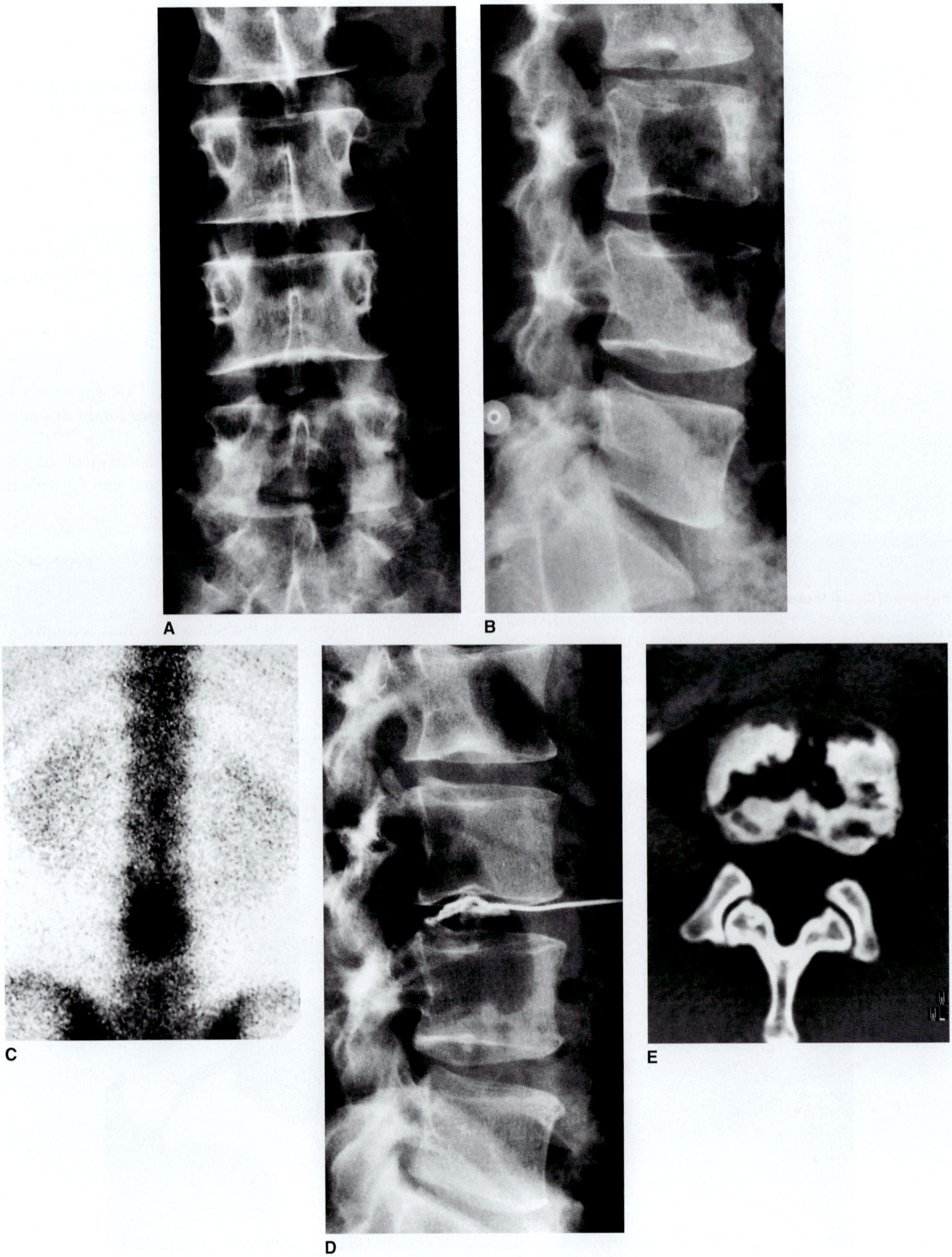

Figure 9.36 ■ **Intervertebral disk infection.** Conventional anteroposterior **(A)** and lateral **(B)** radiographs of the lumbar spine of a 40-year-old man who had back pain for 4 weeks show no definite abnormalities. **C:** Radionuclide bone scan, however, reveals an increased uptake of radiopharmaceutical tracer at the L3–L4 level. **D:** On a subsequent diskogram, using the oblique approach, partial disk destruction is evident. **E:** The extent of destruction is revealed by CT. Bacteriologic examination of aspirated fluid yielded *Escherichia coli*.

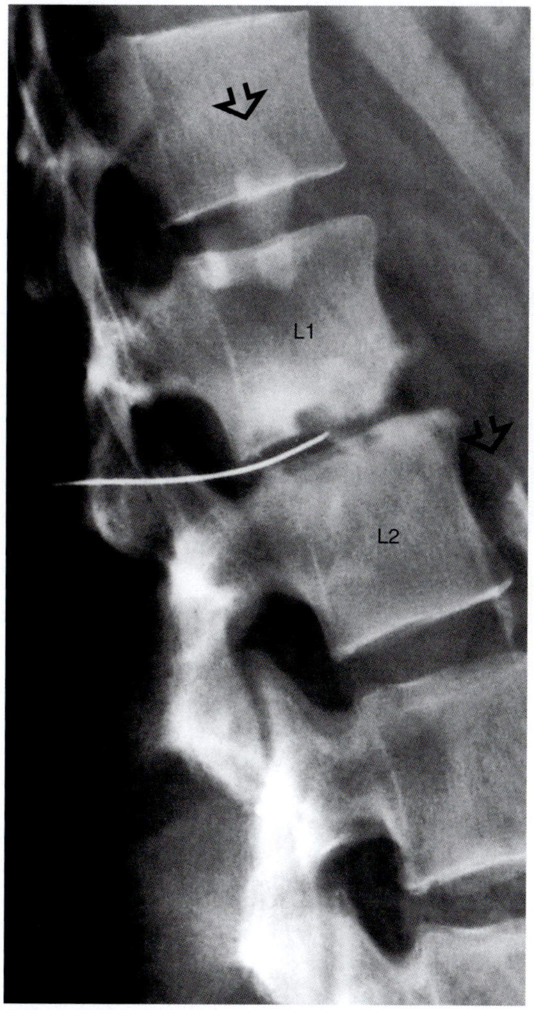

A

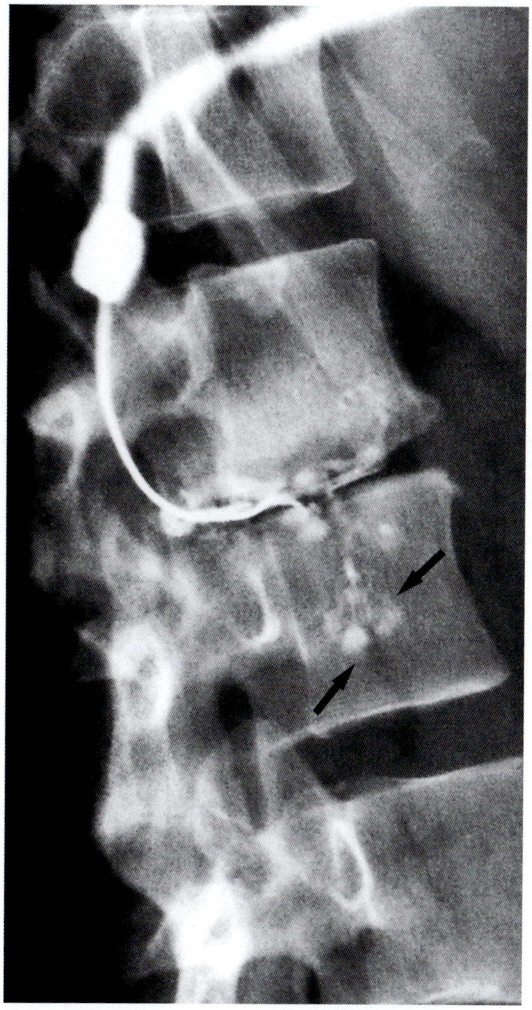

B

Figure 9.37 ■ **Disk space infection and vertebral osteomyelitis.** A 22-year-old intravenous drug user with back pain for 2 months was diagnosed with an intervertebral disk infection. A diskogram was performed primarily to aspirate fluid for bacteriologic examination, which revealed *Pseudomonas aeruginosa.* Before the puncture, the patient received an intravenous injection of iodine contrast agent to visualize the kidneys, as a precautionary step before spine biopsy at that level. **A:** Lateral radiograph of the lumbar spine shows narrowing of the disk space at L1–L2 and destruction of the adjacent vertebral end plates. The spinal needle is located in the center of the disk. The *open arrows* point to opacified calyces of kidney. **B:** Lateral radiograph obtained during the injection of metrizamide demonstrates extension of the contrast into the body of L2 (*arrows*), indicating the presence of vertebral osteomyelitis.

and upper lumbar vertebrae being the preferred sites of infection. The disease constitutes 25% to 50% of all cases of skeletal tuberculosis. The clinical features are very similar to those described for pyogenic spine infection (see prior text).

Histopathologic examination reveals a granulomatous inflammatory reaction with many tubercles composed of microscopic aggregates of epithelioid histiocytes and giant cells, enclosed within a rim of fibrosis infiltrated by lymphocytes and plasma cells (Fig. 9.40). The tubercles show central liquefaction necrosis and coalesce to form areas of caseating necrosis.

The imaging features of tuberculous infection of the spine are similar to those seen in pyogenic infections. There is disk space narrowing, and the vertebral end plates adjacent to the involved disk show evidence of destruction. A paraspinal mass is common (Fig. 9.41). Rarely, the infectious process may destroy a single vertebra or part of a vertebra (pedicle) without invasion of the disk.

Tuberculosis of the spine may cause collapse of a partially or completely destroyed vertebra, leading to kyphosis and a gibbous formation (Fig. 9.42). Extension of infection to the adjacent ligaments and soft tissues is also rather frequent; the psoas muscles are often the sites of secondary tuberculous infections, commonly called "cold" abscesses (Fig. 9.43). The most common complication of tuberculous spondylitis, however, is compression of the thecal sac and spinal cord with resulting paraplegia. Myelography (Fig. 9.44) and MRI are very helpful diagnostically if compression is suspected.

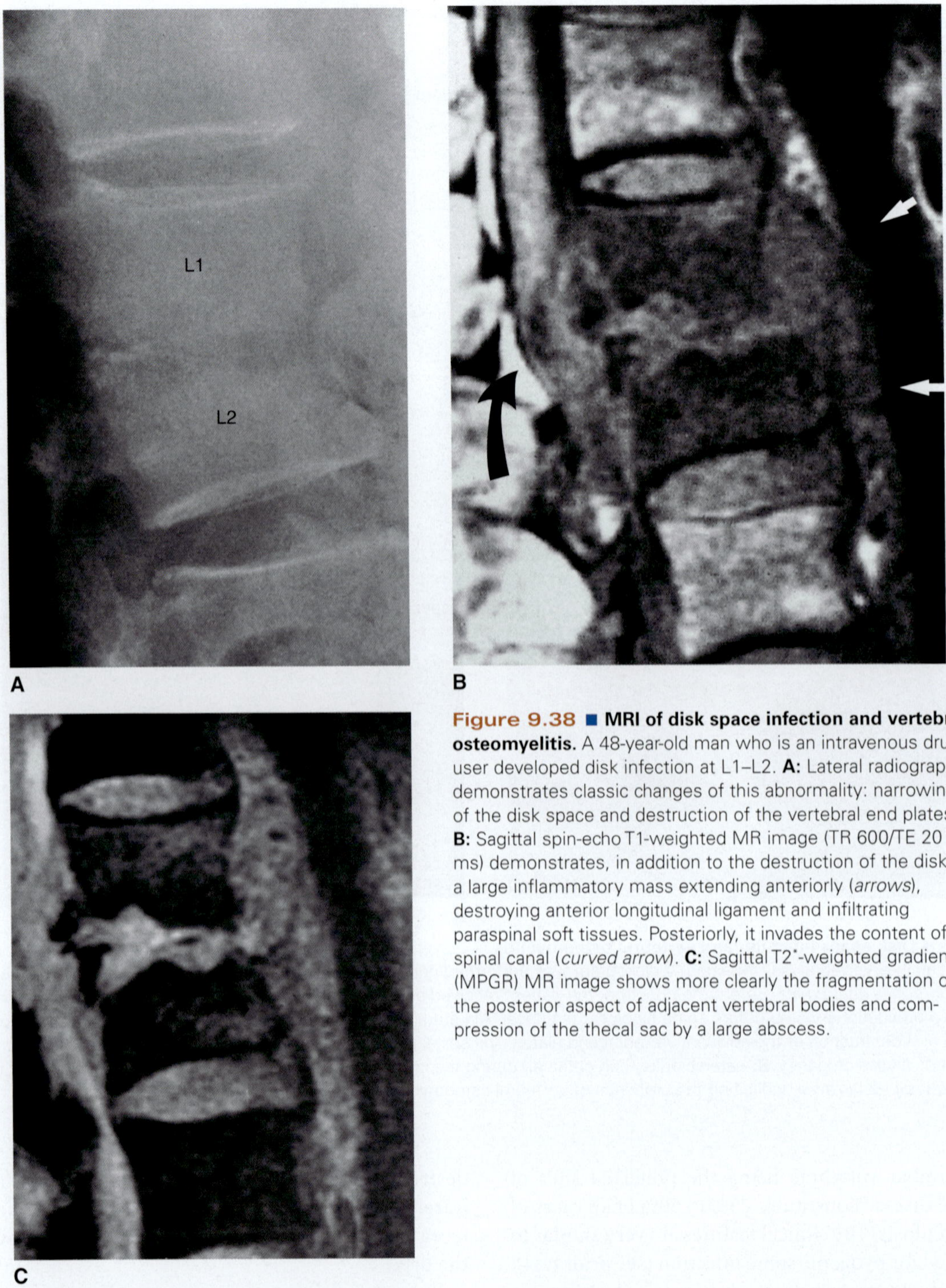

Figure 9.38 ■ **MRI of disk space infection and vertebral osteomyelitis.** A 48-year-old man who is an intravenous drug user developed disk infection at L1–L2. **A:** Lateral radiograph demonstrates classic changes of this abnormality: narrowing of the disk space and destruction of the vertebral end plates. **B:** Sagittal spin-echo T1-weighted MR image (TR 600/TE 20 ms) demonstrates, in addition to the destruction of the disk, a large inflammatory mass extending anteriorly (*arrows*), destroying anterior longitudinal ligament and infiltrating paraspinal soft tissues. Posteriorly, it invades the content of spinal canal (*curved arrow*). **C:** Sagittal T2*-weighted gradient (MPGR) MR image shows more clearly the fragmentation of the posterior aspect of adjacent vertebral bodies and compression of the thecal sac by a large abscess.

The treatment is similar to that described for tuberculous arthritis. Consultation with infectious disease specialist is mandatory.

Coccidioidomycosis

Coccidioidomycosis often involves the vertebral appendages, and paraspinal soft tissue extension is common. Disk space narrowing secondary to spondylodiskitis and gibbous deformity, although occasionally present (Fig. 9.45), are unusual findings in coccidioidomycosis, whereas both these findings are common in tuberculosis. Involvement of the spine most commonly manifests as vertebral osteomyelitis including punched-out and permeative lesions within the vertebral bodies. In most severe cases, almost complete vertebral destruction can occur (Fig. 9.46). The treatment of spinal coccidioidomycosis combines medical management with antifungal medications and surgery including spinal fusion.

(Continued on page 356)

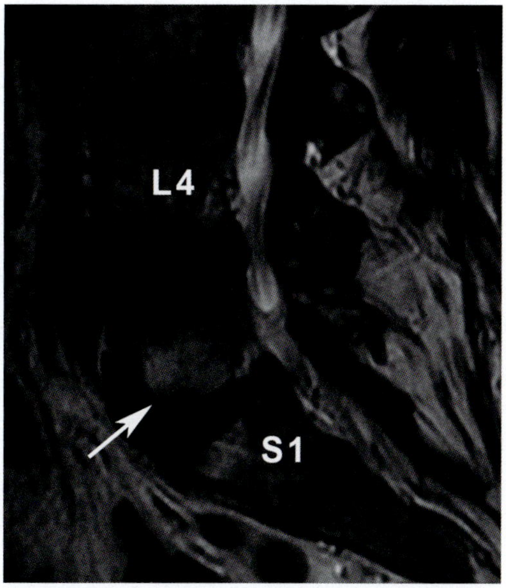

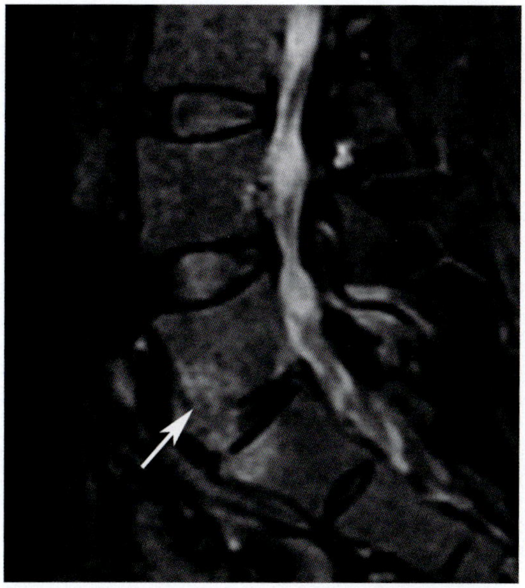

Figure 9.39 ■ **MRI of disk space infection and vertebral osteomyelitis.** Sagittal T2-weighted **(A)** and STIR MR **(B)** images of the lumbar spine of a 53-year-old man show a focal area of decortication of the inferior end plate of L5 (*arrows*) representing osteomyelitis, with bone marrow edema of the inferior aspect of the L5 vertebral body and superior aspect of the S1 vertebral body. There is swelling and high signal intensity of the anterior aspect of the intervertebral disk with mild prevertebral soft tissue edema. There are no signs of epidural abscess.

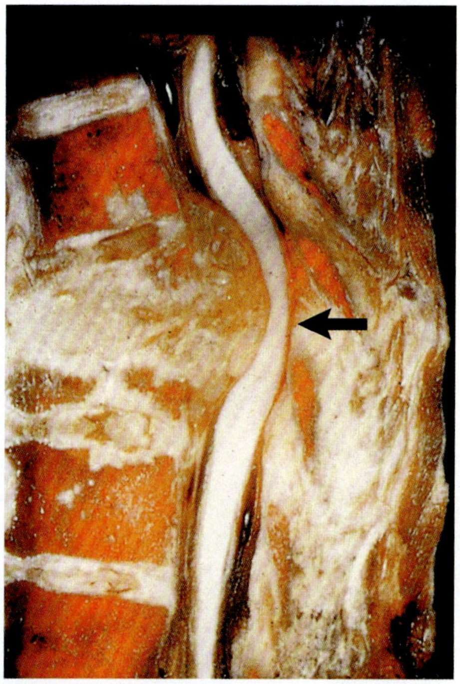

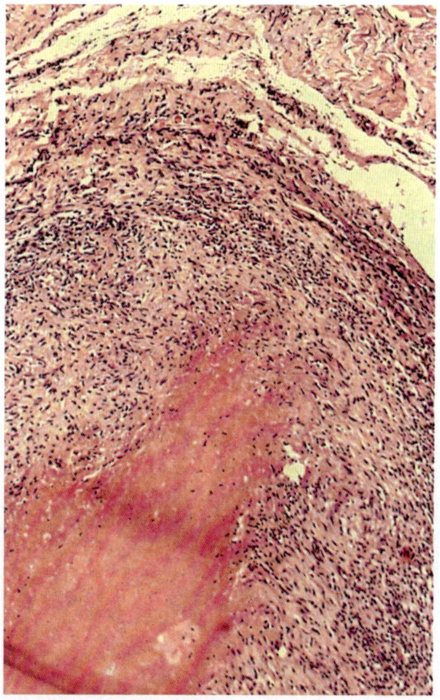

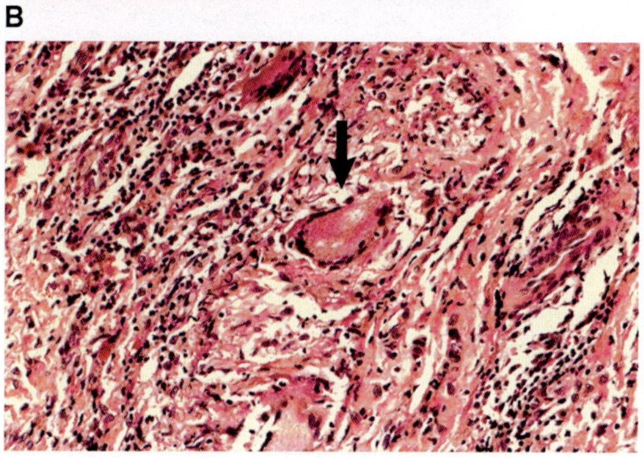

Figure 9.40 ■ **Pathology of tuberculous spondylitis.** **A:** Photograph of a sagittal section of the thoracic spine shows complete destruction of two of the vertebral bodies including the intervertebral disk. The tuberculous abscess has extended anteriorly and posteriorly, causing compression of the spinal cord (*arrow*). **B:** Photomicrograph of a tuberculous granuloma shows central caseation necrosis surrounded by inflammatory tissue (H&E, original magnification ×80). **C:** A high-power view shows a characteristic for tuberculosis Langhans giant cell with a horseshoe-shaped distribution of nuclei (*arrow*), surrounded by a palisade of epithelioid histiocytes and chronic inflammatory cells including lymphocytes and plasma cells (H&E, original magnification ×450). (Modified from Bullough PG, Boachie-Adjei O. *Atlas of Spinal Diseases.* New York, NY: JB Lippincott Company/Gower Medical Publishing; 1988, Figs. 12.19–12.21, pp. 167–168.)

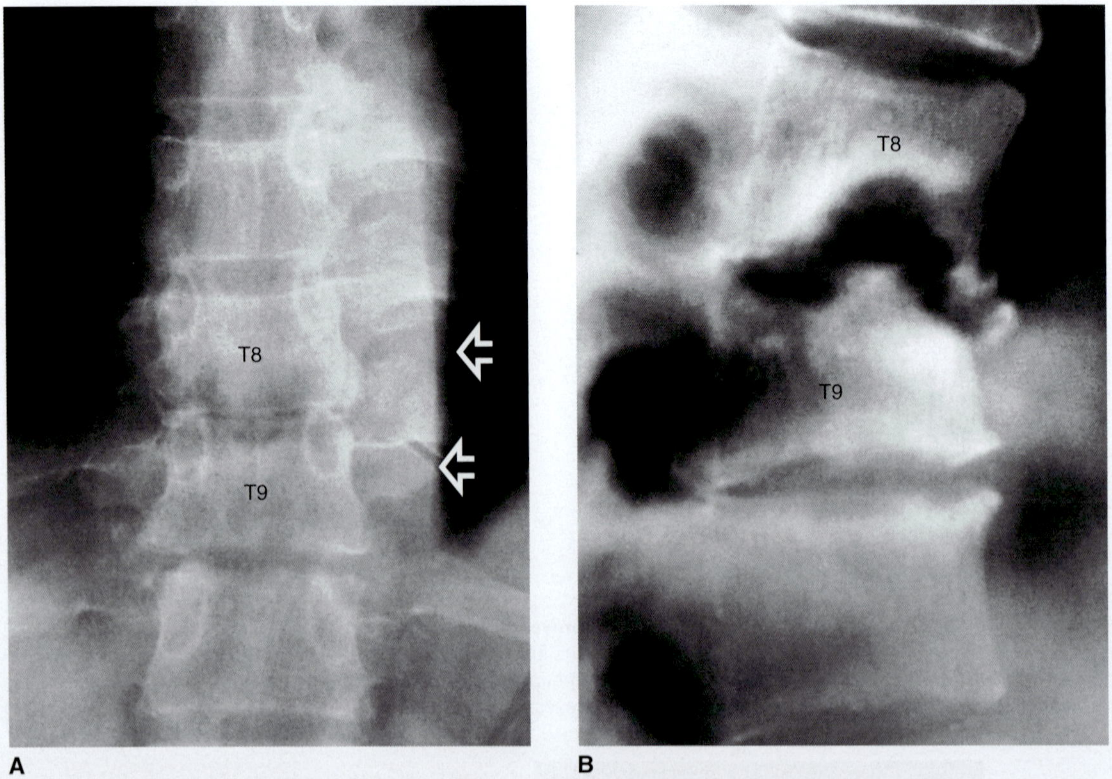

Figure 9.41 ■ **Tuberculous spondylitis. A:** Anteroposterior radiograph of the thoracic spine in a 50-year-old man shows narrowing of the T8–T9 disk space, associated with a paraspinal mass on the left side (*open arrows*). **B:** Lateral conventional tomogram shows destruction of the disk and extensive erosions of the inferior aspect of the body of T8 and the superior end plate of T9.

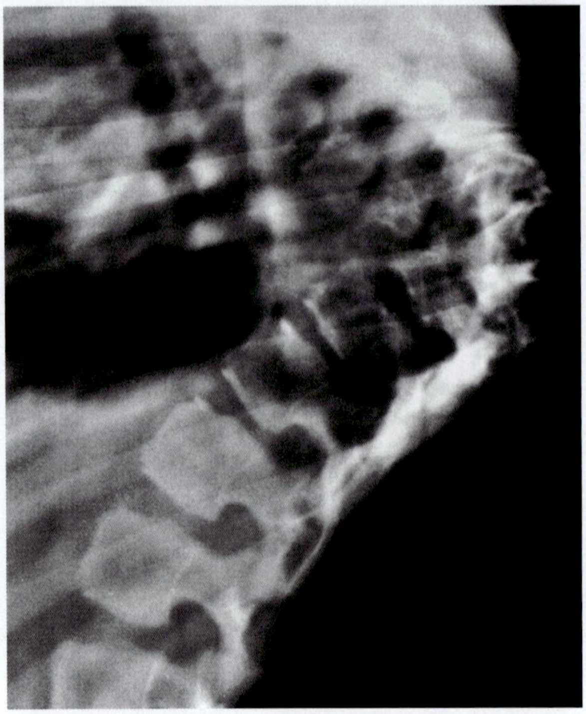

Figure 9.42 ■ **Tuberculous spondylitis.** Lateral radiograph of the lower thoracic spine of a 12-year-old boy with long-standing pulmonary and spinal tuberculosis shows severe kyphosis with a gibbous formation at the site of a collapsed vertebra, a common complication of this condition.

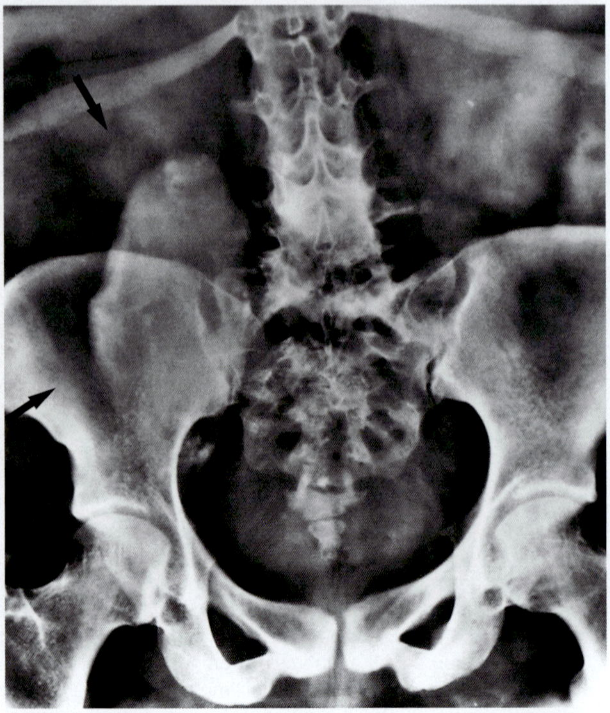

Figure 9.43 ■ **Tuberculous "cold" abscess.** Anteroposterior radiograph of the pelvis in a 35-year-old woman with spinal tuberculosis shows an oval radiodense mass with spotted calcifications overlapping the medial part of the ilium and right sacroiliac joint (right psoas muscle) (*arrows*). This is the typical appearance of a "cold" abscess.

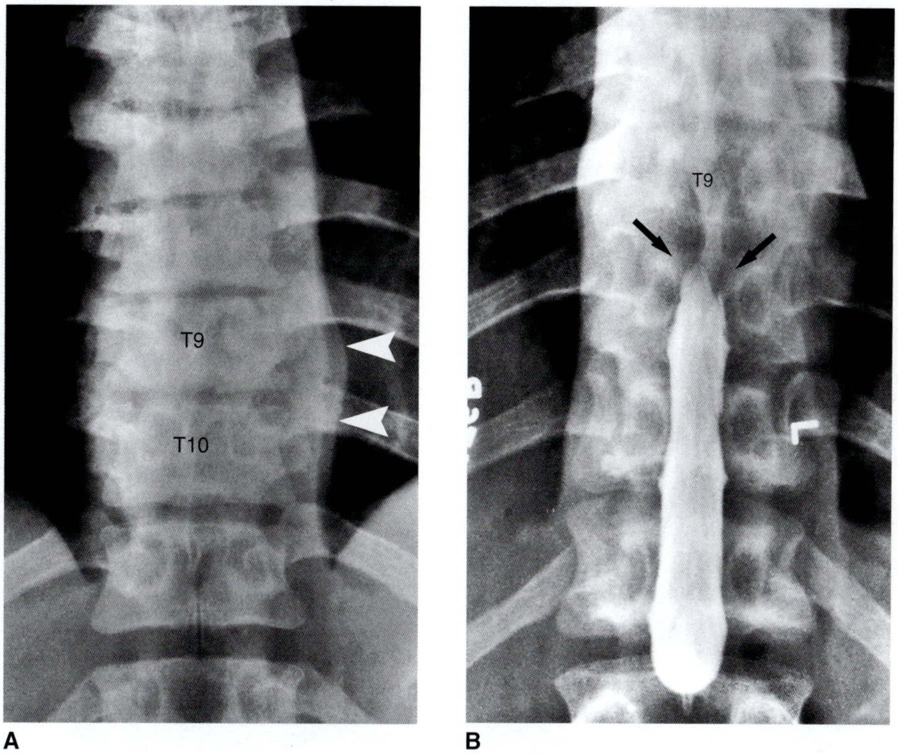

Figure 9.44 ■ **Myelography of tuberculous diskitis.** A 39-year-old man with a history of pulmonary tuberculosis had neurologic symptoms of spinal cord compression. **A:** Anteroposterior radiograph of the lower thoracic spine shows minimal disk space narrowing at T9–T10 and a large left paraspinal mass (*arrowheads*). **B:** A myelogram shows complete obstruction of the flow of contrast in the subarachnoid space at the level of the disk infection (*arrows*).

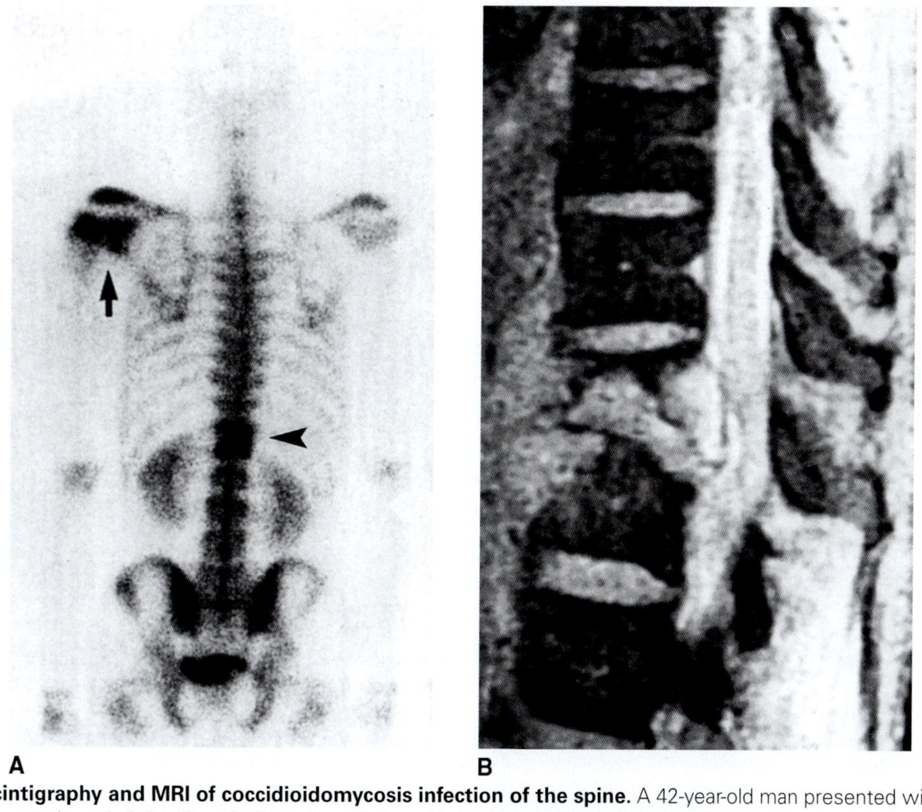

Figure 9.45 ■ **Scintigraphy and MRI of coccidioidomycosis infection of the spine.** A 42-year-old man presented with lower back and left shoulder pain of several weeks' duration. **A:** Posterior scintigraphic image obtained after intravenous administration of 24mCi (891 MBq) of technetium-99m MDP revealed increased uptake of the radiopharmaceutical tracer in the left shoulder (*arrow*) and in the T12 and L1 vertebral bodies (*arrowhead*). **B:** Sagittal MPGR MR image of the thoracolumbar region shows destruction of the disk T12–L1 and adjacent vertebral bodies, associated with a soft tissue mass extending anteriorly and posteriorly, very similar to the abnormalities seen in tuberculous spine infection.

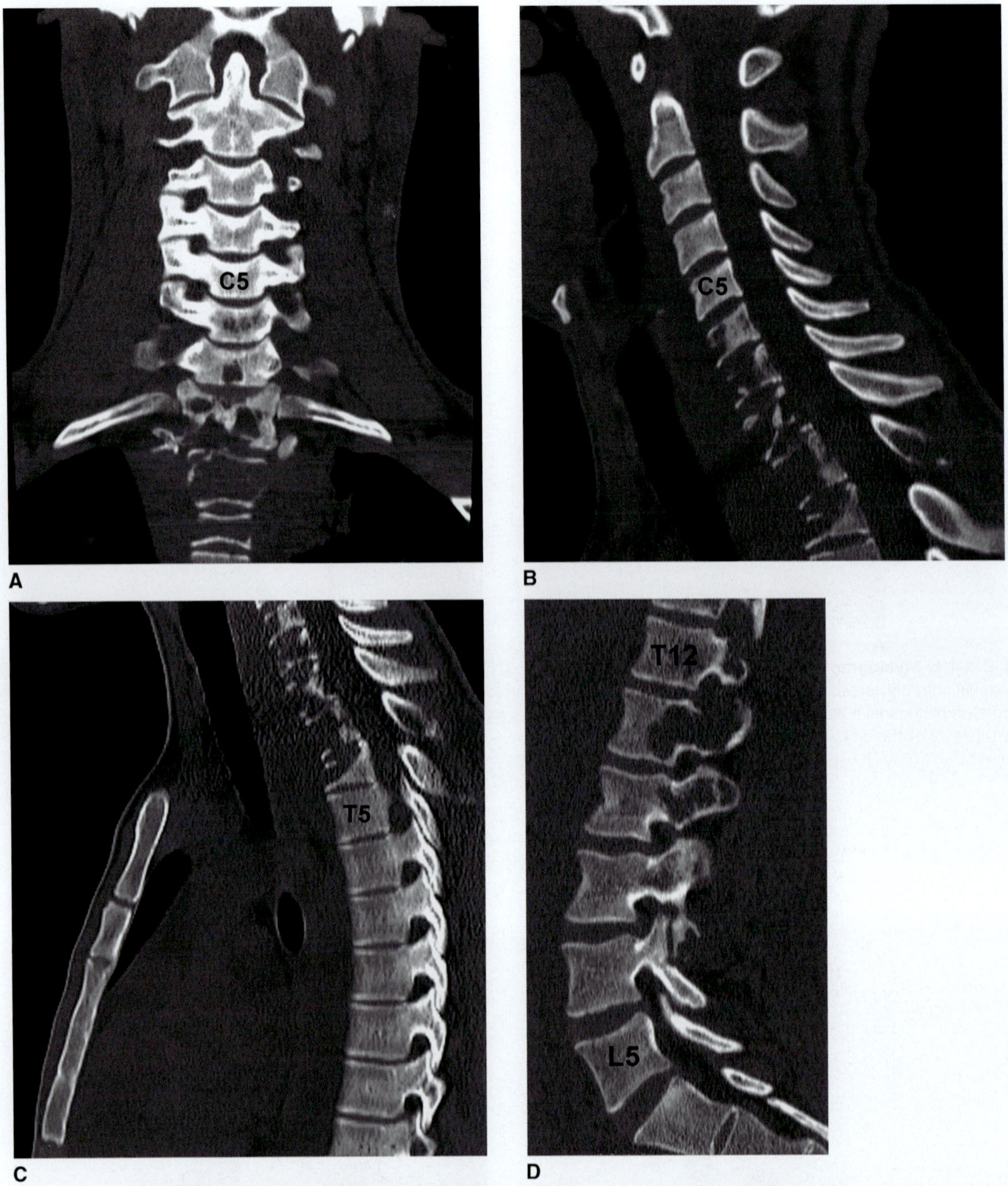

Figure 9.46 ■ **CT of coccidioidomycosis infection of the spine.** Coronal **(A)** and two sagittal **(B, C)** reformatted CT images of the cervical and upper thoracic spine of a 22-year-old man show destruction of several vertebral bodies extending from C6 to T4. **D:** Sagittal reformatted CT image of the lumbar spine of the same patient shows destruction of the vertebral bodies and posterior elements of the L1, L2, and L3 vertebrae. Observe that the intervertebral disk spaces are relatively well preserved.

SUGGESTED READINGS

Abdelwahab IF, Present DA, Zwass A, et al. Tumorlike tuberculosis granulomas of bone. *AJR Am J Roentgenol.* 1987;149:1207–1208.

Adam RD, Elliot SP, Taljanovic MS. The spectrum and presentation of disseminated coccidioidomycosis. *Am J Med.* 2009;122:770–777.

Alazraki NP. Radionuclide imaging in the evaluation of infectious and inflammatory disease. *Radiol Clin North Am.* 1993;31:783–794.

Alexander GH, Mansuy MM. Disseminated bone tuberculosis (so-called multiple cystic tuberculosis). *Radiology.* 1950;55:839–842.

Al-Shahed MS, Sharif HS, Haddad MC, et al. Imaging features of musculoskeletal brucellosis. *Radiographics.* 1994;14:333–348.

Al-Sheikh W, Sfakianakis GN, Mnaymneh W, et al. Subacute and chronic bone infections: diagnosis using In-111, Ga-67 and Tc-99m MDP bone scintigraphy, and radiography. *Radiology.* 1985;155:501–506.

Ampel NM. The treatment of coccidioidomycosis. *Rev Inst Med Trop Sao Paulo.* 2015;57:51–56.

Ampel NM. Coccidioidomycosis: a review of recent advances. *Clin Chest Med.* 2009;30:241–251.

Angus J, Langan SM, Stanway A, et al. The many faces of secondary syphilis: a re-emergence of an old disease. *Clin Exp Dermatol.* 2006;31:741–745.

Armbuster TG, Goergen TG, Resnick D, et al. Utility of bone scanning in disseminated coccidioidomycosis: a case report. *J Nucl Med.* 1977;18: 450–454.

Bancroft LW. MR imaging of infectious processes of the knee. *Radiol Clin North Am.* 2007;45:931–941.

Bassett LW, Gold RH, Webber MM. Radionuclide bone imaging. *Radiol Clin North Am.* 1981;19:675–702.

Bassetti M, Merell M, Di Gregorio F, et al. Higher fluorine-18 fluoroglucose positron emission tomography (FDG-PET) uptake in tuberculous compared to bacterial spondylodiscitis. *Skeletal Radiol* 2017;46:777–783.

Basu S, Chryssikos T, Moghadam-Kia S, et al. Positron emission tomography as a diagnostic tool in infection: present role and future possibilities. *Semin Nucl Med.* 2009;39:36–51.

Baughn RE, Musher DM. Secondary syphilitic lesions. *Clin Microbiol Rev.* 2005;18:205–216.

Bayer AS, Guze LB. Fungal arthritis. II. Coccidioidal synovitis: clinical, diagnostic, therapeutic, and prognostic considerations. *Semin Arthritis Rheum.* 1979;8:200–211.

Becker W, Goldenberg DM, Wolf F. The use of monoclonal antibodies and antibody fragments in the imaging of infectious lesions. *Semin Nucl Med.* 1994;24:142–153.

Behrman RE, Masci JR, Nicholas P. Cryptococcal skeletal infections: case report and review. *Rev Infect Dis.* 1990;12:181–190.

Beltran J, McGhee RB, Shaffer PB, et al. Experimental infections of the musculoskeletal system: evaluation with MR imaging and Tc-99m MDP and Ga-67 scintigraphy. *Radiology.* 1988;161:167–172.

Beltran J, Noto AM, McGhee RB, et al. Infections of the musculoskeletal system: high field-strength MR imaging. *Radiology.* 1987;164:449–454.

Berbari EF, Kanj SS, Kowalski TJ, et al. 2015 Infectious Diseases Society of America (IDSA) guidelines for the diagnosis and treatment of native vertebral osteomyelitis in adults. *Clin Infect Dis.* 2015;61:e26–e46.

Bierry G, Huang AJ, Chanh CY, et al. MRI findings of treated bacterial septic arthritis. *Skeletal Radiol.* 2012;41:1509–1516.

Benninghoven CD, Miller ER. Coccidioidal infection in bone. *Radiology.* 1942;38:663–666.

Birsner JW, Smart S. Osseous coccidioidomycosis: a chronic form of dissemination. *AJR Am J Roentgenol.* 1956;76:1052–1060.

Blauenstein P, Locher JT, Seybold K, et al. Experience with iodine-123 and technetium-99m labeled anti-granulocyte antibody MAb47: a comparison of labeling methods. *Eur J Nucl Med.* 1995;22:690–698.

Bleeker-Rovers CP, Rennen HJ, Boerman OC, et al. 99mTc-labeled interleukin 8 for the scintigraphic detection of infection and inflammation: first clinical evaluation. *J Nucl Med.* 2007;48:337–343.

Bocanegra TS, Espinosa LR, Bridgeford LR, et al. Reactive arthritis due to parasitic infection. *Ann Intern Med.* 1981;94:207–209.

Bockenstadt LK. Lyme disease. In: Imboden JB, Hellmann DB, Stone JH, eds. *Current Diagnosis and Treatment. Rheumatology*. 3rd ed. New York, NY: McGraw Hill; 2013:357–367.

Brodie BC. An account of some cases of chronic abscess of the tibia. *Trans Med Chir Soc.* 1832;17:238–239.

Brown R, Wilkinson T. Chronic recurrent multifocal osteomyelitis. *Radiology.* 1988;166:493–496.

Bruno MS, Silverberg TN, Goldstein DH. Embolic osteomyelitis of the spine as a complication of infection of the urinary tract. *Am J Med.* 1960;29:865–878.

Bullough PG. *Atlas of Orthopedic Pathology with Clinical and Radiologic Correlation.* 2nd ed. New York, NY: Gower Medical Publishing; 1992.

Bullough PG, Boachie-Adjei O. *Atlas of Spinal Diseases.* New York, NY: JB Lippincott Company/Gower Medical Publishing; 1988.

Calabresco LH, Naides SJ. Viral arthritis. *Infect Dis Clin North Am.* 2005;19:963–980.

Carter RA. Infectious granulomas of bones and joints, with special reference to coccidioidal granuloma. *Radiology.* 1934;23:1–16.

Chang MC, Wu HTH, Lee CH, et al. Tuberculous spondylitis and pyogenic spondylitis: comparative magnetic resonance imaging features. *Spine.* 2006;31:782–788.

Chelboun J, Sydney N. Skeletal cryptococcosis. *J Bone Joint Surg Am.* 1977;59A:509–514.

Cremin BJ, Fisher RM. The lesions of congenital syphilis. *Br J Radiol.* 1970;43:333–341.

Crim JR, Seeger LL. Imaging evaluation of osteomyelitis. *Crit Rev Diagn Imaging.* 1994;35:201–256.

Crum NF, Lederman ER, Stafford CM, et al. Coccidioidomycosis: a descriptive survey of a reemerging disease – clinical characteristics and current controversies. *Medicine.* 2004;83:149–175.

Cuellar ML, Silveira LH, Citera G, et al. Other fungal arthritides. *Rheum Dis Clin North Am.* 1993;19:439–455.

Dagirmanjian A, Schills J, McHenry M, et al. MR imaging of vertebral osteomyelitis revisited. *AJR Am J Roentgenol.* 1996;167:1539–1543.

Dalinka MK, Greendyke WH. The spinal manifestations of coccidioidomycosis. *J Can Assoc Radiol.* 1971;22:93–99.

Datz FL. The current status of radionuclide infection imaging. In: Freeman LM, ed. *Nuclear Medicine Annual.* New York, NY: Raven Press; 1993:47–76.

Datz FL. Indium-111-labeled leukocytes for the detection of infection: current status. *Semin Nucl Med.* 1994;24:92–109.

Datz FL, Morton KA. New radiopharmaceuticals for detecting infection. *Invest Radiol.* 1993;28:356–365.

David R, Barron BJ, Madewell JE. Osteomyelitis, acute and chronic. *Radiol Clin North Am.* 1987;25:1171–1201.

De Vuyst D, Vanhoenacker F, Gielen J, et al. Imaging features of musculoskeletal tuberculosis. *Eur Radiol.* 2003;13:1809–1819.

Diaz LA, Foss CA, Thornton K, et al. Imaging of musculoskeletal bacterial infections by [^{124}I] FIAU-PET/CT. *PLoS One.* 2007;2:e1007.

Doury P. Parasitic rheumatism. *Arthritis Rheum.* 1981;24:638–639.

Drutz DJ, Catanzaro A. Coccidioidomycosis. Part I. *Am Rev Respir Dis.* 1978;117:559–585.

Drutz DJ, Catanzaro A. Coccidioidomycosis. Part II. *Am Rev Respir Dis.* 1978;117:727–771.

Duncan GJ, Tooke SM. Echinococcus infestation of the biceps brachii. A case report. *Clin Orthop Relat Res.* 1990;261:247–250.

Eberst-Ledoux J, Tournadre A, Mathieu S, et al. Septic arthritis with negative bacteriological findings in adult native joints: a retrospective study of 74 cases. *Joint Bone Spine.* 2012;79:156–159.

Ehrlich I, Kricum ME. Radiographic findings in early acquired syphilis: case report and critical review. *AJR Am J Roentgenol.* 1976;127:789–792.

Elgafy H, Miller J, Meyers S, et al. Disseminated coccidioidomycosis of the spine. *Spine J.* 2015;15:1478–1479.

Erdman WA, Tamburro F, Jayson HT, et al. Osteomyelitis: characteristics and pitfalls of diagnosis with MR imaging. *Radiology.* 1991;180:533–539.

Ferguson PJ, Sandu M. Current understanding of the pathogenesis and management of chronic recurrent multifocal osteomyelitis. *Curr Rheumatol Rep.* 2012;14:130–141.

Fletcher BD, Scoles PV, Nelson AD. Osteomyelitis in children: detection by magnetic resonance. *Radiology.* 1984;150:57–60.

Fox IN, Zeiger L. Tc-99m-HMPAO leukocyte scintigraphy for the diagnosis of osteomyelitis in diabetic foot infections. *J Foot Ankle Surg.* 1993;32:591–594.

Galgiani JN, Ampel NM, Catanzaro A, et al. Practice guidelines for the treatment of coccidioidomycosis. *Clin Infect Dis.* 2000;30:658–661.

Garrido G, Gomez-Reino JJ, Fernandez-Dapica P, et al. A review of peripheral tuberculous arthritis. *Semin Arthritis Rheum.* 1988;18:142–149.

Gemmel F, Rijk PC, Collins JM, et al. Expanding role of 18F-fluoro-D-deoxyglucose PET and PET/CT in spinal infections. *Eur Spine J.* 2010;19:540–551.

Gilmour WM. Acute haematogenous osteomyelitis. *J Bone Joint Surg Br.* 1962;44B:841–853.

Glaudemans AWJM, Signore A. FDG-PET/CT in infections: the imaging method of choice? *Eur J Nucl Med Mol Imaging.* 2010;37:1986–1991.

Gold RH, Hawkins RA, Katz RD. Bacterial osteomyelitis: findings on plain radiography, CT, MR, and scintigraphy. *AJR Am J Roentgenol.* 1991;157:365–370.

Grados F, Lescure FX, Senneville E, et al. Suggestion for managing pyogenic (non-tuberculous) discitis in adults. *Joint Bone Spine.* 2007;74:133–139.

Graves VB, Schreiber MN. Tuberculosis psoas muscle abscess. *J Can Assoc Radiol.* 1973;24:268–271.

Gray MS, Philp T. Syphilitic arthritis. *Ann Rheum.* 1963:22:19–28.

Graybill JR, Stevens DA, Galgiani JN, et al. Itraconazole treatment of coccidioidimycosis. *Am J Med.* 1990;89:282–290.

Guhlmann A, Brecht-Krauss D, Suger G, et al. Chronic osteomyelitis: detection with FDG PET and correlation with histopathologic findings. *Radiology.* 1998;206:749–754.

Guyot DR, Manoli A II, Kling GA. Pyogenic sacroiliitis in IV drug users. *AJR Am J Roentgenol.* 1987;149:1209–1211.

Harcke HT, Grissom LE. Musculoskeletal ultrasound in pediatrics. *Semin Musculoskel Radiol.* 1998;2:321–329.

Harisinghani M, McLoud T, Shepard J, et al. Tuberculosis from head to toe. *Radiographics.* 2000;20:449–470.

Harkirat S, Anand SS, Indrajit IK, et al. Pictorial essay: PET/CT in tuberculosis. *Indian J Radiol Imaging.* 2008;18:141–147.

Haygood TM, Williamson SL. Radiographic findings of extremity tuberculosis in childhood: back to the future? *Radiographics.* 1994;14:561–570.

Ho J Jr. Infectious disorders. A. Septic arthritis. In: Klippel JH, Stone JH, Crofford LJ, White PH, eds. *Primer on the Rheumatic Diseases.* 13th ed. New York NY: Springer; 2008:271–276.

Ho G Jr. Pseudoseptic arthritis. *R I Med.* 1994;77:7–9.

Ho G Jr. How best to drain an infected joint: will we ever know for certain? *J Rheumatol.* 1993;20:2001–2003.

Hoffer P. Gallium: mechanisms. *J Nucl Med.* 1980;21:282–285.

Hong SH, Kim SM, Ahn JM, et al. Tuberculous versus pyogenic arthritis: MR imaging evaluation. *Radiology.* 2001;218:848–853.

Hopkins KL, Li KC, Bergman G. Gadolinium-DPTA-enhanced magnetic resonance imaging of musculoskeletal infectious processes. *Skeletal Radiol.* 1995;24:325–330.

Ito K, Kubota K, Morooka M, et al. Clinical impact of 18F-FDG PET/CT on the management and diagnosis of infectious spondylitis. *Nucl Med Commun.* 2010;31:691–698.

Jain R, Sawhney S, Berry M. Computed tomography of vertebral tuberculosis: patterns of bone destruction. *Clin Radiol.* 1993;47:196–199.

Jaovisidha S, Chen C, Ryu KN, et al. Tuberculous tenosynovitis and bursitis: imaging findings in 21 cases. *Radiology.* 1996;201:507–513.

Jaramillo D, Treves ST, Kasser JR, et al. Osteomyelitis and septic arthritis in children: appropriate use of imaging to guide treatment. *AJR Am J Roentgenol.* 1995;165:399–403.

Kaandorp CJE, Van Schaardenburg D, Krijnen P, et al. Risk factors for septic arthritis in patients with joint disease: a prospective study. *Arthritis Rheum.* 1995;38:1819–1825.

Kaim A, Maurer T, Ochsner P, et al. Chronic complicated osteomyelitis of the appendicular skeleton: diagnosis with technetium-99m labelled monoclonal antigranulocyte antibody-immunoscintigraphy. *Eur J Nucl Med.* 1997;24:732–738.

Kakarla UK, Kalani MY, Sharma GK, et al. Surgical management of coccidioidomycosis of the spine: clinical article. *J Neurosurg Spine.* 2011; 15:441–446.

Kalicke T, Schmitz A, Risse JH, et al. Fluorine-18 fluorodo-oxyglucose PET in infectious bone diseases: result of histologically confirmed cases. *Eur J Nucl Med.* 2000;27:524–528.

Karchevsky M, Schweitzer ME, Morrison WB, et al. MRI findings of septic arthritis and associated osteomyelitis in adults. *AJR Am J Roentgenol.* 2004;182:119–122.

Kido D, Bryan D, Halpern M. Hematogeneous osteomyelitis in drug addicts. *AJR Am J Roentgenol.* 1973;118:356–363.

Kim H, Kim J, Ihm C. The usefulness of multiplex PCR for the identification of bacteria in joint infection. *J Clin Lab Anal.* 2010;24:175–181.

Kim CW, Perry A, Currier B, et al. Fungal infections of the spine. *Clin Orthop Relat Res.* 2006;444:92–99.

King AD, Peters AM, Stuttle AWJ, et al. Imaging of bone infection with labeled white cells: role of contemporaneous bone marrow imaging. *Eur J Nucl Med.* 1990;17:148–151.

Klein MJ, Bonar SF, Freemont T, et al., eds. *Atlas of Nontumor Pathology. Non-neoplastic Diseases of Bones and Joints.* Washington, DC: The American Registry of Pathology. Armed Forces Institute of Pathology; 2011:411–543.

Kowalski TJ, Layton KF, Berbari EF, et al. Follow-up MR imaging in patients with pyogenic spine infections: lack of correlation with clinical features. *AJNR Am J Neuroradiol.* 2007;28:693–699.

Lammering JC, Iv M, Gupta N, et al. Imaging spectrum of CNS coccidioidomycosis: prevalence and significance of concurrent brain and spinal disease. *AJR Am J Roentgenol.* 2013;200:1334–1346.

Lawson JP, Rahn DW. Lyme disease and radiologic findings in Lyme arthritis. *AJR Am J Roentgenol.* 1992;158:1065–1069.

Lawson JP, Steere AC. Lyme arthritis: radiologic findings. *Radiology.* 1985;154:37–43.

Lazzarini L, Lipsky BA, Mader JT. Antibiotic treatment of osteomyelitis: what have we learned from 30 years of clinical trials? *Int J Infect Dis.* 2005;9:127–138.

Lee SK, Suh KJ, Kim YW, et al. Septic arthritis versus transient synovitis at MR imaging: preliminary assessment with signal intensity alterations in bone marrow. *Radiology.* 1999;211:459–465.

Legius B, Landuyt KV, Verschueren P, et al. Septic arthritis due to Staphylococcus warneri: a diagnostic challenge. *Open Rheumatol J.* 2012;6:310–311.

Lewicky YM, Roberto RF, Curtin SL. The unique complications of coccidioidomycosis of the spine. *Spine.* 2004;29:E435–E441.

Lund PJ, Chan KM, Unger EC, et al. Magnetic resonance imaging in coccidioidal arthritis. *Skeletal Radiol.* 1996;25:661–665.

Malaviya AN, Kotwal PP. Arthritis associated with tuberculosis. *Best Pract Res Clin Rheumatol.* 2003;17:319–343.

Makis W, Abikhzer G, Stern J. Tuberculous synovitis of the hip joint diagnosed by FDG PET-CT. *Clin Nucl Med.* 2009;34:431–432.

Martini M, Ouahes M. Bone and joint tuberculosis: a review of 652 cases. *Orthopedics.* 1988;11:861–866.

Mathew D'Souza M, Sharma R, Tripathi M, et al. F-18 Fluorodeoxyglucose positron emission tomography/computed tomography in tuberculosis of the hip: a case report and brief review of literature. *Indian J Nucl Med.* 2011;26:31–33.

Mathews CJ, Weston VC, Jones A, et al. Bacterial septic arthritis in adults. *Lancet.* 2010;375:846–855.

Matisz CE, McDougall JJ, Sharkey KA, et al. Helminth parasites and the modulation of joint inflammation. *J Parasitol Res.* 2011; http://dx.doi.org/10.1155/2011/942616

May DA, Disler DG. Case 50: primary coccidioidal synovitis of the knee. *Radiology.* 2002;224:665–668.

McGahan JP, Graves DS, Palmer PES. Coccidioidal spondylitis: usual and unusual roentgenographic manifestations. *Radiology.* 1980;136:5–9.

McGahan JP, Graves DS, Palmer PES, et al. Classic and contemporary imaging of coccidioidomycosis. *AJR Am J Roentgenol.* 1981;136:393–404.

McGill PE. Geographically specific infections and arthritis, including rheumatic syndromes associated with certain fungi and parasites, Brucella species and Mycobacterium leprae. *Best Pract Res Clin Rheumatol.* 2003;17:289–307.

McHenry MC, Easley KA, Locker GA. Vertebral osteomyelitis: long-term outcome for 253 patients from 7 Cleveland-area hospitals. *Clin Infect Dis.* 2002;34:1342–1350.

Merkle EM, Schulte M, Vogel J, et al. Musculoskeletal involvement in cystic echinococcosis: report of eight cases and review of the literature. *AJR Am J Roentgenol.* 1997;168:1531–1534.

Miller TT, Randolph DA Jr, Staron RB, et al. Fat-suppressed MR of musculoskeletal infection: fast T2-weighted techniques versus gadolinium-enhanced T1-weighted images. *Skeletal Radiol.* 1997;26:654–658.

Modic MT, Feiglin DH, Piriano DW, et al. Vertebral osteomyelitis: assessment using MR. *Radiology.* 1985;157:157–166.

Modic MT, Pflanze W, Feiglin DHI, et al. Magnetic resonance imaging of musculoskeletal infections. *Radiol Clin North Am.* 1986;24:247–258.

Moon MS. Tuberculosis of the spine. Controversies and a new challenge. *Spine.* 1997;22:1791–1797.

Moore SL, Jones S, Lee JL. Nocardia osteomyelitis in the setting of previously unknown HIV infection. *Skeletal Radiol.* 2005;34:58–60.

Moore S, Rafii M. Imaging of musculoskeletal and spinal tuberculosis. *Radiol Clin North Am.* 2001;39:329–342.

Olson EM, Duberg AC, Herron LD, et al. Coccidioidal spondylitis: MR findings in 15 patients. *AJR Am J Roentgenol.* 1998;171:785–789.

Palestro CJ, Love C, Bhargava KK. Labeled leukocyte imaging: current status and future directions. *Q J Nucl Med Mol Imaging.* 2009;53:105–123.

Palestro CJ, Love C, Tronco GG, et al. Combined labeled leukocyte and technetium 99m sulfur colloid bone marrow imaging for diagnosing musculoskeletal infection. *Radiographics.* 2006;26:859–870.

Palestro CJ, Roumanas P, Swyer AJ, et al. Diagnosis of musculoskeletal infection using combined In-111 labeled leukocyte and Tc-99m SC marrow imaging. *Clin Nucl Med.* 1992;17:269–273.

Paterson DC. Acute suppurative arthritis in infancy and childhood. *J Bone Joint Surg Br.* 1970;52B:474–482.

Patey O, Bouhali R, Brevil J, et al. Arthritis associated with Strongyloides stercoralis. *J Infect Dis.* 1990;22:233–236.

Perronne C, Saba J, Behloul Z, et al. Pyogenic and tuberculous spondylodiskitis (vertebral osteomyelitis) in 80 adult patients. *Clin Infect Dis.* 1994;19:746–750.

Peters AM. The utility of [^{99m}Tc] HMPAO-leukocytes for imaging infection. *Semin Nucl Med.* 1994;24:110–127.

Phemister DB, Hatcher CM. Correlation of pathological and roentgenological findings in the diagnosis of tuberculosis arthritis. *AJR Am J Roentgenol.* 1933;29:736–752.

Plodkowski AJ, Hayter CL, Miller TT, et al. Lamellated hyperintense synovitis: Potential sign of an infected knee arthroplasty. *Radiology.* 2013;266:256–260.

Prasad A, Manchanda S, Sachdev N, et al. Imaging features of pediatric musculoskeletal tuberculosis. *Pediatr Radiol.* 2012;42:1235–1249.

Reach P, Paugam A, Kahan A, et al. Coccidioidomycosis of the spine in an immunocompetent patient. *Joint Bone Spine.* 2010;77:611–613.

Reginato AJ. Syphilitic arthritis and osteitis. *Rheum Dis Clin North Am.* 1993;19:379–398.

Rennen HJ, Boerman OC, Oyen WJ, et al. Specific and rapid scintigraphic detection of infection with ^{99m}Tc-labeled interleukin 8. *J Nucl Med.* 2001;42:117–123.

Rennen HJ, Boerman OC, Oyen WJ, et al. Kinetics of ^{99m}Tc-labeled interleukin 8 in experimental inflammation and infection. *J Nucl Med.* 2003;44:1502–1509.

Resnik CS, Ammann AM, Walsh JW. Chronic septic arthritis of the adult hip: computed tomographic features. *Skeletal Radiol.* 1987;16:513–516.

Resnick D, Niwayama G. Osteomyelitis, septic arthritis, and soft tissue infection: organism. Resnick D, ed. *Diagnosis of Bone and Joint Disorders.* 3rd ed., Vol. 4. Philadelphia, PA: Saunders; 2004:2467–2474.

Ridley N, Shaikh MI, Remedios D, et al. Radiology of skeletal tuberculosis. *Orthopedics.* 1988;21:1213–1220.

Rodin P. Clutton's joints: a brief review of the literature, and an unusual case treated with intra-articular hydrocortisone. *Br J Vener Dis.* 1961;37:204–206.

Ruf J, Oeser C, Amthauer H. Clinical role of anti-granulocyte MoAb versus radiolabeled white blood cells. *Q J Nucl Med Mol Imaging.* 2010;54:599–616.

Ruzbarsky JJ, Gladnick BP, Dodwell E. Diagnosing septic arthritis in the synovial white cell count "gray zone". *HSSJ.* 2016;12:190–192.

Schauwecker D. Osteomyelitis: diagnosis with In-111-labeled leukocytes. *Radiology.* 1989;171:141–146.

Serikawa de Medeiros R, Teles Abdo RC, Cortesi de Paula F, et al. Treatment of spinal tuberculosis: conservative or surgical? *Acta Orthop Bras.* 2007;15(3):128–131.

Shanthi M, Sekar U, Sridharan KS. Septic arthritis of hip caused by Salmonella typhi: a case report. *Case Rep Infect Dis.* 2012; September 9. doi: 10.1155/2012/464527.

Signore A, Soroa VA, Vries EF. Radiolabelled white blood cells or FDG for imaging of inflammation or infection? *Q J Nucl Med Mol Imaging.* 2009;53:23–25.

Skaf GS, Domloj NT, Fehlings MG, et al. Pyogenic spondylodiscitis: an overview. *J Infect Public Health.* 2010;3:5–16.

Sobottke R, Seifert H, Fötkenheuer G, et al. Current diagnosis and treatment of spondylodiscitis. *Dtsch Artztebl Int.* 2008;195:181–187.

Stadalnik RC, Goldstein E, Hoeprich PD, et al. Diagnostic value of gallium and bone scans in evaluation of extrapulmonary coccidioidal lesions. *Am Rev Respir Dis.* 1980;121:673–676.

Stanek G, Strle F. Lyme borreliosis. *Lancet.* 2003;362:1639–1647.

Steere AC, Malawista SE, Snydman DR, et al. Lyme arthritis: an epidemic of oligoarticular arthritis in children and adults in three Connecticut communities. *Arthritis Rheum.* 1977;20:7–17.

Steere AC, Coburn J, Glickstein L. The emergence of Lyme disease. *J Clin Invest* 2004;113:1093–1101.

Stevens DA, Rendon A, Gaona-Flores V, et al. Posaconazole therapy for chronic refractory coccidioidomycosis. *Chest.* 2007;132:952–958.

Teo H, Peh W. Skeletal tuberculosis in children. *Pediatr Radiol.* 2004; 34:853–860.

Theodorou DJ, Theodorou SJ, Kakitsubata Y, et al. Imaging characteristics and epidemiologic features of atypical mycobacterial infections involving the musculoskeletal system. *AJR Am J Roentgenol.* 2001;176:341–349.

Trueta J. The three types of acute, haematogenous osteomyelitis. *J Bone Joint Surg Br.* 1959;41B:671–680.

Toledano TR, Fatone EA, Weis A, et al. MRI evaluation of bone marrow changes in the diabetic foot: a practical approach. *Semin Musculoskelet Radiol.* 2011;15:257–268.

Tsan M. Mechanism of gallium-67 accumulation in inflammatory lesions. *J Nucl Med.* 1985;26:88–92.

Tuli S. General principles of osteoarticular tuberculosis. *Clin Orthop Relat Res.* 2002;398:11–19.

Turecki MB, Taljanovic MS, Stubbs AY, et al. Imaging of musculoskeletal soft tissue infections. *Skeletal Radiol.* 2010;39:957–971.

Vanhoenacker F, Sanghvi D, De Backer A. Imaging features of extraaxial musculoskeletal tuberculosis. *Indian J Radiol Imaging.* 2009;19:176–186.

Van Holsbeeck M, Introcaso JH. *Musculoskeletal Ultrasound.* St. Louis, MO: Mosby-Year Book; 1991:207–229.

van Kuijk AWR, Kerstens PJSM, Perenboom RM, et al. Early-onset polyarthritis as presenting feature of intestinal infection with Strongyloides stercoralis. *Rheumatology.* 2003;42:1419–1420.

Young LW. Neonatal and infantile osteomyelitis and septic arthritis. In: Taveras JM, Ferrucci JT, eds. *Radiology—Diagnosis, Imaging, Intervention*, Vol. 5. Philadelphia, PA: JB Lippincott; 1986:1–15.

Yuh WT, Corson JD, Baraniewski HM, et al. Osteomyelitis of the foot in diabetic patients: evaluation with plain film, ^{99m}Tc-MDP bone scintigraphy, and MR imaging. *AJR Am J Roentgenol.* 1989;152:795–800.

Wallace JO. Diagnosis of syphilis of bones and joints. *J Orthop Surg.* 1919;1:258–293.

Woods CR. Congenital syphilis—persisting pestilence. *Pediatr Infect Dis J.* 2009;28:536–537.

Wrobel CJ, Chappell ET, Taylor W. Clinical presentation, radiological foindings, and treatment results of coccidioidomycosis involving the spine: report on 23 cases. *J Neurosurg.* 2001;95(suppl):33–39.

Zeiger LS, Fox IN. Use of indium-111 labeled white blood cells in the diagnosis of diabetic foot infections. *J Foot Ankle Surg.* 1990;29:46–51.

Zeppa MA, Laorr A, Greenspan A, McGahan JP, Steinbach LS. Skeletal coccidioidomycosis: imaging findings in 19 patients. *Skeletal Radiol.* 1996;25:337–343.

Zhang XM, Zhang HH, McLeroth P, et al. [^{124}I]FIAU: human dosimetry and infection imaging in patients with suspected prosthetic joint infection. *Nucl Med Biol.* 2016;43:273–279.

CHAPTER 10

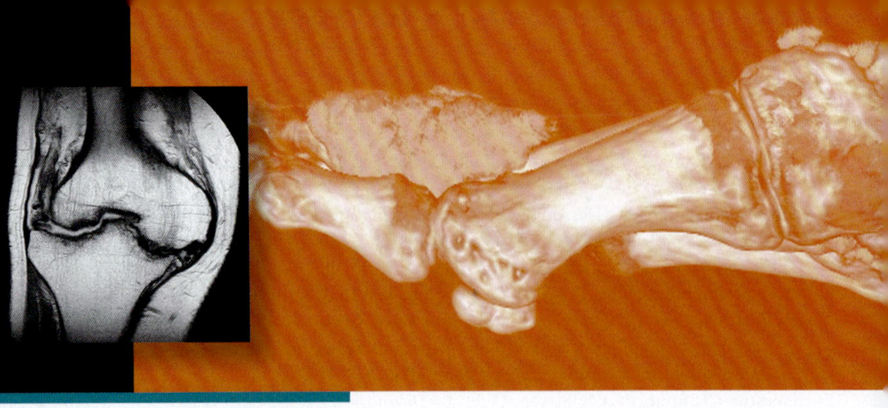

Miscellaneous Conditions

Summary of clinical and imaging features of arthropathies discussed in this chapter is provided in Table 10.1.

AMYLOIDOSIS

Clinical and Pathologic Features

Amyloidosis is a systematic disorder characterized by the infiltration of various organs by a homogeneous eosinophilic material consisting of protein fibers in a ground substance of mucopolysaccharides. There are three major types of systemic amyloidosis: (1) *primary amyloidosis*, the most common form, in which bone marrow produces too much of certain fragments of antibody protein, which builds up in the bloodstream and deposits in the body tissues; (2) *familial (hereditary) amyloidosis*, which is a genetic form, because of mutations in the gene *TTR*, inherited in autosomal dominant manner; and (3) *secondary amyloidosis*, which develops secondary to certain chronic conditions such as tuberculosis or rheumatoid arthritis. Amyloid arthropathy is a sign of acquired idiopathic systemic amyloidosis and is a condition that results in noninflammatory arthropathy. All forms of amyloidosis are characterized pathologically by extracellular deposition of insoluble nonbranching beta-pleated protein fibrils formed as a result of abnormal protein synthesis. Amyloid is seen within the synovium and bone marrow as extensive extracellular deposits of brightly eosinophilic/hyaline amorphous material. Histopathologic sections stained with Congo red have a characteristic apple-green birefringence when examined under polarized light (Fig. 10.1).

Clinically, amyloidosis bears a striking resemblance to rheumatoid arthritis, because the joints are stiff and painful and the arthropathy is bilateral and symmetric. There is a predilection for large joints such as the hips, knees, shoulders, and elbows. Subcutaneous nodules are noted over the extensor surfaces of the forearm and dorsum of the hand, often mimicking the rheumatoid nodules. Another characteristic feature is the massive involvement of the soft tissues, giving the patient an almost pathognomonic appearance known as "shoulder pad sign" or "football player shoulders." Carpal tunnel syndrome is frequently an associated abnormality.

The bone abnormalities and arthropathy associated with deposition of B_2-microglobulin (B_2-MG) amyloid are well-recognized complications of long-term hemodialysis and chronic renal failure. Standard dialysis membranes do not filter B_2-MG, a low molecular weight serum protein. It therefore accumulates in the bones, joints, and soft tissues. Clinically, characteristic pain and decreased joint mobility occur in the affected joints.

Imaging Features

Regardless of cause, imaging studies show massive accumulation of amyloid around the joints, and there is invasion of the periarticular tissue, capsule, and joint. Also, deposits can be seen in the synovium. The articular ends of the bone can be destroyed, and both subluxations and pathologic fractures are frequently encountered. In addition, focal osteolytic lesions, particularly in the bones of the upper extremities (Fig. 10.2) and in the proximal ends of the femora, can be seen. The MRI manifestations of amyloidosis include intermediate-to-low signal intensity deposits of amyloid material in the synovium, ligaments, and tendons with or without erosive changes (Fig. 10.3). Scintigraphy using ^{123}I-serum amyloid P component has been used to identify the systemic distribution of amyloid deposit.

(Continued on page 362)

Table 10.1 MISCELLANEOUS ARTHROPATHIES: CLINICAL AND IMAGING FEATURES

Amyloidosis (M > F)	Large joints (hips, knees, shoulders, elbows)	Articular and periarticular erosions, osteoporosis (periarticular), joint subluxations, pathologic fractures	Standard views of affected joints Radionuclide bone scan (scintigraphy)
Multicentric reticulohistiocytosis (F > M)	Hands (distal and proximal interphalangeal joints) Feet	Soft tissue swelling, articular erosions, lack of osteoporosis	Dorsovolar view Norgaard (ball-catcher) view Dorsoplantar view Oblique view
Sarcoidosis (M = F)	Short tubular bones of hands and feet Cervical spine	Cystic, punch-out lesions, lacy reticulations, honey comb pattern	Standard views of affected joints Magnetic resonance imaging
Hemophilia (M > F)	Large joints (hips, knees, shoulders) Elbows, ankles	Joint effusion, osteoporosis, symmetrical and concentric joint space narrowing, articular erosions, widening of intercondylar notch, squaring of patella; very similar to changes of juvenile rheumatoid arthritis	Standard views of affected joints Magnetic resonance imaging

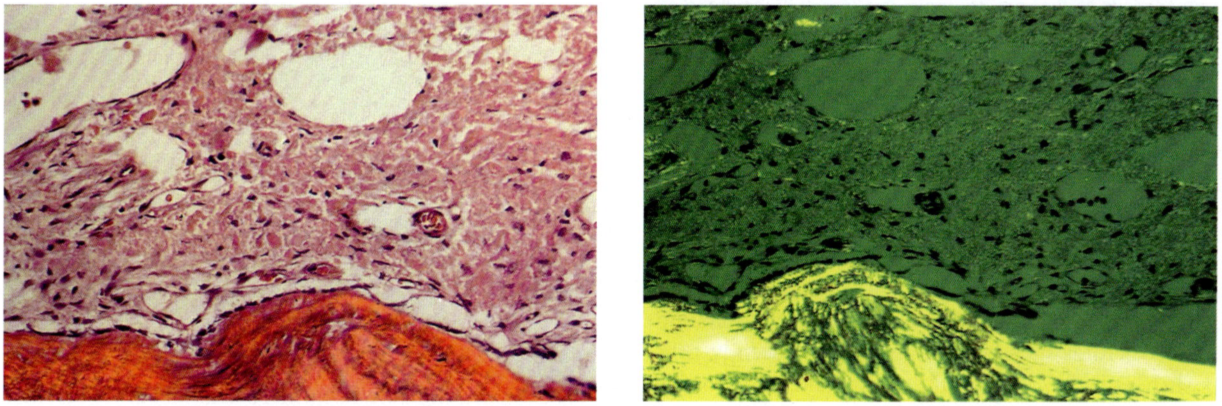

A B

Figure 10.1 ■ **Pathology of amyloidosis. A:** Photomicrograph depicts amyloid deposit in the bone marrow (H&E, original magnification ×10). **B:** Under polarized light, the amyloid deposits are birefringent and apple-green (original magnification ×10). (From Bullough PG. *Atlas of Orthopedic Pathology with Clinical and Radiologic Correlation*, 2nd ed. New York, NY: Gower Medical Publishing, 1992:16.2–16.4., Figs. 8.12 and 8.13, p. 8.6.)

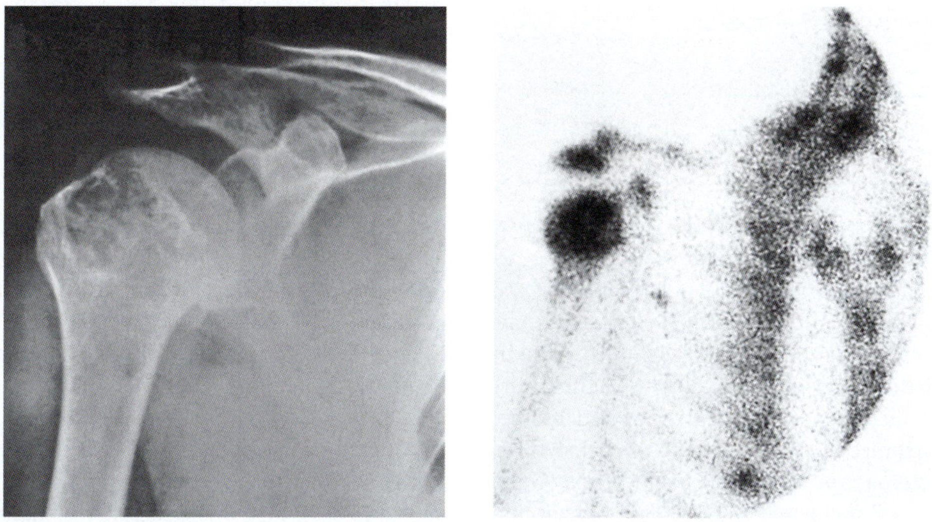

A B

Figure 10.2 ■ **Amyloidosis. A:** Anteroposterior radiograph of the right shoulder of an 80-year-old man demonstrates a moderate degree of juxta-articular osteoporosis, soft tissue swelling, and a large osteolytic lesion in the humeral head. The glenohumeral joint space is relatively well preserved. **B:** Radionuclide bone scan shows an increased uptake of technetium-labeled methylene diphosphonate (MDP) around the shoulder.

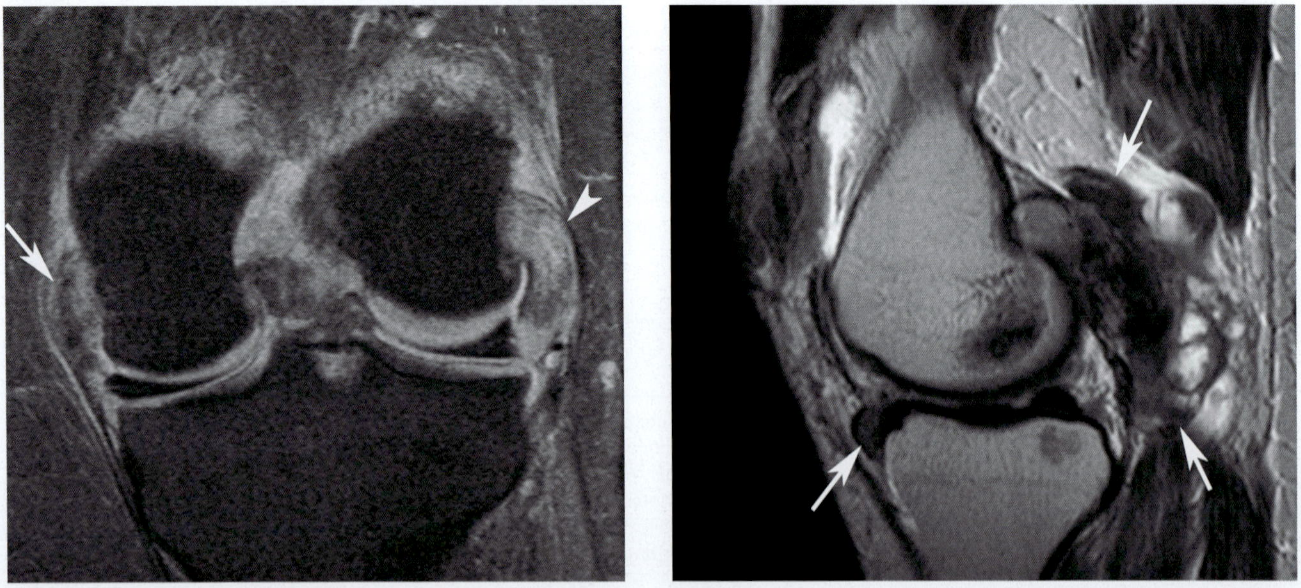

A B

Figure 10.3 ■ MRI of amyloidosis. A: Coronal T2-weighted fat-saturated MRI of the knee in a patient with primary amyloidosis demonstrates thickening of the popliteus tendon (*arrowhead*) and the proximal superficial fibers of the medial collateral ligament (*arrow*) because of extensive deposits of intermediate signal intensity amyloid tissue. Note also amyloid deposition in the intercondylar notch. **B:** Sagittal T2-weighted MRI of the knee shows the hypointense synovial deposits of amyloid tissue (*arrows*).

Treatment

Although there is no cure for amyloidosis, therapy is directed toward relieving the symptoms and limitation of further production of amyloid protein. Treatment includes chemotherapy agents such as melphalan or cyclophosphamide and corticosteroids such as dexamethasone. Recently, other drugs such as bortezomib, thalidomide, and lenalidomide, which are a thalidomide derivative, have been tried with some promising results. In most severe cases, autologous peripheral blood stem cell transplantation using high-dose chemotherapy and transfusion of stem cells has been advocated. Surgical treatment consists of removal of affected organs followed by organ transplantation.

MULTICENTRIC RETICULOHISTIOCYTOSIS (MRH)

Multicentric reticulohistiocytosis (MRH) is a rare systemic granulomatous disorder of unknown cause seen in adulthood and is characterized by the proliferation of the histiocytes (macrophages) in the skin, the mucosa, the subcutaneous tissue, and the synovium. It was first described in 1937 as a nondiabetic cutaneous xanthomatosis. The disorder has been also called lipoid dermatoarthritis, reticulohistiocytoma, lipid rheumatism, giant cell reticulohistiocytosis, giant cell histiocytoma, and giant cell histiocytosis. Goltz and Lymon proposed the name multicentric reticulohistiocytosis for this condition in 1954 because of the multifocal origin and systemic nature of the disease. It usually begins during the fourth decade of life, and women are more commonly affected than men, with ratio 3:1. In ~60% to 70% of patients, polyarthralgia is the first manifestation of the disease. Approximately 25% of cases have been associated with the presence of neoplasia, including all types of cancer, solid and hematologic. MRH frequently coexists with autoimmune diseases, including Sjögren syndrome, systemic lupus erythematosus, scleroderma, and dermatomyositis. Occasionally, nonautoimmune conditions have been associated with MRH, such as diabetes mellitus, thyroid disease, colitis, and dyslipidemia.

Laboratory markers are poorly sensitive and not specific for MRH. About half of the patients show elevated erythrocyte sedimentation rate and C-reactive protein. Serum autoantibodies are only occasionally detected and generally support the coexistence of an autoimmune disorder. Histopathologic findings include histiolymphocytic infiltrate within the dermis with small, sometimes multinucleated histiocytes. These cells are not foamy, which allows distinguishing them from other forms of histiocytic disorders, such as sarcoidosis or xanthogranulomatosis. More advanced dermal lesions are characterized by the pathognomonic multinucleated giant cells with a ground-glass eosinophilic cytoplasm (megalocytes). Additional findings include a strong positivity of histiocytes for periodic acid–Schiff (PAS) and expression of acid phosphatase, nonspecific esterase, and lysozyme. Triglycerides, cholesterol, and phosphate esters appear to be present in the lesion, suggesting either that histiocytes are stimulated to produce these substances or that this is a form of lipid storage disease. Immunohistologically, MRH histiocytes express positivity for tartrate-resistant acid phosphatase (TRAP), CD68, CD45, MAC387, vimentin, lysosome, and human alveolar

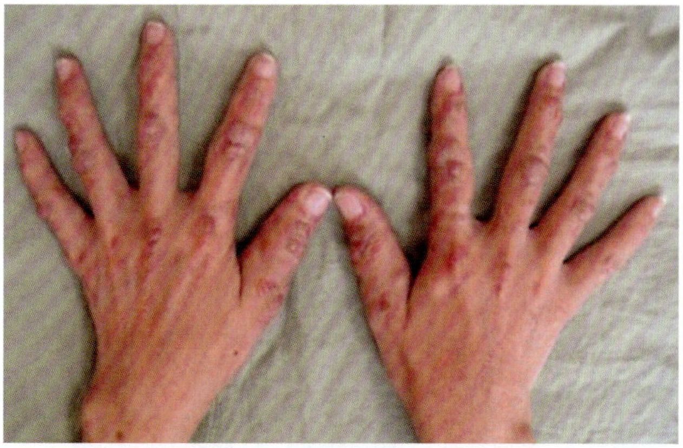

Figure 10.4 ■ Multicentric reticulohistiocytosis. Clinical photograph of the hands of the patient with MRH shows characteristic erythematous nodules on the dorsal aspect of the metacarpophalangeal and interphalangeal joints.

macrophage 56 (HAM-56); however, there is conspicuous negativity for S100 protein, CD1a, and factor XIIIa. Furthermore, the synovial fluid mononuclear cells from patients with MRH express macrophage-specific markers including CD11b, CD14, CD68, and class II HLA DR. Quantitative amounts of proinflammatory cytokines are elevated, including TNF-alpha, IL-6, IL-12, and IL-1-beta. More recent data support the hypothesis that synovial fluid macrophages may differentiate into osteoclasts following RANKL pathway activation or macrophage colony-stimulating factor (M-CSF) as suggested in other inflammatory diseases. Ultrastructurally, the histiocytes resemble type A synoviocytes. The cytoplasm contains osmiophilic membrane-bound lysosomal granules, often closely associated with a single large stellate Golgi apparatus.

Clinical findings include characteristic cutaneous manifestations appearing as translucent brown-reddish to flesh-colored papulonodular lesions of variable sizes (1 mm to 1 cm or larger) (Fig. 10.4). The other clinical features may be very similar to those of rheumatoid arthritis, consisting of soft tissue swelling, stiffness, and tenderness of the joints. Unlike rheumatoid arthritis, however, the distal interphalangeal joints are most frequently affected. Less commonly affected are the proximal interphalangeal, metacarpophalangeal, shoulder, and elbow joints. Occasionally, the articular lesions may be marked by severe destruction similar to arthritis mutilans of rheumatoid arthritis or psoriatic arthritis (Figs. 10.5 and 10.6). The characteristic absence of significant periarticular osteoporosis distinguishes this disorder from the inflammatory arthritides, and there is also no periosteal new bone formation, which distinguishes it from psoriatic arthritis or juvenile idiopathic arthritis. Lack of osteophytes and interphalangeal ankylosis, and the presence of soft tissue nodules and atlantoaxial abnormalities including subluxation and erosion of the odontoid process distinguish this arthropathy from erosive osteoarthritis. At times, the pattern of bone erosions with sclerotic margins and overhanging edges, and the presence of soft tissue masses, may mimic those of gout (Fig. 10.7). Unlike gout, however, there is symmetrical distribution of the lesions in the hands and feet and lack of calcification within soft tissue nodules.

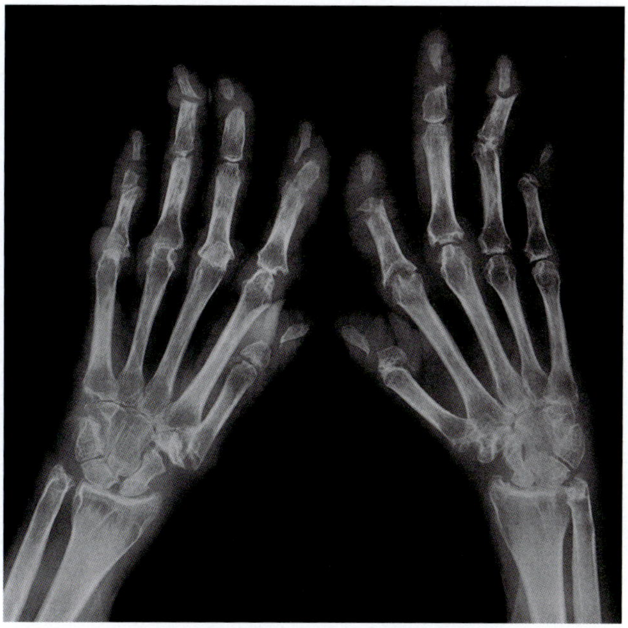

Figure 10.5 ■ Multicentric reticulohistiocytosis. Dorsovolar radiograph of both hands of a 57-year-old woman with long-standing polyarthralgia, soft tissue swelling, and deformities of the fingers demonstrates severe destruction of multiple carpometacarpal, metacarpophalangeal, and interphalangeal joints similar to those seen in rheumatoid or psoriatic arthritis.

Treatment consists of systemic steroids, cytotoxic drugs such as cyclophosphamide, chlorambucil, methotrexate, leflunomide, and infliximab. Bisphosphonates such as alendronate and zoledronate have been reported to improve skin lesions and arthritis.

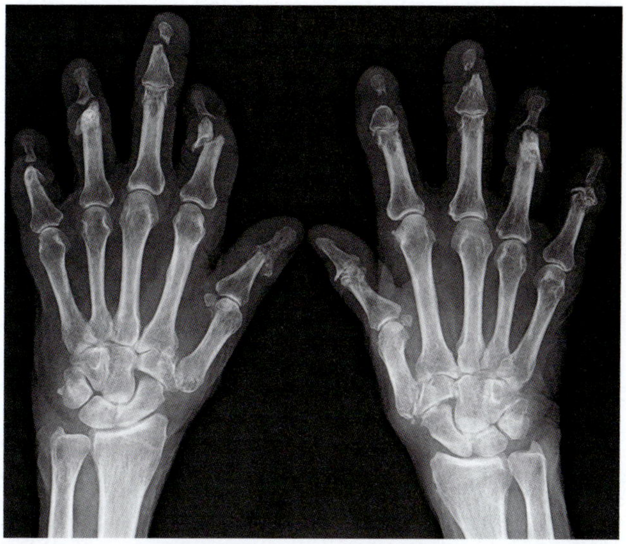

Figure 10.6 ■ Multicentric reticulohistiocytosis. Dorsovolar radiograph of both hands of a 63-year-old man shows arthritis mutilans affecting mainly distal interphalangeal joints.

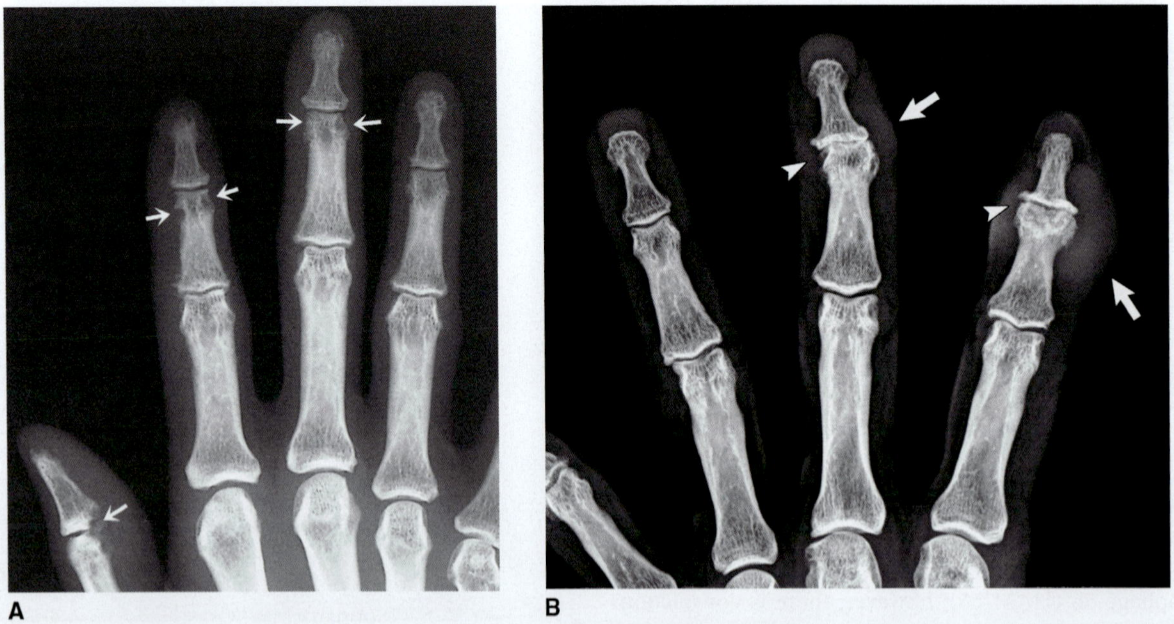

Figure 10.7 ■ **Multicentric reticulohistiocytosis. A:** A 46-year-old woman presented with distal interphalangeal joints pain and soft tissue swelling. Note sharply marginated erosions at the distal interphalangeal joints (*arrows*) resembling gout. **B:** Radiograph of the fingers of the right hand of the 65-year-old woman shows small erosions at the distal interphalangeal joints of the index and middle fingers (*arrowheads*) associated with soft tissue masses (*arrows*) resembling gouty tophi.

SARCOIDOSIS

Sarcoidosis is a systemic inflammatory disorder predominantly affecting young adults, characterized by the presence of noncaseating granulomas in affected organs. The disease has a worldwide distribution, with the greatest incidence in Sweden. Although the etiology still remains unsettled, the evidence that sarcoidosis most commonly involves the lungs, eyes, and skin, focused the search for environmental causes such as exposures to airborne antigens. In fact, some of the earliest studies have reported association of sarcoidosis with exposures irritants found in rural settings, such as emissions from wood-burning stoves and tree pollen. More recently, association of sarcoidosis with exposure to inorganic particles, insecticides, and moldy environments has been suggested. Currently, the investigators found compelling evidence to support the hypothesis implying certain environmental foreign nonparticulates as a plausible cause of this condition in individuals with a genetically based immune dysregulational predisposition. Some researchers suggested that a predisposition to acute sarcoid arthritis is carried by the HLA DQ2-DR3 haplotype that appears to be transmitted as a dominant genetic trait. Many genetic associations have been linked sarcoidosis with genes within the major histocompatibility complex (MHC) locus. Most recent studies suggested the novel gene BTNL2 (butyrophilin-like) has been associated with sarcoidosis of Caucasian patients. The active granulomatous inflammation is associated with a dominant expression of T-helper (Th) 1 cytokines (interferon gamma [IFN-gamma]), interleukin-12 and IL-18, and tumor necrosis factor (TNF).

On histopathologic examination, sarcoid granulomas consist of compact aggregates of epithelioid histiocytes with rare foreign body-type giant cells, encompassed by an outer zone of fibrosis with lymphocytes and plasma cells. Characteristic but not pathognomonic findings include the presence of intracytoplasmic inclusions of two types: laminated concretions composed of calcium and proteins (so-called Schaumann bodies) and stellate inclusions with a central core of degenerating organelles encompassed by multiple rays of collagen filaments (so-called asteroid bodies).

Laboratory findings include anemia, leucopenia, eosinophilia, decrease in serum albumins, elevation of serum globulins, and hypercalcemia.

Clinical presentation varies depending on organs involved. Systemic symptoms such as fatigue, weight loss, and night sweats are common. Dyspnea, cough, and wheezing occur when respiratory system is affected. Soft tissue swelling and cutaneous lesions of the hands and feet can be associated with osseous changes. Maculae, papules, and plaques are common manifestation of skin involvement. The joints are rarely affected and may be present in about 10% to 35% of patients with sarcoidosis. Arthralgia tends to occur in patients with acute presentation of disease that includes a triad of arthritis, erythema nodosum, and bilateral hilar adenopathy (Löfgren syndrome); however, more often, the inflammation is present in the periarticular region (periarthritis). When the skeletal system is affected, cystic, punch-out lesions, lacy reticulations, and honeycomb pattern of destruction are commonly observed in the short tubular bones of the hands and feet (Fig. 10.8). Less frequently, nodular opacities in the medullary portion of these bones and osteosclerosis of the terminal tufts can be seen. Occasionally, generalized osteosclerosis may be present. Involvement of the spinal column is rare, and if present, it is usually limited to the cervical segment (Fig. 10.9).

Corticosteroids, including prednisone, are considered the first line of treatment of sarcoidosis. The antimalarial

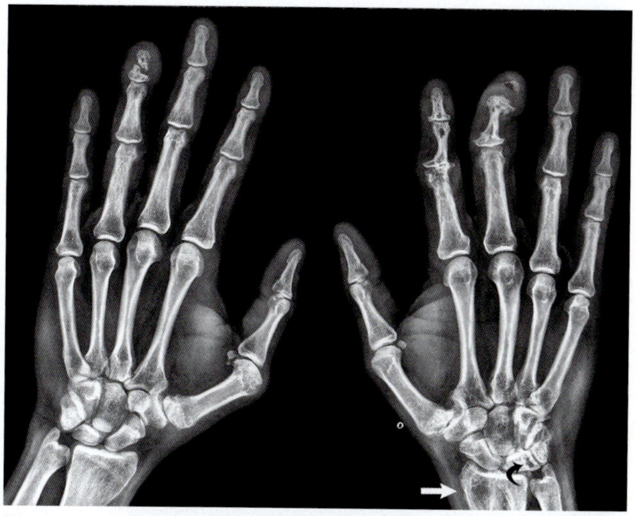

Figure 10.8 ■ Sarcoidosis. Dorsovolar radiograph of the hands of a 55-year-old man shows destructive lesions of the distal phalanx of the ring finger of the right hand and proximal and distal phalanges of the index and middle fingers of the left hand. Note also destructive lesion in the left lunate (*curved arrow*) and in the distal left radius (*arrow*).

drug hydroxychloroquine is effective in patients with dermatologic involvement, joint arthropathy, and hypercalcemia. Some patients benefit from receiving methotrexate, azathioprine, mycophenolate mofetil, leflunomide, and cyclophosphamide.

HEMOPHILIA

Hemophilia A is an inherited bleeding disorder characterized by an anomaly of blood coagulation caused by functional deficiency of antihemophilic factor (AHF) VIII. It is inherited as an X-linked recessive trait and essentially occurs only in males, although female carriers transmit the abnormal gene. In hemophilia B, also known as "Christmas disease," there is a deficiency of plasma thromboplastin component, factor IX. This disorder may also affect females. The articular changes in hemophilia most often occur in the first and second decades of life and are secondary to chronic repetitive bleeding into the joints and bones. Repeated episodes of intra-articular bleeding and inflammatory tissue response cause proliferation of synovium and erosion of cartilage and subchondral bone. Usually, there is no problem in the clinical recognition of this disorder; however, the changes of hemophilic arthropathy may radiographically mimic those of rheumatoid arthritis, particularly juvenile idiopathic arthritis (Fig. 10.10). Cartilage

(Continued on page 367)

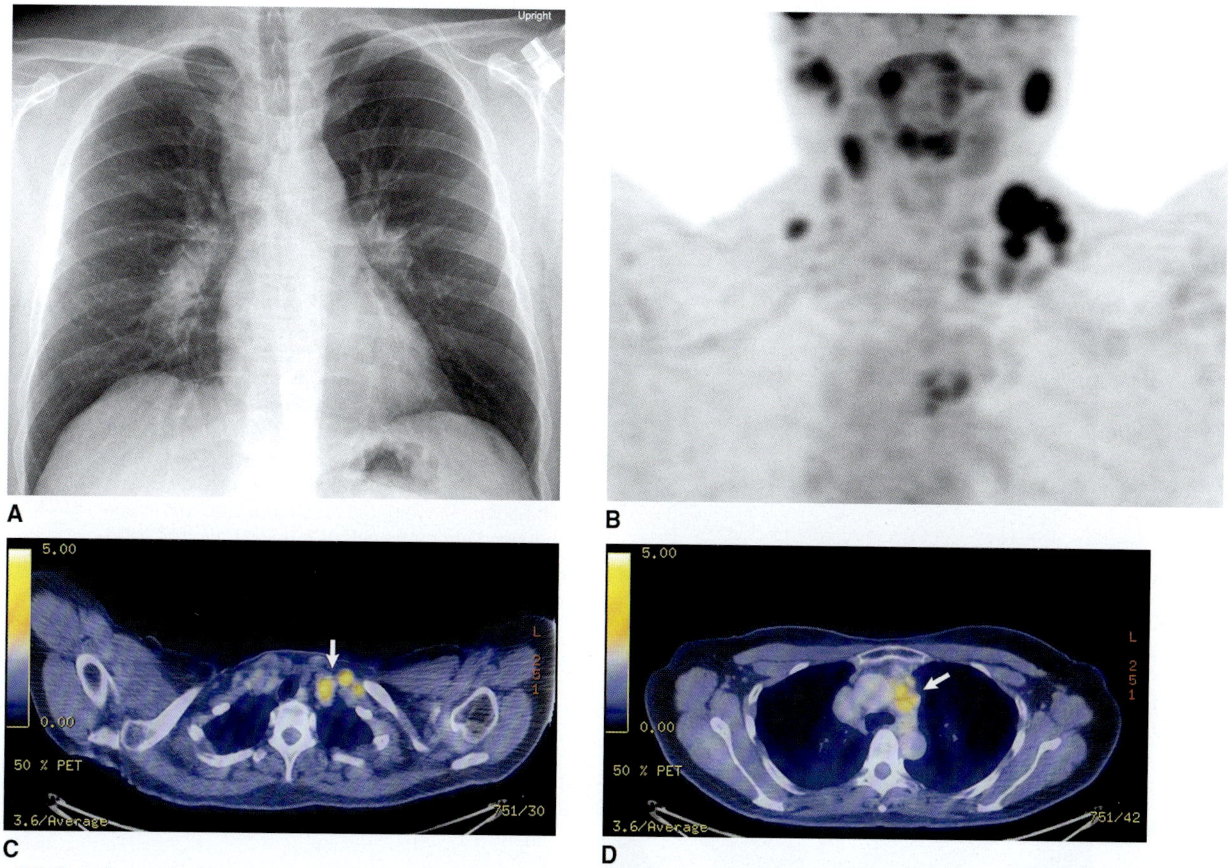

Figure 10.9 ■ Sarcoidosis. A 38-year-old man with known pulmonary sarcoidosis presented with severe neck pain. **A:** Posteroanterior radiograph of the chest shows perihilar and paratracheal adenopathy. **B:** [18]FDG PET scan shows several hypermetabolic foci within neck, supraclavicular, and mediastinal lymph nodes. **C, D:** Two axial fused PET/CT images of the upper chest show hypermetabolic activity within the affected lymph nodes (*arrows*).

(*Continued*)

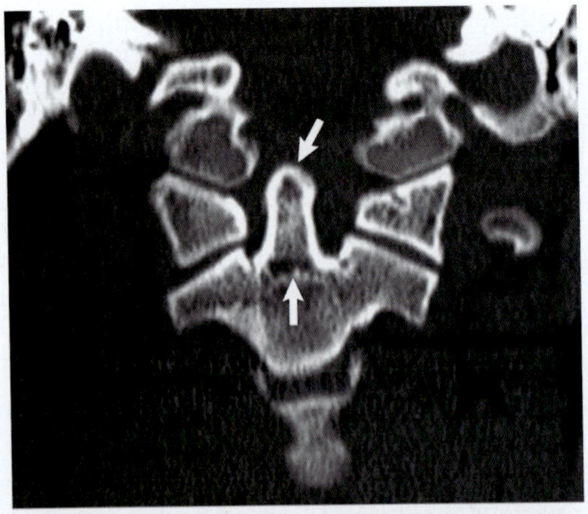

E

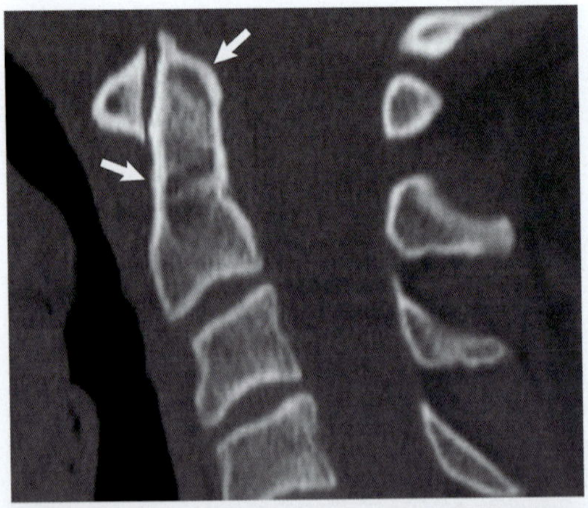

F

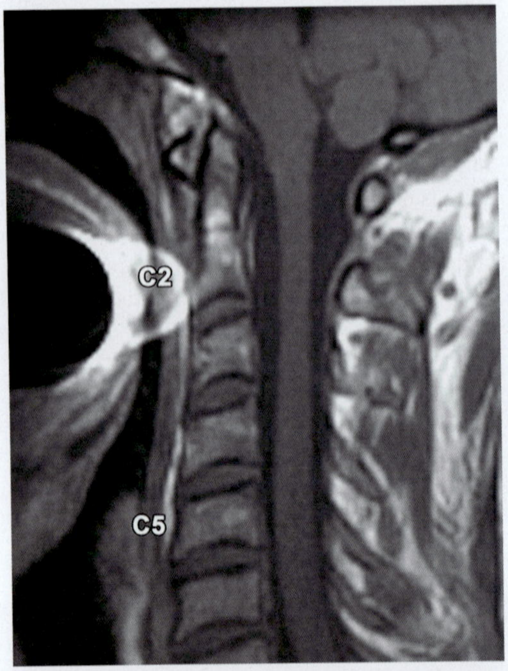

G

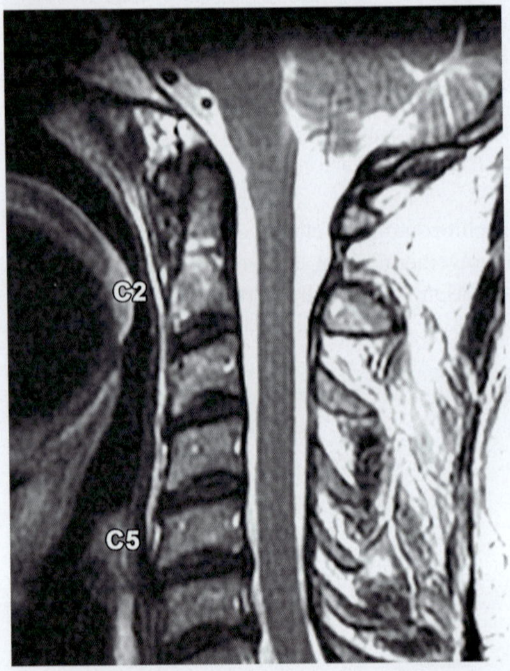

H

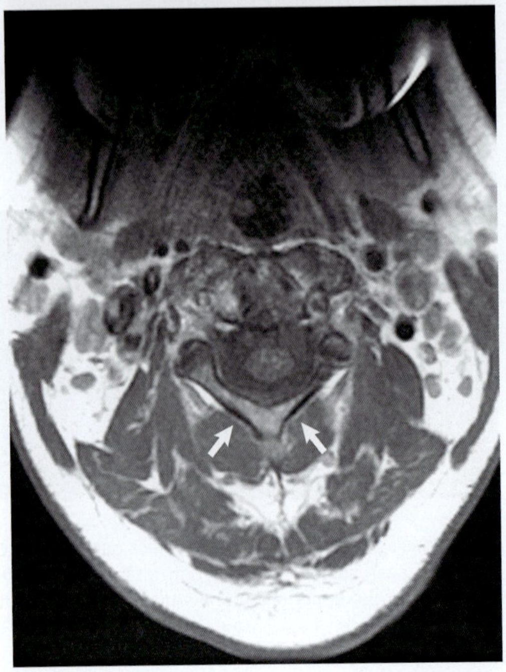

I

Figure 10.9 ■ (*Continued*) Coronal **(E)** and sagittal **(F)** reformatted CT images of the upper cervical spine show two osteolytic lesions in the odontoid process (*arrows*). **G:** Sagittal T2-weighted MR image of the cervical spine shows high signal intensity lesions within the vertebral bodies of C2, C3, and C4. **H:** Sagittal T1-weighted fat-suppressed MR image obtained after intravenous administration of gadolinium shows mild enhancement of the vertebral lesions. **I:** Axial T1-weighted postcontrast MRI shows enhancement of the lesion of the posterior arch of C2 (*arrows*).

destruction, joint space narrowing, and erosions of the subchondral bone are identical to those seen in rheumatoid arthritis (Fig. 10.11). The knee, ankle, and elbow are the most frequently involved articulations, and this involvement is usually bilateral (Figs. 10.12 and 10.13). In the knee, the radiographic features include periarticular osteoporosis, joint effusion (hemarthrosis), overgrowth of femoral condyles with widening of the intercondylar notch, and squaring of the patella. Frequently, multiple subchondral cysts and articular erosions are evident. In the late stages of disease, uniform narrowing of the joint space and secondary osteoarthritic changes may be observed. The differential diagnosis from juvenile idiopathic arthritis is based on evidence that there is no bony ankylosis, no evidence of growth inhibition, and frequent presence of pseudotumors. Recurrent episodes of hemarthrosis of the joint in patients with hemophilia lead to chronic synovitis and deposition of hemosiderin pigment in the synovium and joint capsule. These features are well depicted with MRI (Figs. 10.14 to 10.16, see also Fig. 2.101).

(Continued on page 371)

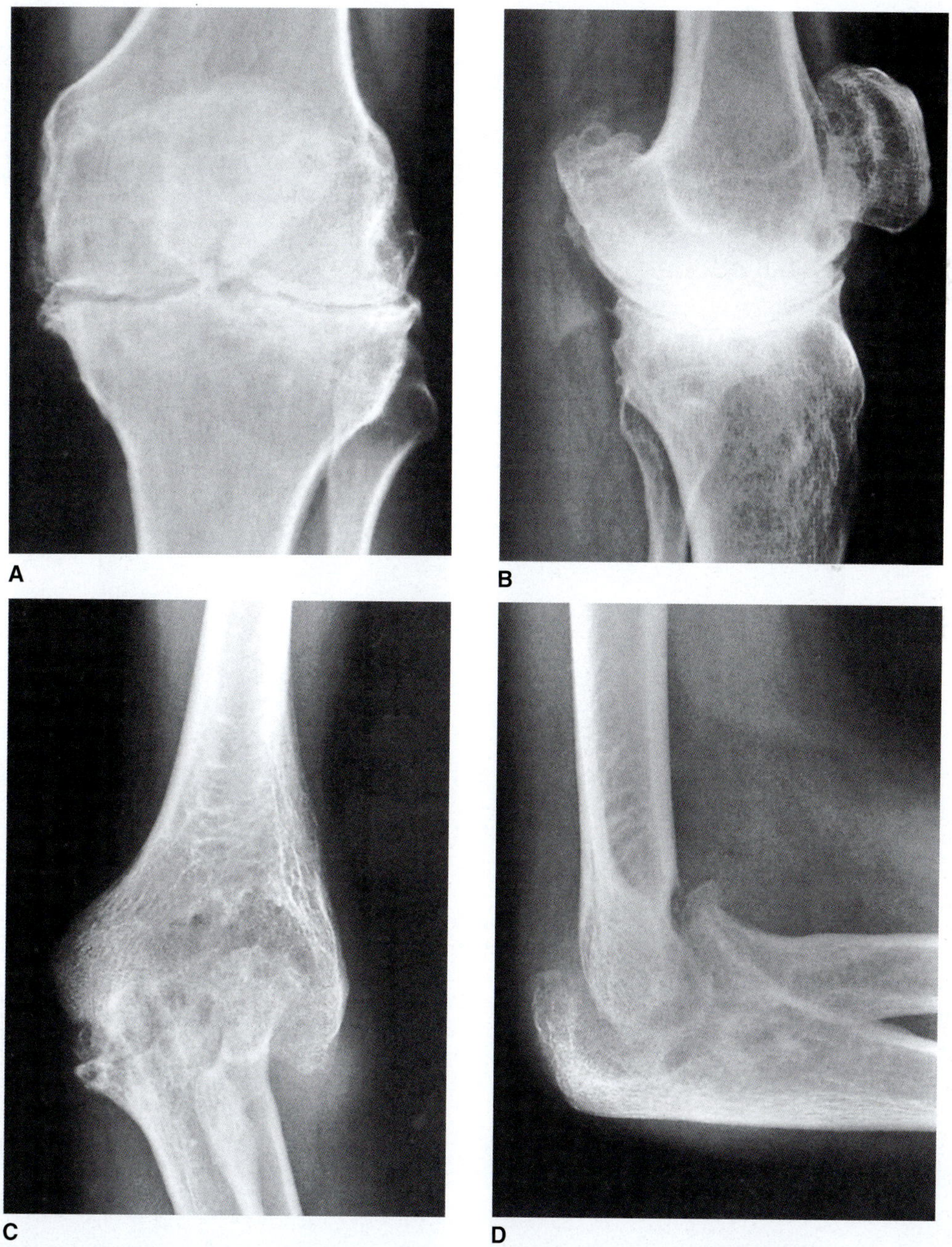

Figure 10.10 ■ Hemophilic arthropathy. A 42-year-old man had several intra-articular bleeding episodes in his life. Anteroposterior **(A)** and lateral **(B)** radiographs of his left knee demonstrate advanced hemophilic arthropathy. Note the involvement of all three joint compartments. Similar destructive changes in the left elbow are demonstrated on anteroposterior **(C)** and lateral **(D)** radiographs of this joint.

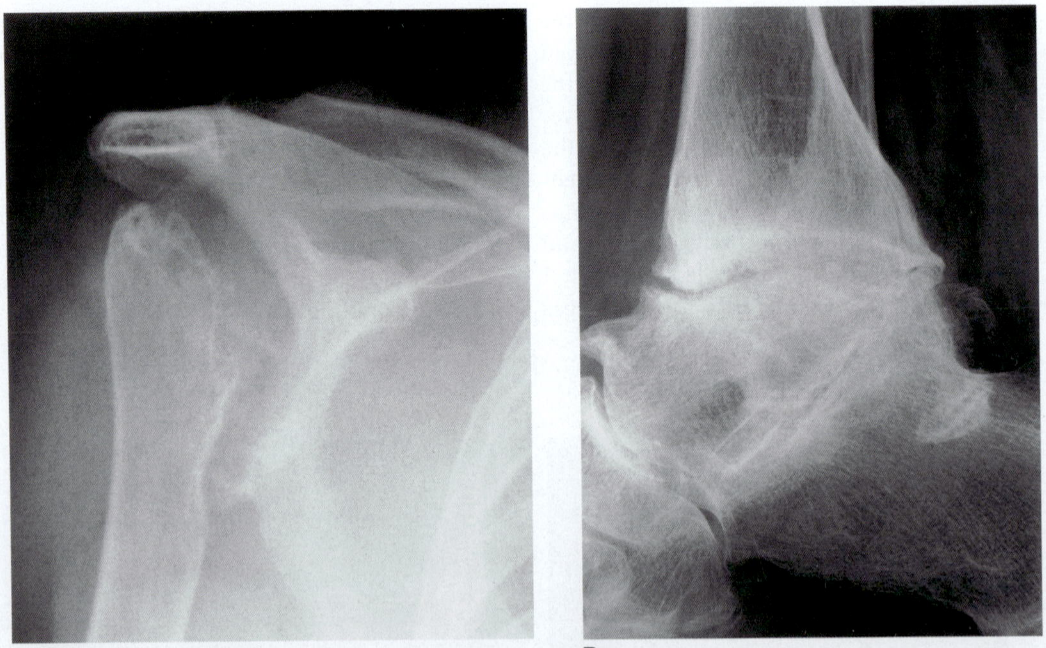

A B

Figure 10.11 ■ **Hemophilic arthropathy.** Anteroposterior radiograph of the right shoulder **(A)** and lateral radiograph of the left ankle **(B)** of a 49-year-old man with hemophilia A show destructive arthropathy of the glenohumeral, ankle, and subtalar joints.

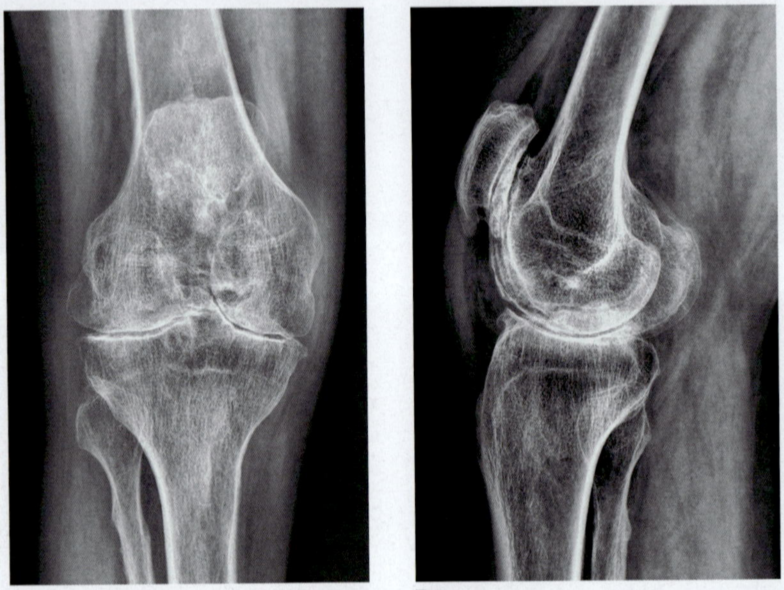

A B

Figure 10.12 ■ **Hemophilic arthropathy.** Anteroposterior **(A)** and lateral **(B)** radiographs of the right knee of a 55-year-old man show uniform destruction of the articular cartilage of all three joint compartments.

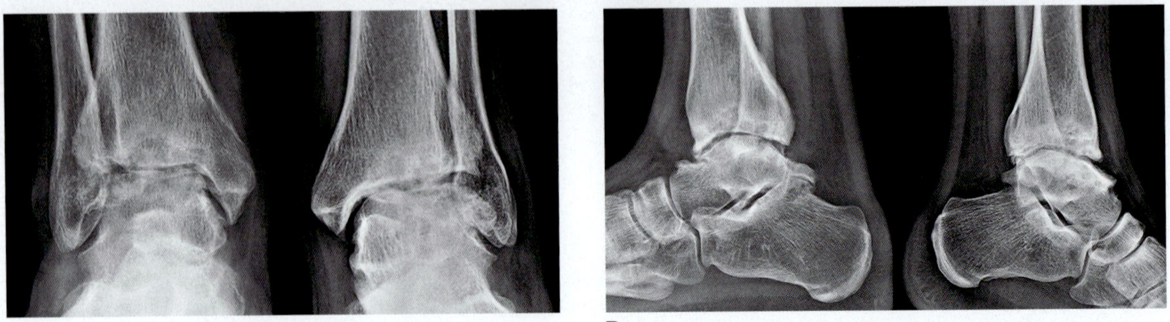

A B

Figure 10.13 ■ **Hemophilic arthropathy.** Anteroposterior **(A)** and lateral **(B)** radiographs of the ankles of a 27-year-old man show uniform destruction of the articular cartilage of the tibiotalar joints.

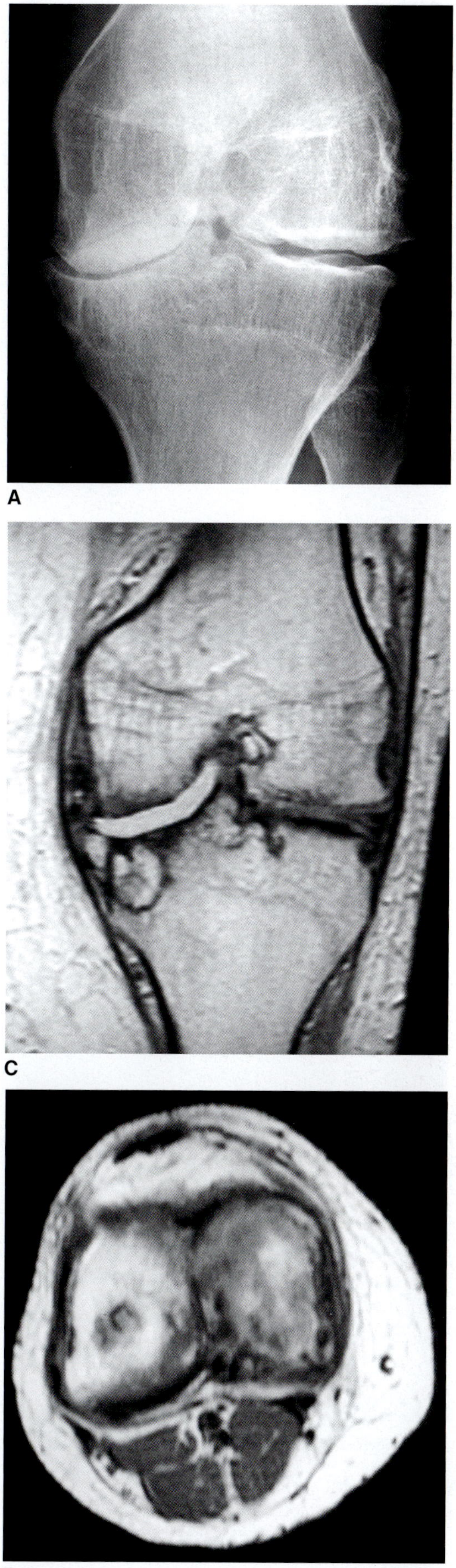

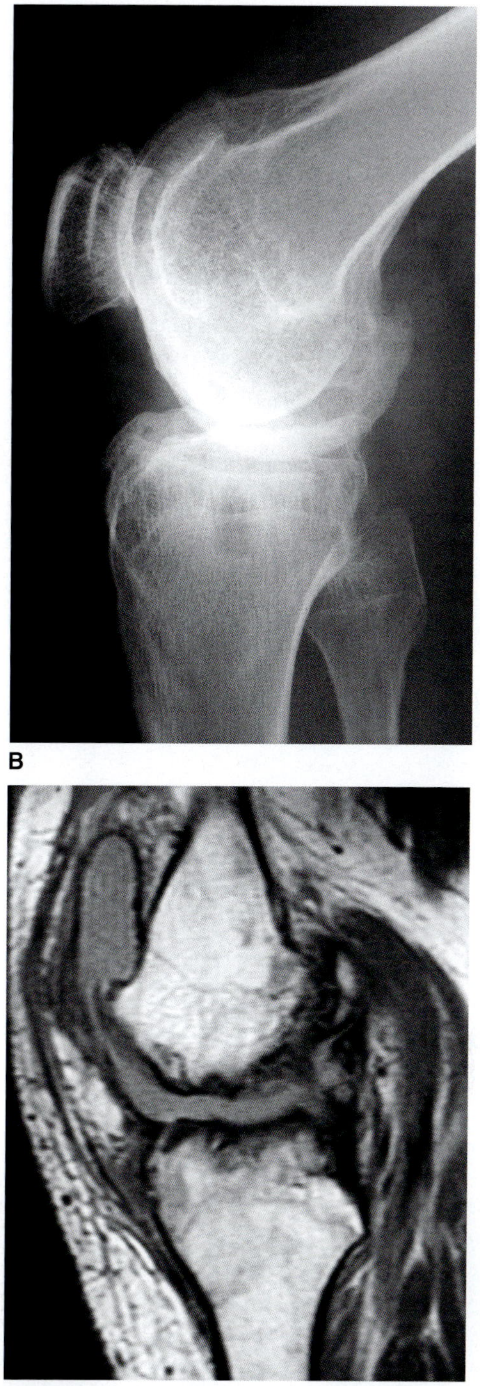

A

B

C

D

E

Figure 10.14 ■ **MRI of hemophilic arthropathy.** A 29-year-old man with hemophilia and multiple episodes of intra-articular bleeding. Anteroposterior **(A)** and lateral **(B)** radiographs of the left knee demonstrate an advanced stage of hemophilia. Abnormalities include periarticular osteoporosis, irregularity of subchondral bone at the tibial plateau and femoral condyles, narrowing of the radiographic joint space, and erosion of the subchondral bone. **C:** Coronal MRI (SE; TR 1900/TE 20 ms) demonstrates, in addition, complete destruction of articular cartilage at the medial joint compartment and a large, subchondral cyst in the proximal tibia, not well appreciated on the radiographic films. **D:** Sagittal MRI (SE; TR 800/TE 20 ms) demonstrates to better advantage the intra-articular blood in the suprapatellar and infrapatellar bursae, displaying intermediate signal intensity. **E:** Axial MRI (TR 400/ TE 20 ms) shows erosive changes of the articular cartilage of the femoral condyles.

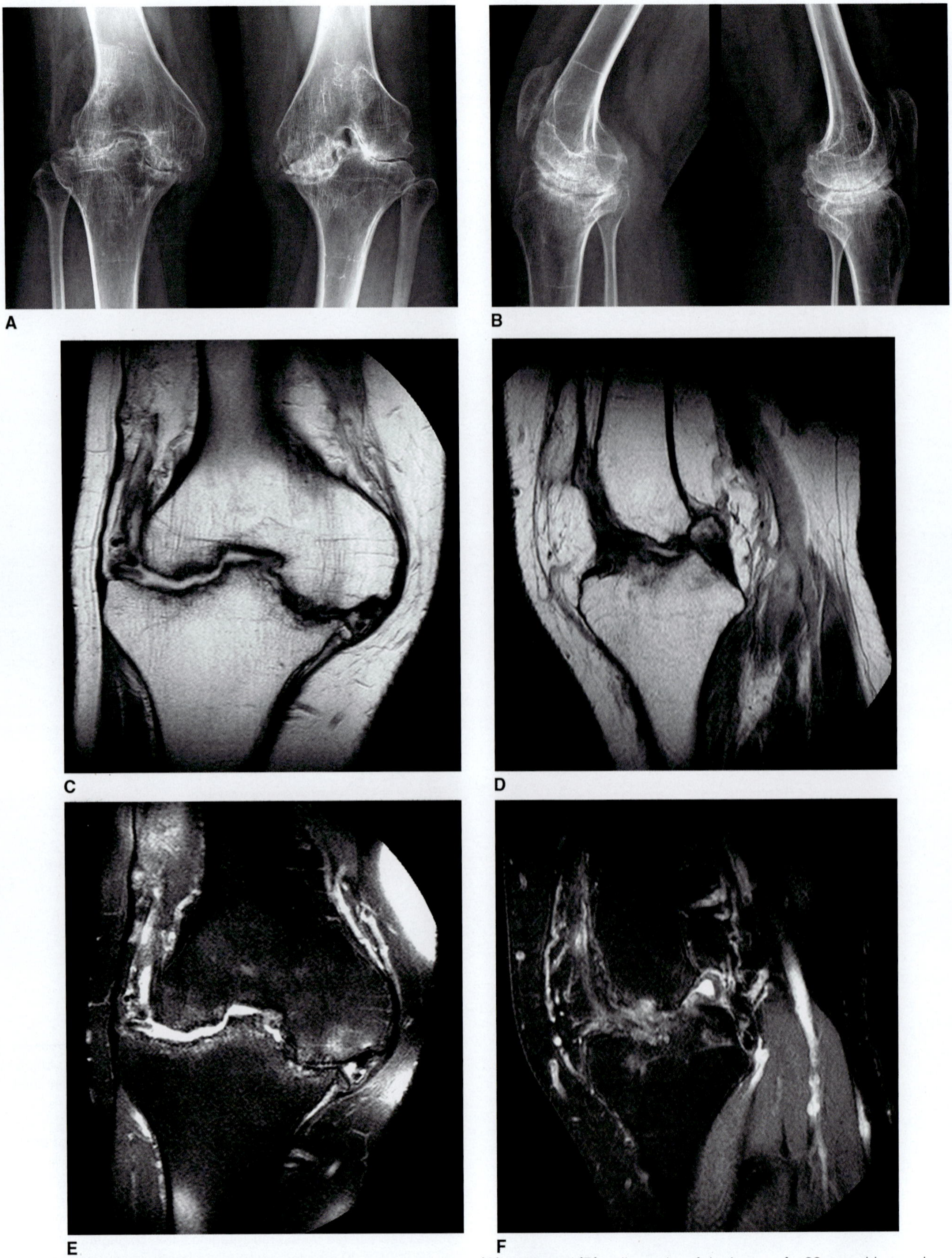

Figure 10.15 ■ **MRI of hemophilic arthropathy.** Anteroposterior **(A)** and lateral **(B)** radiographs of the knees of a 33-year-old man show typical changes of this disorder, including periarticular osteoporosis and severe destruction of the articular cartilage associated with erosive changes of the subchondral bone. Coronal **(C)** and sagittal **(D)** T1-weighted and coronal **(E)** and sagittal **(F)** T2-weighted MR images of the right knee demonstrate in addition the destruction of the lateral and medial menisci and chronic tears of the anterior and posterior cruciate ligaments. There is also small amount of joint fluid.

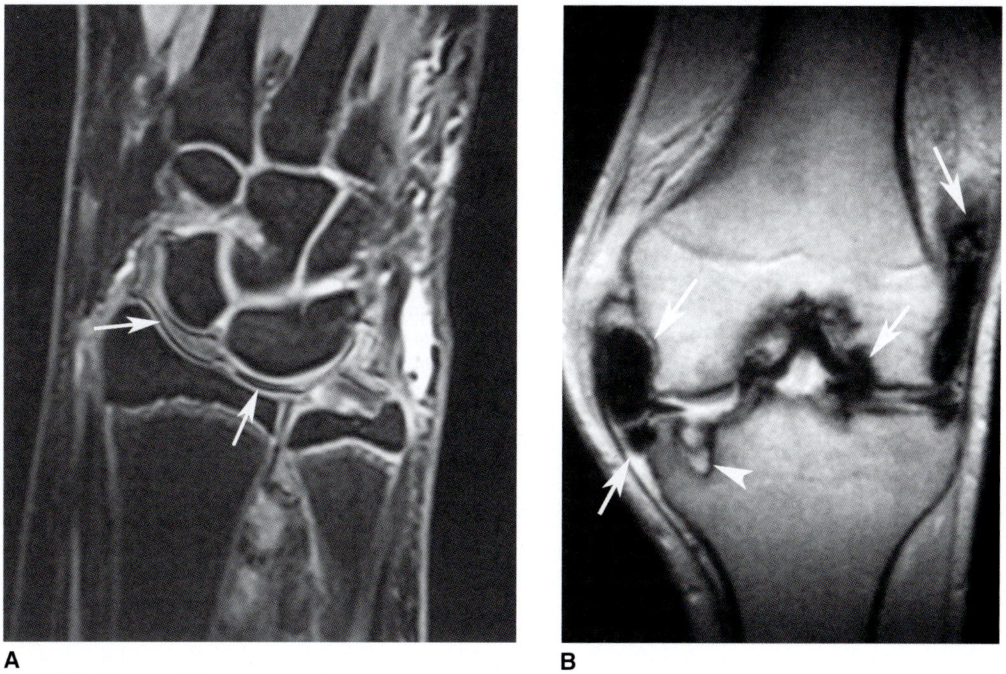

Figure 10.16 ■ MRI of hemophilic arthropathy. A: Coronal T2-weighted fat-saturated MRI of a 10-year-old patient with early hemophilia shows the low signal intensity hemosiderin deposition outlining the synovium in the radiocarpal joint (*arrows*) and the absence of cartilage damage or bone erosions. **B:** Coronal T2-weighted MRI of the knee in a young adult patient with hemophilia demonstrates hemosiderin deposition in the joint space related to repeated episodes of hemarthrosis (*arrows*). Note the articular surface erosion in the medial tibial plateau (*arrowhead*) and the widening of the intercondylar notch.

JACCOUD ARTHRITIS

Jaccoud arthropathy is a deforming, nonerosive form of arthritis initially described in rheumatic fever, but recently observed more frequently in patients with systemic lupus erythematosus and other connective tissue disorders, sarcoidosis, neoplasias, and some infections. Usually, there is complete recovery, but residual stiffness in metacarpophalangeal joints may develop with subsequent attacks. The lesion appears to be periarticular rather than articular, and the changes are caused by mild flexion at the metacarpophalangeal joints with ulnar deviation, most notably in the ring and small fingers, although any finger may be affected. The articular changes are not erosive, and patients can physically correct the deformity, particularly in the early course of the disease. The syndrome is rare and not well recognized in the United States.

ARTHRITIS ASSOCIATED WITH ACQUIRED IMMUNODEFICIENCY SYNDROME

Acquired immunodeficiency syndrome (AIDS) results from infection with human immunodeficiency virus (HIV), resulting in immunodeficiency state and pathologic disorders across multiple organ systems. Recently, an increased prevalence of rheumatologic disorders has been described in patients with HIV infection. Berman and colleagues stated that 71% of patients infected with HIV virus had rheumatic symptoms, including arthralgias, reactive arthritis, psoriatic arthritis, and undifferentiated spondyloarthropathy. The presence of Jaccoud arthropathy as part of an HIV-associated condition has also been occasionally reported. HIV-associated arthropathy can occur at any stage of HIV illness. Solomon et al. found that patients with HIV infection demonstrated a 144-fold increase in the prevalence of reactive arthritis and a 10-fold to 40-fold increase in the prevalence of psoriasis compared with the general population. It is interesting to note that arthritis was seen during various stages of HIV infection and often preceded clinical manifestations of the AIDS. The arthritis was more severe and was unresponsive to conventional treatment with nonsteroidal anti-inflammatory medications. A few hypotheses have been suggested to explain the coexistence of inflammatory arthritis and HIV infection. One is that reactive arthritis entails an interaction between a genetic predisposition (e.g., HLA-B27 locus) and environmental factors, most often venereal infections. The immune system also plays a role in the pathogenesis of reactive arthritis. Likewise, the pathogenesis of psoriatic arthritis may entail genetic predisposition (e.g., HLA-B27 or HLA-B38 loci). Because HIV infection is commonly followed by the development of immunodeficiency, it is possible that the altered immune mechanism noted in patients with AIDS triggered the onset of reactive arthritis or psoriatic arthritis in genetically predisposed patients. The second hypothesis is that HIV-related immunodeficiency causes susceptibility to infection with a variety of bacterial and viral organisms, which in turn trigger the onset of arthritis in a genetically predisposed patient. A third hypothesis is that there may be yet-undiscovered causative factors that predispose an individual to arthritis when exposed to HIV. Finally, the arthritis may reflect the direct action of HIV infection on synovium. As Rosenberg et al. have pointed out, radiographic documentation of seronegative arthritis should raise the possibility of HIV-associated arthritis as part of the differential diagnosis, particularly in patients with known risk factors for HIV infection. Other nonarticular rheumatologic disorders including osteonecrosis, vasculitis, and myositis are well known manifestations of HIV, but are not within the scope of this chapter.

SUGGESTED READINGS

Adizie T, Moots RJ, Hodkinson B, et al. Inflammatory arthritis in HIV positive patients: a practical guide. *BMC Infect Dis.* 2016;16:100–105.

Ali S, Huebner S. Multicentric reticulohistiocytosis. *Skeletal Radiol.* 2013;42:1483–1484.

Allroggen A, Frese A, Rahmann A, et al. HIV associated arthritis: a case report and review of the literature. *Eur J Med Res.* 2005;10:305–308.

Ashrani AA, Key NS, Soucie JM, et al. Septic arthritis in males with haemophilia. *Haemophilia.* 2008;14:494–503.

Ballard M, Meyer O, Adle-Biassette H, et al. Jaccoud's arthropathy with vasculitis and primary Sjögren's syndrome. A new entity. *Clin Exp Rheumatol.* 2006;24:S102–S103.

Barrow MV, Holubar K. Multicentric reticulohistiocytosis. A review of 33 patients. *Medicine.* 1969;48:287–305.

Baughman RP, Lower EE, du Bois RM. Sarcoidosis. *Lancet.* 2003;362: 1111–1118.

Benson MD. The hereditary amyloidoses. In: Picken MM, Dogan A, Herrera GA, eds. *Amyloid and Related Disorders: Surgical Pathology and Clinical Correlations.* New York, NY: Springer, 2012:53.

Benson MD. Amyloidosis. In: Koopman WJ, Moreland LW, eds. *Arthritis and Allied Conditions: a Textbook of Rheumatology.* Philadelphia, PA: Lippincott Williams & Wilkins, 2005:1933–1960.

Berman A, Espinoza LR, Diaz JD. Rheumatic manifestations of human immunodeficiency virus infection. *Am J Med.* 1988;85:59–64.

Booth TC, Chhaya NC, Bell JRG, et al. Update on imaging of non-infectious musculoskeletal complications of HIV infection. *Skeletal Radiol.* 2012;41:1349–1363.

Bradley JD, Pinals RS. Jaccoud's arthropathy in scleroderma. *Clin Exp Rheumatol.* 1984;2:337–340.

Bradley JD. Jaccoud's arthropathy in adult dermatomyositis. *Clin Exp Rheumatol.* 1986;4:273–276.

Bullough PG. *Atlas of Orthopedic Pathology with Clinical and Radiologic Correlation.* 2nd ed. New York, NY: Gower, 1992:16.2–16.4.

Bushara KO, Petermann G, Waclawik AJ, et al. Sarcoidosis of the spinal cord with extensive vertebral involvement: a case report. *Comp Med Imag Graphics.* 1995;19:443–446.

Buskila D, Gladman DD, Langvitz P. Rheumatologic manifestations of infection with the human immunodeficiency virus. *Clin Exp Rheumatol.* 1990;8:567–573.

Buzbaum JN, Tagoe CE. The genetics of the amyloidoses. *Ann Rev Med.* 2000;51:543–569.

Calabrese LH. The rheumatic manifestations of infection with human immunodeficiency virus. *Semin Arthritis Rheum.* 1989;18:225–239.

Campbell SE, Reed CM, Bui-Mansfield LT, et al. Vertebral and spinal sarcoidosis. *AJR Am J Roentgenol.* 2005;184:5.

Cascado E, Tena X, Olive A. HIV infection-associated rheumatic syndromes. *Clin Exper Rheumatol.* 1999;17:633.

Carey RN, Blotzer JW, Wolfe ID, et al. Multicentric reticulohistiocytosis associated with Sjögren's syndrome. *J Rheumatol.* 1985;12:1193–1195.

Chen ES, Moller DR. Cytokines and chemokines in sarcoidosis. In: Baughman R, ed. *Sarcoidosis.* Vol. 210. New York, NY: Taylor & Francis Group, 2006:123–161.

Chen ES. Sarcoidosis. In: Klippel JH, Stone JH, Crofford LJ, White PH, eds. *Primer on the Rheumatic Diseases.* 13th ed. New York, NY: Springer, 2008:514–522.

Cuellar ML, Espinoza LR. Rheumatic manifestations of HIV-AIDS. *Best Prac Res Clin Rheumatol.* 2000;14:579–593.

Cuellar ML, Espinoza LR. Human immunodeficiency virus associated spondyloarthropathy: lessons from the Third World. *J Rheumatol.* 1999;26:2071–2073.

Elsaman AM, Radwan AR, Akmatov MK, et al. Amyloid arthropathy associated with multiple myeloma: a systematic analysis of 101 reported cases. *Sem Arthritis Rheum.* 2013;43:405–412.

Escobedo EM, Hunter JC, Zink-Brody GC, et al. Magnetic resonance imaging of dialysis-related amyloidosis of the shoulder and hip. *Skeletal Radiol.* 1996;25:41–48.

Fox C, Walker-Bone K. Evolving spectrum of HIV-associated rheumatic syndromes. *Best Pract Res Clin Rheumatol.* 2015;29:244–258.

Freemont AJ, Jones CJ, Denton J. The synovium and synovial fluid in multicentric reticulohistiocytosis—a light microscopic, electron microscopic and cytochemical analysis of one case. *J Clin Pathol.* 1983;36:860–866.

Gaary E, Gorlin JB, Jaramillo D. Pseudotumor and arthropathy in the knees of a hemophiliac. *Skeletal Radiol.* 1996;25:85–87.

Gertz MA, Kyle RA. Amyloidosis with IM monoclonal gammopathies. *Semin Oncol.* 2003;30:325–328.

Ginsberg LE, Williams DW, Stanton D. MRI of vertebral sarcoidosis. *J Comput Assist Tomogr.* 1993;17:158–159.

Goldman AB, Pavlov H, Bullough P. Case report 137. Primary amyloidosis involving the skeletal system. *Skeletal Radiol.* 1981;6:69–74.

Goltz RW, Laymon CW. Multicentric reticulohistiocytosis of the skin and synovial; reticulohistiocytoma or ganglioneuroma. *AMA Arch Dermatol Syphilol.* 1954;69:717–731.

Goto H, Inaba M, Kobayashi K, et al. Successful treatment of multicentric reticulohistiocytosis with alendronate: evidence for direct effect of bisphosphonate on histiocytes. *Arthritis Rheum.* 2003;48:3538–3541.

Grahame R, Mitchell AB, Scott JT. Chronic post-rheumatic fever (Jaccoud's) arthropathy. *Ann Rheum Dis.* 1970;29:622–625.

Grossman RE, Hensley GT. Bone lesions in primary amyloidosis. *AJR Am J Roentgenol.* 1967;101:872–875.

Hawkins PN. Amyloidosis. *Blood Rev.* 1995;9:135–142.

Hawkins PN, Lavender JP, Pepys MB. Evaluation of systemic amyloidosis by scintigraphy with 123I-labeled serum amyloid P component. *N Engl J Med.* 1990;323:508–513.

Heffner DK. Review article; the cause of sarcoidosis: the Centurial enigma solved. *Ann Diagnostic Pathol.* 2007;11:142–152.

Iannuzzi MC, Rybicki BA, Teirstein AS. Sarcoidosis. *N Engl J Med.* 2007;357:2153–2165.

Janssen BA, Kencian J, Brooks PM. Close temporal and anatomic relationship between multicentric reticulohistiocytosis and carcinoma of the breast. *J Rheumatol.* 1992;19:322–324.

Kandiah DA. Multicentric reticulohistiocytosis. *Mayo Clin Proc.* 2014;89:e73.

Kaplan H. Sarcoid arthritis. A review. *Arch Intern Med.* 1963;112:924–935.

Kelly D, Zhang QC, Soucie JM, et al. Prevalence of clinical hip abnormalities in haemophilia A and B: an analysis of the UDC database. *Haemophilia.* 2013;19:424–433.

Kovach BT, Calamia KT, Walsh JS, et al. Treatment of multicentric reticulohistiocytosis with etanercept. *Arch Dermatol.* 2004;140:919–921.

Krey PR, Comerford FR, Cohen AS. Multicentric reticulohistiocytosis. Fine structural analysis of the synovium and synovial fluid cells. *Arthritis Rheum.* 1974;17:615–633.

Kumar N, Frohman EM. Spinal neurosarcoidosis mimicking an idiopathic inflammatory demyelinating syndrome. *Arch Neurol.* 2004;61:586–589.

Lee DJ, Sartoris DJ. Musculoskeletal manifestations of human immunodeficiency virus infection: review of imaging characteristics. *Radiol Clin North Am.* 1994;32: 399–411.

Lesher JL Jr, Allen BS. Multicentric reticulohistiocytosis. *J Am Acad Dermatol.* 1984;11:713–723.

Lima I, Ribeiro DS, Cesare A, et al. Typical Jaccoud's arthropathy in a patient with sarcoidosis. *Rheumatol Int.* 2013;33:1615–1617.

Llauger J, Palmer J, Roson N, et al. Nonseptic monoarthritis: imaging features with clinical and histopathologic correlation. *Radiographics.* 2000;20:S263–S278.

Maclachlan J, Gough-Palmer A, Hargunani R, et al. Hemophilia imaging: a review. *Skeletal Radiol.* 2009;38:949–957.

Major NM, Tehranzadeh J. Musculoskeletal manifestations of AIDS. *Radiol Clin North Am.* 1997;35:1167–1189.

McIlwain KL, DiCarlo JB, Miller SB, et al. Multicentric reticulohistiocytosis with prominent cutaneous lesions and proximal muscle weakness masquerading as dermatomyositis. *J Rheumatol.* 2005;32:193–194.

Melton JW III, Irby R. Multicentric reticulohistiocytosis. *Arthritis Rheum.* 1972;15: 221–226.

Miller CH, Benson J, Ellingsen D, et al. F8 and F9 mutations in US haemophilia patients: correlation with history of inhibitor and race/ethnicity. *Haemophilia.* 2012;8:375–382.

Moore SL, Teirstein A, Golimbu C. MRI of sarcoidosis patients with musculoskeletal symptoms. *AJR Am J Roentgenol.* 2005;185:154–159.

Oldenburg J, Zimmermann R, Katsarou O, et al. Controlled, cross-sectional MRI evaluation of joint status in severe haemophilia A patients treated with prophylaxis vs. on demand. *Haemophilia.* 2015;21:171–179.

Ozulker T, Ozulker F, Derin E, et al. The efficacy of magnetic resonance imaging and X-ray in the evaluation of response to radiosynovectomy in patients with hemophilic arthropathy. *Mol Imaging Radionucl Ther.* 2011;20:38–44.

Pacheco-Tena C, Reyes-Cordero G, Ochoa-Albiztegui R, et al. Treatment of multicentric reticulohistiocytosis with tocilizumab. *J Clin Rheumatol.* 2013;19:272–276.

Paredes JG, Lazaro MA, Citera G, et al. Jaccoud's arthropathy of the hands in overlap syndrome. *Clin Rheumatol.* 1997;16:65–69.

Rajkumar SV, Gertz MA. Advances in the treatment of amyloidosis. *N Engl J Med.* 2007;356:2413–2415.

Rapini RP. Multicentric reticulohistiocytosis. *Clin Dermatol.* 1993;11:107–111.

Ribeiro DS, Galvao V, Fernandes JL, et al. Magnetic resonance imaging of Jaccoud's arthropathy in systemic lupus erythematosus. *Joint Bone Spine.* 2010;77:241–245.

Robledo G, vila-Fajardo CL, Marquez A, et al. Association between 174 Interleukin-6 gene polymorphism and biological response to rituximab in several systemic autoimmune diseases. *DNA Cell Biol.* 2012;31:1486–1491.

Rosenberg ZS, Norman A, Solomon G. Arthritis associated with HIV infection: radiographic manifestations. *Radiology.* 1989;173:171–176.

Ross LV, Ross GJ, Mesgarzadeh M, et al. Hemodialysis-related amyloidomas of bone. *Radiology.* 1991;178:263–265.

Sanchorowala V. Light-chain (AL) amyloidosis: diagnosis and treatment. *Clin J Am Soc Nephrol.* 2006;1:1331–1341.

Santiago MB, Galvao V. Jaccoud arthropathy in systemic lupus erythematosus: analysis of clinical characteristics and review of the literature. *Medicine (Baltimore).* 2008;87:37–44.

Schurman M, Reichel P, Muller-Myhsok B, et al. Results from a genome-wide search for predisposing genes in sarcoidosis. *Am J Respir Crit Care Med.* 2001;164:840–846.

Selmi C, Greenspan A, Huntley A, et al. Multicentric reticulohistiocytosis: a critical review. *Curr Rheumatol Rep.* 2015;17:36–44.

Sood SL, Cuker A, Wang C, et al. Similarity in joint function limitation in Type 3 von Willebrand's disease and moderate haemophilia A. *Haemophilia.* 2013;19:595–601.

Steinbach LS, Tehranzadeh J, Fleckenstein J, et al. Human immunodeficiency virus infection: musculoskeletal manifestations. *Radiology.* 1993;186: 833–838.

Stoker DJ, Murray RO. Skeletal changes in hemophilia and other bleeding disorders. *Semin Roentgenol.* 1974;9:185–193.

Tajirian AL, Malik MK, Robinson-Bostom L, et al. Multicentric reticulohistiocytosis. *Clin Dermatol.* 2006;24:486–492.

Tashiro A, Takeuchi S, Nakahara T, et al. Aberrant expression of CD10 in ground-glass-like multinucleated giant cells of multicentric reticulohistiocytosis. *J Dermatol.* 2010;37:995–997.

Tehranzadeh J, Steinbach LS. *Musculoskeletal Manifestations of AIDS.* St. Louis, MO: Warren H. Green; 1994.

Tirumalae R, Rout P, Jayaseelan E, et al. Paraneoplastic multicentric reticulohistiocytosis: a clinicopathologic challenge. *Indian J Dermatol Venereol Leprology.* 2011;77:318–320.

Tishler M, Yaron M. Jaccoud's arthropathy and psoriatic arthritis. *Clin Exp Rheumatol.* 1993;11:663–664.

Torralba KD, Quismorio FP Jr. Sarcoid arthritis: a review of clinical features, pathology and therapy. *Sarcoidosis Vasc Diffuse Lung Dis.* 2003;20: 95–103.

Volpato BR, de Freire CJ. Jaccoud's arthropathy associated with cutaneous polyarteritis nodosa. *Isr Med Assoc J.* 2010;12:514.

Wilcox A, Bharadwaj P, Sharma OP. Bone sarcoidosis. *Curr Opin Rheumatol.* 2000;12:321–330.

Weber FP, Freudenthal W. Nodular non-diabetic cutaneous xanthomatosis with hypercholesterolaemia and atypical histological features. *Proc R Soc Med.* 1937;30:522–526.

Winchester R, Bernstein DH, Fischer HD. The co-occurrence of Reiter's syndrome and acquired immunodeficiency. *Ann Int Med.* 1987;106: 19–26.

Yaghmai I. Radiographic, angiographic, and radionuclide manifestation of osseous sarcoidosis. *Radiographics.* 1983;3:375–396.

Yamada T, Kurohori YN, Kashiwazaki S, et al. MRI of multicentric reticulohistiocytosis. *J Comput Assist Tomogr.* 1996;20:838–840.

Yap FB. Multicentric reticulohistiocytosis in a Malaysian Chinese lady: a case report and review of literature. *Dermatol Online J.* 2009;15:2.

Yeter KC, Arkfeld DG. Treatment of multicentric reticulohistiocytosis with adalimumab, minocycline, methotrexate. *Int J Rheum Dis.* 2013;16:105–106.

Zisman D, Schorr AF, Lynch JP III. Sarcoidosis involving the musculoskeletal system. *Semin Resp Crit Care Med.* 2002;23:555–570.

PART III

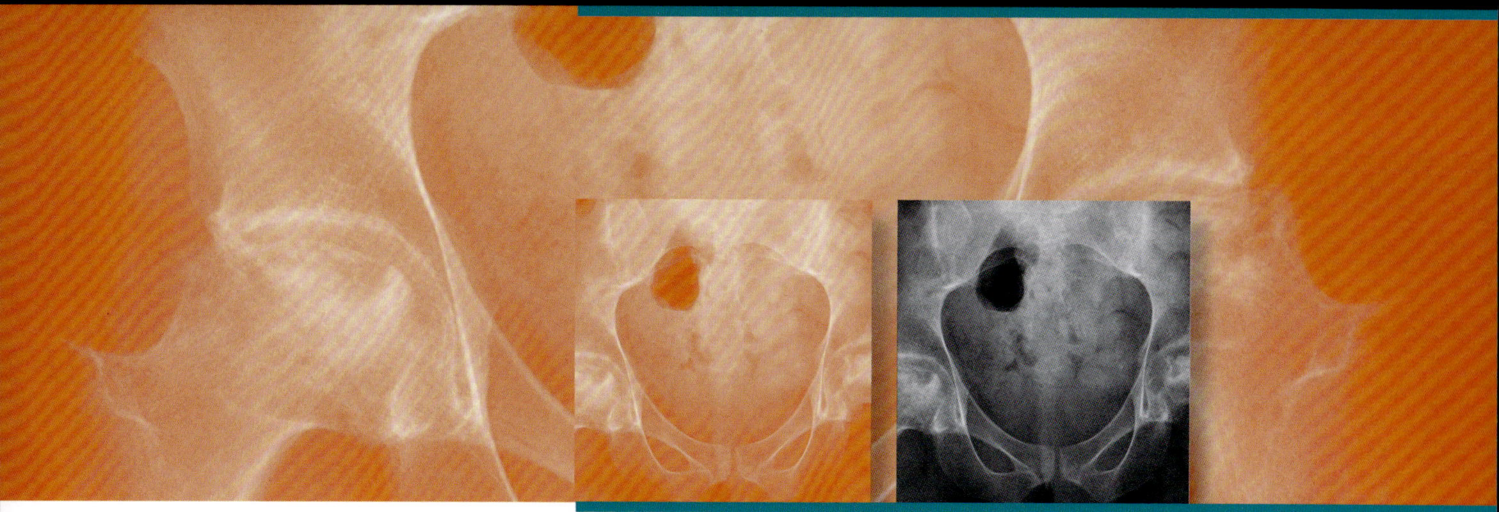

Articular and Periarticular Abnormalities That May Masquerade as Arthritis

In this part, we are discussing some conditions in which the clinical presentation may suggest an arthritic process. In majority of these cases, the imaging features will clarify the true nature of the disease. Because of the constraint of this volume, only some of these abnormalities are included.

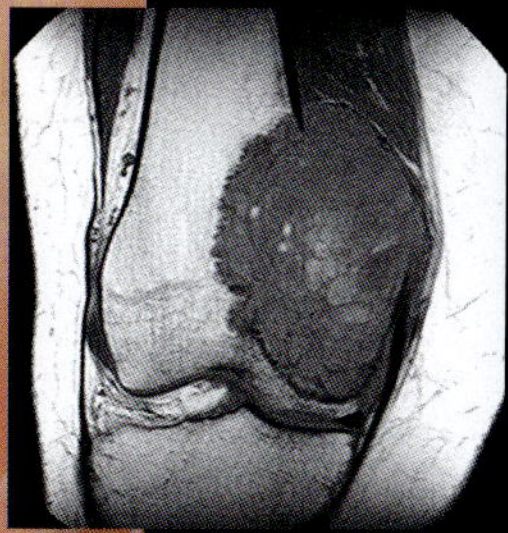

CHAPTER 11

Tumors and Tumor-like Lesions

SYNOVIAL (OSTEO)CHONDROMATOSIS

Synovial (osteo)chondromatosis (also known as synovial chondromatosis or synovial chondrometaplasia) is an uncommon benign disorder marked by the metaplastic proliferation of multiple cartilaginous nodules in the synovial membrane of the joints, bursae, or tendon sheaths. It is almost invariably monoarticular; rarely, multiple joints may be affected. The disorder is twice as common in men as in women and is usually discovered in the third to fifth decade. The knee is a preferential site of involvement, with the hip, shoulder, and elbow accounting for most of the remaining cases. Patients usually report pain and swelling. Joint effusion, tenderness, limited motion in the joint, and a soft tissue mass are common clinical findings, occasionally mistaken for arthritis.

Three phases of articular disease have been identified: an initial phase, characterized by metaplastic formation of cartilaginous nodules in the synovium; a transitional phase, characterized by detachment of those nodules and formation of free intra-articular bodies; and an inactive phase, in which synovial proliferation has resolved but loose bodies remain in the joint, usually with variable amounts of joint fluid.

Gross pathologic findings consist of multiple blue/white ovoid nodules within synovial tissue (Fig. 11.1). By microscopy, these nodules are covered by fibrous tissue with synovial lining and are highly cellular, and the cells themselves may exhibit a moderate pleomorphism, with occasional plump and double nuclei (Figs. 11.2 and 11.3). The cartilaginous nodules, which often are undergoing calcification and endochondral ossification, may detach and become loose bodies. The loose bodies continue to be viable and may increase in size as they receive nourishment from the synovial fluid.

The imaging findings depend on the degree of calcification within the cartilaginous bodies, ranging from merely joint effusion to visualization of many radiopaque joint bodies, usually small and uniform in size (Figs. 11.4 to 11.6). The best proof that the bodies are indeed intra-articular is achieved by arthrography or computed tomography (CT) (Figs. 11.7 and 11.8). These modalities can visualize even noncalcified bodies. Magnetic resonance imaging (MRI) may also be helpful, although MRI appearance is variable and depends on the relative preponderance of synovial proliferation, loose bodies formation, and extent of calcification or ossification. Unmineralized hyperplastic synovial masses exhibit high signal intensity on T2-weighted images, whereas calcifications can be seen as signal void against the high–signal intensity fluid (Figs. 11.9 and 11.10). In addition to revealing loose bodies in the joint, CT and MRI may demonstrate bone erosion.

(Continued on page 381)

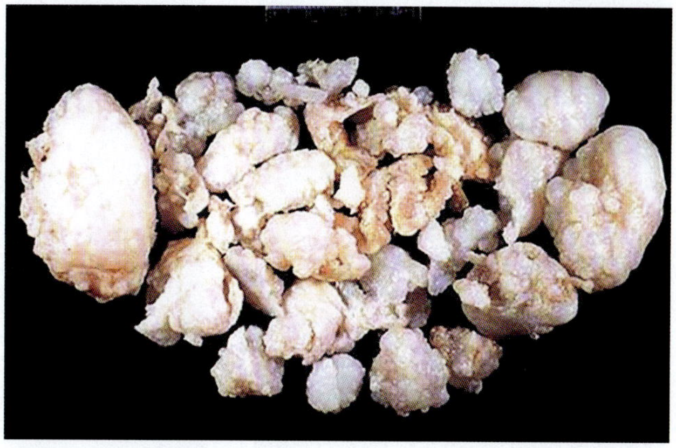

Figure 11.1 ■ Gross pathology of synovial (osteo)chondromatosis. Multiple blue/white ovoid nodules of cartilage are scattered within the synovial tissue.

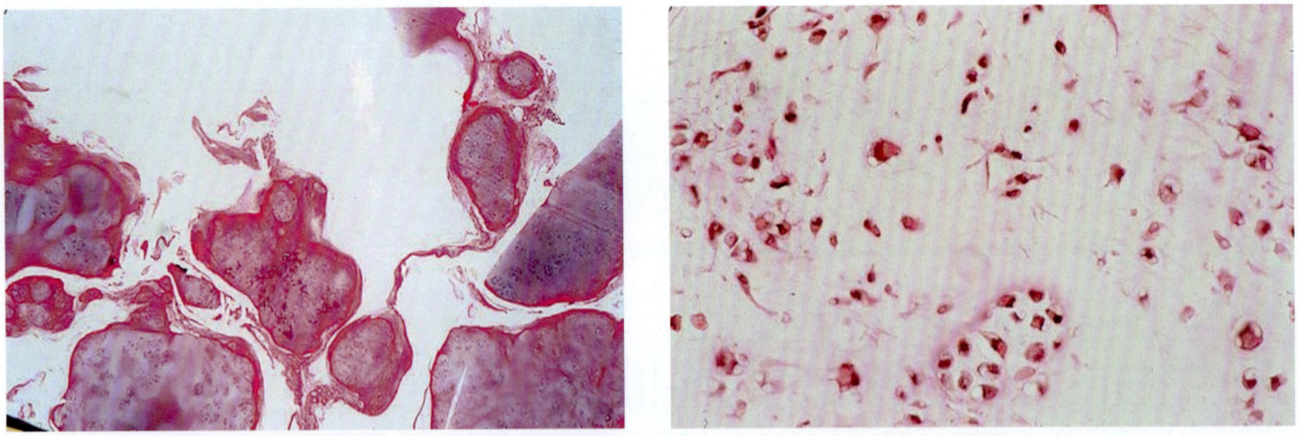

A B

Figure 11.2 ■ Histopathology of synovial (osteo)chondromatosis. A: Photomicrograph of the synovium removed from the knee of a patient with primary synovial (osteo)chondromatosis shows nodules of irregular cellular cartilage covered by a thin layer of synovium (H&E, original magnification ×6). **B:** Higher-power photomicrograph shows cells with double nuclei arranged in clusters (H&E, original magnification ×100).

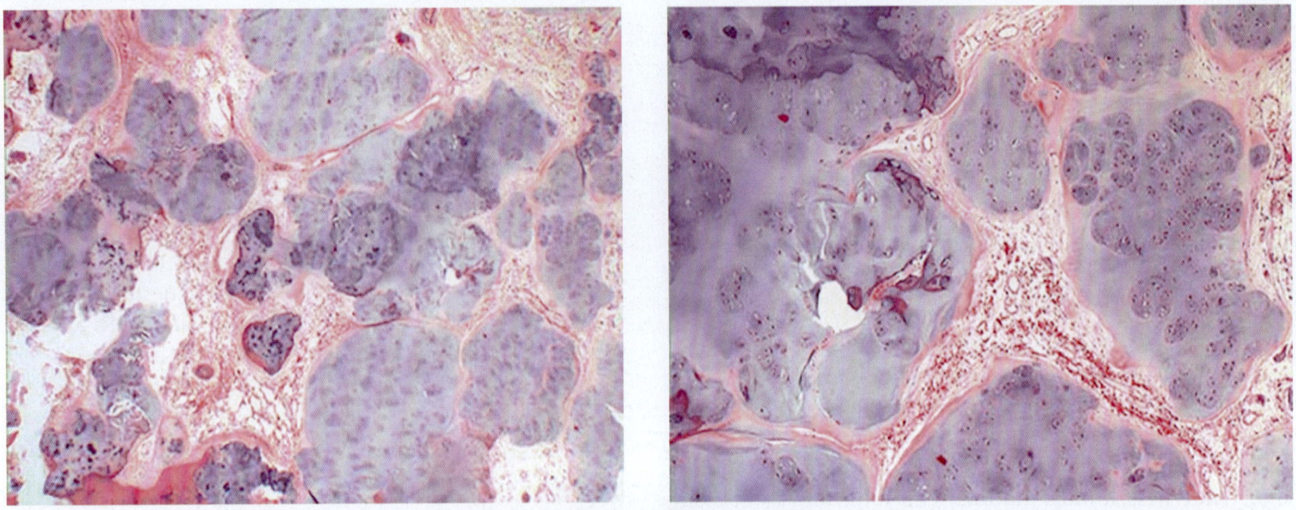

A B

Figure 11.3 ■ Histopathology of synovial (osteo)chondromatosis. A: Variable cartilaginous nodules are covered by synovial tissue (H&E, original magnification ×100). **B:** Higher magnification shows the clusters of chondrocytes with plump nuclei. Some of the cells show binucleation (H&E, original magnification ×200).

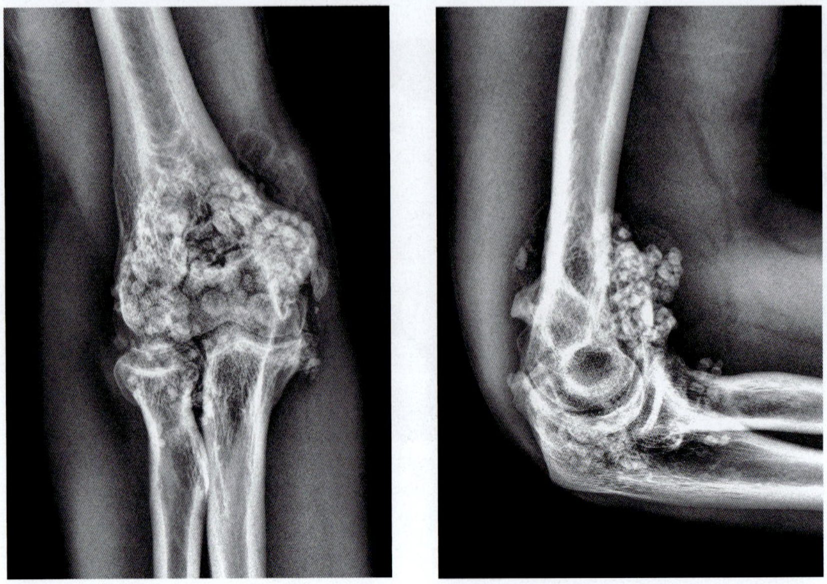

A B

Figure 11.4 ■ Synovial (osteo)chondromatosis. A 27-year-old man reported pain and occasional locking in the elbow joint; he had no history of trauma. Anteroposterior **(A)** and lateral **(B)** radiographs demonstrate multiple osteochondral bodies in the elbow joint, which are regularly shaped and uniform in size.

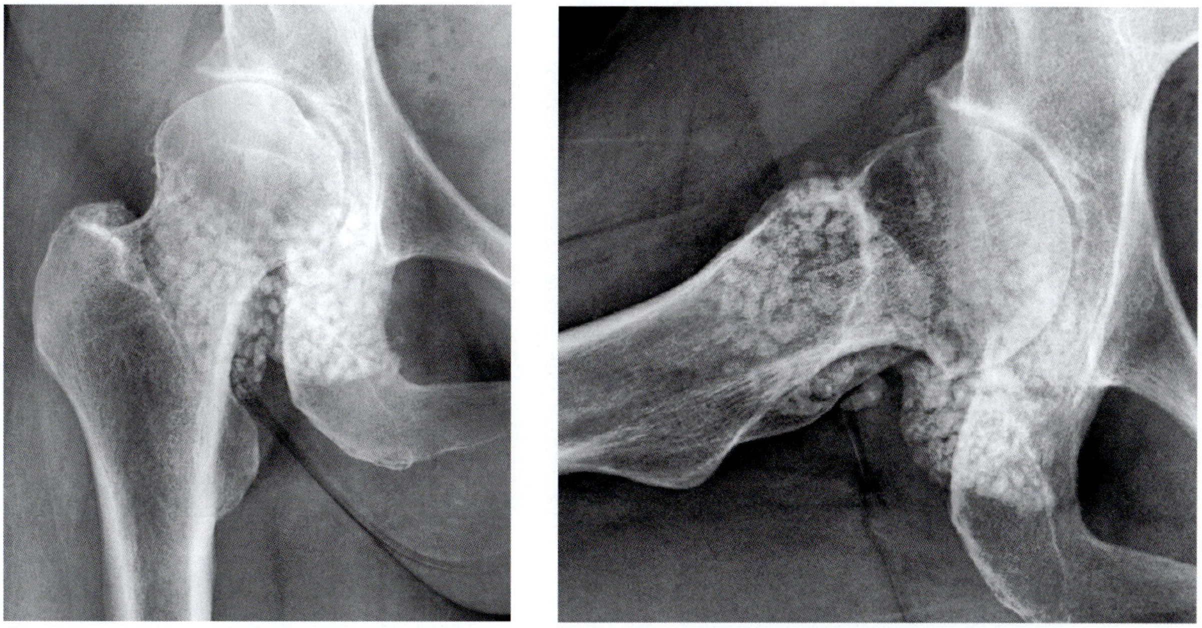

A B

Figure 11.5 ■ **Synovial (osteo)chondromatosis.** Anteroposterior **(A)** and frog-lateral **(B)** radiographs of the right hip of a 59-year-old woman show numerous, uniform in size, intra-articular osteochondral bodies.

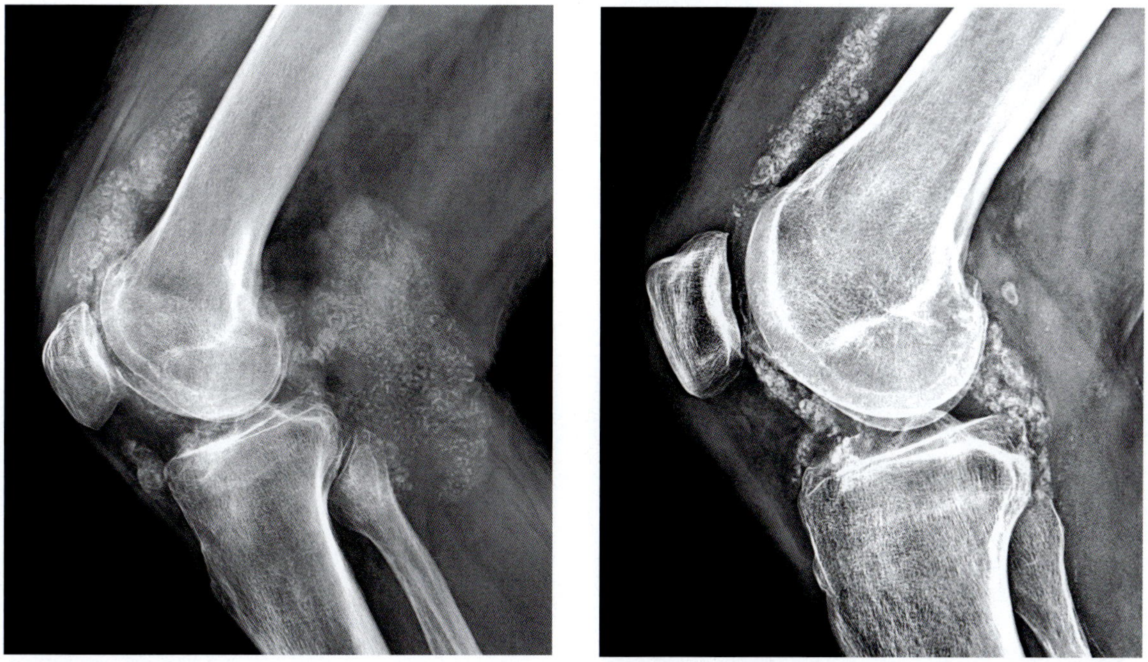

A B

Figure 11.6 ■ **Synovial (osteo)chondromatosis. A:** Lateral radiograph of the knee of a 58-year-old man shows numerous small and uniform in size intra-articular osteochondral bodies. **B:** Lateral radiograph of the knee of another patient, a 45-year-old woman, shows typical appearance of this condition.

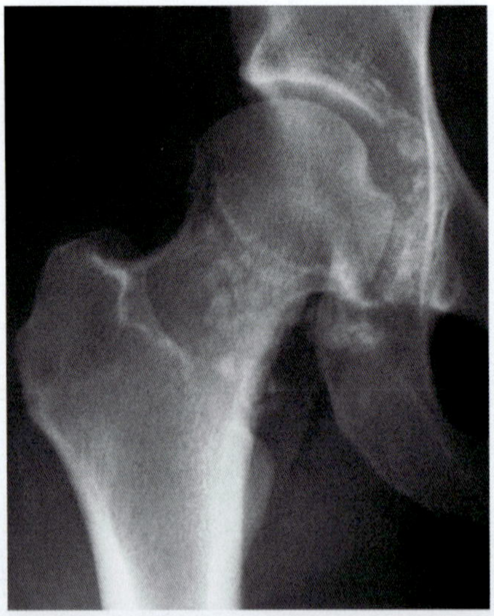

A

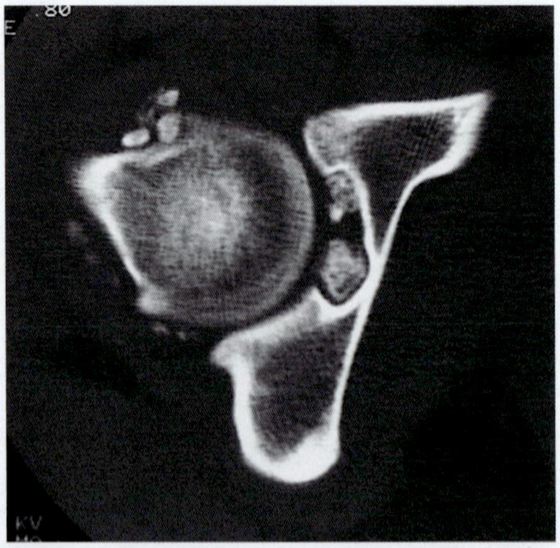

B

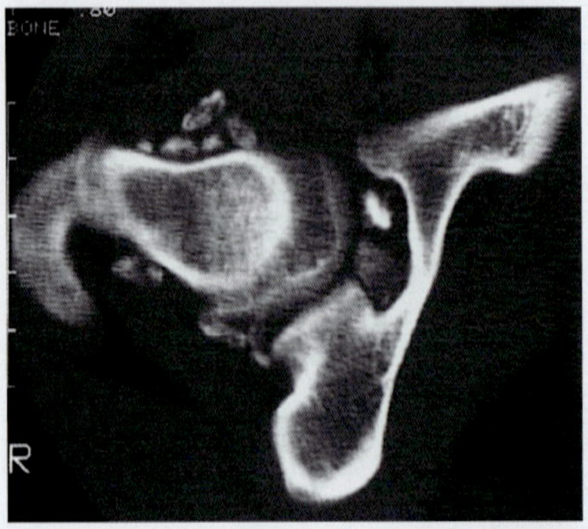

C

Figure 11.7 ■ CT of synovial (osteo)chondromatosis. A: Anteroposterior radiograph of the right hip of a 27-year-old woman shows multiple osteochondral bodies around the femoral head and neck. Note preservation of the joint space, a characteristic feature of synovial (osteo)chondromatosis. **B, C:** Two CT sections, one through the femoral head and another through the femoral neck, demonstrate unquestionably the intra-articular location of multiple osteochondral bodies.

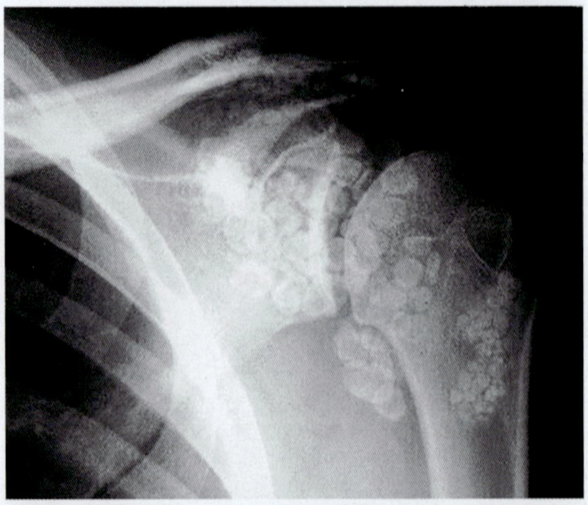

A

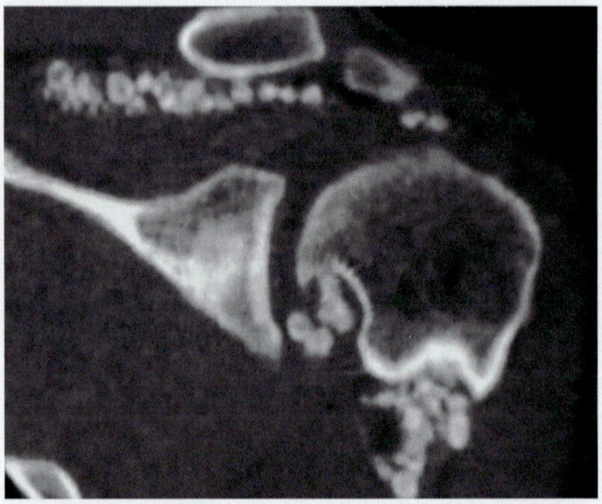

B

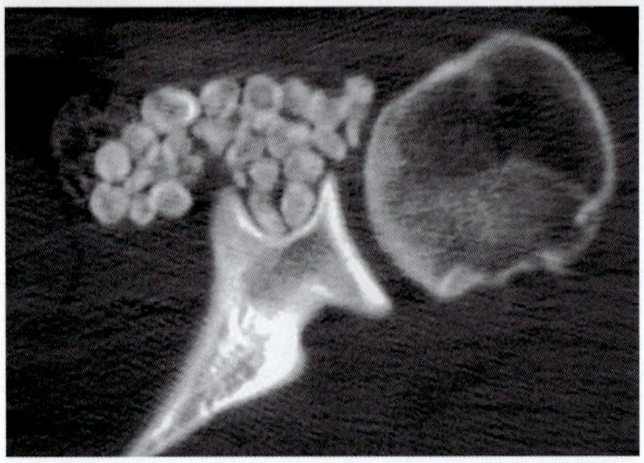

C

Figure 11.8 ■ CT of synovial (osteo)chondromatosis. A: Anteroposterior radiograph of the left shoulder of a 36-year-old man shows multiple osteochondral bodies around the glenohumeral joint. Axial **(B)** and coronal **(C)** reformatted CT sections effectively show the location of the uniform in size calcific bodies in the glenohumeral joint and subacromial bursa.

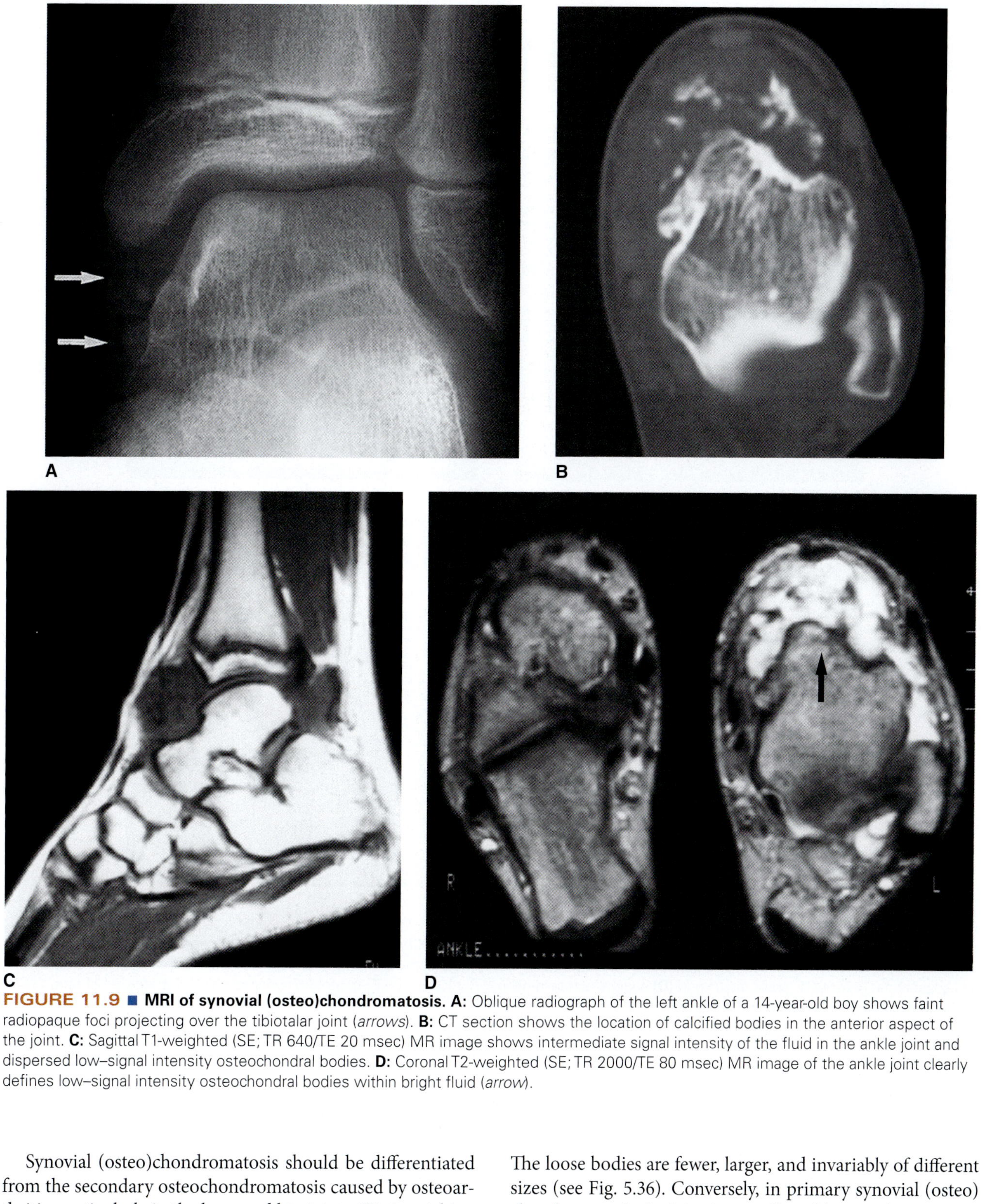

FIGURE 11.9 ■ MRI of synovial (osteo)chondromatosis. A: Oblique radiograph of the left ankle of a 14-year-old boy shows faint radiopaque foci projecting over the tibiotalar joint (*arrows*). **B:** CT section shows the location of calcified bodies in the anterior aspect of the joint. **C:** Sagittal T1-weighted (SE; TR 640/TE 20 msec) MR image shows intermediate signal intensity of the fluid in the ankle joint and dispersed low–signal intensity osteochondral bodies. **D:** Coronal T2-weighted (SE; TR 2000/TE 80 msec) MR image of the ankle joint clearly defines low–signal intensity osteochondral bodies within bright fluid (*arrow*).

Synovial (osteo)chondromatosis should be differentiated from the secondary osteochondromatosis caused by osteoarthritis, particularly in the knee and hip joints. Distinguishing *primary* from *secondary osteochondromatosis* usually presents no problems. In the latter condition, there is invariably radiographic evidence of osteoarthritis with all of its typical features, such as narrowing of the radiographic joint space, subchondral sclerosis, and, occasionally, periarticular cysts or cystlike lesions (see Figs. 5.44 to 5.46 and 5.48 and 5.50). The loose bodies are fewer, larger, and invariably of different sizes (see Fig. 5.36). Conversely, in primary synovial (osteo) chondromatosis the joint is not affected by any degenerative changes. In some cases, however, the bone may show erosions secondary to pressure of the calcified bodies on the outer aspects of the cortex. The intra-articular bodies are numerous, small, and usually of uniform size (see Figs. 11.4 to 11.6).

The other conditions that can radiologically mimic synovial chondromatosis include pigmented villonodular

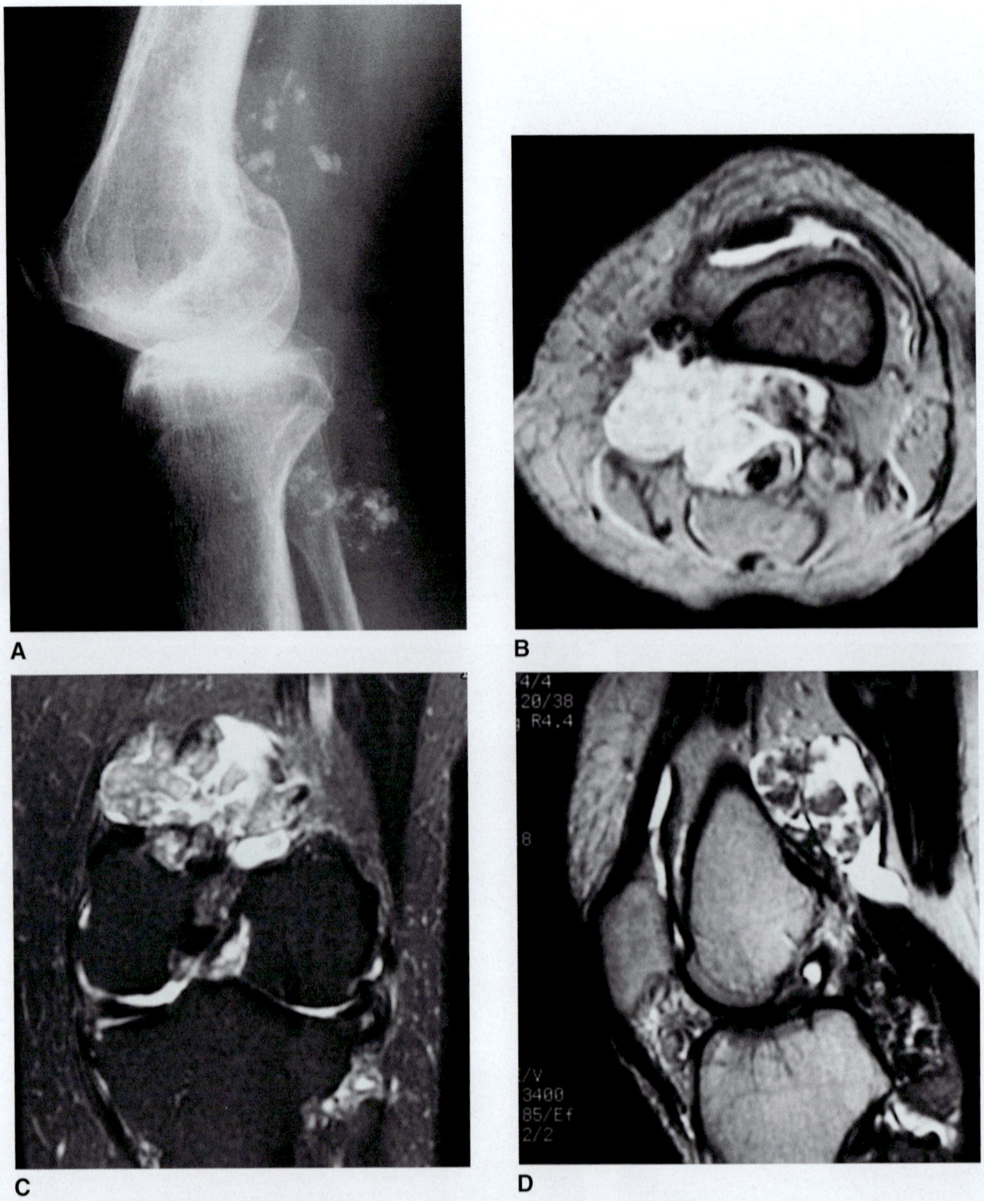

Figure 11.10 ■ **MRI of synovial (osteo)chondromatosis. A:** Lateral radiograph of the left knee of a 50-year-old man shows multiple osteochondral bodies in and around the joint. **B:** Axial T2*-weighted (MPGR; TR 500/TE 20 msec, flip angle 30 degrees) MR image demonstrates high-signal joint effusion and multiple bodies of intermediate signal intensity, primarily located in a large popliteal cyst. **C:** Coronal fast spin-echo (TR 2400/TE 85 Ef msec) and **(D)** sagittal fast spin-echo (TR 3400/TE 85 Ef msec) MR images show to better advantage the distribution of numerous osteochondral bodies.

synovitis (PVNS), synovial hemangioma, and lipoma arborescens. In *pigmented villonodular synovitis* (discussed in detail later in this chapter), the filling defects in the joint are more confluent and less distinct. MRI may show foci of decreased intensity of the synovium in all sequences because of the paramagnetic effects of deposition of hemosiderin (see Figs. 11.15 to 11.17). *Synovial hemangioma* usually presents as a single soft tissue mass. On MRI, T1-weighted images show that the lesion is either isointense or slightly higher (brighter) in signal intensity than surrounding muscles, but much lower in intensity than subcutaneous fat. On T2-weighted images, the mass is invariably much brighter than fat (see Figs. 11.22 to 11.26). Phleboliths and fibrofatty septa in the mass are common findings that show low-signal characteristics. *Lipoma arborescens* is a villous lipomatous proliferation of the synovial membrane. This rare condition usually affects the knee joint but has occasionally been reported in other joints, including the wrist and ankle. The disease has been variously reported to have a developmental, traumatic, inflammatory, or neoplastic origin, but its true cause is still unknown. The clinical findings include slowly increasing but painless synovial thickening as well as joint effusion with sporadic exacerbation. Imaging studies reveal a joint effusion occasionally accompanied by various degrees of osteoarthritis (see Figs. 11.28 to 11.30). Histologic examination demonstrates complete replacement of the subsynovial tissue by mature fat cells and the formation of proliferative villous projections (see text below).

Treatment of synovial chondromatosis usually consists of removal of the intra-articular bodies and synovectomy, but local recurrence is not uncommon.

PIGMENTED VILLONODULAR SYNOVITIS (PVNS)

PVNS is a locally destructive fibrohistiocytic proliferation, characterized by many villous and nodular synovial protrusions, which affects joints, bursae, and tendon sheaths. Jaffe, Lichtenstein, and Sutro first described PVNS in 1941 and used this name to identify the lesion because of its yellow–brown, villous, and nodular appearance. The yellow–brown pigmentation is caused by excessive deposits of lipid and hemosiderin. This condition can be diffuse or localized. When the entire synovium of the joint is affected, and when there is a major villous component, the condition is referred to as *diffuse pigmented villonodular synovitis*. When a discrete intra-articular mass is present, the condition is called *localized pigmented villonodular synovitis*. When the process affects the tendon sheaths, it is called *localized giant cell tumor of the tendon sheaths*. The diffuse form usually occurs in the knee, hip, elbow, or wrist and accounts for 23% of cases. The localized nodular form is often regarded as a separate entity. It consists of a single polypoid mass attached to the synovium. Nodular tenosynovitis is most often seen in the fingers and is the second most common soft tissue tumor of the hand, exceeded only by the ganglion. In the new (2002) revised classification of soft tissue tumors, the World Health Organization (WHO) classifies localized intra-articular and extra-articular lesions as giant cell tumor of tendon sheath, whereas diffuse intra-articular and extra-articular forms are categorized as diffuse-type giant cell tumor (keeping PVNS as a synonym).

Both the diffuse and the localized form of villonodular synovitis usually occur as a single lesion, mainly in young and middle-aged individuals of either gender, with peak incidence in the third and fourth decades. One of the most characteristic findings in PVNS is the ability of the hyperplastic synovium to invade the subchondral bone, producing cysts and erosions. Although the cause is unknown and is often controversial, some investigators have suggested an autoimmune pathogenesis. Trauma is also a suspected cause, because similar effects have been produced experimentally in animals by repeated injections of blood into the knee joint. Some investigators have suggested a disturbance in lipid metabolism as a causative factor. It has also been postulated by Jaffe and colleagues that these lesions may represent an inflammatory response to an unknown agent. Ray, Stout, and Lattes contended that they are true benign neoplasms. Although the latter theory was presumed to be supported by pathologic studies indicating that the histiocytes present in PVNS may function as facultative fibroblasts and that foam cells may derive from histiocytes, thus relating PVNS to a benign neoplasm of fibrohistiocytic origin, these findings do not constitute definite proof that PVNS is a true neoplasm. They are rather indicative of a special form of a chronic proliferative inflammation process, as has already been postulated by Jaffe and colleagues.

Gross pathologic examination shows tan-colored or reddish-brown synovial mass with hypertrophic villi (Fig. 11.11). On histopathologic examination, PVNS reveals a tumor-like proliferation of the synovial tissue. A dense infiltration of mononuclear histiocytes is observed, accompanied by plasma cells, xanthoma cells, lymphocytes, and variable numbers of giant cells (Fig. 11.12). Long-standing lesions show fibrosis and hyalinization.

Clinically, PVNS is a slowly progressive process that manifests as mild pain and joint swelling with limitation of motion, mimicking arthritis. Occasionally, increased skin temperature is noted over the affected joint. The knee joint is most commonly affected and 66% of patients present with a bloody joint effusion. In fact, the presence of a serosanguinous synovial fluid in the absence of a history of recent trauma should strongly suggest the diagnosis of PVNS. The synovial fluid contains elevated levels of cholesterol, and fluid reaccumulates rapidly after aspiration. Other joints may be affected, including the hip, ankle, wrist, elbow, and shoulder. There is a 2:1 predilection for females. Patients range from 4 to 60 years of age, with a peak incidence in the third and fourth decades. The duration of symptoms can range from 6 months to as long as 25 years.

Recently, attention has been drawn to the extra-articular form of diffuse PVNS, also referred to as *diffuse-type giant cell tumor*. This condition is characterized by the presence of an infiltrate and extra-articular mass with or without involvement of the adjacent joint. This presentation of PVNS

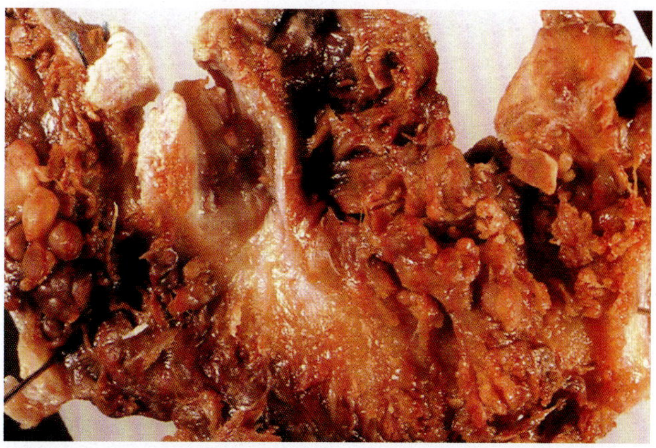

Figure 11.11 ■ Gross pathology of pigmented villonodular synovitis. Photograph of the synovium removed from the knee of a patient with pigmented villonodular synovitis shows reddish brown in color (because of hemosiderin deposition) synovial mass exhibiting hypertrophic villi.

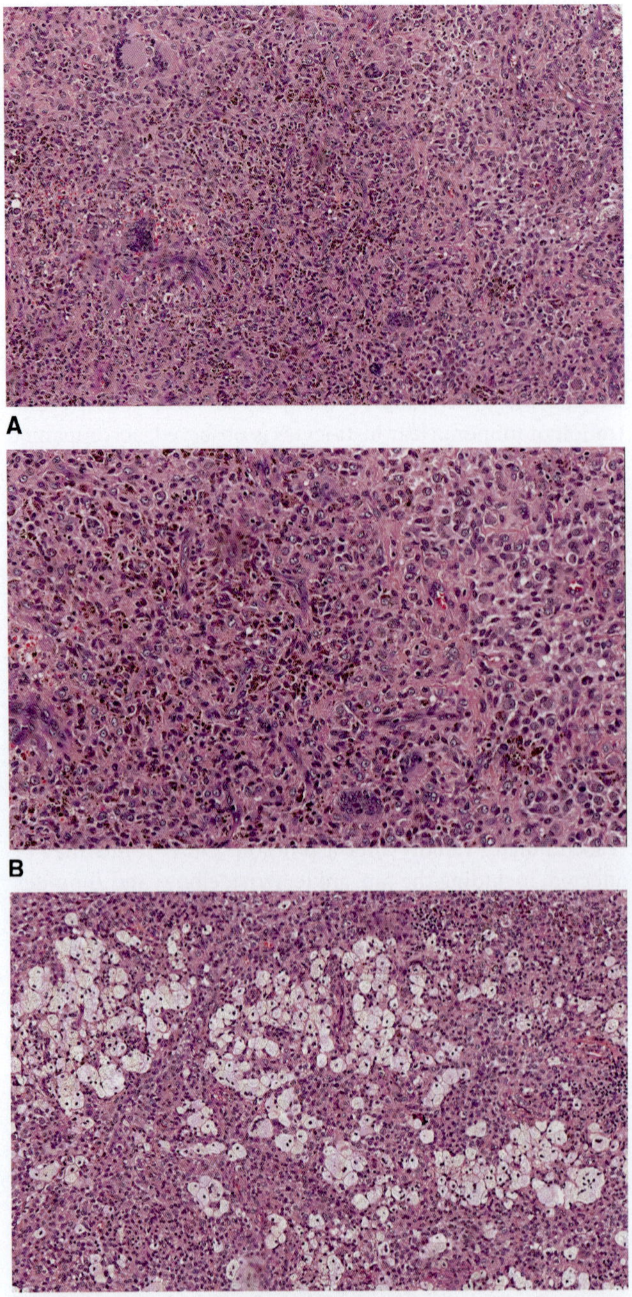

A

B

C

Figure 11.12 ■ Histopathology of pigmented villonodular synovitis. A: Tumor tissue is composed of admixture of small histiocytic-like cells and irregularly distributed osteoclast-like giant cells (H&E, original magnification ×100). **B:** On higher magnification, observe giant cells, small histiocytic cells, and large dendritic cells with abundant cytoplasm and deposits of hemosiderin (*brown foci*) (H&E, original magnification ×200). **C:** On the periphery of the lesion, note the sheets of foamy cells (H&E, original magnification ×200).

creates a real diagnostic challenge for both radiologist and pathologist because its extra-articular location, invasion of the osseous structures, and more varied histologic infiltrative pattern may suggest malignancy.

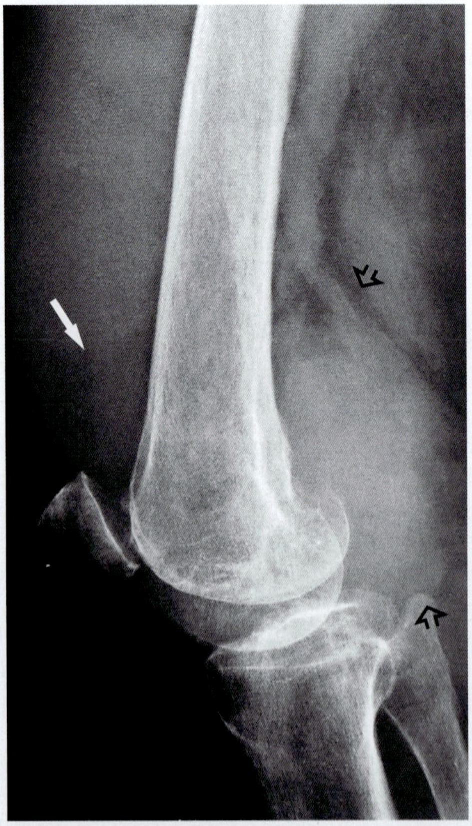

Figure 11.13 ■ Pigmented villonodular synovitis. Lateral radiograph of the knee of a 58-year-old man shows a large suprapatellar joint effusion (*arrow*) and a dense, lumpy soft tissue mass eroding the posterior aspect of the lateral femoral condyle (*open arrows*). Note that posteriorly the density is greater than that of a suprapatellar fluid.

Radiography reveals a soft tissue density in the affected joint, frequently interpreted as joint effusion. However, the density is greater than that of simple effusion, and it reflects not only a hemorrhagic fluid but also lobulated synovial masses (Fig. 11.13). A marginal, well-defined erosion of subchondral bone with a sclerotic margin may be present (incidence reported from 15% to 50%), usually on both sides of the affected articulation. Narrowing of the joint space has also been reported. In the hip, multiple cystlike or erosive areas involving non–weight-bearing regions of the acetabulum, as well as the femoral head and neck, are characteristic. Calcifications are encountered only in exceptional cases.

Arthrography reveals multiple lobulated masses with villous projections, which appear as filling defects in the contrast-filled suprapatellar bursa (Fig. 11.14). CT effectively demonstrates the extent of the disease. The increase in iron content of the synovial fluid results in high Hounsfield values, a feature that can help in the differential diagnosis. MRI is extremely useful in making a diagnosis, because on T2-weighted images the intra-articular masses demonstrate a combination of high–signal intensity areas,

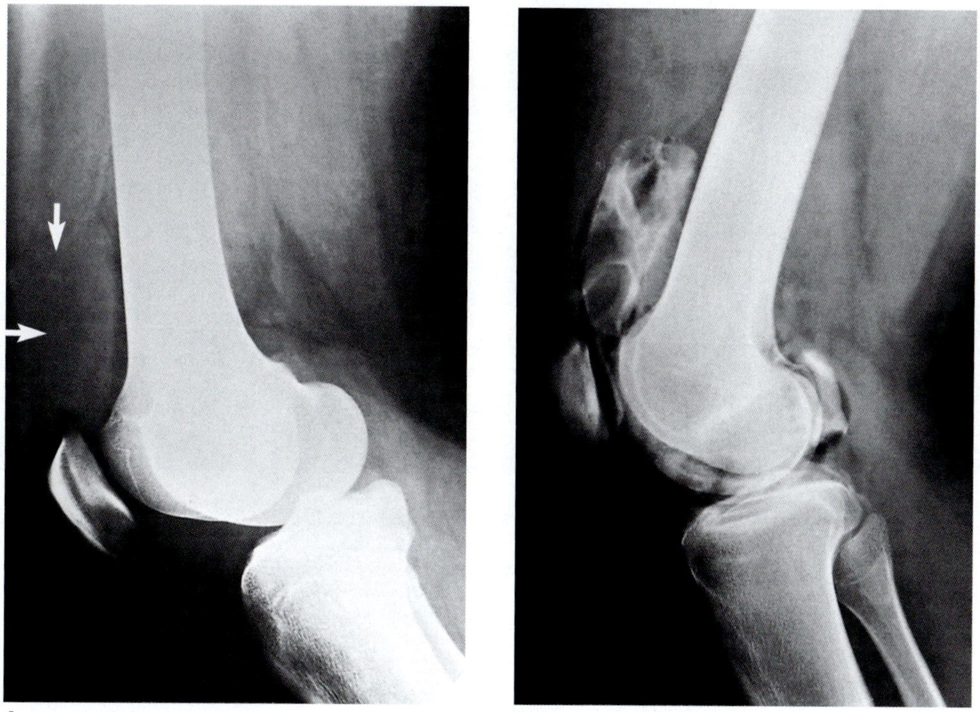

A B

Figure 11.14 ■ Arthrography of pigmented villonodular synovitis. A: Lateral radiograph of another patient shows what appears to be a suprapatellar effusion (*arrows*). The density of the "fluid," however, is increased, and there is some lobulation evident. **B:** Contrast arthrogram of the knee shows lobulated filling defects in the suprapatellar pouch, representing lumpy synovial masses. Joint puncture yielded thick bloody fluid, which explains the increased density of the soft tissue mass seen on the radiograph.

representing fluid and congested synovium, interspersed with areas of intermediate-to-low signal intensity, secondary to random distribution of hemosiderin in the synovium (Fig. 11.15). In general, MRI shows a low signal on T1- and T2-weighted images because of hemosiderin deposition and thick fibrous tissue (Figs. 11.16 to 11.18). In addition, within the mass, signals consistent with fat can be noted, which are caused by clumps of lipid-laden macrophages.

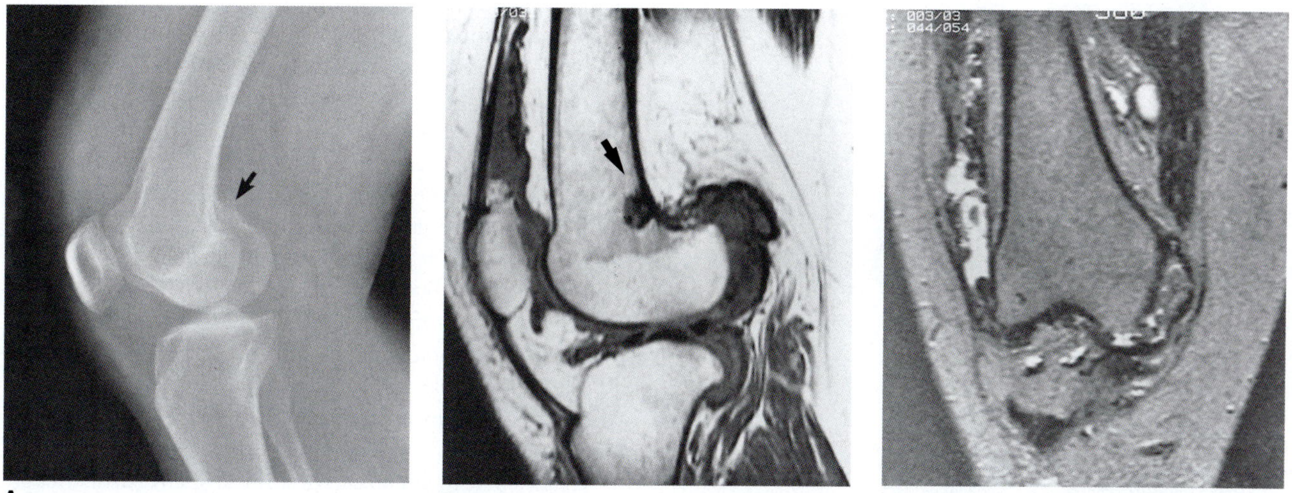

A B C

Figure 11.15 ■ MRI of pigmented villonodular synovitis. A 22-year-old woman had several episodes of knee pain and swelling. Bloody fluid was aspirated from the knee joint on two occasions. **A:** Lateral radiograph of the right knee shows fullness in the suprapatellar bursa that was interpreted as "joint effusion." Note also the increased density in the region of the popliteal fossa and subtle erosion of the posterior aspect of the distal femur (*arrow*). **B:** Sagittal MRI (SE; TR 800/TE 20 msec) shows a lobulated mass in the suprapatellar bursa, extending into the knee joint and invading the infrapatellar fat. Note also the lobulated mass in the posterior aspect of the joint capsule, extending toward the proximal tibia. These masses demonstrate an intermediate-to-low signal intensity. The erosion at the posterior aspect of the distal femur (supracondylar) is clearly demonstrated by an area of low signal intensity (*arrow*). **C:** Coronal MRI (SE; TR 1800/TE 80 msec) demonstrates areas of high signal intensity that represent fluid and congested synovium, interspersed with areas of intermediate-to-low signal intensity, characteristic of hemosiderin deposits.

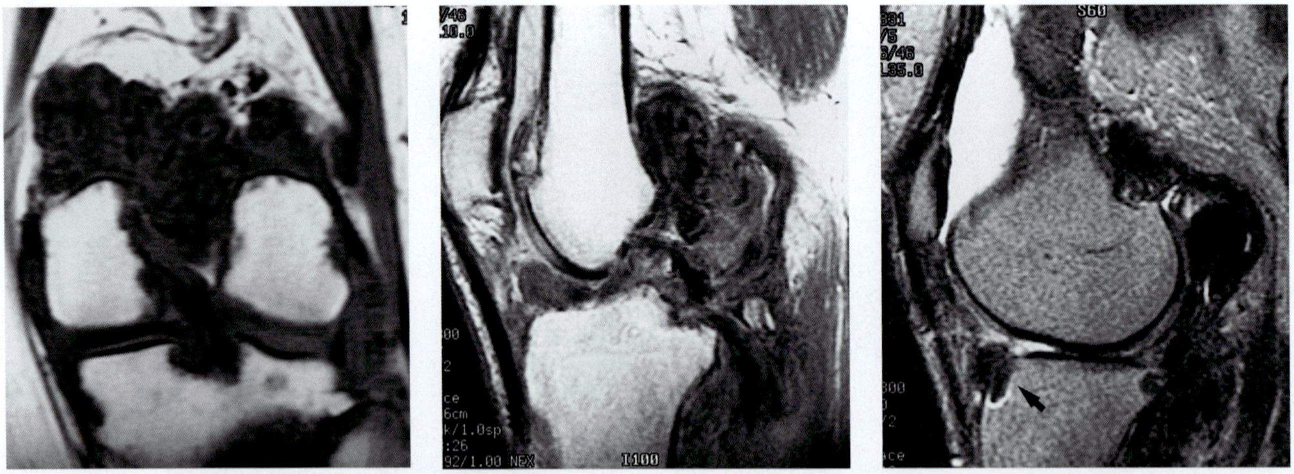

A B C

Figure 11.16 ■ **MRI of pigmented villonodular synovitis.** Coronal **(A)** and sagittal **(B)** T1-weighted MR images of the knee of a 40-year-old man show lobulated low–signal intensity masses mainly localized to the popliteal fossa. **C:** Sagittal T2-weighted MR image shows high-intensity fluid in the suprapatellar bursa. The lobulated masses of PVNS remain of low signal intensity. Note erosion of the anterior tibia (*arrow*).

Other MRI findings include hyperplastic synovium and occasionally bone erosions (see Figs. 11.15A,B and 11.16C). Administration of gadolinium in the form of Gd–DTPA leads to a notable increase in overall heterogeneity, which tends toward an overall increase in signal intensity of the capsule and septae. This enhancement of the synovium allows it to be differentiated from the fluid invariably present, which does not enhance (Fig. 11.18D). Apart from its diagnostic effectiveness, MRI is also useful in defining the extent of the disease.

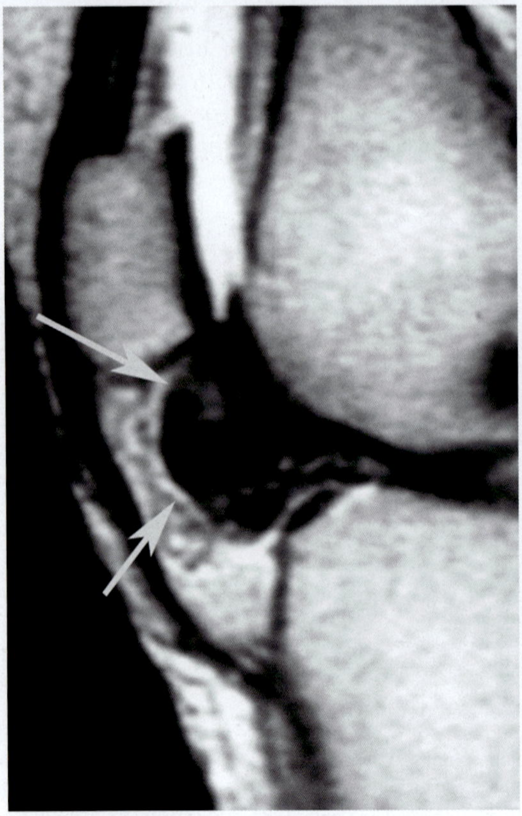

Figure 11.17 ■ **MRI of pigmented villonodular synovitis.** Sagittal T2-weighted MR image of the knee demonstrates a hypointense mass in the anterior aspect of the joint (*arrows*), consistent with hemosiderin deposition in a focal nodule of PVNS.

The most common differential diagnostic possibilities include *hemophilic arthropathy*, *synovial chondromatosis*, *synovial hemangioma*, and *synovial sarcoma*. MRI is very effective in distinguishing these entities because it can reveal hemosiderin deposition in PVNS. Although this feature may also be present in *hemophilic arthropathy*, detection of diffuse hemosiderin clumps, synovial irregularity and thickening, and distention of the synovial sac favors the diagnosis of PVNS. In addition, hemophilia, unlike PVNS, commonly affects multiple joints and is associated with growth disturbance at the articular ends of the affected bones. *Synovial chondromatosis* may manifest with pressure erosions of the bone similar to those of PVNS. However, it can be distinguished by the presence of multiple joint bodies, calcified or uncalcified. *Synovial hemangioma* is commonly associated with the formation of phleboliths. *Synovial sarcoma* tends to have a shorter T1 and longer T2 on MRI compared with PVNS, and when calcifications are present, the latter diagnosis can be excluded.

Treatment usually consists of surgical open or arthroscopic synovectomy. Occasionally, intra-articular radiation synovectomy is used when the abnormal synovial tissue is <5 mm thick. Recently, reports appeared of postsynovectomy adjuvant treatment with external beam radiation therapy or intra-articular injection of radioactive material such as yttrium-90 (^{90}Y). Local recurrence is not uncommon and is reported in ~50% of cases.

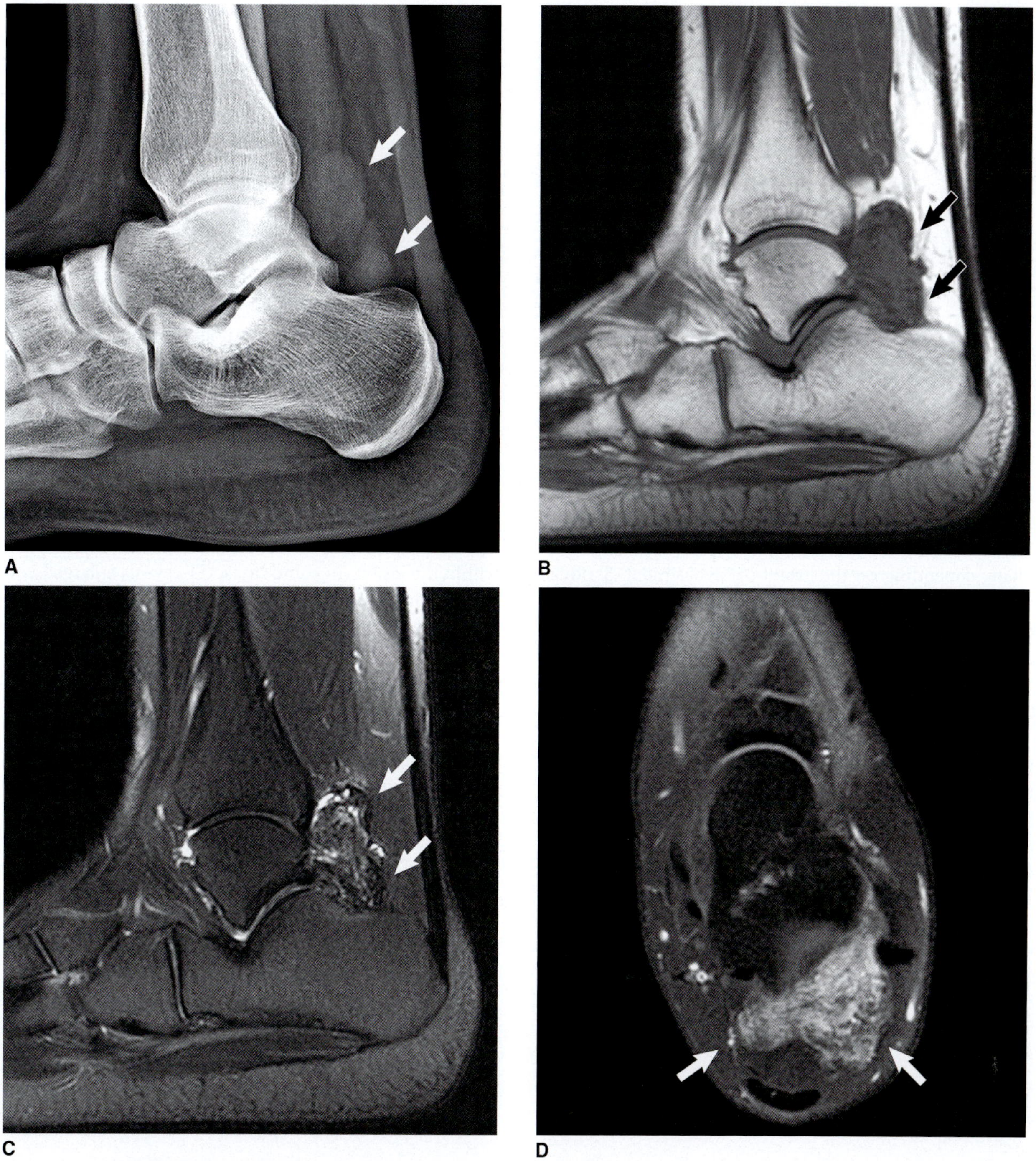

Figure 11.18 ■ **MRI of pigmented villonodular synovitis. A:** Lateral radiograph of the left ankle of an 18-year-old man shows a lobulated dense mass adjacent to the posterior talus and calcaneus, encroaching the Kager fat pad (*arrows*). **B:** Sagittal T1-weighted MR image shows the mass displaying intermediate-to-low signal intensity (*arrows*). **C:** Sagittal T2-weighted MR image shows the mass becoming heterogeneous but predominantly of intermediate signal intensity (*arrows*). Observe small foci of low signal intensity within the mass, representing hemosiderin deposition. **D:** Axial T1-weighted fat-suppressed MR image obtained after intravenous injection of gadolinium shows significant enhancement of the mass (*arrows*).

SYNOVIAL HEMANGIOMA

Synovial hemangioma is a rare benign lesion that most commonly affects the knee joint, usually involving the anterior compartment. This lesion has also been found in the elbow, wrist, and ankle joints, as well as in tendon sheaths. Most cases affect children and adolescents. Almost all patients with synovial hemangioma are symptomatic, frequently presenting with a swollen knee or with mild pain or limitation of movement in the joint. Sometimes, patients report a history of recurrent episodes of joint swelling and various degrees of pain of several years' duration. Synovial hemangioma is

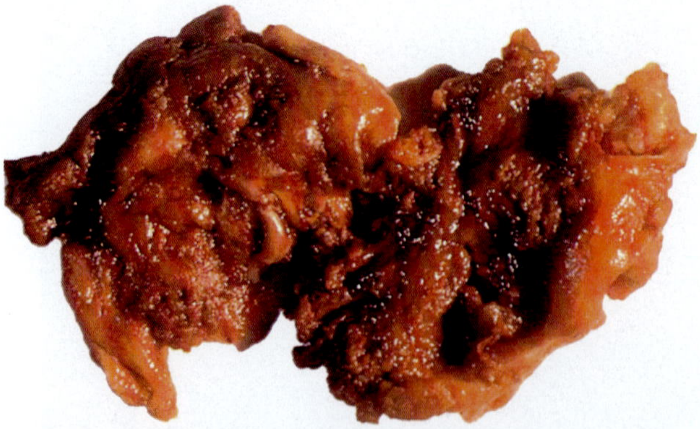

Figure 11.19 ■ Gross pathology of synovial hemangioma. Photograph of the surgical specimen removed from the knee of a patient with synovial hemangioma shows strawberry-like appearance of the synovial lining and marked hemosiderin staining of the tissue.

often associated with an adjacent cutaneous or deep soft tissue hemangioma. For this reason, some investigators classify knee joint lesions as intra-articular, juxta-articular, or intermediate, depending on the extent of involvement. Synovial hemangioma is frequently misdiagnosed. According to one estimate, a correct preoperative diagnosis is made in only 22% of cases.

Originating in the subsynovial layer mesenchyme of the synovial membrane, synovial hemangioma is a vascular lesion that contains variable amounts of adipose, fibrous, and muscle tissue, as well as thrombi in the vessels. When the lesion is completely intra-articular, it is usually well circumscribed and apparently encapsulated, attached to the synovial membrane by a pedicle of variable size, and adherent to the synovium on one or more surfaces by separable adhesions. Grossly, the tumor is a lobulated soft, brown, doughy mass with overlying villous synovium that is often stained mahogany brown by hemosiderin (Fig. 11.19). On microscopic examination, the lesion exhibits arborizing vascular channels of different sizes and a hyperplastic overlying synovium, which may show abundant iron deposition in chronic cases with repeated hemarthrosis (Fig. 11.20).

Until recently, synovial hemangiomas were evaluated by a combination of conventional radiography, arthrography, angiography, and contrast-enhanced CT. Although radiographs appear normal in at least half of the patients, they may reveal soft tissue swelling, a mass around the joint, joint effusion, or erosions (Fig. 11.21). Phleboliths, periosteal thickening, advanced maturation of the epiphysis, and arthritic changes are also occasionally noted on conventional radiographs. Arthrography usually shows nonspecific filling defects with a villous configuration. Angiograms yield much more specific information than radiography. They can often reveal a vascular lesion and can demonstrate pathognomonic features of hemangioma. Contrast-enhanced CT of the joint typically reveals a heterogeneous-appearing soft tissue mass that displays tissue attenuation approximating that of skeletal muscle and containing areas of decreased attenuation, some approaching that of fat. CT is effective for demonstrating phleboliths and revealing patchy enhancement around them, as well as enhancement of tubular areas and contrast pooling within the lesion. In some cases, CT reveals enlarged vessels feeding and draining the mass, as well as enlarged adjacent subcutaneous veins.

At present, MRI has become the modality of choice for the evaluation of hemangiomas because, with this modality, a presumptive diagnosis can be made. The soft tissue mass typically exhibits an intermediate signal intensity on T1-weighted sequences, appearing isointense with or slightly brighter than muscle but much less bright than fat. The mass is usually much brighter than subcutaneous fat on T2-weighted images and on fat suppression sequences (Figs. 11.22 to 11.24) and shows thin, often serpentine, low-intensity septa within it (Fig. 11.25). In general, the signal intensity characteristics of hemangiomas appear to be related to a number of factors, including slow flow, thrombosis, vessel occlusion, and stagnant blood that pools in larger vessels and dilated sinuses, as well as to the variable amounts of adipose tissue in the lesion. After intravenous

(Continued on page 390)

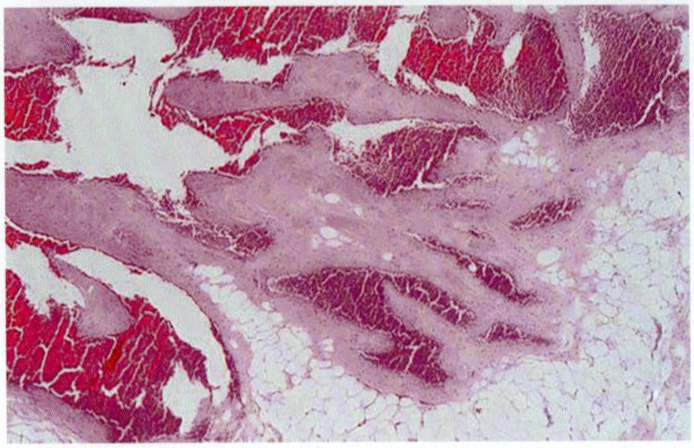

A

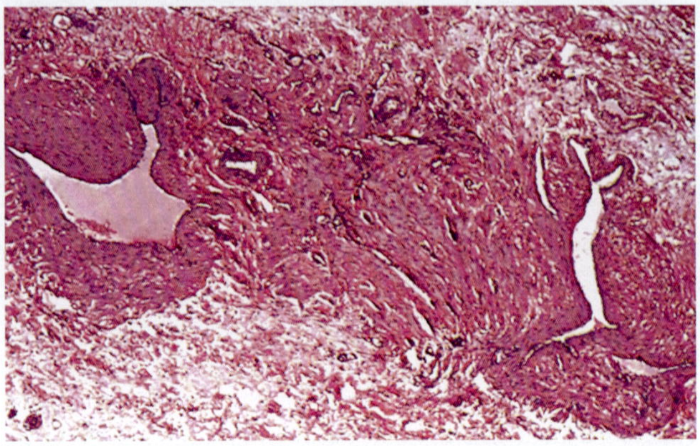

B

Figure 11.20 ■ Histopathology of synovial hemangioma. A: The lesion consists of a network of connected blood-filled spaces within the loose connective tissue of the synovium (H&E, original magnification ×12.5). **B:** Observe prominent vascular spaces, copious hemosiderin deposition, and hyperplastic reactive synovial tissue (H&E, original magnification ×10).

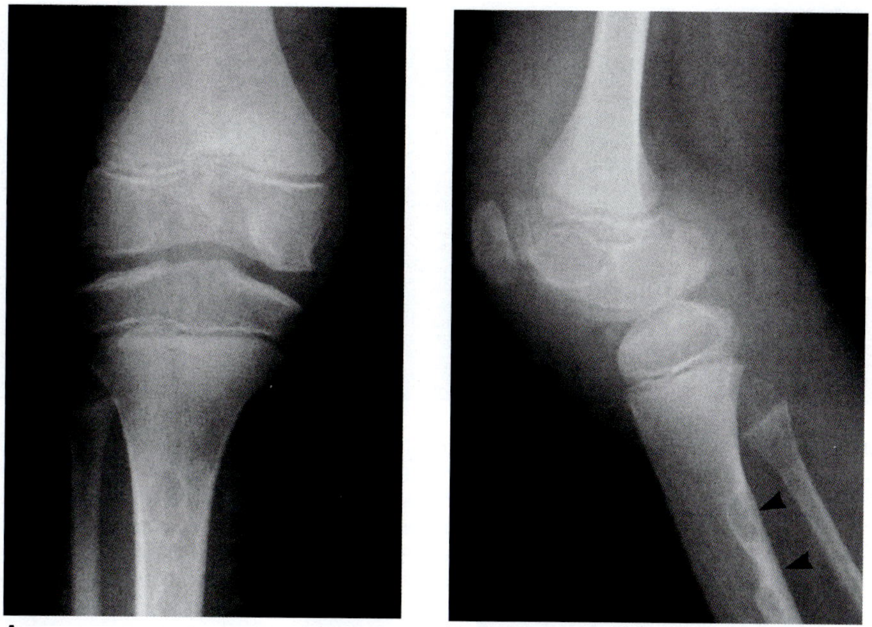

A B

Figure 11.21 ■ Synovial hemangioma. Anteroposterior **(A)** and lateral **(B)** radiographs of the right knee of a 7-year-old boy show articular erosions at femoropatellar and femorotibial joint compartments. Soft tissue masses are seen anteriorly and posteriorly. An incidental finding is a nonossifying fibroma in the posterior tibia (*arrowheads*).

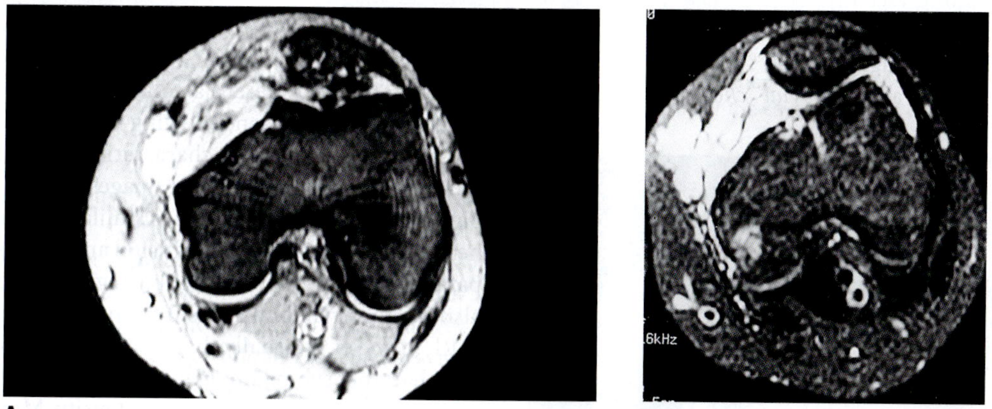

A B

Figure 11.22 ■ MRI of synovial hemangioma. Axial T2*-weighted (MPGR) **(A)** and axial fast spin-echo (FSE) fat-suppressed **(B)** MR images of the left knee of a 16-year-old girl show a large intra-articular lesion exhibiting high signal intensity.

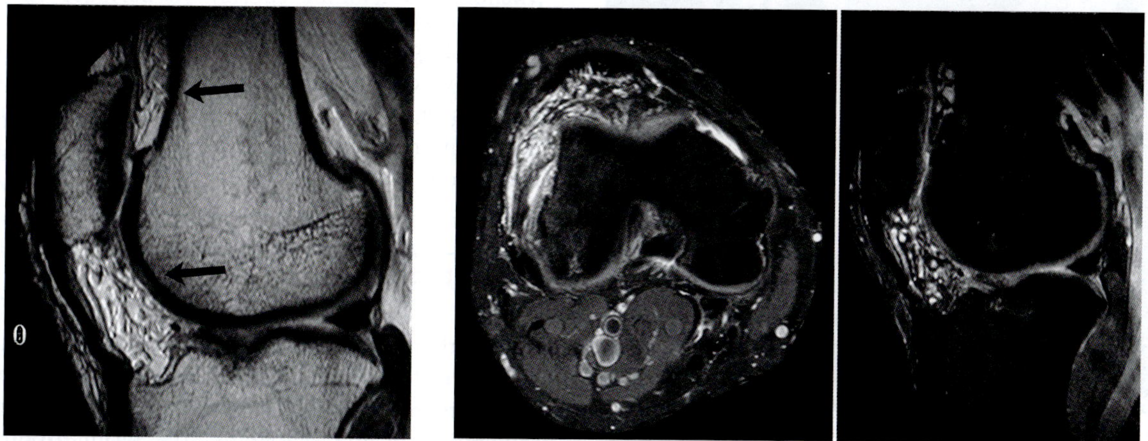

A B

Figure 11.23 ■ MRI of synovial hemangioma. A: Sagittal T1-weighted MR image of the knee of a 34-year-old man shows lacelike pattern of several vascular channels within the femoropatellar joint compartment and in the Hoffa fat pad (*arrows*) exhibiting high signal intensity. **B:** Axial and sagittal T2-weighted MR images confirm the presence of hemangiomas within the synovial membrane. Note the vascular structures exhibiting high signal intensity, separated by low-signal linear structures, representing fibrofatty septa.

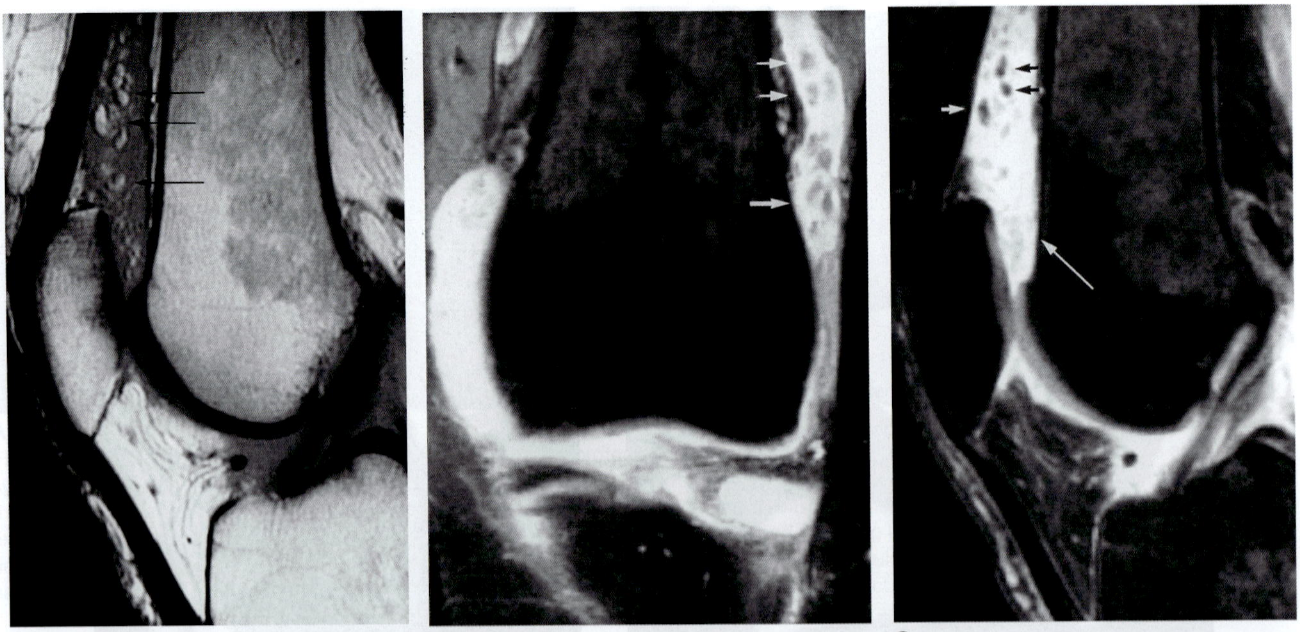

A B C

Figure 11.28 ■ MRI of lipoma arborescens. A 54-year-old woman reports fullness in the left knee for the past 5 months. Conventional radiography (not shown here) revealed knee joint effusion. **A:** Sagittal proton density MRI shows numerous structures within suprapatellar bursa exhibiting signal intensity consistent with fat (*arrows*). Coronal **(B)** and sagittal **(C)** T2-weighted fat-suppressed images demonstrate high–signal intensity joint effusion (*long arrow*). Hypertrophic synovial villa (*short arrows*) again shows signal consistent with fat.

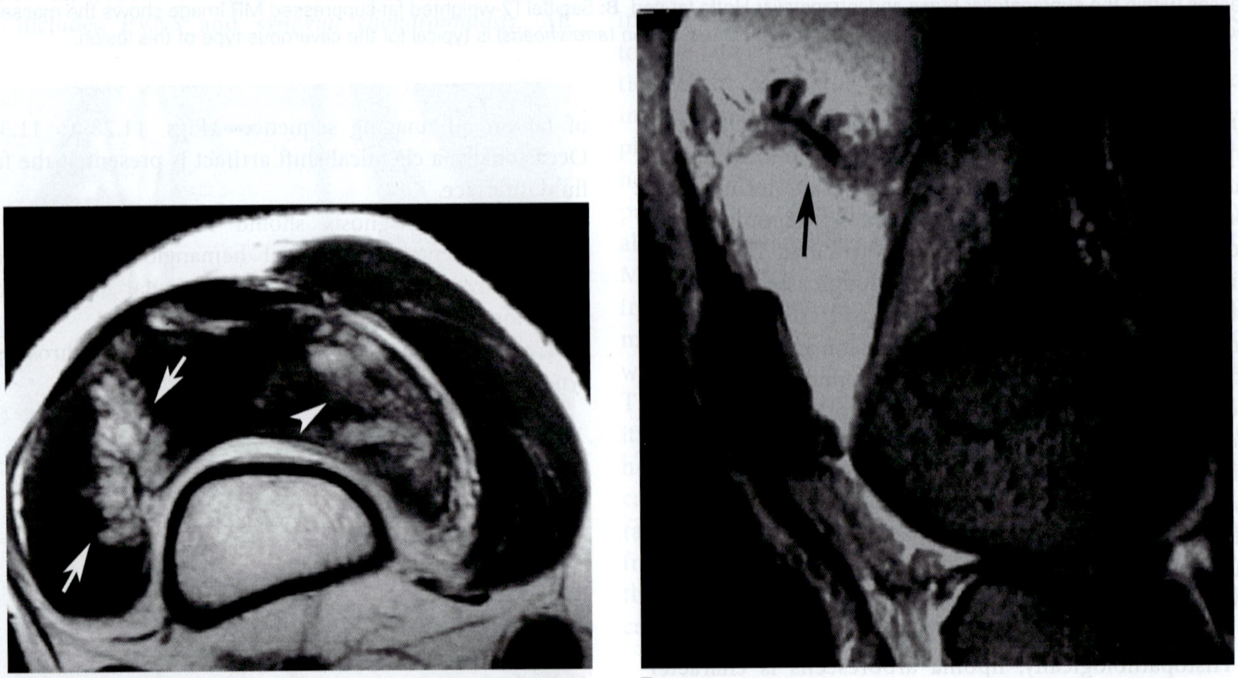

A B

Figure 11.29 ■ MRI of lipoma arborescens. A: Axial T1-weighted MRI demonstrates an intra-articular "treelike" lipomatous mass in the fluid-distended suprapatellar recess (*arrows*). Note additional intra-articular lipomatous growths in the medial aspect of the suprapatellar recess (*arrowhead*). **B:** Sagittal T2-weighted MRI demonstrates the "treelike" lipoma arborescens in the suprapatellar recess (*arrow*).

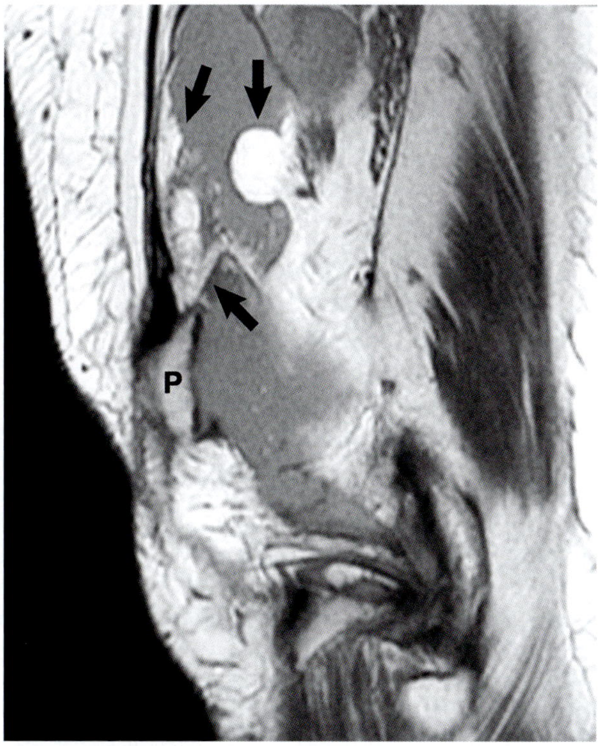

A

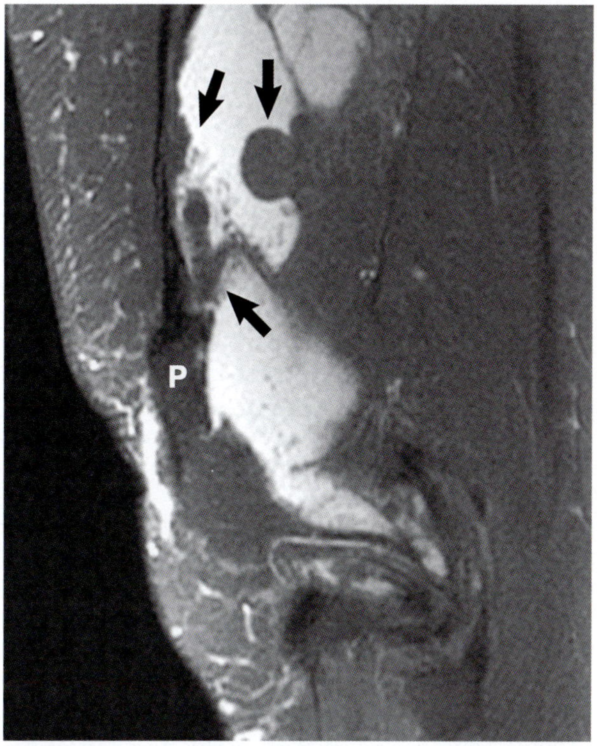

B

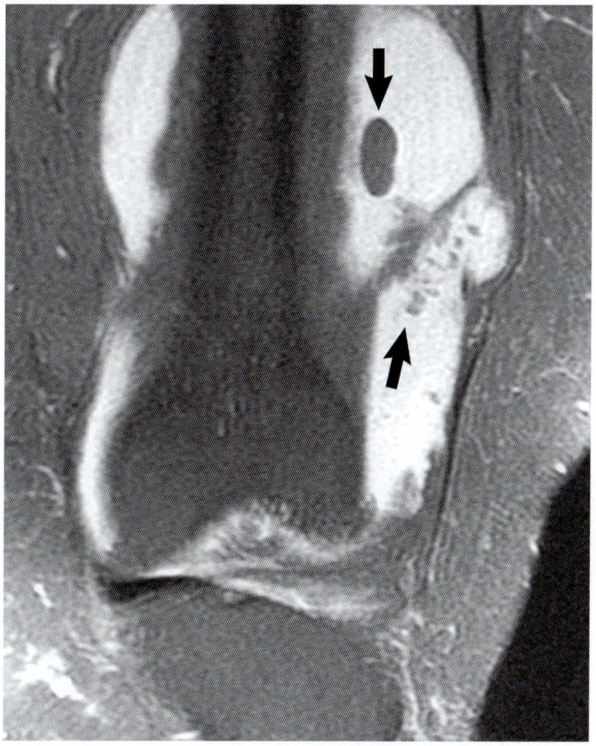

C

Figure 11.30 ■ MRI of lipoma arborescens. A: Sagittal T1-weighted MR image of the left knee of a 60-year-old woman shows high–signal intensity masses (*arrows*) identical in appearance to subcutaneous fat. On sagittal **(B)** and coronal **(C)** proton density-weighted fat-suppressed MR images the masses become of intermediate signal (*arrows*), again following the appearance of subcutaneous fat. P, patella.

JUXTA-ARTICULAR MYXOMA

Juxta-articular myxoma is a rare, benign soft tissue lesion arising close to the large joints such as the knee and the elbow. Shoulder, ankle, and hip joints are less commonly affected. Age of the patients range from 16 to 83 years, with median age of 43 years. Men are more commonly affected than women. Clinical findings are not specific and include the presence of a palpable and painful mass. Histopathologically, the mass resembles cellular form of intramuscular myxoma and is composed of bland-appearing spindle ells embedded in a hypovascular myxoid matrix (Fig. 11.31A). Increased cellularity may be present, but mitotic figures are absent or very rare. Cystic or ganglion-like spaces lined by layer of delicate fibrin or thick collagen are often present (Fig. 11.31B). Immunohistochemistry shows positivity for CD34, vimentin, and actin. Genetics show lack of mutations of the *GNAS1* gene, in contrast to intramuscular myxoma.

Imaging features of the lesion are not specific. MRI shows the mass to be either isointense or slightly brighter than muscles on T1-weighted sequences and of homogeneously high signal intensity on T2 weighting. After intravenous administration of gadolinium, the mass shows heterogeneous enhancement.

Local recurrence after surgical resection was reported in about 34% of cases.

DYSPLASIA EPIPHYSEALIS HEMIMELICA (TREVOR-FAIRBANK DISEASE)

This is a developmental disorder characterized by asymmetric cartilaginous overgrowth of one or more epiphyses in the lower extremity, with a decided preference for the distal

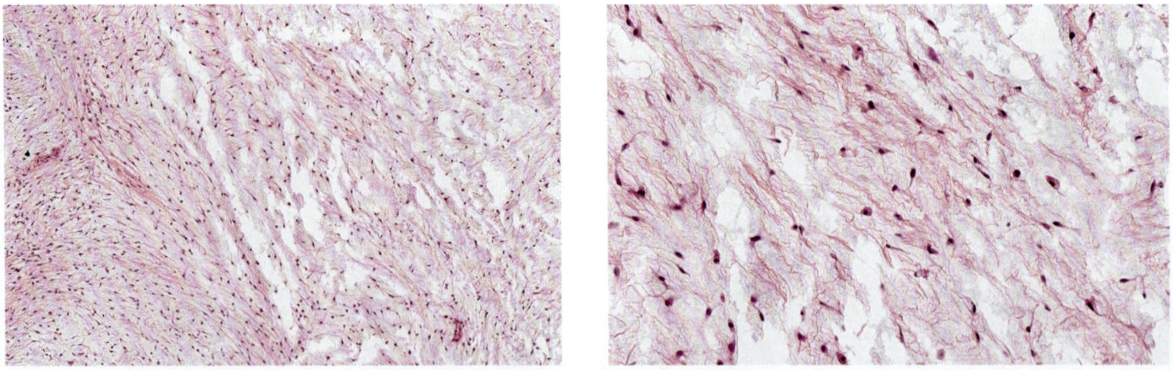

A B

Figure 11.31 ■ Histopathology of juxta-articular myxoma. A: Bland-appearing spindle cells are embedded in hypovascular myxoid stroma (H&E, original magnification ×50). **B:** High-power photomicrograph shows various in size cystic spaces between the sheets of spindle cells (H&E, original magnification ×200).

tibial epiphysis and the talus. The lesion is characteristically found on one side of the affected limb, hence the name *hemimelica*. Moucher and Belot in 1926 reported the first case and used the term *tarsomegalie*. Trevor in 1950 reviewed 10 cases and used the term *tarsoepiphyseal aclasis*. Finally, in 1956, Fairbank reported 14 cases and coined the term *dysplasia epiphysealis hemimelica*. Its cause is unknown, and there is no definite familial or hereditary predilection. Males are affected three times as often as females. Pathologically, the lesion shows similarity to an osteochondroma, and for this reason, it is occasionally referred to as *epiphyseal* or *intra-articular osteochondroma*. Clinically, there is deformity and restricted motion of the affected joint, and pain, particularly around the ankle, is the most frequent presenting symptom in adults. A diagnosis can be established through radiographic and MRI examination. The lesion typically presents as an irregular, bulbous overgrowth of the ossification center or epiphysis on one side, resembling an osteochondroma (Figs. 11.32 to 11.34). Occasionally, the other ossifications centers, particularly at the knee, may be similarly affected in the same patient. Treatment for this condition is individualized according to the amount of deformity and pain; usually, surgical resection of the lesion is required. Recurrences are common.

(Continued on page 396)

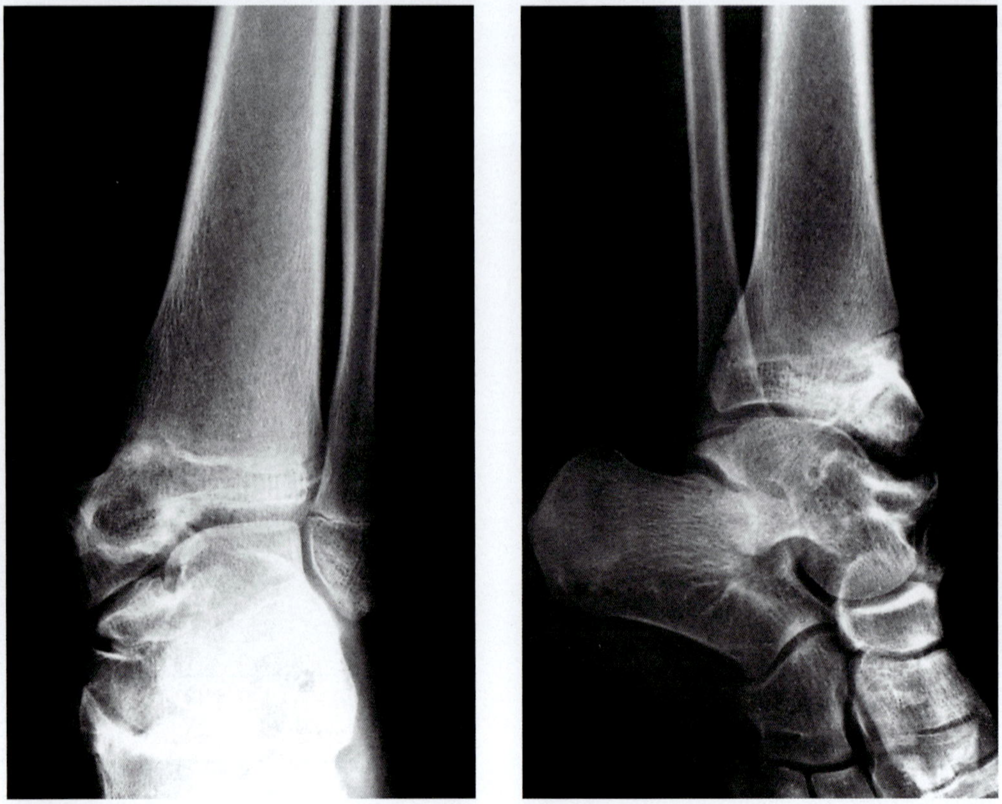

A B

Figure 11.32 ■ Trevor–Fairbank disease. A 12-year-old girl presented with pain and limitation of motion in the ankle joint. Anteroposterior **(A)** and lateral **(B)** radiographs of the ankle demonstrate deformity and enlargement of the medial malleolus, talus, and navicular bone, features typical of dysplasia epiphysealis hemimelica. Note that the growth disturbance is limited to the medial side of the ankle and foot.

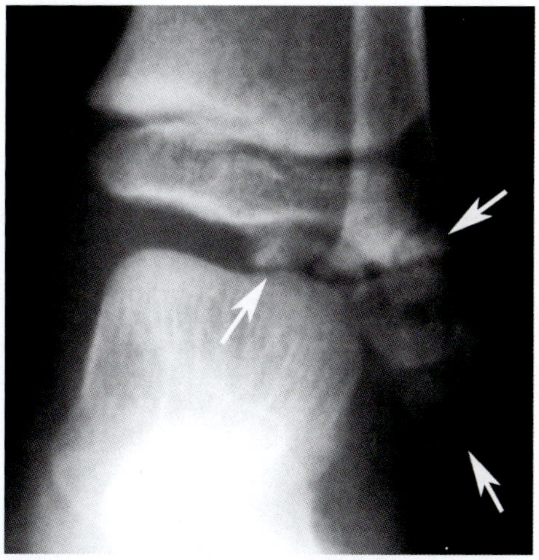

A

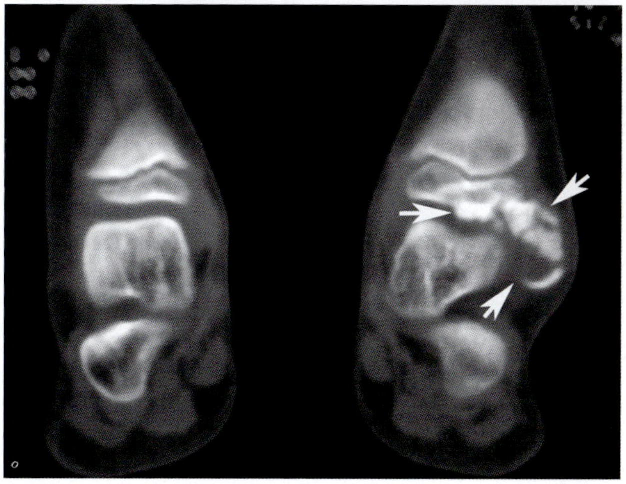

B

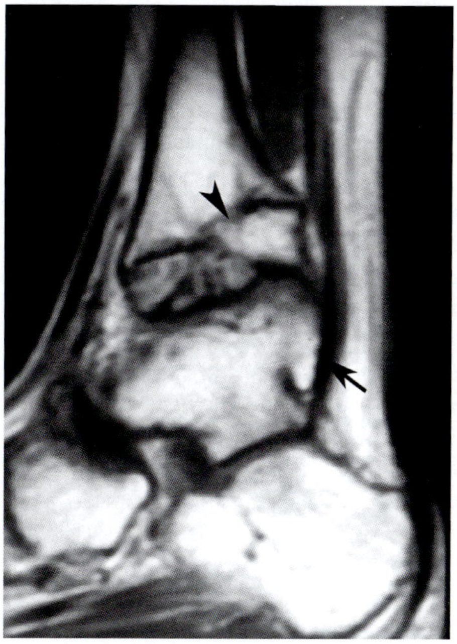

C

Figure 11.33 ■ **CT and MRI of Trevor–Fairbank disease.** **A:** Anteroposterior radiograph of the left ankle of a 7-year-old boy demonstrates an osteochondroma-like mass originated in the distal tibial epiphysis, with intra-articular extension (*arrows*). **B:** Coronal CT of bilateral ankles confirms the origin of the tumor-like excrescence from the distal tibial epiphysis and demonstrates the intra-articular component (*arrows*). Note the deformed and expanded medial malleolus and the chondroid-type calcifications. **C:** Sagittal T1-weighted MRI of the ankle in another patient with Trevor–Fairbank disease demonstrates the osteochondroma originating from the posterior aspect of the talar dome (*arrow*). Note the remodeling deformity of the distal tibial epiphysis (*arrowhead*).

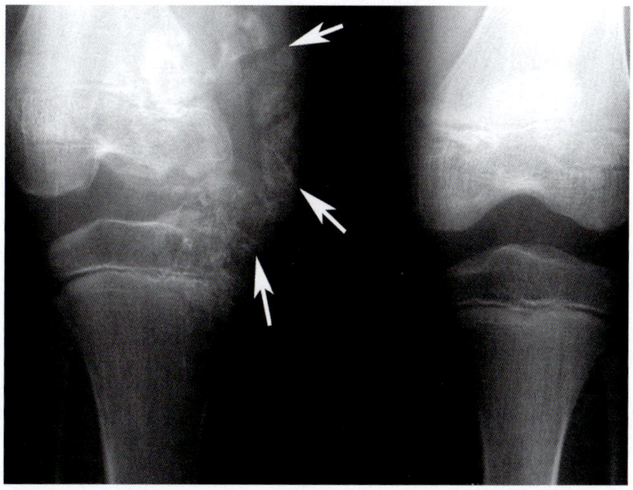

A

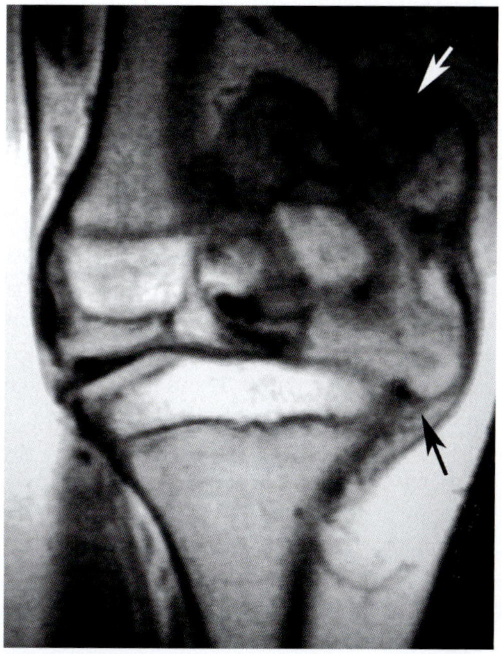

B

Figure 11.34 ■ **MRI of Trevor–Fairbank disease.** **A:** Anteroposterior radiograph of the knees demonstrates a calcified cartilaginous mass extending from the medial epicondyle and medial metaphysis of the right femur to the medial proximal tibial epiphysis (*arrows*). **B:** Coronal T1-weighted MRI of the right knee confirms the extent of involvement of the tumor, "bridging" from the femur to the tibia (*arrows*).

OSTEOID OSTEOMA

Osteoid osteoma is a benign osteoblastic lesion characterized by a nidus of osteoid tissue, which may be purely radiolucent or have a sclerotic center. The nidus has limited growth potential and usually measures <1 cm in diameter. It is often surrounded by a zone of reactive bone formation. Depending on its location in the particular part of the bone, the lesion can be classified as cortical, medullary (cancellous), or subperiosteal. Osteoid osteomas can be further subclassified as extracapsular or intracapsular (intra-articular). These lesions occur in the young, usually between the ages of 10 and 35 years, and their sites of predilection are the long bones, particularly the femur and tibia. Cytogenetic analysis performed in a few cases of this lesion reveled chromosomal alterations involving chromosome 22 [del(22)(q13.1)]. The most important clinical symptom of osteoid osteoma is pain that is more severe at night and is dramatically relieved by salicylates (aspirin) within ~20 to 25 minutes. This typical history holds in more than 75% of cases and serves as an important clue to the diagnosis. It is the intra-articular (intracapsular) location of the lesion that may create a problem in diagnosis and occasionally may be mistaken for arthritis. Moreover, as Norman and associated have pointed out, the intra-articular lesions may result in arthritis of precocious onset. This latter complication may serve as an important diagnostic clue to an osteoid osteoma when a typical history of the condition is elicited from the patient, but the imaging studies may fail to demonstrate the nidus (Fig. 11.35).

Standard radiographs usually demonstrate the lesion, but CT is required to localize it precisely (Figs. 11.36 and 11.37). This technique also has the added advantage of allowing exact measurement of the size of the nidus. Frequently, when the lesion cannot be demonstrated radiographically, a radionuclide bone scan is helpful, because osteoid osteoma invariably shows a marked increase in isotope uptake. This modality can be particularly helpful in cases for which the symptoms are atypical and the initial radiographs appear normal. Radionuclide tracer activity can be observed on both immediate and delayed images.

The suitability of magnetic resonance imaging (MRI) for the detection of osteoid osteoma remains unclear, and published reports have shown mixed results. Goldman and associates reported on four cases of intracapsular osteoid osteoma of the femoral neck, in which the lesions were evaluated with bone scintigraphy, CT, and MRI. Although in all cases abnormal findings were apparent in the MR images, the nidi could not be identified prospectively. On the basis of MRI findings of secondary bone marrow edema or synovitis, several incorrect diagnoses were made, which included Ewing sarcoma, osteonecrosis, stress fracture, and juvenile idiopathic arthritis. In these cases, it is noteworthy that the correct diagnoses were made only after review of the radiographs and thin-section CT studies. However, some reports do suggest the effectiveness of MRI for demonstrating the nidus of osteoid osteoma. For example, Bell and colleagues clearly demonstrated an intracortical nidus on MRI that had not been seen on scintigraphy, angiography, or CT scans. In

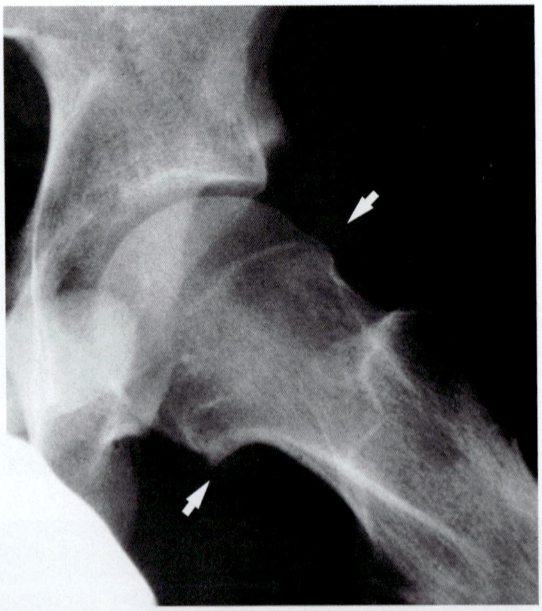

Figure 11.35 ■ Intra-articular osteoid osteoma. A 14-year-old boy presented with pain in the left hip for 8 months; it was more severe at night and was relieved by aspirin within 15 to 20 minutes. Several imaging studies (not shown here) including CT had failed to demonstrate the nidus. On the frog-lateral radiograph of the left hip, no nidus is seen, only periarticular osteoporosis and early osteoarthritic changes in form of osteophyte formation (*arrows*), both presumptive features of osteoid osteoma.

particular, imaging of osteoid osteoma with dynamic gadolinium-enhanced MR technique demonstrated greater conspicuity in detecting the lesion than with nonenhanced MRI.

Gross pathologic specimen shows red, hypervascular well-circumscribed nidus surrounded by sclerotic bone (Fig. 11.38). Histologically, the nidus is composed of osteoid or mineralized immature bone. It is a small, well-circumscribed, and self-limited lesion. Its microtrabeculae and irregular islets of osteoid matrix and bone are surrounded by a richly vascular fibrous stroma in which osteoblastic and osteoclastic activities are often prominent. The perilesional sclerosis is composed of dense bone displaying a variety of maturation patterns (Fig. 11.39).

The treatment of osteoid osteoma consists of complete en bloc resection of the nidus. The resected specimen and the involved bone should be radiographed promptly so as to exclude the possibility of incomplete resection, which can lead to recurrence. A variety of techniques other than en bloc excision have been tried, among them intralesional curettage, excision with trephines after surgical exposure, fluoroscopically guided or CT-guided percutaneous extraction, and percutaneous radiofrequency thermal ablation (RFTA). The latter technique, as suggested by Rosenthal and colleagues, is a promising alternative to surgery in selected patients. It is performed through a small radiofrequency electrode that is introduced into the lesion through the biopsy track with CT guidance to produce thermal necrosis of an ~1-cm sphere of tissue. Several recent reports of successful RFTA of osteoid osteoma confirmed the belief that this technique is an effective method of noninvasive treatment of these lesions.

(*Continued on page 398*)

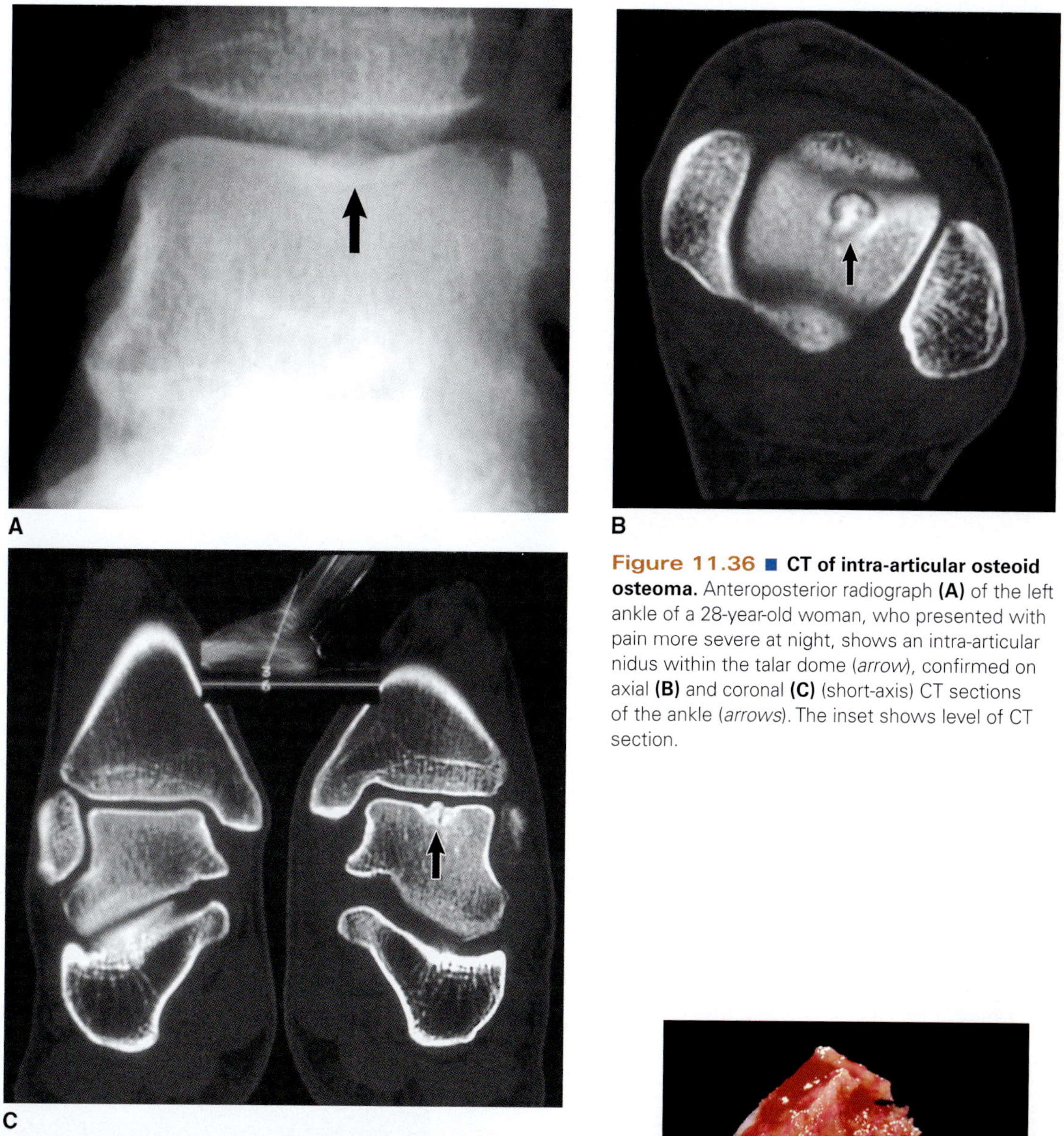

Figure 11.36 ■ **CT of intra-articular osteoid osteoma.** Anteroposterior radiograph **(A)** of the left ankle of a 28-year-old woman, who presented with pain more severe at night, shows an intra-articular nidus within the talar dome (*arrow*), confirmed on axial **(B)** and coronal **(C)** (short-axis) CT sections of the ankle (*arrows*). The inset shows level of CT section.

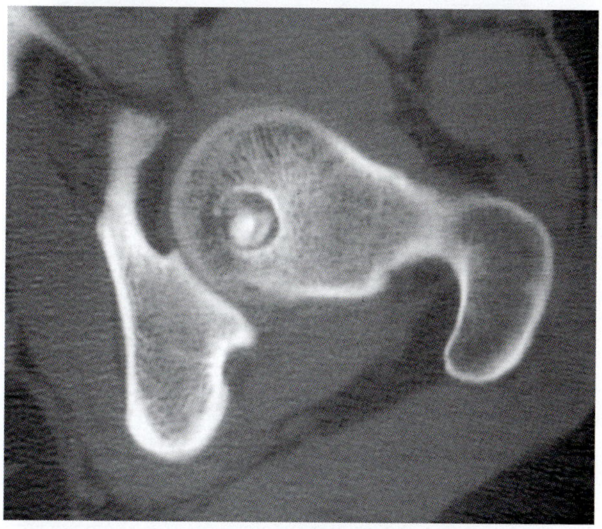

Figure 11.37 ■ **CT of intra-articular osteoid osteoma.** Axial CT section of the left hip of a 20-year-old man shows a low-attenuation lesion with sclerotic center within the femoral head.

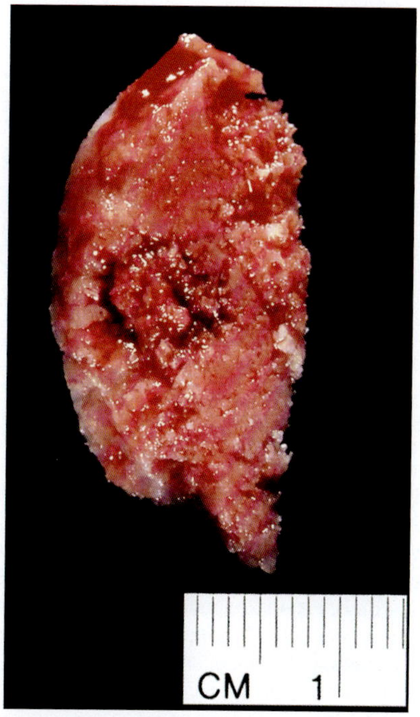

Figure 11.38 ■ **Gross pathology of osteoid osteoma.** The surgical specimen shows red, gritty, round well-circumscribed nidus that exhibits hypervascular zone with surrounding sclerotic rim.

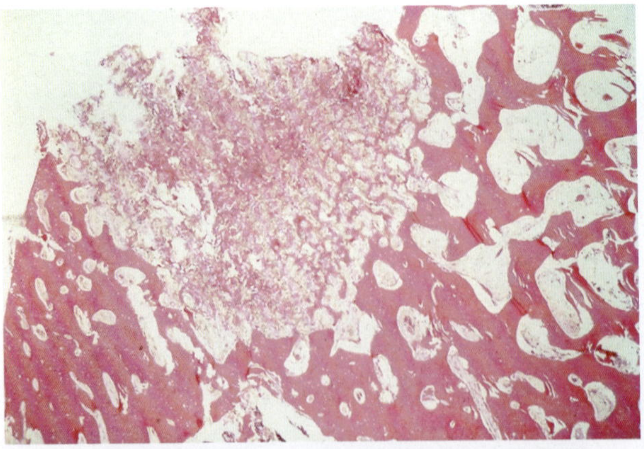

A

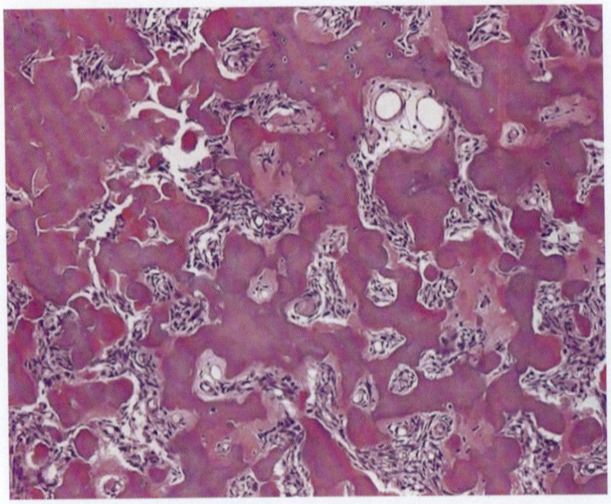

B

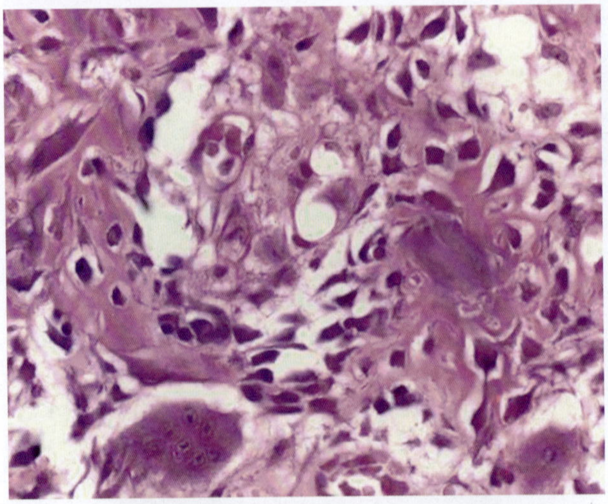

C

Figure 11.39 ■ Histopathology of osteoid osteoma. **A:** Low-power photomicrograph shows a well-demarcated nidus composed of anastomosing bone trabeculae and immature woven bone (center), surrounded by sclerotic reactive bone (H&E, original magnification ×6). **B:** Higher magnification of the center of the nidus shows interconnected, ossified bone trabeculae within areas of vascularized connective tissue, and osteoblastic activity (H&E, original magnification ×100). **C:** High-power photomicrograph of the nidus shows bone trabeculae rimmed by osteoblasts (H&E, original magnification ×400).

CHONDROBLASTOMA

Also known as a Codman tumor, chondroblastoma, representing <1% of all primary bone tumors, is a benign lesion occurring before skeletal maturity, characteristically presenting in the epiphyses of long bones such as the humerus, tibia, and femur. Occasionally, the patella, which is considered equivalent to an epiphysis, is affected. Although the lesion is usually seen in growing bones, some cases have been reported after obliteration of the growth plate. Chondroblastoma is usually located eccentrically, shows a sclerotic border, and often demonstrates scattered calcifications of the matrix (25% of cases) (Fig. 11.40). Brower and colleagues noticed a distinctively

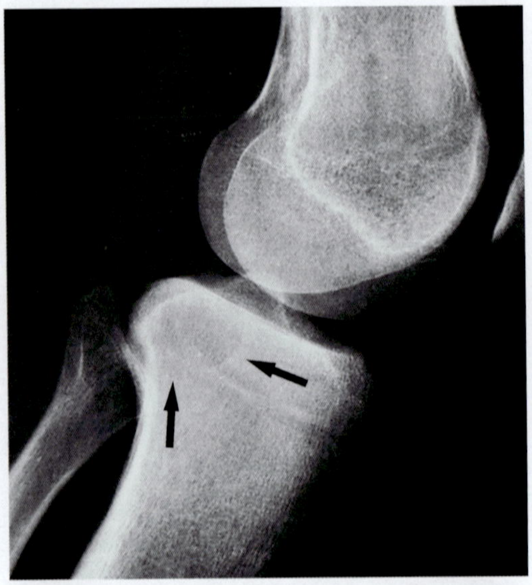

A

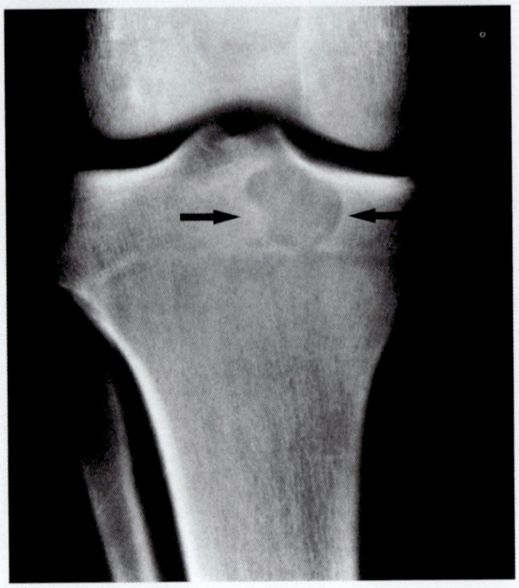

B

Figure 11.40 ■ Chondroblastoma. Lateral radiograph **(A)** and anteroposterior conventional tomogram **(B)** of the right knee of a 15-year-old girl show the typical appearance of this tumor in the proximal epiphysis of the tibia. Note the radiolucent, eccentrically located lesion with a thin sclerotic margin (*arrows*). There are small, scattered calcifications in the center of the lesion.

thick, solid periosteal reaction distal to the lesion in 57% of chondroblastomas in long bones. This most likely represents an inflammatory reaction to the tumor. In most cases, radiography suffices to demonstrate the lesion, but CT scan can help demonstrate the calcifications if they are not visible on the standard radiographs (Fig. 11.41). MRI usually reveals a larger area of involvement than can be seen on radiography, including regional bone marrow and soft tissue edema (Fig. 11.42).

(Continued on page 401)

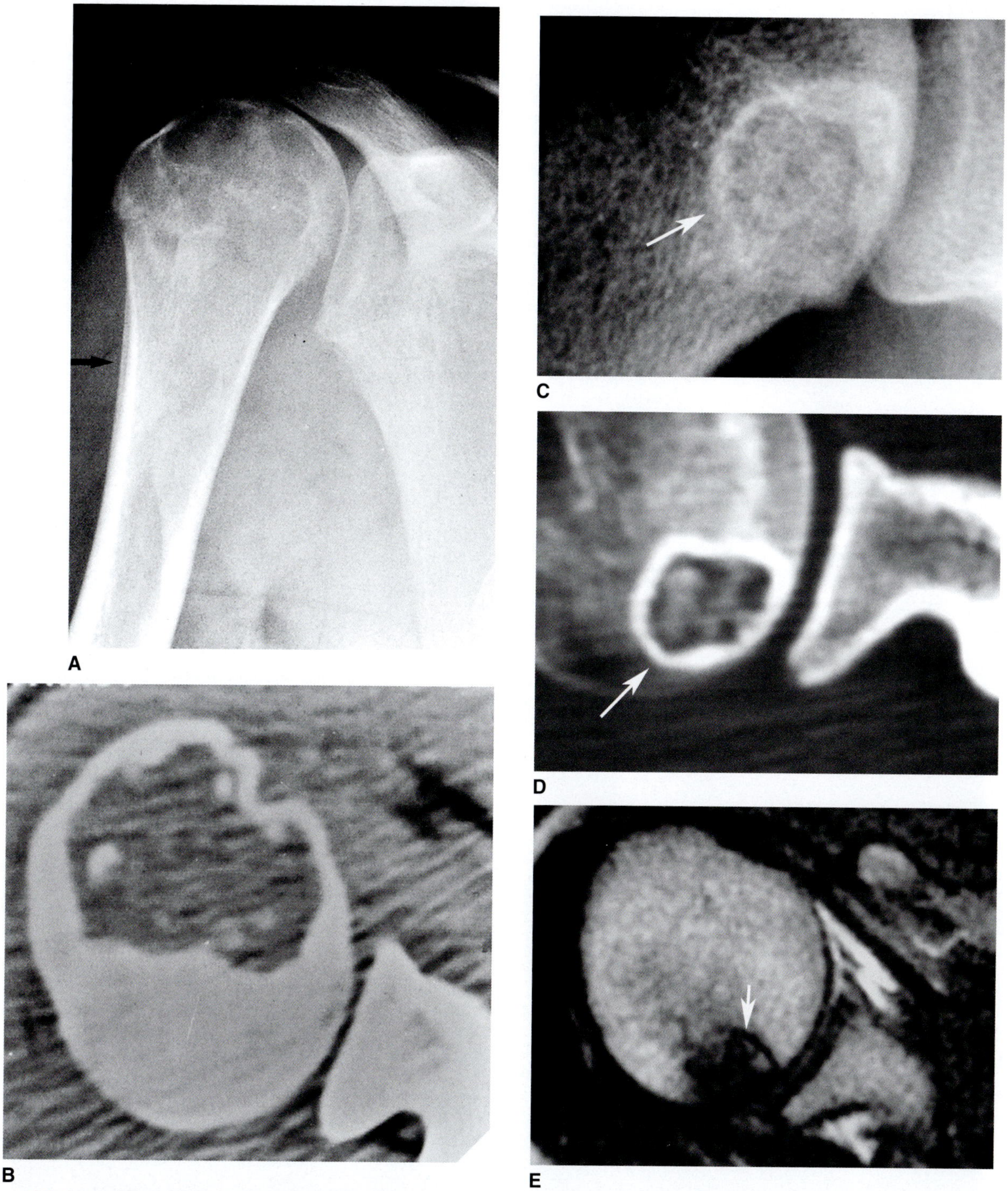

Figure 11.41 ■ **CT and MRI of chondroblastoma. A:** Anteroposterior radiograph of the right shoulder of a 16-year-old boy shows a lesion in the proximal humeral epiphysis, but calcifications are not well demonstrated. Note the well-organized layer of periosteal reaction at the lateral cortex (*arrow*). **B:** CT section shows the calcifications clearly. The tumor was removed by curettage, and a histopathologic examination confirmed the radiographic diagnosis of chondroblastoma. **C:** Anteroposterior radiograph of the shoulder in another patient demonstrates a well-demarcated lesion in the epiphysis of the humerus with a sclerotic rim (*arrow*) and internal calcifications. **D:** Axial CT image shows the sclerotic rim (*arrow*) and chondral calcifications inside the lesion. **E:** Axial T2-weighted MRI demonstrates the tumor (*arrow*) containing low–signal intensity calcified chondral matrix.

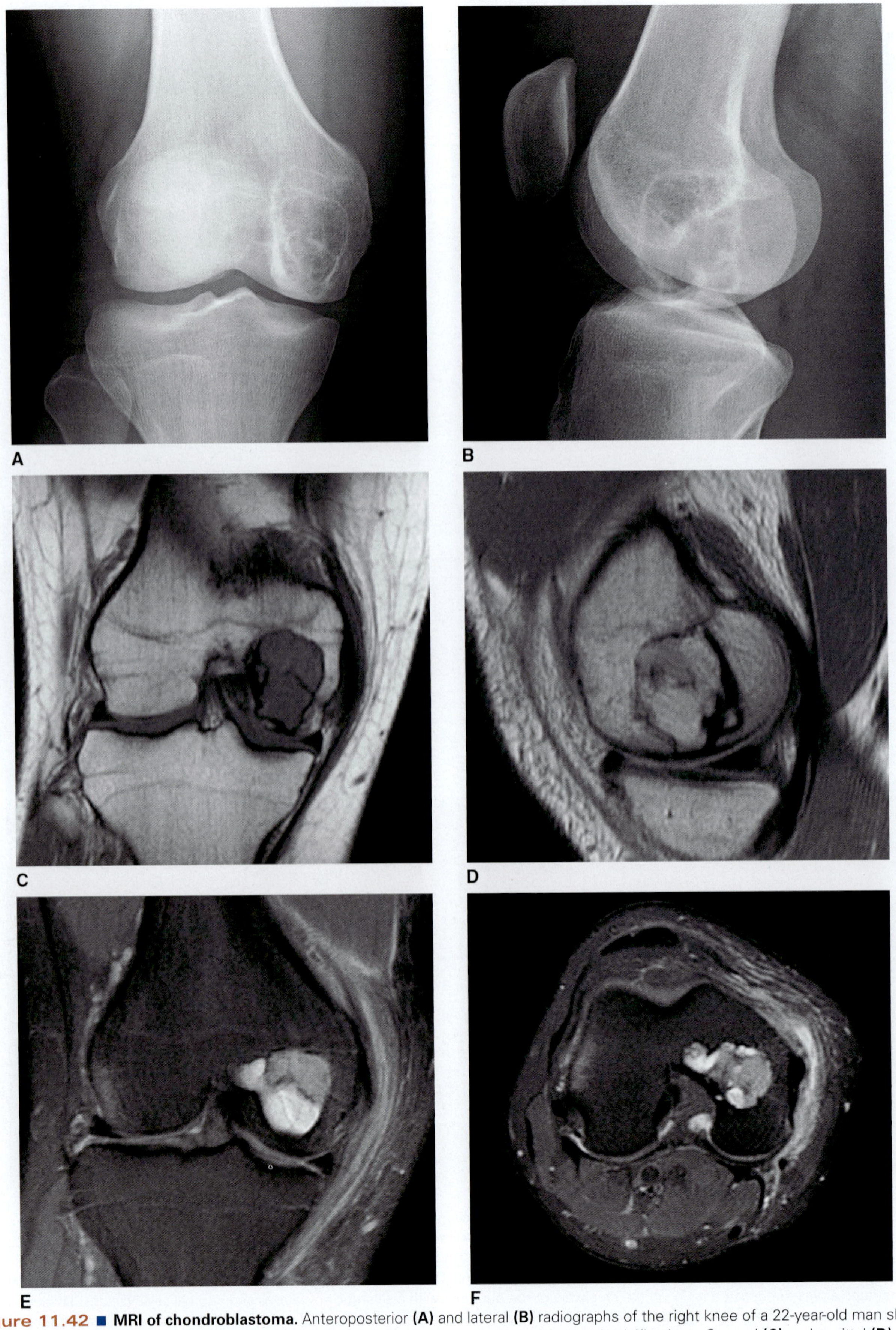

Figure 11.42 ■ **MRI of chondroblastoma.** Anteroposterior **(A)** and lateral **(B)** radiographs of the right knee of a 22-year-old man show a radiolucent lesion within the medial femoral condyle exhibiting sclerotic border and central calcifications. Coronal **(C)** and sagittal **(D)** T1-weighted MR images show the tumor displaying intermediate signal intensity. The sclerotic margin is of low signal intensity. Coronal **(E)** and axial **(F)** fat-suppressed T2-weighted MR images demonstrate heterogeneous but predominantly high signal intensity in the lesion.

Histologically, chondroblastoma is composed of nodules of fairly mature cartilage matrix surrounded by a highly cellular tissue containing uniformly large round cells with ovoid nuclei and clear cytoplasm. Multinucleated osteoclast-like giant cells are a common finding. The matrix shows characteristic lattice-like fine calcifications surrounding apposing chondroblasts, having a spatial arrangement resembling the hexagonal configuration of chicken wire (Fig. 11.43).

Clonal abnormalities in chondroblastoma have been reported, including recurrent structural alterations in chromosomes 5 and 8 with rearrangements of band 8q21 and recurrent breakpoints at 2q35, 3q21-q23, and 18q21.

Chondroblastomas are usually treated by curettage and bone grafting. Only few reported cases have been treated with percutaneous radiofrequency ablation.

In rare cases, pulmonary metastases develop in the absence of any histologic evidence of malignancy in either the primary bone tumor or the pulmonary lesions. Only in exceptional circumstances, pulmonary or widespread metastases led to patient death.

GIANT CELL TUMOR

Also known as osteoclastoma, a GCT of bone is an aggressive lesion characterized by richly vascularized tissue containing proliferating mononuclear stromal cells and numerous uniformly distributed giant cells of osteoclast type. It represents ~5% to 8.6% of all primary bone tumors and ~23% of benign bone tumors; it is the sixth most common primary osseous neoplasm. Sixty percent of these lesions occur in long bones, and almost all are localized to the articular end of the bone. Preferred sites include the proximal tibia, distal femur, distal radius, and proximal humerus. Giant cell tumors are seen almost exclusively after skeletal maturity, when the growth plate is obliterated. Most patients are between ages 20 and 40 years, and there is a female predominance of 2:1.

Clinical symptoms in patients with solitary lesions are nonspecific. They include pain (usually reduced by rest), local swelling, and limitation of range of motion in the adjacent joint and occasionally may mimic arthritis.

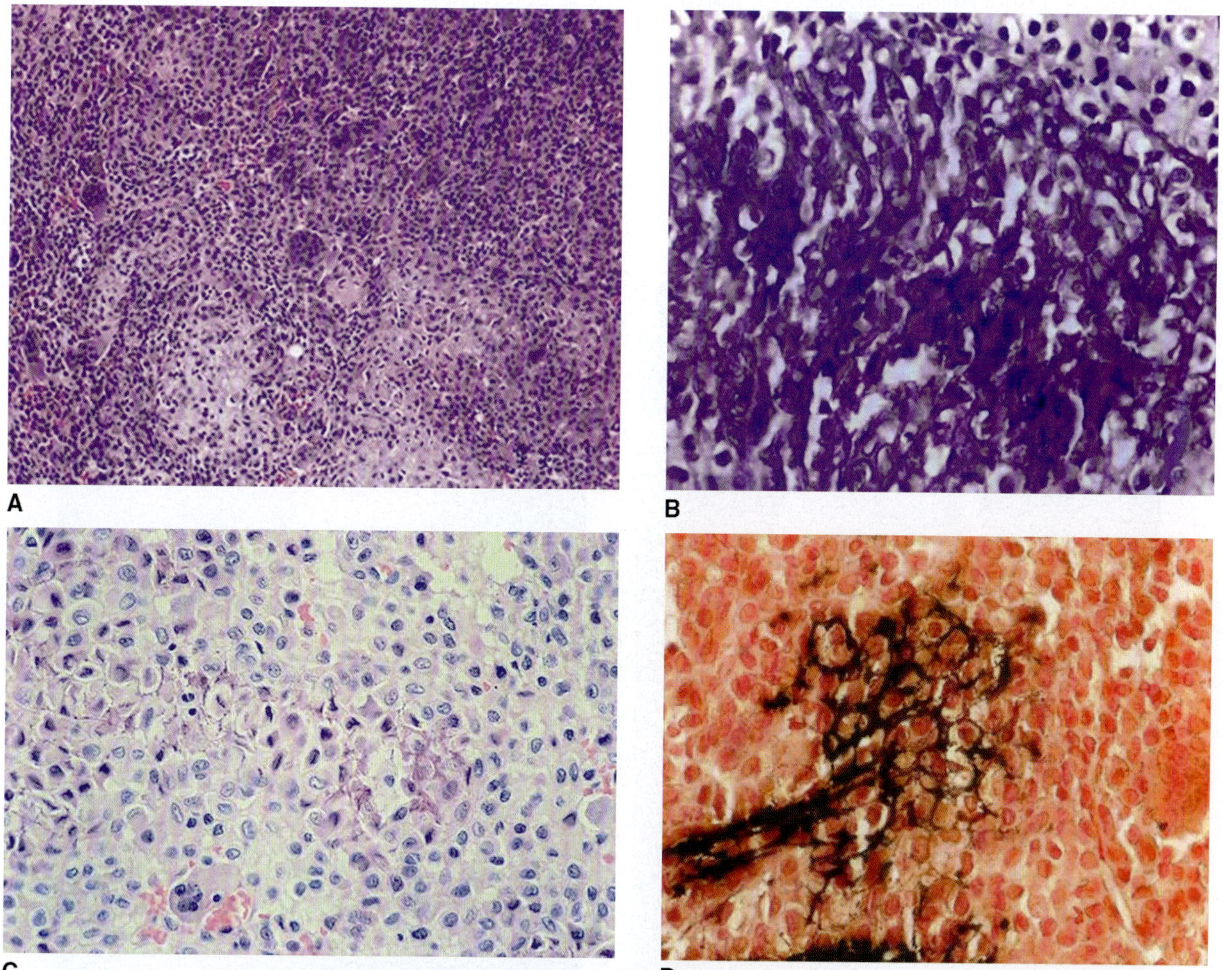

A B C D

Figure 11.43 ■ Histopathology of chondroblastoma. A: Densely cellular tissue is composed of admixture of mononuclear chondroblasts and multinucleated osteoclast-type giant cells (H&E, original magnification ×100). **B:** Higher magnification shows poorly formed primitive cartilaginous matrix with intercellular calcifications in form of chicken wire (H&E, original magnification ×200). **C:** The chondrocytes, some with ovoid and some with elongated nuclei, are embedded in cartilaginous matrix. Surrounding the cells are fine intercellular calcifications, forming chicken wire image (H&E, original magnification ×235). **D:** High magnification shows to better advantage chicken wire calcifications, the hallmark of this tumor (von Kossa, original magnification ×400).

The imaging features of a GCT, however, are characteristic. It is a purely osteolytic, radiolucent lesion with narrow zone of transition lacking sclerotic margins, revealing geographic bone destruction and usually no periosteal reaction (Figs. 11.44 and 11.45). Scintigraphy may show more intense uptake of the tracer around the periphery of the lesion than within the lesion itself, which Hudson calls a "donut configuration," presumably caused by hyperemic changes in the bone surrounding the tumor. A soft tissue mass may also be present, and CT or MRI is usually required for sufficient evaluation (Figs. 11.46 to 11.50). Approximately 5% of GCTs are malignant de novo. Having no characteristic imaging features, however, malignant lesions cannot be diagnosed radiologically (Fig. 11.51, see also Fig. 11.48). It is also well known that benign GCT may evolve into a malignant lesion. Several authors have reported cases of malignant transformation of GCT of bone. In most cases, this transformation occurs after radiation therapy. Only a few cases have been reported of spontaneous malignant transformation after initial surgical therapy. Histologically, the secondary malignancies include malignant fibrous histiocytoma, fibrosarcoma, osteosarcoma, and undifferentiated sarcoma.

Gross specimen of the giant cell tumor shows usually a pinkish-tan hemorrhagic mass (Fig. 11.52). Histopathologically, the tumor is composed of a related dual population of mononuclear stromal cells and multinucleated giant cells (Fig. 11.53). The tumor background contains varying amounts of collagen. Morphologically, the giant cells bear some resemblance to osteoclasts, and they display increased acid phosphatase activity. It is generally accepted that these cells are not neoplastic. The mononuclear cells, however, which arise from primitive mesenchymal stromal cells, represent the neoplastic component. These stromal cells, similar to osteoblasts, express factors necessary for osteoclast formation and differentiation (osteoclast differentiation factor or ODF). They exhibit the characteristics of osteoblast progenitors and express RANKL (receptor activator of nuclear factor kappa B [NF-κB] ligand), a growth factor that is essential for the recruitment of osteoclasts by osteoblasts and their maturation under normal physiologic conditions. *RANKL* gene is located at the chromosome 13q14 locus. In cytogenetic studies of giant cell tumors, telomeric associations (end-to-end fusions of apparently intact chromosomes) involving chromosomes 11p, 13p, 14p, 15p, 19q, 20q, and 21p have been identified as the most commonly occurring chromosomal aberration.

Historically, the imaging appearance and staging of GCTs have not accurately reflected the ultimate clinical outcome, but nevertheless several investigators, including Enneking, Campanacci, and Bertoni, have developed staging systems based on imaging and histologic appearance of this tumor. The stage 1 lesion has an indolent radiographic (well-marginated borders and intact cortex) and benign histologic appearance. The stage 2 lesion demonstrates a more aggressive radiographic appearance, with extensive remodeling of bone, thin cortex but without loss of continuity and intact

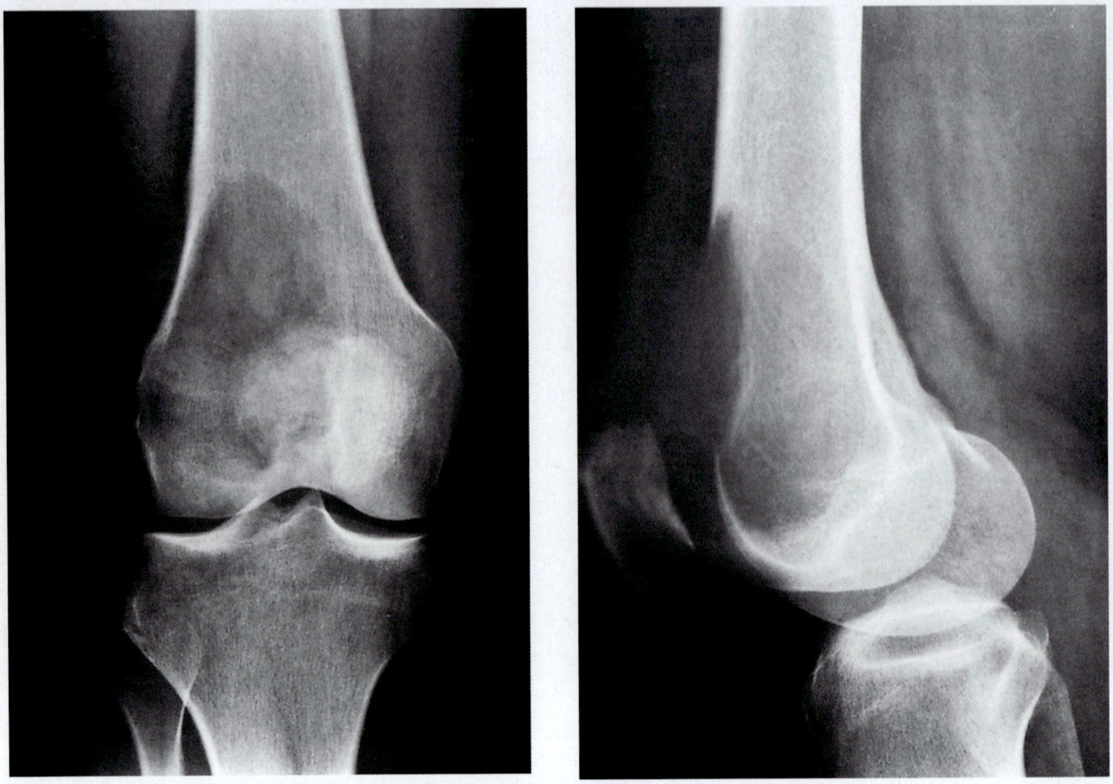

A B

Figure 11.44 ■ **Giant cell tumor.** Anteroposterior **(A)** and lateral **(B)** radiographs of the right knee of a 32-year-old man show a purely osteolytic lesion in the distal end of the femur. Note its eccentric location, the absence of reactive sclerosis, and the extension of the lesion into the articular end of the bone, all characteristic features of this tumor.

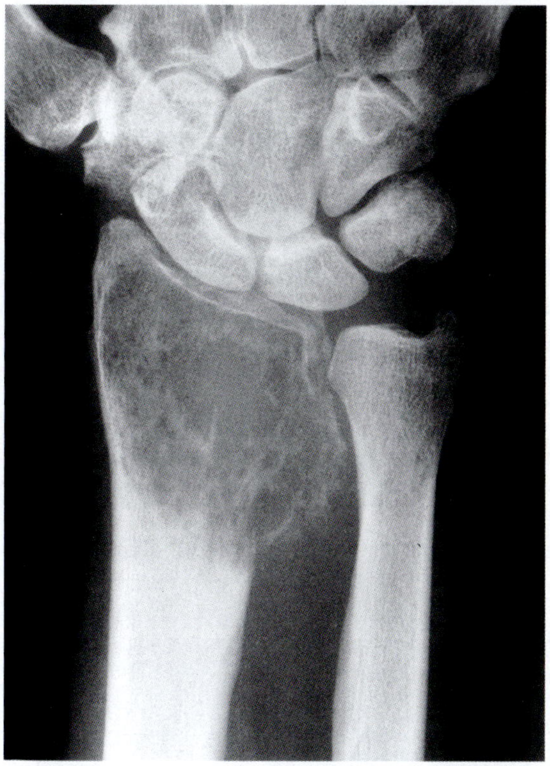

A

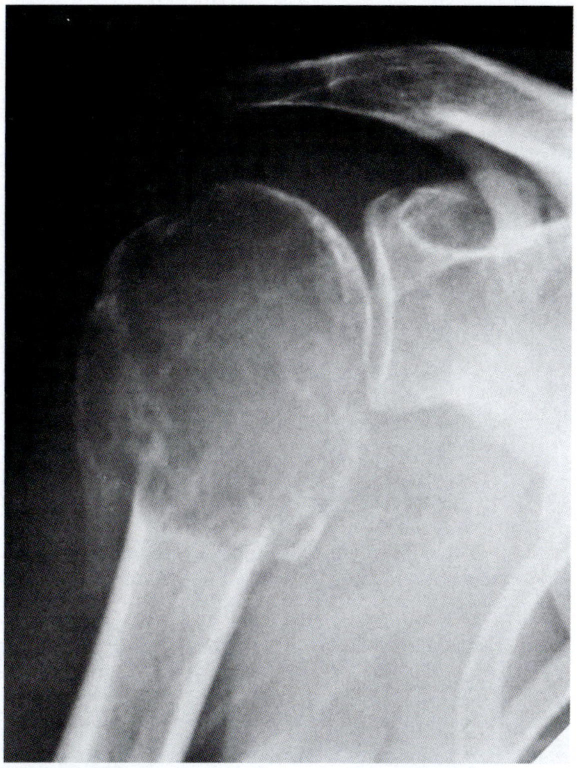

B

Figure 11.45 ■ **Giant cell tumor. A:** Dorsovolar radiograph of the left wrist of a 38-year-old woman shows the classic appearance of this lesion at the distal end of the radius. **B:** Anteroposterior radiograph of the right shoulder of a 27-year-old woman shows an osteolytic lesion affecting almost the entire proximal end of the humerus. **C:** Anteroposterior radiograph of the right knee of a 30-year-old woman shows an eccentric osteolytic lesion affecting proximal end of the tibia.

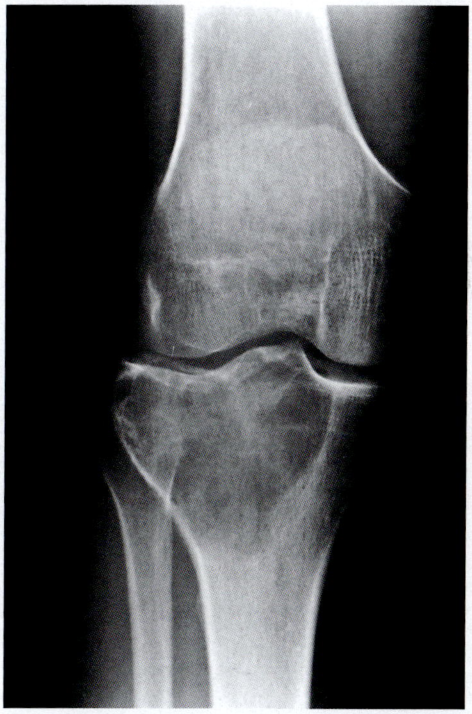

C

periosteum, and benign histologic pattern. Stage 3 GCT reveals aggressive growth with break through the cortex and extension into adjacent soft tissues but remains histologically benign, although distant metastases (predominantly to the lungs) may occur.

The treatment of benign GCTs consists of either surgical curettage and bone grafting or wide resection with secondary implantation of an allograft or an endoprosthesis. Marcove recommended cryosurgery using liquid nitrogen, whereas other authorities recommended heat using methyl methacrylate to pack the tumor bed after intralesional excision. Recurrences are often encountered and are recognized radiographically by resorption of the bone graft and the appearance of radiolucent areas like those in the original tumor. Especially after radiation therapy, recurrent lesions may exhibit malignant transformation to fibrosarcoma, malignant fibrous histiocytoma, or osteosarcoma. Occasionally, even histologically benign lesions produce distant (to the lung) metastases.

Recently, improved understanding of the molecular and cellular biology of this tumor, particularly identification of the osteoclast differentiation factor RANKL, a molecule that is critical to the pathogenesis of giant cell tumor, prompted trials of targeted treatment using a monoclonal antibody denosumab, directed against RANKL. This is a promising therapy in patients with either unresectable or recurrent giant cell tumor.

(Continued on page 408)

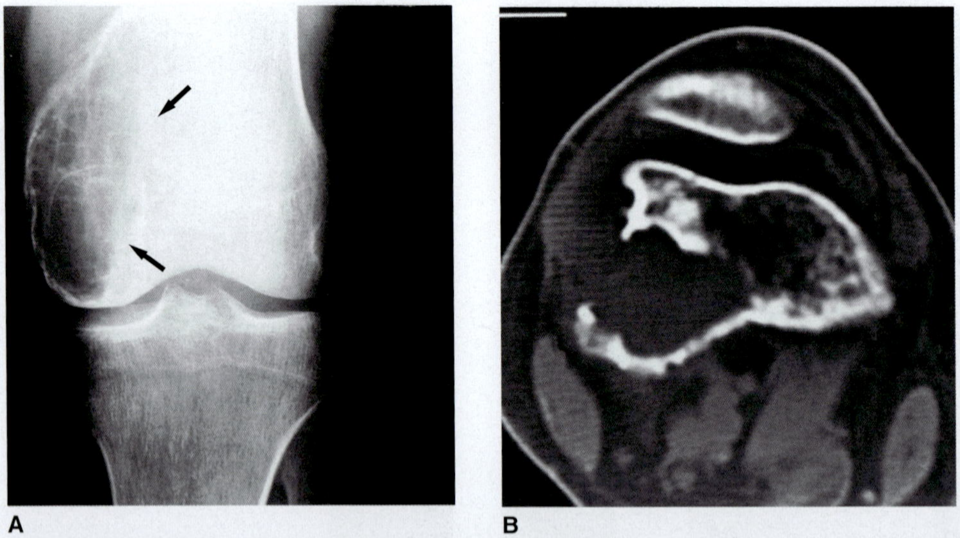

Figure 11.46 ■ **CT of giant cell tumor. A:** Anteroposterior radiograph of the left knee of a 33-year-old woman shows a lytic lesion in the medial femoral condyle (*arrows*). **B:** Axial CT section shows a pathologic fracture and a soft tissue mass.

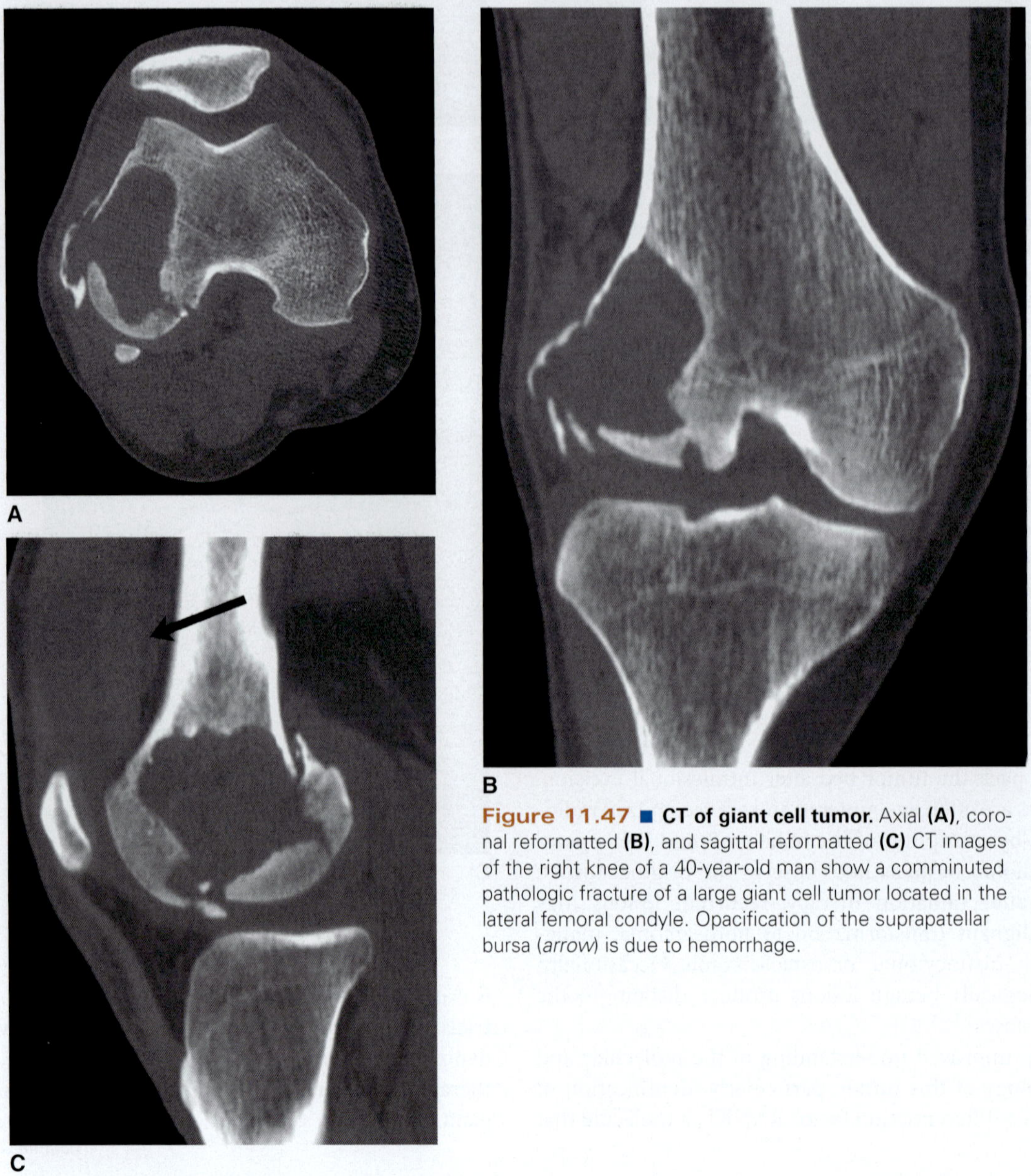

Figure 11.47 ■ **CT of giant cell tumor.** Axial **(A)**, coronal reformatted **(B)**, and sagittal reformatted **(C)** CT images of the right knee of a 40-year-old man show a comminuted pathologic fracture of a large giant cell tumor located in the lateral femoral condyle. Opacification of the suprapatellar bursa (*arrow*) is due to hemorrhage.

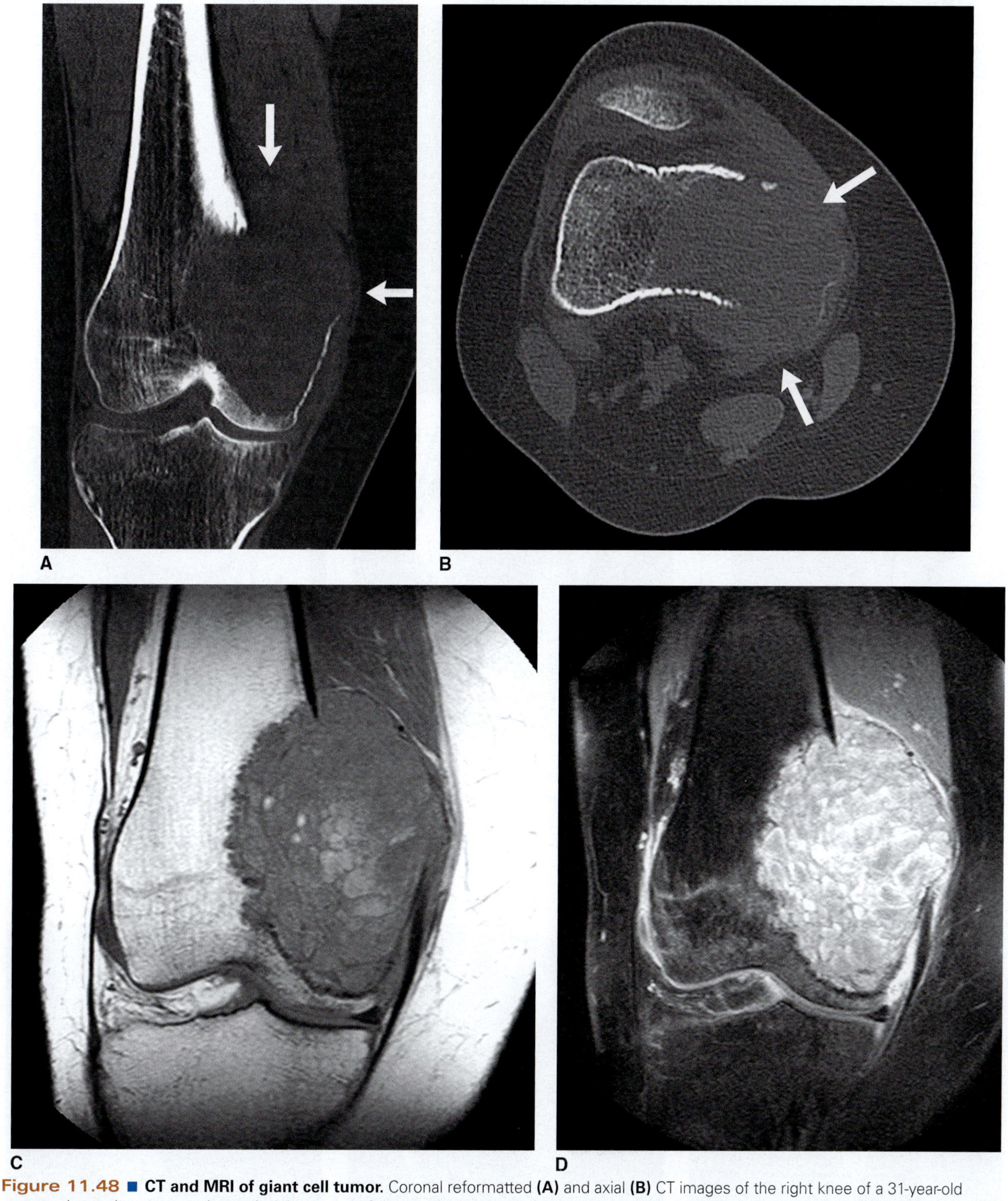

Figure 11.48 ■ **CT and MRI of giant cell tumor.** Coronal reformatted **(A)** and axial **(B)** CT images of the right knee of a 31-year-old woman show a large tumor destroying the cortex of the medial femoral condyle and extending into the soft tissues (*arrows*). **C:** Coronal T1-weighted MR image demonstrates the tumor exhibiting an intermediate, slightly heterogeneous signal because of the bleeding. **D:** Coronal T1-weighted fat-suppressed MR image obtained after intravenous administration of gadolinium shows marked enhancement of the tumor. Histopathologic examination did not reveal any malignant features in the resected specimen.

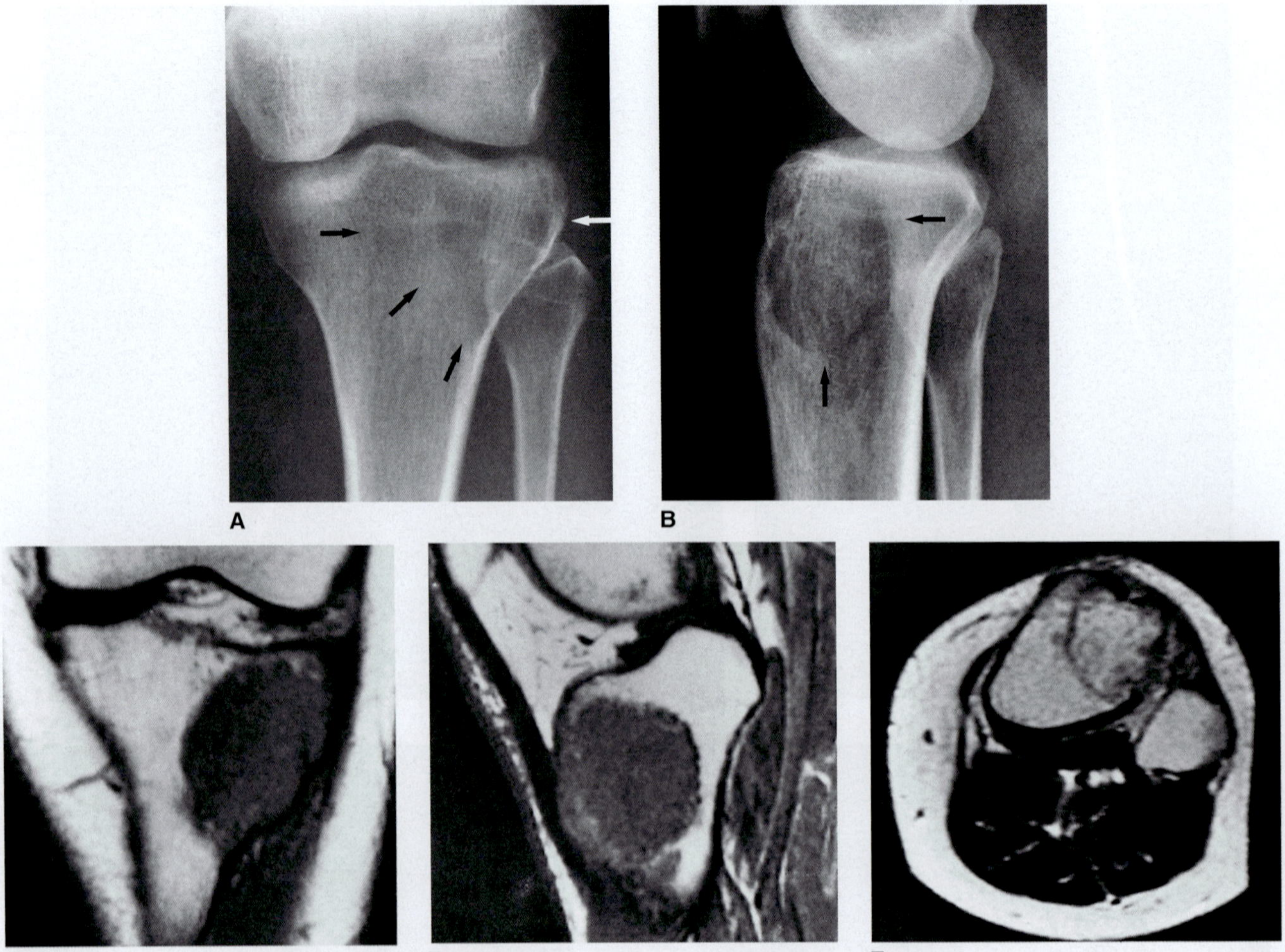

A B C D E

Figure 11.49 ■ **MRI of giant cell tumor.** A 45-year-old woman presented with pain in the left knee of 6 months duration. Anteroposterior **(A)** and lateral **(B)** radiographs demonstrate a radiolucent lesion in the proximal tibia extending to the articular end of the bone (*arrows*). Coronal **(C)** and sagittal **(D)** T1-weighted MR images better outline the tumor, which displays intermediate signal intensity. **E:** Axial proton density-weighted MR image reveals that the lesion, which displays now a heterogeneous but predominantly high signal, penetrates the anterolateral cortex and extends into the soft tissues.

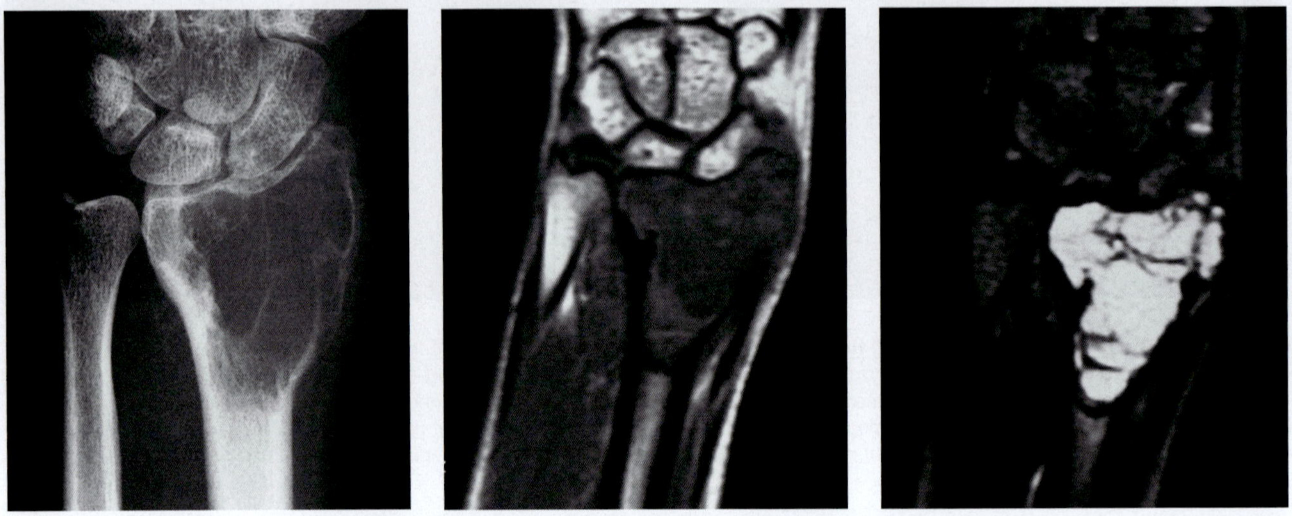

A B C

Figure 11.50 ■ **MRI of giant cell tumor. A:** Dorsovolar radiograph of the right wrist of a 36-year-old woman shows an osteolytic lesion in the distal radius. **B:** Coronal T1-weighted MR image shows the tumor to be of intermediate-to-low signal intensity. **C:** On coronal T2-weighted MR image, the tumor becomes bright displaying low-signal septations.

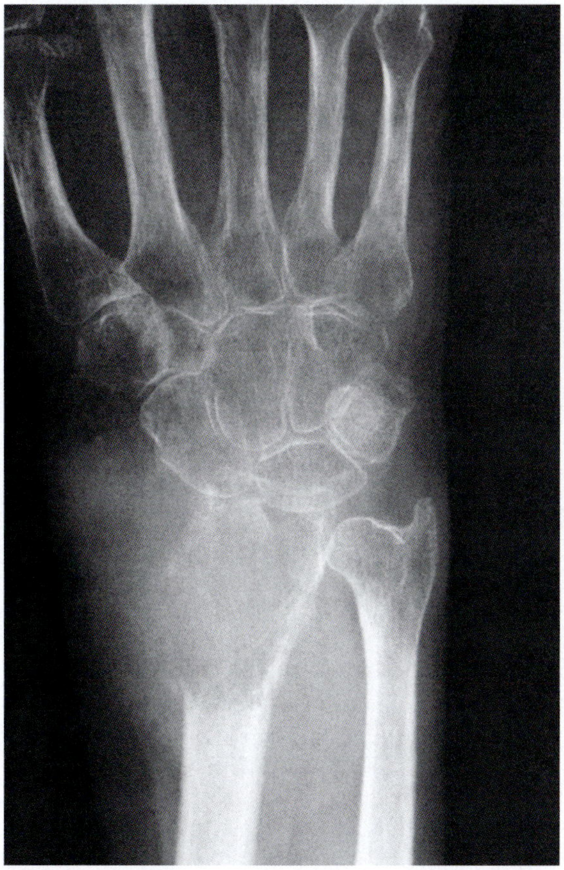

Figure 11.51 ■ Giant cell tumor. Dorsovolar radiograph of the left wrist of a 56-year-old woman shows a lytic lesion of the distal radius that has destroyed the cortex and that extends into the soft tissues. Despite this aggressive radiographic presentation, on histopathologic examination, the tumor had a typically benign appearance, without malignant features. After wide resection, a 5-year follow-up showed no evidence of recurrence or of distant metastases.

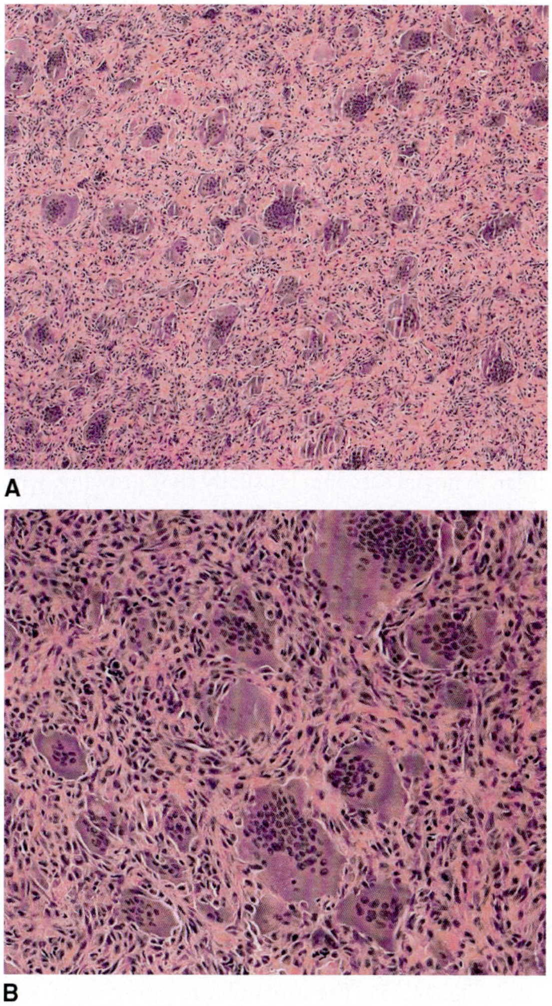

Figure 11.53 ■ Histopathology of giant cell tumor. **A:** A low-power photomicrograph shows dual population of elongated mononuclear stromal cells mixed with numerous evenly distributed osteoclast-like giant cells exhibiting multiple nuclei (H&E, original magnification ×50). **B:** High-power view shows the details of the large giant cells containing numerous nuclei (H&E, original magnification ×200).

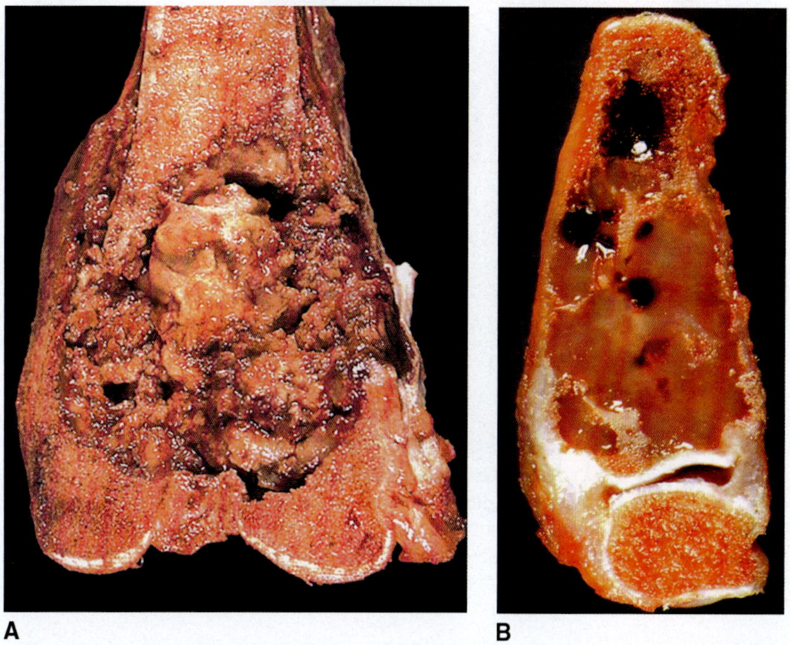

Figure 11.52 ■ Gross pathology of giant cell tumor. **A:** Coronal section of the resected surgical specimen of the distal femur shows a lobulated intramedullary tumor with hemorrhagic foci, extending into the articular end of bone and breaking through the cortex. **B:** Coronal section of surgical specimen of the first metacarpal bone shows pinkish-tan soft intramedullary mass exhibiting foci of hemorrhage. Observe extension of the tumor to the proximal end of bone and preservation of the first carpometacarpal joint.

SYNOVIAL SARCOMA

Synovial sarcoma (synovioma, synovioblastic sarcoma) is an uncommon mesenchymal neoplasm, comprising ~8% to 10% of soft tissue sarcomas. Despite its name (which was designated because of histologic resemblance of synovial sarcoma to normal synovial tissue), it does not arise from synovium, although it may originate from any other structure, including joint capsules, bursae, and tendon sheaths. The tumor usually occurs before age 50, most commonly between ages 15 and 40 years. There is no gender predilection. The extremities account for 80% to 90% of synovial sarcomas, and the most common sites are around the knee and foot. In exceptional instances, the tumor may be intra-articular. Synovial sarcoma is usually slow growing, with an indolent course, although in late stages it may demonstrate aggressiveness. Metastases to the lung by the hematogenous route and to the soft tissue have been reported. Schajowicz cited a local recurrence rate of more than 50%. The clinical symptoms usually include soft tissue swelling or a mass and progressive pain. On physical examination, a diffuse or discrete soft tissue mass is present, usually tender on palpation.

The gross pathology shows a variable in size mass, usually in juxta-articular location, with hemorrhagic foci (Fig. 11.54). On histopathologic examination, several subtypes of synovial sarcoma have been recognized. Among them are biphasic (fibrous and epithelial), monophasic (the most common subtype), and poorly differentiated types. The classical biphasic type exhibits distinct spindle cell and epithelial components arranged in glandular or nestlike patterns (Fig. 11.55). The monophasic synovial sarcoma is

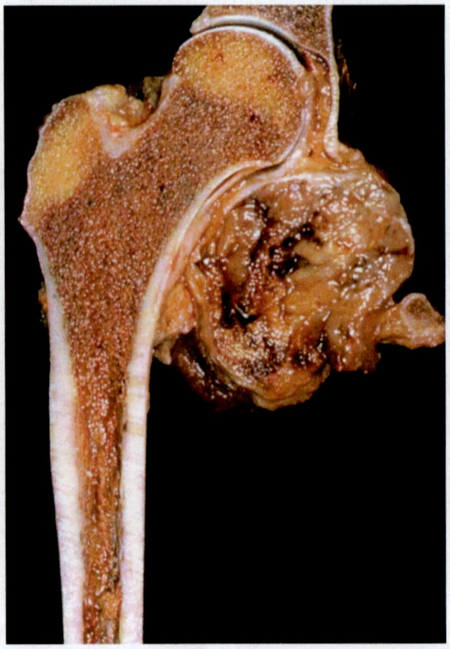

Figure 11.54 ■ Gross pathology of synovial sarcoma. Coronal section of the specimen of the right proximal femur and hip joint shows a large, well-circumscribed tan-yellowish juxta-articular soft tissue mass displaying foci of hemorrhage.

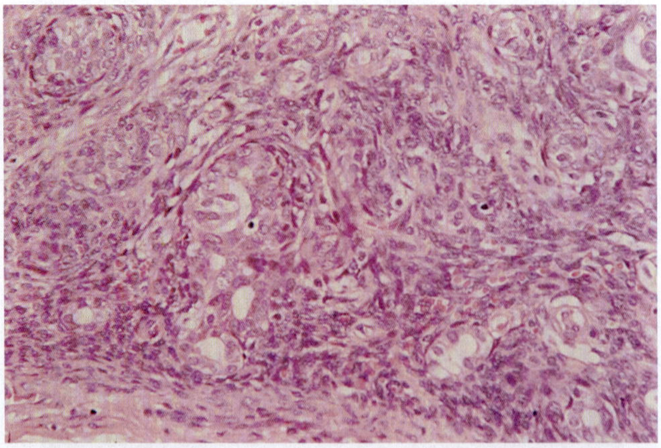

A

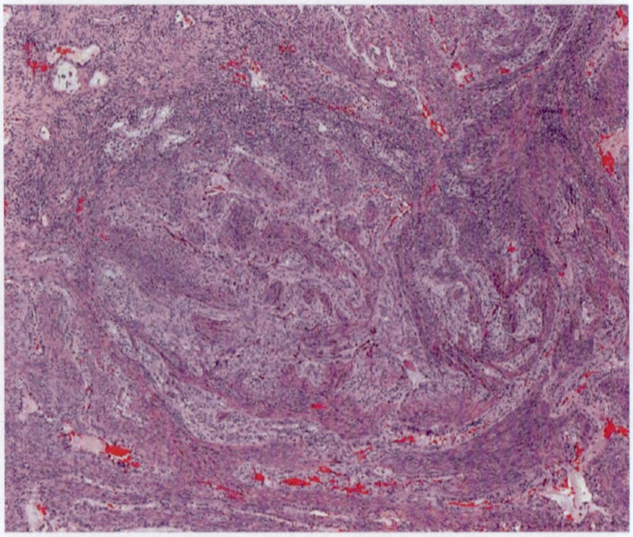

B

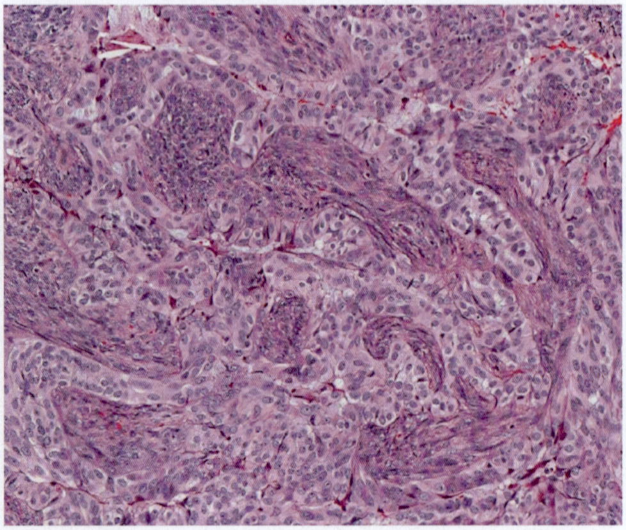

C

Figure 11.55 ■ Histopathology of synovial sarcoma. **A:** Typical biphasic appearance of the tumor with glandlike spaces (left and bottom) side by side with spindle cell sarcomatous areas (H&E, original magnification ×80). **B:** Spindle and epithelioid cells in some areas are arranged in glandlike pattern, in other areas in nestlike pattern (H&E, original magnification ×100). **C:** On higher-magnification photomicrograph, the biphasic arrangement is better appreciated (H&E, original magnification ×200).

composed of interdigitating fascicles and "ball-like" structures formed by the spindle cells (Fig. 11.56A–C). Foci of calcification may also be observed, usually localized in areas of hyalinization within the spindle cell elements of the tumor (Fig. 11.56D, E). A consistent finding, present in about 90% of tumors, is a cytogenetic aberration of translocation involving chromosomes X and 18 [t(x;18)(p11.2;q11.2)], resulting in fusion of *SYT* gene (also known as *SS18* or *SSXT*, encoding 55 kDa protein) to either *SSX1* or *SSX2*. Minorities of cases have a gene rearrangement involving *SSX4*.

The imaging features of synovial sarcoma include a soft tissue mass, usually in close proximity to a joint (Fig. 11.57) and occasionally associated with bone invasion. A periosteal

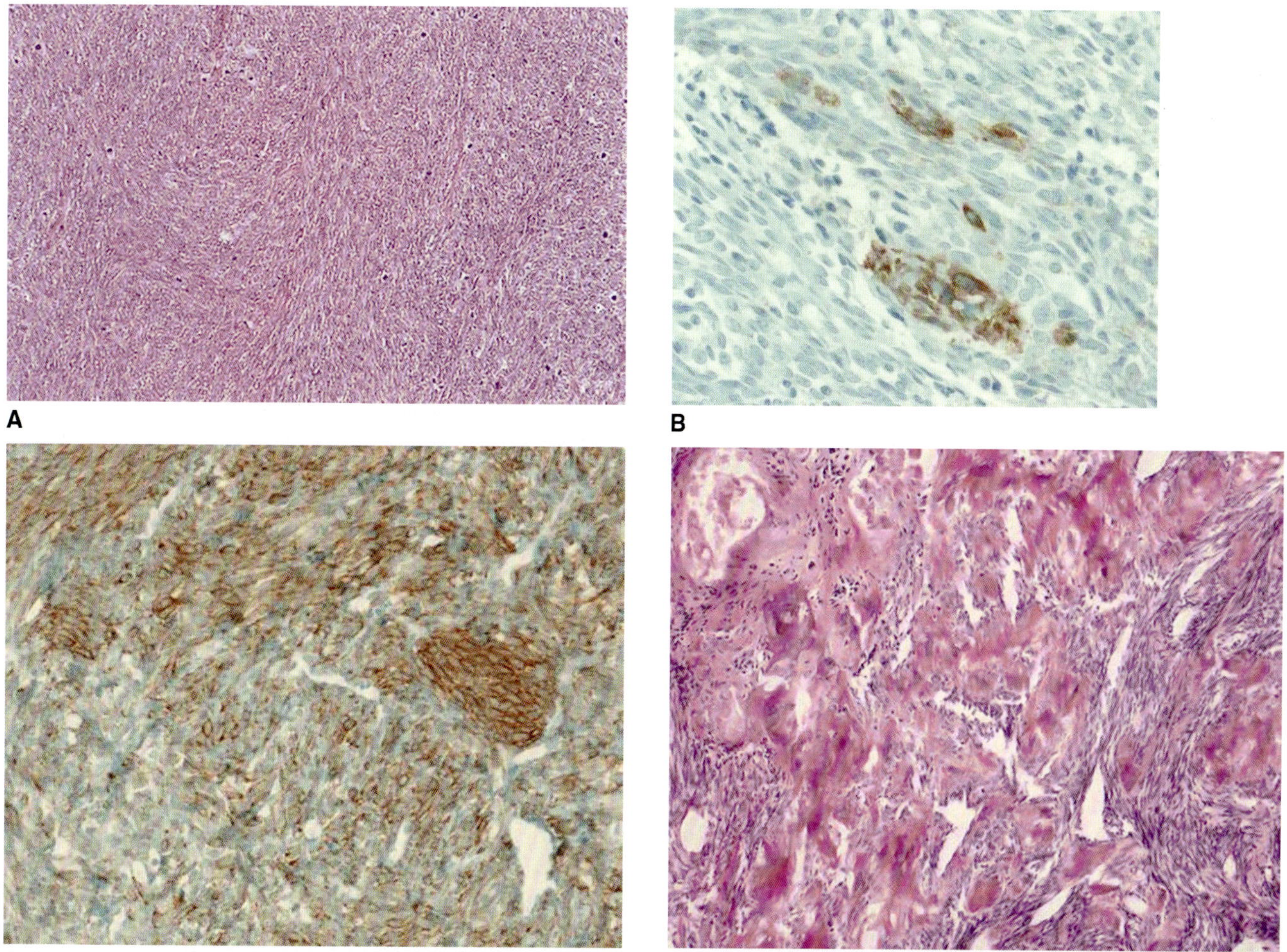

A B C D

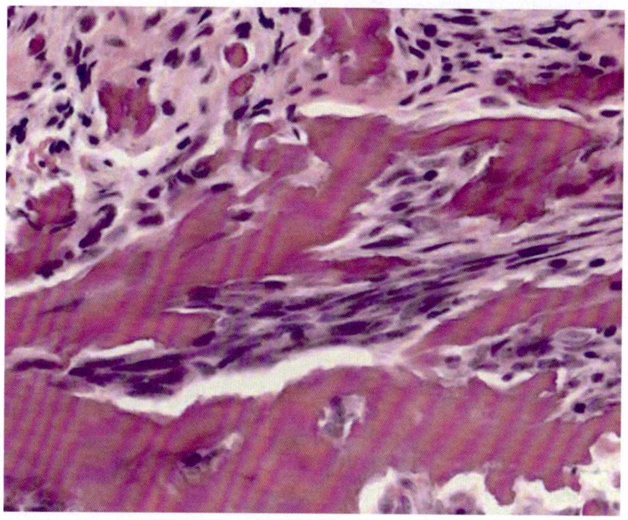

E

Figure 11.56 ■ Histopathology of synovial sarcoma. **A:** Monophasic variant exhibits dense arrangements of spindle cells resembling fibrosarcoma (H&E, original magnification ×50). **B:** Monophasic fibrous variant shows focal positivity for epithelial membrane antigen (EMA) (biotin–avidin–peroxidase, original magnification ×400). **C:** In addition to positivity for CD99 and cytokeratins (not shown here), synovial sarcoma is also positive for BCL-2 (biotin–avidin–peroxidase, original magnification ×200). **D:** Calcifying type of the tumor exhibits extensive mineralization (H&E, original magnification ×100). **E:** At high magnification, observe uniformity of the spindle cells with only mild pleomorphism surrounding areas of mineralization (H&E, original magnification ×400).

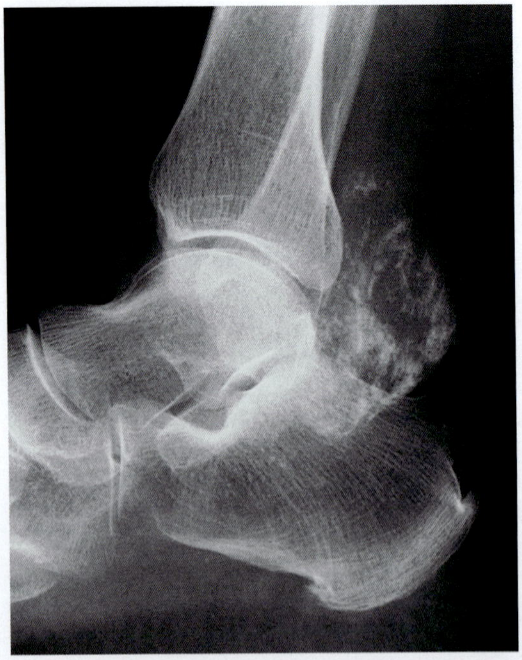

Figure 11.57 ■ Synovial sarcoma. Lateral radiograph of the left ankle of a 71-year-old woman shows a large calcified mass located in the soft tissues anteriorly to the Achilles tendon, not affecting the adjacent bones.

reaction may also be observed. The soft tissue calcifications, usually amorphous in type, are present in ~25% to 30% of cases, commonly located at the periphery of the tumor. Less frequently a central punctuate calcific pattern may be seen. Rarely, extensive calcifications or ossifications resembling an osteoid matrix or bone can be present. This presentation may lead to erroneous diagnosis including soft tissue osteosarcoma or chondrosarcoma, synovial chondromatosis, myositis ossificans, or tumoral calcinosis.

Scintigraphic evaluation reveals increased uptake of radiopharmaceutical agent on blood flow and blood pool images consistent with increased vascularity of these tumors (see Fig. 11.58B, C). CT effectively demonstrates the extent of the soft tissue mass, calcifications, and bone invasion. This modality also is effective to assess the chest for pulmonary metastases. MRI shows the tumor to be heterogeneous, multilobulated septated mass of low-to-intermediate signal intensity with infiltrative margins on T1-weighted sequences, displaying a high signal on T2 weighting (Fig. 11.58) and diffuse but heterogeneous enhancement after administration of gadolinium (Figs. 11.59 and 11.60). The most extensive to date MRI study of synovial sarcoma in 34 patients reported by Jones and associates showed that it tends to be deep, large (85% were >5 cm in diameter), and located in the extremities, with epicenter close to the joint. The lesion was usually heterogeneous on T2-weighted images and was clearly delineated from surrounding tissues. Forty-four percent of the cases had a high signal on both T1- and T2-weighted sequences, consistent with hemorrhage within the tumor. Several investigators consider so-called "triple signal intensity" sign, because of a combination of cystic and solid elements, fibrous tissue, hemorrhage, and hemosiderin deposition, as the most characteristic for this tumor (see Figs. 11.59 and 11.60). Some multilobulated tumors may contain septa and fluid–fluid levels, creating the "bowl of grapes" sign. During the slow growth phase, synovial sarcoma may exhibit a relatively "benign" appearance on MRI, with a low-signal intensity capsule and relatively uniform signal intensity of the tumor, resembling benign tumors such as schwannoma (Fig. 11.61).

Treatment includes a wide local resection, followed with adjuvant chemotherapy with combination of Adriamycin, cisplatin, vincristine, doxorubicin, and ifosfamide. Postoperative radiation therapy is reserved for the patients in whom surgical intervention was not able to ascertain clear margins of resection. In some cases, amputation of a limb remains a treatment of choice. Local recurrences and metastatic spread of the tumor are common complications.

SYNOVIAL CHONDROSARCOMA

Synovial chondrosarcoma is a rare tumor that originates from the synovial membrane. It may arise as a primary synovial tumor, or it may develop as a malignant transformation of synovial (osteo)chondromatosis. The concept of malignant degeneration of synovial chondromatosis is still controversial and the entity is rare, with fewer than 40 well-documented cases on record.

Most synovial chondrosarcomas are located in the knee joint. Rarely, other joints such as the hip, elbow, or ankle are affected. Involvement of the small joints of the hands is exceedingly rare. These malignancies show a slight predominance in men, and patients range in age from 25 to 70 years. The symptoms include pain and swelling, with duration in most patients exceeding 12 months. In patients with primary synovial (osteo)chondromatosis, malignant transformation to synovial chondrosarcoma should be clinically suspected if there is development of soft tissue mass at the site of the affected joint.

Radiologically, the presence of chondroid calcifications within the joint, destruction of the adjacent bones, and a soft tissue mass are highly suggestive of a synovial chondrosarcoma. In a few documented cases, MR showed lobular soft tissue masses within the joint exhibiting heterogeneous but predominantly isointense to muscle signal on T1- and hyperintense signal on T2-weighted images. In patients with documented primary synovial (osteo)chondromatosis, a soft tissue mass and destructive changes in the joint should suggest the development of a secondary synovial chondrosarcoma (Fig. 11.62). Note, however, that frequently both uncomplicated synovial chondromatosis and synovial chondrosarcoma may exhibit similar features on radiography and MRI.

The histopathologic distinction between primary synovial chondromatosis and secondary malignancy in

(Continued on page 413)

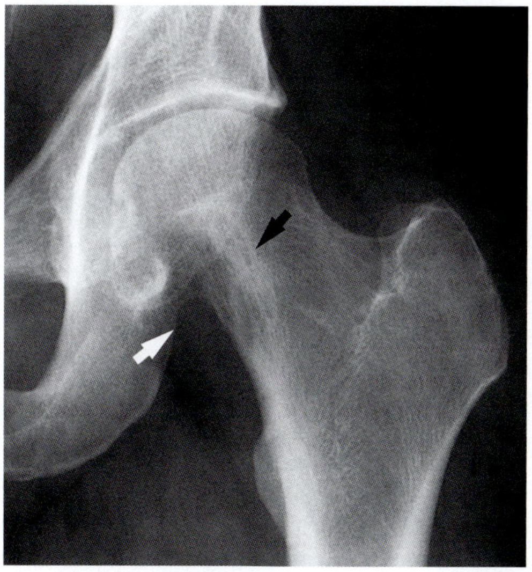

A

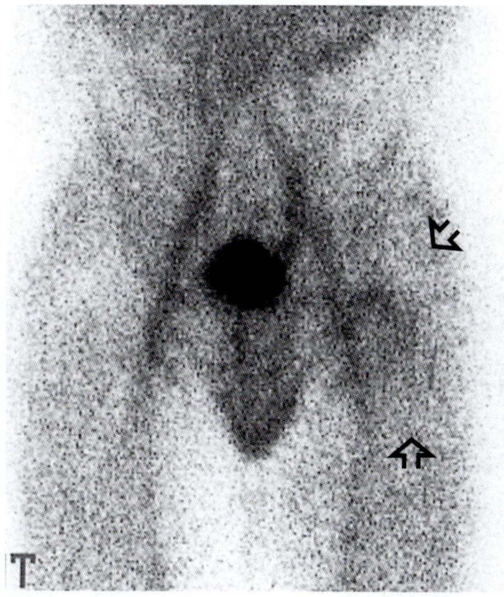

B

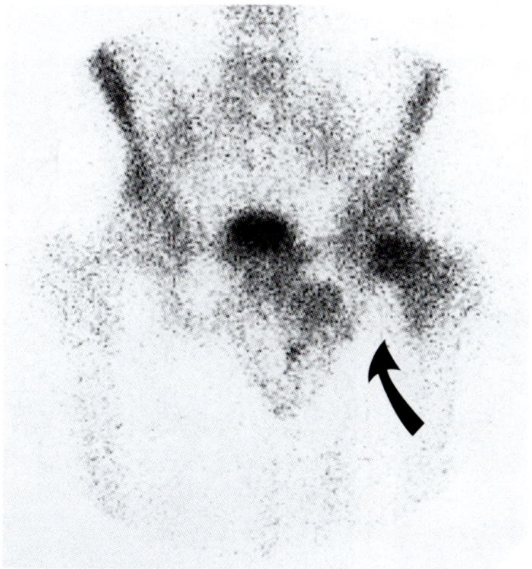

C

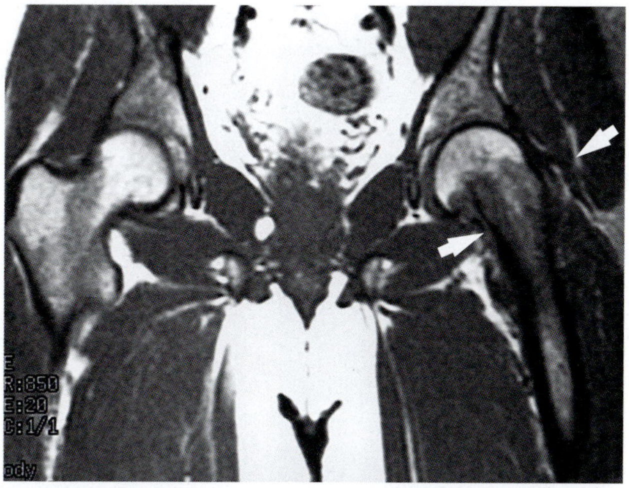

D

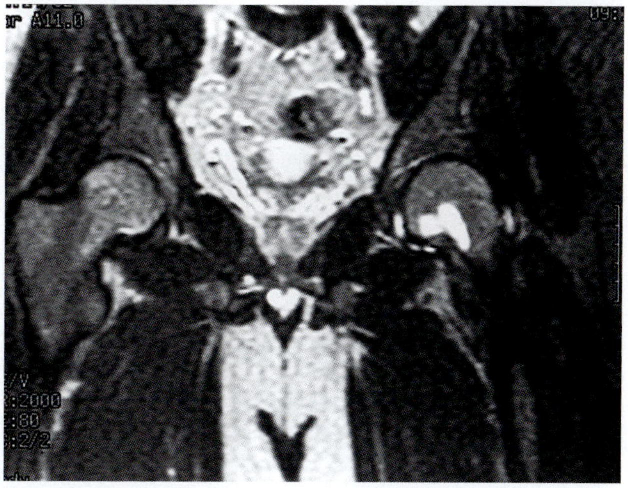

E

Figure 11.58 ■ **Scintigraphy and MRI of synovial sarcoma. A:** Anteroposterior radiograph of the left hip of a 37-year-old man shows an osteolytic lesion in the femoral neck bordered laterally by sclerotic margin (*arrows*). **B:** Scintigraphic (blood pool) examination demonstrates increased vascularity to the left hip joint (*open arrows*). **C:** Delayed radionuclide bone scan with ^{99m}Tc methylene diphosphonate (MDP) shows increased uptake of the radiopharmaceutical tracer in the femoral head and neck and around the hip joint (*curved arrow*). **D:** Coronal T1-weighted (SE; TR 850/TE 20 msec) MR image shows a low–signal intensity lesion affecting the medial aspect of the left femoral neck (*arrows*). **E:** Coronal T2-weighted (SE; TR 2000/TE 80 msec) MR image demonstrates increased signal in the femoral neck and in the medial and lateral aspects of the hip joint. Excision biopsy revealed intra-articular synovial sarcoma.

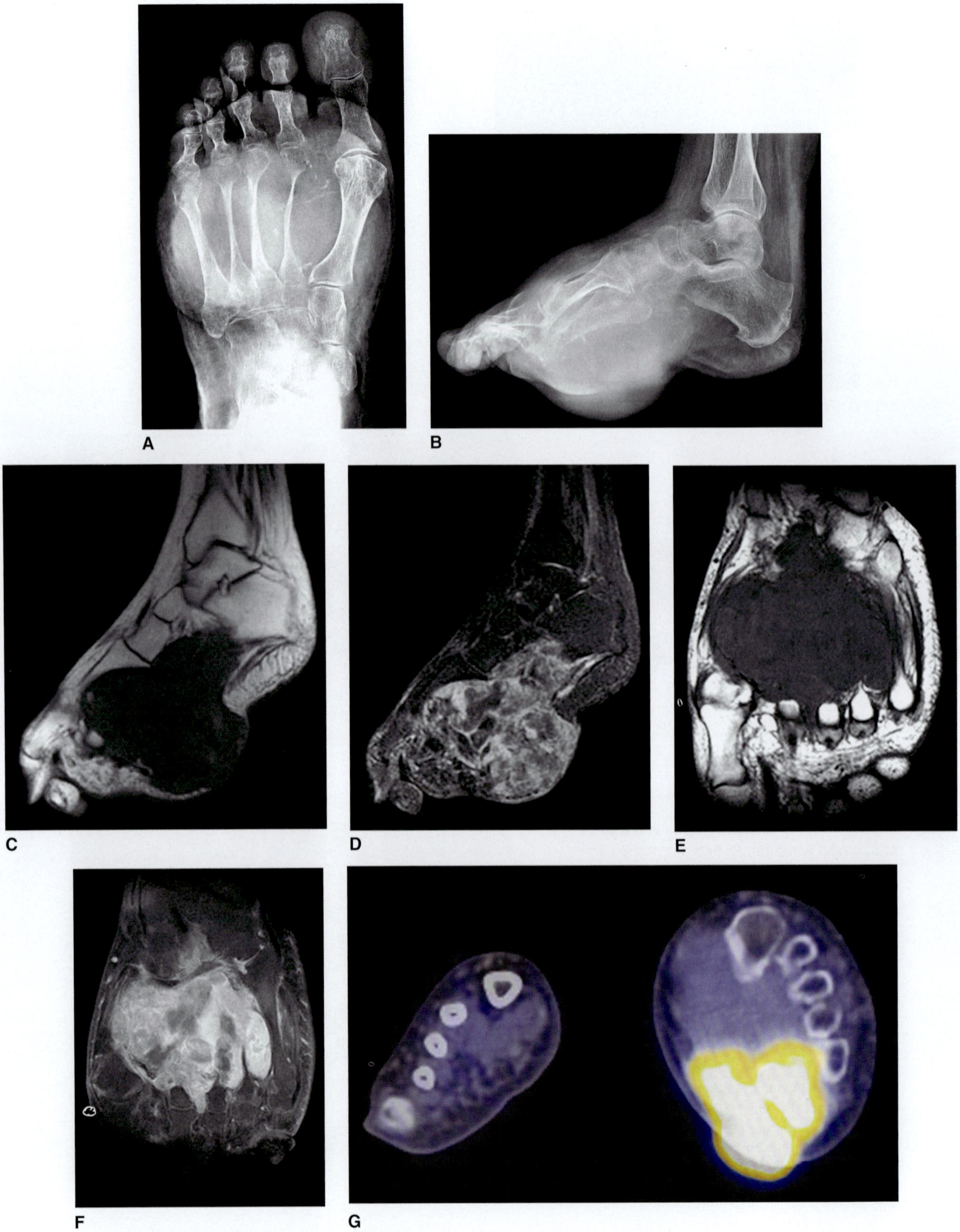

Figure 11.59 ■ MRI and PET/CT of synovial sarcoma. Anteroposterior **(A)** and lateral **(B)** radiographs of the right foot of a 57-year-old woman show a large soft tissue mass containing calcifications, affecting mainly the plantar aspect of the foot. Observe erosions of the second, third, and fourth metatarsal bones. **C:** Sagittal T1-weighted MRI shows the mass to be of intermediate-to-low signal intensity. **D:** Sagittal inversion recovery (IR) MR image shows the heterogeneous mass exhibiting mixtures of low, intermediate, and high signal intensities (triple signal intensity sign). Axial (long-axis) T1-weighted MR image **(E)** and one obtained after intravenous administration of gadolinium **(F)** demonstrate heterogeneous enhancement of the tumor. **G:** Axial fused PET/CT image of both feet reveals a large hypermetabolic tumor in the soft tissues of the left foot. Excision biopsy confirmed the diagnosis of synovial sarcoma.

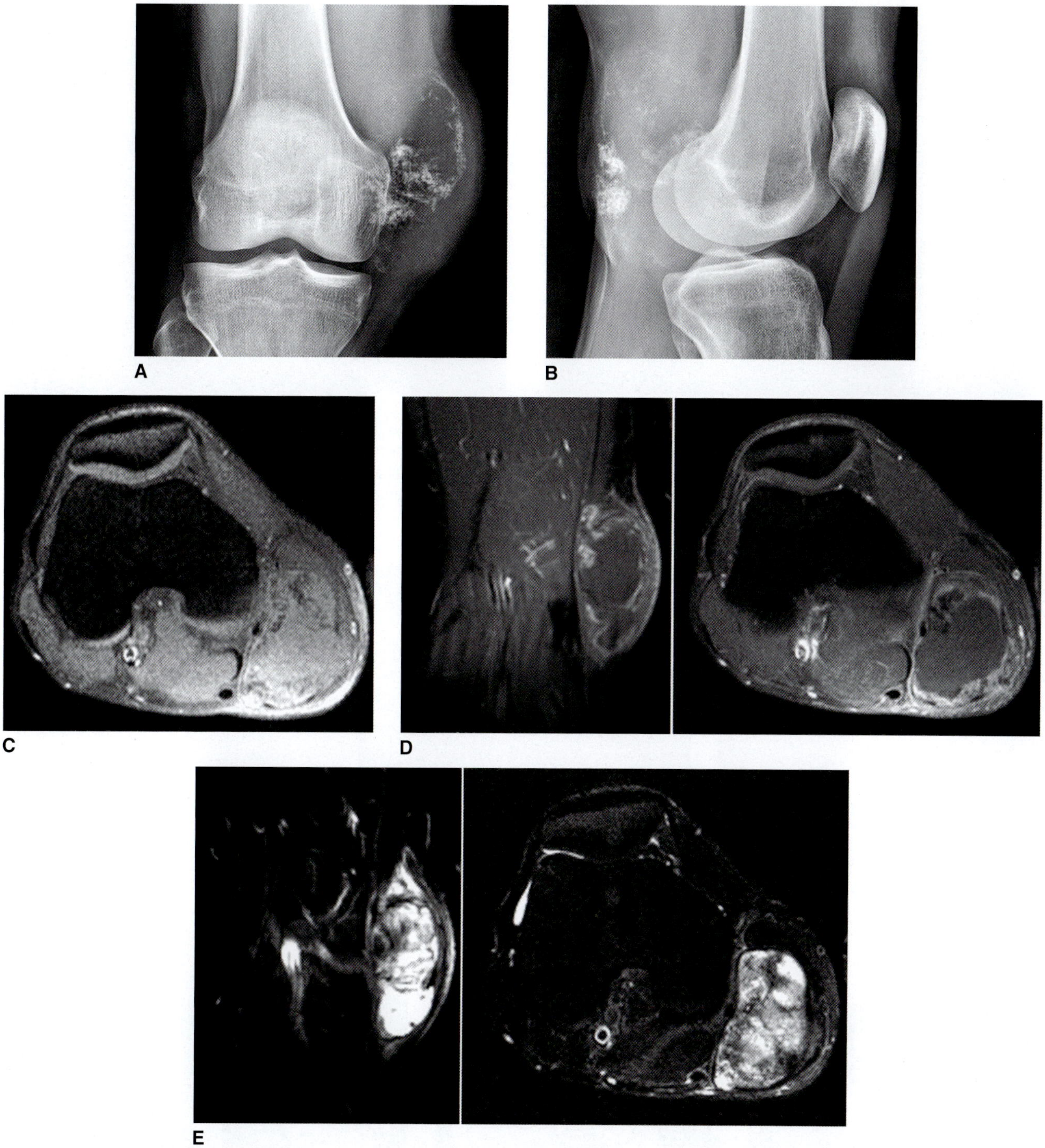

Figure 11.60 ■ MRI of synovial sarcoma. Anteroposterior **(A)** and lateral **(B)** radiographs of the left knee of a 34-year-old man show a large soft tissue mass adjacent to the posterolateral aspect of the medial femoral condyle containing calcifications. The osseous structures are not invaded. **C:** Axial T1-weighted MRI shows the mass to be predominantly of intermediate signal intensity. **D:** Coronal and axial T1-weighted MR images obtained after intravenous administration of gadolinium show peripheral enhancement of the tumor. **E:** Coronal and axial T2-weighted MR images demonstrate heterogenous tumor exhibiting mixture of high, intermediate, and low signal intensity (triple signal intensity sign), characteristic of synovial sarcoma. The diagnosis was confirmed by excision biopsy.

synovial chondromatosis has been a matter of dispute. Manivel and associates suggested that histologic features equivalent to those of grade 2 or 3 central chondrosarcoma must be present before chondrosarcoma arising in synovial chondromatosis can be diagnosed (Fig. 11.63). Occasional foci of increased cellularity showing hyperchromatic atypical cells, consistent with grade 1 chondrosarcoma, should not be sufficient evidence for a malignant change in synovial chondromatosis. However, evidence of aggressive growth (invasion) and a lesion's lack of attachment to the synovial

(Continued on page 415)

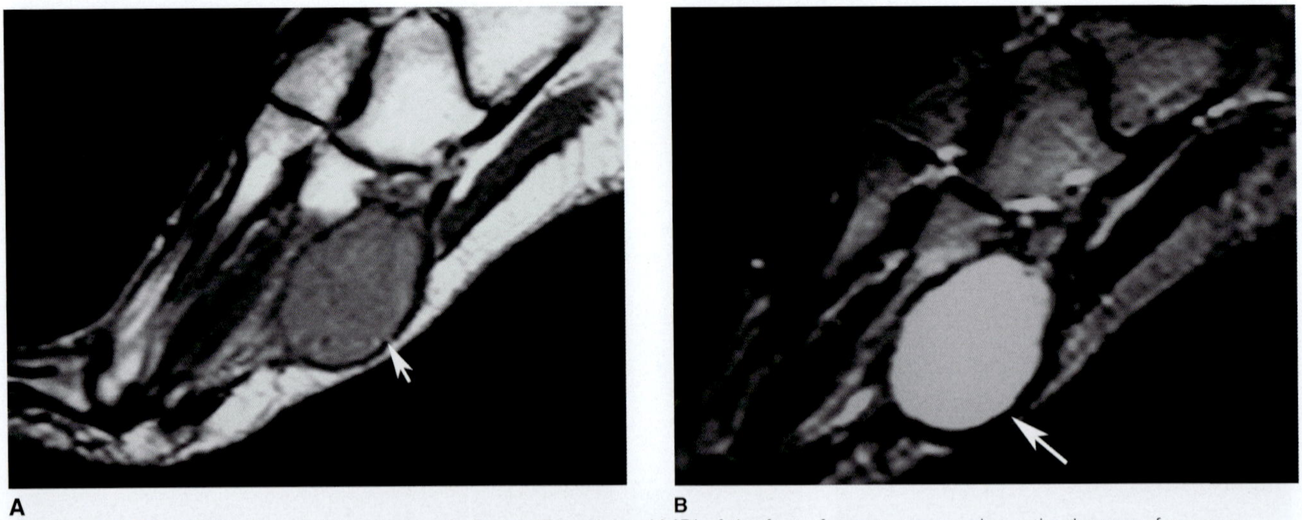

Figure 11.61 ■ **MRI of synovial sarcoma. A:** Sagittal T1-weighted MRI of the foot of a young man, who noticed a mass for over a year in the plantar lateral aspect of the foot, shows well-circumscribed hypointense tumor exhibiting a low–signal intensity capsule (*arrow*). **B:** Sagittal T2-weighted MR image demonstrates uniform high signal intensity of the well-encapsulated lesion (*arrow*). The preoperative diagnosis was neurinoma or schwannoma. The final histologic diagnosis was synovial sarcoma.

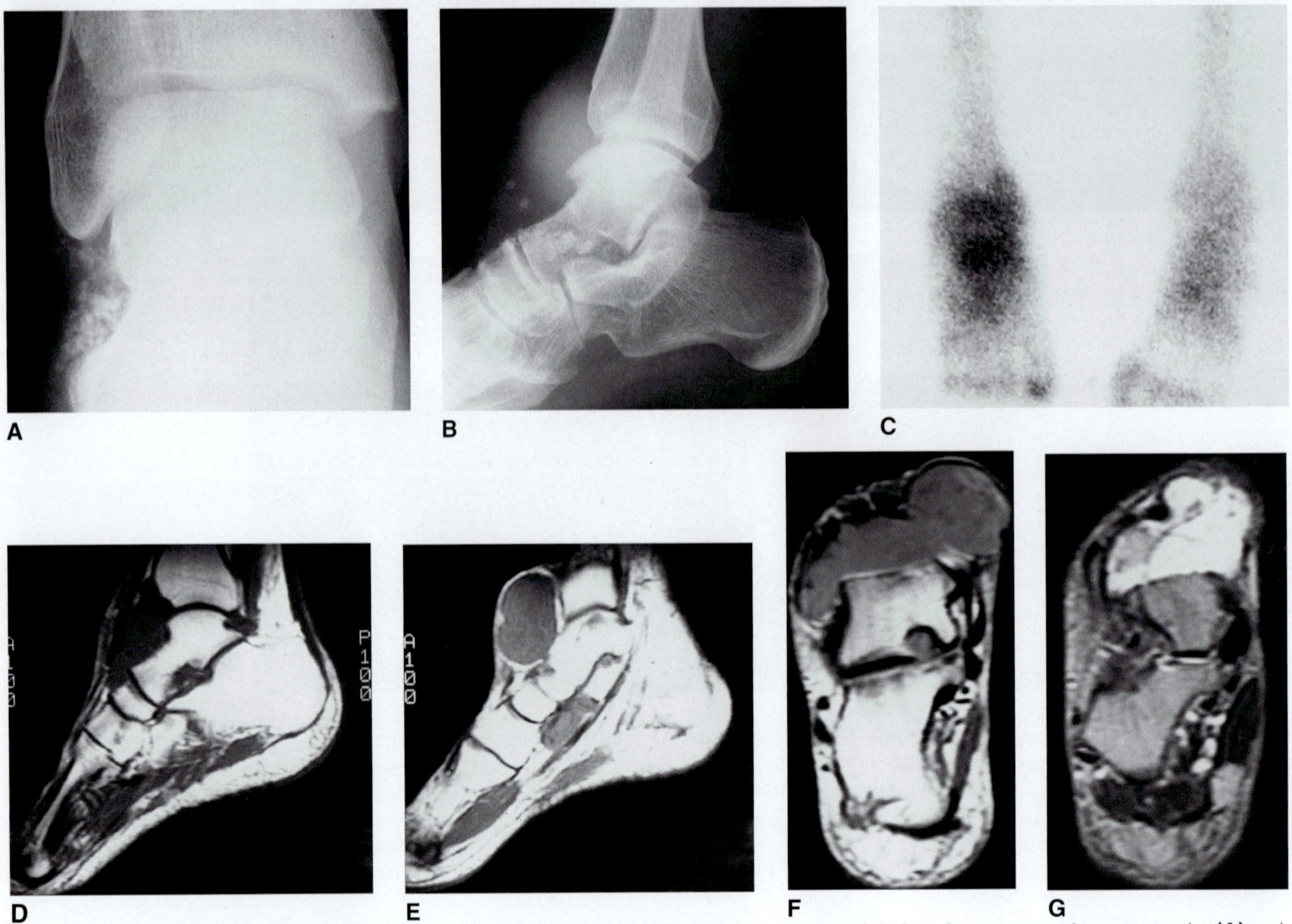

Figure 11.62 ■ **Malignant transformation of synovial osteochondromatosis to synovial chondrosarcoma.** Anteroposterior **(A)** and lateral **(B)** radiographs of the right ankle of a 64-year-old man with a long history of synovial chondromatosis show a large soft tissue mass on the dorsal aspect of the ankle joint, eroding the talus. Multiple calcifications, uniform in size and shape, are noted laterally. **C:** After injection of 15 mCi (555 MBq) of ^{99m}Tc-labeled MDP, there is increased uptake of radiopharmaceutical tracer in the right ankle. **D:** Sagittal T1-weighted MR image shows the mass displaying intermediate signal intensity, isointense with the muscles. **E:** Parasagittal T1-weighted MR image demonstrates the mass to be well encapsulated. **F:** Coronal proton density-weighted MR image shows that the mass is continuous with the ankle joint. **G:** Coronal T2-weighted MR image demonstrates the mass to be of high signal intensity. Punctate areas of low signal intensity within the mass represent calcifications.

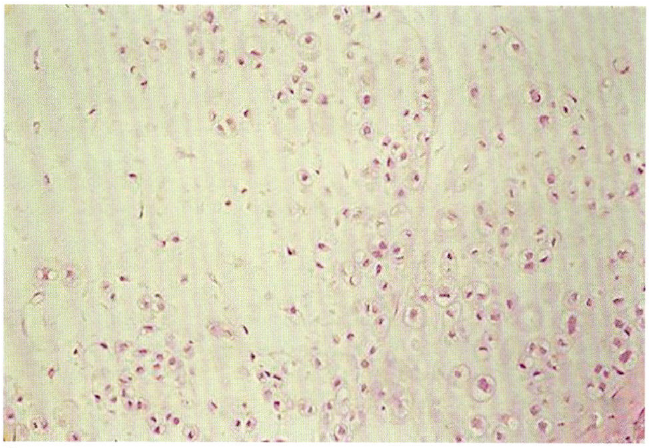

A

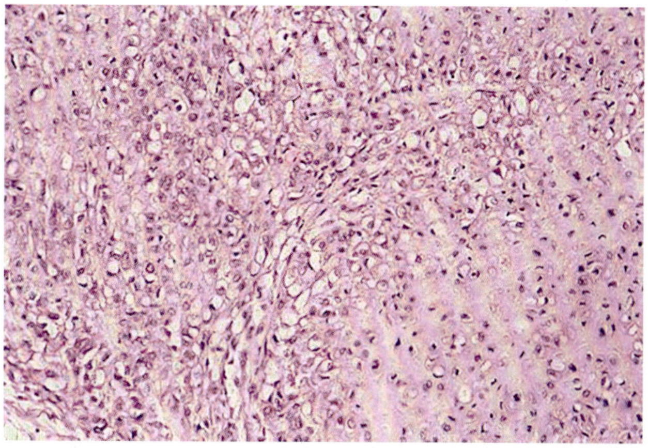

B

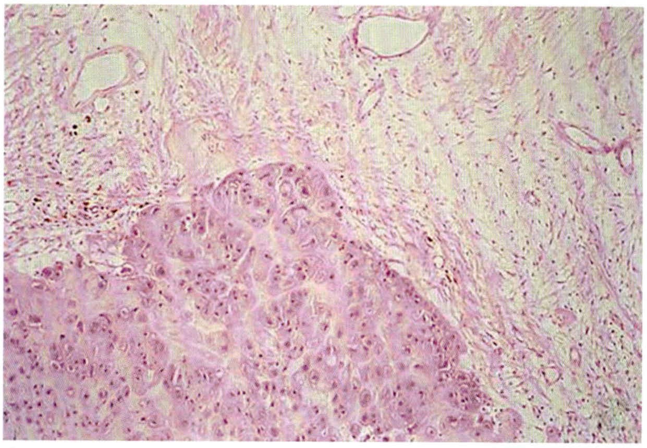

C

Figure 11.63 ■ Histopathology of chondrosarcoma developing in synovial (osteo)chondromatosis. A: The chondrocytes with clearly pleomorphic and occasionally large nuclei (lower right corner) are unevenly distributed. This appearance of nuclear size and structure not necessarily indicate malignancy and may be the feature of uncomplicated synovial (osteo)chondromatosis (H&E, original magnification ×50). **B:** Smaller part of benign synovial lesion (lower right) borders the cell-rich tissue of grade 2 to 3 secondary chondrosarcoma (H&E, original magnification ×50). **C:** At the proliferation line of the tumor against the fibrous connective tissue, there is more cartilaginous matrix formation by the tumor cells (H&E, original magnification ×25).

lining, combined with hypercellularity and pleomorphisms of the cells, should support the diagnosis of malignancy. Bertoni and coworkers have attempted to develop criteria for making this crucial distinction. They identified several microscopic features indicative of malignancy. The distinguishing features of synovial chondrosarcoma include the following: tumor cells arranged in sheets, myxoid changes in the matrix, hypercellularity with crowding and spindling of nuclei at the periphery, necrosis, and permeation of bone trabeculae. Remarking on the danger of misinterpreting synovial chondromatosis as chondrosarcoma on both radiographic and histopathologic examination, Bertoni and colleagues singled out pulmonary metastases as the only distinguishing feature.

The main differential diagnosis is between synovial chondrosarcoma and synovial (osteo)chondromatosis. Frequently, the imaging findings in both conditions are similar, although the development of destructive changes around the affected joint favors synovial chondrosarcoma. However, these destructive changes should be differentiated from periarticular erosions occasionally present in synovial chondromatosis. PVNS can usually be excluded without much difficulty, because it does not exhibit calcifications and, in addition, shows rather characteristic MRI features (see previous text).

MALIGNANT PVNS

Recently, Kalil and Unni reported a case of malignancy in PVNS and cited eight other cases from the literature. Enzinger and Weiss defined malignant PVNS as a malignant lesion occurring with concomitant or previously documented benign PVNS at the same location. Bertoni and coworkers documented histologic evolution from benign to malignant PVNS in three cases. The malignancy in PVNS is an extremely rare occurrence, yet this is a controversial issue, mainly because other synovium-centered lesions, such as clear cell sarcoma or epithelioid sarcoma, may be mistaken for malignant PVNS.

INTRA-ARTICULAR LIPOSARCOMA

Although liposarcomas of the soft tissues are not uncommon malignant tumors, accounting for ~16% of all soft tissue sarcomas, the intra-articular location is extremely rare. Intra-articular low-grade myxoid liposarcoma and high-grade intra-articular liposarcoma, both tumors located within the knee joint, have been reported. The MR imaging features of intra-articular tumors are quite similar to those in the extra-articular location, namely, heterogenous but mostly intermediate signal intensity on T1-weighted images and heterogenous intermediate-to-high signal intensity on T2 weighting.

SUGGESTED READINGS

Abdelwahab IF, Kenan S, Steiner GC, Abdul-Quader M. True bursal pigmented villonodular synovitis. *Skeletal Radiol.* 2002;31:354–358.

Abrahams TG, Pavlov H, Bansal M, Bullough P. Concentric joint space narrowing of the hip associated with hemosiderotic synovitis (HS) including pigmented villonodular synovitis (PVNS). *Skeletal Radiol.* 1988;17:37–45.

Ackerman LV. Extra-osseous localized non-neoplastic bone and cartilage formation (so-called myositis ossificans). Clinical and pathological confusion with malignant neoplasms. *J Bone Joint Surg Am.* 1958;40A: 279–298.

Adams ME, Saifuddin A. Characterisation of intra-articular soft tissue tumours and tumour-like lesions. *Eur Radiol.* 2007;17:950–958.

Aglietti P, Di Muria GV, Salvati EA, Stringa G. Pigmented villonodular synovitis of the hip joint (review of the literature and report of personal case material). *Ital J Orthop Traumatol.* 1983;9:487–496.

Arkun R, Memis A, Akalin T, et al. Liposarcoma of soft tissue: MRI findings with pathologic correlation. *Skeletal Radiol.* 1997;26:167–172.

Armstrong SJ, Watt I. Lipoma arborescens of the knee. *Br J Radiol.* 1989;62:178–180.

Assoun J, Railhac JJ, Bonnevialle P, et al. Osteoid osteoma: percutaneous resection with CT guidance. *Radiology.* 1993;188:541–547.

Assoun J, Richardi G, Railhac JJ, et al. Osteoid osteoma: MR imaging versus CT. *Radiology.* 1994;191:217–223.

Aoki J, Tanikawa H, Ishii K, et al. MR findings indicative of hemosiderin in giant-cell tumor of bone: frequency, cause, and diagnostic significance. *AJR Am J Roentgenol.* 1996;166:145–148.

Atar D, Lehman WB, Grant AD. Tips of the trade: computerized tomography—guided excision of osteoid osteoma. *Orthop Rev.* 1992;21:1457–1458.

Athanasou NA, Bliss E, Gatter KC, et al. An immunohistological study of giant-cell tumor of bone: evidence for an osteoclast origin of the giant cells. *J Pathol.* 1985;147:153–158.

Atmore WG, Dahlin DC, Ghormley RK. Pigmented villonodular synovitis; a clinical and pathologic study. *Minn Med.* 1956;39:196–202.

Bahk W-J, Lee H-Y, Kang Y-K, et al. Dysplasia epiphysealis hemimelica: radiographic and magnetic resonance imaging features and clinical outcome of complete and incomplete resection. *Skeletal Radiol.* 2010;39: 85–90.

Baker ND, Klein JD, Weidner N, et al. Pigmented villonodular synovitis containing coarse calcifications. *AJR Am J Roentgenol.* 1989;153:1228–1230.

Balsara ZN, Staiken BF, Martinez AJ. MR image of localized giant cell tumor of the tendon sheath involving the knee. *J Comput Assist Tomogr.* 1989;13:159–162.

Baruffi MR, Volpon JB, Neto JB, Casartelli C. Osteoid osteoma with chromosome alteration involving 22q. *Cancer Genet Cytogenet.* 2001;124: 127–131.

Bauer TW, Zehr RJ, Belhobek GH, Marks KE. Juxta-articular osteoid osteoma. *Am J Surg Pathol.* 1991;15:381–387.

Bejia I, Younes M, Moussa A, et al. Lipoma arborescens affecting multiple joints. *Skeletal Radiol.* 2005;34:536–538.

Bell RS, O'Conner GD, Waddell JP. Importance of magnetic resonance imaging in osteoid osteoma: a case report. *Can J Surg.* 1989;32: 276–278.

Bertoni F, Bacchini P, Staals EL. Malignancy in giant cell tumor. *Skeletal Radiol.* 2003;32:143–146.

Bertoni F, Present D, Enneking WF. Giant cell tumor of bone with pulmonary metastases. *J Bone Joint Surg Am.* 1985;67A:890–900.

Bertoni F, Present D, Sudanese A, et al. Giant cell tumor of bone with pulmonary metastases: six case reports and a review of the literature. *Clin Orthop.* 1988;237:275–285.

Bertoni F, Unni KK, Beabout JW, Sim FH. Chondrosarcomas of the synovium. *Cancer.* 1991;67:155–162.

Bertoni F, Unni KK, Beabout JW, Sim FH. Malignant giant cell tumor of the tendon sheaths and joints (malignant pigmented villonodular synovitis). *Am J Surg Pathol.* 1997;21:153–163.

Besette PR, Cooley PA, Johnson RP, Czarnecki DJ. Gadolinium-enhanced MRI of pigmented villonodular synovitis of the knee. *J Comput Assist Tomogr.* 1992;16:992–994.

Bixby SD, Hettmer S, Taylor GA, Voss SD. Synovial sarcoma in children: imaging features and common benign mimics. *AJR Am J Roentgenol.* 2010;195:1026–1032.

Blacksin MF, Ghelman B, Freiberger RH, Salvata E. Synovial chondromatosis of the hip: evaluation with air computed arthrotomography. *Clin Imaging.* 1990;14:315–318.

Bravo SM, Winalski CS, Weissman BN. Pigmented villonodular synovitis. *Radiol Clin North Am.* 1996;34:311–326.

Brodsky AE. Synovial hemangioma of the knee joint. *Bull Hosp Jt Dis Orthop Inst.* 1956;17:58–69.

Bullough PG. *Atlas of Orthopedic Pathology with Clinical and Radiologic Correlations.* 2nd ed. New York, NY: Gower; 1992:17.25–17.28.

Burnstein MI, Fisher DR, Yandow DR, et al. Case report 502. Intra-articular synovial chondromatosis of shoulder with extra-articular extension. *Skeletal Radiol.* 1988;17:458–461.

Cadman NL, Soule EH, Kelly PJ. Synovial sarcoma: an analysis of 134 tumors. *Cancer.* 1965;18:613–627.

Campanacci M. *Bone and Soft-Tissue Tumors.* New York, NY: Springer-Verlag; 1990:998–1012.

Campanacci M, Giunti A, Olmi R. Giant-cell tumors of bone: a study of 209 cases with long-term follow-up in 130. *Ital J Orthop Traumatol.* 1975;1:249–277.

Carter TR. Osteoid osteoma of the hip: an alternate method of excision. *Orthop Rev.* 1990;19:903–905.

Cassar-Pullicino VN, McCall IW, Wan S. Intra-articular osteoid osteoma. *Clin Radiol.* 1992;45:153–160.

Caudell JJ, Ballo MT, Zagars GK, et al. Radiotherapy in the management of giant cell tumor of bone. *Int J Radiat Oncol Biol Phys.* 2003;57:158.

Chen DY, Lan JL, Chou SJ. Treatment of pigmented villonodular synovitis with yttrium-90: changes in immunologic features. Tc-99m uptake measurements, and MR imaging of one case. *Clin Rheumatol.* 1992;11:280–285.

Corbett JM, Wilde AH, McCormack LJ, Evarts CM. Intra-articular osteoid osteoma: a diagnostic problem. *Clin Orthop.* 1974;98:225–230.

Cotten A, Flipo R-M, Chastanet P, et al. Pigmented villonodular synovitis of the hip: review of radiographic features in 58 patients. *Skeletal Radiol.* 1995;24:1–6.

Cotten A, Flipo RM, Herbaux B, et al. Synovial haemangioma of the knee: a frequently misdiagnosed lesion. *Skeletal Radiol.* 1995;24:257–261.

Crotty JM, Monu JUV, Pope TL Jr. Synovial osteochondromatosis. *Radiol Clin North Am.* 1996;34:327–342.

Dahlin DC. Giant cell tumor of bone: highlights of 407 cases. *AJR Am J Roentgenol.* 1985;144:955–960.

Dahlin DC, Unni KK. Chondrosarcoma. In: *Bone Tumors. General Aspects and Data on 8,542 Cases.* 4th ed. Springfield, IL: Charles C. Thomas; 1986:227–259.

De Beuckeleer L, De Schepper A, De Belder F, et al. Magnetic resonance imaging of localized giant cell tumour of the tendon sheath (MRI of localized GCTTS). *Eur Radiol.* 1997;7:198–201.

De St. Aubain Sommerhausen N, Dal Cin P. Giant cell tumour of tendon sheath. In: Fletcher CDM, Unni KK, Mertens F, eds. *World Health Organization Classification of Tumours. Pathology and Genetics. Tumours of Soft Tissue and Bone.* Lyon, France: IARC Press; 2002:110–111.

De St. Aubain Sommerhausen N, Dal Cin P. Diffuse-type giant cell tumour. In: Fletcher CDM, Unni KK, Mertens F, eds. *World Health Organization Classification of Tumours. Pathology and Genetics. Tumours of Soft Tissue and Bone.* Lyon, France: IARC Press; 2002:112–114.

Devaney K, Vinh TN, Sweet DE. Synovial hemangioma: report of 20 cases with differential diagnostic considerations. *Hum Pathol.* 1993;24: 737–745.

Dorwart RH, Genant HK, Johnston WH, Morris JM. Pigmented villonodular synovitis of synovial joints: clinical, pathologic, and radiologic features. *AJR Am J Roentgenol.* 1984;143:877–885.

Doyle AJ, Miller MV, French JG. Lipoma arborescens in the bicipital bursa of the elbow: MRI findings in two cases. *Skeletal Radiol.* 2002;31:656–660.

Doyle T, King K. Percutaneous removal of osteoid osteomas using CT control. *Clin Radiol.* 1989;40:515–517.

Dunn EJ, McGavran MH, Nelson P, Greer RB III. Synovial chondrosarcoma. Report of a case. *J Bone Joint Surg Am.* 1974;56A:811–813.

Ebrahim FS, Jacobson JA, Lin J, et al. Intraarticular osteoid osteoma: sonographic findings in three patients with radiographic, CT, and MR imaging correlation. *AJR Am J Roentgenol.* 2001;177:1391–1395.

Ehara S, Rosenthal DI, Aoki J, et al. Peritumoral edema in osteoid osteoma on magnetic resonance imaging. *Skeletal Radiol.* 1999;28:265–270.

Enzinger FM, Weiss SW. Benign tumors and tumor-like lesions of synovial tissue. In: *Soft Tissue Tumors*. St. Louis, MO: CV Mosby; 1988:638–658.

Enzinger FM, Weiss SW. *Soft Tissue Tumors*. 3rd ed. St. Louis, MO: CV Mosby, 1995:749–751, 757–786.

Eustace SE, Harrison M, Srinivasen U, Stack J. Magnetic resonance imaging in pigmented villonodular synovitis. *Can Assoc Radiol J.* 1994;45:283–286.

Evans HL. Synovial sarcoma: a study of 23 biphasic and 17 probably monophasic examples. *Pathol Annu.* 1980;15:309–313.

Fairbank TJ. Dysplasia epiphysealis hemimelica (tarso-epiphysial aclasis). *J Bone Joint Surg [Br].* 1956;38-B:237–257.

Falappa P, Garganese MC, Crocoli A, et al. Particular imaging features and customized thermal ablation treatment for intramedullary osteoid osteoma in pediatric patients. *Skeletal Radiol.* 2011;40:1523–1530.

Fechner RE, Mills SE. *Tumors of the Bones and Joints*. Washington, DC: Armed Forces Institute of Pathology; 1993.

Flanagan AM, Delaney D, O'Donnell P. The benefits of molecular pathology in the diagnosis of musculoskeletal disease. Part I of a two-part review: soft tissue tumors. *Skeletal Radiol.* 2010;39:105–115.

Fletcher AG Jr, Horn RC Jr. Giant-cell tumor of tendon sheath origin: a consideration of bone involvement and report of 2 cases with extensive bone destruction. *Ann Surg.* 1951;133:374–385.

Georgen TG, Resnick D, Niwayama G. Localized nodular synovitis of the knee: a report of two cases with abnormal arthrograms. *AJR Am J Roentgenol.* 1976;126:647–650.

Goldman RL, Lichtenstein L. Synovial chondrosarcoma. *Cancer.* 1964;17:1233–1240.

Goldman AB, Schneider R, Pavlov H. Osteoid osteoma of the femoral neck: report of four cases evaluated with isotopic bone scanning, CT, and MR imaging. *Radiology.* 1993;186:227–232.

Greenfield GB, Arrington JA, Kudryk BT. MRI of soft tissue tumors. *Skeletal Radiol.* 1993;22:77–84.

Greenspan A. Benign bone-forming lesions: osteoma, osteoid osteoma, and osteoblastoma. *Skeletal Radiol.* 1993;22:485–500.

Greenspan A, Azouz EM, Matthews J II, Décarie J-C. Synovial hemangioma: imaging features in eight histologically proved cases, review of the literature, and differential diagnosis. *Skeletal Radiol.* 1995;24:583–590.

Greenspan A, Borys D. *Radiology and Pathology Correlation of Bone Tumors. A Quick Reference and Review*. Philadelphia, PA: Wolters Kluwer; 2016:353–380.

Greenspan A, Jundt G, Remagen W. *Differential Diagnosis in Orthopaedic Oncology*. 2nd ed. Philadelphia, PA: Lippincott Williams & Wilkins; 2007:158–256; 387–431; 481–518.

Greenspan A, Steiner G, Sotello D, et al. Mixed sclerosing bone dysplasias coexisting with dysplasia epiphysealis hemimelica (Trevor-Fairbanks disease). *Skeletal Radiol.* 1986;15:452–454.

Grieten M, Buckwalter KA, Cardinal E, Rougraff B. Case report 873. Lipoma arborescens (villous lipomatous proliferation of the synovial membrane). *Skeletal Radiol.* 1994;23:652–655.

Haldar M, Randall RL, Capecchi MR. Synovial sarcoma: from genetics to genetic-based animal modeling. *Clin Orthop Relat Res.* 2008;466:2156–2167.

Hallel T, Lew S, Bansal M. Villous lipomatous proliferation of the synovial membrane (lipoma arborescens). *J Bone Joint Surg Am.* 1988;70A:264–270.

Hamilton A, Davis RI, Hayes D, Mollan RA. Chondrosarcoma developing in synovial chondromatosis. A case report. *J Bone Joint Surg Br.* 1987;69B:137–140.

Hermann G, Abdelwahab IF, Klein MJ, et al. Synovial chondromatosis. *Skeletal Radiol.* 1995;24:298–300.

Hermann G, Klein MJ, Abdelwahab IF, Kenan S. Synovial chondrosarcoma arising in synovial chondromatosis of the right hip. *Skeletal Radiol.* 1997;26:366–369.

Hisoaka M, Matsuyama A, Shimajiri S, et al. Ossifying synovial sarcoma. *Pathol Res Pract.* 2009;205:195–198.

Huang G-S, Lee C-H, Chan WP, et al. Localized nodular synovitis of the knee: MR imaging appearance and clinical correlates in 21 patients. *AJR Am J Roentgenol.* 2003;181:539–543.

Hudson TM, Schiebler M, Springfield DS, et al. Radiology of giant cell tumors of bone: computed tomography, arthrotomography, and scintigraphy. *Skeletal Radiol.* 1984;11:85–95.

Hudson TM. *Radiologic Pathologic Correlation of Musculoskeletal Lesions*. Baltimore, MD: Williams & Wilkins; 1987:209–237; 249–252; 261–265; 287–303; 359–397; 421–440.

Hughes TH, Sartoris DJ, Schweitzer ME, Resnick DL. Pigmented villonodular synovitis: MRI characteristics. *Skeletal Radiol.* 1995;24:7–12.

Ishida T, Iijima T, Moriyama S, et al. Intra-articular calcifying synovial sarcoma mimicking synovial chondromatosis. *Skeletal Radiol.* 1996;25:766–769.

Jaffe HL, Lichtenstein L, Sutro CJ. Pigmented villonodular synovitis, bursitis and tenosynovitis. *Arch Pathol Lab Med.* 1941;31:731–765.

Jelinek JS, Kransdorf MJ, Shmookler BM, et al. Giant cell tumor of the tendon sheath: MR findings in nine cases. *AJR Am J Roentgenol.* 1994;162:919–922.

Jelinek JS, Kransdorf MJ, Utz JA, et al. Imaging of pigmented villonodular synovitis with emphasis on MR imaging. *AJR Am J Roentgenol.* 1989;152:337–342.

Jones BC, Sundaram M, Kransdorf MJ. Synovial sarcoma: MR imaging findings in 34 patients. *AJR Am J Roentgenol.* 1993;161:827–830.

Jones FE, Soule EM, Coventry MB. Fibrous xanthoma of synovium (giant-cell tumor of tendon sheath, pigmented nodular synovitis). A study of 118 cases. *J Bone Joint Surg Am.* 1969;51A:76–86.

Kaiser TE, Ivins JC, Unni KK. Malignant transformation of extra-articular synovial chondromatosis: report of a case. *Skeletal Radiol.* 1980;5:223–226.

Kakkar N, Vasishta RK, Anand H. Pathological case of the month. Synovial lipomatosis. *Arch Pediatr Adolesc Med.* 1999;153:203–204.

Kalil RK, Unni KK. Malignancy in pigmented villonodular synovitis. *Skeletal Radiol.* 1998;27:392–395.

Kallas KM, Vaughan L, Haghighi P, Resnick D. Pigmented villonodular synovitis of the hip presenting as retroperitoneal mass. *Skeletal Radiol.* 2001;30:469–474.

Karasick D, Karasick S. Giant cell tumor of tendon sheath: spectrum of radiologic findings. *Skeletal Radiol.* 1992;21:219–224.

Kawai A, Woodruff J, Healey JH, et al. SYT-SSX gene fusion as a determinant of morphology and prognosis in synovial sarcoma. *N Engl J Med.* 1998;338:153–160.

Kettelkamp DB, Campbell CJ, Bonfiglio M. Dysplasia epiphysealis hemimelica. A report of fifteen cases and a review of the literature. *J Bone Joint Surg Am.* 1966;48-A:746–766.

Khan AM, Cannon S, Levack B. Primary intra-articular liposarcoma of the knee. *J Knee Surg.* 2003;16:107–109.

Khan S, Neumann CH, Steinback LS, Harrington KD. MRI of giant cell tumor of tendon sheath of the hand: a report of three cases. *Eur Radiol.* 1995;5:467–470.

Kindblom LG, Gunterberg B. Pigmented villonodular synovitis involving bone. Case report. *J Bone Joint Surg Am.* 1978;60A:830–832.

King JW, Spjut HJ, Fechner RE, Vanderpool DW. Synovial chondrosarcoma of the knee joint. *J Bone Joint Surg Am.* 1967;49A:1389–1396.

Kloen P, Keel SB, Chandler HP, et al. Lipoma arborescens of the knee. *J Bone Joint Surg Br.* 1998;80-B:298–301.

Krall RA, Kostinovsky M, Patchefsky AS. Synovial sarcoma: a clinical, pathological, and ultrastructural study of 26 cases supporting the recognition of monophasic variant. *Am J Surg Pathol.* 1981;5:137–151.

Kransdorf MJ, Jelinek JS, Moser RP, et al. Soft-tissue masses: diagnosis using MR imaging. *AJR Am J Roentgenol.* 1989;153:541–547.

Kransdorf MJ, Stull MA, Gilkey FW, Moser RP Jr. Osteoid osteoma. *Radiographics.* 1991;11:671–696.

Krause FG, Wroblewski JA, Younger ASE. Pigmented villonodular synovitis in both hindfeet. *Can J Surg.* 2009;52:E38–E39.

Laorr A, Helms CA. *MRI of Musculoskeletal Masses: A Practical Text and Atlas.* New York, NY: Igaku-Shoin; 1997.

Laorr A, Peterfy CG, Tirman PF, Rabassa AE. Lipoma arborescens of the shoulder: magnetic resonance imaging findings. *Can Assoc Radiol J.* 1995;46:311–313.

Lee M, Mahroof S, Pringle J, et al. Diffuse pigmented villonodular synovitis of the foot and ankle treated with surgery and radiotherapy. *Int Orthop.* 2005;29:403–405.

Lin J, Jacobson JA, Jamadar DA, Ellis JH. Pigmented villonodular synovitis and related lesions: the spectrum of imaging findings. *AJR Am J Roentgenol.* 1999;172:191–197.

Llauger J, Monill JM, Palmer J, Clotet M. Synovial hemangioma of the knee: MRI findings in two cases. *Skeletal Radiol.* 1995;24:579–581.

Llauger J, Palmer J, Rosón N, et al. Pigmented villonodular synovitis and giant cell tumors of the tendon sheath: radiologic and pathologic features. *AJR Am J Roentgenol.* 1999;172:1087–1091.

Mahajan H, Lorigan JG, Shirkhoda A. Synovial sarcoma: MR imaging. *Magn Reson Imaging.* 1989;7:211–216.

Malawer MM, Bickels J, Meller I, et al. Cryosurgery in the treatment of giant cell tumor. A long term followup study. *Clin Orthop Relat Res.* 1999;359:176–188.

Marcove RC, Lynden JP, Huvos AG, Bullough PG. Giant cell tumor treated by cryosurgery. *J Bone Joint Surg Am.* 1973;55-A:1633–1644.

Marui T, Yamamoto T, Yoshihara H, et al. De novo malignant transformation of giant cell tumor of bone. *Skeletal Radiol.* 2001;30:104–108.

Mazoyer JF, Kohler R, Bossard D. Osteoid osteoma: CT-guided percutaneous treatment. *Radiology.* 1991;181:269–271.

McDonald DJ, Sim FH, McLeod RA, Dahlin DC. Giant cell tumor of bone. *J Bone Joint Surg Am.* 1986;68A:235–242.

McGrath J. Giant-cell tumour of bone: an analysis of fifty-two cases. *J Bone Joint Surg Br.* 1972;54B:216–229.

McMaster PE. Pigmented villonodular synovitis with invasion of bone. Report of six cases. *J Bone Joint Surg Am.* 1960;42A:1170–1183.

Miettinen M, Virtanen I. Synovial sarcoma—a misnomer. *Am J Pathol.* 1984;117: 18–25.

Morton MJ, Berquist TH, McLeod RA, et al. MR imaging of synovial sarcoma. *AJR Am J Roentgenol.* 1991;156:337–340.

Mullins F, Berard CW, Eisenberg SH. Chondrosarcoma following synovial chondromatosis. A case study. *Cancer.* 1965;18:1180–1188.

Murphey MD, Gibson MS, Jennings BT, et al. From the archives of the AFIP: Imaging of synovial sarcoma with radiologic-pathologic correlation. *Radiographics.* 2006;26:1543–1565.

Murphey MD, Vidal JA, Fanburg-Smith JC, Gajewski DA. Imaging of synovial chondromatosis with radiologic-pathologic correlation. *Radiographics.* 2007;27:1465–1488.

Myers BW, Masi AT. Pigmented villonodular synovitis and tenosynovitis, a clinical epidemiologic study of 166 cases and literature review. *Medicine.* 1980;59:224–238.

Nascimento AG, Huvos AG, Marcove RC. Primary malignant giant cell tumor of bone: a study of eight cases and review of the literature. *Cancer.* 1979;44:1393–1402.

Nassar WAM, Bassiony AA, Elghazaly HA. Treatment of diffuse pigmented villonodular synovitis of the knee with combined surgical and radiosynovectomy. *HSS J.* 2009;5:19–23.

Norman A. Persistence or recurrence of pain: a sign of surgical failure in osteoid osteoma. *Clin Orthop.* 1978;130:263–266.

Norman A, Steiner GC. Bone erosion in synovial chondromatosis. *Radiology.* 1986;161:749–752.

Norman A, Abdelwahab IF, Buyon J, Matzkin E. Osteoid osteoma of the hip stimulating an early onset of osteoarthritis. *Radiology.* 1986;158:417–420.

Ontell F, Greenspan A. Chondrosarcoma complicating synovial chondromatosis: findings with magnetic resonance imaging. *Can Assoc Radiol J.* 1994;45:318–323.

O'Sullivan PJ, Harris AC, Munk PL. Radiological features of synovial cell sarcoma. *Br J Radiol.* 2008;81:346–356.

Parsonage S, Mehr A, Davies MD. Lipoma arborescens: a definitive MR imaging diagnosis. *Osteol Közlem.* 2001;9:80–82.

Peh WCG, Shek TWH, Davies AM, et al. Osteochondroma and secondary synovial osteochondromatosis. *Skeletal Radiol.* 1999;28:169–174.

Perry BE, McQueen DA, Lin JJ. Synovial chondromatosis with malignant degeneration to chondrosarcoma. Report of a case. *J Bone Joint Surg Am.* 1988;70A:1259–1261.

Pradhan S, Nayak BP, Padhi T, Sethy M. Bullous erythema nodosum leprosum masquerading as systemic onset juvenile idiopathic arthritis: a case report. *Lepr Rev.* 2015;86:387–390.

Prud'homme C, Nueffer J-P, Runge M, et al. Prospective pilot study of CT-guided microwave ablation in the treatment of osteoid osteoma. *Skeletal Radiol.* 2017;46:315–323.

Rao AS, Vigorita VJ. Pigmented villonodular synovitis (giant-cell tumor of the tendon sheath and synovial membrane). A review of eighty-one cases. *J Bone Joint Surg Am.* 1984;66A:76–94.

Resnick D, Oliphant M. Hemophilia-like arthropathy of the knee associated with cutaneous and synovial hemangiomas. *Radiology.* 1975;114: 323–326.

Rock MG, Pritchard DJ, Unni KK. Metastases from histologically benign giant-cell tumor of bone. *J Bone Joint Surg Am.* 1984;66A:269–274.

Rock MG, Sim FH, Unni KK, et al. Secondary malignant giant-cell tumor of bone. Clinicopathological assessment of nineteen patients. *J Bone Joint Surg Am.* 1986;68A:1073–1079.

Rosenthal DI, Aronow S, Murray WT. Iron content of pigmented villonodular synovitis detected by computed tomography. *Radiology.* 1979;133:409–411.

Rosenthal DI, Hornicek FJ, Wolfe MW, et al. Percutaneous radiofrequency coagulation of osteoid osteoma compared with operative treatment. *J Bone Joint Surg Am.* 1998;80A:815–821.

Rosenthal DI, Springfield DS, Gebhardt MC, et al. Osteoid osteoma: percutaneous radiofrequency ablation. *Radiology.* 1995;197:451–454.

Roux S, Mariette X. RANK and RANKL expression in giant-cell tumour of bone. *Lancet Oncol.* 2010;11:514.

Rubin BP. Tenosynovial giant cell tumor and pigmented villonodular synovitis: a proposal for unification of these clinically distinct but histologically and genetically identical lesions. *Skeletal Radiol.* 2007;36:267–268.

Rybak LD, Khaldi L, Wittig J, Steiner GC. Primary synovial chondrosarcoma of the hip joint in a 45-year-old male: case report and literature review. *Skeletal Radiol.* 2011;40:1375–1381.

Ryu KN, Jaovisidha S, Schweitzer M, et al. MR imaging of lipoma arborescens of the knee joint. *AJR Am J Roentgenol* 1996;167:1229–1232.

Salerno M, Avnet S, Alberghini M, et al. Histogenetic characterization of giant cell tumor of bone. *Clin Orthop Relat Res.* 2008;466:2081–2088.

Sánchez Reyes JM, Alcaraz Mexia M, Quiñones Tapia D, Aramburu JA. Extensively calcified synovial sarcoma. *Skeletal Radiol.* 1997;26:671–673.

Sanerkin NG. Malignancy, aggressiveness and recurrence in giant cell tumor of bone. *Cancer.* 1980;46:1641–1649.

Schajowicz F. Synovial chondromatosis. In: *Tumors and Tumorlike Lesions of Bones and Joints.* New York, NY: Springer-Verlag; 1981:541–545.

Shaerf DA, Mann B, Alorjani M, et al. High-grade intra-articular liposarcoma of the knee. *Skeletal Radiol.* 2011;40:363–365.

Shanmugapriya V, Subashini B, Brindha K, Shobhana S. A "benign" condition masquerading as arthritis. *BMJ Case Rep.* 2013; doi:10.1136/bcr-2013-010518.

Sharma H, Jane MJ, Reid R. Pigmented villonodular synovitis of the foot and ankle: forty years of experience from the Scottish Bone Tumor Registry. *Foot Ankle Surg.* 2006;45:329–336.

Sheldon PJ, Forrester DM, Learch TJ. Imaging of intraarticular masses. *Radiographics.* 2005;25:105–119.

Shen M, Ng SC. Multiple myeloma masquerades as rheumatic diseases. *Proc Singapore Health.* 2013;22:64–69.

Sherry JB, Anderson W. The natural history of pigmented villonodular synovitis of tendon sheath. *J Bone Joint Surg Am.* 1956;37A: 1005–1011.

Singh AS, Chawla NS, Chawla SP. Giant-cell tumor of bone: treatment options and role of denosumab. *Biologics.* 2015;9:69–74.

Skubitz KM, Cheng EY, Clohisy DR, et al. Gene expression in giant-cell tumors. *J Lab Clin Med.* 2004;144:193–200.

Smith LT, Mayerson J, Nowak NJ, et al. 20q11.1 amplification in giant-cell tumor of bone: array CGH, FISH, and association with outcome. *Genes Chromosomes Cancer.* 2006;45:957–966.

Sommerhausen NSA, Fletcher CDM. Diffuse-type giant cell tumor. Clinicopathologic and immunohistochemical analysis of 50 cases with extraarticular disease. *Am J Surg Pathol.* 2000;24:479–492.

Soule EH. Synovial sarcoma. *Am J Surg Pathol.* 1986;10:78–82.

Stacy GS, Peabody TD, Dixon LB. Pictorial essay. Mimics on radiography of giant cell tumor of bone. *AJR Am J Roentgenol.* 2003;181: 1583–1589.

Steiner GC, Ghosh L, Dorfman HD. Ultrastructure of giant cell tumor of bone. *Hum Pathol.* 1972;3:569–586.

Stout AP, Lattes R. Tumors of the soft tissue. In: *Atlas of Tumor Pathology*, 2nd series, fascicle 1. Washington, DC: Armed Forces Institute of Pathology; 1967.

Strickland B, Mackenzie DH. Bone involvement in synovial sarcoma. *J Fac Radiol.* 1959;10:64–72.

Thomas D, Henshaw R, Skubitz K, et al. Denosumab in patients with giant-cell tumor of bone: an open-label, phase 2 study. *Lancet Oncol.* 2010;11:275.

Tubbs WS, Brown LR, Beabout JW, et al. Benign giant-cell tumor of bone with pulmonary metastases: clinical findings and radiologic appearance of metastases in 13 cases. *AJR Am J Roentgenol.* 1992;158:331–334.

Ushijima M, Hashimoto H, Tsuneyoshi M, Enjoji M. Giant cell tumor of the tendon sheath (nodular tenosynovitis). A study of 207 cases to compare the large joint group with the common digit group. *Cancer.* 1986;57:875–884.

van Rijswijk CSP, Hogendoorn PCW, Taminiau AHM, Bloem JL. Synovial sarcoma: dynamic contrast-enhanced MR imaging features. *Skeletal Radiol.* 2001;30:25–30.

Vengadakrishnan K, Saraswat PK, Mathur PC. A study of rheumatological manifestations of leprosy. *Indian J Dermatol Venereol Leprol.* 2004;70:76–78.

Vergara-Lluri ME, Stohr BA, Puligandla B, et al. A novel sarcoma with dual differentiation: clinicopathologic and molecular characterization of a combined synovial sarcoma and extraskeletal myxoid chondrosarcoma. *Am J Surg Pathol.* 2012;36:1093–1098.

von Borstel D, Taguibao RA, Strle NA, Burns JE. Giant cell tumor of bone: aggressive case initially treated with denosunab and intralesional surgery. *Skeletal Radiol.* 2017;46:571–578.

White EA, Omid R, Mateuk GR, et al. Lipoma arborescens of the biceps tendon sheath. *Skeletal Radiol.* 2013; 42:1461–1464.

Wilkerson BW, Crim JR, Hung M, Layfield LJ. Characterization of synovial sarcoma calcification. *AJR Am J Roentgenol.* 2012;199:W730–W734.

Winnepenninckx V, De Vos R, Debiec-Rychter M, et al. Calcifying/ossifying synovial sarcoma shows t(x;18) with SSX2 involvement and mitochondrial calcifications. *Histopathology.* 2001;38:141–145.

Wittkop B, Davies AM, Mangham DC. Primary synovial chondromatosis and synovial chondrosarcoma: a pictorial review. *Eur Radiol.* 2002;12:2112–2119.

Wright PH, Sim FH, Soule EH, Taylor WF. Synovial sarcoma. *J Bone Joint Surg Am.* 1982;64A:112–122.

CHAPTER 12

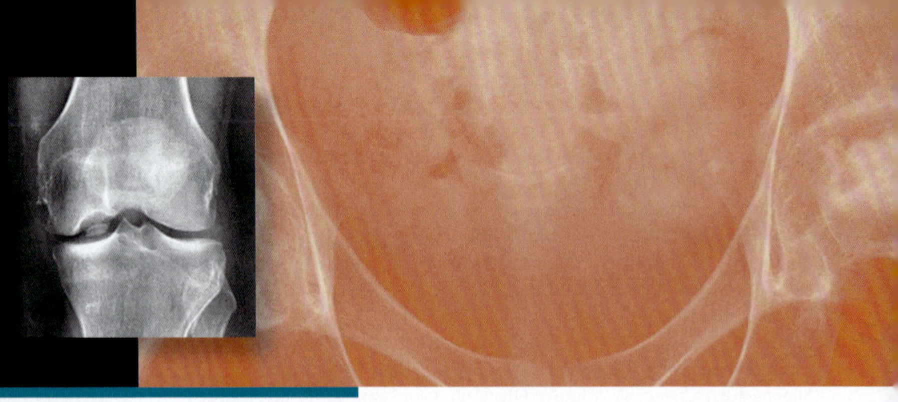

Trauma and Trauma-Related Conditions

COMPLEX REGIONAL PAIN SYNDROME (CRPS)/REFLEX SYMPATHETIC DYSTROPHY SYNDROME (RSDS)

Known also as *reflex sympathetic dystrophy syndrome* and *Sudeck atrophy*, CRPS is a clinical syndrome of variable course and unknown cause, characterized by disabling pain, swelling, and vasomotor dysfunction of an extremity. CRPS represents a vastly overdiagnosed illness. There are no specific diagnostic tests, and the diagnosis is based on clinical history, clinical examination, and supportive laboratory findings. There is also no single pathophysiologic mechanism that can explain the diversity and heterogeneity of the symptoms. It can occur following trauma that includes a neurologic injury, and the patient may present with pain and hyperesthesia, diffuse soft tissue swelling, joint stiffness, vasomotor instability, and dystrophic skin changes. There are no acceptable classifications. In 1993, International Association for Study of Pain (IASP) designated a task force to review the nomenclature and develop diagnostic criteria of CRPS. In 1994, at a consensus workshop in Florida, the task force developed the nomenclature (CRPS) and proposed the diagnostic criteria. Furthermore, they subdivided CRPS into types I and II. In CRPS type I, there is no clinically significant neurologic injury, whereas CRPS type II is a classic abnormality first described during civil war that is characterized by well-defined neurologic injury. Some researches have even claimed that the symptoms can spread throughout the body, a claim neither with scientifically proven data nor, even more importantly, with any biologic or medical plausibility. Occasionally, CRPS may be mistakenly diagnosed as arthritis, which can lead to overprescription of pain medication.

Three stages of this condition have been identified. The initial (or acute) inflammatory stage lasts from 1 to 7 weeks and is characterized by diffuse regional pain, inflammation, edema, and hypothermia or hyperthermia. In the second (or dystrophic) stage, which lasts from 3 to 24 months, the clinical findings include pain on exercise, increased sensitivity of the skin to pressure and temperature changes, and skin and muscle atrophy. In the final (or atrophic) stage, irreversible scleroderma-like skin changes and aponeurotic and tendinous retraction may occur.

On the radiographs, RSDS is characterized by soft tissue swelling and severe, patchy osteoporosis that progresses rapidly (Fig. 12.1). Bone densitometry shows a lowered bone mineral density content in affected limb. Three-phase technetium bone scan may show increased blood flow, blood pool, and periarticular increased uptake in the affected areas (Fig. 12.2), although these findings are not specific and can be present in patients with other bone abnormalities. The above-listed findings are seen in ~ 60% of affected patients that truly have CRPS.

The clinical management of patients with CRPS is a nearly daily challenge to rheumatologists, neurologists, neurosurgeons, orthopedic surgeons, and pain specialists. The aim of the treatment is pain control and recovery of limb function. Physical therapy is the first line of treatment. Pharmacologic therapy and selection of the drugs are determined by the severity of the pain and include NSAIDs and COX-2 inhibitors. Metamizol and controlled release opioids (such as hydrocodone or oxycodone) are considered in patients with more severe pain that is not responding to other measures. Recently, neuromodulation of central pain pathways by delivery of an electrical current or chemical application to the central neural axis has been tried with promising results.

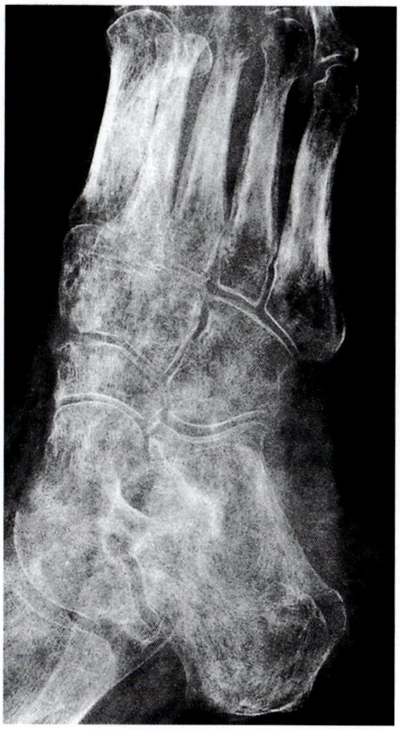

Figure 12.1 ■ **Reflex sympathetic dystrophy syndrome.** A 35-year-old man sustained fractures of the tibia and fibula, which eventually have healed. Subsequently, he reported weakness, stiffness, and pain in his foot. Radiographic examination showed changes typical of this condition, including rapidly progressive, patchy osteoporosis associated with marked soft tissue swelling.

TRANSIENT REGIONAL OSTEOPOROSIS

Transient regional osteoporosis is a collective term for a group of conditions that have one feature in common: rapidly developing osteoporosis that usually affects the periarticular regions and has no definite etiology such as trauma or immobilization. It is a self-limited and reversible disorder, of which three subtypes have been described. *Transient osteoporosis of the hip* is seen predominantly in pregnant women and in young and middle-aged men. Its primary manifestation is local osteoporosis involving the femoral head, femoral neck, and the acetabulum (Fig. 12.3). Regional migratory osteoporosis, which affects the knee, the ankle, and the foot, is mainly seen in men in their fourth and fifth decades. This migratory condition is characterized by pain and swelling around the affected joints and can mimic arthritis. It develops rapidly and subsides in about 6 to 9 months; there may be subsequent recurrence and involvement of other joints. *Idiopathic juvenile osteoporosis* is commonly seen during or just before puberty and typically regresses spontaneously. Skeletal involvement is often symmetrical and osteoporosis is generally juxta-articular in location. Spine is occasionally affected, and the vertebral body compression fractures may be encountered.

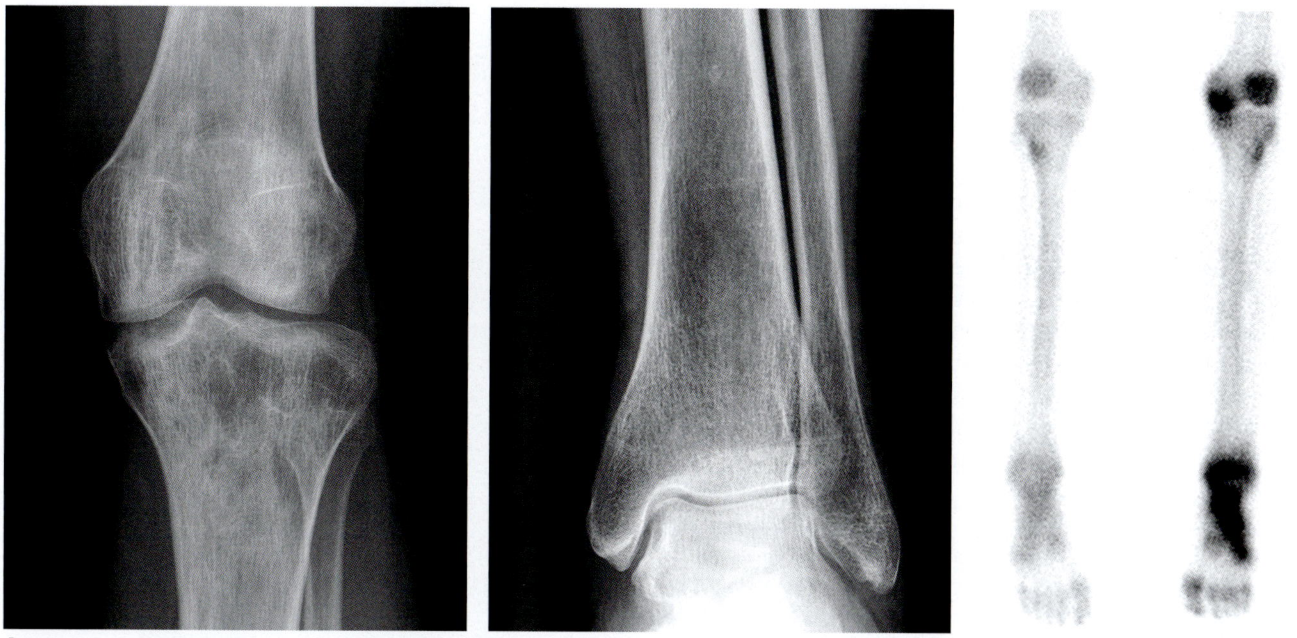

A B C

Figure 12.2 ■ **Scintigraphy of reflex sympathetic dystrophy syndrome.** A 52-year-old man, who sustained a fracture of the left femur 2 years previously, presented with history of pain and edema in the left lower extremity exaggerated by exercise, as well as increased sensitivity of the skin to pressure and temperature changes. Anteroposterior radiographs of the left knee **(A)** and left ankle **(B)** show diffuse periarticular osteoporosis. **C:** A radionuclide bone scan of both legs obtained after intravenous administration of 15 mCi of ^{99m}Tc-labeled MDP shows increased uptake of a radiopharmaceutical tracer in the region of the left knee and left ankle. In addition, there was typical for this condition an increase activity in the blood flow and blood pool phases of scintigraphy of this extremity (not shown here).

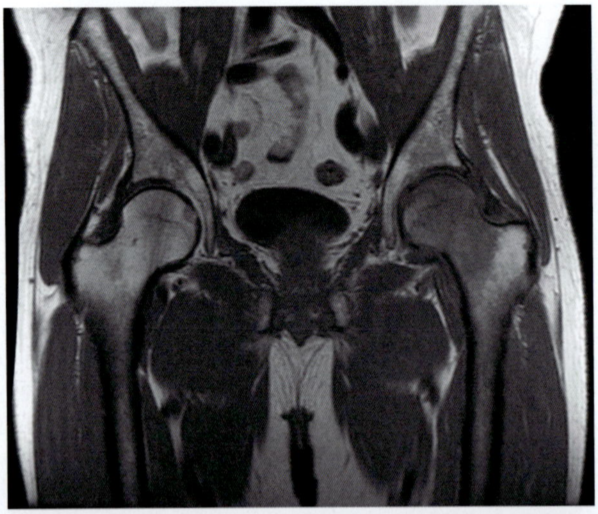

A

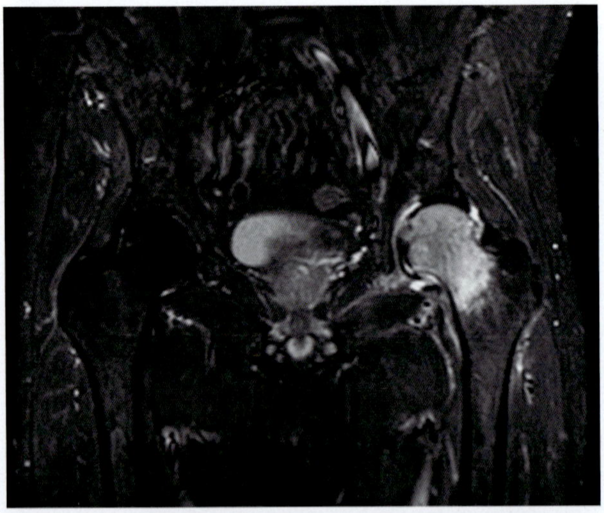

B

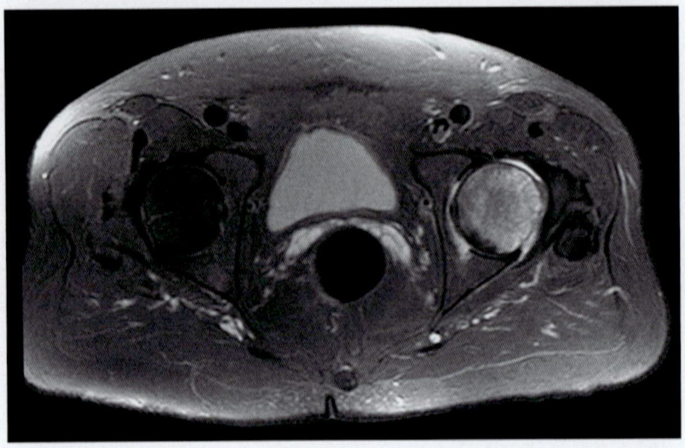

C

Figure 12.3 ■ MRI of transient osteoporosis of hip. A 50-year-old man presented with left hip pain. Conventional radiographs (not shown here) were unremarkable. **A:** Coronal T1-weighted MR image of the pelvis and hip joints shows decreased signal intensity in the left femoral head and neck. Coronal short time inversion recovery (STIR) **(B)** and axial T2-weighted **(C)** MR images demonstrate high signal intensity in the same sites.

POSTTRAUMATIC MYOSITIS OSSIFICANS

Occasionally, after a fracture, dislocation, or even minor trauma to the soft tissues, an enlarging, well-circumscribed painful mass develops at the site of injury. Clinically, pain and swelling at this site persist for many days. The pain tends to become more localized and may increase in intensity for up to 4 to 6 weeks. The characteristic feature of this lesion includes the clearly recognizable pattern of its evolution, which correlates well with the lapse of time after the trauma. Thus, by the 3rd or 4th week, calcifications and ossifications in the mass begin to develop (Fig. 12.4), and by the 6th to 8th week, the periphery of the mass shows definite, well-organized cortical bone (Fig. 12.5). The important radiographic hallmark of this complication is the presence of the so-called *zonal phenomenon*. On the radiograph, this phenomenon is characterized by a radiolucent area in the center of the lesion, indicating the formation of an immature bone, and by a dense zone of mature ossification at the periphery (myositis ossificans circumscripta). In addition, a thin radiolucent cleft separates the ossific mass from the adjacent cortex (Fig. 12.6). These important features help differentiate this condition from juxtacortical osteosarcoma, which

(Continued on page 424)

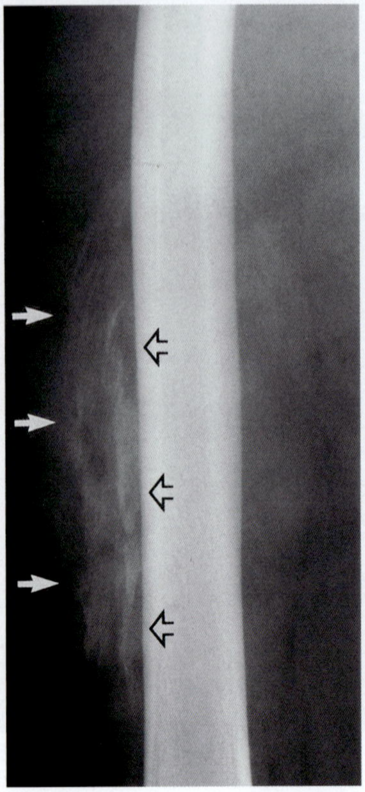

Figure 12.4 ■ Myositis ossificans. Maturation of myositis ossificans in a 28-year-old woman who sustained an injury to her thigh 5 weeks before this radiograph was obtained. Note the formation of peripheral ossification (*arrows*) and the presence of a radiolucent cleft (*open arrows*).

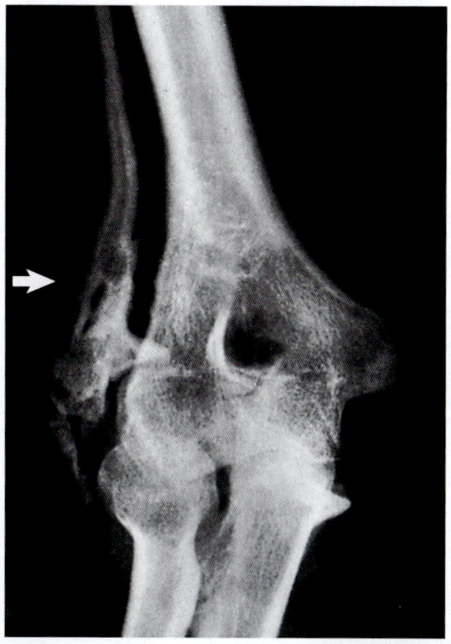

Figure 12.5 ■ **Myositis ossificans.** Anteroposterior radiograph of the right elbow of a 27-year-old man, who 1 year previously had sustained an injury to this site, shows a well-organized mature focus of myositis ossificans circumscripta. Note the well-developed cortex at the periphery of the osseous mass (*arrow*), and the radiolucent gap separating the lesion from the cortex of the humerus.

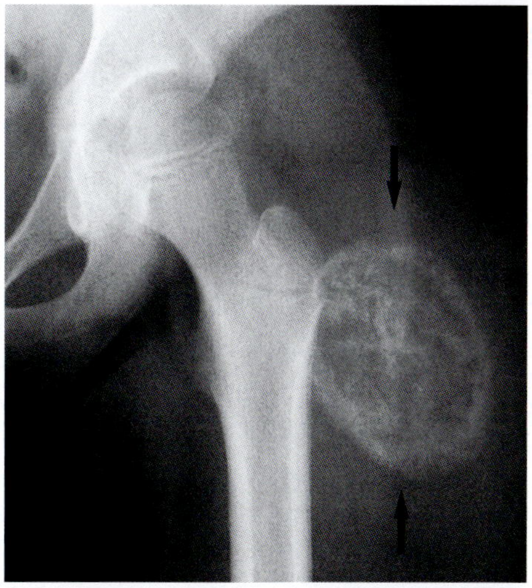

A

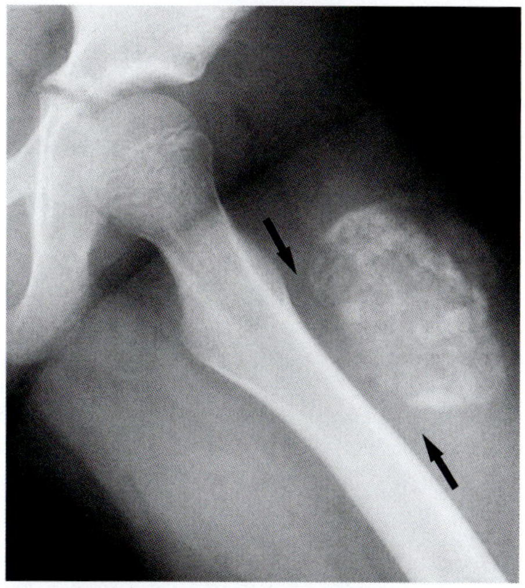

B

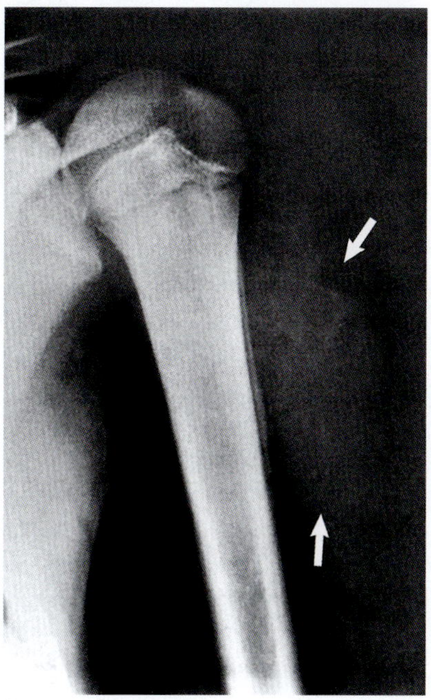

C

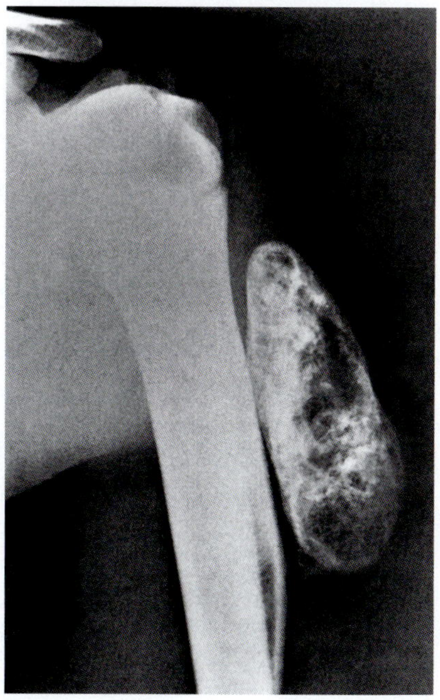

D

Figure 12.6 ■ **Myositis ossificans.** **A:** Anteroposterior radiograph of the left hip of a 7-year-old boy, who presented with a history of trauma 6 weeks before this radiographic examination, demonstrates a soft tissue lesion that exhibits features of zonal phenomenon (*arrows*). **B:** Frog-lateral projection shows radiolucent cleft (*arrows*) separating ossific mass from the posterolateral cortex of the femur. **C:** Three weeks after injury to the left upper arm, a well-organized periosteal reaction is seen along the lateral aspect of the proximal humeral diaphysis of an 11-year-old boy. Soft tissue mass adjacent to the cortex (*arrows*) shows evidence of early mineralization. **D:** Ten weeks after injury, the soft tissue mass shows well-organized peripheral ossifications with radiolucencies in the center, typical of zoning phenomenon.

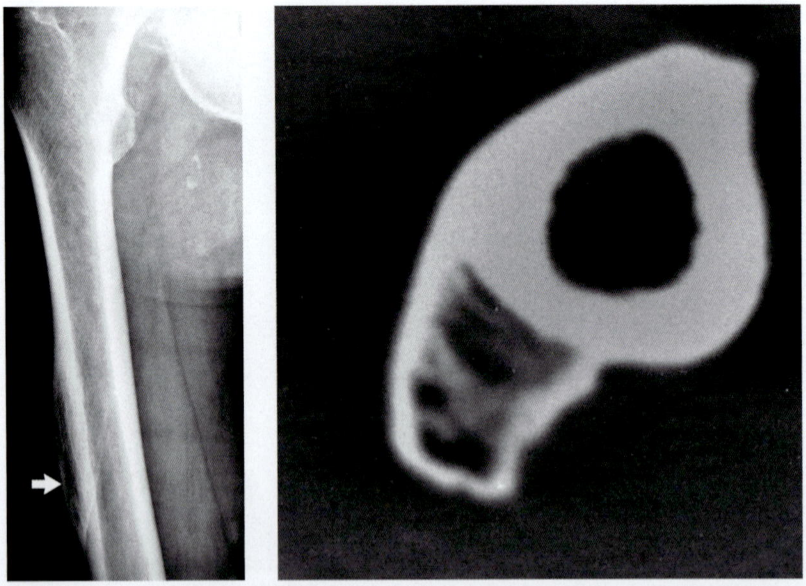

A B

Figure 12.7 ■ CT of myositis ossificans. A 52-year-old man sustained an injury to the lateral aspect of the right thigh 6 months previously. **A:** The anteroposterior radiograph of the proximal femur shows an ossific mass adherent to the lateral cortex (*arrow*). **B:** Axial CT section demonstrates the classic zonal phenomenon of this lesion, namely, the radiolucent center surrounded by mature cortex.

may, at times, appear very similar. It must be stressed, however, that occasionally, the focus of myositis ossificans may adhere and fuse with the cortex, mimicking parosteal osteosarcoma on radiographs. In these cases, CT may provide additional information, such as the presence of the zonal phenomenon characteristic of myositis ossificans (Fig. 12.7). The MRI appearance of myositis ossificans depends on the stage of maturation of the lesion. In the early stage, T1-weighted sequences usually show a mass that lacks definable borders with homogeneous intermediate signal intensity, slightly higher than that of adjacent muscle. T2-weighted images show the lesion to be of high signal intensity. The more mature lesions show intermediate signal intensity on T1-weighted sequences isointense with adjacent muscle, surrounded by a rim of low signal intensity, which corresponds to peripheral bone maturation. On T2 weighting, the lesion is generally of high signal intensity but may appear heterogeneous. The rim of low signal is seen at the periphery. Sometimes, the focus of myositis ossificans (whether immature or mature) may contain a fatty component, giving the lesion a high-intensity signal on T1-weighted images (Fig. 12.8). After an intravenous administration of gadopentetate dimeglumine, T1-weighted images show a well-defined peripheral rim of contrast enhancement, but the center of the lesion does not enhance (Fig. 12.9).

(Continued on page 426)

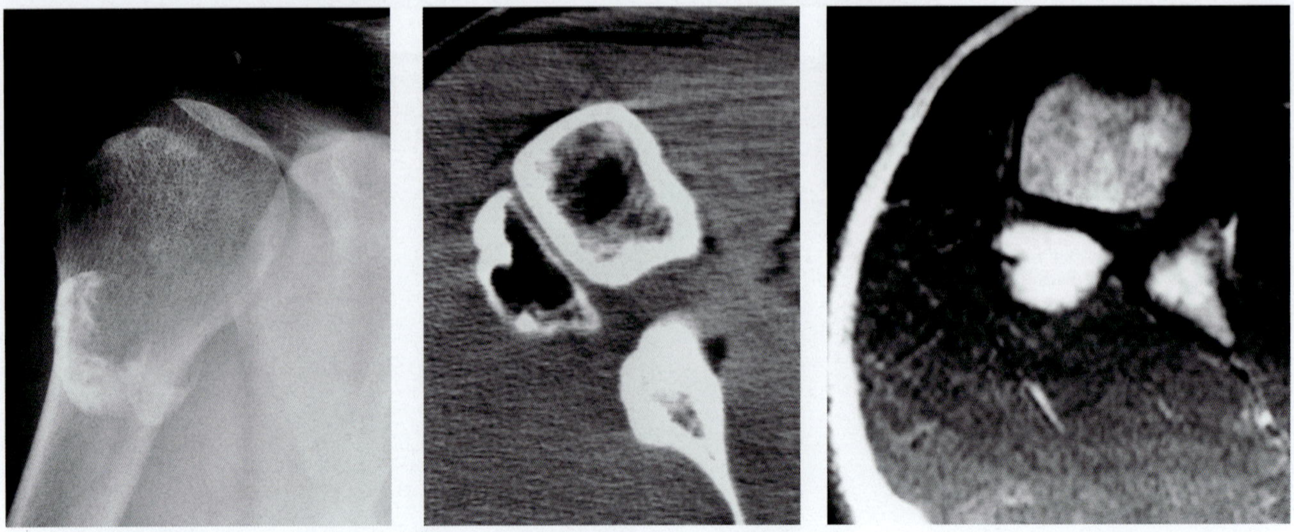

A B C

Figure 12.8 ■ CT and MRI of myositis ossificans. A 41-year-old man presented with palpable mass over posterior aspect of the proximal right humerus. **A:** Anteroposterior radiograph of the right shoulder shows calcifications and ossifications overlying the proximal humerus. **B:** Axial CT section demonstrates the zonal phenomenon typical for myositis ossificans circumscripta. The center of the lesion shows a low-attenuation area cased by fatty changes. The cleft separates the mass from the humeral cortex. **C:** Axial T1-weighted MR image shows the center of the lesion to be of high signal intensity representing fat, whereas the periphery of the lesion exhibits intermediate-to-low signal consistent with ossification.

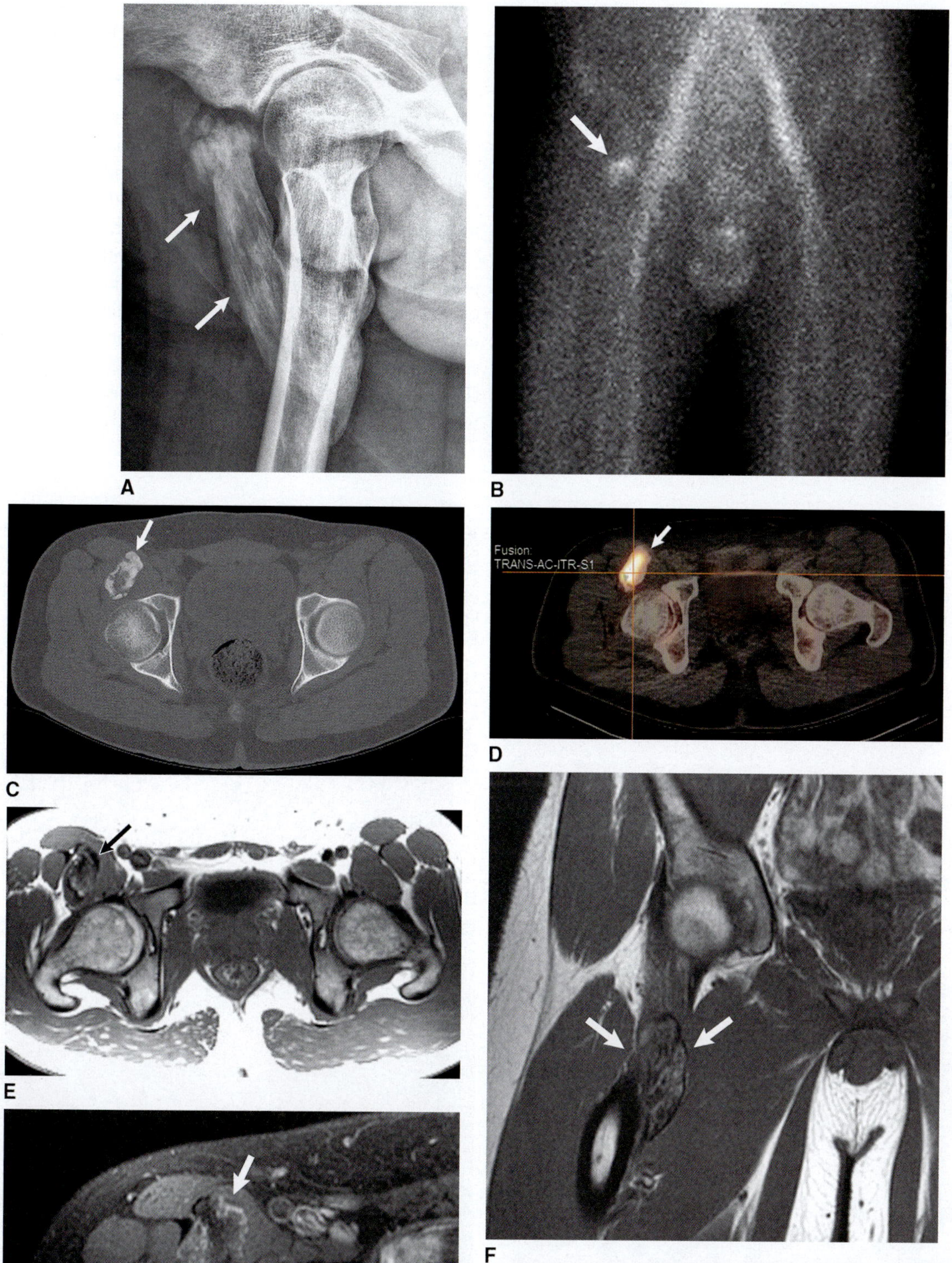

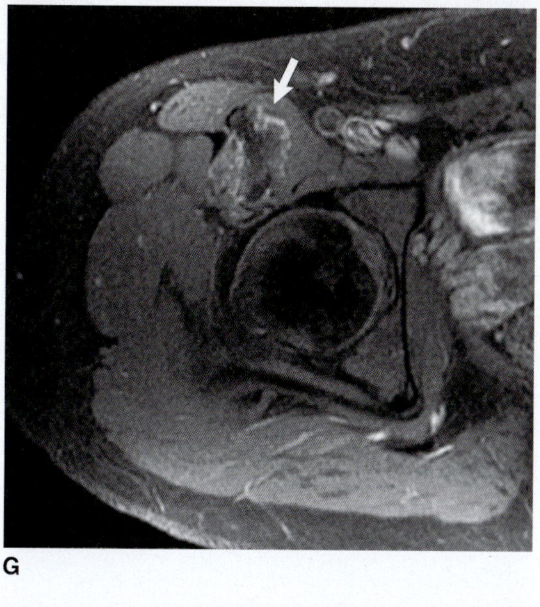

Figure 12.9 ■ **Scintigraphy, CT, PET/CT, and MRI of myositis ossificans. A:** Frog-lateral radiograph of the right hip of a 20-year-old man shows ossific soft tissue mass adjacent to the proximal femur and hip joint (*arrows*). **B:** Blood pool phase of the radionuclide bone scan shows accumulation of the radiopharmaceutical agent in the region of the mass (*arrow*). **C:** Axial CT image of the hip joints shows the mass (*arrow*) displaying low attenuation in the center and high attenuation at the periphery, characteristic features of zonal phenomenon. **D:** Fused PET/CT image shows the mass (*arrow*) exhibiting higher metabolic activity in the center and much lower activity in the periphery of the lesion, again, typical for zonal phenomenon. Axial **(E)** and coronal **(F)** T1-weighted MR images show the mass (*arrows*) displaying heterogeneous but predominantly low signal intensity. **G:** Axial T1-weighted MR image obtained after intravenous administration of gadolinium shows peripheral enhancement of the mass (*arrow*).

The histopathologic features are pathognomonic and consist of the least mature tissue in the center of the lesion and more mature at the periphery, corresponding to the radiographic zonal phenomenon. In the central portion of the lesion, noted are increased cellularity and the presence of immature fibroblastic cells, whereas at the periphery, microtrabeculae with peripheral appositional osteoblasts are present (Fig. 12.10). Biopsy of the lesion in its early stage may lead to erroneous diagnosis of malignancy.

The treatment of myositis ossificans varies with each case. In most cases, so-called "wait and watch" approach is advisable, because the lesion may shrink in time and became asymptomatic. Complete surgical excision is performed after full maturation of the lesion. Nonsurgical treatment with shock waves has been occasionally tried.

POSTTRAUMATIC OSTEOLYSIS OF THE DISTAL CLAVICLE

After injury to the shoulder, such as sprain of the acromioclavicular joint, resorption of the distal (acromial) end of the clavicle may occasionally occur. At times, this abnormality may be mistaken for resorption of the acromial end of the clavicle occurring in rheumatoid arthritis or in the primary hyperparathyroidism. The osteolytic process, which is associated with mild-to-moderate pain, usually begins within 2 months after injury. The initial radiographic findings consist of soft tissue swelling and periarticular osteoporosis associated with slightly irregular contour of acromial end of the clavicle (Fig. 12.11). Later, small erosions may develop (Fig. 12.12). MRI findings comprise increased signal intensity on water-sensitive sequences of the acromial end of the clavicle related

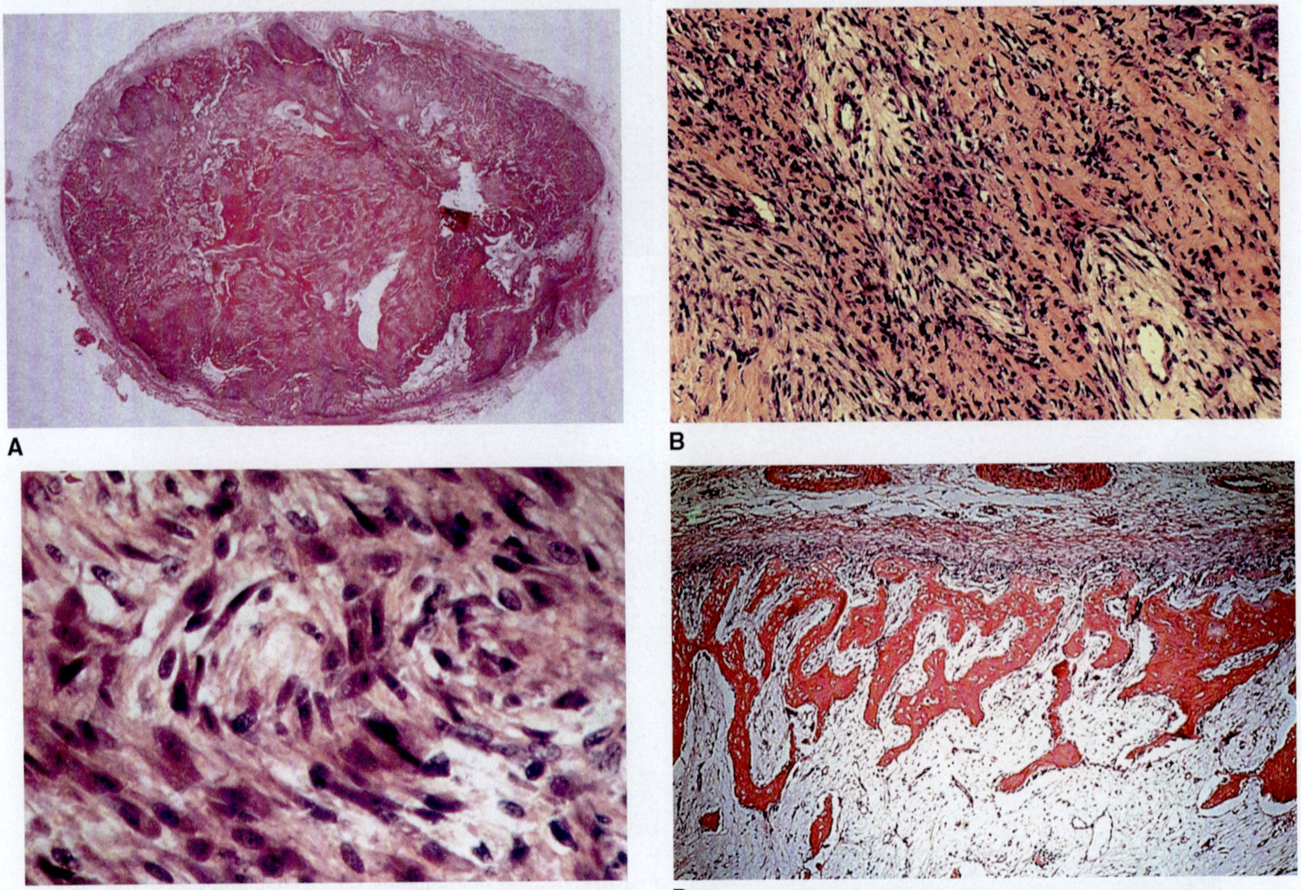

A B C D

Figure 12.10 ■ **Histopathology of myositis ossificans. A:** Photomicrograph of the entire resected lesion shows the fibrous cellular center and more mature bone at the periphery (H&E, original magnification ×1). **B:** Histologic section taken from the central portion of the lesion shows immature bone matrix formation (H&E, original magnification ×25). **C:** Higher-power photomicrograph of the same areas shows spindle-cell features. The cells have a disorderly arrangement and are producing collagen (H&E, original magnification ×40). **D:** Histologic section taken from the periphery of the lesion demonstrates mature bone formation (H&E, original magnification ×10). (From Bullough PG. *Atlas of Orthopedic Pathology with Clinical and Radiologic Correlation.* 2nd ed. New York, NY: Gower Medical Publishing, 1992. Figs. 18.35, 18.33, 18.32, and 18.34, pp. 18.14–18.15.)

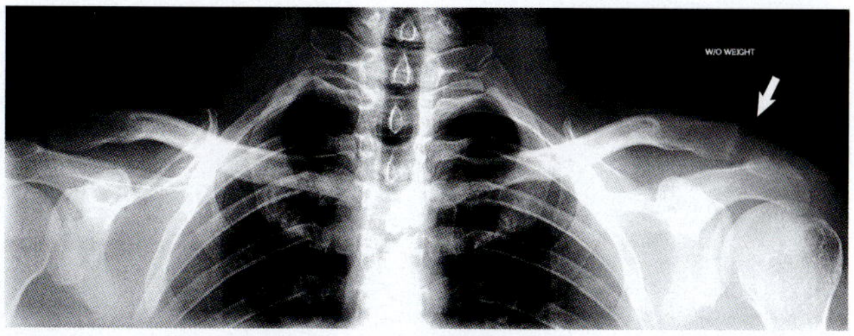

A

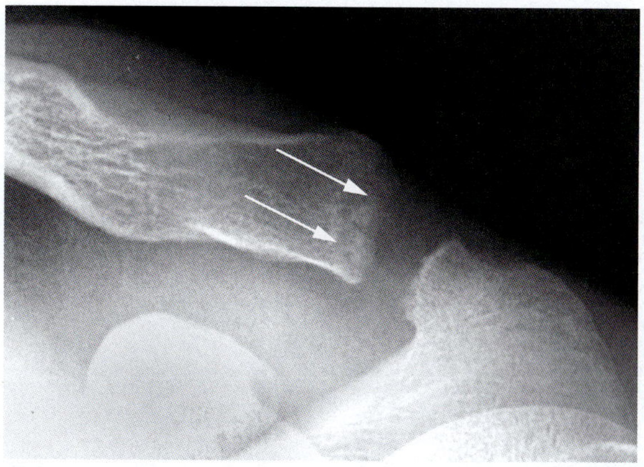

B

Figure 12.11 ■ Posttraumatic osteolysis of the distal clavicle. **A:** Anteroposterior radiograph of both clavicles shows slight widening of the left acromioclavicular joint (*arrow*). **B:** A magnified coned-down view of the left acromioclavicular joint shows periarticular osteoporosis and irregular contour of acromial end of the clavicle associated with small radiolucent foci (*arrows*).

to bone marrow edema, marginal irregularity of the bone outline, and fluid within the acromioclavicular joint (Fig. 12.13). In its late stage, resorption of the distal end of the clavicle results in marked widening of the acromioclavicular joint (Fig. 2.14).

SHOULDER IMPINGEMENT SYNDROME

Impingement syndrome of the shoulder refers to a condition in which the supraspinatus tendon and subacromial bursa are chronically entrapped between the humeral head inferiorly and the anterior acromion itself, spurs of the anterior acromion or acromioclavicular joint, or the coracoacromial ligament (coracoacromial arc) superiorly. Early diagnosis and treatment of impingement syndrome are critical to improve shoulder function and prevent the progression of this condition. Frequently, however, clinical signs and symptoms are nonspecific and may mimic arthritis, and the diagnosis is often delayed until a full-thickness tear in the rotator cuff has developed. Only rarely it can be definitely diagnosed based on the clinical findings, characterized by severe pain during abduction and external rotation of the arm. More reliable are imaging findings associated with this abnormality, including subacromial proliferation of bone, spurring at the inferior aspect of the acromion, and degenerative changes of the humeral tuberosities at the insertion of the rotator cuff.

Neer described three progressive stages of impingement syndrome apparent clinically and at surgery. Stage I consists of edema and hemorrhage and is reversible with conservative therapy. It typically occurs in young individuals engaged in sport activities requiring excessive use of the arm above the head (i.e., swimming). Stage II consists of fibrosis and thickening of the subacromial soft tissues, rotator cuff tendinitis, and sometimes a partial tear of the rotator cuff. It is manifested clinically by recurrent pain and is often seen in patients 25 to 40 years old. Stage III represents complete rupture of the rotator cull and is associated with progressive disability. It is usually seen in patients older than 40 years of age. Because of its high soft tissue contrast resolution and multiplanar imaging capabilities, MRI is the only technique that can accurately image the early changes of this condition, in particular bursal thickening and effusion (subacromial bursitis), edema, and inflammatory changes of the rotator cuff and its tendons (Fig. 12.15A, B), and later changes consisting of partial- and full-thickness tear of the rotator cuff (Fig. 12.15C, D).

(Continued on page 430)

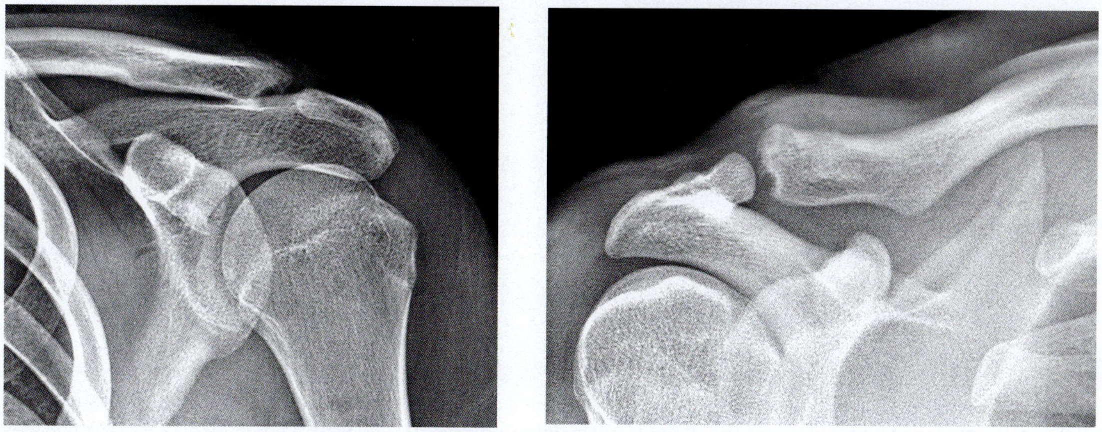

A B

Figure 12.12 ■ Posttraumatic osteolysis of the distal clavicle. **A:** Anteroposterior radiograph of the left shoulder of a 20-year-old man, who presented with shoulder pain following a football injury 5 months previously, shows erosion of the acromial end of the clavicle. **B:** Anteroposterior radiograph of the right acromioclavicular joint (obtained with a 15-degree cephalad angulation of the radiographic tube) of a 22-year-old rugby player, who presented with shoulder pain of 6 months duration, shows similar erosion of the distal end of the clavicle.

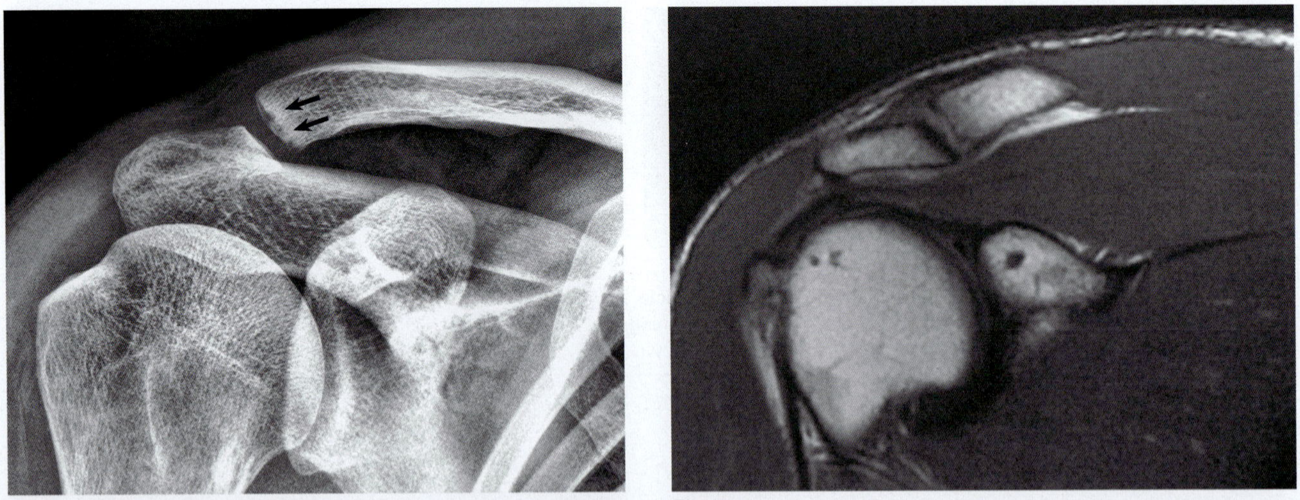

A

B

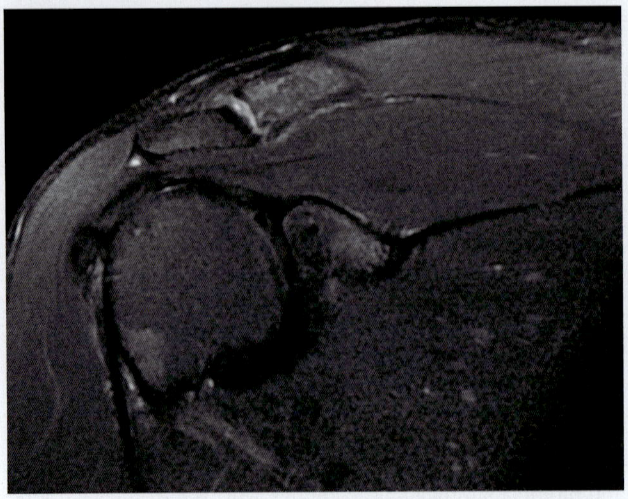

C

Figure 12.13 ■ MRI of posttraumatic osteolysis of the distal clavicle. A 32-year-old weight lifter presented with right shoulder pain for the past 4 months. **A:** Anteroposterior radiograph shows subtle erosions in the acromial end of the clavicle (*arrows*). **B:** Coronal T1-weighted MR image shows irregular contour of the distal clavicle. **C:** Coronal proton density–weighted fat-suppressed MR image shows in addition an increased signal within the distal end of the clavicle and fluid within the acromioclavicular joint.

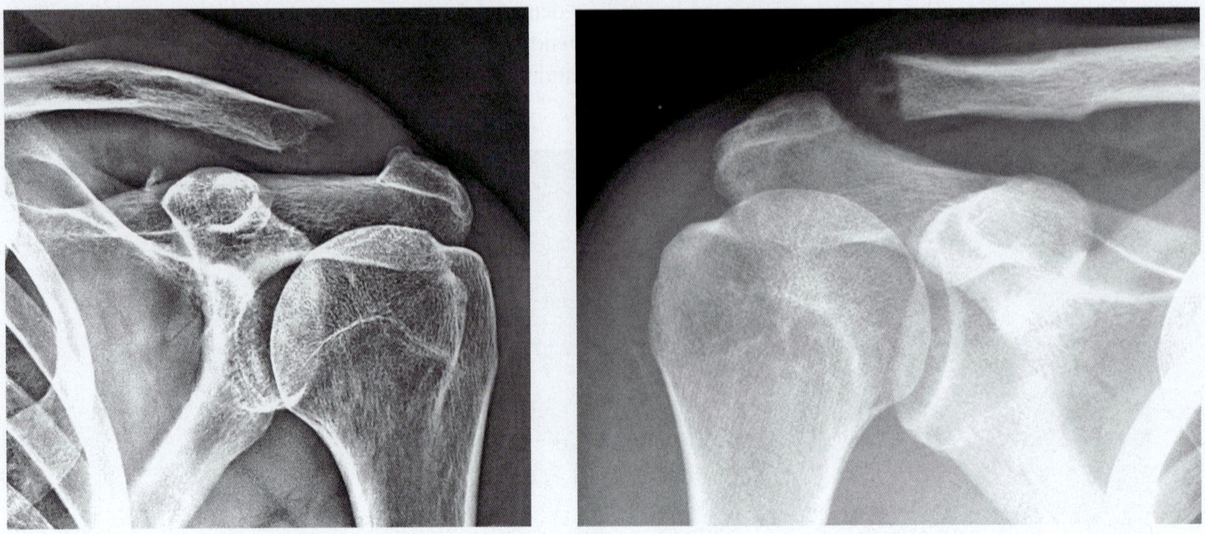

A B

Figure 12.14 ■ Posttraumatic osteolysis of the distal clavicle, late findings. A: A 59-year-old man who 12 months previously had injured the left shoulder in a fall presented with symptoms of pain while playing tennis. Anteroposterior radiograph of the left shoulder shows marked widening of the acromioclavicular joint secondary to resorption of the distal end of the clavicle—radiographic features typical of posttraumatic osteolysis. **B:** Similar osteolysis of the acromial end of the right clavicle is seen in this 21-year-old man, who 14 months previously sustained injury to the right shoulder.

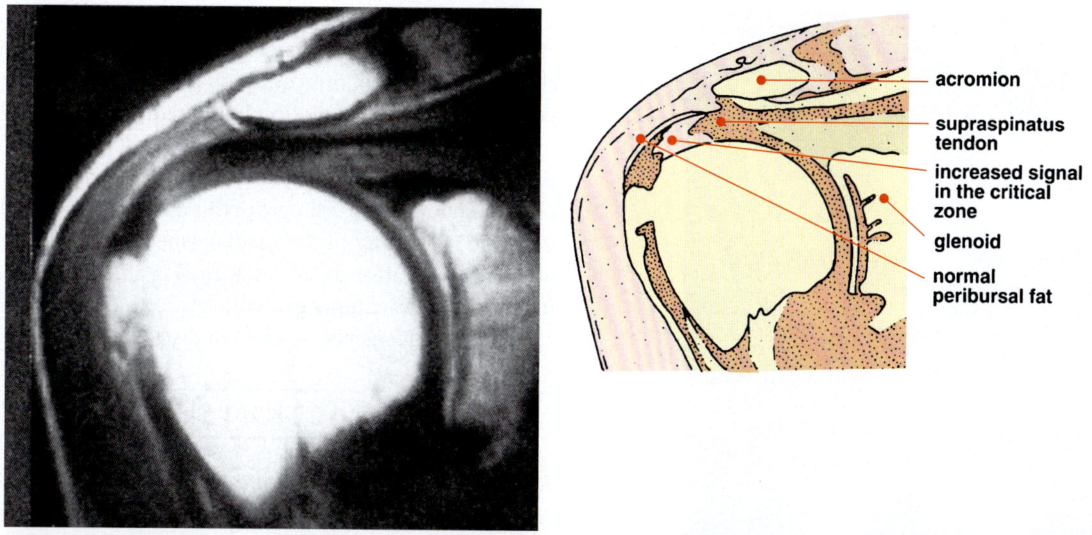

A

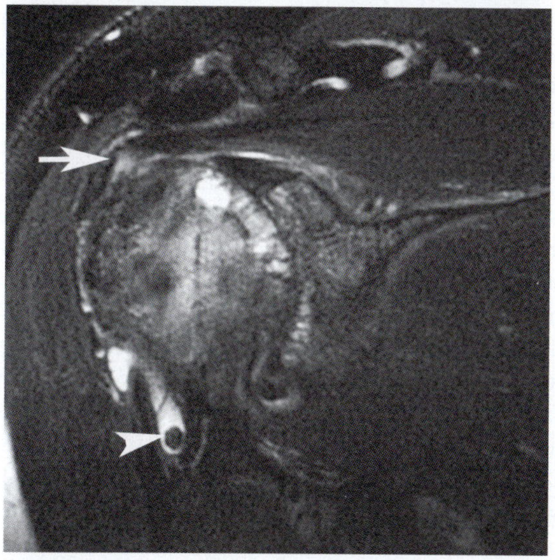

B

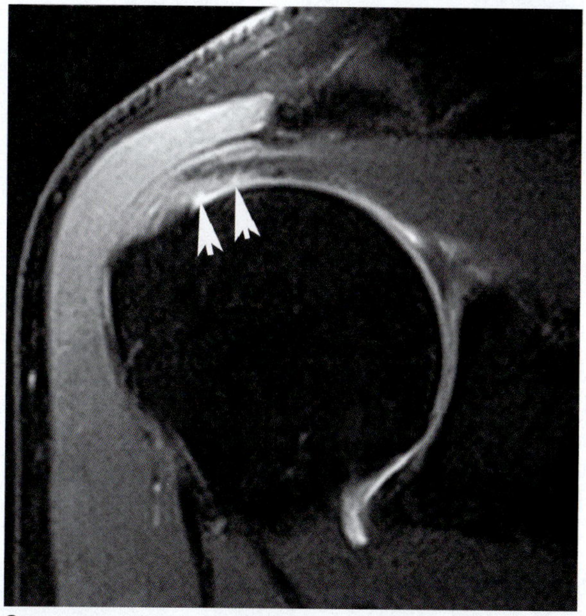

C

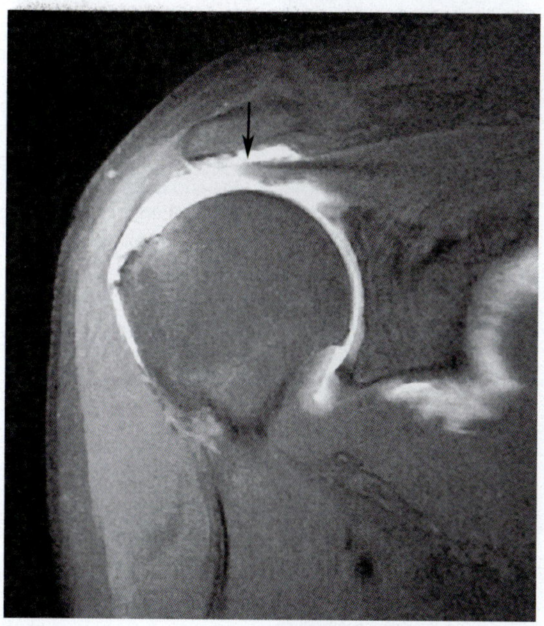

D

Figure 12.15 ■ **MRI of shoulder impingement syndrome. A:** Oblique coronal T1-weighted MR image of early stage of the impingement syndrome. There is slightly increased signal in the critical zone of the supraspinatus tendon. Peribursal fat demarcating the subacromial subdeltoid bursa complex is still intact. **B:** Oblique coronal T2-weighted MR image of stage II impingement syndrome shows a focus of intermediate signal (*arrow*) of the supraspinatus tendon. Note the advanced degenerative changes of the glenohumeral joint and an intra-articular loose body (*arrowhead*). **C:** Oblique coronal T1 fat-saturated MRA of stage II impingement syndrome demonstrates surface fibrillation of the articular fibers of the supraspinatus tendon (*arrows*), representing a partial tear. **D:** Oblique coronal T1-weighted fat-saturated MRA demonstrates a full-thickness tear of the rotator cuff (*arrow*), corresponding to a stage III impingement syndrome. (**A**, From Holt RG, Helms CA, Steinbach L, et al. Magnetic resonance imaging of the shoulder: rationale and current applications. *Skeletal Radiol* 1990;19:5–14.)

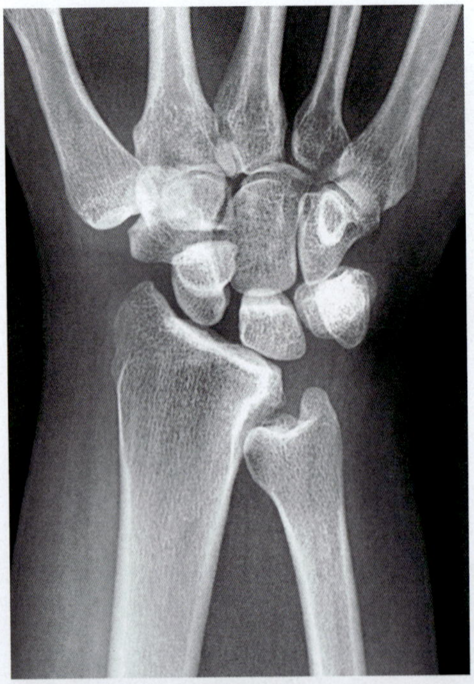

Figure 12.16 ■ Ulnar impingement syndrome. Posteroanterior radiograph of the right wrist shows a negative ulnar variance. The distal ulna impinges on the medial cortex of distal radius.

ULNAR IMPINGEMENT SYNDROME

A short distal ulna that impinges on the distal radius proximal to the sigmoid notch causes ulnar impingement syndrome. A short ulna may represent a congenital anomaly, such as a negative ulnar variance, or may be the result of premature fusion of the distal ulnar growth plate secondary to previous trauma. In most cases, however, it is caused by surgical procedures that involve a resection of the distal ulna secondary to trauma, rheumatoid arthritis, or correction of Madelung deformity. The clinical symptoms of this condition consist of ulnar-sided wrist pain and limitation of motion in the radiocarpal joint that can mimic arthritis. In addition, patients experience discomfort during pronation and supination of the forearm. On radiography, the characteristic changes of this abnormality include short ulna and scalloping of the medial aspect of the distal radius, in cases of negative ulnar variance (Fig. 12.16) or premature fusion of the distal ulnar growth plate, or radial scalloping and radioulnar convergence, in cases of distal ulna resection.

ULNAR IMPACTION SYNDROME

Also known as the *ulnolunate abutment syndrome* or *ulnocarpal loading*, the ulnar impaction syndrome is a well-recognized entity clinically characterized by ulnar-sided wrist pain and limitation of motion in the radiocarpal joint, occasionally mistaken for arthritis. It is commonly associated with the positive ulnar variance. The pathologic mechanism of this syndrome is linked to altered and increased force transmitted across the ulnar side of the wrist, leading to a compression of the distal ulna on the medial surface of the lunate bone. This causes the development of degenerative changes in the cartilage covering both bones. In addition, frequent association of the tear of the triangular fibrocartilage complex (TFCC) has been reported. In cases of excessive ulnar length, dorsal subluxation of the ulna is present compromising supination of the forearm. The conventional radiography shows a positive ulnar variance associated with significantly decreased ulnolunate interval and occasionally foci of sclerosis or cystic changes in the lunate (Fig. 12.17). MRI is the most effective technique for the diagnosis of this

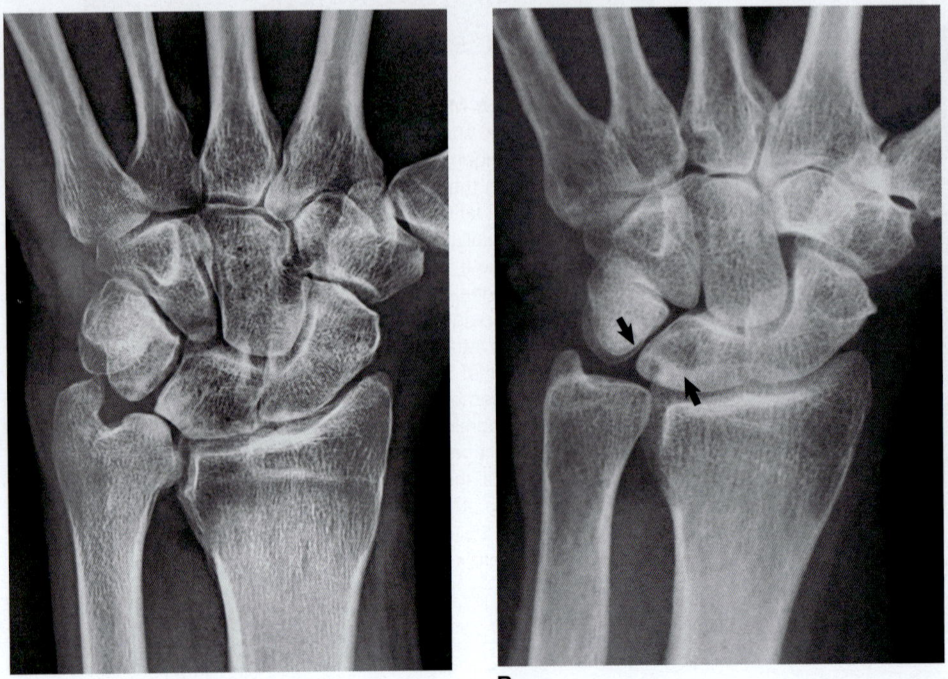

A

B

Figure 12.17 ■ Ulnar impaction syndrome. A: Posteroanterior radiograph of the left wrist shows a positive ulnar variance. The ulnolunate interval is significantly decreased and there is sclerosis of the distal ulna and medial aspect of the lunate. **B:** In another patient, note the cystic changes in the lunate (*arrows*).

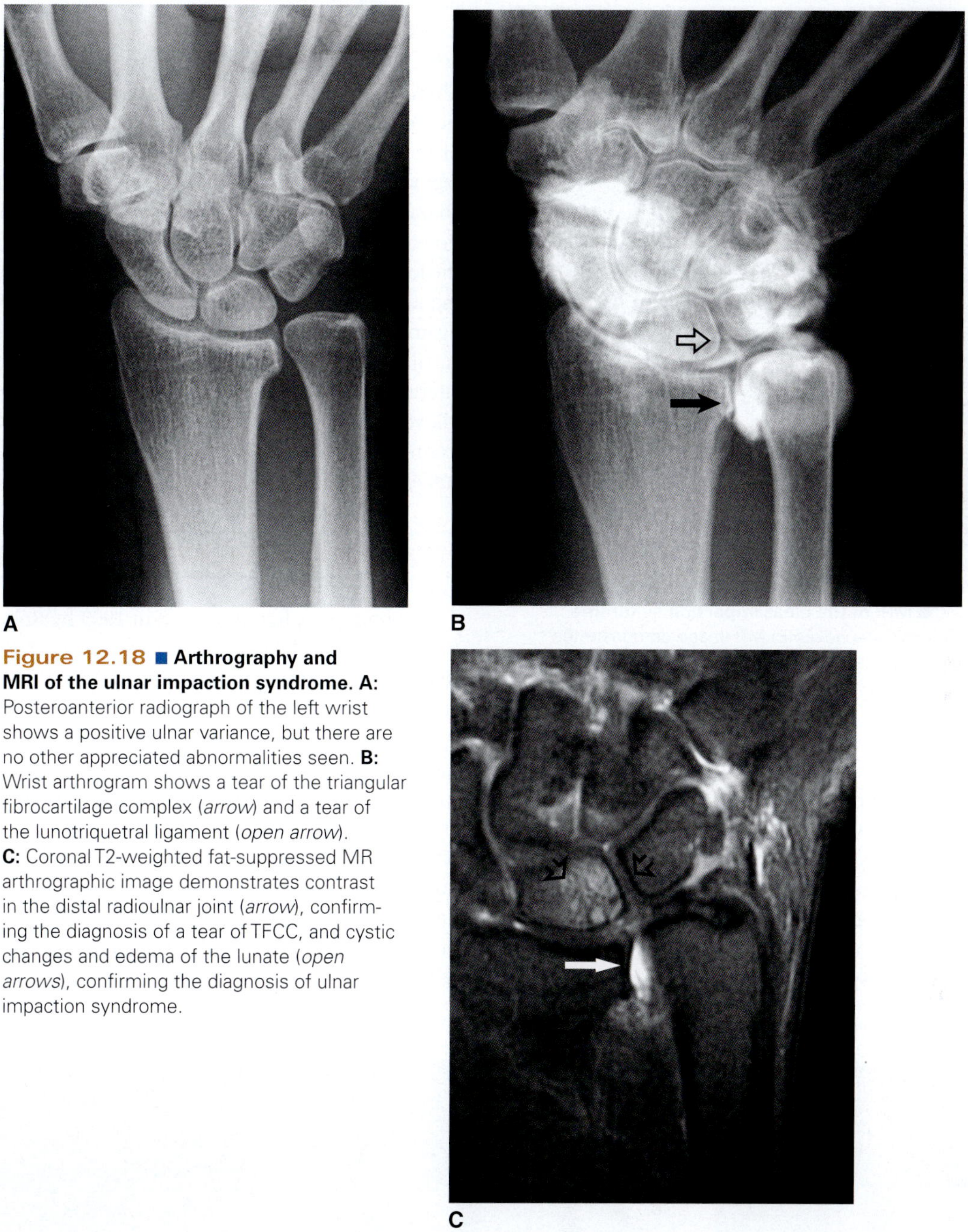

Figure 12.18 ■ Arthrography and MRI of the ulnar impaction syndrome. A: Posteroanterior radiograph of the left wrist shows a positive ulnar variance, but there are no other appreciated abnormalities seen. **B:** Wrist arthrogram shows a tear of the triangular fibrocartilage complex (*arrow*) and a tear of the lunotriquetral ligament (*open arrow*). **C:** Coronal T2-weighted fat-suppressed MR arthrographic image demonstrates contrast in the distal radioulnar joint (*arrow*), confirming the diagnosis of a tear of TFCC, and cystic changes and edema of the lunate (*open arrows*), confirming the diagnosis of ulnar impaction syndrome.

syndrome and demonstration of pathologic changes in the affected bones and surrounding soft tissues. MRI reveals bone marrow edema of the distal ulna and lunate, subchondral sclerosis, cyst formation, and destruction of the cartilage. Associated abnormalities, such as tears of the TFCC and lunotriquetral ligament, are also well imaged (Figs. 12.18 to 12.20). Treatment of this condition includes TFCC debridement and ulnar shortening.

HAMATOLUNATE IMPACTION SYNDROME

Recently described painful condition of the ulnar side of the wrist, hamatolunate impaction syndrome results from an anatomic variant of the lunate bone that has an "extra" facet articulating with the hamate bone (so-called type II lunate bone). The repeated contact of these two bones when the wrist is in ulnar deviation leads to bone marrow edema, chondromalacia, and, occasionally, erosive changes of the proximal pole of the hamate effectively demonstrated by MRI (Fig. 12.21).

CYCLIST'S WRIST

This lesion that can mimic wrist arthritis represents an ulnar neuropathy, known as *handlebar palsy*. It is caused by compression of the ulnar nerve at the hand and wrist as a result of direct pressure on the nerve from the grip on the handlebars.

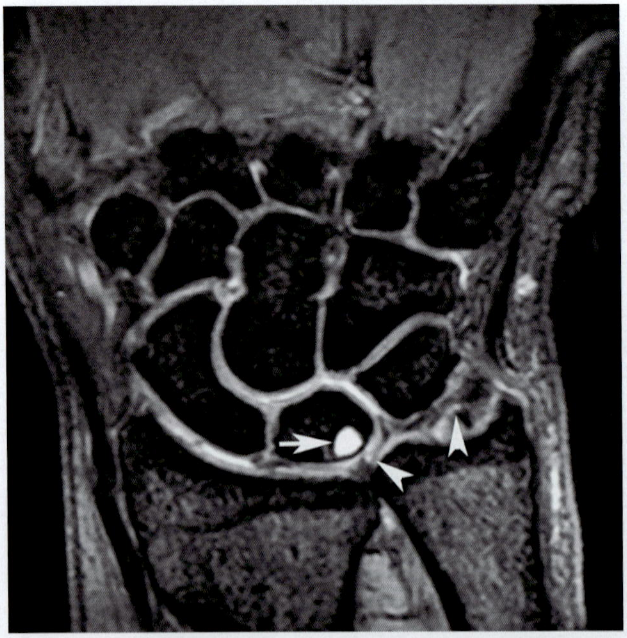

Figure 12.19 ■ MRI of the ulnar impaction syndrome. Coronal gradient-recalled echo (GRE) MR image demonstrates ulnar positive variance. There is complete tear of the TFCC (*arrowheads*) and subchondral cyst in the ulnar aspect of the lunate (*arrow*).

Often, the nerve may be stretched or hyperextended when a drop-down handlebar is held in the lower position. The pressure placed on the ulnar nerve results in numbness and tingling in the ring and small fingers or hand weakness or both. Occasionally, compression of the median nerve can also occur by pressure against the handle bar, with development of carpal tunnel syndrome (Fig. 12.22).

SINDING-LARSEN-JOHANSSON DISEASE

This condition seen predominantly in adolescents is now considered to be related to trauma. It occurs at the proximal end of the patellar ligament, where it attaches to the lower pole (apex) of the patella. Sinding-Larsen-Johansson disease is characterized clinically by local pain and tenderness on palpation and radiographically by separation and fragmentation of the lower pole of the patella, associated with soft tissue swelling and, occasionally, calcifications at the site of the patellar ligament. The condition is caused by persistent traction at the cartilaginous junction of the patella and patellar ligament. The lateral radiograph of the knee, preferably obtained with a low-kilovoltage/soft tissue technique, is the single most important examination (Fig. 12.23). In combination with a positive clinical examination, it usually establishes the diagnosis.

OSGOOD-SCHLATTER DISEASE

This abnormality, first described in 1903 by Robert Osgood of Boston and Carl Schlatter of Zurich, occurs three times more frequently in adolescent boys than adolescent girls and is characterized by fragmentation of the tibial tuberosity, soft tissue swelling, and thickening at the insertion of the patellar ligament, as well as inflammation of the deep infrapatellar bursa. In 25% to 33% of all reported cases, the condition is bilateral and occasionally can mimic juvenile idiopathic arthritis. As in Sinding-Larsen-Johansson disease, the lateral radiograph of the knee obtained using a soft tissue technique is effective in demonstrating this abnormality (Fig. 12.24). However, an accurate diagnosis is based on both imaging and clinical findings. Soft tissue swelling and deep infrapatellar bursitis and/or fibrosis are

(*Continued on page 435*)

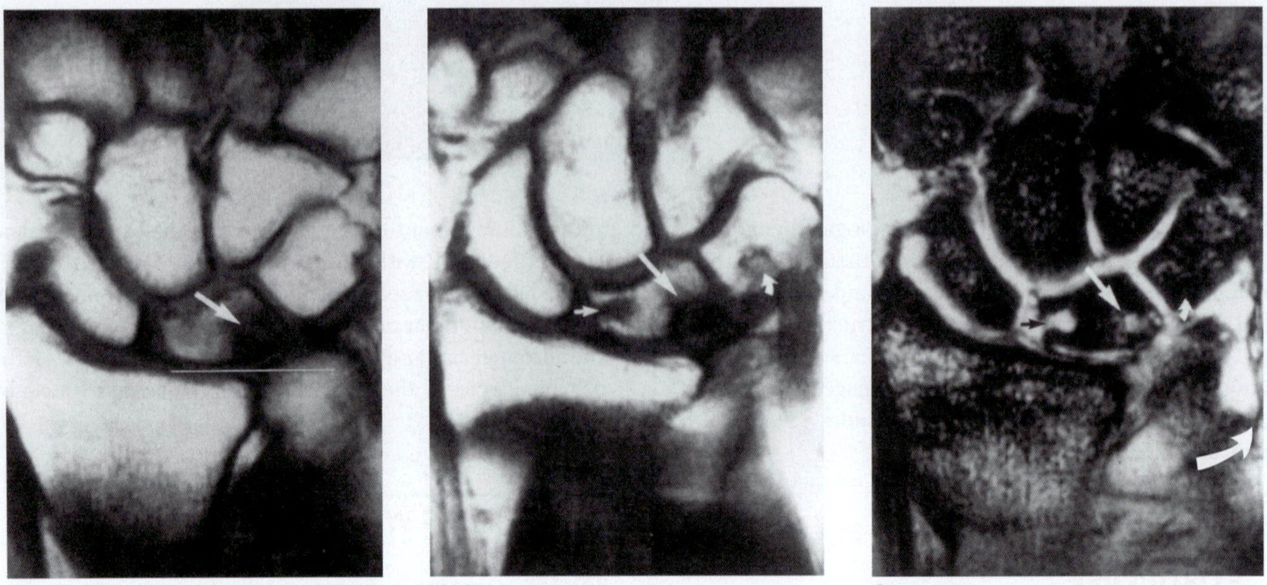

Figure 12.20 ■ MRI of the ulnar impaction syndrome. A: Coronal T1-weighted MR image shows a positive ulnar variance and sclerosis of the proximal aspect of the lunate (*arrow*). Coronal T1-weighted MR image **(B)** obtained slightly more volarly, and corresponding T2*-weighted image **(C)** shows subchondral cysts (*straight arrows*) and involvement of the triquetrum (*small curved arrow*). Note also the disruption of the triangular fibrocartilage (*large curved arrow*).

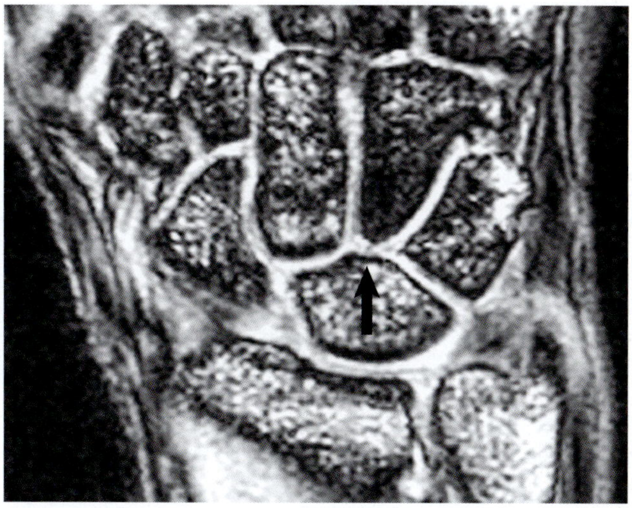

A

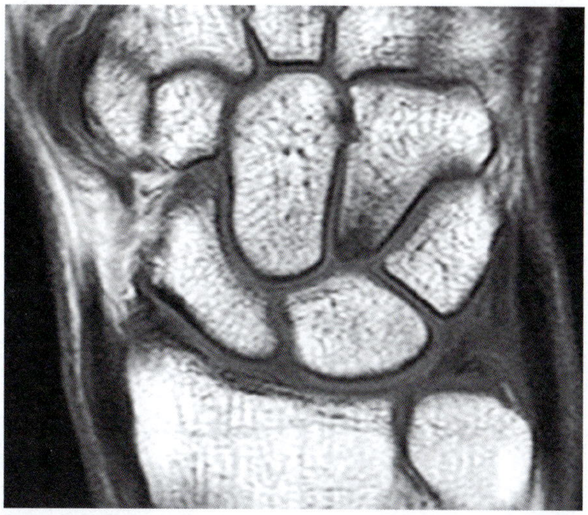

B

Figure 12.21 ■ **MRI of the hamatolunate impaction syndrome. A:** Coronal 3D gradient-echo MR image shows a type II lunate articulating with the hamate (*arrow*). Note decreased signal intensity within the most proximal aspect of the hamate bone. Coronal T1-weighted **(B)** and coronal T2-weighted **(C)** fat-suppressed MR images demonstrate the erosion of the articular cartilage (*arrow*) and edematous changes of the hamate, diagnostic features of hamatolunate impaction syndrome.

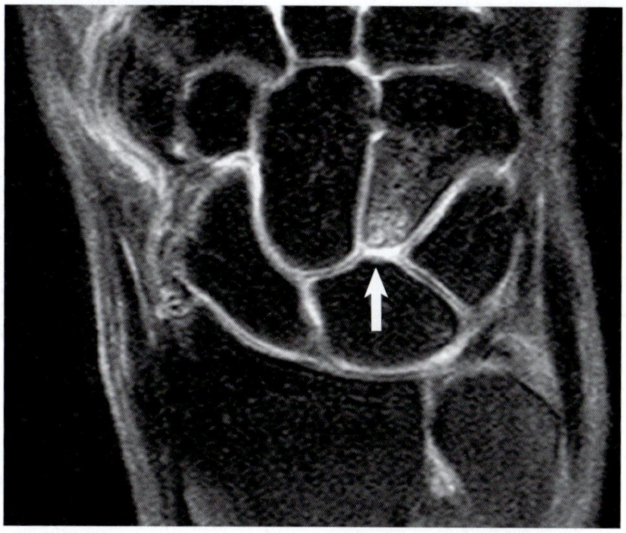

C

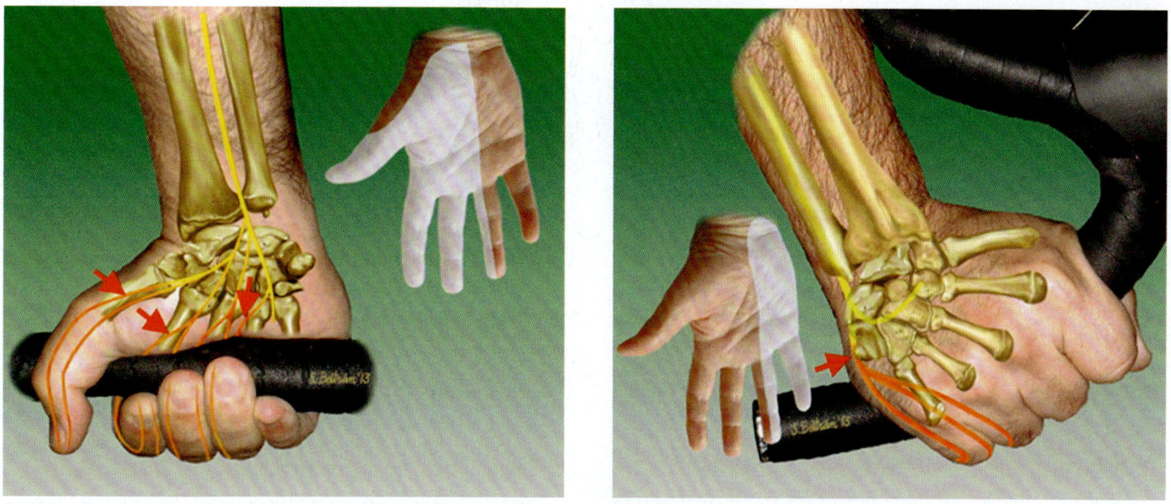

A B

Figure 12.22 ■ **Cyclist's wrist, mechanism of injury. A:** Gripping of the drop-down handlebar held in upper position may produce compression of the digital branches of the median nerve (*arrows*) leading to sensory deficit of the innervated area (*white region in the hand*). **B:** Gripping of the drop-down handlebar held in the lower position may produce compression of the sensory branch of the ulnar nerve (*arrow*), leading to sensory deficit of the innervated area (*white region of the hand*). This is also known as *Guyon canal syndrome*.

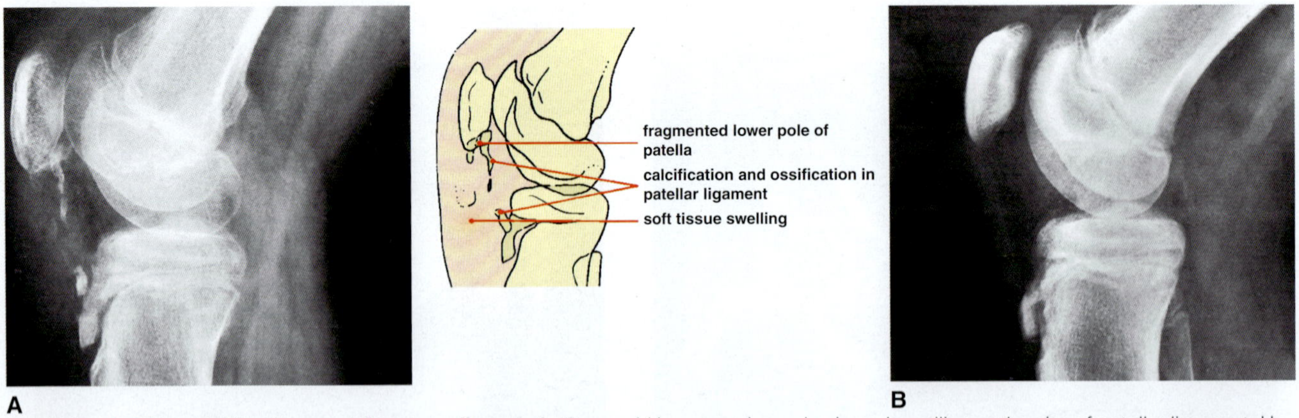

Figure 12.23 ■ **Sinding-Larsen-Johansson disease.** A 13-year-old boy experienced pain and swelling at the site of patellar ligament. He had no history of acute trauma. **A:** Lateral radiograph of the right knee shows fragmentation of the lower pole of the patella and significant soft tissue swelling associated with calcifications and ossifications of the patellar ligament. **B:** The normal left knee is shown for comparison.

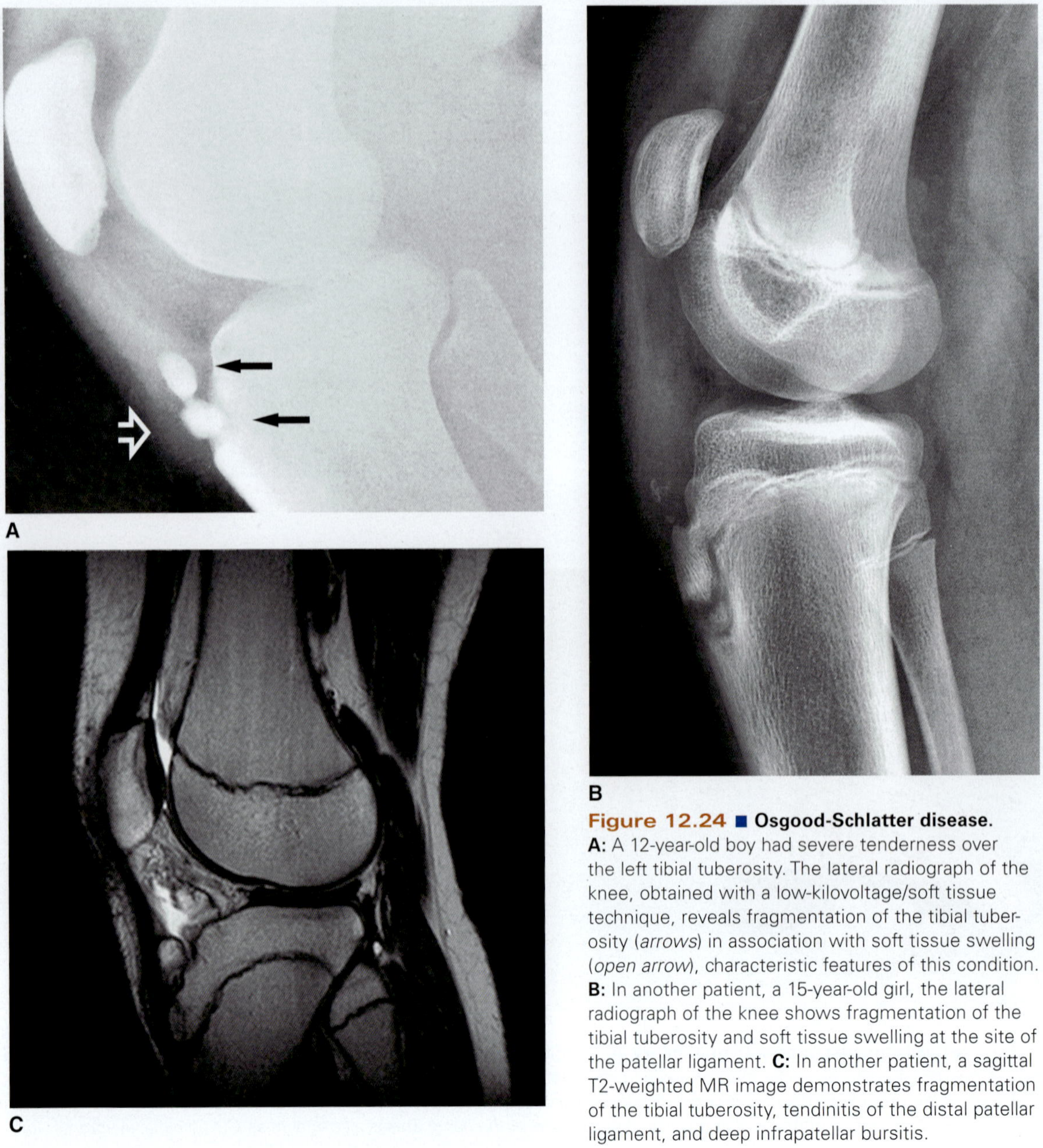

Figure 12.24 ■ **Osgood-Schlatter disease.** **A:** A 12-year-old boy had severe tenderness over the left tibial tuberosity. The lateral radiograph of the knee, obtained with a low-kilovoltage/soft tissue technique, reveals fragmentation of the tibial tuberosity (*arrows*) in association with soft tissue swelling (*open arrow*), characteristic features of this condition. **B:** In another patient, a 15-year-old girl, the lateral radiograph of the knee shows fragmentation of the tibial tuberosity and soft tissue swelling at the site of the patellar ligament. **C:** In another patient, a sagittal T2-weighted MR image demonstrates fragmentation of the tibial tuberosity, tendinitis of the distal patellar ligament, and deep infrapatellar bursitis.

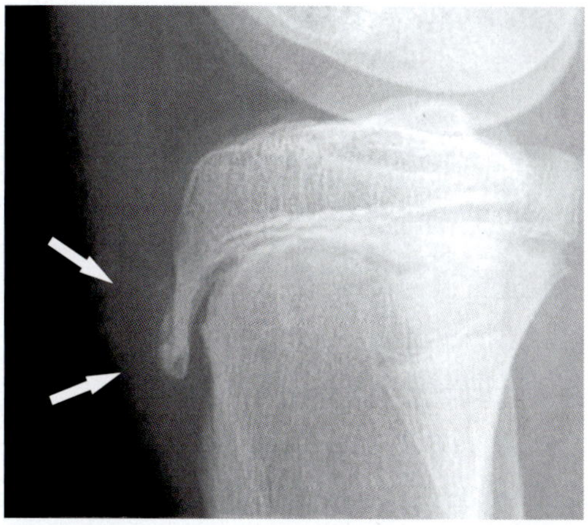

A

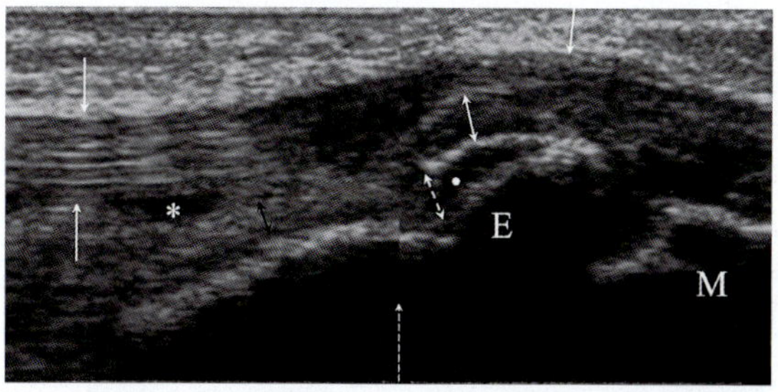

B

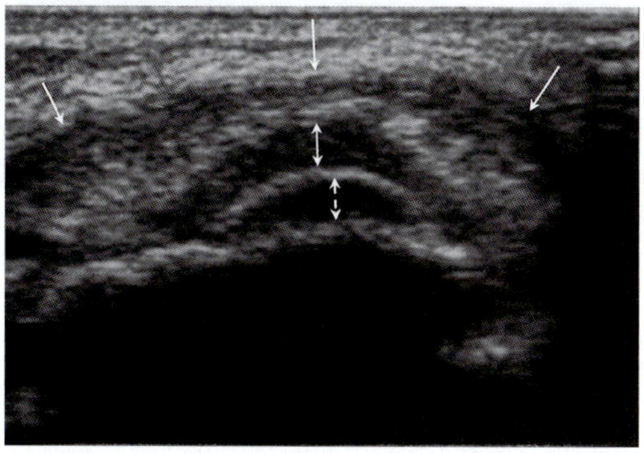

C

Figure 12.25 ■ US of Osgood-Schlatter disease. An 11-year-old boy presented with pain and swelling in the region of tibial tuberosity for several weeks. **A:** Lateral radiograph shows soft tissue swelling and small calcifications at the site of ossification center of tibial tuberosity (*arrows*). Longitudinal **(B)** and transverse **(C)** ultrasound images showa a fracture and delamination of the cartilaginous portion of the ossification center of tibial tuberosity. *Arrows* point to the margin of the patellar ligament; *double solid arrow* indicates the thickness of cartilage between the ossification center and patellar ligament insertion; *double dashed arrow* indicates delamination thickness within the ossification center; *double black arrow* indicates fibrosis within deep infrapatellar bursa; *asterisks* marks effusion within deep infrapatellar bursa; *dot* indicates ossification center. E, epiphysis; M, metaphysis.

fundamental diagnostic features. Ultrasound of the tibial tuberosity complex is an effective method to demonstrate all features of the Osgood-Schlatter disease because it provides excellent visualization of the fine structures of the patellar ligament, and superficial and deep infrapatellar bursae, as well as the status of the cartilage of the ossification center of the tibial tuberosity (Fig. 12.25). On MRI, T1-weighted images show replacement of the normal high-signal infrapatellar fat with an area of decreased signal adjacent to the patellar ligament insertion. The ligament itself may show focal areas of increased signal on water-sensitive sequences, depending on the degree of associated tendinitis (Figs. 12.26 and 12.27).

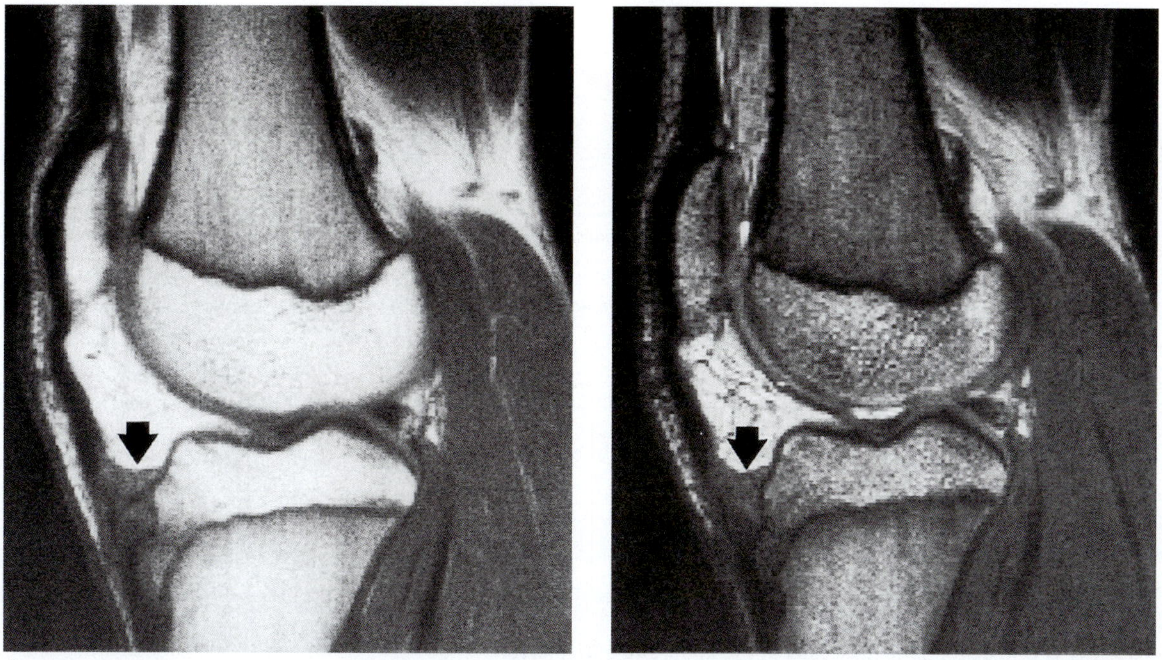

A B

Figure 12.26 ■ MRI of Osgood-Schlatter disease. T1-weighted **(A)** and T2*-weighted **(B)** sagittal MR images of the knee demonstrate focus of decreased signal within normal V-shaped area formed by the patellar ligament and anterior tibia (*arrows*).

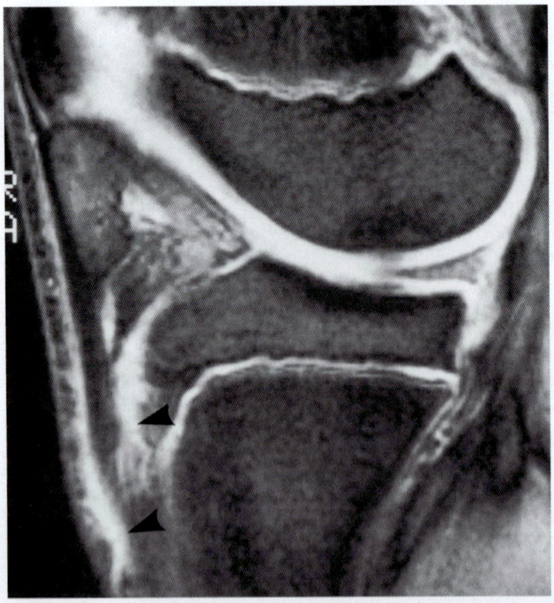

Figure 12.27 ■ MRI of Osgood-Schlatter disease. A sagittal T2-weighted image of the knee of a 14-year-old boy shows inflammatory changes along the distal patellar ligament (*arrowheads*).

Occasionally, Sinding-Larsen-Johansson and Osgood-Schlatter diseases may coexist. It is important to remember that the presence of multiple ossifications centers in the tibial tuberosity, and lower pole of the patella may at times mimic these conditions. However, the absence of soft tissue swelling in such cases allows the distinction to be made.

Conservative treatment is usually recommended until the tibial growth plate fuses, including decrease physical activity and limit movements that aggravate the pain. Long immobilization, however, seems potentially harmful, as it creates muscle atrophy and contracture. Nonsteroidal anti-inflammatory drugs may help with symptoms. Occasionally, surgical excision of painful ossicles may be performed in skeletally mature patients.

OSTEOCHONDRITIS DISSECANS

Osteochondritis dissecans is a relatively common condition seen predominantly in adolescents and young adults, and more often in males than females. Recently, this abnormality has come to be considered a form of osteochondral fracture caused not by acute but chronic injury. Shearing or rotary forces applied to the articular surface of the femur result in detachment of a fragment of articular cartilage, often together with a segment of subchondral bone.

Aichroth has pointed out that the separated segment is avascular and this feature distinguishes osteochondritis from acute osteochondral fracture. In a clinical survey of osteochondritis dissecans in 200 patients, he also determined the distribution of the lesion. The most common location was the non–weight-bearing segment at the lateral aspect of the medial femoral condyle; other sites were less commonly affected (Fig. 12.28). The degree of damage to the

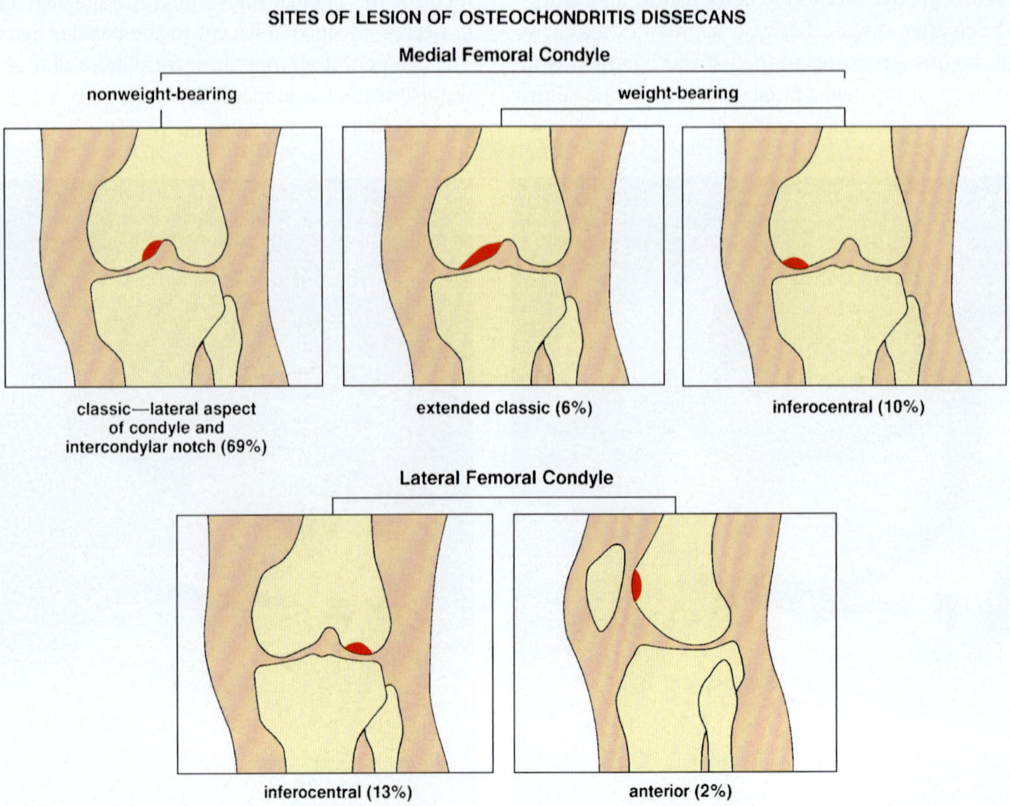

Figure 12.28 ■ Osteochondritis dissecans of the knee, site of the lesion. Osteochondritis dissecans most frequently affects the medial femoral condyle, the non–weight-bearing portion (the lateral aspect and the intercondylar notch), which is the most common site of the lesion. The lateral femoral condyle is much less commonly involved. (Modified from Aichroth P. Osteochondritis dissecans of the knee: a clinical survey. *J Bone Joint Surg [Br]*. 1971;53B:440–447.)

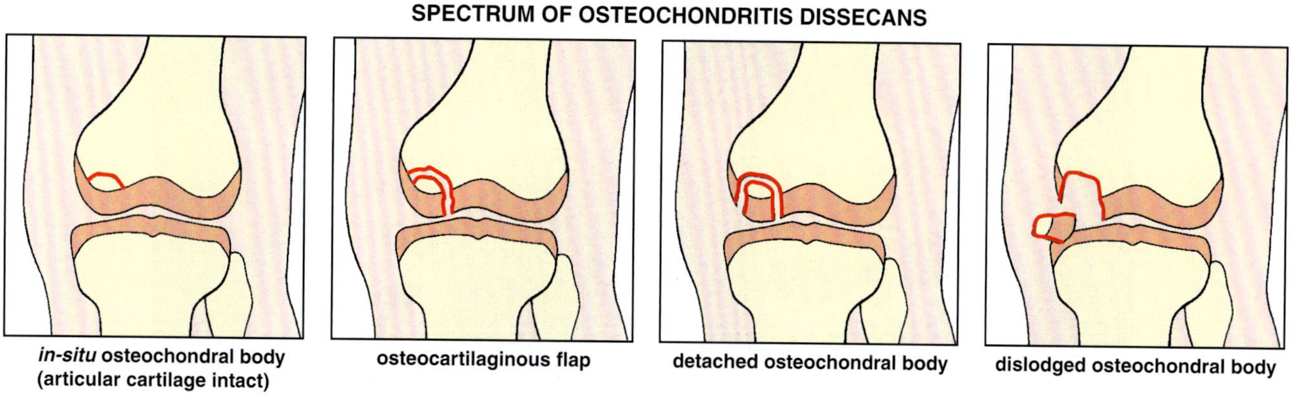

Figure 12.29 ■ Stages of osteochondritis dissecans. The spectrum of chronic injury to the articular end of the distal femur ranges from an *in situ* lesion to a defect in the subchondral bone associated with a dislodged osteochondral body.

articular cartilage varies from an *in situ* osteochondral body to an osteocartilaginous flap to complete detachment of an osteochondral segment (Fig. 12.29).

In early stages of the disease, conventional radiographs in the standard projections usually show no abnormalities. The only positive finding may be joint effusion. In more advanced stages of the disease, radiolucent line is seen separating the osteochondral body from the femoral condyle (Fig. 12.30). For the orthopedic management of this condition, it is important to evaluate the status of the articular cartilage. In the past, double-contrast arthrography was an examination of choice to differentiate an *in situ* lesions from more advanced lesions, where the osteochondral body is partially or completely detached from its bed (Fig. 12.31). Currently, MRI is routinely performed, alone or in conjunction with arthrography. T1- and T2-weighted images in coronal and sagittal planes are most effective (Fig. 12.32). The lesion usually displays intermediate signal intensity on all sequences and is separated by a narrow zone of low signal intensity from the viable bone (Figs. 12.33 and 12.34). The disruption of articular cartilage is best seen on T2 or T2* (gradient-echo) images (Fig. 12.35). When osteochondral body is separated from the host bone by a rim of high signal intensity on water-sensitive sequences (a phenomenon that denotes a fluid or granulation tissue), it usually signifies loosening or complete detachment of the necrotic fragment (Fig. 12.36).

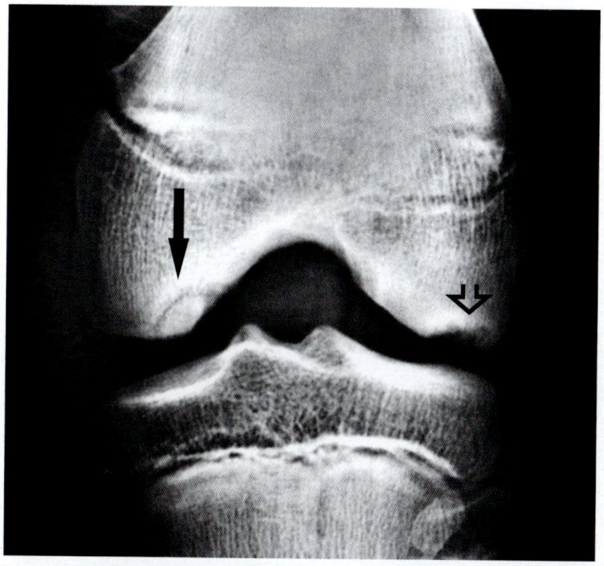

Figure 12.30 ■ Osteochondritis dissecans. An 11-year-old boy presented with pain in his right knee for 3 months. Posteroanterior (tunnel) radiograph of the knee shows the typical lesion of osteochondritis dissecans in the medial femoral condyle (*arrow*). A radiolucent line separates the oval *in situ* body from the femoral condyle. Incidentally, the lateral femoral condyle shows an irregular outline of the weight-bearing segment (*open arrow*). This finding represents a developmental variant in ossification and is of no further consequence.

Treatment of osteochondritis dissecans of the knee depends largely on the age of the patient, symptomatology, and status of osteochondral segment. Children and skeletally immature patients who do not have loose bodies may be initially treated conservatively. This therapy includes limitation of activity and protection of weight bearing to allow healing of the lesion and to prevent further separation. After 3 months, symptomatic patients should be offered surgical intervention. Depending on imaging findings, surgical therapy includes the following procedures: arthroscopic subchondral drilling to create channels that link the subchondral bone to the osteochondral fragment; arthroscopic debridement and fragment stabilization; arthroscopic excision and curettage; open surgery to remove the loose body or bodies, reconstruction of the base of the crater, and mosaicplasty for fragment healing; autologous chondrocyte transplantation; and removal of loose body and sclerotic bone with bone grafting of the defect and autologous chondrocyte transplantation.

(Continued on page 441)

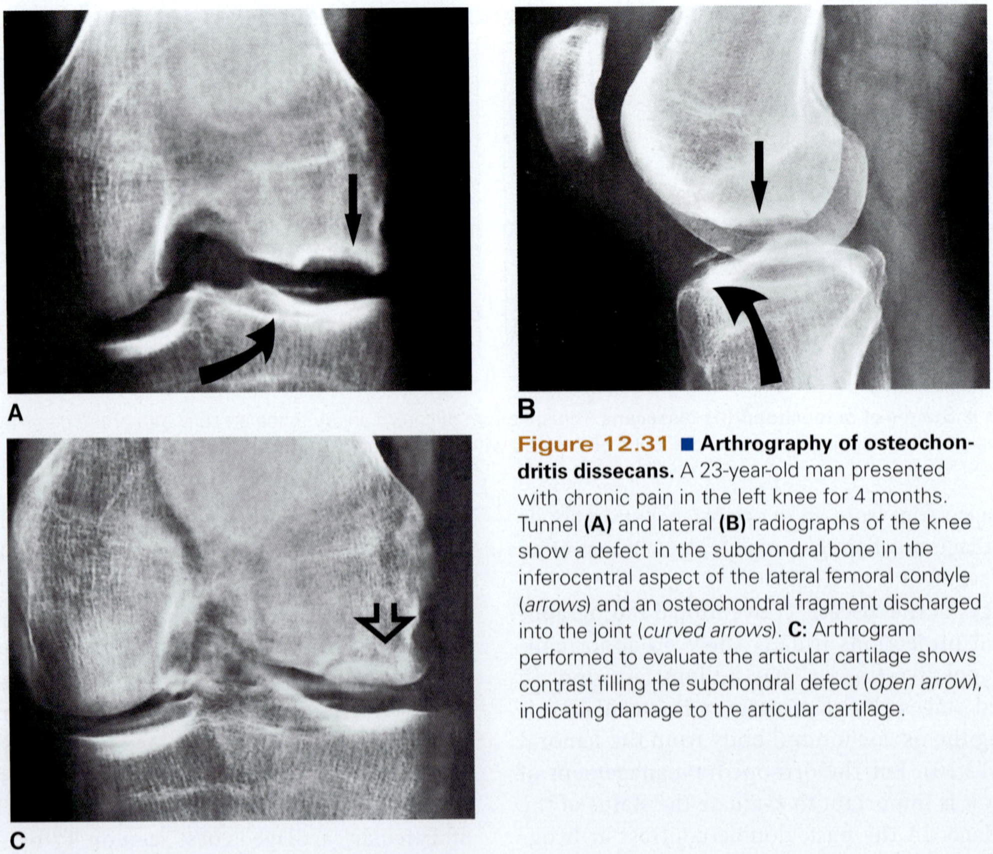

Figure 12.31 ■ **Arthrography of osteochondritis dissecans.** A 23-year-old man presented with chronic pain in the left knee for 4 months. Tunnel **(A)** and lateral **(B)** radiographs of the knee show a defect in the subchondral bone in the inferocentral aspect of the lateral femoral condyle (*arrows*) and an osteochondral fragment discharged into the joint (*curved arrows*). **C:** Arthrogram performed to evaluate the articular cartilage shows contrast filling the subchondral defect (*open arrow*), indicating damage to the articular cartilage.

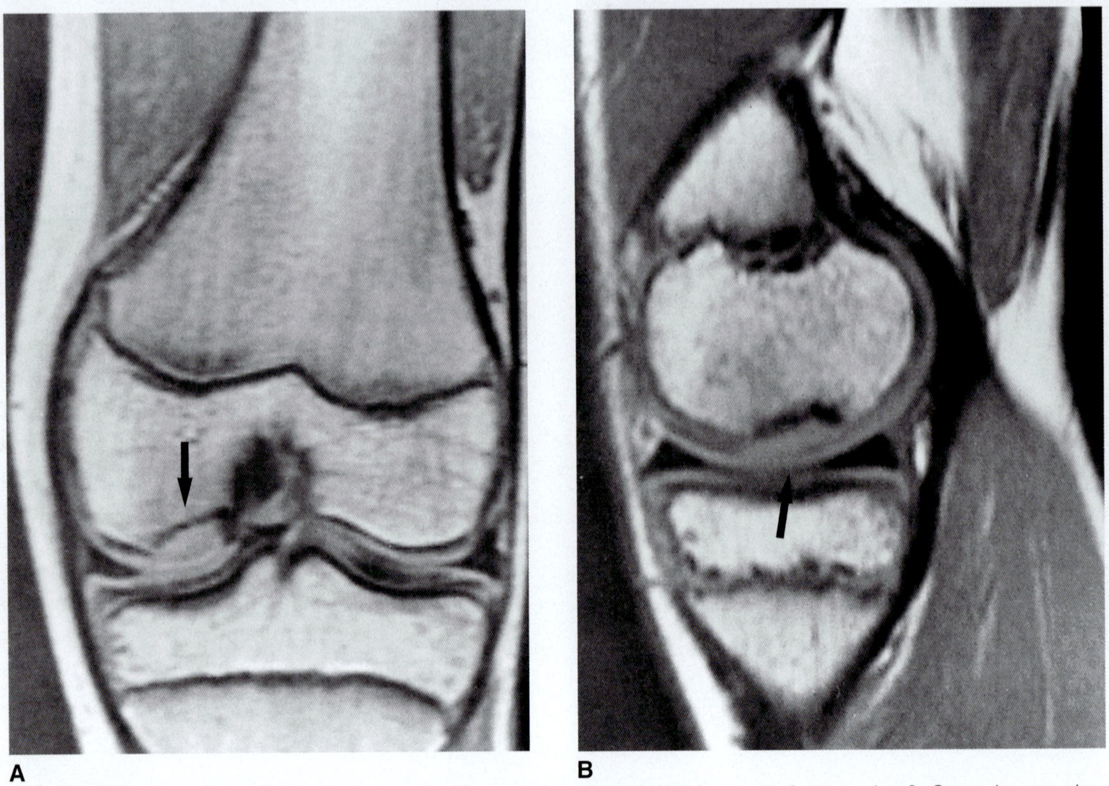

Figure 12.32 ■ **MRI of osteochondritis dissecans.** An 11-year-old boy experienced knee pain for 3 weeks. **A:** Coronal proton density–weighted MR image shows osseous fragment well separated from the medial femoral condyle by the low–signal intensity line (*arrow*). **B:** Sagittal proton density–weighted MR image demonstrates intact articular cartilage overlying the separated fragment (*arrow*), indicating an *in situ* lesion.

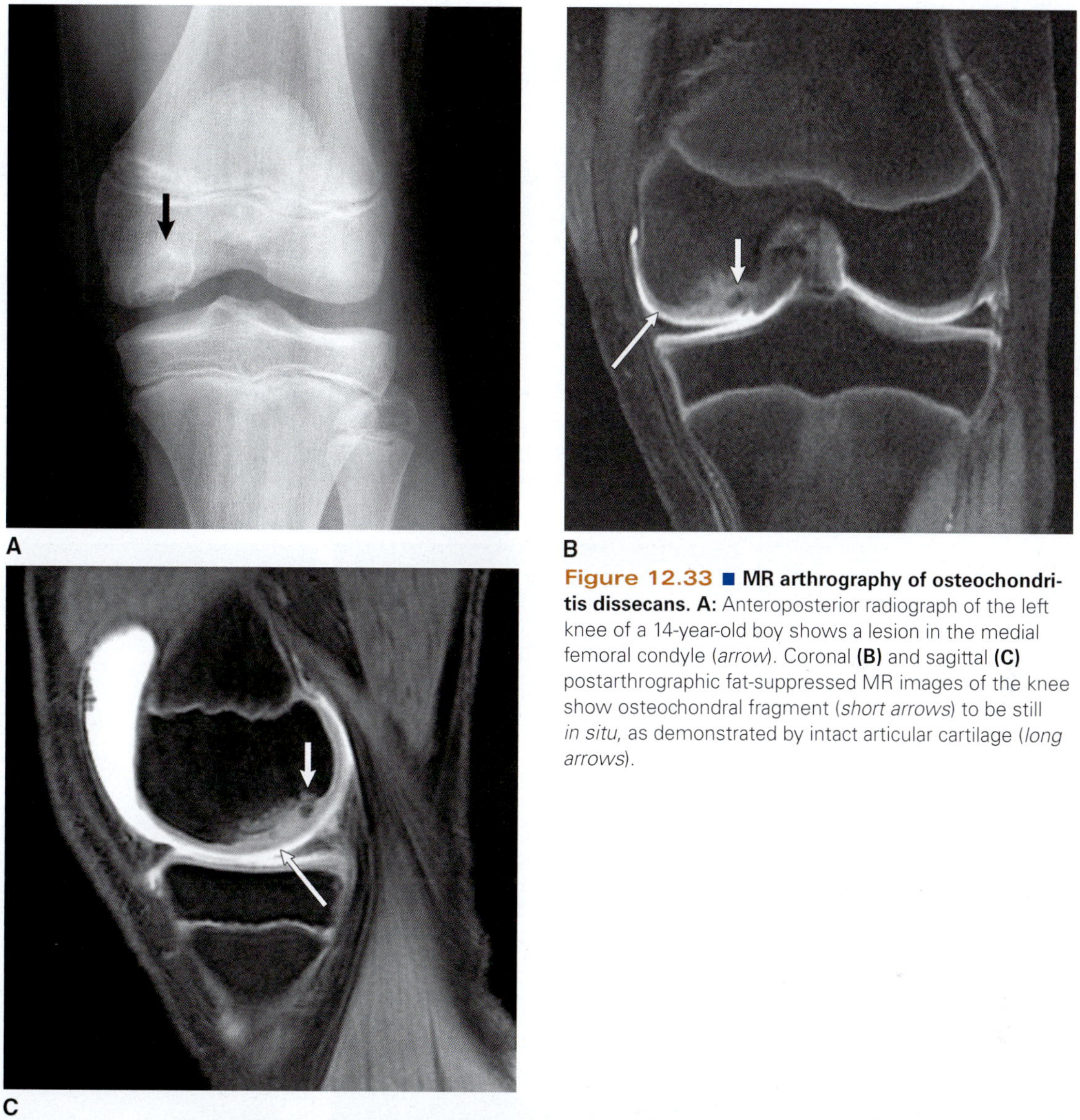

Figure 12.33 ■ **MR arthrography of osteochondritis dissecans. A:** Anteroposterior radiograph of the left knee of a 14-year-old boy shows a lesion in the medial femoral condyle (*arrow*). Coronal **(B)** and sagittal **(C)** postarthrographic fat-suppressed MR images of the knee show osteochondral fragment (*short arrows*) to be still *in situ*, as demonstrated by intact articular cartilage (*long arrows*).

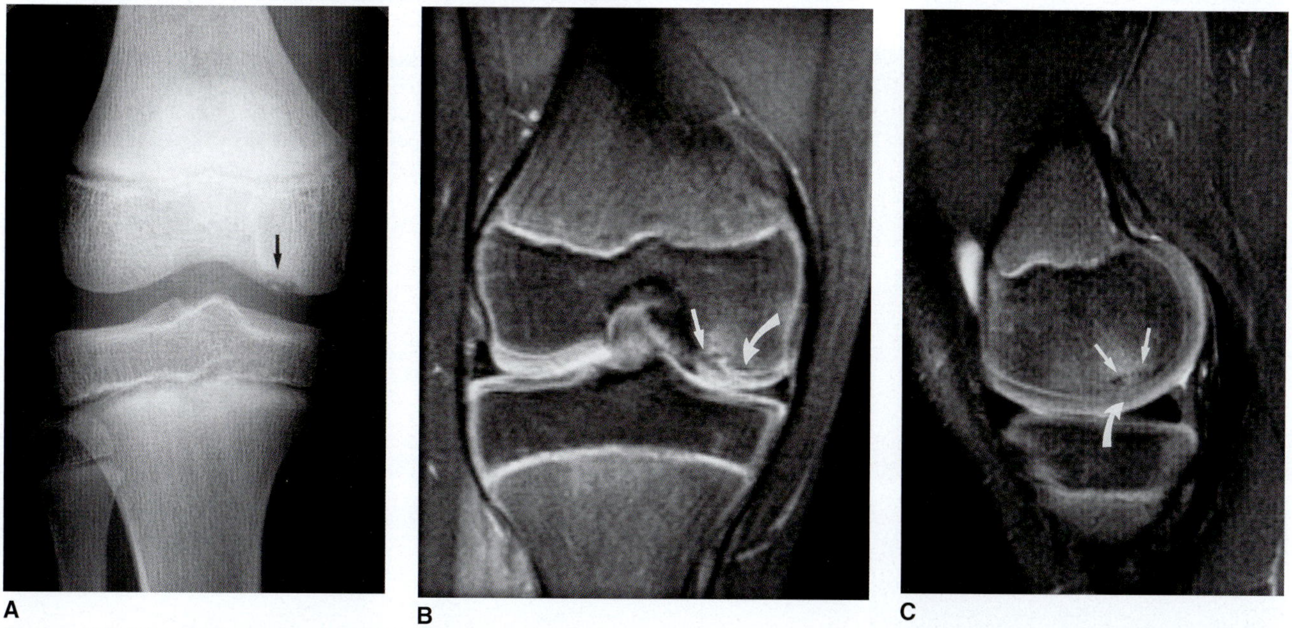

Figure 12.34 ■ **MRI of osteochondritis dissecans. A:** Anteroposterior radiograph of the right knee shows a lesion in the femoral condyle (*arrow*). Coronal **(B)** and sagittal **(C)** T2-weighted fat-suppressed MR images demonstrate the osteochondral body being still *in situ* (*arrows*), although the articular cartilage is already damaged (*curved arrows*).

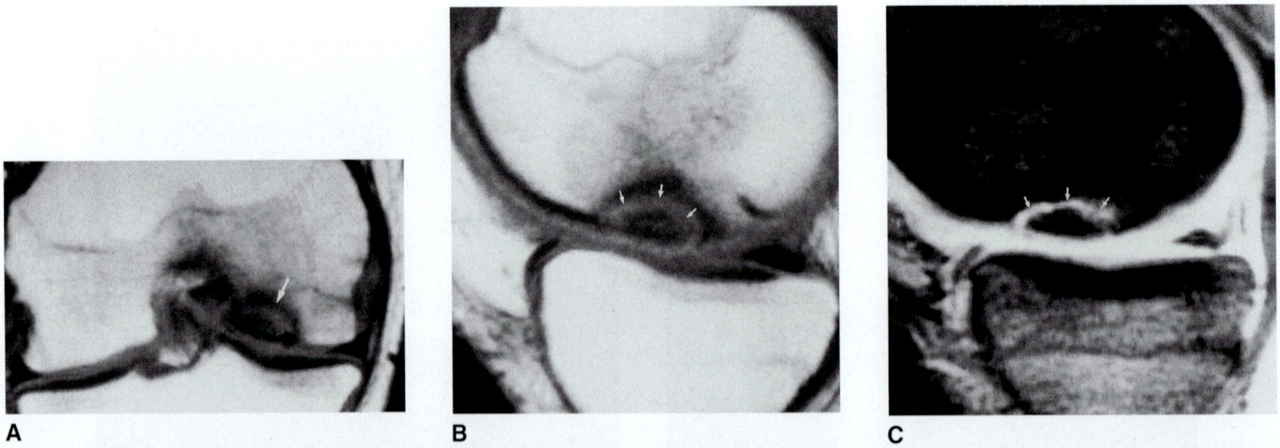

Figure 12.35 ■ MRI of osteochondritis dissecans. A loose osteochondral body in the medial femoral condyle is seen on T1-weighted coronal **(A)** and sagittal **(B)** MR images (*arrows*). **C:** On the sagittal T2*-weighted sequence, high–signal intensity fluid (*arrows*) separates the loose fragment from the viable bone.

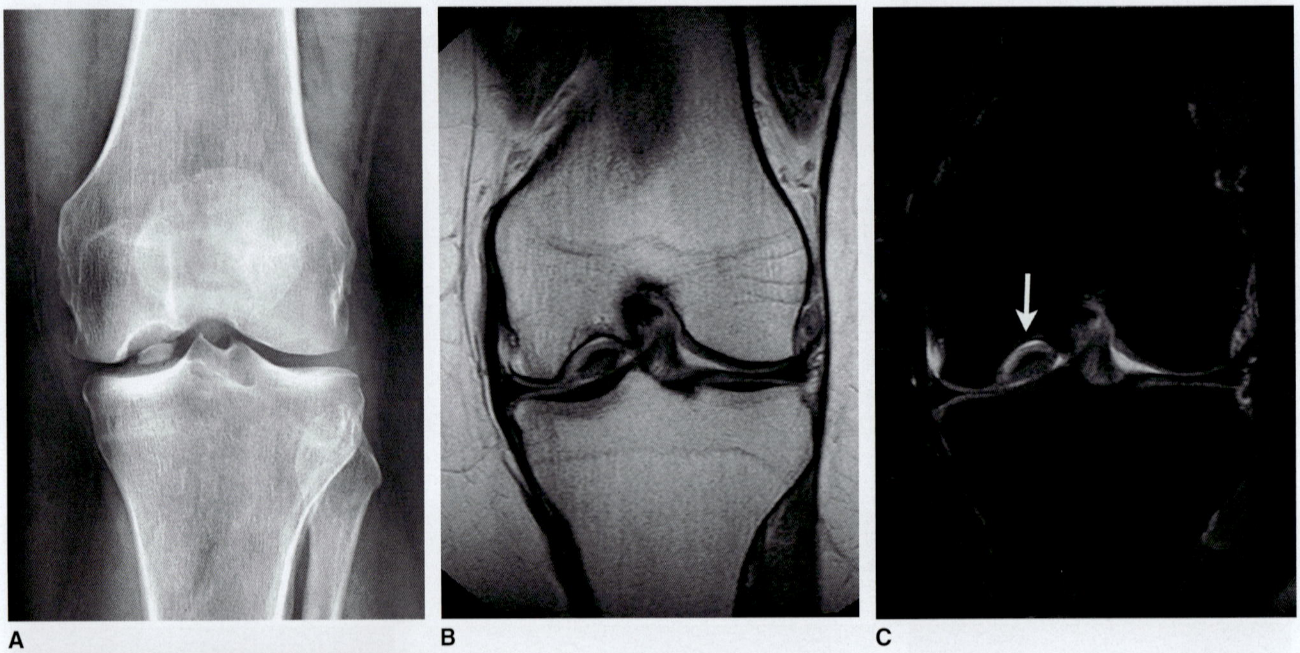

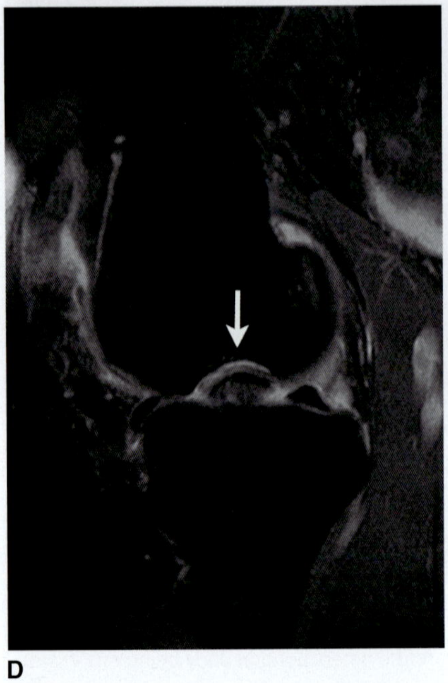

Figure 12.36 ■ MRI of osteochondritis dissecans. A: Anteroposterior radiograph of the left knee of a 23-year-old man shows an osteochondral body within the subchondral defect in the medial femoral condyle. Coronal proton density–weighted fat-suppressed **(B)** and sagittal proton density–weighted fat-suppressed **(C, D)** MR images show that the osteochondral fragment is separated from the host bone by fluid (*arrows*) and flipped vertically, a diagnostic sign of instability.

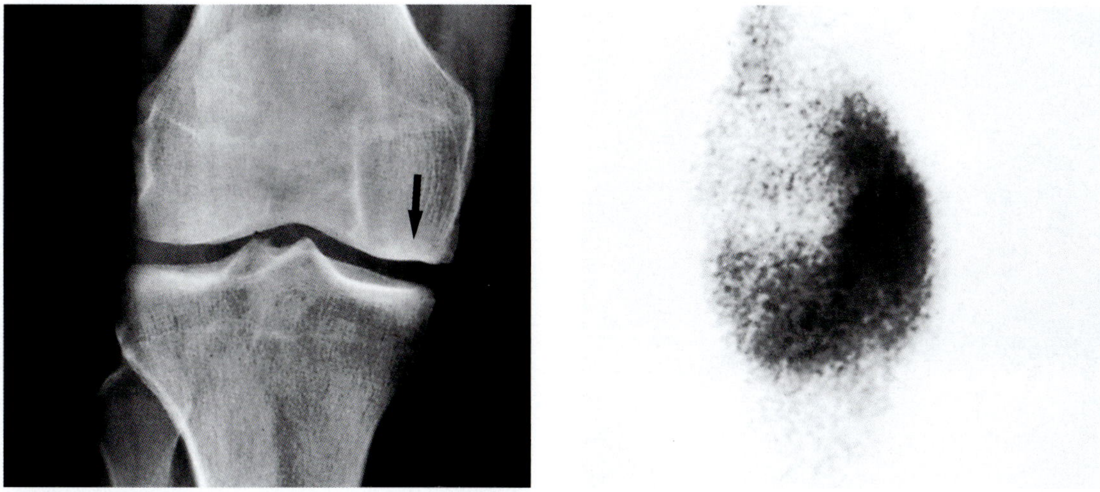

A B

Figure 12.37 ■ **SONK/SIFK.** A 58-year-old man felt a sharp pain in the right knee when he stepped off a curb. The pain subsided after 1 week but recurred soon afterward. **A:** Anteroposterior radiograph of the right knee shows flattening of the medial femoral condyle (*arrow*). **B:** Technetium radionuclide bone scan shows marked increase in uptake of the radiopharmaceutical tracer in the area of the medial femoral condyle.

SPONTANEOUS OSTEONECROSIS OF THE KNEE (SONK)/SUBCHONDRAL INSUFFICIENCY FRACTURE OF THE KNEE (SIFK)

Characterized by acute onset of pain, SONK is a distinct clinicopathologic entity with a predilection for the weight-bearing segment of the medial femoral condyle, first described by Ahlbäck et al. in 1968. It occurs in older adults, frequently in their sixths and seventh decade of life, and may at times be mistaken for arthritis. Although the cause is obscure, certain factors such trauma, intra-articular injections of steroids, and possible tear of the meniscus may play a role in the pathogenesis of this condition. Current concepts indicate that this condition represents a subchondral insufficiency fracture.

The earliest radiologic sign of this abnormality is an increased uptake of isotope on radionuclide bone scans; radiographically, the earliest indication is a minimal degree of flattening of the femoral condyle (Fig. 12.37). Later, usually 1 to 3 months after the sudden onset of symptoms, radiographs may show a subchondral focus of radiolucency. As the condition progresses, the lesion may be seen radiographically as a subchondral osteolytic (necrotic) focus surrounded by a sclerotic margin representing a zone of repair (Fig. 12.38).

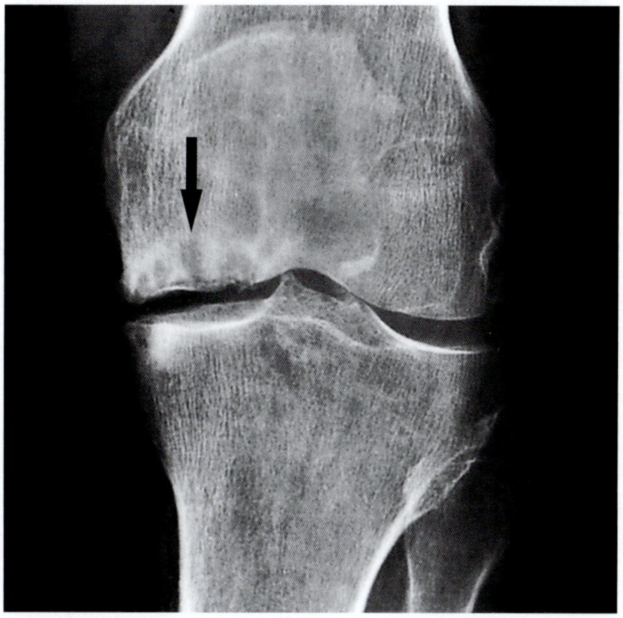

Figure 12.38 ■ **SONK/SIFK.** A 74-year-old man stepped off a curb and felt a sharp pain in the left knee. Radiographs obtained on the next day showed no abnormalities. The pain subsided after 10 days, but 2 months later, joint effusion developed, which was aspirated. The patient was given a series of intra-articular injections of hydrocortisone, after which most of the symptoms subsided. At that time, the conventional radiographs of the knee were repeated. Anteroposterior radiograph shows a large radiolucent defect in the weight-bearing segment of the medial femoral condyle, surrounded by zone of sclerosis (*arrow*). The lesion represents an insufficiency fracture.

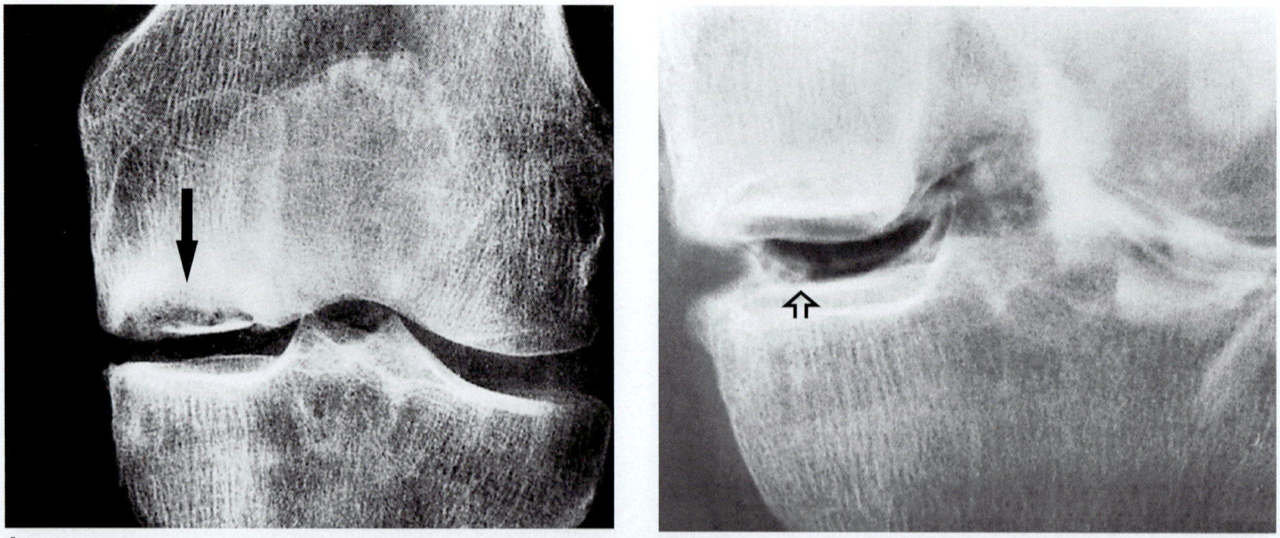

A B

Figure 12.39 ■ **Arthrography of SONK/SIFK.** A 63-year-old woman missed a step while descending the staircase and felt a pain in the left knee. The radiographic examination performed 3 days later showed only moderate periarticular osteoporosis, which was not related to trauma. Three months later, she was re-examined for persistent pain and accumulation of joint fluid. **A:** Anteroposterior radiograph of the left knee shows insufficiency fracture in the weight-bearing portion of the medial femoral condyle (*arrow*). **B:** Double-contrast arthrogram demonstrates a vertical tear of the medial meniscus at the site of insufficiency fracture (*open arrow*).

Frequently, these lesions are accompanied by meniscal tears, and, for this reason, contrast arthrography is used to be performed in the past (Fig. 12.39). Currently, MRI is the procedure of choice (Fig. 12.40). In the early stages, before collapse of the subchondral bone plate, this modality demonstrates the subchondral insufficiency fracture with surrounding edema (Fig. 12.41). Unless the knee is protected from weight bearing, the lesion will progress, and the subchondral bone plate will collapse (Fig. 12.42).

Initially, majority of patients are treated conservatively with nonsteroidal anti-inflammatory drugs (NSAIDs), analgesics, and bisphosphonates. Those patients who do not respond to these measures may be offered a surgical treatment, consisting of a variety of procedures, such as arthroscopic debridement, core decompression, allografting, mosaicplasty, or unicompartmental or total knee arthroplasty, depending upon the stage of disease.

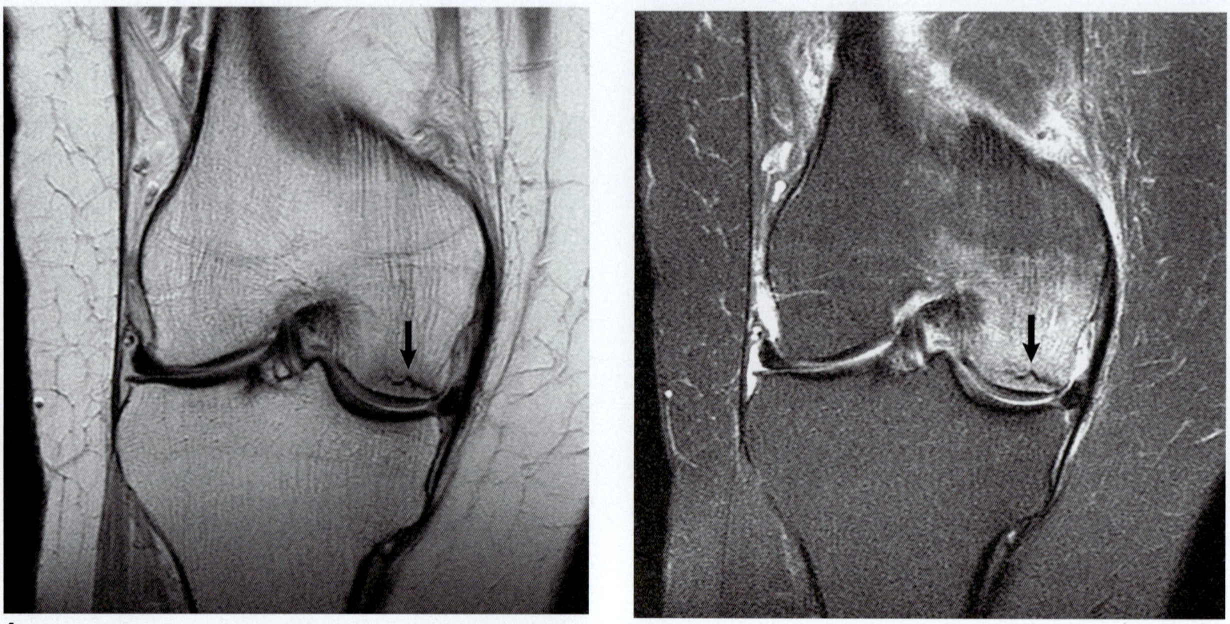

A B

Figure 12.40 ■ **MRI of SONK/SIFK.** A 78-year-old woman felt a sudden sharp pain in her right knee while crossing the street. Coronal T1-weighted **(A)** and coronal proton density–weighted **(B)** fat-suppressed MR images of the right knee show typical subchondral insufficiency fracture at the medial femoral condyle (*arrows*).

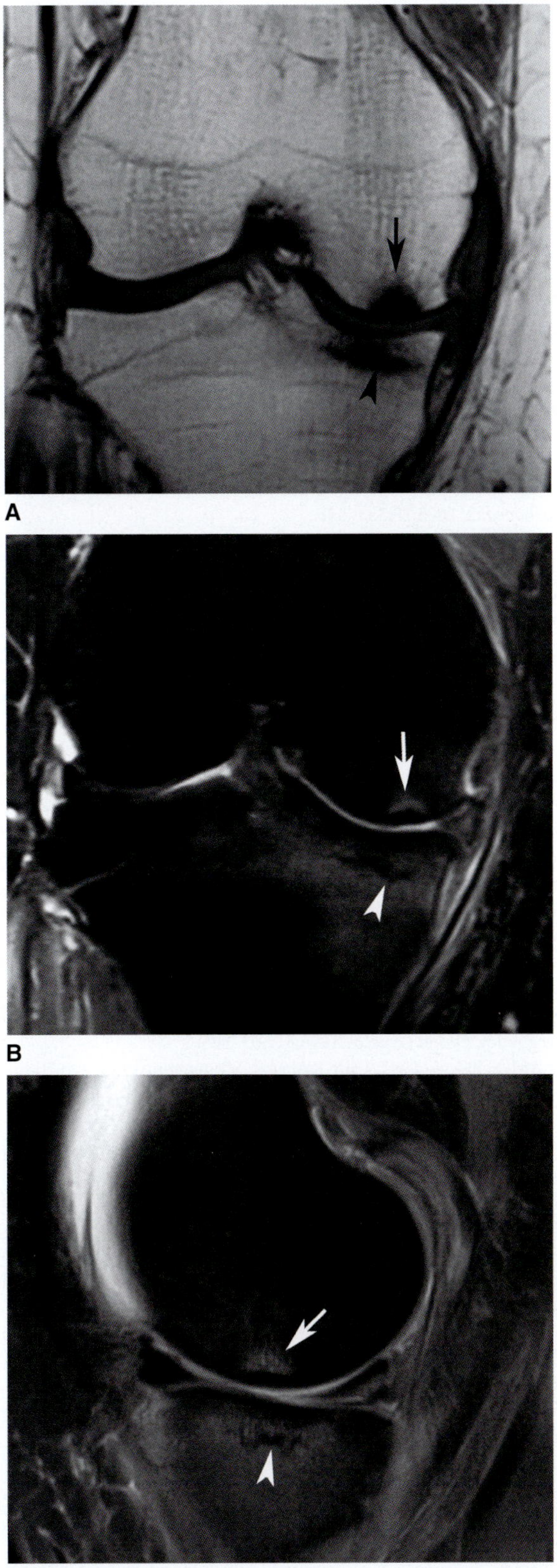

Figure 12.41 ■ **MRI of SONK/SIFK.** Coronal T1-weighted **(A)** and coronal **(B)** and sagittal **(C)** proton density–weighted fat-suppressed MR images of the right knee of an 85-year-old man with acute onset of knee pain demonstrate a nondepressed subchondral insufficiency fracture in the medial femoral condyle with a halo of surrounding bone marrow edema (*arrows*). Note also presence of second insufficiency fracture at the proximal medial tibia with surrounding bone marrow edema (*arrowheads*).

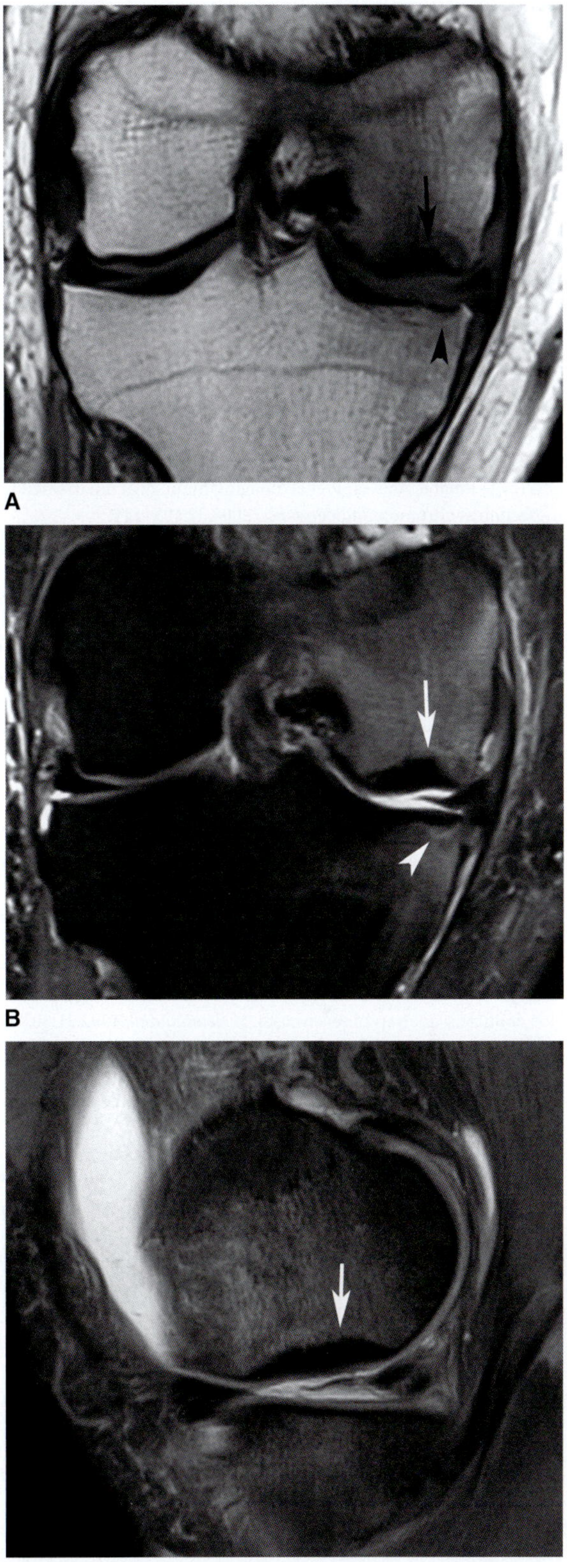

Figure 12.42 ■ **MRI of SONK/insufficiency fracture.** Coronal T1-weighted **(A)** and coronal **(B)** and sagittal **(C)** proton density–weighted fat-suppressed MR images of the right knee of a 63-year-old man with acute onset of knee pain demonstrate a depressed subchondral insufficiency fracture in the medial femoral condyle (*arrows*) with extensive surrounding bone marrow edema. There is also a smaller insufficiency fracture of the medial tibial plateau (*arrowheads*). Note in addition a tear of the posterior horn of the medial meniscus.

SUGGESTED READINGS

Ahlbäck S, Bauer GCH, Bohne WH. Spontaneous osteonecrosis of the knee. *Arthritis Rheum.* 1968;11:705–733.

Aichroth P. Osteochondritis dissecans of the knee: a clinical survey. *J Bone Joint Surg Br.* 1971;53:440–447.

Borchers AT, Gershwin ME. Complex regional pain syndrome: a comprehensive and critical review. *Autoimmun Rev.* 2014;13:242–265.

Borchers AT, Gershwin ME. The clinical relevance of complex regional pain syndrome type I: the emperor's new clothes. *Autoimmun Rev.* 2017;16:22–33.

Bullough PG. *Atlas of Orthopedic Pathology with Clinical and Radiologic Correlations.* 2nd ed. New York, NY: Gower Medical Publishing; 1992:18.12–18.14.

Buselli P, Coco V, Notarnicola A, et al. Shock waves in the treatment of post-traumatic myositis ossificans. *Ultrasound Med Biol.* 2010;36:397–409.

Cakmak S, Tekin L, Akarasu S. Long-term outcome of Osgood–Schlatter disease: not always favorable. *Rheumatol Int.* 2014;34:135–136.

Cerezal L, del Pinal F, Abascal F, et al. Imaging findings in ulnar-sided wrist impaction syndromes. *Radiographics.* 2002;22:105–121.

Cone RO, Resnick D, Danzig L. Shoulder impingement syndrome: radiologic evaluation. *Radiology.* 1984;150:29–33.

Cooper T, Boyles A, Samora WP, et al. Prevalence of bilateral JOCD of the knee and associated risk factors. *J Pediatr Orthop.* 2015;35:507–510.

Czyrny Z. Osgood–Schlatter disease in ultrasound diagnostics—a pictorial essay. *Med Ultrason.* 2010;12:323–335.

Czyrny Z, Greenspan A. Osgood–Schlatter disease: a new perspective and classification based on ultrasonography. *Ultrasonografia.* 2009;38:55–70.

DeFlaviis L, Nessi R, Scagione P, et al. Ultrasonic diagnosis of Osgood–Schlatter and Sinding–Larsen–Johansson disease of the knee. *Skeletal Radiol.* 1989;18:193–197.

De Smet AA, Fisher DR, Graf BK, et al. Osteochondritis dissecans of the knee: value of MR imaging in determining lesion stabilization and presence of articular cartilage defects. *AJR Am J Roentgenol.* 1990;155:549–553.

De Smet AA, Alahi OA, Graf BK. Reassessment of the MR criteria for stability of osteochondritis dissecans in the knee and ankle. *Skeletal Radiol.* 1996;25:159–163.

DeSmet AA, Norris MA, Fisher DR. Magnetic resonance imaging of myositis ossificans: analysis of seven cases. *Skeletal Radiol.* 1992;21:503–507.

De Smet L. Ulnar variance: fact and fiction, review article. *Acta Orthop Belg.* 1994;60:1–9.

Dunningham TH. The treatment of Sudeck's atrophy in the upper limb by sympathetic blockade. *Injury.* 1980;12:139–144.

Ellermann J, Johnson CP, Wang L, et al. Insight into the epiphyseal cartilage origin and subsequent osseous manifestation of juvenile osteochondritis dissecans with a modified clinical MR imaging protocol: a pilot study. *Radiology.* 2017;282:798–806.

Ellermann J,Donald B, Rohr S, et al. Magnetic resonance imaging of osteochondritis dissecans: validation study for ICRS classification system. *Acad Radiol.* 2016;23:724–729.

Escobedo EM, Bergman AG, Hunter JC. MR imaging of ulnar impaction. *Skeletal Radiol.* 1995;24:85–90.

Genant HK, Kozin F, Bekerman C, et al. The reflex sympathetic dystrophy syndrome. *Radiology.* 1975;117:21–32.

Grimm NL, Weiss JM, Kessler JI, et al. Osteochondritis dissecans of the knee: pathoanatomy, epidemiology, and diagnosis. *Clin Sports Med.* 2014;33:181–188.

Gupta RC, Popoutzer MM, Huffer WE, et al. Regional migratory osteoporosis. *Arthritis Rheum.* 1973;16:363–368.

Hangody L, Fules P. Analogous osteochondral mosaicplasty for the treatment of full-thickness defects of weight-bearing joints: ten years of experimental and clinical experience. *J Bone Joint Surg Am.* 2003;85-A(suppl 2): 25–32.

Herrmann LG, Reinecke HG, Caldwell JA. Post-traumatic painful osteoporosis: a clinical and roentgenological entity. *AJR Am J Roentgenol.* 1942;47:353–361.

Heywood CS, Benke MT, Brindle K, et al. Correlation of magnetic resonance imaging to arthroscopic findings of stability in juvenile osteochondritis dissecans. *Arthroscopy.* 2011;27:194–199.

Houang MTW, Brenton DP, Renton P, et al. Idiopathic juvenile osteoporosis. *Skeletal Radiol.* 1978;3:17–21.

Hughston JC, Hergenroeder PT, Courtenay BG. Osteochondritis dissecans of the femoral condyles. *J Bone Joint Surg Am.* 1984;66A:1340–1348.

Jacobs JC Jr, Archibald-Seiffer N, Grimm NL, et al. A review of arthroscopic classification systems for osteochondritis dissecans of the knee. *Orthop Clin North Am.* 2015;46:133–139.

Kabiri L, Tapley H, Tapley S. Evaluation and conservative treatment of Osgood–Schlatter disease: a critical review of the literature. *Int J Ther Rehabil.* 2014;21:91–96.

Kaplan PA, Resnick D. Stress-induced osteolysis of the clavicle. *Radiology.* 1986;158:139–140.

Kattapuram TM, Kattapuram SV. Spontaneous osteonecrosis of the knee. *Eur J Radiol.* 2008;67:42–48.

Kidwai AS, Hemphill SD, Griffiths HJ. Radiologic case study. Spontaneous osteonecrosis of the knee reclassified as insufficiency fracture. *Orthopedics.* 2005;28:333–336.

Kijowski R, Blankenbaker DG, Shinki K, et al. Juvenile versus adult osteochondritis dissecans of the knee: appropriate MR imaging criteria for instability. *Radiology.* 2008;248:571–578.

Koch E, Hofer HO, Sialer G, et al. Failure of MR imaging to detect reflex sympathetic dystrophy of the extremities. *AJR Am J Roentgenol.* 1991;156:113–115.

Kozin F. Reflex sympathetic dystrophy syndrome: a review. *Clin Exp Rheumatol.* 1992;10:401–409.

Kransdorf MJ, Meis JM, Jelinek JS. Myositis ossificans: MR appearance with radiologic-pathologic correlation. *AJR Am J Roentgenol.* 1991;157:1243–1248.

Krause BI, Williams JP, Caterall A. Natural history of Osgood–Schlatter disease. *J Pediatr Orthop.* 1990;10:63–68.

Lafforgue P, Daumen-Legre V, Clairet D, et al. Insufficiency fractures of the medial femoral condyle. *Rev Rhum Engl Ed.* 1996;63:262–269.

Laurin NR, Powe JE, Pavlosky WF, et al. Multimodality imaging of early heterotopic bone formation. *J Can Assoc Radiol.* 1990;41:93–95.

Linden B. The incidence of osteochondritis dissecans in the condyles of the femur. *Acta Orthop Scand.* 1976;47:640–667.

Longstreth PL, Malinak LR, Hill CS. Transient osteoporosis of the hip in pregnancy. *Obstet Gynecol.* 1973;41:563–565.

Malik AM, Schweitzer ME, Culp RW, et al. MR imaging of the type II lunate bone: frequency, extent, and associated findings. *AJR Am J Roentgenol.* 1999;173:335–338.

Malizos K, Zibis A, Dailiana Z. MR imaging findings in transient osteoporosis of the hip. *Eur J Radiol.* 2004;50:238–244.

Medlar RC, Lynce ED. Sinding–Larsen–Johansson disease. Its etiology and natural history. *J Bone Joint Surg Am.* 1978;60A:1113–1116.

Meier C, Kraenzlin C, Friederich NF, et al. Effect of ibandronate on spontaneous osteonecrosis of the knee: a randomized, double-blind, placebo-controlled trial. *Osteoporos Int.* 2014;25:359–366.

Melenevsky Y, Yablon CM, Ramappa A, et al. Clavicle and acromial joint injuries: a review of imaging, treatment, and complications. *Skeletal Radiol.* 2011;40:831–842.

Michael JW, Wurth A, Eysel P, et al. Long-term results after operative treatment of osteochondritis dissecans of the knee joint—30 years results. *Int Orthop.* 2008;32:217–221.

Miller AE, Davis BA, Beckley OA. Bilateral and recurrent myositis ossificans in an athlete: a case report and review of treatment options. *Arch Phys Med Rehabil.* 2006;87:286–290.

Miyanishi K, Yamamoto T, Motomura G. Subchondral changes in transient osteoporosis of the hip. *Skeletal Radiol.* 2001;30:255–261.

Mont MA, Marker DR, Zywiel MG, et al. Osteonecrosis of the knee and related conditions. *J Am Acad Orthop Surg.* 2011;19:482–494.

Neer CS II. Impingement lesions. *Clin Orthop.* 1983;173:70–77.

Norman A, Baker ND. Spontaneous osteonecrosis of the knee and medial meniscal tears. *Radiology.* 1978;129:653–660.

Norman A, Dorfman HD. Juxtacortical circumscribed myositis ossificans. Evolution and radiographic features. *Radiology.* 1970;96:301–306.

Nuovo MA, Norman A, Chumas J, et al. Myositis ossificans with atypical clinical, radiographic, or pathologic findings: a review of 23 cases. *Skeletal Radiol.* 1992;21:87–101.

Ogden JA, Southwick WO. Osgood–Schlatter's disease and tibial tuberosity development. *Clin Orthop.* 1976;116:180–189.

Osgood RB. Lesions of the tibial tubercle occurring during adolescence. *Boston Med Surg J.* 1903;148:114–117.

Palmer WE, Brown JH, Rosenthal DI. Rotator cuff: evaluation with fat-suppressed MR arthrography. *Radiology.* 1993;188:683–687.

Pascual-Garrido C, Moran CJ, Green DW, et al. Osteochondritis dissecans of the knee in children and adolescents. *Curr Opin Pediatr.* 2013;25: 46–51.

Peh WCG, Farmer THR, Totty WG. Acromial arch shape: assessment with MR imaging. *Radiology.* 1995;195:501–505.

Petrini F, Amoroso L, Carotti L, et al. Myositis ossificans circumscripta: computerized tomography and magnetic resonance findings. *Radiol Med.* 1995;90:492–494.

Ramnath RR, Kattapuram SV. MR appearance of SONK-like subchondral abnormalities in the adult knee: SONK redefined. *Skeletal Radiol.* 2004;33:575–581.

Recht MP, Resnick D. Magnetic resonance imaging studies of the shoulder. Diagnosis of lesions of the rotator cuff. *J Bone Joint Surg Am.* 1993;75-A:1244–1253.

Rosenberg ZS, Kawelblum M, Cheung YY, et al. Osgood–Schlatter lesion: fracture or tendinitis? Scintigraphic, CT, and MR imaging features. *Radiology.* 1992;185:853–858.

Sebastin SJ. Complex regional pain syndrome. *Indian J Plast Surg.* 2011;44:298–307.

Shirkhoda A, Armin A-R, Bis KG, et al. MR imaging of myositis ossificans: variable patterns at different stages. *J Magn Reson Imaging.* 1995;5:287–292.

Sokoloff RM, Farooki S, Resnick D. Spontaneous osteonecrosis of the knee associated with ipsilateral tibial plateau stress fracture: report of two patients and review of the literature. *Skeletal Radiol.* 2001;30:53–56.

Thompson MJ, Rivara FP. Bicycle-related injuries. *Am Fam Physician.* 2001;63:2007–2015.

Torrance DA, deGraauw C. Treatment of post-traumatic myositis ossificans of the anterior thigh with extracorporeal shock wave therapy. *J Can Chiropr Assoc.* 2011;55:241.

Tuompo P, Landtman M, Sandelin J, et al. Operative treatment of osteochondritis dissecans of the knee: a retrospective comparison of fixation with autologous bone pegs vs. bioabsorbable rods. *Knee.* 2000;7:31–38.

Tyler P, Saifuddin A. The imaging of myositis ossificans. *Semin Musculoskelet Radiol.* 2010;14:201–216.

Van Heest A, James MA, Lewica A, et al. Posterior elbow capsulotomy with triceps lengthening for treatment of elbow extension contracture in children with arthrogryposis. *J Bone Joint Surg Am.* 2008;90-A:1517–1523.

Victoroff BN, Marcus RE, Deutsch A. Arthroscopic bone peg fixation in the treatment of osteochondritis dissecans in the knee. *Arthroscopy.* 1996;12:506–509.

Yamamoto T, Bullough PG. Spontaneous osteonecrosis of the knee: the result of subchondral insufficiency fracture. *J Bone Joint Surg Am.* 2000;82-A:858–866.

Yamamoto T, Bullough PG. Subchondral insufficiency fracture of the femoral head and medial femoral condyle. *Skeletal Radiol.* 2000;29:40–44.

Yanow J, Pappagallo M, Pillai L. Complex regional pain syndrome (CRPS/RSD) and neuropathic pain: role of intravenous bisphosphonates as analgesics. *Sci World J.* 2008;8:229–236.

Wall EJ, Polousky JD, Shea KG, et al. Novel radiographic feature classification of knee osteochondritis dissecans: a multicenter reliability study. *Am J Sports Med.* 2015;43:303–309.

Williams JL, Cliff MM, Bonakdarpour A. Spontaneous osteonecrosis of the knee. *Radiology.* 1973;107:15–19.

Wnorowski DC, Mosher JF. Carpal collapse and Sudeck's atrophy. *J Hand Surg [Am].* 1992;17:773–776.

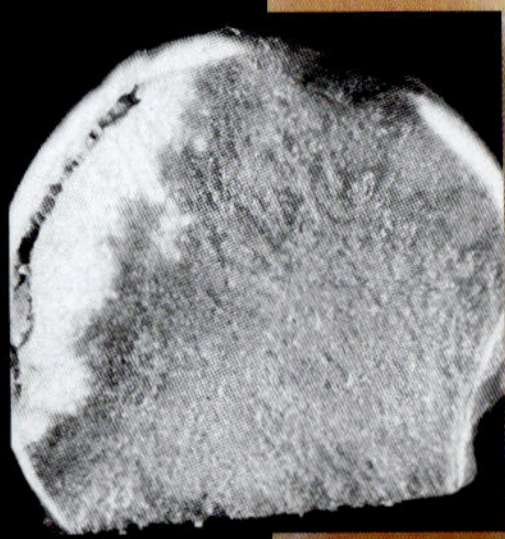

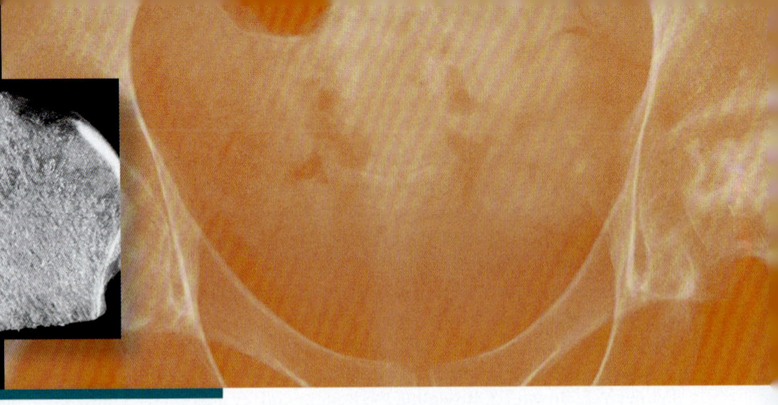

CHAPTER 13

Osteonecrosis (Ischemic or Avascular Necrosis)

Osteonecrosis, the cellular death of bone tissue, may occur after a fracture or dislocation when the bone is deprived of a sufficient supply of arterial blood. However, it is important to recognize that this condition may also develop as a result of factors unrelated to mechanical trauma, particularly from the use of corticosteroids and from alcohol abuse (Table 13.1). Regardless of cause, the pathomechanism of osteonecrosis includes intraluminal vascular obstruction, vascular compression, or disruption of a blood vessel. Among the reported mechanisms of osteonecrosis (other than a fracture or dislocation) are the following:

1. *Embolization of arteries.* This may occur in a variety of conditions. It is seen, for example, in certain hemoglobinopathies, such as sickle cell disease, in which arteries are occluded by abnormal red blood cells; in decompression states of dysbaric conditions, such as caisson disease, in which embolization by nitrogen bubbles occurs; or in chronic alcoholism and pancreatitis, when fat particles embolize arteries.
2. *Vasculitis.* Inflammation of the blood vessels may lead to interruption of the supply of arterial blood to the bone, as seen in collagen disorders such as systemic lupus erythematosus (SLE). However, the use of steroids in these conditions is a major cofactor and may be even more contributing determinant than the primary disease.
3. *Abnormal accumulation of cells.* In Gaucher disease, which is characterized by the abnormal accumulation of lipid-containing histiocytes in the bone marrow, or after steroid therapy, which can lead to an increase of fat cells, sinusoidal blood flow may be compromised, resulting in a deprivation of blood supply to the bone.
4. *Elevated intraosseous pressure.* This theory, championed by Hungerford and Lennox, suggests that any acute or chronic pathologic process that results in increased pressure within the femoral head (which is essentially a sphere of cancellous bone, marrow, and fat surrounded by a cortical shell) may compromise the blood flow and lead to osteonecrosis. The use of steroids and alcohol abuse falls into this category, as well as chronic tobacco use, although the latter addiction plays relatively minor role compared with the two formerly mentioned.
5. *Inhibition of angiogenesis.* Osteonecrosis may result from compromise of normal angiogenesis that occurs consistently in bone tissue. Smith and coworkers recently introduced this new hypothesis, supported by the fact that a number of drugs and mediators, including glucocorticoids, interferons, and other endogenously produced cytokines, inhibit angiogenesis. A similar effect was observed in the angiographic studies of the femoral head after the administration of steroids.
6. *Mechanical stress.* This causative factor was occasionally attributed to nontraumatic osteonecrosis of the femoral head. The weight-bearing segment of the femoral head is the anterior–superior quadrant and, therefore, is under a large mechanical strain. Occlusion of the vessels in this region of the femoral head might be the result of cartilage breakdown secondary to excessive mechanical stress. Support for this hypothesis stems from experiments on rats by Iwasaki et al. and Suehiro et al.
7. *Radiation exposure.* Exposure to radiation may result in damage to the vascularity of a bone.
8. *Idiopathic.* Often, no definite cause can be established, as in the case of certain conditions such as Legg-Calvé-Perthes disease involving the femoral head or Freiberg disease affecting the head of the second metatarsal. This diagnosis is usually made when the osteonecrosis affects only one bone and should only be entertained when all other etiologic factors are excluded.

The degree to which genetics and the environment play the role in the pathogenesis of nontraumatic osteonecrosis is the subject of an ongoing investigation. Single nucleotide polymorphisms have been noted in a number of genes that may be associated with osteonecrosis. It has been argued that endothelial nitric oxide synthase is an important player in the development of this condition. Nitric oxide may have beneficial effects on three systems involved in osteonecrosis, namely, skeletal, vascular, and thrombotic. Each of these may be a target for proposed mechanisms of pathogenesis. A comparative analysis of the 26-base pair repeats polymorphism in intron 4 and the Glu298Asp polymorphism in exon 7 of the *eNOS* gene in patients with idiopathic, steroid-induced, alcohol-induced, and normal control subjects was performed. The frequency of the homozygous 4a allele was found to be higher in patients with idiopathic osteonecrosis compared with control subjects, and the frequency of the 4a/b allele was found to be higher in all types of osteonecrosis when compared with control subjects. The 4a allele is known to be associated with reduced synthesis of endothelial nitric oxide synthase, suggesting that nitric oxide may play a protective role against the development of osteonecrosis.

Forty-one percent of patients with osteonecrosis compared with only 20% of controls were homozygous for the 4G/4G mutation in the plasminogen activator inhibitor-1 gene. This mutation causes increased hypofibrinolytic plasminogen activator inhibitor activity, resulting in decreased stimulated plasminogen activator activity. This observation lends support to the theory that procoagulants may play a significant role in the pathogenesis of osteonecrosis. A polymorphism in the plasminogen activator inhibitor-1 (*PAI-1*) gene has also been reported to be predictive of osteonecrosis in children with acute lymphoblastic leukemia.

OSTEONECROSIS OF FEMORAL HEAD

Although osteonecrosis of the femoral head is a common complication after an intracapsular fracture of the femoral neck (60% to 75%), dislocation in the hip joint (25%), and slipped capital femoral epiphysis (15% to 40%), there are other causes of this abnormality (see Table 13.1).

Clinical Features

Pain is almost always the presenting symptom. The pain may be mild initially or vague in cases of insidious onset, when the diagnosis is not suspected. Conversely, severe pain can develop rapidly in cases in which trauma is the obvious cause. Rarely, pain can be very intense, particularly when caused by large infarcts such as those that occur in Gaucher disease, dysbarism, or hemoglobinopathy. The pain is located most commonly in the groin or anterior thigh and is almost always unilateral to begin with; however, in ~55% of cases, the opposite hip becomes involved within 2 years. Usually, pain increases with use of the extremity, ultimately appears even at rest, and frequently requires analgesics for relief. Range of motion is well preserved at the beginning of the disease but gradually deteriorates.

Table 13.1 DISEASES OR CONDITIONS ASSOCIATED WITH OR LEADING TO OSTEONECROSIS

Diseases or Conditions
Trauma
Fracture of femoral head and neck
Dislocation of the femoral head
Proximal femoral epiphysiolysis
Slipped capital femoral epiphysis
Epiphyseal compression
Fracture of talus
Fracture of scaphoid
Kienböck disease
Vascular injury
Burns
Radiation exposure
Hemoglobinopathies
Sickle cell disease
Hb S/C hemoglobinopathy
Hb S thalassemia
Polycythemia
Congenital and Developmental Conditions
Congenital dysplasia of the hip
Ehlers-Danlos syndrome
Hereditary dysostosis
Legg-Calvé-Perthes disease
Fabry disease
Local Infiltrative Lesions
Gaucher disease
Neoplastic conditions
Lymphoproliferative disorders
Metabolic Conditions
Hypercortisolism
Corticosteroid medications
Cushing disease
Hyperlipidemia
Hyperparathyroidism
Dysbaric Disorders
Caisson disease
Infectious and Inflammatory Conditions
Osteomyelitis
Pancreatitis
Giant cell arteritis
Systemic lupus erythematosus
Acquired immunodeficiency syndrome
Meningococcemia
Miscellaneous Factors
Alcohol consumption
Cigarette smoking
Chronic renal failure
Hemodialysis
Intravascular coagulation
Organ transplantation
Pregnancy
Idiopathic

Note: Some of the listed conditions have been reported to be associated with osteonecrosis, whether or not the direct cause has been definitively established.

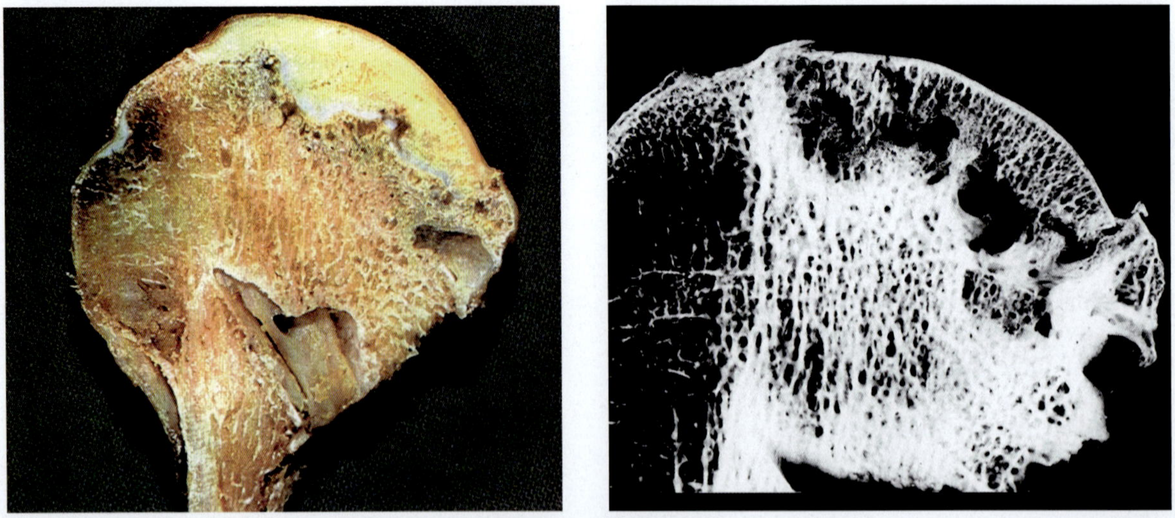

A B

Figure 13.1 ■ Gross pathology of osteonecrosis, early stage. A: Photograph of a coronal section of the femoral head specimen shows subchondral triangular, opaque-yellow area representing infracted bone. **B:** Radiograph of the same specimen shows the radiolucent area at the base of the infarction resulting from fibrous granulation tissue invading the necrotic bone. The viable bone is dense, because of formation of new bone in this area by the process of creeping substitution. (From Bullough PG. *Atlas of Orthopedic Pathology with Clinical and Radiologic Correlations*, 2nd ed. New York, NY: Gower Medical Publishing; 1992. Figs. 10.43 and 10.44, p. 10.15.)

Pathology

In the early stage of the disease, on the cut section of the specimen, the necrotic zone can be seen in subarticular location as wedge-shaped region in which bone marrow is dull yellow, chalky, and opaque. This region is well demarcated and is separated from the surrounding unaffected bone marrow by a thin, red hyperemic border (Fig. 13.1). At this stage, changes in the trabecular architecture are not appreciable. On microscopic examination, the subchondral bone is necrotic. The marrow elements are replaced by granular, eosinophilic material lacking cellular elements. There may be also cysts of lipid material present together with extensive calcification (Fig. 13.2). The osteocytic lacunae in the bone may be empty, may contain cellular debris, or may have a pale-staining nucleus. In more advanced stage of the disease, the gross pathologic specimen shows fracture and collapse of subchondral bone (Fig. 13.3). The linear fracture in subchondral bone corresponds to the radiolucent zone, referred to as the "crescent sign" seen on the radiographs (see Fig. 13.5). The subchondral infarct is demarcated from the viable bone by zone of hyperemia. The crescent represents a space between the articular cartilage and the underlying infracted subchondral bone. On microscopy, at the margin of the infarct, there is increased osteoclastic activity. Focal fat necrosis and fibroblastic and vascular proliferation into the marrow spaces are the common findings (Fig. 13.4).

Imaging Features

In its very early stages, radiographs may appear completely normal; however, radionuclide bone scan may show first decreased and later increased isotope uptake at the site of the lesion, which is a very valuable indication of abnormality. The

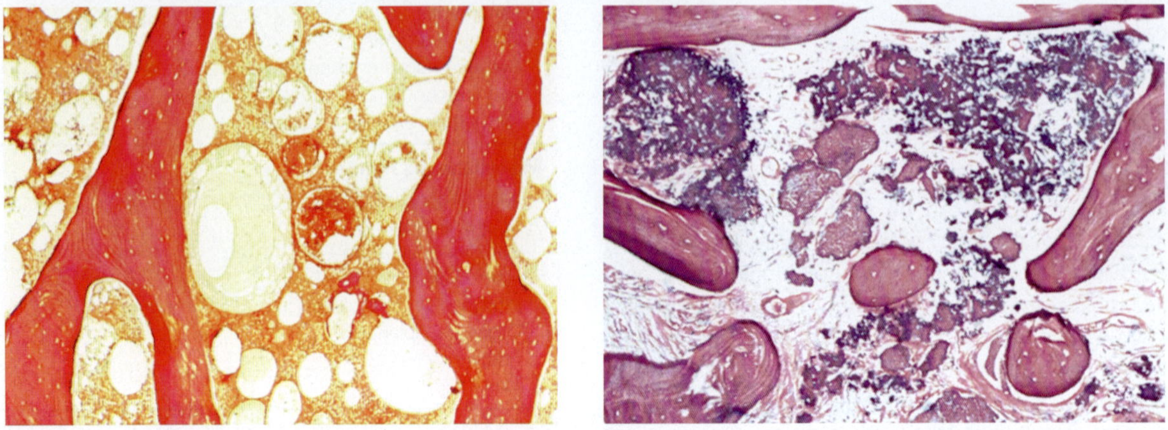

A B

Figure 13.2 ■ Histopathology of osteonecrosis, early stage. A: Photomicrograph of infracted bone and bone marrow reveals the acellular nature of the tissue and a large fat cysts, characteristic feature of infracted bone marrow (phloxine and tartrazine, original magnification ×4). **B:** Calcifications are seen in the infracted bone marrow, occasionally a prominent feature (H&E, original magnification ×4). (From Bullough PG. *Atlas of Orthopedic Pathology with Clinical and Radiologic Correlations*. 2nd ed., Figs. 10.35 and 10.36, p. 10.12.)

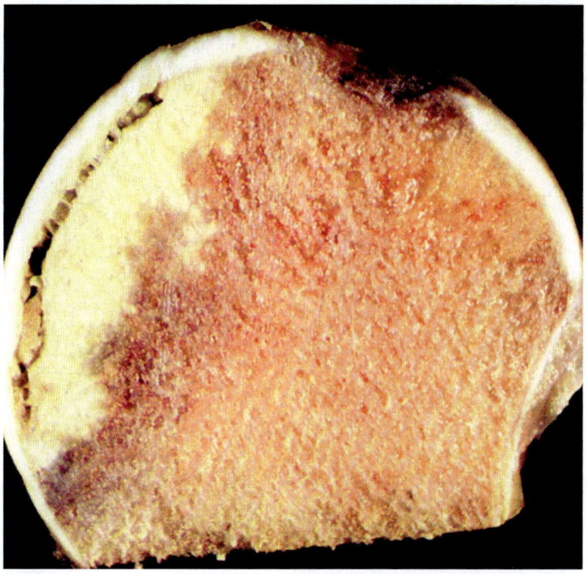

A

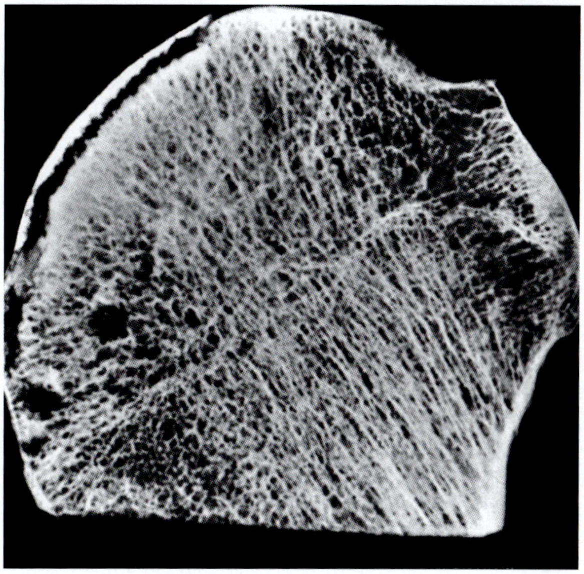

B

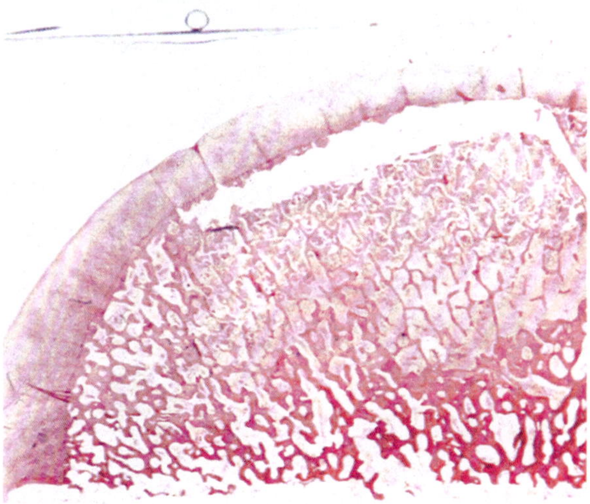

C

Figure 13.3 ■ **Gross pathology and histopathology of osteonecrosis, late stage. A:** Photograph of coronal section of the femoral head specimen shows the subchondral infarct (*yellow*) demarcated from the viable bone by a zone of hyperemia (*red*). Note the crescent representing subchondral bone collapse. **B:** Radiograph of the same specimen shows the crescent sign. **C:** Photomicrograph of a histologic preparation of the femoral head shows space between the articular cartilage and subchondral bone. Observe the thickened trabeculae of the viable bone (H&E, original magnification ×1). (From Bullough PG. *Atlas of Orthopedic Pathology with Clinical and Radiologic Correlations*. 2nd ed., Figs. 10.52, 10.53, and 10.54, p. 10.18.)

earliest radiographic sign of this condition is the presence of a radiolucent crescent, which may be seen as early as 4 weeks after the initial injury. This phenomenon, as Norman and Bullough have pointed out, is secondary to the subchondral structural collapse of the necrotic segment and is visible as a narrow radiolucent line parallel to the articular surface of the bone. Radiographically, the sign is most easily demonstrated on the frog-lateral view of the hip (Figs. 13.5 and 13.6). Because the necrotic process most of the time does not affect the articular cartilage, the width of the joint space (i.e., the radiographic joint space: the width of the articular cartilage of adjoining bones plus the actual joint cavity) is preserved. Preservation of the joint space helps to differentiate this condition from osteoarthritis. In its later stage, osteonecrosis can be readily identified on the anteroposterior view of the hip by a flattening of the articular surface and the dense appearance of the femoral head (Figs. 13.7 and 13.8). The density is secondary to the compression of bony trabeculae after a microfracture of the nonviable bone, calcification of the dendritic marrow, and repair of the necrotic area by the deposition of a new bone, the so-called *creeping substitution*. CT examination frequently helps to delineate the details of this condition (Figs. 13.9 and 13.10). Ficat and Arlet proposed a

(Continued on page 452)

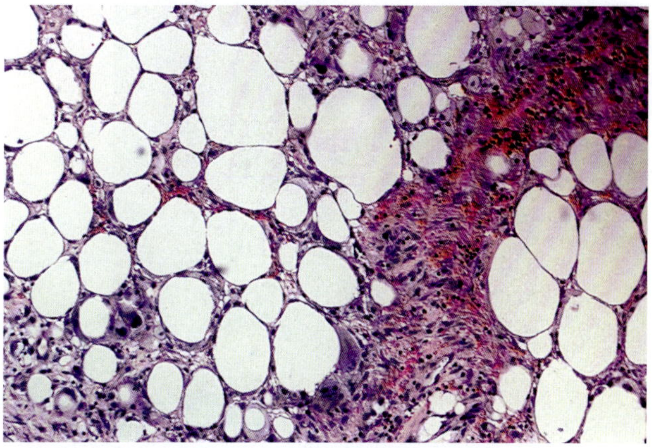

Figure 13.4 ■ **Histopathology of osteonecrosis, late stage.** Photomicrograph shows focal fat necrosis as well as fibroblastic and vascular proliferation at the margin of the infracted area (H&E, original magnification ×10). (From Bullough PG. *Atlas of Orthopedic Pathology with Clinical and Radiologic Correlations*. 2nd ed., Fig. 10.40, p. 10.14.)

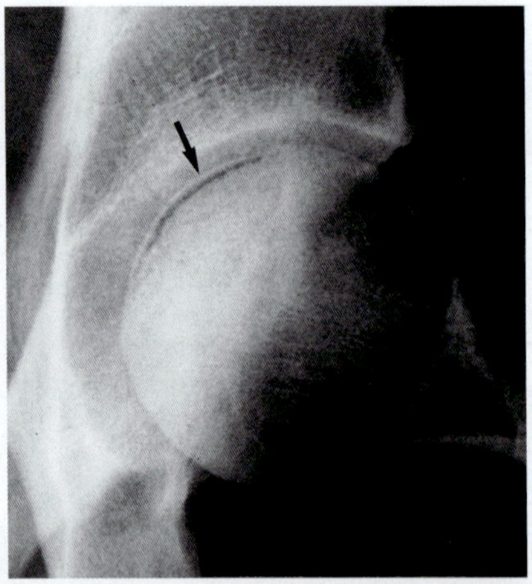

Figure 13.5 ■ Osteonecrosis of the femoral head. The frog-lateral view of the left hip shows the crescent sign (*arrow*) in a 45-year-old woman who sustained a hip dislocation 5 weeks earlier.

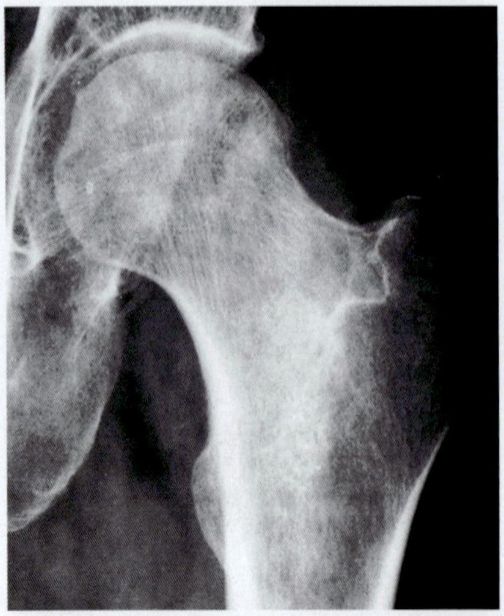

A

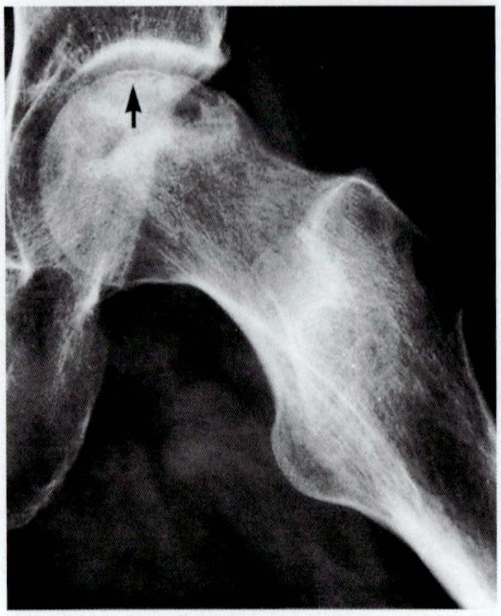

B

Figure 13.6 ■ Osteonecrosis of the femoral head. A: A 41-year-old man presented with a history of traumatic dislocation in the left hip joint. On frontal projection, the increased density of the femoral head suggests osteonecrosis, but a definite diagnosis cannot be made. **B:** The frog-lateral view demonstrates a thin radiolucent line parallel to the articular surface of the femoral head (*arrow*). This represents the crescent sign, a radiographic hallmark of osteonecrosis.

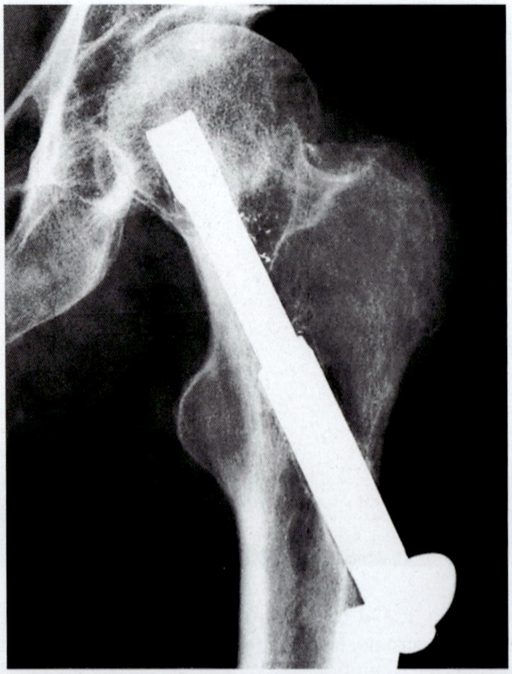

Figure 13.7 ■ Osteonecrosis of the femoral head. A 56-year-old woman sustained an intracapsular fracture of the left femoral neck, which healed after surgical treatment by open reduction and internal fixation. The anteroposterior radiograph shows a Smith-Peterson nail inserted into the femoral neck and head. The fracture line is obliterated. The dense (sclerotic) appearance of the femoral head indicates the development of osteonecrosis.

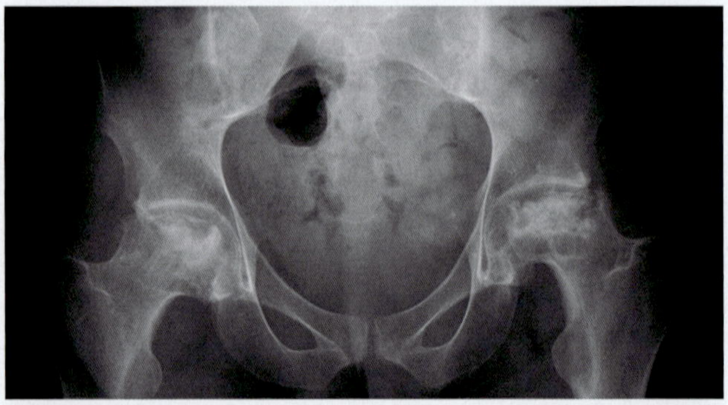

A

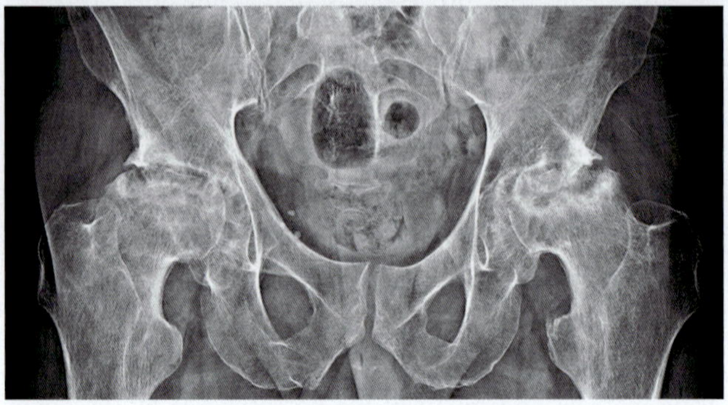

B

Figure 13.8 ■ Osteonecrosis of the femoral head.
A: Anteroposterior radiographs of the hip joints of a 40-year-old man demonstrate more advanced stage of osteonecrosis of both femoral heads showing subchondral collapse. **B:** Similar changes are seen affecting both femoral heads of a 50-year-old man.

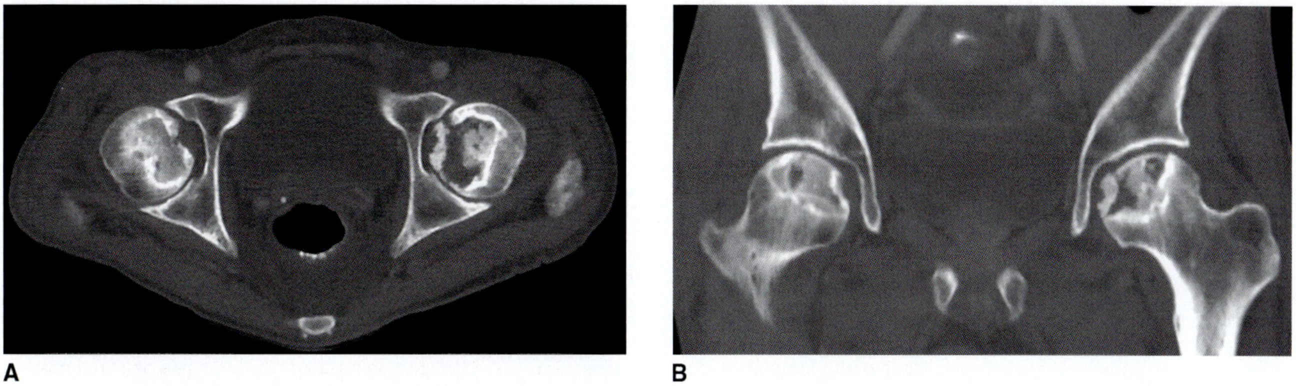

Figure 13.9 ■ **CT of osteonecrosis of the femoral head.** Axial **(A)** and coronal **(B)** reformatted CT images of both hip joints of a 65-year-old man show subchondral sclerosis and fragmentation of the femoral heads. Note that despite advanced osteonecrotic changes, the hip joint space is well preserved.

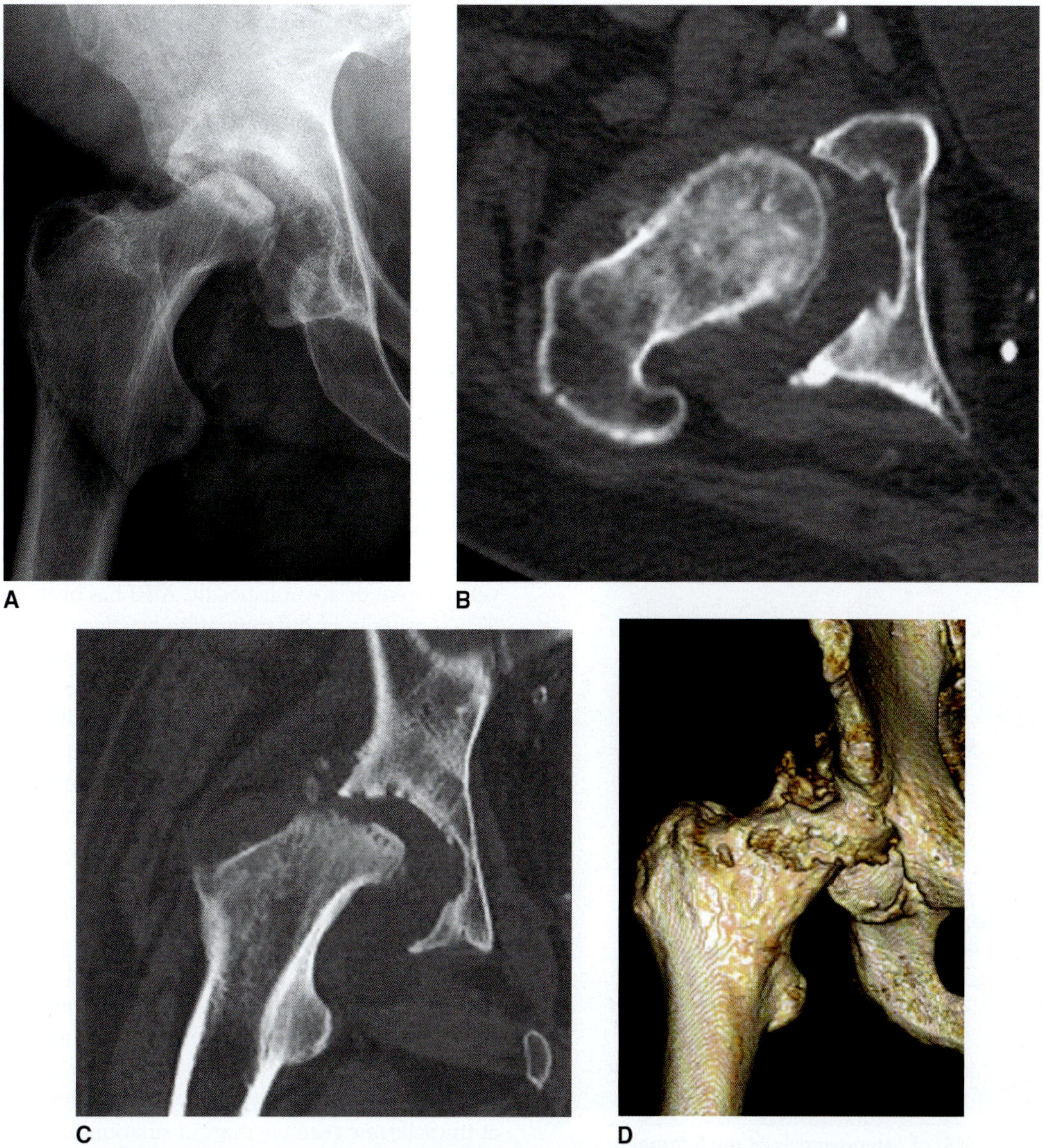

Figure 13.10 ■ **CT and 3D CT of osteonecrosis of femoral head. A:** Anteroposterior radiograph of the right hip shows sclerotic changes and subchondral radiolucency of the deformed femoral head, indicative of advanced osteonecrosis. Observe also superolateral subluxation of the femoral head. All these features are more effectively demonstrated on axial **(B)**, coronal reformatted **(C)**, and 3D reconstructed **(D)** CT images.

Table 13.2 OSTEONECROSIS OF FEMORAL HEAD: CORRELATION OF CLINICAL SYMPTOMS AND IMAGING FINDINGS WITH HISTOPATHOLOGIC CHANGES BASED ON FICAT AND ARLET CLASSIFICATION

Stage	Clinical Symptoms	Radiographic Findings	Scintigraphy	Pathologic Changes	Biopsy
1	None	Normal	Normal	Infarction of weight-bearing segments	Necrotic marrow and osteoblasts
2	Mild pain	Increased density of femoral head and normal joint space	Increased uptake	Spontaneous repair	New bone deposition
3	Mild-to-moderate pain	Loss of sphericity, collapse of the femoral head, and crescent sign	Increased uptake	Subchondral fracture with collapse, impaction, and fragmentation of the necrotic segment	Dead bone trabeculae and dead marrow cells on both sides of the fracture line
4	Moderate pain, assistive devices needed	Joint space narrowing and acetabular changes	Increased uptake	Osteoarthritis	Degenerative changes in articular cartilage

Modified from Assouline-Dayan Y, Chang C, Greenspan A, et al. Pathogenesis and natural history of osteonecrosis. *Semin Arthritis Rheum*. 2002;32:94–124.

classification system of osteonecrosis of the femoral head consisting of four stages, based on radiographic, hemodynamic, and symptomatic criteria (Table 13.2). A significant breakthrough in identifying osteonecrosis in patients who had normal bone scan and normal conventional radiographs was achieved with MRI. Currently, this modality is considered the most sensitive and specific for the diagnosis and evaluation of osteonecrosis (Fig. 13.11). Its characteristic MRI appearance consists of a serpentine band of low–signal intensity rim in the femoral head (Fig. 13.12A). This rim corresponds to the interface of repair between ischemic and normal bone consisting mainly of sclerosis and fibrosis. On T2-weighted images, a second inner rim of high signal has been observed (the double-line sign) (Fig. 13.12B). It is believed that this appearance represents fibrovascular tissue in the reparative zone. Many authors hypothesize that this finding is pathognomonic for osteonecrosis. Other authors have played down the importance of this finding, claiming that it may be largely artifactual, representing the so-called *chemical shift*. Bone marrow edema and joint effusion are frequently associated with osteonecrosis (Fig. 13.12C). Once the subchondral fracture occurs, the femoral head will collapse (Fig. 13.12D), and eventually, the hip joint will develop secondary osteoarthritis. Intravenous injection of gadolinium can help to delineate the extension of the osteonecrosis and determine if there are areas of residual viable tissue (Fig. 13.12E). Several reports have established the diagnostic sensitivity of MRI in the early stages of osteonecrosis, when radiographic changes are not yet apparent or are nonspecific. MRI has been shown to have 97% sensitivity in differentiating osteonecrotic femoral head from normal femoral head and 85% sensitivity in differentiating osteonecrotic femoral head from other disorders of the femoral head, with an overall sensitivity of 91%. MRI appears to be a better predictive test for subsequent femoral head collapse than radionuclide bone scans. The narrow bandlike area of low signal intensity that traverses the femoral head in midcoronal sections present on MRI was a significant indicator of subsequent collapses.

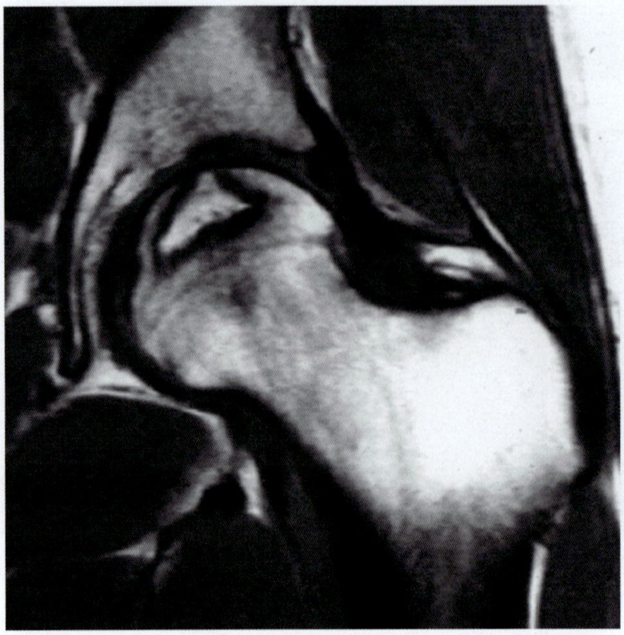

Figure 13.11 ■ MRI of osteonecrosis of the femoral head. Coronal T2-weighted MRI in an 18-year-old woman with SLE demonstrates a focal area of osteonecrosis of the femoral head.

MRI is indispensable in the accurate staging of osteonecrosis because it reflects the size of the lesion and roughly the stage of the disease. Mitchell and colleagues have described a classification system of osteonecrosis based on alterations in the central region of MR signal intensity in the osteonecrotic focus (Table 13.3). In early stages (class A or fatlike), there is preservation of a normal fat signal, except at the sclerotic reactive margin surrounding the lesion, that manifests as a central region of high signal intensity on short spin-echo (SE) repetition time (TR)/echo time (TE)

(Continued on page 454)

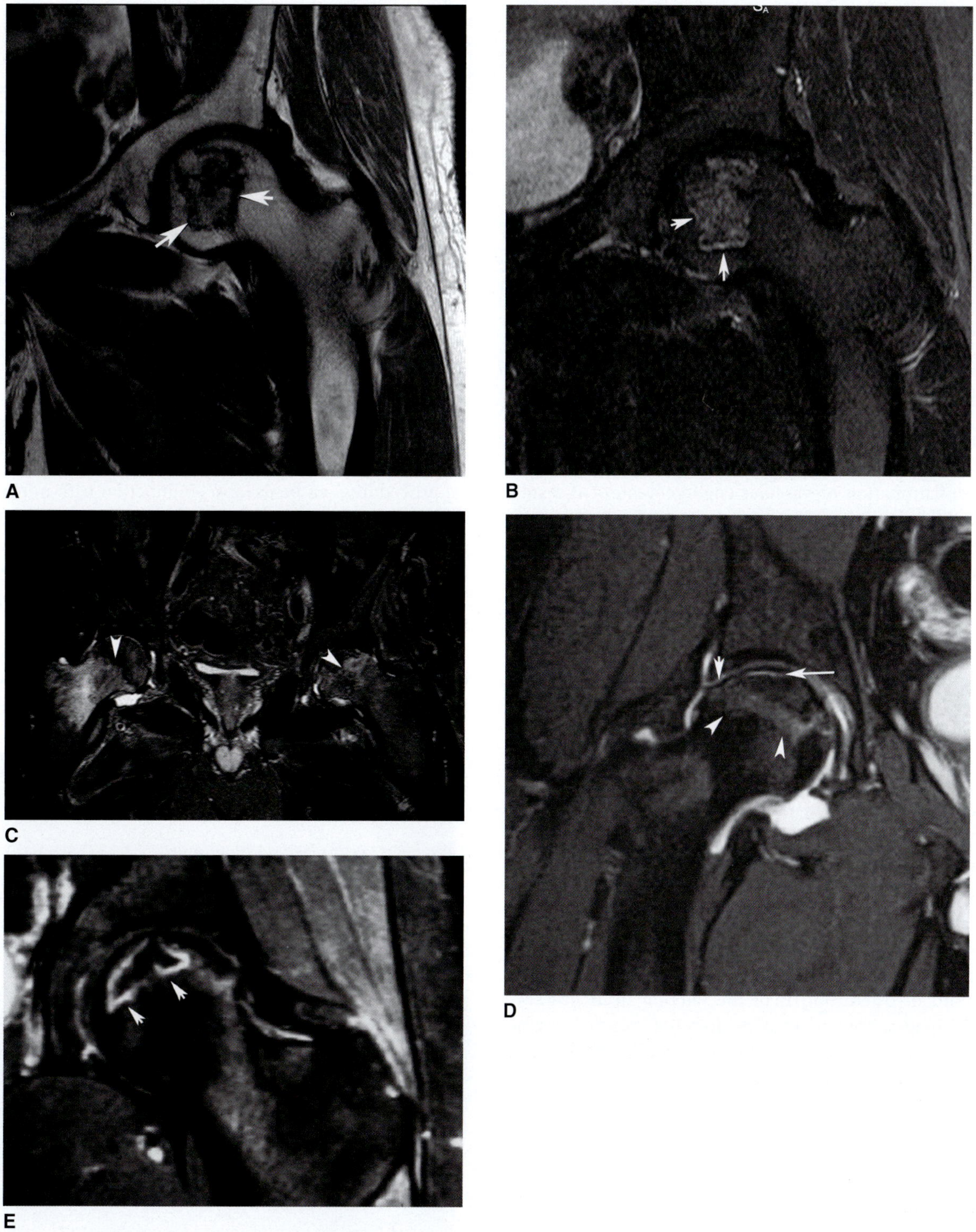

Figure 13.12 ■ **MRI of osteonecrosis of the femoral head. A:** Coronal T1-weighted image shows a serpentine band of low signal intensity (*arrows*) representing the reactive interface surrounding the central area of bone necrosis. **B:** Coronal STIR pulse sequence MR image shows a serpentine low–signal intensity line adjacent to a high–signal intensity line (so-called *double-line sign*) (*arrows*). **C:** Coronal T2-weighted fat saturated MR image demonstrates osteonecrosis of both femoral heads (*arrowheads*), with prominent bone marrow edema in the right femoral neck and joint effusions. The presence of bone marrow edema and joint effusion is frequently associated with osteonecrosis and correlates clinically with pain. **D:** Coronal STIR pulse sequence MR image shows osteonecrosis of the right femoral head (*arrowheads*) with a subchondral hyperintense line (*long arrow*) representing the subchondral fracture. This finding correlates with the crescent sign seen on the conventional radiographs (see Figs. 13.5 and 13.6). Note the early collapse of the lateral aspect of the femoral head (*short arrow*) and the presence of a high-signal joint effusion. **E:** T1-weighted fat-suppressed coronal MR image following intravenous administration of gadolinium shows enhancement of the reactive interface (*arrowheads*) but no enhancement of the necrotic area.

Table 13.3 CORRELATION OF MAGNETIC RESONANCE IMAGING FINDINGS WITH HISTOLOGIC CHANGES

Class	Magnetic Resonance Imaging Findings	Appearance	Histology
A	Normal fat signal except at the sclerotic margin surrounding the lesion	Fatlike	Premature conversion to fatty marrow within the femoral neck or intertrochanteric region
B	High signal intensity of the inner border and low signal intensity of the surrounding rim	Bloodlike	Bone resorption and replacement by vascular granulation tissue
C	Diffusely decreased signal on T1 and high signal on T2 weighting	Fluid-like	Bone marrow edema
D	Decreased signal on T1- and T2-weighted images	Fibrous	Sclerosis from reinforcement of existing trabeculae at the margin of a live bone (i.e., repair tissue interface)

Modified from Assouline-Dayan Y, Chang C, Greenspan A, et al. Pathogenesis and natural history of osteonecrosis. *Semin Arthritis Rheum.* 2002;32:94–124.

images (T1 weighted) and intermediate signal intensity on long TR/TE images (T2 weighted). Later, when there is sufficient inflammation or vascular engorgement, or if a subacute hemorrhage is present (class B or bloodlike), high signal intensity is noted on short and long TR/TE images. This signal is similar to that of a subacute hemorrhage. If there is enough inflammation, hyperemia, and fibrosis present to replace the fat content of the femoral head (class C or fluid-like), a low-intensity signal with short TR/TE and a high-intensity signal with long TR/TE are seen. Finally, in advanced stages, where fibrosis and sclerosis predominate (class D or fibrous-like), low signal intensity is present on both short and long TR/TE images. MRI findings correlate well with histologic changes. The central region of high signal intensity corresponds to necrosis of the bone and marrow. The low signal of the peripheral band corresponds to the sclerotic margin of reactive tissue at the interface between necrotic and viable bones. The advanced stages of osteonecrosis may be further complicated by development of secondary osteoarthritis of the hip joint (Figs. 13.13 and 13.14). As Seiler and coworkers have pointed out, MRI evaluation of osteonecrosis of the femoral head has several advantages: it is noninvasive, does not require ionizing radiation, provides multiplanar images, reflects physiologic changes in the bone marrow, provides excellent resolution of surrounding soft tissues, and makes it possible to evaluate the contralateral femoral head simultaneously.

Treatment

When the involved segment is smaller than 15% and is far from the weight-bearing region, conservative measures, such as medicating for pain relief and limited weigh bearing, may be beneficial, but they do not generally prevent disease progression. A number of newer modes of pharmacologic therapeutic agents including growth and differentiation factors, cytokines, angiogenic factors, and bone morphogenic proteins have theoretical promise in the treatment of this condition. Most of the patients with osteonecrosis of the femoral head ultimately require surgical intervention.

There are various surgical techniques ranging from core decompression to total hip replacement. Sometimes, surgical procedures can be used in conjunction with nonsurgical approaches. The more advanced the disease is, the more extensive surgery is performed. The surgical procedures include core decompression, structural bone grafting, vascularized fibula grafting, osteotomy, resurfacing arthroplasty, hemiarthroplasty, and total hip arthroplasty.

Ficat in 1962 first introduced core decompression procedure. The goal of this approach is to reduce the elevated

(Continued on page 456)

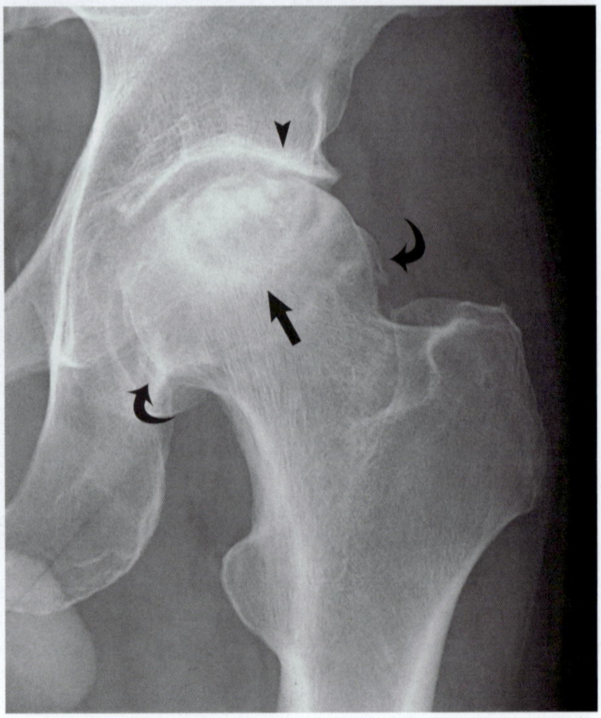

Figure 13.13 ■ Osteonecrosis of the femoral head complicated by secondary osteoarthritis. Anteroposterior radiograph of the left hip of a 39-year-old chronic alcoholic man shows advanced osteonecrosis of the femoral head (*arrow*). Secondary osteoarthritis is manifested by subchondral sclerosis and segmental narrowing of the weight-bearing portion of the hip joint (*arrowhead*) and osteophyte formation (*curved arrows*).

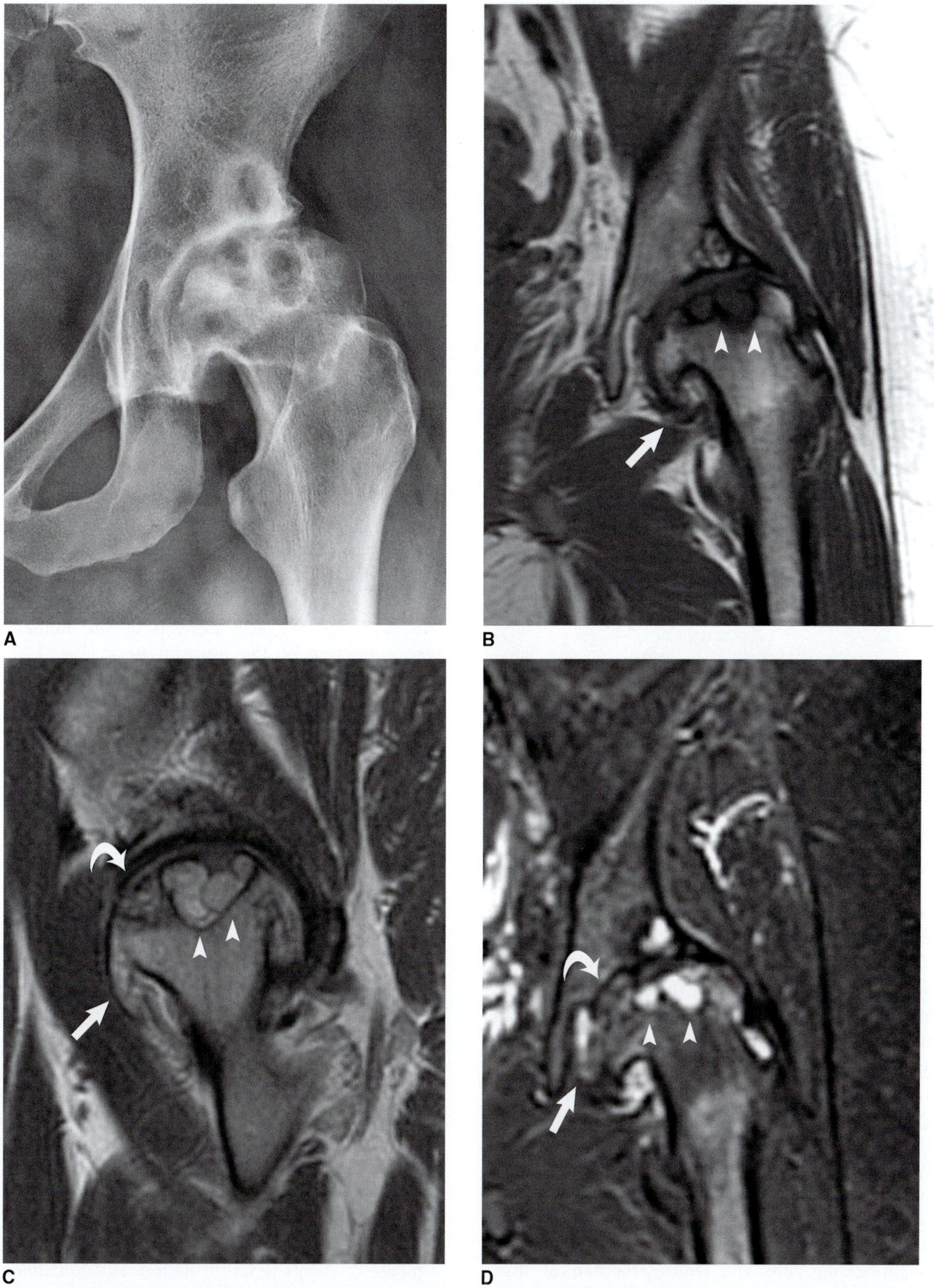

Figure 13.14 ■ MRI of osteonecrosis of the femoral complicated by secondary osteoarthritis. A: Anteroposterior radiograph of the left hip of a 23-year-old woman with systemic lupus erythematosus shows advanced osteonecrosis of the femoral head. The secondary osteoarthritic changes are characterized by narrowing of the joint space, subchondral cysts, and formation of the osteophytes. Coronal T1-weighted **(B)**, sagittal proton density–weighted **(C)**, and coronal STIR **(D)** MR images show osteonecrosis (*curved arrows*), osteophytes (*arrows*), and degenerative cysts (*arrowheads*).

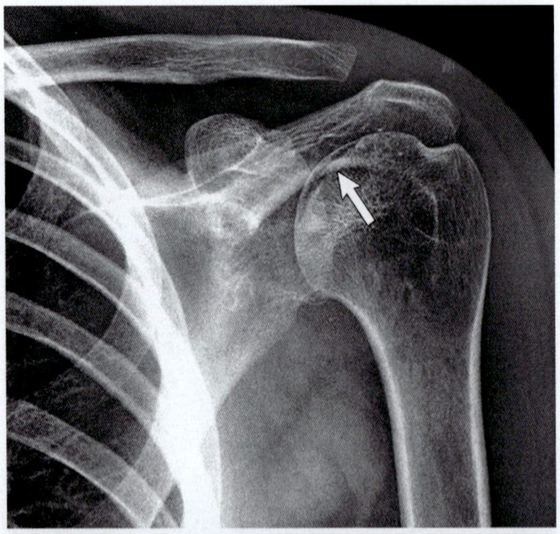

A

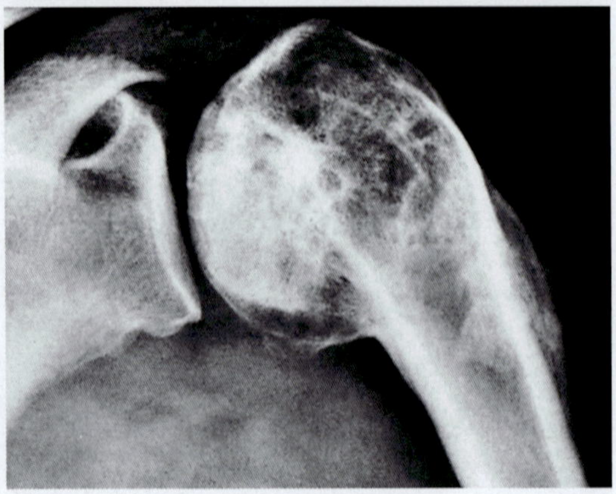

B

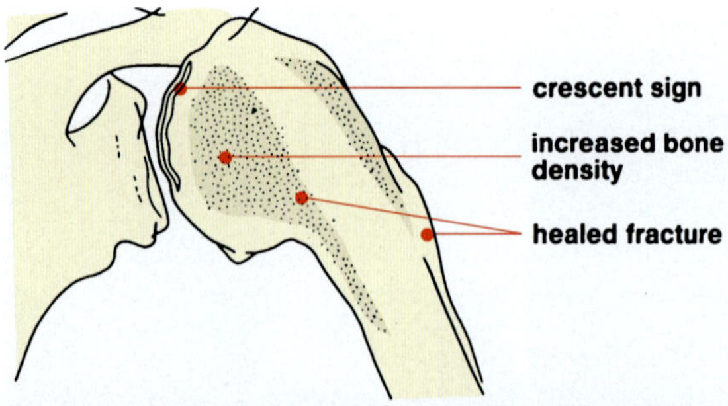

Figure 13.15 ■ Osteonecrosis of the humeral head. **A:** Anteroposterior radiograph of the left shoulder of a 28-year-old woman diagnosed with systemic lupus erythematosus shows a radiolucent crescent sign in subchondral bone of the humeral head (*arrow*) pathognomonic for osteonecrosis. **B:** Six months after sustaining a fracture of the left humeral neck that united, a 62-year-old man developed osteonecrosis of the humeral head, evident on the radiograph from the increased bone density and the collapse of the subchondral segment.

intramedullary pressure within the femoral head and to interrupt the cycle that results in worsening of the ischemia. The procedure also provides immediate and dramatic pain relief. Core decompression yields the best results when performed in early stages of the disease.

Various types of bone graft procedures have been used to provide mechanical support for the affected joint and to delay the need for arthroplasty. These include autogenous and allogenous cortical bone grafts of ilium, fibula, or tibia, alone or in combination with core decompression, osteochondral grafts, muscle pedicle bone grafts, and free vascularized bone grafts. Cortical bone grafts are simple to perform, but long-term outcome are not encouraging, with a success rate of only 25%. A combination of cortical bone graft and core decompression is a safe procedure and the outcomes are better in young patients with Ficat stage II and III disease.

Osteotomy shifts the necrotic bone segment away from the weight-bearing zone and reduces mechanical stress. Once the femoral head has collapsed, the treatment of choice is reconstructive surgery. The procedures most commonly performed are resurfacing or conventional hemiarthroplasty. Occasionally, the total hip arthroplasty is performed. The decision to select one of these procedures over another depends on the stage and the extent of the disease.

OSTEONECROSIS OF HUMERAL HEAD

Osteonecrosis may also develop in the humeral head after a fracture of the humeral neck (Fig. 13.15), but this complication is infrequently seen. A majority of osteonecrosis of the humeral head is either idiopathic or related to connective tissue disorders or treatment with steroids (Fig. 13.16).

KIENBÖCK DISEASE

Single or repeated trauma to the lunate or dislocation of the bone may impair its blood supply and cause it to become necrotic. However, the development of Kienböck disease, as this form of osteonecrosis affecting the lunate is known, may not be solely attributable to extrinsic trauma. Whether the natural history begins with a single simple transverse fracture or numerous compression fractures from repeated compressive strains is still the subject of speculation. An interesting but controversial hypothesis links this condition with negative ulnar variance in individuals whose ulna projects more proximally. They may be predisposed to Kienböck disease because of compression of the lunate against the irregular radioulnar articular surface created by the discrepancy in radial and ulnar length.

Once lunate necrosis begins, an established progressive sequence of events is set in motion. Lunate flattening and elongation, proximal migration of the capitate, scapholunate dissociation, and, finally, osteoarthritis of the radiocarpal joint mark the progression of this abnormality. This series of changes also forms the basis for classification of Kienböck disease (Fig. 13.17). Clinically, stage I is indistinguishable from a wrist sprain. Wrist radiographs may be completely

(Continued on page 458)

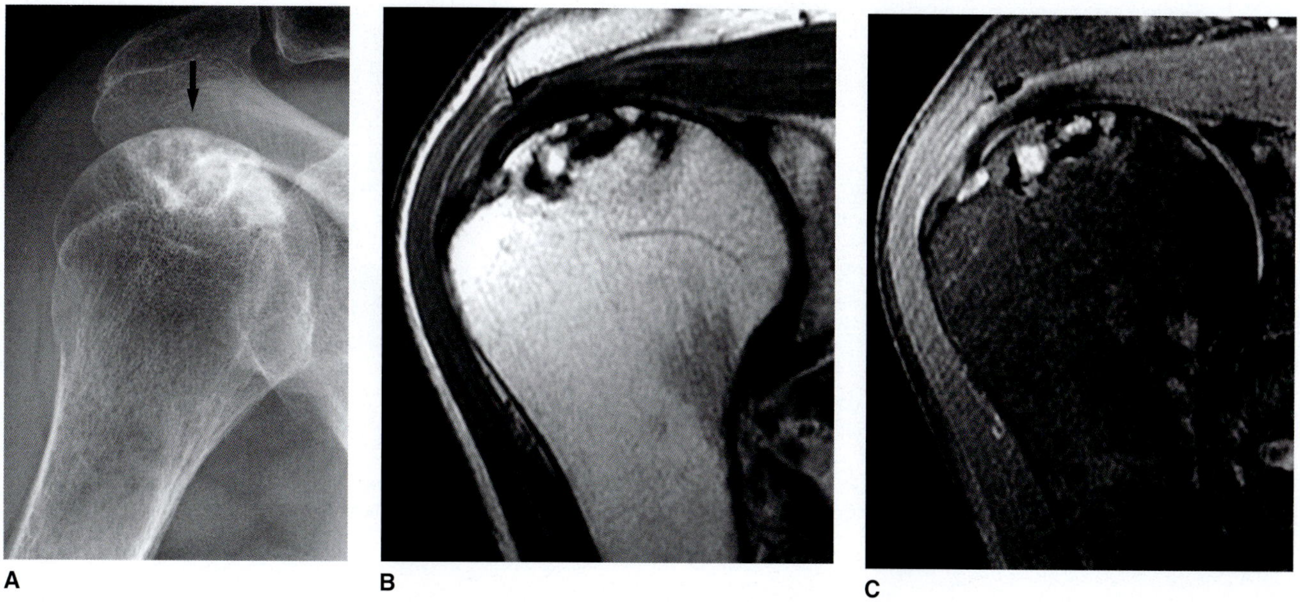

Figure 13.16 ■ **MRI of osteonecrosis of the humeral head.** A 58-year-old woman presented with right shoulder pain for several weeks after an apparent dislocation in the glenohumeral joint, which was spontaneously reduced. She also gives a history of SLE treated with corticosteroids. Radiograph of the right shoulder **(A)** shows a classic appearance of osteonecrosis of the humeral head (*arrow*), a diagnosis that was confirmed on coronal proton density–weighted **(B)** and coronal proton density–weighted **(C)** fat-suppressed MR images. Osteonecrosis was more likely secondary to SLE and the treatment with steroids rather than due to traumatic event.

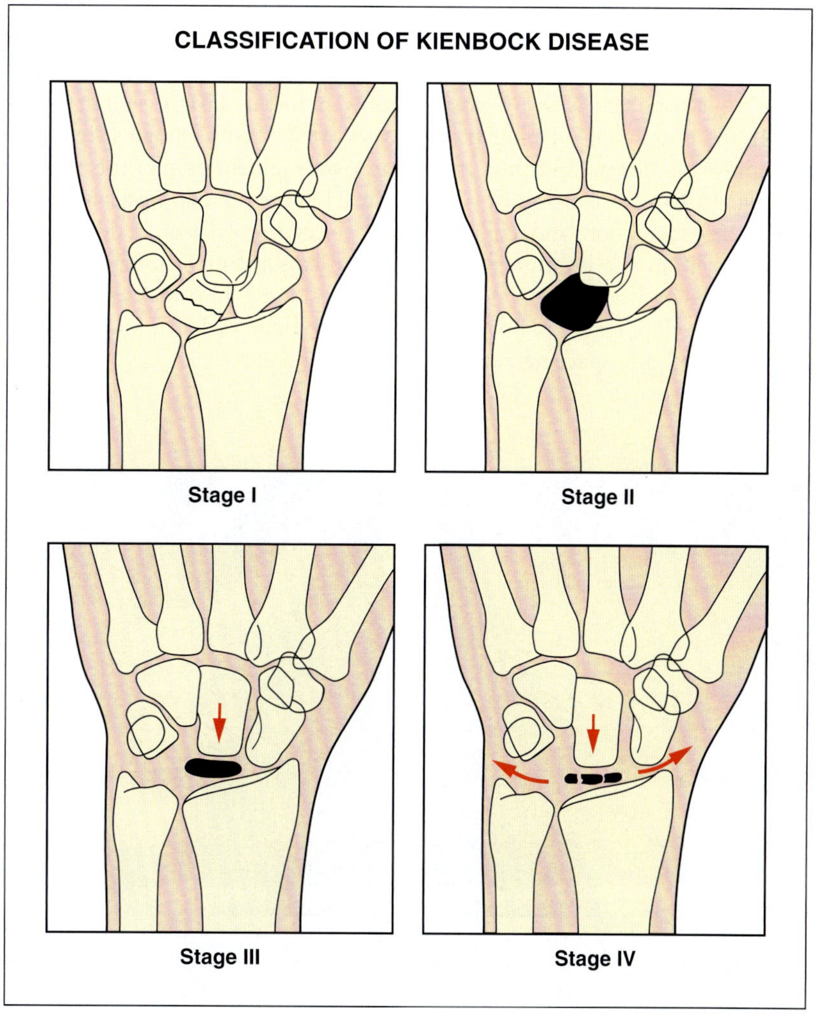

Figure 13.17 ■ **The four stages of Kienböck disease.** Proximal migration of the capitate is seen in stages III and IV (*vertical arrows*). Lateral and medial migration of the fractured fragments of the lunate is seen in stage IV (*curved horizontal arrows*). (Modified from Gelberman RH, Szabo RM. Kienböck's disease. *Orthop Clin North Am.* 1984;15:355–367.)

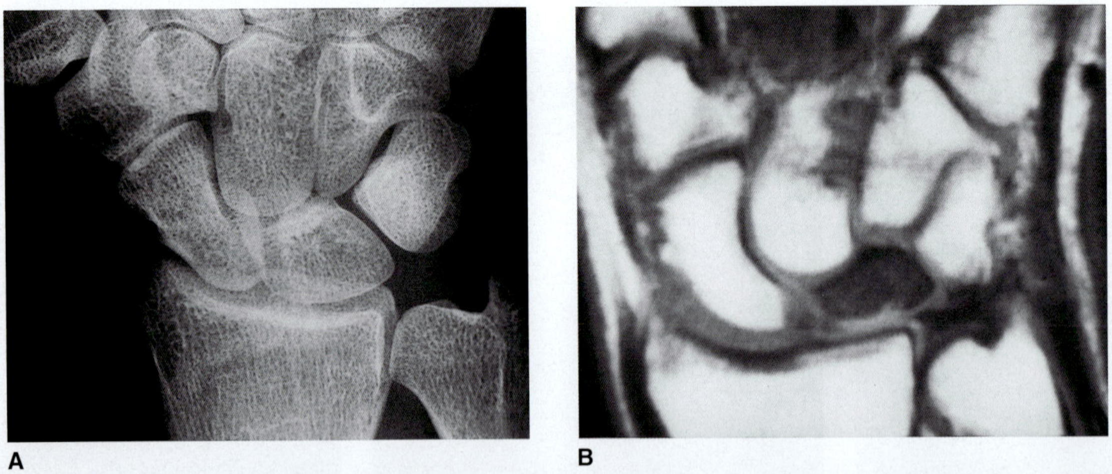

Figure 13.18 ■ **MRI of Kienböck disease.** A 35-year-old man presented with wrist pain of 2 months duration. **A:** Conventional dorsovolar radiograph of the left wrist is normal. **B:** Coronal T1-weighted MR image shows low signal intensity of the lunate consistent with osteonecrosis.

normal, and only CT or MRI may detect a subtle linear fracture. Skeletal scintigraphy may show an increased uptake of a radiopharmaceutical tracer by the lunate. MRI invariably demonstrates the abnormality, displaying decreased signal intensity of lunate on T1-weighted sequences (Fig. 13.18). As the condition progresses (stage II), the conventional radiographs show increased density of the lunate accompanied by some degree of flattening on the radial side of this bone (Fig. 13.19). The radionuclide bone scan is always positive in this stage. In stage III, the radiographs demonstrate marked decrease in the height of the lunate and proximal migration of the capitate (Fig. 13.20). Necrotic and cystic changes may lead to further fragmentation and collapse (Fig. 13.21). Scapholunate dissociation is a prominent feature of this stage. Stage IV is marked by almost complete disintegration of the lunate and the development of radiocarpal osteoarthritis with typical changes of joint space narrowing, osteophyte formation, subchondral sclerosis, and degenerative cysts (Fig. 13.22).

Merely diagnosing Kienböck disease is not sufficient from the orthopedic point of view; rather, it is essential for the radiologist to demonstrate the integrity of the lunate. The reason for this is that at early stage of the disease, in the absence of fracture or fragmentation, a revascularization procedure aimed at restoring circulation to this bone may prevent further progression of the necrotic process and eventual collapse of the lunate (Fig. 13.23). In the event of a fracture or fragmentation of the lunate, which is best diagnosed on CT, alternative to revascularization procedures—such as silastic arthroplasty or, in the absence of a collapse deformity, ulnar lengthening or radial shortening—would then have to be considered. In some cases, the latter procedures restoring neutral ulnar variance may allow spontaneous healing of a lunate fracture.

(Continued on page 460)

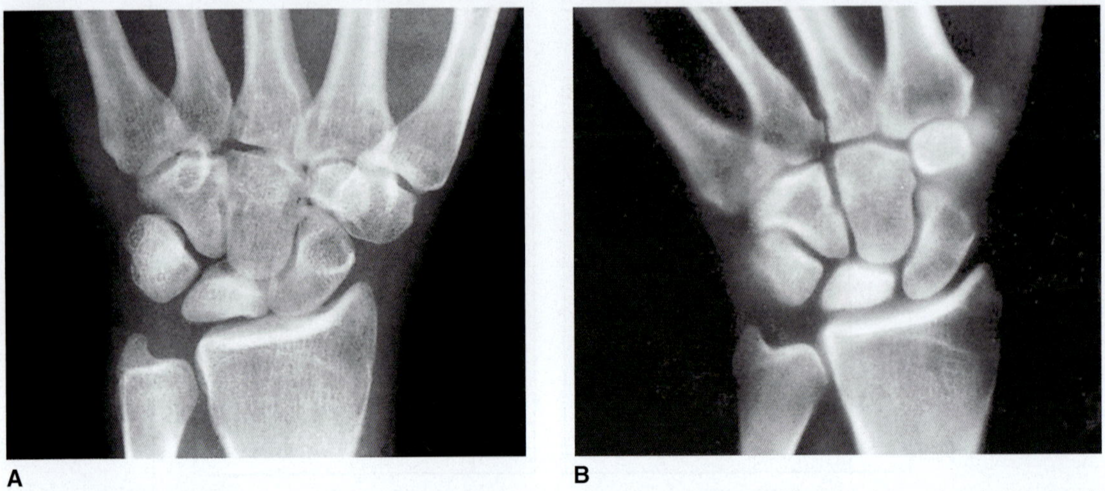

Figure 13.19 ■ **Kienböck disease.** Dorsovolar radiograph **(A)** and conventional tomogram **(B)** of the right wrist of a 32-year-old woman show the dense, flattened appearance of the lunate characteristic for this abnormality. Note the presence of negative ulnar variance, a possible predisposing factor in this condition.

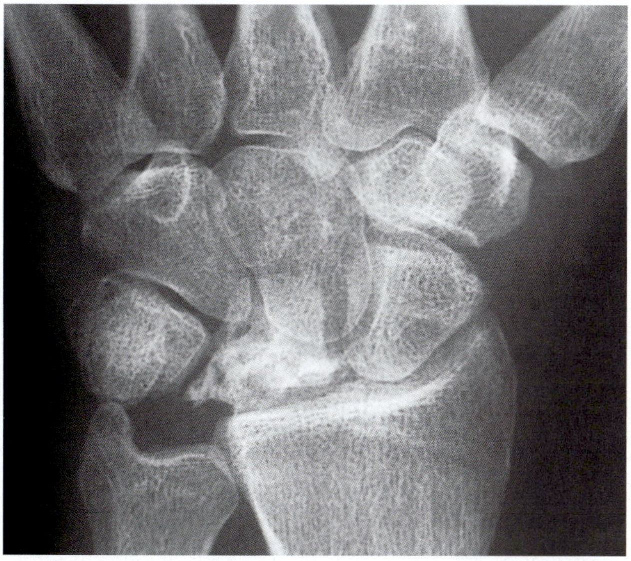

Figure 13.20 ■ **Kienböck disease.** A 21-year-old man presented with long-standing wrist pain. Dorsovolar radiograph of the left wrist show stage III of Kienböck disease. Note the collapse of osteonecrotic lunate and proximal migration of the capitate.

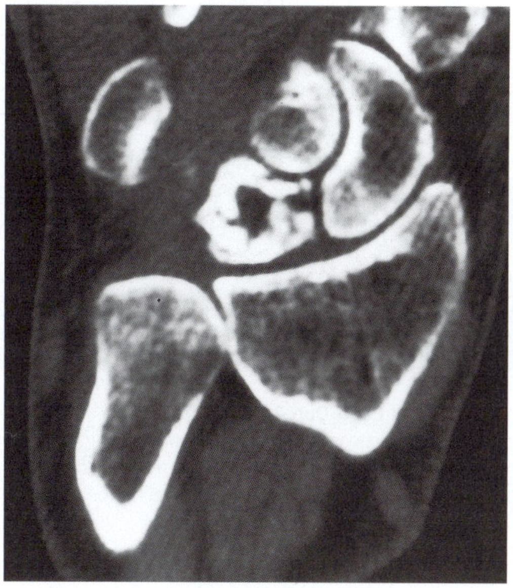

Figure 13.21 ■ **CT of Kienböck disease.** Coronal reformatted CT image of the right wrist reveals cystic changes of the osteonecrotic lunate associated with a pathologic fracture.

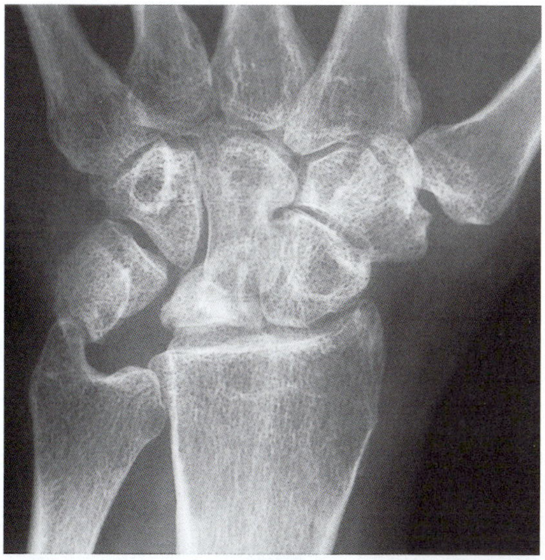

Figure 13.22 ■ **Kienböck disease.** Stage IV is marked by fragmentation and collapse of the lunate, proximal migration of the capitate, rotary subluxation of the scaphoid, and osteoarthritis of the radiocarpal joint.

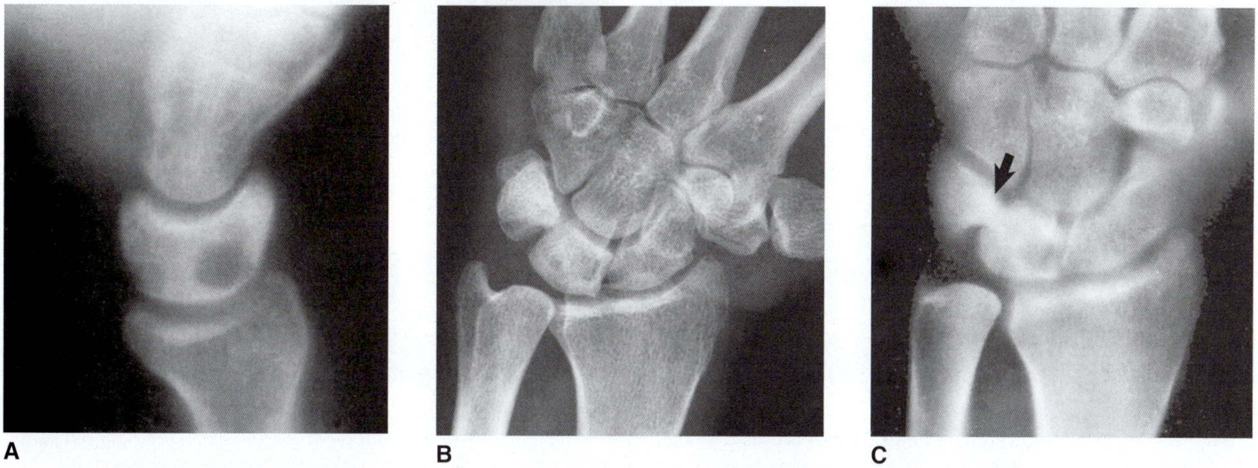

Figure 13.23 ■ **Kienböck disease. A:** Lateral conventional tomogram of the left wrist shows the dense appearance of the lunate characteristic of osteonecrosis; there is also evidence of cystic degeneration, but no apparent fracture is present. After triquetrolunate arthrodesis, the dorsovolar radiograph of the wrist in radial deviation **(B)** and a trispiral tomogram **(C)** demonstrate the vascular bone flap (*arrow*) bridging the triquetrum and lunate.

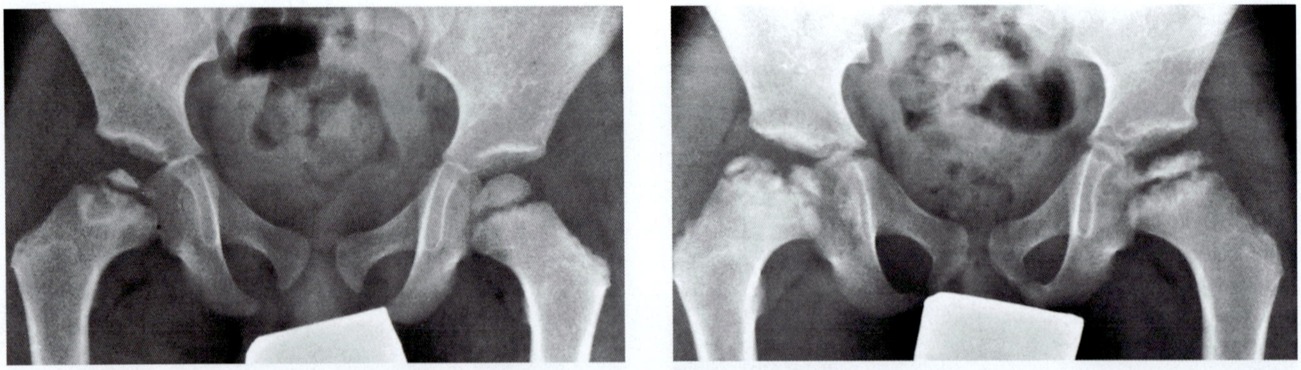

A B

Figure 13.24 ■ Legg-Calvé-Perthes disease. A 5-year-old boy presented with pain in the right hip for several months. **A:** Anteroposterior radiograph of the pelvis and hips show advanced stage of this condition affecting the right hip, where osteonecrosis and collapse of the capital femoral epiphysis are apparent, as are extensive changes in the metaphysis. Note lateral subluxation in the hip joint. The left hip is normal. **B:** Three years later, the left hip also became affected. Note progression of osteonecrotic changes in the right femoral epiphysis.

LEGG-CALVÉ-PERTHES DISEASE

Clinical Features

This condition, also known as *coxa plana*, represents the osteonecrosis (ischemic necrosis) of the proximal epiphysis of the femur. Recent genetic studies suggest that beta fibrinogen gene *G-455-A* polymorphism is a risk factor for this disease. The anomaly occurs five times more often in boys than in girls, usually between the ages of 4 and 8 years. Its appearance at an early age is usually associated with a better prognosis. Either hip can be affected, and bilateral involvement, which is successive rather than simultaneous, is seen in ~10% of cases. The clinical symptoms consist of pain, limping, and limitation of motion. Not infrequently, the pain is localized not to the involved hip but to the ipsilateral knee. It is a self-limiting disorder that eventually heals, but because of the progressive deformity of the femoral head and neck, it often leads to precocious osteoarthritis of the hip joint. The cause of this anomaly has been the subject of debates. Some investigators consider it a type of idiopathic osteonecrosis, but trauma or repeated microtrauma may play a role in compromising the circulation of blood to the femoral capital epiphysis. Trueta has suggested that the blood supply to the femoral head is deficient between the ages of 4 and 8 years and that this might be a factor in the development of the condition.

Imaging Features

Imaging is essential for diagnosing Legg-Calvé-Perthes disease and for identifying its prognostic signs. Conventional radiography is adequate for evaluating most of the features of the disease (Fig. 13.24), whereas arthrography (Fig. 13.25) or MRI (see Fig. 13.29) helps in the assessment of the

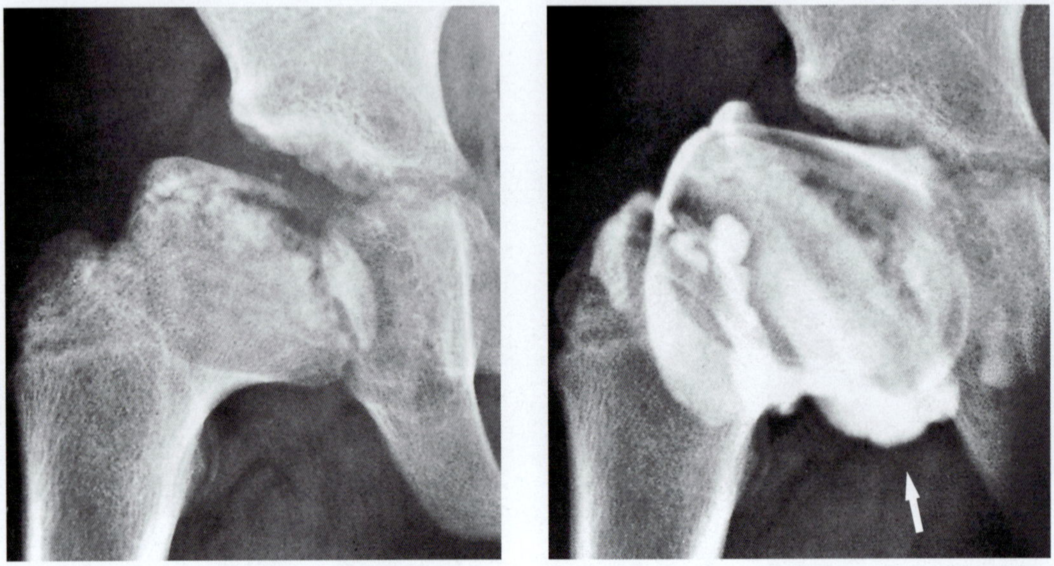

A B

Figure 13.25 ■ Arthrography of Legg-Calvé-Perthes disease. A 6-year-old boy presented with progressive pain in the right hip joint and a limp for the previous 8 months. **A:** Anteroposterior radiograph shows a dense, flattened, and deformed femoral epiphysis, with subchondral collapse and fragmentation, diffuse metaphyseal changes, broadening of the femoral neck, and lateral subluxation. **B:** Contrast arthrogram demonstrates flattening of the articular cartilage at the lateral aspect of the femoral head and a relatively smooth contour of the cartilage at the anteromedial aspect. The pulling of the contrast medially (*arrow*) indicates lateral subluxation.

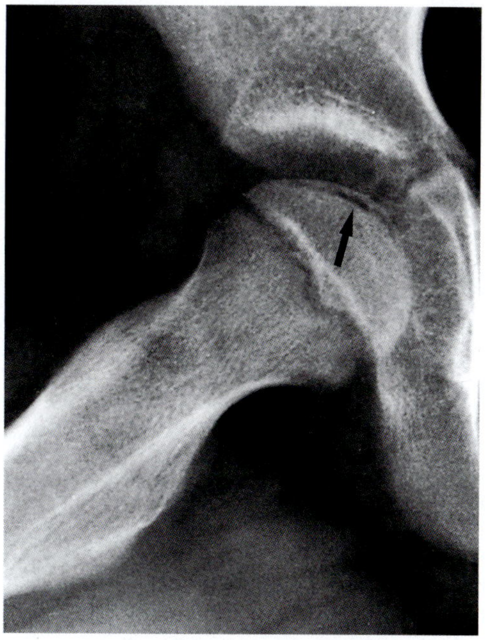

Figure 13.26 ■ Legg-Calvé-Perthes disease. Frog-lateral view of the right hip of a 7-year-old girl shows the crescent sign (*arrow*), one of the earliest radiographic features of osteonecrosis.

acetabular congruity, the thickness of the articular cartilage, and the degree of subluxation. The earliest indication of this condition is demonstrated on radionuclide bone scan by a decreased uptake of the radiopharmaceutical tracer in the hips caused by a deficient blood supply. However, with progression of the disease, an increased uptake is seen, which reflects reparative processes. The earliest radiographic sign is periarticular osteoporosis and periarticular soft tissue swelling, with distortion of the pericapsular and iliopsoas fat planes. There may be also a discrepancy in the size of the ossification centers of the capital epiphyses. Later, lateral displacement of the affected ossification center produces widening of the medial aspect of the joint. The presence of the crescent sign (which at times may be detected only on the frog-lateral projection of the hip) (Fig. 13.26), or of radiolucent fissures in the epiphysis, indicates progression of the disease. At a more advanced stage, flattening and sclerosis of the capital femoral epiphysis become apparent and are associated with an increased density of the femoral head secondary to necrosis of the bone, microfractures, and reparative changes known as *creeping substitution*. A vacuum phenomenon may occasionally be seen, caused by nitrogen gas released into the fissures in the capital epiphysis. Cystic changes may also be encountered in the metaphyseal segment. Later, there may be broadening of the femoral neck. Throughout the course of the disease, the joint space is remarkably well preserved because the articular cartilage is not affected. Only in the end stage of Legg-Calvé-Perthes disease, when secondary osteoarthritis develops, does the joint become compromised as in primary degenerative joint disease.

One of the radiographic features of advanced Legg-Calvé-Perthes disease is the so-called *sagging rope sign*. It consists of a thin, curved, U-shaped opaque line in the proximal femoral metaphysis, extending laterally from the inferior border of the femoral neck (Fig. 13.27).

The Moss technique is used to determine the degree of deformity of the femoral head. This consists of overlaying the anteroposterior radiograph of the hip with a template having concentric circles spaced 2 mm apart. If the concentricity of the femoral head deviates by more than two of the 2-mm circles, then the result is rated "poor," deviation equal to one 2-mm circle is "fair," and no deviation is rated "good." Lateral subluxation can be measured by means of the C–E angle of Wiberg (Fig. 13.28). It must be stressed that both measurements do not correlate well with development of secondary osteoarthritis, the main complication of Legg-Calvé-Perthes disease.

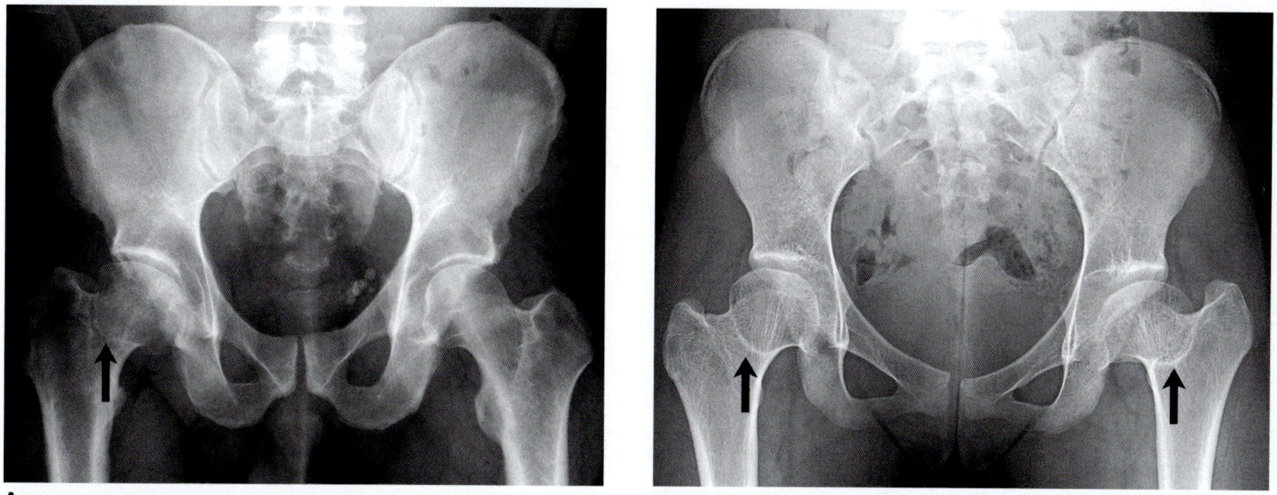

A B

Figure 13.27 ■ Legg-Calvé-Perthes disease. A: Anteroposterior radiograph of the pelvis of a 30-year-old man shows enlargement of the right femoral head (*coxa magna*), and flattening of the articular aspect with deformity, consistent with osteonecrosis. The *arrow* points to the sagging rope sign. **B:** Anteroposterior radiograph of the pelvis of a 17-year-old girl shows bilateral osteonecrosis of femoral head in late reparative stage. Note bilateral sagging rope sign (*arrows*), characteristic for this condition.

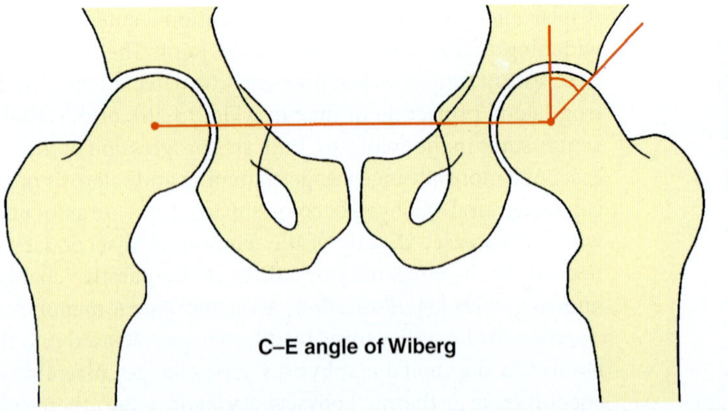

Age (years)	Lowest Normal Value of C–E Angle
5–8	19°
9–12	12°–25°
13–20	26°–30°

Figure 13.28 ■ Angle of Wiberg. The C–E angle of Wiberg is helpful in evaluating the development of the acetabulum and its relation to the femoral head. A baseline is projected, connecting the centers of the femoral heads. The C–E angle is formed by two lines originating in the center of the femoral head, one drawn perpendicular to the baseline into the acetabulum and the other connecting the center of the femoral head with the superior acetabular lip. Values below the lowest normal value given for each age group indicate hip dysplasia.

Several investigators have recently stressed the applicability of MRI for early detection of Legg-Calvé-Perthes disease and for evaluation of cartilaginous and synovial changes. This technique also has proved valuable for determination of the cartilaginous shape of the femoral head. MRI allows preoperative and postoperative assessment of containment of the femoral head and enables its medial aspect to be visualized. The advantage of MRI over arthrography is noninvasiveness, the ability to obtain images in several imaging planes (i.e., axial, coronal, and sagittal), and lack of exposure to the side effects of radiation and injection of intra-articular contrast (Fig. 13.29).

Classification

Several classification systems and prognostic indicators have been developed for the evaluation of Legg-Calvé-Perthes disease. Waldenström proposed a three-stage system based on the progression of the osteonecrotic process. The first stage is marked by changes in the blood supply to the femoral epiphysis, with secondary alteration in the shape and density of the femoral head. In the second stage, revascularization takes place, and sclerotic bone is replaced by new bone (creeping substitution). The third stage represents a healing phase of the disease in which reconstruction of the femoral epiphysis may result either in congruency of the joint or in incongruence because of deformity of the femoral head (coxa magna), with a predisposition to degenerative changes.

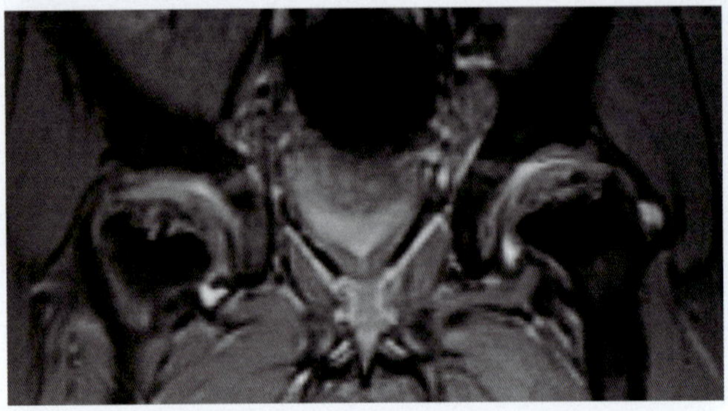

Figure 13.29 ■ MRI of Legg-Calvé-Perthes disease. Coronal gradient-recalled echo (GRE) MR image demonstrates osteonecrosis of both femoral heads with flattening and fragmentation of the proximal femoral epiphyses and irregular growth plates.

The Catterall classification, which has better prognostic value, divides the anomaly into four groups based on radiographic findings:

Group 1: The anterior portion of the epiphysis is involved; there is no evidence of subarticular collapse or fragmentation of the femoral head (see Fig. 13.26). The prognosis is good, and patients do well even without treatment, particularly those younger than 8 years of age.

Group 2: The anterior portion of the epiphysis is more severely affected, but the medial and lateral segments are still preserved (Fig. 13.30). Small cystic changes may be seen

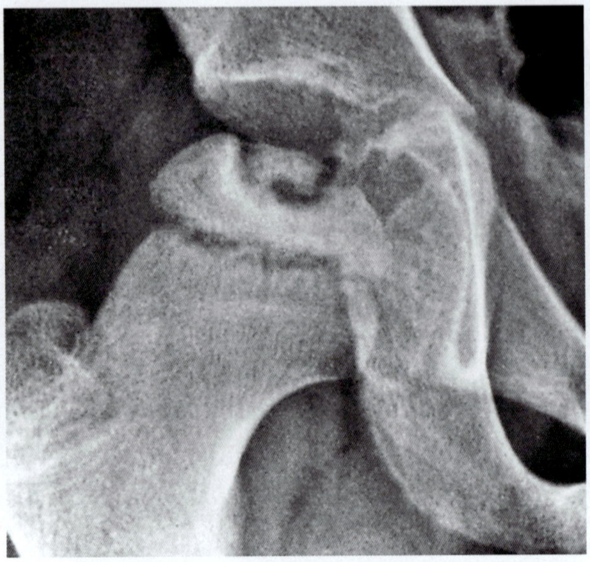

Figure 13.30 ■ Legg-Calvé-Perthes disease. Anteroposterior radiograph of the right hip of a 9-year-old boy shows a central defect in the femoral epiphysis, with preservation of the lateral and medial buttresses (Catterall group 2).

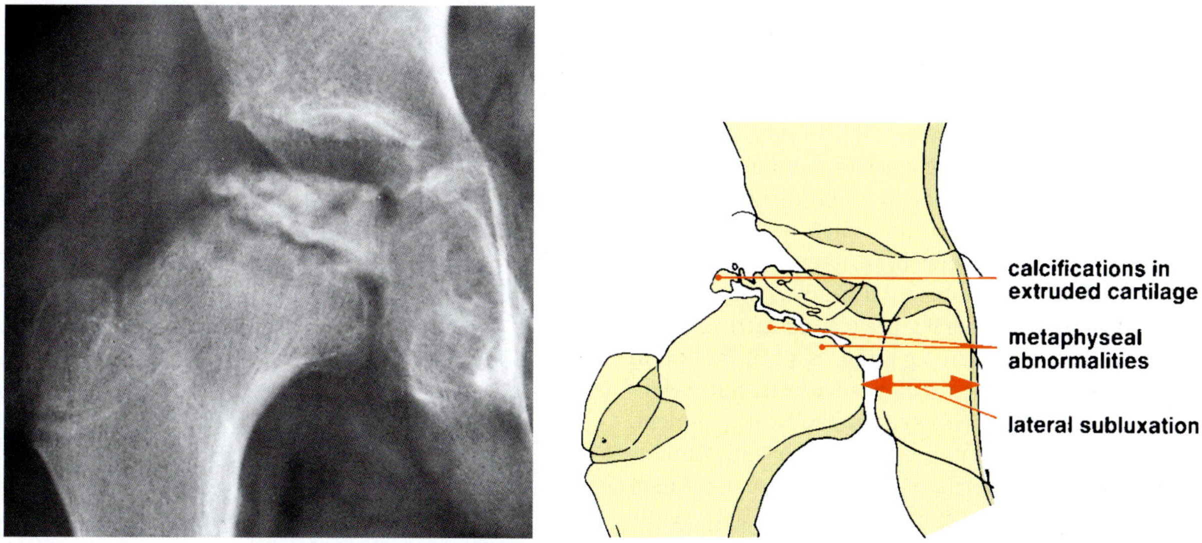

Figure 13.31 ■ **Legg-Calvé-Perthes disease.** Anteroposterior radiograph of the right hip of an 8-year-old girl with advanced disease (Catterall group 4) shows increased density and fragmentation of the entire femoral epiphysis. "Head-at-risk" signs are apparent in the metaphyseal changes and the lateral subluxation. Calcifications lateral to the epiphysis represent extruded cartilage and indicate pressure on the head from the lateral edge of the acetabulum.

in the metaphysis. The prognosis is worse than of patients in group 1, but healing may occur, particularly in children younger than 5 years of age.

Group 3: The entire epiphysis appears dense, yielding a "head-within-a-head" phenomenon. The changes are more generalized, and the femoral neck becomes widened (see Fig. 13.25A). The prognosis is poor, and more than 70% of patients require surgical intervention.

Group 4: There is marked flattening and "mushrooming" of the femoral head, eventually leading to its complete collapse; the metaphyseal changes are extensive (Fig. 13.31). The prognosis is much worse than in the previous groups.

Subsequently, Catterall improved this classification by introducing four "head-at-risk" signs that signify a poor prognosis; these features can be demonstrated on the anteroposterior radiographs of the hip joint:

1. Gage sign—a radiolucent, V-shaped osteoporotic segment in the lateral portion of the femoral head (Fig. 13.32).
2. Calcification lateral to the epiphysis, representing extruded cartilage and indicating pressure on the femoral head from the lateral edge of the acetabulum (see Fig. 13.24).
3. Lateral subluxation of the femoral head (see Figs. 13.25 and 13.31).
4. Horizontal inclination of the growth plate, indicating physeal growth closure.
5. Recently, Murphy and Marsh added a fifth sign to this group of indicators—diffuse metaphyseal changes (see Fig. 13.24).

Patients in any of the four groups who have two or more "head-at-risk" signs have a significantly worsened prognosis. Moreover, the prognosis is poor when disease is in a late stage at the time of diagnosis and when the patient is older than 6 years of age.

Differential Diagnosis

The differential diagnosis of this condition should include other causes of osteonecrosis, for example, Gaucher disease and sickle cell anemia. Patients with congenital hypothyroidism may present with fragmentation of the femoral head, which however is not the result of osteonecrosis but the result of femoral epiphyses ossifying from numerous ossification centers.

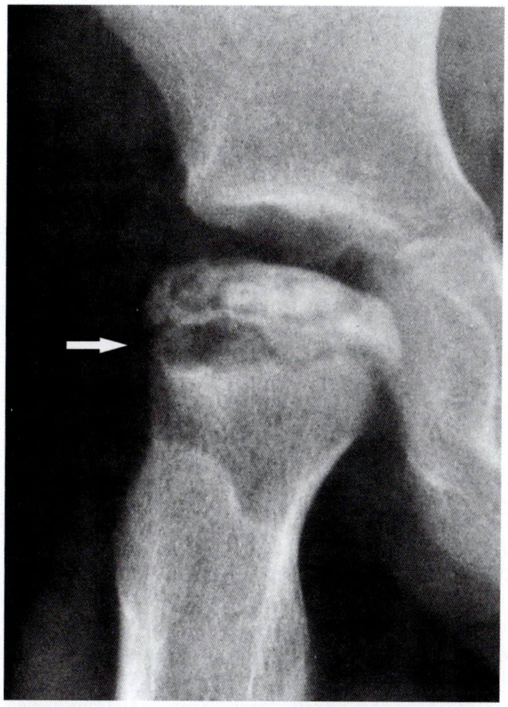

Figure 13.32 ■ **Legg-Calvé-Perthes disease.** A V-shape radiolucent defect in the lateral aspect of the physis, known as a Gage sign (*arrow*), indicating a "head-at-risk" is demonstrated in this 7-year-old girl.

Treatment

The therapy is individualized on the basis of the clinical and imaging findings, including the age of onset, the range of motion in the hip joint, the extent of femoral head abnormalities, and the present or absence of femoral deformity and lateral subluxation. Although some orthopedic surgeons have suggested eliminating weight bearing to prevent deformity of the femoral head, prevention requires measures that maintain the femoral head within the acetabulum (containment), thereby preventing extrusion and subluxation, as well as obtaining a full range of motion in the hip joint. In this respect, Salter advocated full weight bearing together with containment methods of treatment. To minimize synovitis and its sequelae of pain and stiffness, a combination of non–weight bearing, traction, treatment with nonsteroidal anti-inflammatory agents, and gentle range-of-motion exercises is used to enhance molding of the femoral head by acetabulum. The surgical treatment consists of femoral (varus derotational) or pelvic (innominate bone) osteotomy, aimed at covering the femoral head with the acetabulum.

SUGGESTED READINGS

Adelberg JS, Smith GH. Corticosteroid-induced avascular necrosis of the talus. *J Foot Surg.* 1991;30:66–69.

Allard JC, Porter G, Ryerson RW. Occult posttraumatic avascular necrosis of hip revealed by MRI. *Magn Reson Imaging.* 1992;10:155–159.

Assouline-Dayan Y, Chang C, Greenspan A, et al. Pathogenesis and natural history of osteonecrosis. *Semin Arthritis Rheum.* 2002;32:94–124.

Athanasian G, Wickiewicz T. Osteonecrosis of the femoral condyle after arthroscopic reconstruction of a cruciate ligament. *J Bone Joint Surg Am.* 1995;77A:1418–1421.

Beltran J, Burk JM, Herman LJ, et al. Avascular necrosis of the femoral head: early MRI detection and radiological correlation. *Magn Reson Imaging.* 1987;5:531–542.

Beltran J, Herman LJ, Burk JM, et al. Femoral head avascular necrosis: MR imaging with clinical-pathologic and radionuclide correlation. *Radiology.* 1988;166:215–220.

Beltran J, Knight CT, Zuelzer WA, et al. Core decompression for avascular necrosis of the femoral head: correlation between long-term results and preoperative MR staging. *Radiology.* 1990;175:533–536.

Castro FP Jr, Barrack RL. Core decompression and conservative treatment for avascular necrosis of the femoral head: a meta-analysis. *Am J Orthop.* 2000;29:187–194.

Chan WP, Liu Y-J, Huang G-S, et al. MRI of joint fluid in femoral head osteonecrosis. *Skeletal Radiol.* 2002;31:624–630.

Chang CC, Greenspan A, Gershwin ME. Osteonecrosis: current perspectives on pathogenesis and treatment. *Semin Arthritis Rheum.* 1993;23:47–69.

Coleman BG, Kressel HY, Dalinka MK, et al. Radiographically negative avascular necrosis: detection with MR imaging. *Radiology.* 1988;168: 525–528.

Colwell CW, Robinson C. Osteonecrosis of the femoral head in patients with inflammatory arthritis on asthma receiving corticosteroid therapy. *Orthopedics.* 1996;19:941–946.

Cushner FO, Friedman RJ. Osteonecrosis of the femoral head. *Orthop Rev.* 1988;17:29–34.

Davidson JK. Dysbaric disorders. Aseptic bone necrosis in tunnel workers and divers. *Clin Rheumatol.* 1989;3:1–23.

Davidson JK, Briggs JD. Osteonecrosis and fracture following renal transplantation. *Clin Radiol.* 1985;36:27–35.

Drery P, Sartoris DJ. Osteonecrosis in the foot. *J Foot Surg.* 1991;30:477–483.

Dubois E, Cosen L. Avascular necrosis associated with lupus erythematosus. *JAMA.* 1960;174:966–971.

Ferlic OC, Morin P. Idiopathic avascular necrosis of the scaphoid—Preiser's disease? *J Hand Surg.* 1989;14:13–16.

Ficat RP. Idiopathic bone necrosis of the femoral head: early diagnosis and treatment. *J Bone Joint Surg Br.* 1985;67-B:3–9.

Ficat RP. Treatment of avascular necrosis of the femoral head. In: Hungerford DS, ed. *The Hip: Proceedings of the Eleventh Open Meeting of the Hip Society.* St. Louis, MO: CV Mosby, 1983:279–295.

Ficat RP, Arlet J. Ischemia and necrosis of bone. In: Hungerford DS, ed. *Ischemia and Necrosis of Bone.* Baltimore, MD: Williams & Wilkins, 1980:196.

Ficat RP, Arlet J. Treatment of bone ischemia and necrosis. In: Hungerford DS, ed. *Ischemia and Necrosis of Bone.* Baltimore, MD: Williams & Wilkins, 1980:171–182.

French D, Hamilton LH, Mattano LA Jr, et al. A PAI-1 (SERPINE 1) polymorphism predicts osteonecrosis in children with acute lymphoblastic leukemia: a report from the Children's Oncology Group. *Blood.* 2008;111:4496–4499.

Frostick SP, Wallace WP. Osteonecrosis of the humeral head. *Clin Rheumatol.* 1989;3:651–657.

Gelberman RH, Szabo RM. Kienböck's disease. *Orthop Clin North Am.* 1984;15:355–367).

Glueck CJ, Fontaine RN, Gruppo R, et al. The plasminogen activator inhibitor-1 gene, hypofibrinolysis, and osteonecrosis. *Clin Orthop Relat Res.* 1999;366:133–146.

Haajanen J, Saarinen O, Laasonen L, et al. Steroid treatment and aseptic necrosis of the femoral head in renal transplant recipients. *Transplant Proc.* 1984;16:1316–1319.

Hungerford DS, Lennox DW. The importance of increased intraosseous pressure in the development of osteonecrosis of the femoral head: implications for treatment. *Orthop Clin North Am.* 1985;16:635–654.

Hungerford DS, Zizic TM. Alcoholism associated ischemic necrosis of the femoral head. *Clin Orthop.* 1978;130:144–153.

Hungerford DS. Response: the role of core decompression in treatment of ischemic necrosis of the femoral head. *Arthritis Rheum.* 1989;32: 801–806.

Imhof H, Breitenseher M, Trattnig S, et al. Imaging of avascular necrosis of bone. *Eur Radiol.* 1997;7:180–186.

Iwasaki K, Hirano T, Sagara K, et al. Idiopathic necrosis of the femoral epiphyseal nucleus in rats. *Clin Orthop.* 1992;277:31–40.

Jergesen HE, Khan AS. The natural history of untreated asymptomatic hips in patients who have nontraumatic osteonecrosis. *J Bone J Surg [Am].* 1997;79A:359–363.

Jones JP, Engleman GP, Najarian JS. Systemic fat embolism after renal transplantation and treatment with corticosteroids. *N Engl J Med.* 1965;273:1453–1458.

Kay NRM, Park WM, Bark MB. The relationship between pregnancy and femoral head necrosis. *Br J Radiol.* 1972;45:828–831.

Khanna A, Yoon T, Mont M, et al. Femoral head osteonecrosis: detection and grading by using a rapid MR imaging protocol. *Radiology.* 2000;217:188–192.

Koo K-H, Lee JS, Lee YJ, et al. Endothelial nitric oxide synthase gene polymorphism in patients with nontraumatic femoral head osteonecrosis. *J Orthop Res.* 2006;24:1722–1728.

Koo K-H, Ahn I-O, Kim R, et al. Bone marrow edema and associated pain in early stage osteonecrosis of the femoral head: prospective study with serial MR images. *Radiology.* 1999;213:715–722.

Lafforgue P, Dahan P, Chagnaud C, et al. Early-stage avascular necrosis of the femoral head: MR imaging for prognosis in 31 cases with at least 2 years of follow-up. *Radiology.* 1993;187:199–204.

Lang P, Jergesen HE, Moseley ME, et al. Avascular necrosis of the femoral head: high-field-strength MR imaging with histologic correlation. *Radiology.* 1988;169:517–524.

Langevitz P, Baskila O. Osteonecrosis in patients receiving dialysis: report of two cases and review of the literature. *J Rheumatol.* 1990;17:402–406.

Lotke PA, Geker ML. Osteonecrosis of the knee. *J Bone Joint Surg Am.* 1988;70A:470–473.

Mankin HJ. Nontraumatic necrosis of bone (osteonecrosis). *N Engl J Med.* 1992;326:1473–1479.

Marcus NO, Enneking WF. The silent hip in idiopathic aseptic necrosis. *J Bone Joint Surg Am.* 1973;55A:1351–1366.

Markisz JA, Knowles RJR, Altchek DW, et al. Segmental patterns of avascular necrosis of the femoral heads: early detection with MR imaging. *Radiology.* 1987;162:717–720.

McDougall IR, Rieser RP. Scintigraphic techniques in musculoskeletal trauma. *Radiol Clin North Am.* 1989;27:1003–1011.

Mirzai A, Chang CC, Greenspan A, et al. The pathogenesis of osteonecrosis and the relationship to corticosteroids. *J Asthma.* 1999;36:77–95.

Mirzai R, Chang CC, Greenspan A, et al. Avascular necrosis. *Comp Ther.* 1998;24:251–255.

Mitchell DG, Joseph PM, Fallon M, et al. Chemical-shift MR imaging of the femoral head: an in vitro study of normal hips and hips with avascular necrosis. *AJR Am J Roentgenol.* 1987;148:1159–1164.

Mitchell DG, Kressel HY, Arger PH, et al. Avascular necrosis of the femoral head: morphologic assessment by MR imaging, with CT correlation. *Radiology.* 1986;161:739–742.

Mitchell DG, Kundel JL, Steinberg MF. Avascular necrosis of the hip: comparison of MR, CT and scintigraphy. *AJR Am J Roentgenol.* 1986;147:67–71.

Mitchell DG, Rao VM, Dalinka MK, et al. Femoral head avascular necrosis: correlation of MR imaging, radiographic staging, radionuclide imaging, and clinical findings. *Radiology.* 1987;162:709–715.

Montella BJ, Nunley JA, Urbaniak JR. Osteonecrosis of the femoral head associated with pregnancy. A preliminary report. *J Bone Joint Surg Am.* 1999;81-A:790–798.

Moran MC. Osteonecrosis of the hip in sickle cell hemoglobinopathy. *Am J Orthop.* 1995;24:18–24.

Norman A, Bullough P. The radiolucent crescent line—an early diagnostic sign of avascular necrosis of the femoral head. *Bull Hosp Joint Dis.* 1963;24:99–104.

Ohzono K, Saito M. The fate of nontraumatic avascular necrosis of the femoral head: a radiologic classification to formulate prognosis. *Clin Orthop.* 1992;277:73–78.

Ono K, Tohjima T. Risk factors of avascular necrosis of the femoral head in patients with systemic lupus erythematosus under high-dose corticosteroid therapy. *Clin Orthop.* 1992;277:89–97.

Pappas JN. The musculoskeletal crescent sign. *Radiology.* 2000;217:213–214.

Patton RW, Evans DIK. Silent avascular necrosis of the femoral head in haemophilia. *J Bone Joint Surg Br.* 1988;70-B:737–739.

Seiler JG III, Christie MJ, Homra L. Correlation of the findings of magnetic resonance imaging with those of bone biopsy in patients who have stage I or II ischemic necrosis of the femoral head. *J Bone Joint Surg Am.* 1989;71A:28–32.

Shimizu K, Moriya H, Akita T, et al. Prediction of collapse with magnetic resonance imaging of avascular necrosis of the femoral head. *J Bone Joint Surg Am.* 1994;76A:215–223.

Shinoda S, Hasegawa Y, Kawasaki S, et al. Magnetic resonance imaging of osteonecrosis in divers: comparison with plain radiographs. *Skeletal Radiol.* 1997;26:354–359.

Smith DW. Is avascular necrosis of the femoral head the result of inhibition of angiogenesis? *Med Hypotheses.* 1997;49:497–500.

Sonoda K, Motomura G, Kawanami S, et al. Degeneration of articular cartilage in osteonecrosis of the femoral head begins at the necrotic region after collapse: a preliminary study using T1 rho MRI. *Skeletal Radiol.* 2017;46:463–467.

Stevens K, Tao C, Lee S-V, et al. Subchondral fractures in osteonecrosis of the femoral head: comparison of radiography, CT, and MR imaging. *AJR Am J Roentgenol.* 2003;180:363–368.

Suehiro M, Hirano T, Mihara K, et al. Etiologic factors in femoral head osteonecrosis in growing rats. *J Orthop Sci.* 2000;5:52–56.

Sugimoto H, Okubu RS, Ohsawa T. Chemical shift and the double-line sign in MRI of early femoral avascular necrosis. *J Comput Assist Tomogr.* 1992;16:727–730.

Szabo RM, Greenspan A. Diagnosis and clinical findings of Keinböck's disease. *Hand Clin.* 1993;9:399–407.

Takatori Y, Kokubo T, Ninomiya S, et al. Avascular necrosis of the femoral head: natural history and magnetic resonance imaging. *J Bone Joint Surg Br.* 1993;75B:217–221.

Thickman D, Axel L, Kressel HY, et al. Magnetic resonance imaging of avascular necrosis of the femoral head. *Skeletal Radiol.* 1986;15: 133–140.

Thometz JG, Lamdan R. Osteonecrosis of the femoral head after intramedullary nailing of a fracture of the femoral shaft in an adolescent. *J Bone Joint Surg Am.* 1995;77A:1423–1426.

Trumble TE. Avascular necrosis after scaphoid fracture: a correlation of magnetic resonance imaging and histology. *J Hand Surg [Am].* 1990;15: 557–564.

Urbaniak JR, Coogan PG, Gunneson EB, et al. Treatment of osteonecrosis of the femoral head with free vascularized fibular grafting. A long-term follow-up study of one hundred and three hips. *J Bone Joint Surg Am.* 1995;77-A:681–694.

Vande Berg B, Malghem J, Labaisse MA, et al. Avascular necrosis of the hip: comparison of contrast-enhanced and nonenhanced MR imaging with histologic correlation. *Radiology.* 1992;182:445–450.

Williams ES, Khreisat S, Ell PJ, et al. Bone imaging and skeletal radiology in dysbaric osteonecrosis. *Clin Radiol.* 1987;38:589–592.

Zurlo JV. The double-line sign. *Radiology.* 1999;212:541–542.

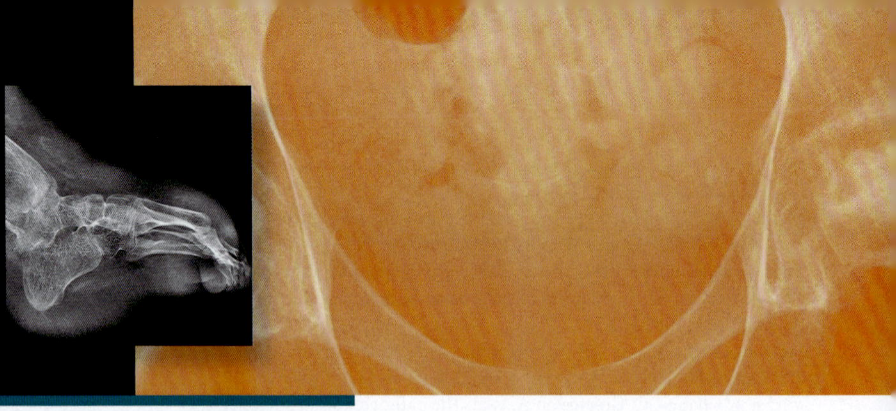

CHAPTER 14

Miscellaneous Conditions

BLOUNT DISEASE (CONGENITAL TIBIA VARA)

This anomaly predominantly affects the medial portion of the proximal tibial growth plate, as well as the medial segment of the tibial metaphysis and epiphysis, resulting in a varus deformity at the knee joint. The cause of this condition is unknown, but it is probably a multifactor disorder with genetic, humoral, biomechanical, and environmental factors. Bateson has demonstrated convincingly that Blount disease and physiologic bowleg deformity are part of the same condition, which is influenced by early weight-bearing and racial factors. On the basis of a study of South African black children, among whom there is an increased incidence of this disorder, Bathfield and Beighton have suggested that its cause might be related to the custom of mothers carrying children on their backs. The child's thighs are abducted and flexed, and the flexed knees gripping the mother's waist are forced to assume a varus configuration.

Two forms of Blount disease have been identified: *infantile tibia vara*, which is usually bilateral and affects children younger than 10 years of age, with onset most commonly between ages 1 and 3 years, and *adolescent tibia vara*, which is usually unilateral and occurs in children between the ages 8 and 15 years. The course of the adolescent form of disease is less severe and its incidence less frequent than that of the infantile form. Regardless of its variants, Blount disease must be differentiated from other causes of genu varum, such as in variety of arthritides.

Imaging Features

Radiographically, the early stages of Blount disease are marked by hypertrophy of the nonossified cartilaginous portion of the tibial epiphysis and hypertrophy of the medial meniscus, which represent compensatory changes secondary to growth arrest at the medial aspect of the physis. The medial aspect of the tibial metaphysis is characteristically depressed, exhibiting an abrupt angulation and formation of a beaklike prominence, which is associated with cortical thickening of the medial aspect of the tibia. Similar changes are seen in the medial aspect of the tibial epiphysis. Because of the sharp angulation of the metaphysis and adduction of the diaphysis, the tibia assumes a varus configuration (Fig. 14.1). In most instances, the lateral cortex of the tibia remains relatively straight. As the metaphysis and growth plate become depressed, the cartilage decreases in height. In advanced stages of the disease, there is premature fusion of the growth plate on the medial side (Fig. 14.2). The presence of fusion is important information for surgical planning because either resection of the bony bridge or epiphysiodesis (fusion of the physis) would be required in addition to corrective osteotomy. In the past, double-contrast arthrography was a valuable technique in the imaging evaluation of Blount disease, because it permitted visualization of nonossified cartilage of the medial plateau (Fig. 14.3) and associated abnormalities of the medial meniscus (Fig. 14.4). Currently, MRI is the imaging of choice to visualize the condition of the growth plate, the epiphyseal cartilage, and the degree of deformity of the epiphysis and menisci (Fig. 14.5). This information is valuable for preoperative assessment.

Classification

Based on the progression of imaging changes in Blount disease, Langenskiöld divided congenital tibia vara into six stages as a guideline for prognosis and treatment:

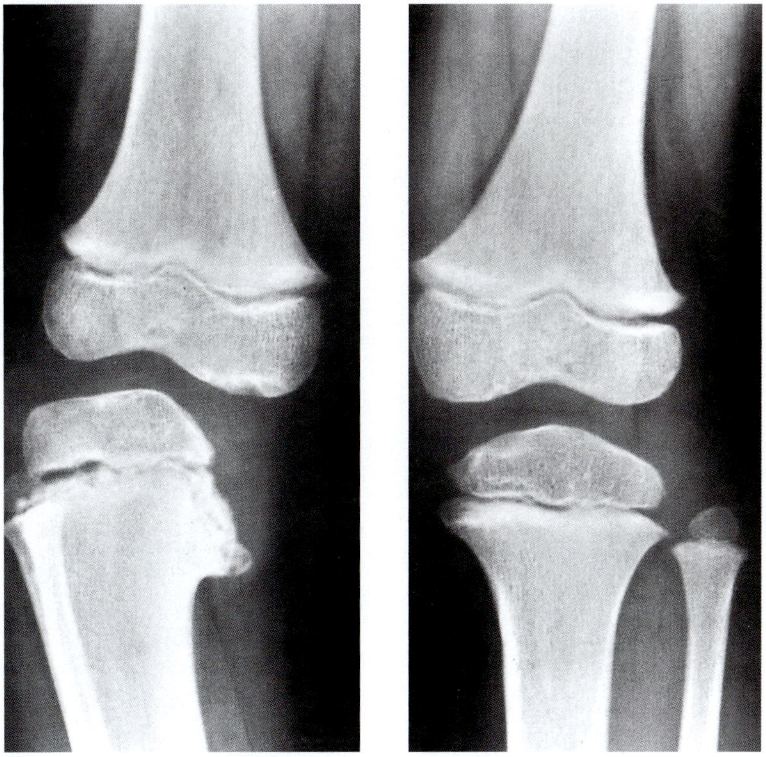

Figure 14.1 ■ **Blount disease. A:** Anteroposterior radiograph of the right knee of a 4-year-old girl with unilateral congenital tibia vara shows depression of the medial tibial metaphysis associated with a beak formation and medial slant of the tibial epiphysis. **B:** The left knee is normal.

Stage I. A varus deformity of the tibia, associated with irregularity of the growth plate and a small beak at the medial metaphysis; usually seen in children from 2 to 3 years of age.

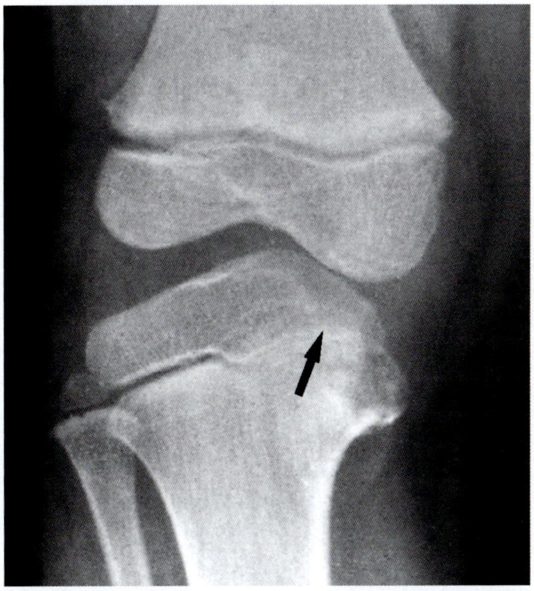

Figure 14.2 ■ **Blount disease.** Anteroposterior radiograph of the right knee of an 8-year-old girl shows the typical changes of congenital tibia vara. There is, in addition, a fusion of the medial portion of the growth plate (*arrow*).

Stage II. A definite depression of the medial portion of the metaphysis, associated with slanting of the medial aspect of the epiphysis; usually seen in children from 2 to 4 years of age.

Stage III. Progression of the varus deformity and a very prominent beak, with occasional fragmentation of the medial portion of the metaphysis; seen in children between 4 and 6 years of age.

Stage IV. Marked narrowing of the growth plate and severe slanting of the medial aspect of the epiphysis, which shows an irregular border; usually seen in children between 5 and 10 years of age.

Stage V. Marked deformity of the medial epiphysis, which is separated into two parts by a clear band, the distal part having a triangular shape; seen in children between 9 and 11 years of age.

Stage VI. An osseous bridge between the epiphysis and metaphysis and possible fusion of the triangular fragment of the separated medial epiphysis to the metaphysis; seen in children between 10 and 13 years of age.

Stages V and VI represent phases of irreparable structural damage.

Recently, Smith introduced a simplified classification of Blount disease in attempt to relate the grade of deformity to the need for treatment. His scheme comprises four grades: grade A, potential tibia vara; grade B, mild tibia vara; grade C, advanced tibia vara; and grade D, physeal closure.

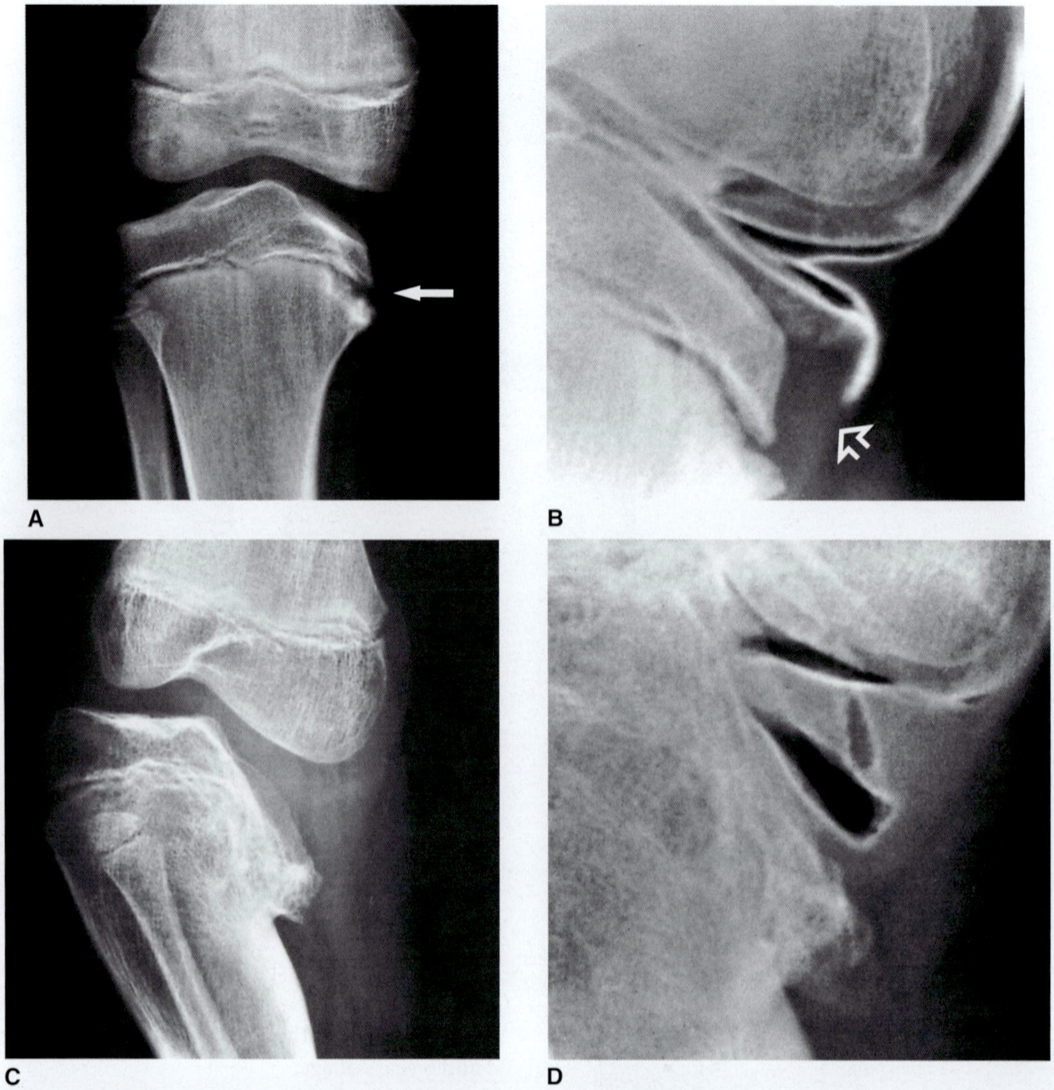

Figure 14.3 ■ Arthrography of Blount disease. A: Anteroposterior radiograph of the right knee of a 10-year-old boy demonstrates the classic appearance of this condition, as evident in the depression of the medial metaphysis associated with a beak formation and slanting of the medial tibial epiphysis (*arrow*). **B:** Arthrographic spot film shows contrast outlining the thickened nonossified cartilage of the medial tibial plateau (*open arrow*). The medial meniscus shows no abnormalities. **C:** Anteroposterior radiograph of the right knee of a 4-year-old boy shows more advanced deformities of the medial tibial epiphysis and metaphysis. **D:** Double-contrast arthrogram shows hypertrophy of the medial meniscus and thick nonossified articular cartilage at the medial aspect of the proximal tibial epiphysis.

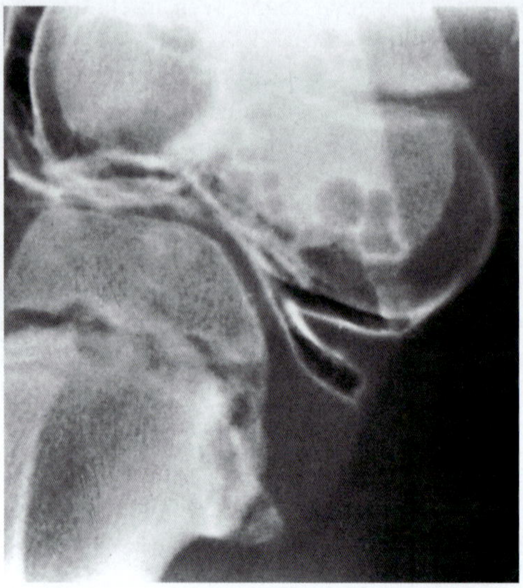

Figure 14.4 ■ Arthrography of Blount disease. Fluoroscopic spot film of a knee arthrogram in a 4-year-old girl shows hypertrophy of the medial aspect of the proximal tibial articular cartilage and an enlarged medial meniscus.

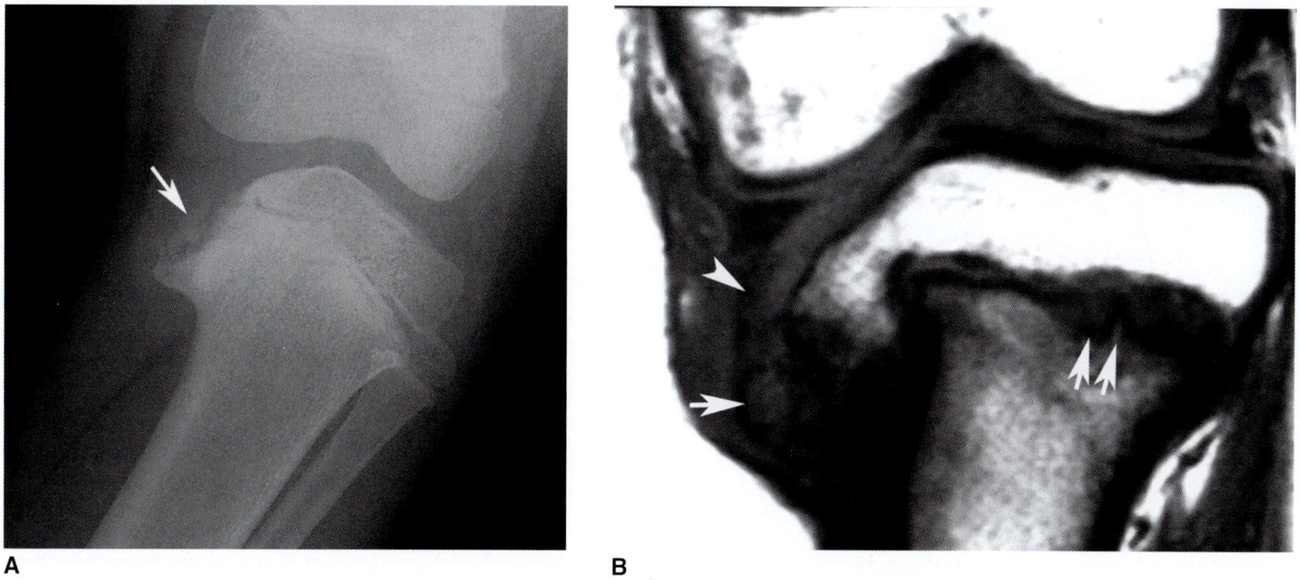

Figure 14.5 ■ **MRI of Blount disease. A:** Anteroposterior radiograph of the left knee demonstrates the characteristic depression of the medial tibial plateau and medial epiphyseal fragmentation (*arrow*). **B:** Coronal T1-weighted image demonstrates the irregular, depressed epiphyseal cartilage of the medial tibial plateau (*arrowhead*) with partial calcification and fragmentation of the depressed medial epiphyseal cartilage (*arrow*). Note the irregularity and widening of the growth plate, not evident on the radiograph (*double arrows*).

Treatment

Blount disease is usually treated conservatively with braces. If the deformity continues to progress despite such treatment, a high valgus tibial osteotomy may be required to achieve normal alignment of the limb; usually, correction of a rotary deformity requires an osteotomy of the proximal fibula as well. MRI may be required before surgery to determine the status of the tibial articular cartilage, information necessary in planning the degree of angular correction necessary to eliminate the deformity.

SLIPPED CAPITAL FEMORAL EPIPHYSIS (SCFE)

Clinical Features

SCFE is a disorder of adolescence in which the femoral head gradually slips posteriorly, medially, and inferiorly with respect to the femoral neck. Boys are affected more often than girl, and children of both genders with this disorder are often overweight. In boys, the left hip is involved twice as often as the right, whereas in girls, both hips are affected with equal frequency. Bilateral involvement occurs in 20% to 40% of patients.

Although the specific cause of SCFE is obscure, its onset, which is usually insidious and without history of trauma, commonly coincides with the growth spurt at puberty. Studies by Harris have suggested that an imbalance between growth hormone and sex hormones weaken the growth plate, rendering it more vulnerable to the shearing forces of weight bearing and injury. Pain in the hip, or occasionally in the knee, is often the presenting symptom of this condition, and physical examination may reveal shortening of the involved extremity and limitation of abduction, flexion, and internal rotation in the hip joint.

Imaging Features

The radiographic abnormalities that may be seen in SCFE depend on the degree of displacement of the capital epiphysis. The anteroposterior radiograph of the hip, supplemented by a frog-lateral view, is usually sufficient to make a correct diagnosis. Several diagnostic indicators of SCFE have been identified on the anteroposterior radiograph of the hip (Fig. 14.6). The triangle sign of Capener may be of value in recognizing early SCFE. On conventional radiograph of the normal adolescent hip, an intracapsular area at the medial aspect of the femoral neck is seen overlapping the posterior wall of the acetabulum, creating a dense triangular shadow; in most cases of SCFE, this triangle is lost (Fig. 14.7). In a later stage, periarticular osteoporosis becomes apparent, as do widening and blurring of the physis and a decrease in height of the epiphysis. Moreover, as the disease progresses, slippage of the capital epiphysis can be identified by the absence of an intersection of the epiphysis with a line drawn tangentially to the lateral cortex of the femoral neck (Fig. 14.8). The frog-lateral projection of the hip reveals slippage more readily (Fig. 14.8B), and comparison radiographs of the opposite side are helpful. Chronic stages of this disorder exhibit reactive bone formation along the superolateral aspect of the femoral neck, along with remodeling; this creates a protuberance and broadening of the femoral neck, which gives it a "pistol-grip" appearance known as a *Herndon hump* (Fig. 14.9).

(Continued on page 472)

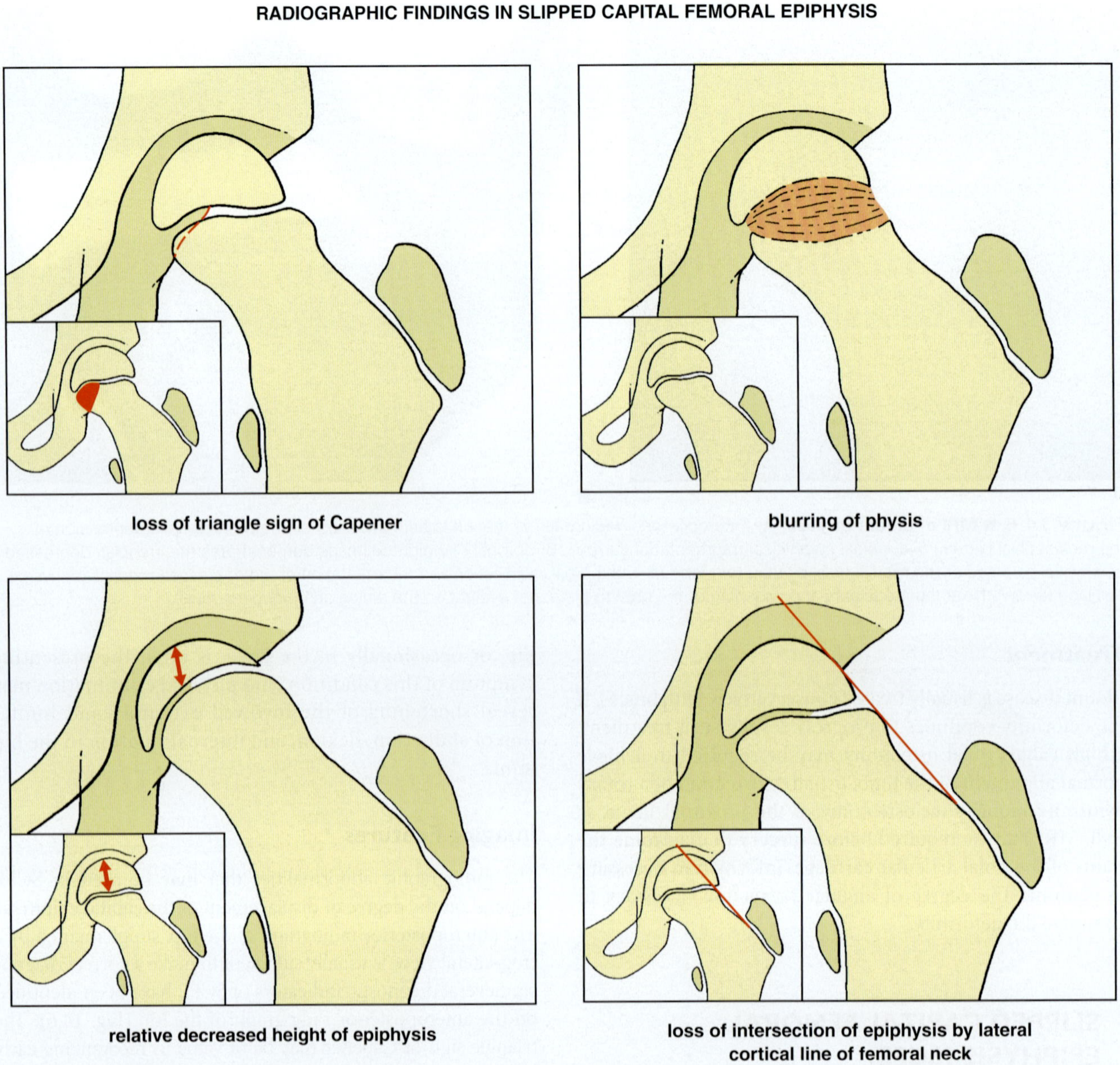

Figure 14.6 ■ **Slipped capital femoral epiphysis.** Various radiographic findings have been identified as diagnostic clues to SCFE. The insets show the normal appearance.

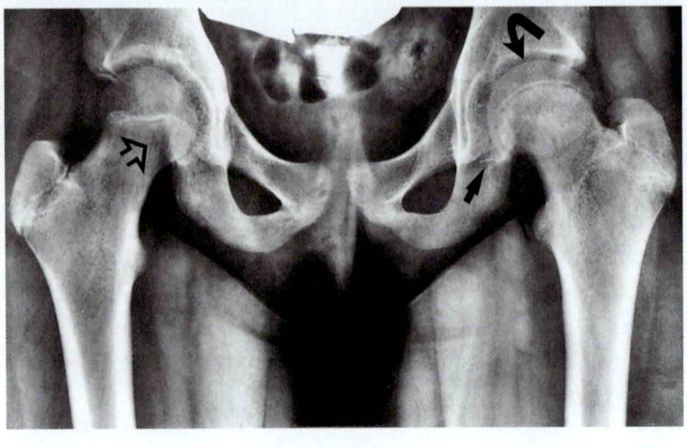

Figure 14.7 ■ **Slipped capital femoral epiphysis.** Anteroposterior radiograph of the hips of a 12-year-old girl shows the absence of a triangular density in the area of overlap of the medial segment of the femoral metaphysis with the posterior wall of the acetabulum (Capener sign) (*arrow*). The triangle is clearly seen in the normal right hip (*open arrow*). Note also relative decreased height of left femoral epiphysis (*curved arrow*).

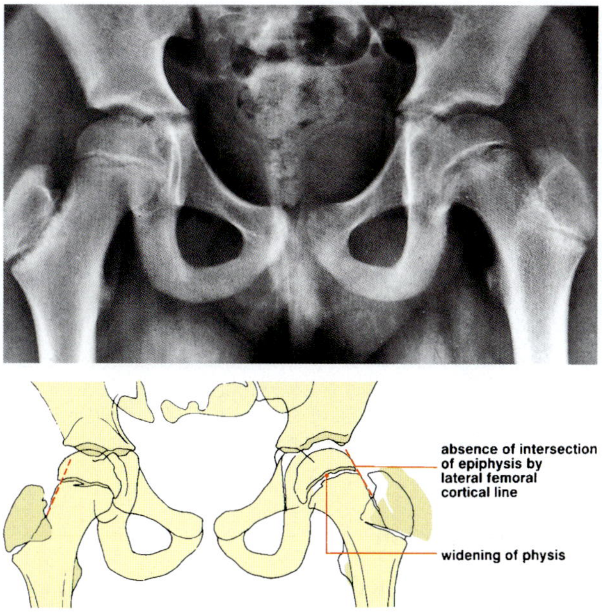

A

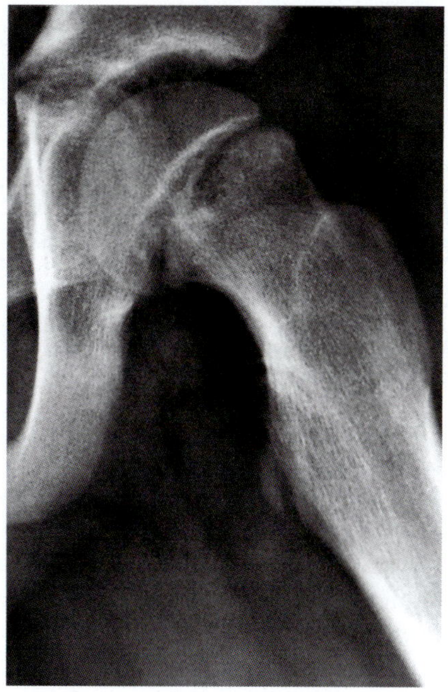

B

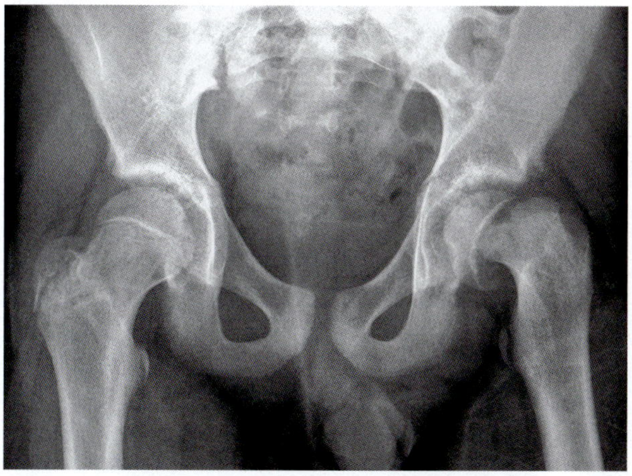

C

Figure 14.8 ■ **Slipped capital femoral epiphysis.** A 9-year-old girl presented with pain in the left hip and knee for 4 months. On physical examination, there was slight limitation of abduction and internal rotation in the hip joint. **A:** Anteroposterior radiograph of the pelvis demonstrates a minimal degree of periarticular osteoporosis of the left hip, widening of the growth plate, and a slight decrease in the height of the epiphysis. Note the lack of intersection of the epiphysis by the lateral cortical line of the femoral neck. **B:** Frog-lateral view of the left hip shows posteromedial slippage of capital epiphysis. **C:** More obvious slip of the left femoral epiphysis is seen in this 12-year-old boy.

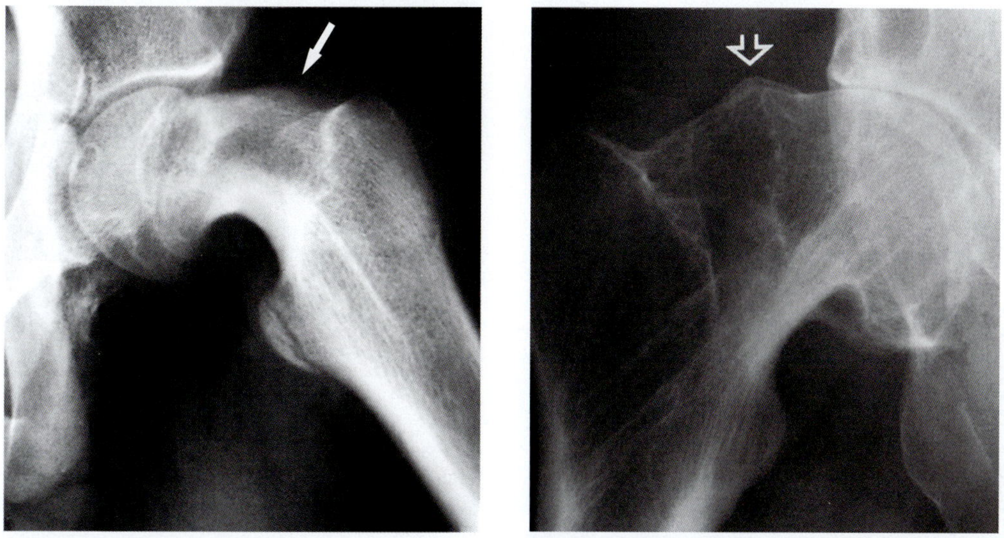

A B

Figure 14.9 ■ **Slipped capital femoral epiphysis. A:** A 14-year-old boy with a 14-month history of chronic pain in the left hip was examined by a pediatrician because of significant foreshortening of the left leg and a limp. Frog-lateral view of the left hip shows changes typical of chronic SCFE. There is a moderate degree of osteoporosis and a remodeling deformity of the femoral neck, known as a Herndon hump (*arrow*). **B:** Anteroposterior radiograph of the right hip of a 20-year-old man who had an SCFE treated with pins demonstrates a Herndon hump (*open arrow*) and secondary osteoarthritis.

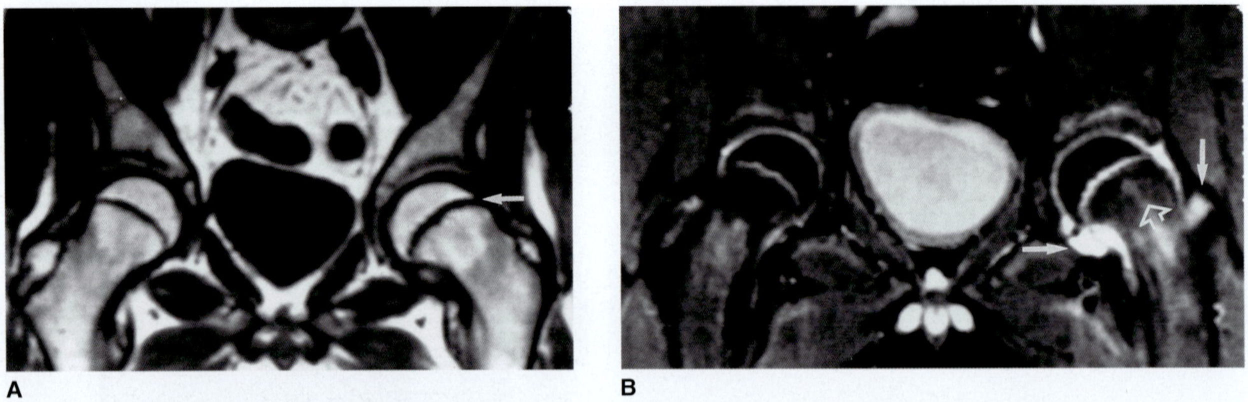

Figure 14.10 ■ MRI of slipped capital femoral epiphysis. **A:** Coronal T1-weighted MRI of the hips in a 14-year-old boy shows slipped femoral epiphysis on the left side (*arrow*). The right hip is normal. **B:** Coronal T2-weighted fat-suppressed image reveals joint effusion (*arrows*) and marrow edema in the metaphysis (*open arrow*).

MRI is a useful technique in the evaluation of SCFE. This modality, in addition to findings revealed by radiography, may show bone marrow edema of the affected femur and early imaging manifestations of SCFE and pre-SCFE (Figs. 14.10 and 14.11).

Treatment

SCFE is treated surgically by closed or open reduction of the slippage and internal fixation using various types of nails, screws, wires, and pins to prevent further slippage and to induce closure of the physis. Complications of the treatment

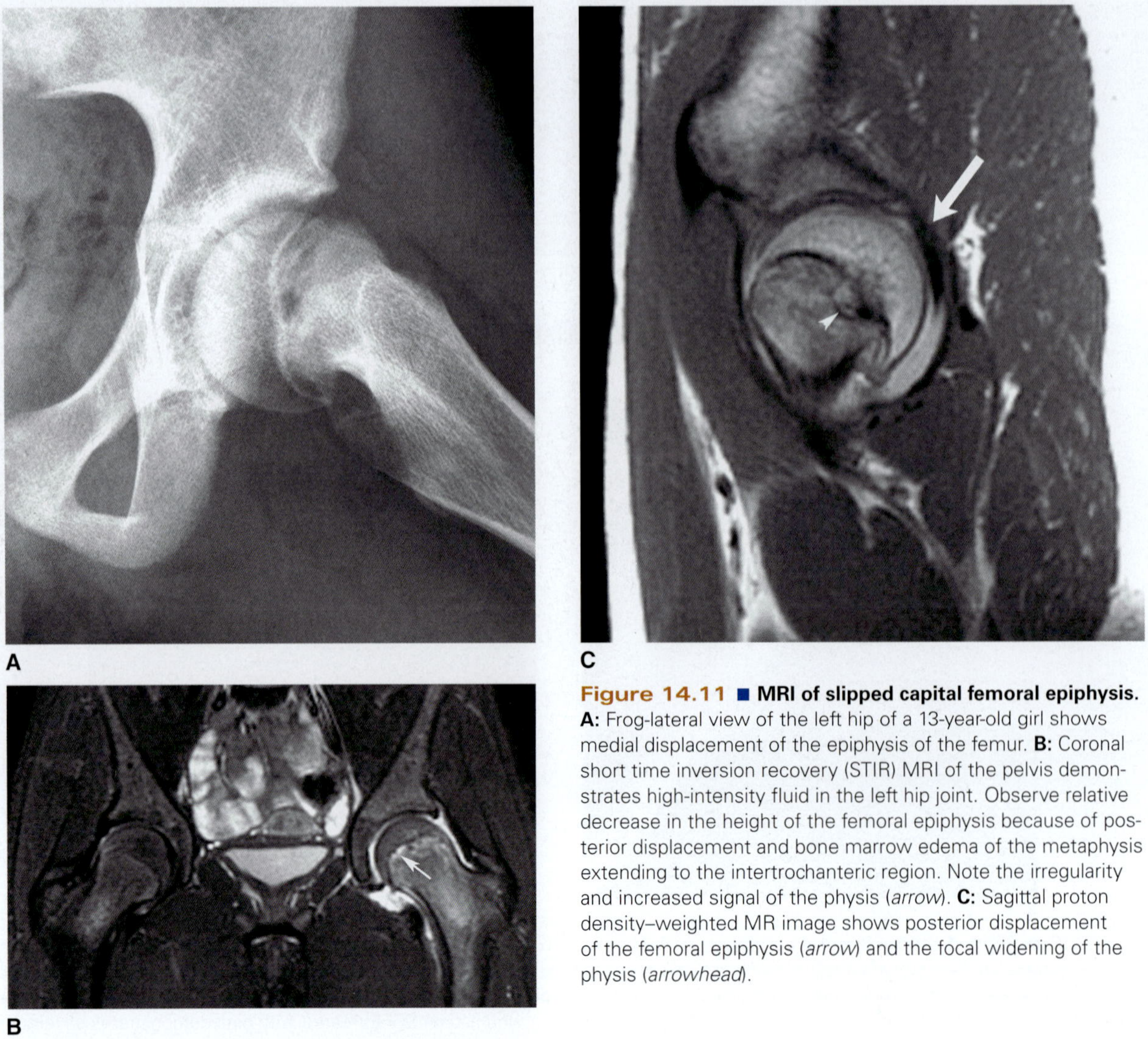

Figure 14.11 ■ MRI of slipped capital femoral epiphysis. **A:** Frog-lateral view of the left hip of a 13-year-old girl shows medial displacement of the epiphysis of the femur. **B:** Coronal short time inversion recovery (STIR) MRI of the pelvis demonstrates high-intensity fluid in the left hip joint. Observe relative decrease in the height of the femoral epiphysis because of posterior displacement and bone marrow edema of the metaphysis extending to the intertrochanteric region. Note the irregularity and increased signal of the physis (*arrow*). **C:** Sagittal proton density–weighted MR image shows posterior displacement of the femoral epiphysis (*arrow*) and the focal widening of the physis (*arrowhead*).

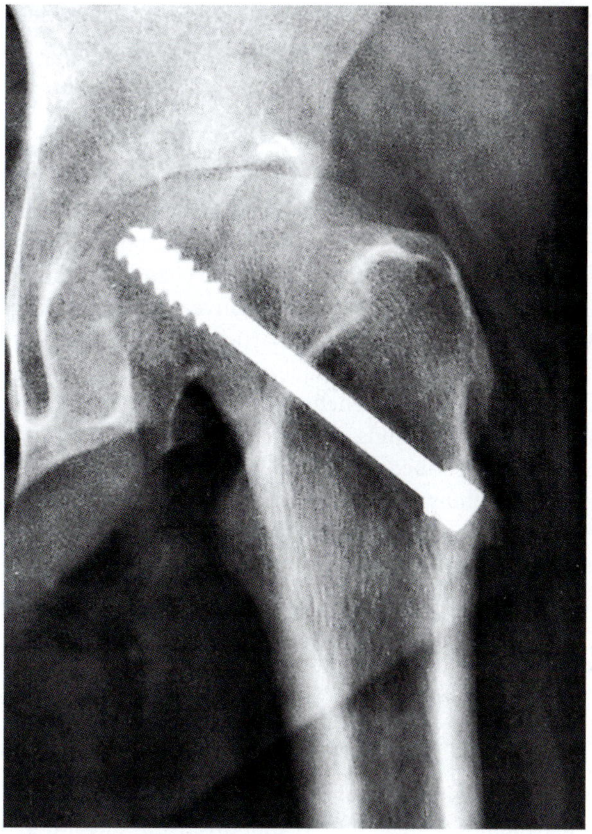

Figure 14.12 ■ Complication of slipped capital femoral epiphysis. Anteroposterior radiograph of the left hip of a 13-year-old girl who 1 year earlier had been treated for SCFE shows narrowing of the joint secondary to chondrolysis, a complication of this condition.

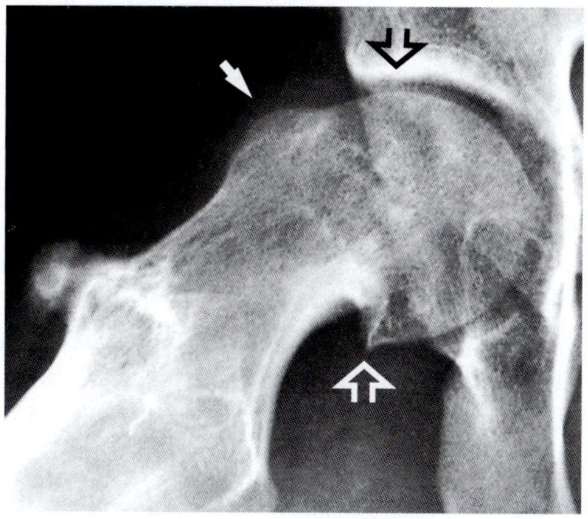

Figure 14.14 ■ Complication of slipped capital femoral epiphysis. Frog-lateral radiograph of the right hip of a 14-year-old boy who had acute slippage of the capital epiphysis at age 9 years demonstrates narrowing of the joint space and osteophytosis (*open arrows*), characteristic features of a secondary osteoarthritic process. Note the presence of a Herndon hump (*arrow*).

include chondrolysis, which is observed in about 30% to 35% of patients with SCFE. It usually occurs within 1-year after the treatment and is evident by gradually narrowing of the joint space (Fig. 14.12). Osteonecrosis secondary to the precarious blood supply to the femoral head and the vulnerability of the epiphyseal vessels has been reported in ~25% of patients with SCFE (Fig. 14.13). Secondary osteoarthritis may also occur, and it can be recognized by a typical narrowing of the joint space, subchondral sclerosis, and marginal osteophyte formation (Fig. 14.14, see also Fig. 14.12).

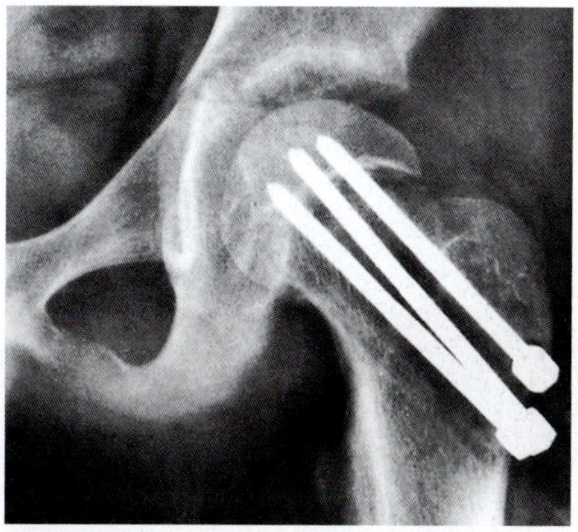

A

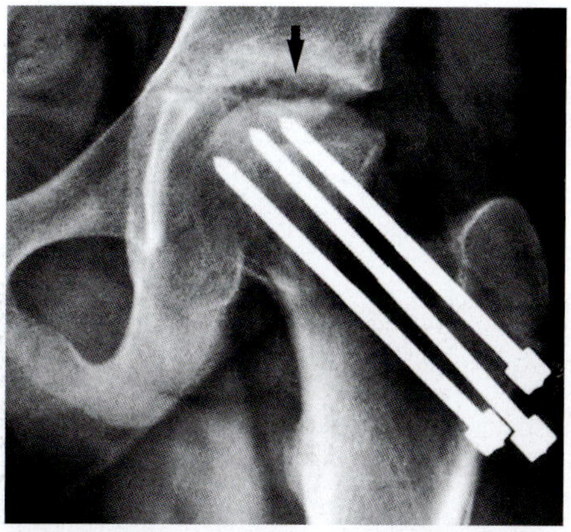

B

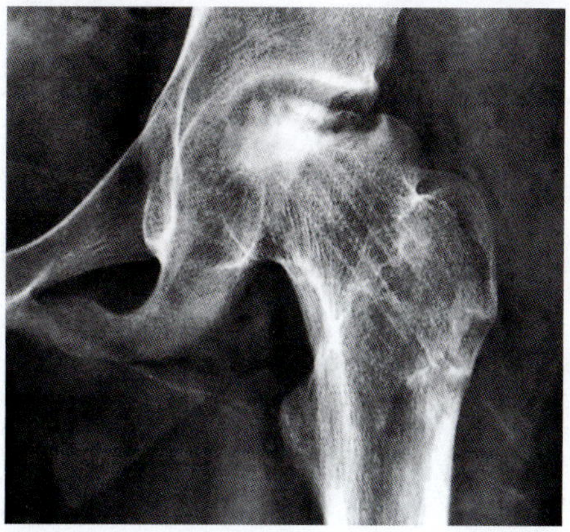

C

Figure 14.13 ■ Complication of slipped capital femoral epiphysis. A: A 12-year-old boy was treated by the insertion of three Knowles pins into the femoral head. Six months later, a repeat film **(B)** shows minimal flattening of the weight-bearing segment of the femoral epiphysis (*arrow*), an early sign suggesting osteonecrosis. The pins were removed. **C:** On a radiograph obtained 1 year later, there is an increase in density of the femoral head together with fragmentation of the epiphysis and subchondral collapse, features of advanced osteonecrosis.

A severe varus deformity of the femoral neck, known as *coxa vara*, may also be encountered.

MELORHEOSTOSIS

A rare condition of unknown cause, melorheostosis (Leri disease) shows no evidence of hereditary features. It belongs to a group of bone disorders called the mixed sclerosing dysplasias, which combine characteristics of both endochondral and intramembranous failure of ossification. It has been postulated that the disease develops due to a loss-of-function mutation in *LEMD3* gene. This gene, also known as *MAN1*, encodes for an integral protein of the inner nuclear membrane. Happle suggested that melorheostosis originates from an early mutation event with loss of the corresponding wild-type allele at gene locus of osteopoikilosis. Recently, however, some investigators concluded that mutation in the *LEMD3* gene does not cause isolated melorheostosis. Laboratory abnormalities affect osteoblastic specific factor-2 (osf-2), osteonectin, fibronectin, transforming growth factor beta (TGF-beta), and fibroblast growth factor 23 (FGF-23).

Clinical Features

The presenting symptom is pain intensified by activity. Limitation of joint motion and stiffness are common, because of contractures, soft tissue fibrosis, and periarticular bone formation in the soft tissues. The condition may be monostotic (*forme fruste*), affecting only one bone; monomelic, affecting one limb; or polyostotic, with generalized affection of the skeleton. Long bones are most commonly affected, with other sites including the pelvis, and short tubular bones of the hands and feet. The ribs and the bones of the skull are rarely affected. Melorheostosis affecting thoracic vertebrae complicated by involvement of the facet joints has recently been reported.

Pathology

Microscopic examination of melorheostotic specimens reveals nonspecific, hyperostotic periosteal bone formation with thickened trabeculae and fibrotic changes in the marrow spaces. The bone appears primitive and consists largely of primary haversian systems, particularly on the periosteal surface, that are almost completely obliterated by the deposition of sclerotic, thickened, and somewhat irregular lamellae (Fig. 14.15). Islands of cartilage in periarticular lesions have been described, with evidence of both endochondral and intramembranous bone formation within the cellular fibrous tissue, and osteoblastic activity along the margins of osteons.

Imaging Features

Conventional radiography is sufficient to make a diagnosis. The lesion is characterized by a wavy hyperostosis that resembles melted wax dripping down the side of a candle, the feature from which the disease derives its name (Greek *melos* [member]; *rhein* [flow]); moreover, only one side of the bone is usually involved (Figs. 14.16 and 14.17). Associated joint abnormalities are also well delineated on standard radiographs. The involvement of soft tissues is not rare, and the ossified masses are often present around the hip and knee joints (Fig. 14.18). CT effectively reveals involvement of the cortex and the medullary cavity, and clear demarcation of normal from abnormal bone (Fig. 14.19A). MRI shows low signal intensity localized to the affected areas on all pulse sequences (Figs. 14.19–14.21). This technique

(Continued on page 477)

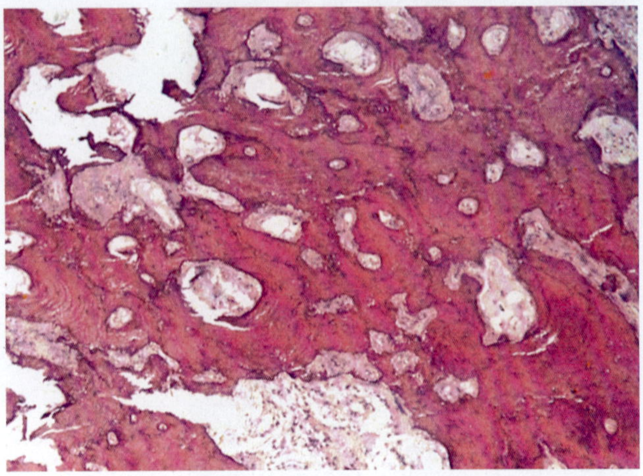

A

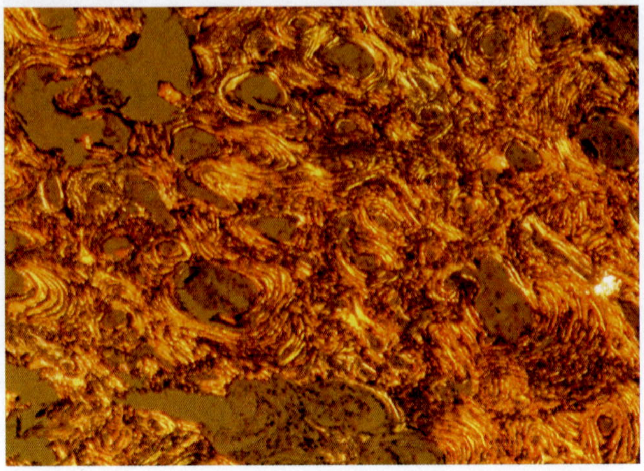

B

Figure 14.15 ■ Histopathology of melorheostosis. A: Biopsy specimen from melorheostotic focus reveals markedly irregular bone trabeculae with relatively little cellular activity (H&E, original magnification ×4). **B:** The same histologic field photographed with polarized light shows mixture of irregular trabeculae of lamellar and woven bone. (From Bullough PG. *Atlas of Orthopedic Pathology with Clinical and Radiologic Correlations*, 2nd ed. New York, NY: Gower Medical Publishing; 1992. Fig. 14.53 and 14.54, p. 14.18.)

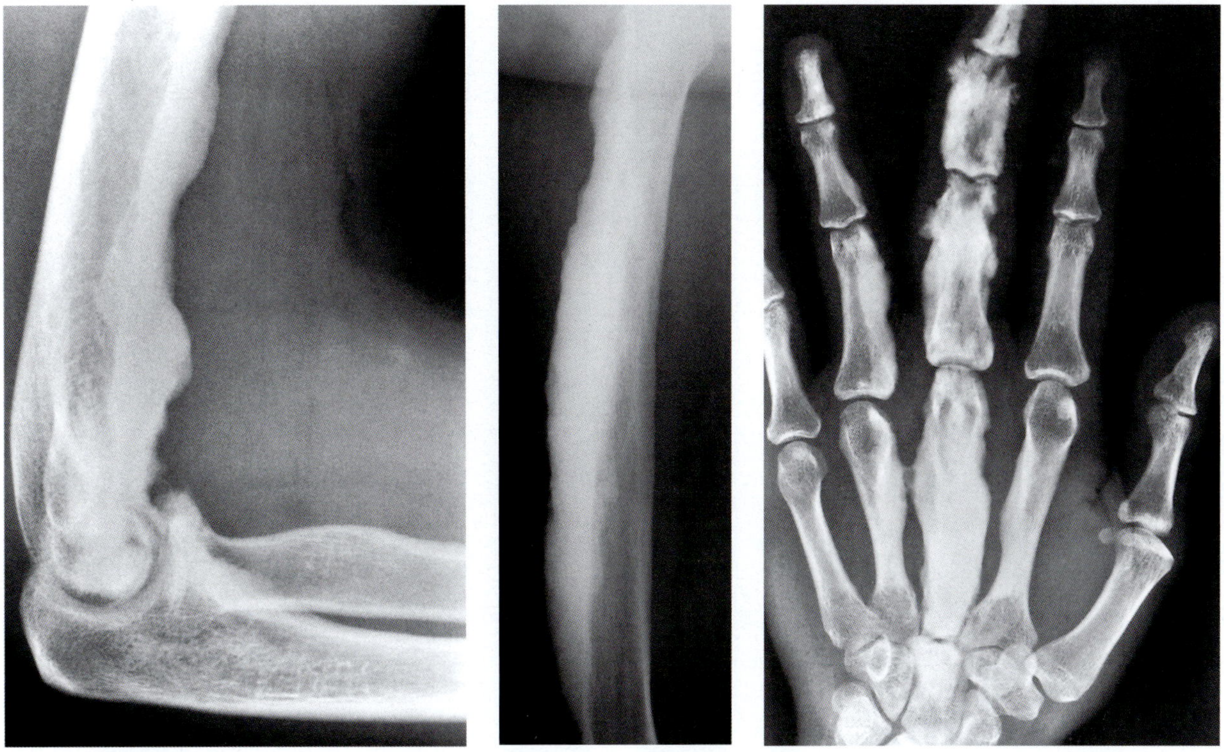

A B C

Figure 14.16 ■ **Melorheostosis.** A 28-year-old man presented with pain in the right elbow and an enlargement of the middle finger of his right hand. **A:** Lateral radiograph of the elbow demonstrates a flowing hyperostosis of the anterior cortex of the distal humerus, typical of melorheostosis. Note the bridging of the joint by the lesion and the involvement of the coronoid process of the ulna. **B:** The radiograph of the right femur shows involvement of only the anterolateral aspect of the bone. **C:** Dorsovolar radiograph of the right hand shows marked hypertrophy of the middle digit. The cortices (the sites of intramembranous ossification) are involved, as are the articular ends of the bones (the sites of endochondral ossification). This is characteristic of mixed sclerosing dysplasias.

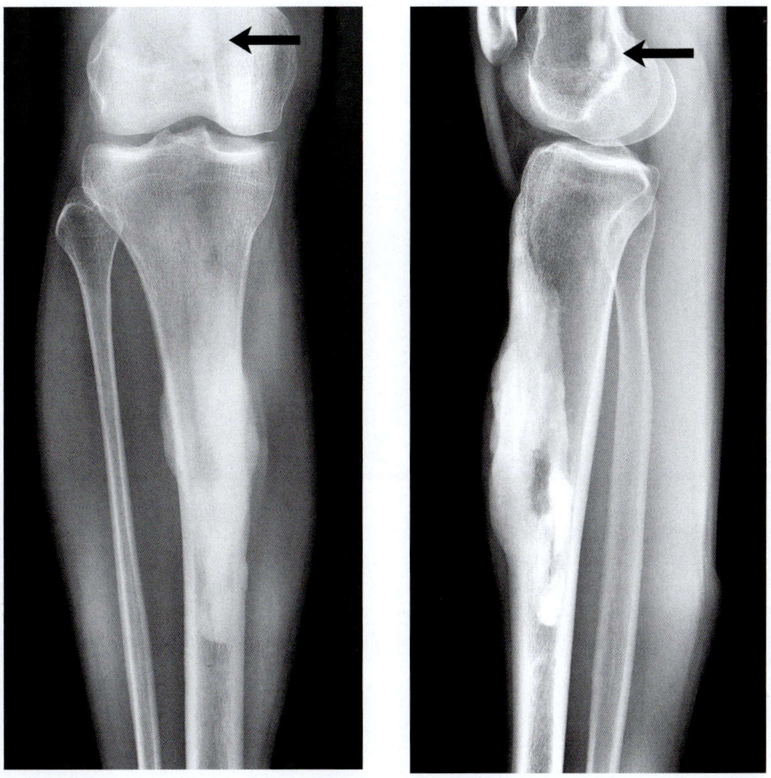

A B

Figure 14.17 ■ **Melorheostosis.** Anteroposterior **(A)** and lateral **(B)** lateral radiographs of the right leg of a 31-year-old woman show sclerotic changes affecting predominantly anterior aspect of the tibia. Note also a medullary focus of melorheostosis in the distal femur (*arrows*).

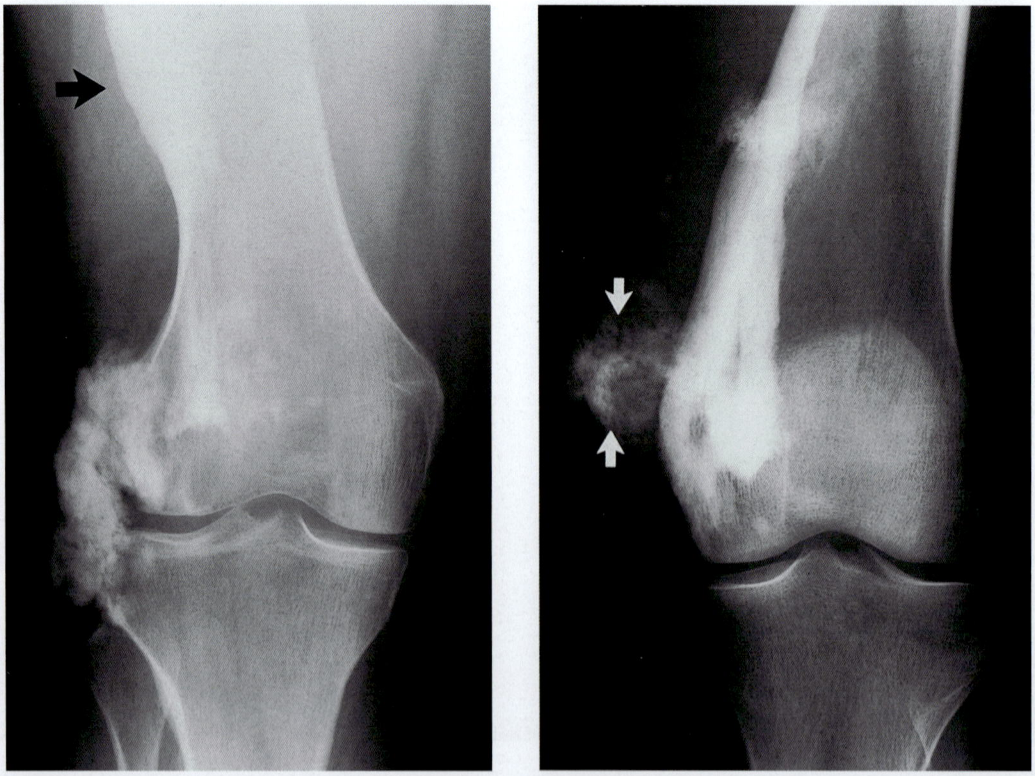

A B

Figure 14.18 ■ Melorheostosis. A: Anteroposterior radiograph of the right knee in a 46-year-old woman shows ossifications of the soft tissues at the lateral aspect of the knee joint. The femoral cortex is also affected (*arrow*). **B:** A radiograph of the left knee in a 25-year-old woman shows involvement of the medial femoral cortex extending into the soft tissues (*arrows*).

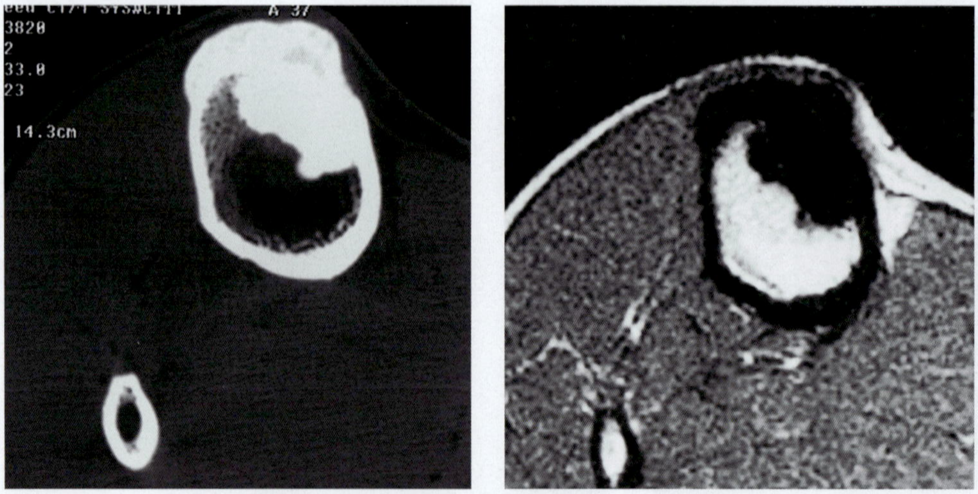

A B

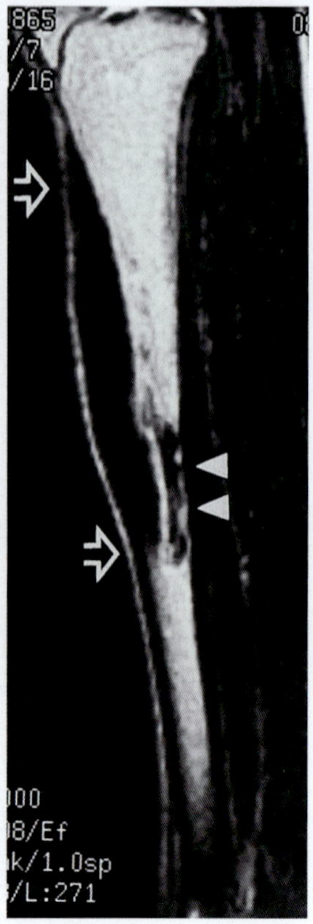

C

Figure 14.19 ■ CT and MRI of melorheostosis. A: CT section through the middle segment of tibia in a 30-year-old woman shows involvement of the anterior cortex and anteromedial portion of medullary cavity. **B:** An axial T1-weighted MR image shows the lesion to be of low signal intensity, which is the same as the cortical bone. The uninvolved bone marrow exhibits high signal similar to the subcutaneous fat. **C:** A sagittal T2-weighted MR image shows that the lesion remains of low signal intensity (*open arrows*). *Arrowheads* point to the medullary involvement.

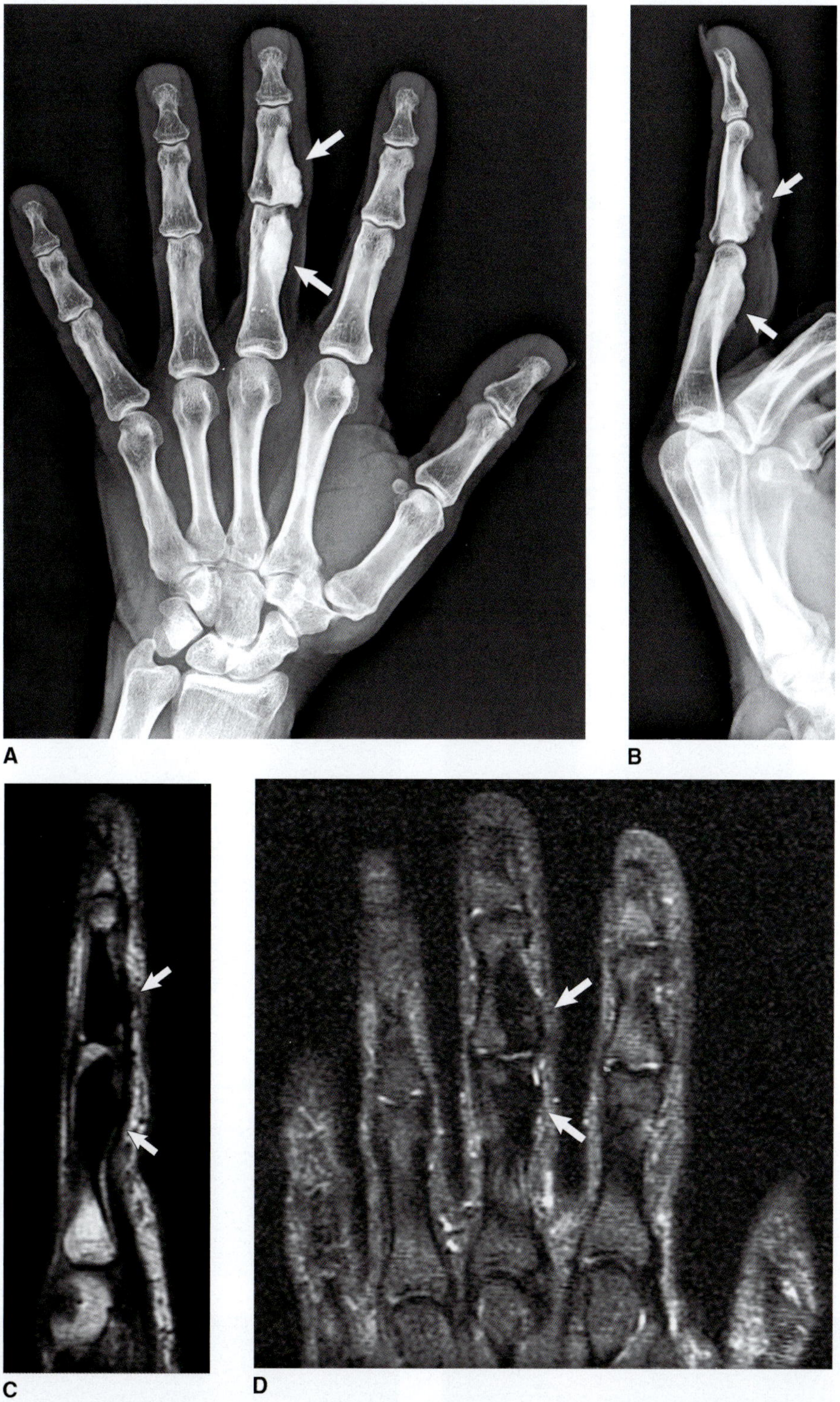

Figure 14.20 ■ MRI of melorheostosis. Dorsovolar radiograph of the right hand **(A)** and lateral radiograph of the middle finger **(B)** of a 30-year-old woman show flowing cortical hyperostosis affecting radial and volar aspects of the proximal and middle phalanges (*arrows*). Sagittal T1-weighted MR image of the middle finger **(C)** and coronal T2-weighted MR image **(D)** show the foci of melorheostosis exhibiting low signal intensity on both pulse sequences (*arrows*).

is also helpful for imaging of soft tissue involvement. In one study reported by Judkiewicz and associates, soft tissue masses were heterogeneous on all MRI pulse sequences with signal void in areas corresponding to mineralization on conventional radiographs. Most of the soft tissue masses exhibited ill-defined margins, were contiguous or adjacent to areas of osseous hyperostosis, and demonstrated enhancement after administration of gadolinium–DTPA. PET/CT images demonstrate increased metabolic activity within the lesion (Fig. 14.22). Radionuclide bone scan can determine other sites of skeletal involvement by demonstrating abnormal uptake of radiopharmaceutical tracer

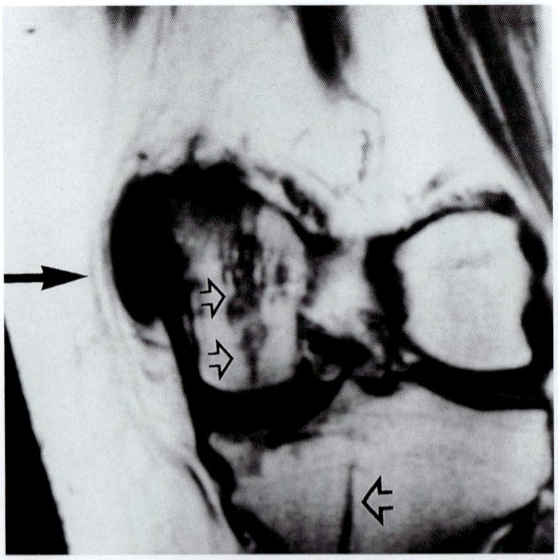

Figure 14.21 ■ **MRI of melorheostosis.** A coronal T1-weighted image of the knee in a 20-year-old man shows low signal intensity of the ossific mass attached to the femoral condyle (*arrow*) as well as in the medullary foci of melorheostosis (*open arrows*).

(Fig. 14.23). The factors responsible for increased uptake include the increased mass of the cortex, osteoblastic activity, and local hyperemia.

The disorder is chronic and occasionally debilitating. Conservative treatment with bisphosphonate (pamidronate) infusion has been tried occasionally, with mixed results. Surgical treatment consists of soft tissue procedures such as tendon lengthening, excision of fibrous and osseous tissue, fasciotomy, and capsulotomy. Other procedures include corrective osteotomies, excision of hyperostotic bone, and even amputations in severely affected and painful limbs caused by vascular ischemia. Recurrences are common.

FIBRODYSPLASIA OSSIFICANS PROGRESSIVA (MYOSITIS OSSIFICANS PROGRESSIVA)

Fibrodysplasia ossificans progressiva is a rare systemic autosomal dominant disorder with variable expressivity

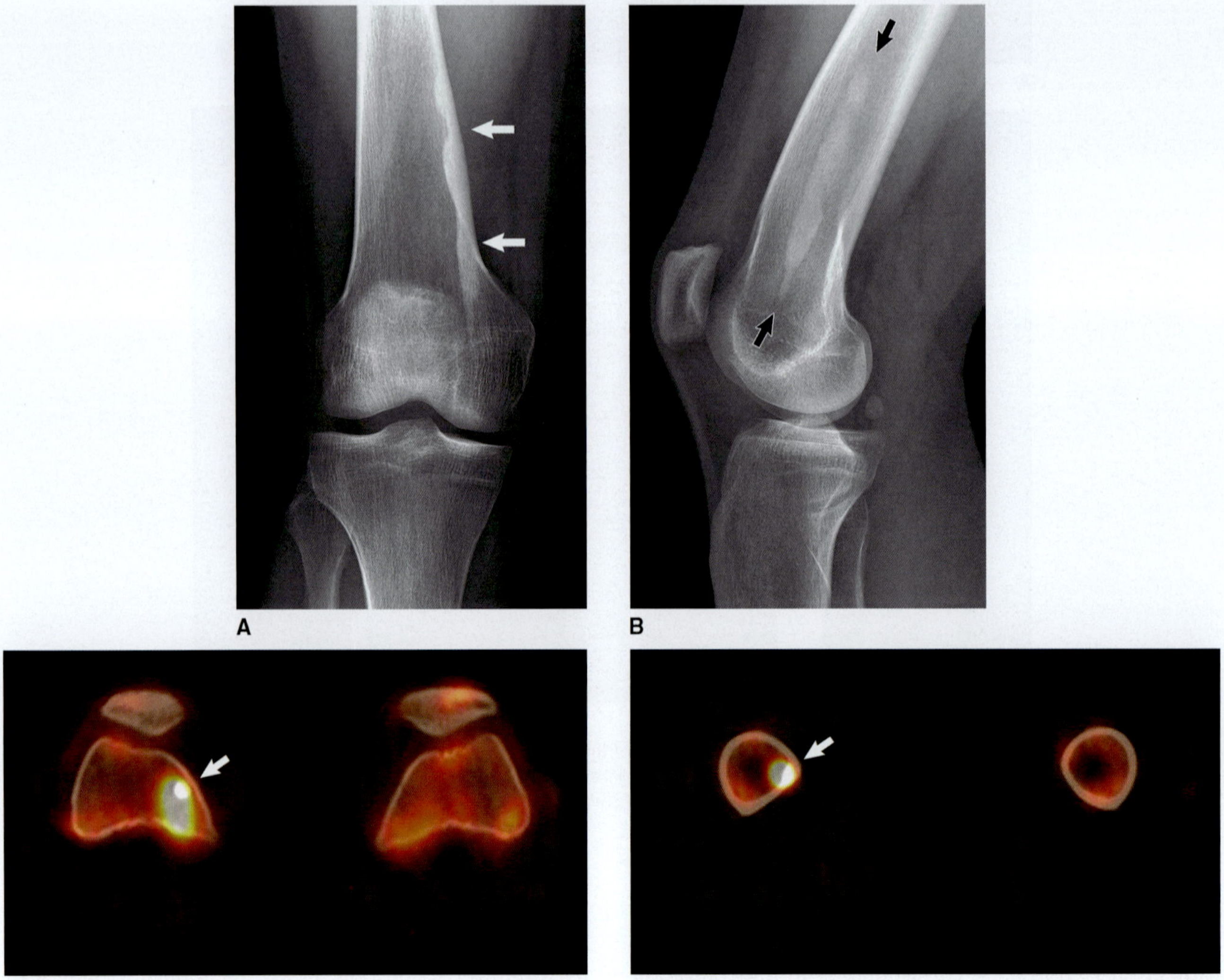

A B C D

Figure 14.22 ■ **PET/CT of melorheostosis.** Anteroposterior **(A)** and lateral **(B)** radiographs of the right knee of a 21-year-old man show wavy cortical hyperostosis affecting medial aspect of the distal femur (*arrows*). Axial fused PET/CT images, one obtained through the knee joints **(C)** and the other through the distal femora **(D)**, show metabolic hyperactivity of the lesion (*arrow*).

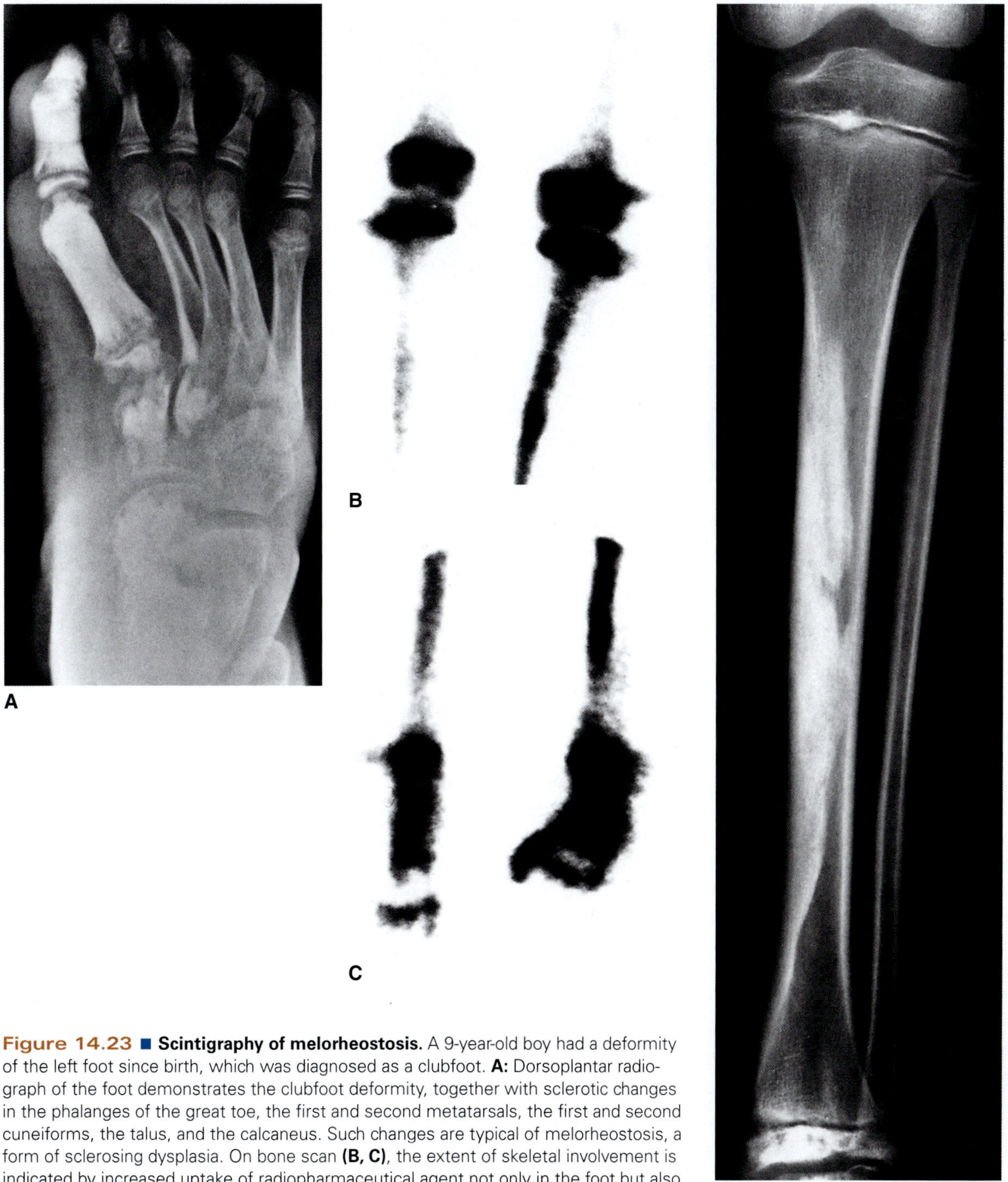

A

B

C

D

Figure 14.23 ■ Scintigraphy of melorheostosis. A 9-year-old boy had a deformity of the left foot since birth, which was diagnosed as a clubfoot. **A:** Dorsoplantar radiograph of the foot demonstrates the clubfoot deformity, together with sclerotic changes in the phalanges of the great toe, the first and second metatarsals, the first and second cuneiforms, the talus, and the calcaneus. Such changes are typical of melorheostosis, a form of sclerosing dysplasia. On bone scan **(B, C)**, the extent of skeletal involvement is indicated by increased uptake of radiopharmaceutical agent not only in the foot but also in the left tibia, which is confirmed on a subsequent radiograph of the left leg **(D)**.

and complete penetrance. The responsible *ACVR1* gene has recently been mapped to chromosome 17q21-22, and another study has localized it to chromosome 4q21-31. In most cases, only a single family member is affected. This suggests the involvement of a sporadic mutation.

Clinical Features

Most patients are affected early in life (from birth to age 5 years), and there is no gender predominance. The earliest clinical symptom is the appearance of painful nodules and masses in the subcutaneous tissue, particularly around the head and neck, with associated stiffness and limitation of movement. Subsequently, excessive ossification of muscles, ligaments, and fascia occur, with the predominant sites of involvement in the head and neck, the dorsal paraspinal muscles, the shoulder girdles, and the hips. Involvement of intercostal musculature interferes with respiration. Clinically, the condition progresses from the shoulder girdle to the upper arms, spine, and pelvis. The natural history is one of remissions and exacerbations; death secondary to respiratory failure caused by constriction of the chest wall

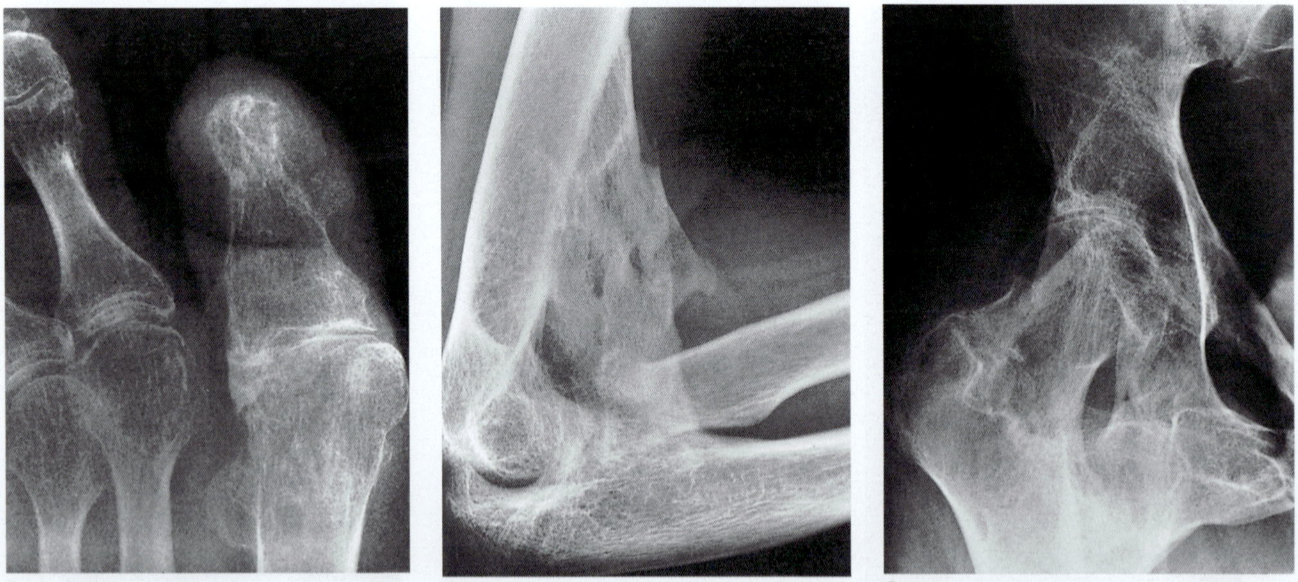

A B C

Figure 14.24 ■ Fibrodysplasia ossificans progressiva. A 28-year-old man was diagnosed with fibrodysplasia ossificans progressiva at age 3 years. **A:** Microdactyly of the great toe is a frequent feature of this disorder. **B:** Lateral radiograph of the elbow shows extensive ossification in the soft tissues, bridging the distal humerus to the radius and ulna. **C:** Massive ossification around the hip accompanies the ankylosis of the hip joint.

is an almost inevitable outcome. No effective treatment is known to date.

Pathology

The primary histopathologic abnormality is in the connective tissues. The pathologic abnormalities are similar to those of myositis ossificans circumscripta, but the zoning phenomenon of centripetal ossification is absent. The earliest histologic changes are edema and inflammatory exudate, followed by mesenchymal proliferation and formation of a large mass of collagen. This collagen is capable of accepting the deposition of calcium salts. Eventually, the lesion is transformed into irregular masses of lamellar and woven bone.

Imaging Features

Abnormalities of the thumb and great toe are present at birth and precede the soft tissue ossification. The characteristic radiologic changes consist of agenesis, microdactyly, or congenital hallux valgus, occasionally with fusion at the metacarpophalangeal or metatarsophalangeal joints (Fig. 14.24A). Short big toes and short thumbs may be associated with clinodactyly of the fifth finger, as well as with brachydactyly. In the soft tissues, extensive ossifications are seen, along with bridging osseous masses in the cervical and thoracic spine, the thorax, and the extremities (Fig. 14.24B). Involvement of the insertions of ligaments and tendons occasionally produces osseous excrescences mimicking exostoses. Joint ankylosis results most often from ossification of the surrounding soft tissue, but a true intra-articular fusion may occur (Figs. 14.24C and 14.25). CT provides accurate anatomic localization of preosseous lesions. MRI, particularly contrast-enhanced studies, may further characterize soft tissue abnormalities. Early-stage lesions exhibit low signal intensity on T1-weighted sequences and high signal intensity on T2-weighted images, accompanied by marked homogeneous enhancement on postgadolinium studies.

ARTHROGRYPOSIS (ARTHROGRYPOSIS MULTIPLEX CONGENITA)

Arthrogryposis is a congenital anomaly consisting of joint contractures in two or more areas of the body. The term "arthrogryposis" comes from the Greek words *arthron* for joint and *gruposis* for crooked. This disorder consists of several conditions of different etiology and mixed clinical features. Three groups of this disorder have been identified: amyoplasia, characterized by severe joint contractures and muscle weakness; distal arthrogryposis, an autosomal dominant disorder also known as Sheldon-Hall syndrome, mainly affecting the hands and feet; and syndromic arthrogryposis, presenting with neurologic abnormalities. The characteristic features of Sheldon-Hall syndrome, beside permanently bent fingers and toes (camptodactyly), overlapping fingers, and ulnar deviation of the wrist, also include distinctive facial features, such as triangular face, nasolabial folds, and a small mouth with a high arched palate.

Although the etiology of arthrogryposis is still unclear, several genetic factors have been implicated as a cause

(Continued on page 482)

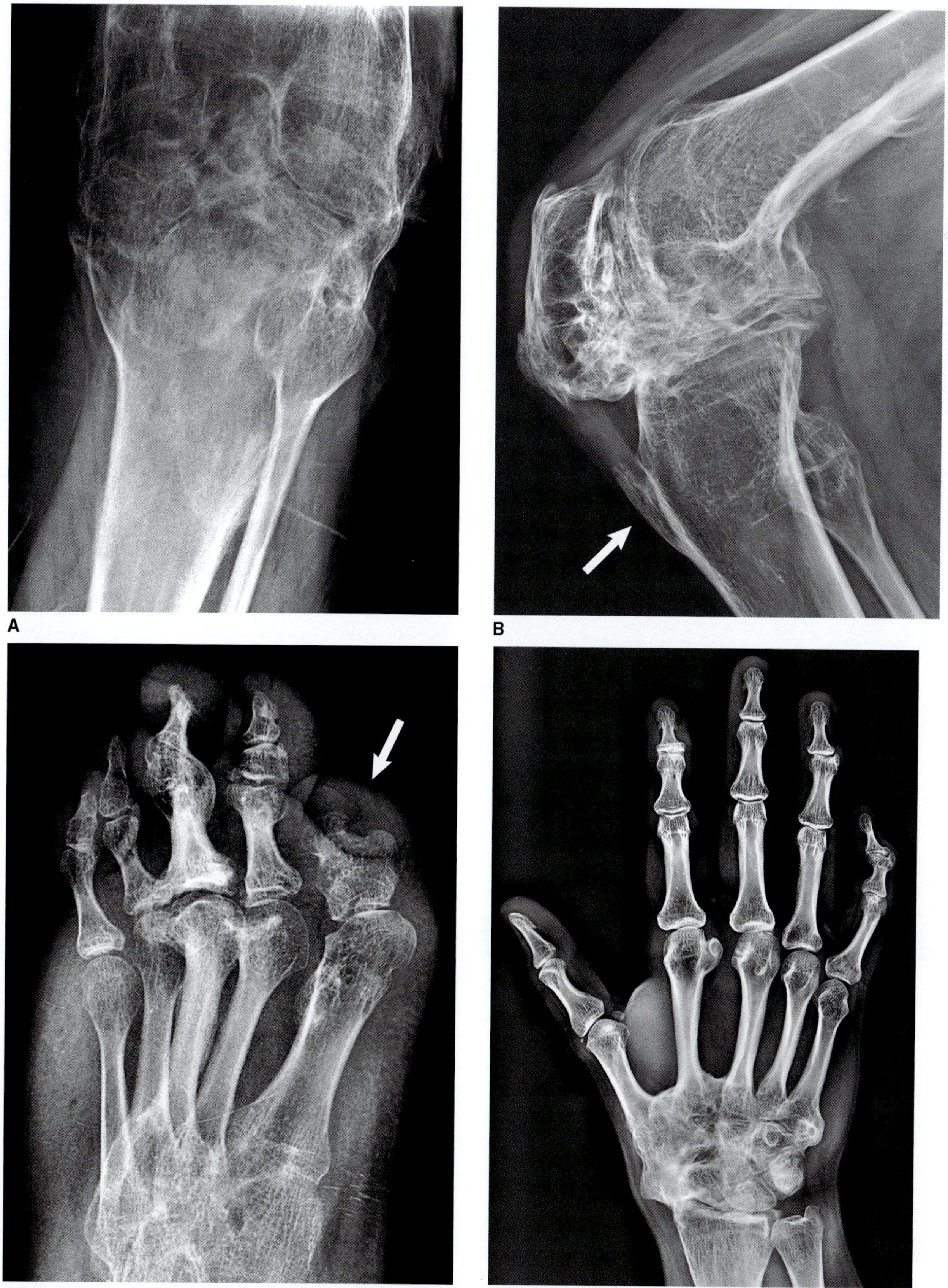

A B C D

Figure 14.25 ■ Fibrodysplasia ossificans progressiva. Anteroposterior **(A)** and lateral **(B)** radiographs of the left knee of a 35-year-old woman show osseous bridging of all three joint compartments. The *arrow* points to ossification of the patellar ligament. **C:** Dorsoplantar radiograph of the right foot shows characteristic deformity of the great toe (*arrow*). Observe also osseous fusion of the metatarsophalangeal joints and interphalangeal joints of the third toe. **D:** Dorsovolar radiograph of the left hand shows osseous fusion of the intercarpal and carpometacarpal joints.

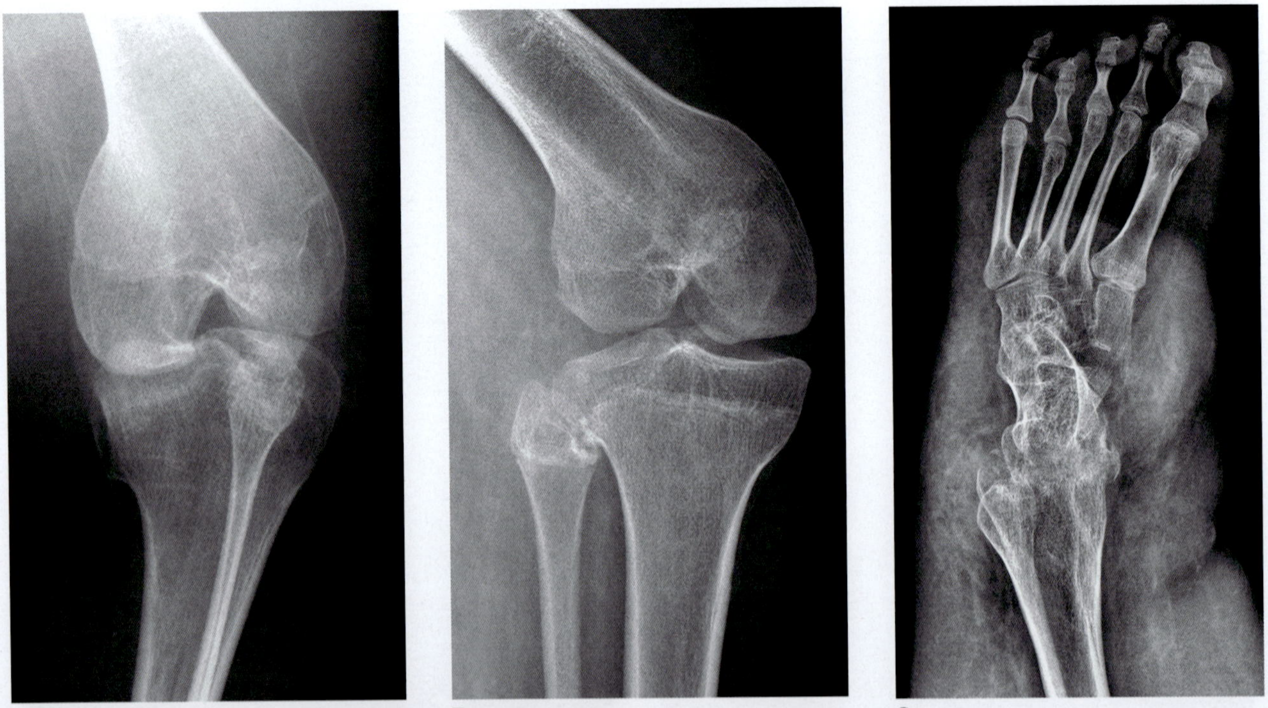

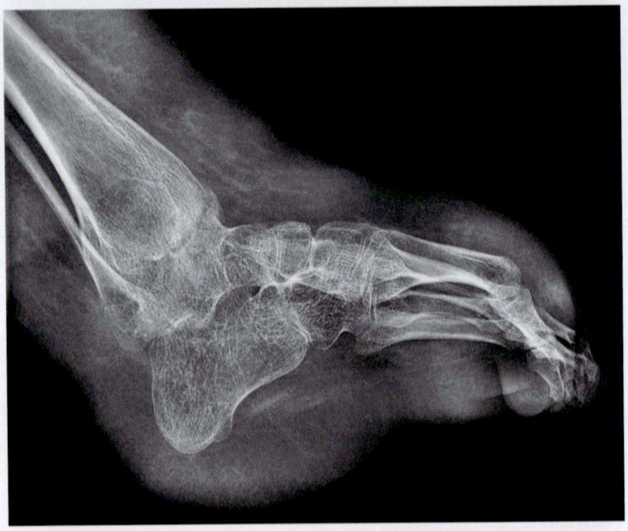

Figure 14.26 ■ **Arthrogryposis. A, B:** Two radiographs of the right knee of a 16-year-old girl show flexion contracture in the femorotibial joint and deformity of the distal femur. Dorsoplantar **(C)** and lateral **(D)** radiographs of the right foot show flexion contractures of the toes and fatty atrophy of the muscles.

of this disorder, including single-gene defects (X-linked recessive, autosomal recessive, and autosomal dominant), mitochondrial defects, and chromosomal disorders, such as trisomy 18. Mutations in at least five genes, *TNN12*, *TNNT3*, *TPM2*, *MYH3*, and *MYH8*, might be the cause of distal arthrogryposis. Some researches suggested that the malformations of arthrogryposis could be secondary to environmental factors such as decreased intrauterine movement, oligohydramnios, and defects in the fetal blood supply.

Imaging features are not specific and include contractures in various joints, muscle atrophy, and occasionally congenital fusion of the joints (Figs. 14.26–14.28).

Treatment of arthrogryposis is individualized and is based on the signs and symptoms present in each patient and the severity of the condition. Physical therapy to stretch contractures can improve the range of motion of affected joints, and occupational therapy has proven beneficial in improving muscle strength. Hands and feet deformities can be surgically corrected.

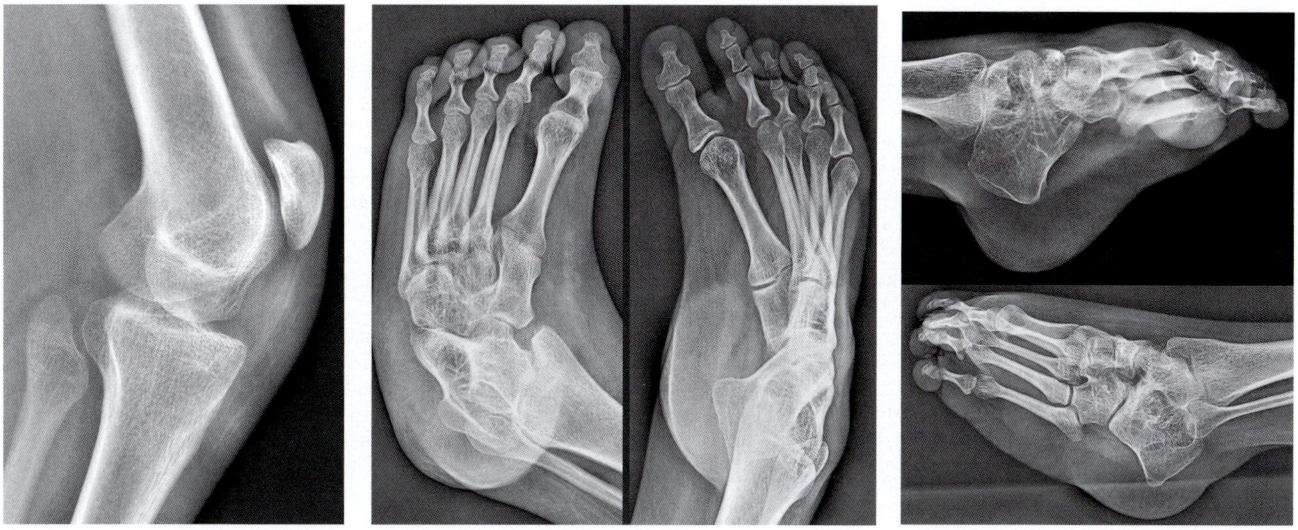

A B C

Figure 14.27 ■ **Arthrogryposis. A:** Lateral radiograph of the knee of a 41-year-old woman shows flexion contracture in the femorotibial joint and fatty atrophy of the muscles. Note also a high position of the patella (patella alta). Dorsoplantar **(B)** and lateral **(C)** radiographs of the feet show clubfoot deformity consisting of equinus position of the heel, varus position of the hindfoot, and adduction, supination, and varus position of the forefoot. Observe also osseous fusions of the mid- and hindfeet.

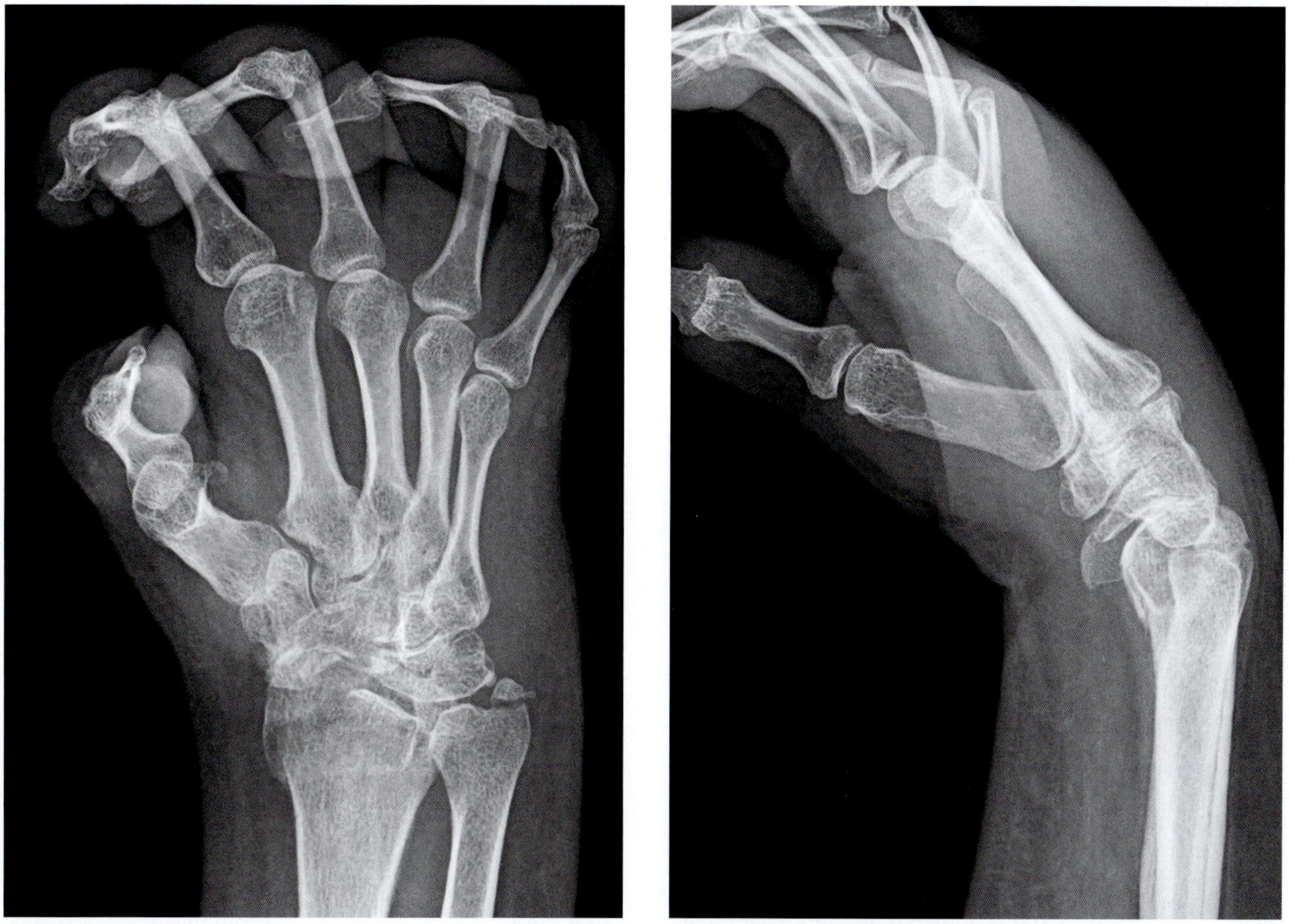

A B

Figure 14.28 ■ **Arthrogryposis.** Dorsovolar **(A)** and lateral **(B)** radiographs of the left hand of a 36-year-old woman show flexion contractures of the fingers and fatty atrophy of the muscles.

SUGGESTED READINGS

Apley AG, Wientrob S. The sagging rope sign in Perthes disease and allied disorders. *J Bone Joint Surg [Br]*. 1981;63-B:43–47.

Attali R, Warwar N, Israel A, et al. Mutation of SYNE-1, encoding an essential component of the nuclear lamina, is responsible for autosomal recessive arthrogryposis. *Hum Mol Genet*. 2009;18:3462–3469.

Bamshad M, Jorde LB, Carey JC. A revised and extended classification of the distal arthrogryposes. *Am J Med Genet*. 1996;65:277–281.

Bamshad M, Van Heest AE, Pleasure D. Arthrogryposis: a review and update. *J Bone Joint Surg [Am]*. 2009;91-A(suppl 4):40–46.

Barnes JM. Premature epiphyseal closure in Perthes' disease. *J Bone Joint Surg [Br]*. 1980;62-B:432–437.

Bateson EM. The relationship between Blount's disease and bow leg. *Br J Radiol*. 1968;41:107–114.

Bathfield CA, Beighton PH. Blount disease. A review of etiological factors in 110 patients. *Clin Orthop*. 1978;135:29–33.

Bellyei A, Mike G. Weight bearing in Perthes' disease. *Orthopedics*. 1991;14:19–22.

Bennett JT, Mazurek RT, Cash JD. Chiari's osteotomy in the treatment of Perthes' disease. *J Bone Joint Surg [Br]*. 1991:73-B:225–228.

Bernstein RM. Arthrogryposis and amyoplasia. *J Am Acad Orthop Surg*. 2002;10:417–424.

Bevan WP, Hall JG, Bamshad M, et al. Arthrogryposis multiplex congenita (amyoplasia): an orthopaedic perspective. *J Pediatr Orthop*. 2007;27:594–600.

Bloomberg TJ, Nuttall J, Stocker DJ. Radiology in early slipped femoral capital epiphysis. *Clin Radiol*. 1978;29:657–667.

Blount WP. Tibia vara. Osteochondrosis deformans tibiae. *J Bone Joint Surg*. 1937;19:1–29.

Boehm S, Limpaphayom N, Alaee F, et al. Early results of the Ponseti method for the treatment of clubfoot in distal arthrogryposis. *J Bone Joint Surg [Am]*. 2008;90-A:1501–1507.

Boyer DW, Mickelson MR, Ponseti IV. Slipped capital femoral epiphysis—long-term follow-up study of 125 patients. *J Bone joint Surg [Am]*. 1981;63-A:85–95.

Brown RR, Steiner GC, Lehman WB. Melorheostosis: case report with radiologic-pathologic correlation. *Skeletal Radiol*. 2000;29:548–552.

Caron KH, DiPietro MA, Aisen AM, et al. MR imaging of early fibrodysplasia ossificans progressiva. *J Comput Assist Tomogr*. 1990;14:318–321.

Catterall A. *Legg-Calvé-Perthes' Disease*. New York, NY: Churchill Livingstone, 1982.

Catterall A. The natural history of Perthes' disease. *J Bone Joint Surg [Br]*. 1971:53-B:37–53.

Cheema JI, Grissom LE, Harcke HT. Radiographic characteristics of lower-extremity bowing in children. *Radiographics*. 2003;23:871–880.

Connor J, Evans DA. Genetic aspects of fibrodysplasia ossificans progressiva. *J Med Genet*. 1982;19:35–39.

Connor J, Evans DA. Fibrodysplasia ossificans progressiva: the clinical features and natural history of 34 patients. *J Bone Joint Surg [Br]*. 1982;64-B:76–83.

Craig JG, van Holsbeeck M, Zaltz I. The utility of MR in assessing Blount disease. *Skeletal Radiol*. 2002;31:208–213.

Cremin B, Connor J, Beighton P. The radiologic spectrum of fibrodysplasia ossificans progressiva. *Clin Radiol*. 1982;33:499–508.

Dalinka MK, Coren G, Hensinger R, Irani RN. Arthrography in Blount's disease. *Radiology*. 1974;113:161–164.

Diaz A, Sia D, Sia VMG, et al. Magnetic resonance imaging confirmed clinical diagnosis of amyoplasia in two infants with arthrogryposis multiplex congenita. *IJCRI*. 2013; doi:10.5348/ijcri-2013-01-248-CS-2.

Dillman JR, Hernandez R. MRI of Legg-Calvé-Perthes disease. *AJR Am J Roentgenol*. 2009;193:1394–1407.

Ducou le Ponte H, Mousselard H, Rudell A, et al. Blount's disease: magnetic resonance imaging. *Pediatric Radiol*. 1995;25:12–14.

Egund N, Wingstrand H. Legg-Calvé-Perthes disease: imaging with MR. *Radiology*. 1991;179:89–92.

Evans IK, Deluca PA, Gage JR. A comparative study of ambulation–abduction bracing and varus derotation osteotomy in the treatment of severe Legg-Calvé-Perthes disease in children over 6 years of age. *J Pediatr Orthop*. 1988;8:676–682.

Eyring EJ, Bjornson DR, Peterson CA. Early diagnosis and prognostic signs in Legg-Calvé-Perthes disease. *AJR Am J Roentgenol*. 1965;93:382–387.

Gallagher JM, Weiner DS, Cook AJ. When is arthrography indicated in Legg-Calvé-Perthes disease? *J Bone Joint Surg [Am]*. 1983;65-A:900–905.

Gissen P, Johnson CA, Morgan NV, et al. Letter. Mutations in VPS33B, encoding a regulator of SNARE-dependent membrane fusion, cause arthrogryposis-renal dysfunction-cholestasis (ACR) syndrome. *Nature Genet*. 2004;36:400–404.

Goldman AB, Schneider R, Martel W. Acute chondrolysis complicating slipped capital femoral epiphysis. *AJR Am J Roentgenol*. 1978;130:945–950.

Greenspan A, Steiner G, Sotello D, et al. Mixed sclerosing bone dysplasias coexisting with dysplasia epiphysealis hemimelica (Trevor-Fairbanks disease). *Skeletal Radiol*. 1986;15:452–454.

Greenspan A. Sclerosing bone dysplasias—a target-site approach. *Skeletal Radiol*. 1991;20:561–583.

Greenspan A, Azouz EM. Bone dysplasias series. Melorheostosis: review and update. *Canad Assoc Radiol J*. 1995;46:368–379.

Guidera KJ, Drennan JC. Foot and ankle deformities in arthrogryposis multiplex congenita. *Clin Orthop Rel Res*. 1985;194:93–98.

Hall JG. Arthrogryposis multiplex congenital: etiology, genetics, classification, diagnostic approach, and general aspects. *J Pediatr Orthop*. 1997;6:159–166.

Happle R. Melorheostosis may originate as a type 2 segmental manifestation of osteopoikilosis. *Am J Med Genet*. 2004;125A:221–223.

Hasegawa S, Kanda S, Imada H, et al. Melorheostosis with recurrent soft-tissue components: a histologically confirmed case. *Skeletal Radiol*. 2017;46:339–404.

Herring JA. Current concept review. The treatment of Legg-Calvé-Perthes disease. A critical review of the literature. *J Bone Joint Surg [Am]*. 1994;76-A:448–458.

Herring JA, Neustadt JB, Williams JJ, et al. The lateral pillar classification of Legg-Calvé-Perthes disease. *Pediatr Orthop*. 1992;12:143–150.

Judkiewicz AM, Murphey MD, Resnick D, et al. Advanced imaging of melorheostosis with emphasis on MRI. *Skeletal Radiol*. 2001;30:447–453.

Kalampokas E, Kalampokas T, Sofoudis C, et al. Diagnosing arthrogryposis multiplex congenita: a review. *ISRN Obstetrics Gyn*. 2012; doi: 10.5402/2012/264918.

Kaplan FS, Chakkalakal SA, Shore EM. Fibrodysplasia ossificans progressiva: mechanism and model of skeletal metamorphosis. *Dis Model Mech*. 2012;5:756–762.

Kelly FB Jr, Canale ST, Jones RR. Legg-Calvé-Perthes disease. Long-term evaluation of non-containment treatment. *J Bone Joint Surg [Am]*. 1980;62-A:400–407.

Kim HT, Eisenhauer E, Wenger DR. The "sagging rope sign" in avascular necrosis in children's hip disease—confirmation by 3D CT studies. *Iowa Orthop J*. 1995;15:101–111.

Langenskiöld A. Tibia vara (osteochondrosis deformans tibiae): a survey of seventy-one cases. *Acta Chir Scan*. 1952;103:1–22.

Langenskiöld A, Riska EB. Tibia vara (osteochondrosis deformans tibiae). *J Bone Joint Surg [Am]*. 1964;46-A:1405–1420.

Lloyd-Reberts GC, Catterall A, Salamon PB. A controlled study of the indications for and the results of femoral osteotomy in Perthes disease. *J Bone joint Surg [Am]*. 1976;58-A:31–36.

Lowe HG. Necrosis of articular cartilage after slipping of capital femoral epiphysis. Report of six cases with recovery. *J Bone Joint Surg [Br]*. 1970;52-B:108–118.

Mahoney J, Achong DM. Demonstration of increased bone metabolism in melorheostosis by multiple bone scanning. *Clin Nucl Med*. 1991;16:847–848.

Martinez AG, Weinstein SL, Dietz FR. The weight-bearing abduction brace for the treatment of Legg-Perthes disease. *J Bone Joint Surg [Am]*. 1992;74-A:12–21.

Maxted MJ, Jackson RK. Innominate osteotomy in Perthes disease: a radiological survey of results. *J Bone Joint Surg [Br]*. 1985;67-B:399–401.

Mennen U, van Heest A, Ezaki M-B, et al. Arthrogryposis multiplex congenital. *J Hand Surg*. 2005;30:468–474.

Rink BD. Arthrogryposis: a review and approach to prenatal diagnosis. *Obstet Gyn Surv*. 2011;66:369–377.

Salter RB. Current concept review. The present status of surgical treatment for Legg-Perthes disease. *J Bone Joint Surg [Am]*. 1984;66-A:961–966.

Salter RB. Legg-Perthes disease. The scientific basis for methods for treatment and their indications. *Clin Orthop*. 1980;150:8–11.

Salter RB, Thompson GH. Legg-Calvé-Perthes disease. The prognostic significance of the subchondral fracture and a two-group classification of the femoral head involvement. *J Bone Joint Surg [Am]*. 1984;66-A:479–489.

Scham SM. The triangular sign in the early diagnosis of slipped capital femoral epiphysis. *Clin Orthop*. 1974;103:16–17.

Shingade VU, Song H-R, Lee S-H, et al. The sagging rope sign in achondroplasia—different from Perthes' disease. *Skeletal Radiol*. 2006;35: 923–928.

Silbert JR, Bray PT. Probable dominant inheritance in Blount disease. *Clin Genet*. 1977;11:394–396.

Smith CF. Current concept review. Tibia vara (Blount's disease). *J Bone Joint Surg [Am]*. 1982;64-A:603–632.

Van Heest A, James MA, Lewica A, Anderson KA. Posterior elbow capsulotomy with triceps lengthening for treatment of elbow extension contracture in children with arthrogryposis. *J Bone Joint Surg [Am]*. 2008;90-A:1517–1523.

Werner CML, Ramseier LE, Ruckstuhl T, et al. Normal values of Wiberg's lateral center-edge angle and Lequesne's acetabular index—a coxometric update. *Skeletal Radiol*. 2012;41:1273–1278.

Index

Page numbers followed by "f" refer to figures and those followed by "t" refer to tables.

B

C

D

E

F

G

H

J

K

L

M

N

O

P

R

S

T

U